KOCHAR'S CONCISE TEXTBOOK OF MEDICINE

Third Edition

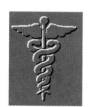

KOCHAR'S CONCISE TEXTBOOK OF MEDICINE

Third Edition

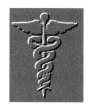

Editor-in-Chief
Kesavan Kutty, MD
Professor of Medicine
Medical College of Wisconsin
Academic Chairman of Medicine
St. Joseph's Hospital
Milwaukee, Wisconsin

Editors
James L. Sebastian, MD
Associate Professor of Medicine
Medical College of Wisconsin
Clement J. Zablocki VA Medical Center
Milwaukee, Wisconsin

Beth A. Mewis, MD
Formerly, Assistant Clinical Professor of Medicine
Medical College of Wisconsin
Milwaukee, Wisconsin

Dale D. Berg, MD
Formerly, Assistant Professor of Medicine
Medical College of Wisconsin
Milwaukee, Wisconsin

Consulting Editor
Mahendr S. Kochar, MD
Professor of Medicine and Pharmacology
Associate Dean, Graduate Medical Education, Medical College of Wisconsin
Associate Chief of Staff for Education
Clement J. Zablocki VA Medical Center
Milwaukee, Wisconsin

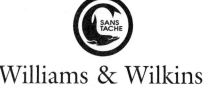

Williams & Wilkins
A WAVERLY COMPANY

BALTIMORE • PHILADELPHIA • LONDON • PARIS • BANGKOK
BUENOS AIRES • HONG KONG • MUNICH • SYDNEY • TOKYO • WROCLAW

Editor: Elizabeth A. Nieginski
Managing Editor: Crystal Taylor
Development Editors: Alice Tufel, Mike Bokulich
Marketing Manager: Christine Kushner
Design Coordinator: Mario Fernandez
Illustrations: Lavery Illustration, Joy Marlowe, and Chansky, Inc.
Printer/Binder: World Color, Inc.

351 West Camden Street
Baltimore, Maryland 21201-2436 USA

Rose Tree Corporate Center
1400 North Providence Road
Building II, Suite 5025
Media, Pennsylvania 19063-2043 USA

Printed in the United States of America

First Edition, 1982   Second Edition, 1990

Library of Congress Cataloging-in-Publication Data

Kochar's concise textbook of medicine   /   editors, Kesavan Kutty ... [et
al.]. — 3rd ed.
       p.   cm.
   Rev. ed. of: Concise textbook of medicine /   edited by Mahendr S.
Kochar, Kesavan Kutty. 2nd. ed. c–1990.
   Includes bibliographical references and index.
   ISBN 0-683-04798-1
   1. Internal medicine.   I. Kutty, Kesavan.   II. Kochar, Mahendr
S., 1943–   .   III. Concise textbook of medicine.
   [DNLM: 1. Internal Medicine.   WB 115 K76 1998]
RC46.T328   1998
616—dc21
DNLM/DLC
for Library of Congress   97-42621
                                                               CIP

*The publishers have made every effort to trace the copyright holders for borrowed material.
If they have inadvertently overlooked any, they will be pleased to make the necessary
arrangements at the first opportunity.*

To purchase additional copies of this book, call our customer service department at **(800)
638-0672** or fax orders to **(800) 447-8438.** For other book services, including chapter reprints
and large quantity sales, ask for the Special Sales department.

Canadian customers should call **(800) 268-4178**, or fax **(905) 470-6780.** For all other calls
originating outside of the United States, please call **(410) 528-4223** or fax us at **(410) 528-8550.**

Visit *Williams & Wilkins* on the *Internet*: http://www.wwilkins.com or contact our customer
service department at **custserv@wwilkins.com**. Williams & Wilkins customer service
representatives are available from 8:30 am to 6:00 pm, EST, Monday through Friday, for
telephone access.

                                                        98 99
                                    1 2 3 4 5 6 7 8 9 10

To our families and friends

Foreword

This is the third edition of *Kochar's Concise Textbook of Medicine*. The book is an ambitious undertaking. The authors are clinically active physicians, and the text is written for the "student" of clinical medicine, particularly medical students and house officers. Most (although not all) of the authors are faculty of the Department of Medicine at The Medical College of Wisconsin, reflecting the enthusiasm and commitment of the Department to medical education.

The book is informative without being overwhelming. Pathophysiology is presented in a manner that focuses on clinical implications, and practical approaches to the evaluation and management of patients are described. In addition to providing factual information, the authors share their own philosophies and values as they relate to the practice of medicine. The first part, "The Art and Science of Medicine," includes a discussion of the interface of the traditional role of the physician as a provider of care with newer forms of reimbursement for care and the use of expanded information systems. Subsequent parts cover the broad spectrum of topics usually included in a medicine text.

The editors of this text are to be commended for their foresight and clarity of purpose in introducing and, subsequently, updating this text. All are highly regarded as teachers and are committed to the education of future and current physicians. Dr. Mahendr Kochar served as editor and co-editor for the first and second editions,

respectively. Dr. Kochar is Associate Dean for Graduate Medical Education at The Medical College of Wisconsin. Dr. Kesavan Kutty also served as co-editor of the second edition and is the editor-in-chief of this edition. In addition to his faculty appointment at The Medical College of Wisconsin, Dr. Kutty is the Academic Chairman of Medicine and Director of the Transitional Year Residency Program at St. Joseph's Hospital in Milwaukee, and has been the recipient of several teaching awards. Drs. Beth Mewis, Dale Berg and James Sebastian have also served as editors of this third edition. Dr. Mewis is a former Chief Resident of our Medicine Residency Program. She is currently practicing General Internal Medicine in Fort Worth, Texas. Dr. Dale Berg has been Course Director for "Advanced Physical Diagnosis," an elective course for senior medical students. Dr. James Sebastian is Director of the "Introduction to Clinical Examination" course for sophomore students, and also serves as Director of Undergraduate Education for the Department of Medicine. Both Drs. Berg and Sebastian have received numerous teaching awards from medical students and house staff.

I would also like to acknowledge each of the authors for their contributions to the text and for their dedicated service as teachers of medicine.

Theodore A. Kotchen, MD
Professor and Chairman, Department of Medicine
The Medical College of Wisconsin

Preface

It has been said, with some degree of seriousness that, the more things change, the more they remain the same. The face of medicine, in as short a spell as within the last decade, has been beset with series of changes. Irrespective of whether or not one considers it consoling that medicine was not singled out for the change, things have hardly remained the same; in fact, these changes will fundamentally alter the practice of medicine for generations to come.

In a sense, besides death and taxes, change remains the only other certainty because change is the "mother's milk" of progress. However, not all change is for the better, and every change involves some inconvenience–even when it is for the better. A healthy attitude toward change revolves around two concepts: one, of exercising a sufficient degree of healthy skepticism toward it; the other, one of accepting it after one's skepticism is resolved. Both are lessons learned during a clerkship in Internal medicine. However, one also needs to pit a new concept or a new approach against the backdrop of one's fundamental concepts and understanding; such a basis is required for furthering one's learning. With the passage of time and gaining of practical experience, new concepts not only get contrasted against one's knowledge, but also get reshaped on the anvil of one's own experience through contemplation and reflection.

Medical students decide their future career(s) rather early during their medical education. Although inherent pros and cons to this early decision making do exist, a thorough basis in internal medicine is essential to the practice of any specialty. The recent "discovery" of primary care underscores this even more, regardless of one's concepts as to the origins of this discovery. It is the essential underpinning of all medical specialties. It teaches the concept of getting the facts straight, assembling the possibilities, integrating the facts against the possibilities and getting a match, generating a hypothesis, and finally, employing a minimum number of specific tests to confirm or refute one's hypothesis. The integration of physiology and pathophysiology are essential components of this process. The scenes and actors change, but the principles remain the same.

That the medical student need not learn a "standard" textbook of medicine cover to cover during a medicine clerkship or more importantly, fails predictably in that mission, was known to us a long time ago; it formed the impetus for the first edition of this textbook. The manner in which it was accepted by both students and critics made us confident of our assessment; the appearance of similar books in the marketplace merely conferred accuracy on our assessment. The doubling of editors through these three editions also signifies our own appreciation of both the length and breadth of internal medicine, and reflects the courage of our conviction that despite our constant involvement with undergraduate education, an optimum number of editors is a prerequisite to conveying our thoughts and concepts in a balanced manner.

In this edition, a number of changes have been made. Although the authors have maintained the emphasis of conciseness in conveying their ideas, they have added a large complement of tables, figures, and line diagrams to convey their ideas effectively and to make the product visually appealing. Almost three-fourths of the authors are new and belong to various divisions of internal medicine and departments of the Medical College of Wisconsin. They are both accomplished teachers and fine clinicians, who have been "in the trenches." Much of the text has been rewritten and where it was only revised, every effort has been made to incorporate current concepts and information. A number of new multiple-choice questions have been provided at the end of every part to help drive the concepts home. Some of these questions involve pictorial material representing actual situations that have confronted many house officers. A completely revised list of references follow as a guide to further reading.

The work on this has been exhilarating as we found our own concepts challenged and consolidated during its development and as we saw the horizons of our own knowledge widening. While we appreciate the help and support of the editorial staff at Williams & Wilkins in making this publication a reality, we also wish to take this opportunity to thank our senior colleague, Dr. Mahendr Kochar, for the confidence and trust he placed in us to continue a project and a fine tradition that he both founded and nurtured.

Samuel Johnson wrote: "The greatest part of a writer's time is spent in reading, in order to write: a man will turn over half a library to make one book." As this textbook made its way from concept to reality, we authors and editors have come to appreciate the enormity of and the truth behind this statement. As we burned our midnight oil "turning over" our libraries, our families and colleagues watched us and encouraged us, which only confirmed we were doing the right thing.

Kesavan Kutty
James Sebastian
Beth Mewis
Dale Berg
June 1998

Preface to the Second Edition

onventional wisdom tells us that the clinician arrives at a bedside diagnosis by careful history taking, thorough clinical examination, assimilation of the available information, and finally, by reflective reshaping of the resultant product on the anvil of prior experience. However, as stated by Dr. Roman Yanda, experience alone is a poor teacher: by the time one has enough, success or failure no longer matters. The background of organized learning—theoretical knowledge— should supplement experience if one were to succeed. Providing that necessary supplementation is the prime function of a textbook. As was the case with the first edition, published as *Textbook of General Medicine*, our objective in writing and editing this second edition is to provide the student with a course in internal medicine that could be read cover to cover during a 12-week rotation in medicine and to acquire knowledge in that field considered essential to graduation from medical school. Even though the book is directed to medical students, it will also serve as a quick reference source for internal medicine and family practice residents as well as nurses and other health professionals. The success of the first edition indicated that we had attained our objective. Its reviews in peer reviewed journals were extremely favorable, and we came to the inescapable conclusion that a second edition was in order.

Once again each chapter begins with an outline that defines the scope of the subject matter presented and ends with multiple choice questions meant to assist in self-evaluation. Liberal use of headings and use of simple, yet precise, language should make it easier to read. Almost half the contributors to the second edition are new. As was the case with the first edition, they are among today's leading teachers of medicine, all being board certified in their specialties and, where applicable, in the respective subspecialties as well.

Two new chapters, Psychiatry and Medical Genetics, have been added, and a whole section on alcoholism and substance abuse has been added to the chapter on clinical toxicology.

To say that medical practice is being reshaped is perhaps an understatement. At times it is hard to discern whether technology is driving medicine or vice versa. Medicine has made tremendous strides and seen new developments since 1983 when the first edition was published—the advent of magnetic resonance imaging, proliferation of antibiotics, calcium channel blockers, entry of AIDS as the greatest scourge of humankind, refinements in critical care and fibrinolytic therapy, just to name a few. To reflect the current advances, every chapter in the book has been thoroughly revised to reflect the current understanding of the subject, yet at the same time the book has been kept concise and the price affordable to the student.

The use of detailed references has been deliberately avoided, but a selected bibliography is provided at the end of each chapter for further reading. If the reader wishes to study a subject in greater detail, after studying the relevant portion from Concise Textbook of Medicine, he or she is encouraged to seek from a medical library an up-to-date computer printout of recent literature on the subject and then to read the most recent review articles on the subject.

Mahendr S. Kochar
Kesavan Kutty
October 1989

Preface to the First Edition

"To study the phenomena of disease without books is to sail an uncharted sea; while to study books without patients is not to go to sea at all," wrote Sir Williams Osler in 1901.[1]

There is only one way to learn clinical medicine, and that is at the bedside participating in diagnosis and treatment of the patient's illness; however no one can expect to acquire even the essential knowledge of internal medicine without books. With intensive biomedical research, there has been a knowledge explosion in medicine in the last three decades; there is too much to learn in a limited amount of time. It is impossible for a medical student to read the standard textbooks of medicine from beginning to end, but the student must acquire knowledge of the essentials of internal medicine in order to become a Doctor of Medicine.

The purpose of this book is to provide the student with a course in internal medicine that can be read from cover to cover during an 8- to 12-week rotation in medicine; it contains the essentials of internal medicine that the student must know before graduating. The book will also serve as a source of concise information for family practice and internal medicine residents desiring a rapid review of internal medicine. Allied health professionals, particularly nurse practitioners and physicians' assistants, will find the book readable and understandable.

Each chapter begins with an outline that defines the scope of the subject matter that one needs to learn and ends with multiple-choice questions, which should help in recapitulating what has been learned. Liberal use of headings and use of simple yet precise language should make the reading of this book an enjoyable experience.

This text has been written by specialists who are among today's leading teachers of internal medicine. All of the authors are board certified in both internal medicine and their subspecialties and have written their chapters with the objective of presenting all relevant information in the most lucid manner. The use of references has been deliberately avoided, but a selected bibliography is provided at the end of each chapter for further reading.

I would like to take this opportunity to thank Danial J. McCarty, MD, Professor and Chairman of the Department of Medicine at the Medical College of Wisconsin, Milwaukee, for writing the foreword to this book.

Mahendr S. Kochar
September 1982

[1]Olsen W. Books and men. Boston Med Surg J 1901; 144:60–62.

Acknowledgments

Because it is almost impossible to list the names and contributions of all those who have assisted in the preparation and publication of this book, this summation of acknowledgments is only a partial list.

First and foremost, we express our appreciation to the contributors and their secretaries who have worked hard and patiently in getting this book to fruition. We gratefully acknowledge the Medical Media Service, Echocardiography laboratory, and the Radiology Museum at St. Joseph's Hospital for their services. We are extremely grateful to Mrs. Maxine Cowell and Mrs. Catherine Ruchti for their excellent secretarial support and proofreading skills. Each section was reviewed by several reviewers and we thank them for their time, constructive suggestions, and encouraging remarks. The editorial staff at Williams & Wilkins, including Tim Satterfield, Crystal Taylor, Lisa Franko, Nancy Evans, and Jane Velker deserve our thanks for their undivided attention toward bringing out this third edition. We are especially grateful to the Development Editors, Alice Tufel and Michael Bokulich, for their very careful review of the manuscript and suggestions to make the text more readable and simple to follow. We would also like to take this opportunity to thank Dr. Theodore A. Kotchen, Chairman, Department of Medicine, Medical College of Wisconsin, for reviewing the manuscript and writing the Foreword to our textbook. Last but not least, we gratefully acknowledge the gentle encouragement, constructive criticism, and timely suggestions we have received from our friend, colleague, and the previous senior editor, Dr. Mahendr Kochar, whose name this textbook bears and without whose help this book may not have seen the light of the day. We are indebted to our families for their selfless devotion and love.

Kesavan Kutty
James L. Sebastian
Beth Mewis
Dale Berg

Contributors

Tom Anderson, MD
Professor of Medicine
Medical College of Wisconsin
Chief, Division of Hematology and Oncology
Froedtert Memorial Lutheran Hospital
Milwaukee, Wisconsin

George L. Bakris, MD
Associate Professor of Preventive and Internal Medicine
Rush Medical College
Director, Hypertension Research Fellowship Program
Presbyterian-St. Luke's Medical Center
Chicago, Illinois

Virinderjit S. Bamrah, MD
Professor of Medicine, Cardiology Division
Medical College of Wisconsin
Chief, Cardiology Section
VA Medical Center
Milwaukee, Wisconsin

Dale D. Berg, MD
Formerly Assistant Professor of Medicine
Medical College of Wisconsin
Milwaukee, Wisconsin

Jeffrey Binder, MD
Associate Professor of Neurology
Medical College of Wisconsin
Director, Stroke and Neurobehavioral Program
MCW Clinic at Froedtert Hospital
Milwaukee, Wisconsin

Theresa M. Braun, MD
Assistant Professor of Neurology
Medical College of Wisconsin
Director, Movement Disorders Program
MCW Clinic at Froedtert Hospital
Milwaukee, Wisconsin

Mary E. Cohan, MD
Assistant Professor of Medicine
Division of Geriatrics and Gerontology
Medical College of Wisconsin
Froedtert Memorial Lutheran Hospital
Milwaukee, Wisconsin

Hugh L. Davis, MD
Professor of Medicine
Medical College of Wisconsin
VA Medical Center
Milwaukee, Wisconsin

Vincents J. Dindzans, MD
Associate Clinical Professor of Medicine
University of Wisconsin, Milwaukee Clinical Campus
Assistant Clinical Professor of Medicine
Medical College of Wisconsin
Milwaukee, Wisconsin

Kulwinder S. Dua, MD
Assistant Professor of Medicine
Division of Gastroenterology and Hepatology
Medical College of Wisconsin
Chief of Endoscopy
VA Medical Center
Milwaukee, Wisconsin

Edmund H. Duthie Jr., MD
Professor of Medicine
Medical College of Wisconsin
Chief, Division of Geriatrics and Gerontology
VA Medical Center
Milwaukee, Wisconsin

Janet A. Fairley, MD
Professor of Dermatology
Medical College of Wisconsin
Milwaukee, Wisconsin

Robert H. Fisher, MD
Assistant Clinical Professor of Medicine
Medical College of Wisconsin
Chairman, Allergy Section and Subspecialty Medicine
Medical Associates of Menomonee Falls
Menomonee Falls, Wisconsin

Jerome L. Gottschall, MD
Associate Clinical Professor of Pathology
Medical College of Wisconsin
Medical Director, Clinical Laboratories Transfusion
    Services
The Blood Center of Southeastern Wisconsin
Milwaukee, Wisconsin

Paul B. Halverson, MD
Professor of Medicine
Division of Rheumatology
Medical College of Wisconsin
St. Joseph's Hospital
Milwaukee, Wisconsin

Janet R. Hosenpud, MD
Assistant Professor of Medicine
Division of Hematology and Oncology
Medical College of Wisconsin
Froedtert Memorial Lutheran Hospital
Milwaukee, Wisconsin

Safwan Jaradeh, MD
Associate Professor of Neurology
Medical College of Wisconsin
MCW Clinic at Froedtert Hospital
Milwaukee, Wisconsin

Albert L. Jochen, MD
Associate Professor of Medicine
Division of Endocrinology, Metabolism and Clinical
 Nutrition
Medical College of Wisconsin
VA Medical Center
Milwaukee, Wisconsin

Carl L. Junkerman, MD
Professor Emeritus of Medicine
Assistant Director, Center for Study of Bioethics
Medical College of Wisconsin
Milwaukee, Wisconsin

Mahendr S. Kochar, MD
Professor of Medicine and Pharmacology
Associate Dean, Graduate Medical Education
Medical College of Wisconsin
Associate Chief of Staff for Education
VA Medical Center
Milwaukee, Wisconsin

Kesavan Kutty, MD
Professor of Medicine
Medical College of Wisconsin
Academic Chairman of Medicine
St. Joseph's Hospital
Milwaukee, Wisconsin

James P. Lash, MD
Assistant Professor of Medicine
Division of Nephrology
University of Illinois at Chicago College of Medicine
Chicago, Illinois

David Letzer, DO
Assistant Clinical Professor of Medicine
Medical College of Wisconsin
Infectious Diseases Section
Medical Associates of Menomonee Falls
Menomonee Falls, Wisconsin

Albert Liebman, MD
Assistant Clinical Professor of Medicine and
 Psychiatry
Medical College of Wisconsin
Milwaukee, Wisconsin

Lorri J. Lobeck, MD
Assistant Professor of Neurology
Medical College of Wisconsin
Director, Multiple Sclerosis Clinic
MCW Clinic at Froedtert Hospital
Milwaukee, Wisconsin

Diana L. Maas, MD
Assistant Professor of Medicine
Division of Endocrinology, Metabolism and Clinical
 Nutrition
Medical College of Wisconsin
VA Medical Center
Milwaukee, Wisconsin

Eric F. Maas, MD, PhD
Associate Professor of Neurology
Neuro-ophthalmology
Medical College of Wisconsin
MCW Clinic at Froedtert Hospital
Milwaukee, Wisconsin

Kevin S. Madigan, MD
Fellow in Transfusion Medicine
The Blood Center of Southeastern Wisconsin
Milwaukee, Wisconsin

Melinda McCord, MD
Resident in Dermatology
Medical College of Wisconsin
Milwaukee, Wisconsin

Beth A. Mewis, MD
Formerly Assistant Clinical Professor of Medicine
Medical College of Wisconsin
Medical Clinics of North Texas
Fort Worth, Texas

Irene M. O'Shaughnessy, MD
Associate Professor of Medicine
Division of Endocrinology, Metabolism and Clinical
    Nutrition
Medical College of Wisconsin
VA Medical Center
Wauwatosa, Wisconsin

Anthony V. Pisciotta, MD
Robert A. Uihlein, Jr. Professor Emeritus
    of Hematologic Research
Division of Hematology and Oncology
Medical College of Wisconsin
Froedtert Memorial Lutheran Hospital
Milwaukee, Wisconsin

David L. Schiedermayer, MD
Associate Professor of Medicine
Division of General Internal Medicine
Medical College of Wisconsin
Froedtert Memorial Lutheran Hospital
Milwaukee, Wisconsin

James L. Sebastian, MD
Associate Professor of Medicine
Medical College of Wisconsin
VA Medical Center
Milwaukee, Wisconsin

Konrad H. Soergel, MD
Professor of Medicine and Physiology
Division of Gastroenterology and Hepatology
Medical College of Wisconsin
Froedtert Memorial Lutheran Hospital
Milwaukee, Wisconsin

L. Cass Terry, MD, PhD
Professor and Chairman of Neurology
Medical College of Wisconsin
Chief of Staff
Froedtert Memorial Lutheran Hospital
Milwaukee, Wisconsin

Basil Varkey, MD
Professor of Medicine
Medical College of Wisconsin
VA Medical Center
Milwaukee, Wisconsin

David K. Wagner, MD
Associate Professor of Medicine
Division of Infectious Diseases
Medical College of Wisconsin
VA Medical Center
Milwaukee, Wisconsin

Rebekah Wang-Cheng, MD
Associate Professor of Medicine and Psychiatry
Division of General Internal Medicine
Medical College of Wisconsin
Froedtert Memorial Lutheran Hospital
Milwaukee, Wisconsin

Russell Wilke, MD, PhD
Resident in Medicine
University of Wisconsin Hospital and Clinics
Madison, Wisconsin

John C. Wynsen, MD
Associate Professor of Medicine
Division of Cardiovascular Medicine
Medical College of Wisconsin
Director, Coronary Care Unit,
VA Medical Center
Milwaukee, Wisconsin

Contents

VII GASTROENTEROLOGY AND DISEASES OF THE LIVER

XI KIDNEY DISEASES, ELECTROLYTE DISORDERS, AND HYPERTENSION

Kidney Diseases

Fluid, Electrolyte, and Acid-Base Disorders

Hypertension

XII NEUROLOGIC DISORDERS

XIII   ONCOLOGY

XIV   PULMONARY DISEASES

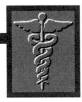

PART I

ART AND SCIENCE OF MEDICINE

Kesavan Kutty
Beth Mewis
Dale D. Berg
James L. Sebastian
Mahendr S. Kochar

with a chapter on
Medical Ethics by
Carl L. Junkerman
David L. Schiedermayer

edicine is both an art and a science. The diagnosis of illness is based on clinical methods and laboratory tests, supplemented when necessary by the application of the most modern technology. Eliciting a good history, performing a thorough physical examination, and selecting the most crucial laboratory tests without subjecting the patient to undue risk or expense—and then synthesizing the resulting information—require skill. Laboratory tests, diagnostic imaging, endoscopic studies, and electrophysiologic tests are all examples of the application of science in medicine. However, extracting the relevant information from a mass of conflicting physical signs and laboratory data to arrive at the correct diagnosis is an art that requires experience and judgment. Similarly, whereas pharmaceutical modalities and surgical procedures are a highly developed science, knowing when and how to use them is an art.

■ The Changing Face of Medicine

The dual aspect of medicine as both an art and a science has become more important than ever over the last decade, a time of dramatic change for the medical profession. Three major factors—all related to medicine as "art" —have fueled this change: 1) the development and implementation of diagnosis-related groups (DRGs); 2) the rapid spread of managed care, caused by the escalation in the cost of medical care; and 3) finally, the explosive growth of, and almost instant availability of, medical information (see chapter 2). Prior to the DRG method of reimbursement, hospitals had little incentive to control medical care costs. The latest, and often very expensive, equipment was installed, and physicians were encouraged to use it.

Under the DRG system of payment, hospitals receive a fixed amount, depending on the discharge diagnosis, regardless of the length of stay. In managed care systems, the patient chooses a primary care physician who is responsible for the ongoing health care of that patient in a cost-effective manner. Reducing costs is emphasized: only necessary treatments and/or tests are allowed or ordered; the least expensive medications are used; and patients are treated expeditiously, thus causing early discharges from the hospital. Because no two patients are alike, this emphasis on cost-cutting (what is permitted) is sometimes at odds with what is appropriate or necessary—although the rational application of information often enables the physician to make the right choice in such situations. Predetermined practice guidelines and

clinical pathways are promulgated to standardize managed care as much as possible. For more information on managed care, see chapter 2.

Another way in which medicine is changing is that an ever-increasing number of illnesses are now diagnosed and treated in outpatient settings. Thus, patients who are hospitalized are more ill on average and require more attention from physicians, nurses, and other hospital personnel. Providing care to hospitalized patients is becoming increasingly difficult for physicians because their offices and clinic schedules require them to be present there. As a result, some internists—called "hospitalists," connoting hospital-based specialists—confine their practices to hospitals.

■ Approach to the Patient

In practicing the art of medicine, physicians must approach patients with empathy and tact. The patient should never be regarded as a case with a collection of symptoms, signs, physical examination results, and abnormal laboratory and diagnostic indications, but rather as an individual who is seeking relief and reassurance. The physician is expected to be knowledgeable, courteous, and wise. In addition, patients want a physician who can assist their decision making by clearly communicating the diagnosis, treatment options, and potential outcomes. This can help allay the fear of dependence, disability, or death resulting from the illness. The patient groups described in the following paragraphs may require additional attention and skills.

Adolescent patients

Adolescent patients often receive primary care from a general internist. These patients are generally healthy and usually present to the physician for a required physical examination or a minor illness. In adolescence, prevention can have a significant impact on health, but teenagers are often reluctant to discuss their lifestyle. Physicians should encourage and welcome questions with the assurance of confidentiality, using this office time as an opportunity to discuss the risks associated with driving, smoking, alcohol and drug use, and, for sexually active adolescents, sex education, birth control, and sexually transmitted diseases (STDs).

Alcohol and drug-dependent patients

Alcohol and drug abuse (substance abuse) are common problems in the United States. Because such problems eventually lead to physical and emotional problems, primary care physicians will certainly see these patients in their practices. Denial is a common component of substance abuse problems, and few patients will come forward on their own to request help. If they do, the physician can be most helpful by assisting admission to a detoxification and rehabilitation program. The physician should discuss suspected substance abuse with the patient in an understanding and nonaccusatory manner, helping the patient to realize that the abuse problem is real and requires intervention. When intervention is unsuccessful, the physician must set limits with the patient regarding prescription writing, frequency of office visits, and accepting phone calls. This firmness may allow the patient to eventually realize the severity of his or her problem. (Alcoholism and substance abuse are further discussed in part III, Behavioral Medicine.)

Geriatric patients

Old age is often associated with illness, frailty, and greater dependency, but the physician's attitude toward the elderly should be respectful and supportive. The effects of aging on the body must be differentiated from those caused by illness (see the part Multisystem Changes Due to Aging in Geriatric Medicine). The patient's capacity and views rather than his or her age should be the deciding factors in determining the extent of diagnostic evaluation and treatment.

Terminally ill patients

Diagnosing and then caring for a terminally ill patient can be stressful, yet satisfying, for the physician. A supportive relationship among the patient, family, and physician can be sustaining for all during this difficult time. The physician should counsel the patient and the family about the terminal nature of the disease, thus allowing them to prepare themselves for the inevitable. (See chapter 7, Medical Ethics, for a discussion of cardiopulmonary resuscitation, pain control, and the withdrawal of artificial life-support in this setting.) In instances of terminal illness due to accidents, the idea of organ donation should be carefully broached with the next-of-kin.

■ Approach to the Patient's Family and Significant Others

The patient's well-being is directly related to his or her relationships with others. Therefore, the primary care physician should know about the significant individuals in each patient's life. With the patient's concurrence, the physician should include significant others in communications with the patient, seeking their support in restoring the patient to health and comforting them when the patient is seriously ill. When a patient dies, the physi-

cian's responsibility is to inform the loved ones gently, offering support when possible. Finally, if an autopsy is contemplated, the physician should tactfully seek the family's permission, explaining the reasons for the autopsy.

■ Maintenance of Health and Prevention of Disease: Health Education

The physician who is only diagnosing and treating established illnesses is ignoring medicine as an "art" and is, therefore, only partially effective. A good clinician can foster behavioral change in asymptomatic persons when necessary and helping them to overcome the social, economic, and geographic barriers to disease prevention. Few aspects of medicine benefit any one person or the community more than maintaining health and preventing illness. A family's participation is often necessary in obtaining the maximum benefit from counseling the patient. (Prevention and screening are discussed in chapter 5.)

■ Physician as a Healer: Iatrogenic Disorders

With advances in therapeutics, potent medications are now available for the treatment of many illnesses that could only be treated symptomatically in the past. These drugs, however, are potentially harmful and can cause disease (iatrogenic disorders); therefore, the physician must take precautions to minimize such dangers. Drugs or surgery alone—the "science of medicine"—can seldom provide maximal benefit. Physicians must learn to treat the patient, not the illness. Patients should ideally feel that their individuality is respected and appreciated. The caring attitude of the physician should supplement and complement the drugs and/or surgical procedures used in restoring the patient to health and happiness. The patient's spouse, family, or significant other can often help provide information on the use of prescribed and over-the-counter drugs and herbs the patient is taking.

■ Consultants

Physicians who are unsure of a diagnosis or prognosis should be honest about their uncertainty and consult with a specialist. No physician loses respect or confidence by admitting ignorance and seeking help. The physician should make use of this opportunity to learn from the consultant the latest advances in treating the illness in question and other related matters. Whenever the patient wants another opinion, the physician should respect that wish and assist in obtaining a second opinion without hesitation. Such requests do not necessarily imply the patient's lack of confidence in the physician.

The role of the consultant includes determining the

specific question being addressed (which may not be obvious); establishing the urgency of the consultation; gathering appropriate data; making specific recommendations; providing contingency plans; offering educational information; communicating directly, briefly, and succinctly with the referring physician; and discussing with the patient the essence of the consultation, detailing specific areas at the patient's request. The communication with the patient must be in clear and understandable lay terms.

Just as other physicians, consulting physicians should serve both the primary physician and the patient. Consultants should be both honest and tactful, and they must be confident without conveying a superiority over the primary physician. They should answer all questions from the patient that relate to the issue at hand. If the primary care physician has made errors in diagnosis and treatment, the consultant must courteously and tactfully point these out to the primary care physician and suggest corrective measures. If the patient asks questions whose answers might embarrass the primary care physician, the consultant should answer them honestly and tactfully, keeping the primary care physician fully informed. A consultant should continue to conduct follow-up consultations with the patient as long as the referring physician and the patient want.

CHAPTER 2 — PHYSICIAN AND THE MEDICAL ENVIRONMENT

■ Larger Environment of Medicine: Allied Health Care Professionals in Medical Practice

Because of increasing demands from patients and society at large—and fueled by technologic advances and social changes—a variety of trained professionals other than physicians and nurses are involved in health care. These professionals include physician's assistants, dietitians, physical therapists, respiratory therapists, biochemists, psychologists, and others. Both the patient and the primary care physician can greatly benefit from such collaboration, but the physician must maintain responsibility as the team leader; be familiar with the techniques, skills, and objectives of the allied health care professionals; and oversee the total care delivered to the patient.

■ Multispecialty Clinics and Health Maintenance Organizations

In the past, medical care was provided by solo practitioners, but market forces and the growth of managed care have led to the formation of group practices and multispecialty clinics. Increasing numbers of patients are cared for by groups of physicians, clinics, hospitals, and health maintenance organizations (HMOs) rather than by solo practitioners. Even if patient care is rendered in a clinic setting, the identity of the physician who is primarily and continuously responsible for each patient must be clearly defined. The primary care physician is responsibile for overseeing the patient's total care.

Traditional health care in the United States reimburses hospitals and physicians on the basis of use or provision of services—the so-called fee-for-service system. This system implicitly provides hospitals and physicians with a monetary incentive to perform as many services as possible. Because the potential for abuse in a fee-for-service system is high and the incentive for controlling the patient's costs is small, alternate health insurance plans offer prepaid care as "capitation" by the subscriber (enrollee or the employer, depending on the plan). The emphasis is on providing low-cost medical care, with cost-cutting resulting from diminished hospital use. Dr. Paul Ellwood, a Minnesota pediatrician, called such a prepaid plan a **health maintenance organization** (HMO). Studies have shown that the quality of care in a properly managed HMO—managed care system—can be comparable to that in a fee-for-service system.

The HMO movement has gained momentum throughout the United States. The chief attraction of HMOs to employers, who often pay the premiums (or part thereof), is the predictability of costs. Patients receiving health care through HMOs are assigned or select a primary care physician who acts as a "gatekeeper," thereby controlling the use of services. However, HMOs can, and sometimes do, reduce costs by demanding deep discounts from physicians and hospitals, by denying services to patients, or by insuring only healthy people. Another concept, which evolved in the 1980s to 1990s, is **managed competition,** born out of the perceived need to manage managed care itself. This concept promotes open but regulated competition among all health care plans—both fee-for-service and prepaid types. In this setting, the employer or a government agency (sponsor) provides a number of standardized benefit packages in a way that fosters comparison shopping for subscribers, pays the insurer an amount commensurate with the risk of the enrolled population, and develops enough disincentives to prevent plans from insuring only the healthy, through "skimming" the population. In other words, it depends on the strengths of a free-market system.

A **preferred provider organization** (PPO) is a hospital, clinic, or a group of physicians who may agree to provide health care services to a company's employees or group of individuals at lower fees. Conceptually, it is a hybrid of HMOs and fee-for-service plans. An **independent practice association** (IPA) is a group of physicians, usually members of a certain hospital's medical staff, who agree to comply with such contractual agreements regarding their fees.

■ Specific Aspects of Today's Medical Environment

Medical records

The medical record is essentially a road map, depicting a factual portrayal of the patient's medical condition and its evolution over time. The medical record has value only if all pertinent data relating to the patient's clinical and laboratory examinations and treatment are permanently recorded promptly, accurately, and completely. In hospitalized patients, rapid changes in condition and multisystem illnesses are common as is the provision of medical care by more than one physician and one allied health care professional. Such patients necessitate careful, prompt, and thorough recording of the initial observations. This information should be updated several times during a 24-hour period, the frequency being determined by the rate the patient's condition changes. The concept is the same in physicians' offices and clinics; only the periodicity of follow-up is different.

Given the increased mobility of patients and physicians, timeliness is important in completing medical records. Delays can result in the loss of important information, caused by caregivers' forgetfulness. Incomplete medical records, especially summaries of hospital records, impose a needless financial burden on hospitals because financial reimbursement is not possible if records remain incomplete. Finally, the content and organization of medical records provide a good approximation of the quality of medical care. Careful documentation of the care of patients not only can help elucidate the underlying processes involved in complex medical illnesses, but it can also help avoid malpractice cases.

Computers in medicine

The need to manage information has become critical—whether one is in academic medicine or private practice. The explosion of knowledge in medicine and the increasing number of people who must have access to medical records have fueled this need. An obvious solution is the application of computer technology since its use in managing the economics of medical practice is well established. The application of information technology to medicine has led to the development of a specialty called "medical informatics."

Organizing unprocessed information—name, address, and other personal information regarding the patient, laboratory data, and radiographic images—and making it easily retrievable represents perhaps the earliest and most "primitive" (data-based) application of computer technology in medicine. In contrast, information-based applications—such as the patient's clinical records, on-line bibliographic systems, and computer-assisted learning—are more sophisticated. The most widely used information-based application is MEDLINE, a compilation of peer-reviewed medical literature, which is available on-line through several systems, the National Library of Medicine, and also on CD-ROM (Compact Disc Read-Only-Memory). Knowledge-based applications are those in which the preprogrammed computer adds integrated information—for example, the reminder about specific drug allergies when a patient receives an inappropriate prescription due to an oversight, or reminders about important drug interactions. The fundamental objective is the ability of such systems to improve quality of care. The final frontier is the use of artificial intelligence to help diagnose disorders.

With more than 600,000 medical articles published yearly, for any physician to remain up-to-date with the entire literature of medicine is impossible. The evolution of the MEDLINE system and its indexing strategy has been invaluable in managing this information and making it rapidly accessible. Computerization of the medical record, aided by the Unified Medical Language System (UMLS), is another development on the horizon. In the past, computers have been capable of only a minor application in medicine—storing raw data; however, the advent of medical informatics will bring a more integrated and comprehensive application of computer technology to the practice of medicine. Increasingly, many medical schools are promoting computer literacy for medical students by teaching them data-management skills, word processing, and information retrieval from on-line medical literature databases.

Two potential dangers of computers are their capacity to subvert the patient's right to confidentiality and their ability to destroy what remains of the patient-physician relationship. While encouraging the use of computers to enhance patient care, physicians must guard against potential misuse. Some physicians take the opposite point of view and, with a patient's permission, put his or her medical information on the World Wide Web (WWW) for ready retrieval by any provider of care so that regardless of where the patient travels, his or her medical information is readily available. Such a patient knows his or her WWW address and permits the provider to access it and retrieve the necessary information.

Accountability in medical practice

Increasingly, physicians are being held accountable for their actions regarding the quality and cost-effectiveness of care. Review of medical records, mandatory continuing education for relicensing, and recertification by examination are examples of regulatory measures by lawmakers and voluntary efforts by physicians to ensure and demonstrate competence. For the patient, reducing costly hospital admissions as much as possible and keeping the cost of medical care affordable have become essential. In the final analysis, the medical profession must guide the public in matters of health-related legislation. While maintaining concern for the welfare of their patients, physicians must also make every possible effort to alleviate the socioeconomic problems of health care delivery through civic activism and political awareness.

Human research

If the science of medicine is to progress, research must be done on human beings. Physicians engaged in research on humans must explain to each patient, in clear and understandable language, the nature, risks, and benefits of all diagnostic and therapeutic procedures that are not well established or are considered experimental, and obtain the patient's informed consent. When conducting research, the physician must take extraordinary precautions to protect the patient's interests and to minimize risks. Only by using these safeguards can human research be undertaken for the progress of medicine without jeopardizing the patient's health.

Physicians' responsibilities to themselves, their families, and the community

The conflict between meeting one's personal and family responsibilities and addressing the needs of one's patients is a perennial one. This conflict and the rapid pace of the practice of medicine impose tremendous stress on physicians; the suicide rate among physicians is one of the highest compared with that of other professionals. To relieve stress, every physician must devote time to recreation and family and engage regularly in physical exercise.

Physicians also have a responsibility to the community. As is true for all citizens, regular participation in civic affairs and public elections is important, requiring the intelligent prioritization of professional and leisure time. Physicians who work all the time are not serving their patients well.

CHAPTER 3 | # BEDSIDE TECHNIQUES

Clinical information comes from the patient's history, physical examination results, and investigations such as laboratory tests, imaging studies, and other applicable procedures. Information thus obtained enables the physician to make a diagnosis, to decide on the best therapy, and to determine a prognosis. The term "clinical methods" encompasses all the ways of obtaining clinical information, and "bedside methods"—history taking and physical examination—represent the cornerstone of this process. Bedside methods are inexpensive but extremely productive ways to obtain relevant information about the patient's illness, and they also provide a way to interact with the patient.

The physician should be meticulous when taking a history and conducting a physical examination, devoting enough time to analyzing and contemplating all the information obtained before ordering potentially hazardous, unnecessary, and expensive tests. A focused history and a physical examination are crucial to selectively apply the endless number of available studies and tests within the context of the patient's illness; tests should never be ordered based on a knee-jerk reaction. Despite such technological marvels as computed tomographic (CT) scanning and magnetic resonance imaging (MRI), the bedside evaluation remains the most important and cost-effective way to diagnose illnesses.

■ History

The key to diagnosis is an accurate and comprehensive medical history; its importance cannot be overemphasized. The history summarizes the evolution of the patient's illness and describes symptoms; it should suggest certain diagnostic possibilities, aid in excluding others, and help determine which studies are necessary. At times, the history might be the only clue to a diagnosis. The physician must adopt a form and style for the medical history, adhering to this pattern until it becomes habitual. The advantages of establishing such a regimen are that no analytical effort is then needed for the act of history taking, no topic is overlooked, and full attention is directed toward interpreting the meaning of each response. The information to be gathered in a history, as often used by most physicians, is provided in the sections that follow. Obtaining a more detailed history after the physical examination and laboratory tests are performed may be necessary if unexpected findings are detected.

Demographic information

Demographic information includes the patient's name, age, race, sex, marital status, address, phone number, hospital (medical record) number, date of examination, and source and reliability of the informant.

Chief "complaint" or principal reason for seeking care

Identifying the major reason for the patient's clinic visit, hospitalization, or visit to the emergency department is important. The term "chief complaint" is a misnomer because it implies that the patient complained about something and it presupposes that all patients are capable of expressing their reasons for seeking medical attention. This is often not the case, and the physician must determine the reason for the visit. In other cases, hospitalization is necessitated by a discovery (e.g., thrombocytopenia or a massive pleural effusion) detected during a workup of the patient's symptoms and may explain the patient's initial concerns. Perhaps a better term would be "principal reason" for seeking medical care or for consulting a physician. Traditional teaching emphasizes identification of the chief complaint first; in practice, however, it is best to conduct the full interview and synthesize all the issues, at which point the principal reason for the visit might become apparent. Identification of the principal reason for a medical visit is important because it not only addresses the patient's concerns but also provides a framework for a plan, which is essential in today's practice of medicine.

Other symptoms and complaints must also be elicited since they need to be addressed as well. Those that are relevant to the history of the present illness are included there; others are recorded in the review of systems.

History of present illness

Information concerning the patient's present illness should be written as an orderly and chronological account. Lucid and succinct, this account should detail the chief complaint and progress logically. If the patient is not sure when the illness began, the physician should ask, "When did you last feel well or normal?" Each symptom should be described in detail (e.g., pain), including specifics about intensity and location, accompanying symptoms, factors that relieve or aggravate the symptom, and the symptom's course (progression or regression). When a symptom is suggestive of several conditions, statements detailing the lack of usual concomitant symptoms should be included.

If the present illness has progressed in attacks separated by symptom-free intervals, a typical attack should be described in terms of onset, duration, and associated symptoms. In both acute and chronic illnesses, the date that the patient stopped work or began bed rest should be noted. When a conspicuous disturbance of a particular organ or system exists, direct questions should be asked about all possible symptoms relating to the particular organ system. Specific inquiry should be made of past affliction of the specific organ system that is implicated in the present illness. The patient's previous treatment should be noted, including the use of over-the-counter medications. Constitutional symptoms such as chills, fever, night sweats, and weight loss should be noted. Finally, the patient's level of activity at work and during leisure time should be reported. Current medications and their dosages are ideally listed at the end of the history of the present illness, which fulfills a dual role: first, if medication is causing the present illness, the diagnosis of an iatrogenic illness will be easier, and second, the evolution of the present illness might necessitate an adjustment of medication dose and frequency.

Past medical history

The patient's history includes a description of previous illnesses, general health, operations, injuries, hospitalizations, and allergies, which are all unrelated to the present illness. This information should be listed chronologically.

Family history

The family history includes a statement concerning any similar illness or symptoms in the family or the lack thereof; it notes the age and state of health of parents, siblings, and children, or the causes of their deaths and their ages at death. The family history of common heritable diseases such as diabetes, hypertension, heart disease, kidney disease, cancer, allergies, and mental illness is also included. Diagraming a family tree is helpful if several members of the family have had the same illness.

Personal and social history

Personal and social history includes information on diet and nutrition, smoking, alcohol consumption, use of illicit drugs (cocaine, marijuana, amphetamines, etc.), sleep and exercise habits, education, occupation, marital status, sex life, and home and environmental conditions. An occupational history, chronologically arranged starting with the first job held, is sometimes useful.

Review of systems

The patient should be asked about salient symptoms pertaining to each organ system. All the symptoms reported by the patient should be described and the lack of significant symptoms noted.

■ Physical Examination

The physical examination is conducted by means of the four basic methods of **inspection, palpation, percussion,** and **auscultation.** Often, some aspects of the patient's illness are revealed only by physical examination; therefore, thoroughness is essential. Physical examination is indispensable in obtaining the following information about a patient: general appearance, including mental status; vital signs (temperature, pulse rate, respiratory rate, blood pressure); visible lesions on the body; palpable lesions, such as masses, local tenderness, deformities, and pulsations; signs of respiratory difficulty; auscultatory findings, such as murmurs, friction rubs, and alteration in breath and/or bowel sounds; and neurologic signs.

The environment in which the patient is examined should be quiet and well lighted, preferably by daylight. The physician should be considerate when examining the patient, respecting the patient's need for privacy and avoiding discomfort to the patient as much as possible. A systematic approach is essential. The physician's aim is to maintain objectivity and record observations instead of interpreting them. For the routine physical examination, a full complement of equipment includes stethoscope,

TABLE 3.1 Outline of a Physical Examination
General appearance and vital signs
Skin
Lymph nodes
Head
Eyes
Ears
Nose
Mouth and throat
Neck
Back
Thorax
Breasts
Heart
Abdomen
Genitalia
Rectum
Limbs and musculoskeletal system
Neurologic system

penlight, tongue blades, otoscope and ophthalmoscope, reflex hammer, sphygmomanometer, tuning fork, gloves, lubricating jelly, guaiac test reagents (Hemoccult), and a pelvic speculum. Infection control precautions—use of gloves, gowns, and masks—should be used as appropriate. Hand-washing is essential following hand contact with the patient, patient's fomites, or personal effects. An outline for performing the physical examination and recording the findings appears in Table 3.1.

 **CHAPTER 4** DIAGNOSTIC STUDIES

■ Laboratory Diagnosis

Laboratory tests cannot supplant a careful history and physical examination, but tests do provide diagnostic information not obtainable by other means. Skills in making effective use of the laboratory are developed through training and experience. Physicians must acquire the ability to integrate laboratory data with other clinical information.

Laboratory data can be useful for a number of purposes, as follows:

Screening. Application of laboratory tests for screening is discussed in chapter 5.

Diagnosis. The most common and important use of laboratory tests is diagnostic. Physicians use them as aids in selecting the most likely diagnosis from a list of several possibilities that may have been suggested by the history and physical examination—that is, tests are used in

making the **differential diagnosis.** Further laboratory testing can help the physician reach a precise diagnosis or limit the differential diagnosis.

Selection of therapy. Laboratory studies can help the physician select the appropriate mode of therapy. Antimicrobial susceptibility tests used in selecting the most effective antibiotic for bacterial infections are a prime example. Other examples are blood grouping and cross matching before blood transfusion and tissue typing before tissue transplantation.

Follow-up. Because many laboratory tests are more objective than the history and physical examination and because they provide quantitative information, they have proved useful in following the course of a disease and determining the effectiveness of therapy.

Prevention. Tests used in genetic counseling to detect carrier states are an excellent example of using the laboratory in the prevention of diseases.

Medico-legal uses. Legal evidence is collected, for example, by examining fingerprints or dried blood on clothing, by examining body fluids of rape victims, or by performing autopsies. Other applications include drug screens of urine and serum.

Environmental protection. Microbiologic and toxicologic surveillance is commonly used by environmental protection specialists.

Therapeutic drug monitoring. Serum levels of drugs such as gentamicin, phenytoin, theophylline, and digoxin are commonly used to ensure adequate therapy.

The following considerations apply in various applications of laboratory data:

Qualitative versus quantitative testing. Qualitative data are descriptive and include information regarding the presence or absence of a particular finding. For example, qualitative data include a statement on the presence or absence of sugar in the urine. Qualitative data are often expressed in semiquantitative terms. On the other hand, quantitative data are expressed in numbers, such as blood sugar levels and blood counts.

Sensitivity versus specificity. Sensitivity indicates that the result of the test is positive in the presence of the disease, whereas specificity indicates that it is negative in healthy persons and/or persons who do not have that particular disease. An ideally sensitive test is one in which all patients with a disease show positive results. A highly sensitive test is used to exclude a diagnosis, and a specific test is used to confirm it. For example, a perfusion lung scan is highly sensitive, and results of this test will be positive in all patients with clinically significant pulmonary embolism. A normal perfusion scan in a patient suspected of pulmonary embolism excludes this diagnosis. However, a positive scan does not automatically indicate pulmonary embolism. On the other hand, positive findings on a pulmonary angiogram are highly specific for pulmonary embolism and confirm the diagnosis. Usually, as the specificity of the test increases, the sensitivity diminishes, and as the sensitivity increases, the specificity declines.

Precision versus accuracy (reliability versus validity). A precise, reliable test is one that is highly reproducible. An accurate, valid test is one that gives a true measurement of the tested variable. A precise test is not necessarily accurate. Accuracy and precision in clinical laboratories are continually monitored by in-house, regional, and national laboratory proficiency surveys.

Normal ranges for laboratory values. Normal ranges for quantitative test results allow for both the biologic variability in the normal population and the analytic imprecision of the method. Imprecise methods produce wider normal ranges. Nearly all clinical labora-

tories have a list of normal values that were established by doing the tests on a large number of healthy persons and calculating values from these tests.

Errors in Laboratory Testing. Errors can occur in clinical laboratories during the collection of specimens, during performance of the tests, and in the interpretation of the test results. The physician must appreciate the inherent limitations of laboratory tests and be aware that misleading or diagnostically useless information may be obtained if inappropriate tests are ordered. Incorrect handling of the specimen often leads to errors, an example being incorrect use of anticoagulants in tubes used for collecting blood. Improperly handled or inadequate specimens are a common problem. Technical and clerical errors in the laboratory are additional sources of errors. Although laboratory errors do occur, they are not common; therefore, one should not routinely attribute an unanticipated result to laboratory error. When the physician suspects a laboratory error, the test should be repeated and, if the results are the same as before, they should not be ignored. Medications can interfere with laboratory tests; however, this is not a common occurrence, despite combination drug therapy. The ultimate value of the laboratory test depends on the physician's appreciation of the limitations and capabilities of the clinical laboratory.

■ Diagnostic Imaging

Imaging using x-rays, ultrasound, radioactive isotopes, and magnetic resonance has an increasingly important role in diagnosis today.

Diagnostic roentgenography

Diagnostic roentgenography supplements the physical examination. Chest x-ray examination (CXR) is the most common radiographic study. A peripheral lung cancer can be detected in its early stages by CXR. Plain x-ray films (without the use of radio-opaque contrast material) are also widely used in evaluating bones and detecting radio-densities in soft tissues. Contrast radiography is used to delineate soft tissue organs, to study the function of certain organs such as the kidneys, and to observe bloodflow patterns using angiography. The most commonly used contrast agents are compounds of iodine and barium, which absorb more x-rays than do soft tissues. Iodine-containing contrast materials are usually injected intravenously; when ingested orally, they are absorbed into the bloodstream through the gastrointestinal tract. Barium, on the other hand, is used only for gastrointestinal examinations and is not absorbed through the gastrointestinal tract. Contrast materials can be used to study almost all the organ systems of the body.

The request for a radiographic imaging study should always be accompanied by a brief clinical summary and the reason for requesting the procedure. If more than one procedure is available to accomplish the objective, the radiologist might use this information to determine the best procedure to provide the required information; the information is integrated into the interpretation of the imaging studies. In many instances, direct communication between the clinician and the radiologist before the x-ray study not only helps the radiologist provide the maximum information but also minimizes the radiation exposure to the patient since the radiologist would then perform only the necessary procedures. The clinician must personally review the radiographs and must not be satisfied simply by reading the radiologist's report. Consultation with a radiologist when interpreting the films often benefits patient care, and the exchange of information is educational for both the clinician and the radiologist. Since prolonged or frequent exposure to x-rays can be a health hazard, only essential diagnostic radiographic examinations should be performed.

Computed tomography

Computed (axial) tomography (CAT or CT scanning) has added a new dimension to radiographic diagnosis and is one of the most remarkable applications of computers in medicine. When x-ray beams pass through organs of varying tissue density in the body, they are subject to different degrees of attenuation. By analyzing such attenuations and reconstructing an image of the various organs based on this analysis, a computer provides an image of a transverse slice of the body, of variable thickness. The examination is done at multiple levels, and images generated after administration of radiographic contrast media help distinguish vascular from nonvascular structures. Valuable information may be obtained concerning the density of a particular organ or tissue—for example, solid, cystic, and metallic (calcification). Organs that could not previously be visualized on x-ray examination can now be studied using this technique. CT scanning with or without contrast enhancement can help physicians make an early diagnosis with the least amount of discomfort and risk to the patient. CT scanning is invaluable in the evaluation and staging of neoplasms and in the diagnosis of intracranial and intra-abdominal lesions. Availability of CT scans has greatly reduced the need for angiographic examinations and exploratory surgery.

Because of the cost and radiation exposure, this technique should be reserved for conditions in which plain x-ray films and routine contrast studies do not reveal sufficient information for a diagnosis. As with many such procedures, before ordering a CT scan, one should consider both the expense involved and how the information gained would facilitate decision making.

Diagnostic ultrasound

Ultrasonography is a noninvasive, painless technique that has no known harmful effects. A pulse of high-frequency sound waves (1 to 20 million Hz, which is well above 20,000 Hz, the upper limit of human hearing) is emitted from a transducer placed on the body surface over the organs to be studied. The sound waves are reflected in the form of echoes that are converted electronically into a display on a cathode ray oscilloscope. Acoustic interfaces occur whenever a substance changes in acoustic density. Larger reflections occur when the acoustic density difference is greater. Because the sound is well transmitted through fluid, a large reflection occurs when sound passes from fluid to soft tissues.

Ultrasound examination has widespread applications. It can detect fluid (as it occurs in pancreatic pseudocysts, renal cysts, and pericardial effusion), facilitate a diagnosis of gallstones, or help determine the diameter of the biliary ducts (bile duct obstruction) or the size of abdominal aortic aneurysms. Other examples of its application include locating appropriate areas for prostate biopsy through **transrectal ultrasound,** detecting atheromatous plaques (when peripheral vascular disease is suspected, especially in the carotid system), and imaging the kidneys in renal failure to determine kidney size (acute versus chronic renal failure) and **hydronephrosis** (diagnosis of obstructive uropathy). Ultrasound is used to diagnose intrauterine pregnancy and, later, to identify the gender of the fetus and/or location of the placenta. **Echocardiography,** a specialized application, has proven to be invaluable in the noninvasive diagnosis of heart disease; it is described in greater detail in part 4.

Radionuclide imaging

Various applications of radionuclide imaging are summarized in Table 4.1.

Magnetic resonance imaging

Magnetic resonance imaging (MRI) is a relatively new diagnostic technique that has rapidly gained acceptance in clinical applications. Based on the theory that, when radio frequency (RF) signals are applied to protons situated in a strong external magnetic field, the protons become "energized" and emit weak RF signals, the MRI uses nuclear resonance induced by RF signals rather than ionizing radiation to detect contrast and spatial resolutions between tissues. The most common application of the technique is in the investigation of central nervous system lesions, especially those involving the posterior cranial fossa and spinal cord. Cardiac imaging, using rapid sequence (cine) MRI is also now available at many

TABLE 4.1	Clinical Applications of Radionuclide Imaging	
Type	**Purpose**	**Clinical Setting**
Perfusion (Q) scan	diagnosis	pulmonary embolism
Ventilation (V) lung scan	diagnosis	sometimes combined with Q scans
Bone scan	diagnosis	osteomyelitis and bony metastases from cancer
Cardiac imaging	diagnosis	myocardial ischemia or infarction
	evaluation	ventricular performance
Tagged RBC scan	localization	intestinal bleeding
Tagged WBC scan	diagnosis and localization	localized pus collections (abscess)

teaching hospitals. In addition, reports suggest that MRI may be superior to CT scanning in diagnosing soft tissue trauma, infections, tumors, and some metabolic disorders. Because no ionizing radiation is involved, the MRI offers a major advantage in the workup of pelvic disorders in pregnant women and children. No known hazards exist, but extreme caution is required in patients with pacemakers, surgical clips, and metallic prostheses.

■ Other Diagnostic Modalities

In the last three decades, numerous diagnostic modalities have been developed. **Fiberoptic endoscopy,** for example, permits visualization of areas of the gastrointestinal tract and bronchi that were previously inaccessible for inspection. Through endoscopes, removing biopsy specimens for histopathologic evaluation is now possible. **Electrocardiography** and **electroencephalography** are examples of diagnostic electrophysiologic procedures that have been used for decades. **Radioimmunoassay** techniques, which permitted measurement of hormone levels in picogram quantities, have been supplanted by newer, more precise techniques, such as **polymerase chain reaction** (PCR). These techniques have been immensely helpful in clarifying the normal milieu and physiology of various organs, often aiding diagnosis.

■ The Art of Diagnosis

Experienced clinicians use the following six steps, in the order listed, to determine a diagnosis: 1) aggregating groups of findings into patterns, 2) selecting a "pivotal" or key finding, 3) generating a list of causes, 4) pruning the cause list, 5) selecting a diagnosis, and 6) validating the diagnosis. The cause is almost invariably one of the following: infection/infestation, physical/traumatic, immunologic, neoplastic, genetic/metabolic, iatrogenic, psychosomatic, or idiopathic. (These categories are perhaps best remembered using the following mnemonic device: I-PING I-PI.)

CHAPTER 5	PREVENTION AND SCREENING

■ Basic Tenets and Definitions

Prevention consists of evaluation, intervention, and/or lifestyle modification to prevent or delay the onset of pathologic processes or illnesses or to modify the course of established disease in an individual. In some instances, this may require intervention in asymptomatic individuals to prevent future disease.

Prevention has three guiding tenets: 1) it must provide benefit to the individual without causing actual or potential harm (e.g., some vitamins in high doses can cause severe disease without any known benefit; flexible proctosigmoidoscopy, while valuable, can cause complications if used indiscriminately); 2) its goal must not be to postpone the aging process or the inevitable mortality to which all living beings are destined although individuals can certainly attempt to live as long and as full a life as possible; and 3) it must rely on the individual patient's full motivation, understanding, and commitment. The individual must be capable of making informed, common-sense decisions based on the best information available and be prepared to make lifestyle changes that at times may be painful and difficult.

When specific measures are adopted to prevent the development of a specific disorder—for example, vaccination against poliomyelitis—the process is called **primary prevention.** The course of a disease that is present without manifestations might be modified through early detection. Early detection of disease in asymptomatic individuals is termed **screening** and is synonymous with **secondary prevention**—for example, mammograms to detect breast cancer and fecal occult blood testing to detect colon carcinoma. Finally, the disease may already be clinically evident and treated (but not cured), in which case an attempt must be made to delay its progression. This is **tertiary prevention**—for example, the patient who recently underwent coronary artery bypass surgery and is now asymptomatic but needs to modify lifestyle and risk factors to prevent new disease.

As the prescriber, the physician must know the effectiveness of each measure in the detection and/or prevention of disease. Although the effectiveness of immunizations in the primary prevention of many infectious diseases (diphtheria, polio, and smallpox) is proven, it is debatable in many other instances and, as such, fraught with controversy. The physician must also know the natural history of a disorder, which can be achieved through early detection by screening. Screening for hypertension, for example, has been successful in detecting treatable disease and preventing complications and premature death. Our knowledge regarding screening, however, is far from complete.

Information concerning methods of prevention often comes from recommendations by expert committees. The three commonly quoted and studied are those of the Canadian Task Force on the Periodic Health Examination, the United States Preventive Services Task Force, and the American College of Physicians. Although not edicts, these recommendations will undoubtedly evolve as new information and methods become available.

■ **Strategies for Prevention**

The practicing physician can implement prevention by using one of the following strategies. The **periodic health examination** is a comprehensive history and physical examination, accompanied in the same visit by counseling, if unhealthy behaviors are detected; immunizing, if required; and performing indicated screening procedures (e.g., cervical Papanicolaou smear, breast examination, and flexible sigmoidoscopy). Another method, endorsed by the Canadian Preventive Task Force, is the performance of a limited number of preventive interventions at each patient visit—a strategy known as **case finding.** Advocates of case finding argue that the patient load is already too high for primary care physicians to permit adequate periodic health examinations on numerous patients. In addition, office visits by the general population are sufficiently frequent that preventive interventions can be provided longitudinally over several office visits.

Physicians practicing in primary care specialties have the unique opportunity to implement a variety of primary, secondary, and tertiary preventive interventions, depending on the segment of the population they encounter. The following interventions are applicable to adults.

Primary prevention

A prerequisite to prevention is a knowledge of the pathophysiology and the risk factors for development of the disease. An understanding of the pathophysiology of a disease enables the physician to intervene and block the activity of specific, disease-causing agents before they lead to disease development. Vaccinations and immunizations best exemplify the primary prevention of infectious diseases. When administered to an individual, a vaccine, which is a derivative from protein components of a microbe, stimulates the individual's immune system to form antibodies against that microbe, providing protection from disease by infection with that microbe. The process is effective in preventing specific infectious diseases (e.g., tetanus, pneumococcal pneumonia from certain strains, mumps, measles, rubella, hepatitis B, influenza, and rabies). Many of the primary immunizations have been conducted on individuals early in life—that is, younger than age 6. However, adults who have not received primary immunizations need them and, for those previously immunized, booster immunization is sometimes necessary (e.g., to prevent tetanus and hepatitis).

Immunizations

Table 5.1 describes the recommendations for routine booster and primary immunizations in adults; some adults who have not already been vaccinated commonly require primary immunizations. The currently recommended immunizations fulfill the basic tenets of preventive medicine, efficacy, and cost-effectiveness in prevention and safety. Controversy concerning the pertussis vaccine exists because a small but significant percentage of individuals given this vaccine develop neurologic sequelae and the vaccine's effectiveness is far from uniform. As such, the recommendations for pertussis are in a state of flux.

Modification of risk factors

In addition to pathophysiology, an understanding of the risk factors of disease is also required to modify their influence and thereby decrease the risk of disease development. This modification of risk factors is another exciting example of primary prevention. By working with the patient to modify a lifestyle habit, the physician can positively intervene to prevent the development of disease. This is perhaps no better demonstrated than with

TABLE 5.1	Adult Immunizations: Current Recommendations
Vaccine	**Indications and Comments**
Influenza vaccine	All individuals > age 65. Patients at high risk for significant morbidity and mortality (diabetes mellitus, heart disease, pulmonary disease, renal diseases, and the immunocompromised). Health care personnel. Contraindicated when there is a history of allergy to egg yolk. Vaccine is usually available in the autumn and should be used yearly.
Pneumoccocal vaccine	Similar to those for influenza vaccine. Other indications are asplenia (anatomical or functional), alcoholism, sickle cell disease, Hodgkin's disease, nephrotic syndrome. Vaccine may be administered year-round but only once in the lifetime for each individual. Egg yolk allergy is not a contraindication.
Tetanus toxoid	A must for all adults once every 10 years.
Hepatitis B vaccine	Individuals with high risk of exposure (health care workers, individuals at biomedical research laboratories, homosexually active men, and intravenous drug abusers). Recombinant, inactivated vaccine. Over 95% of healthy individuals given vaccine develop immunity. Duration of immunity has not been clearly defined.
Measles vaccine	Individuals born after 1956 who lack evidence of immunity.
Rubella vaccination	Women of childbearing age who lack proof of immunity. CDC recommends health care workers, military recruits, and college students. Recipient has to agree not to become pregnant in the 3 months to follow. Pregnancy is an absolute contraindication.

TABLE 5.2	Risk Factors for Atherosclerosis

Established factors
Cigarette smoking
Hypertension
Hypercholesterolemia
Old age
Male gender

Hypothesized factors
Diabetes mellitus
Family history of premature coronary artery disease
Reduced high-density lipoprotein (HDL) cholesterol level
Pronounced obesity
Sedentary lifestyle
Stress and personality
Increased Apolipoprotein A (LpA)
Increased homocystine level

atherosclerosis, of which we now have a basic understanding. Specific risk factors for atherosclerosis are listed in Table 5.2. Convincing evidence indicates that modifying risk factors does, indeed, slow the development of atherosclerosis and prevent premature morbidity and mortality from many of its clinical syndromes, such as myocardial infarction and stroke. Other examples of disease prevention through lifestyle modifications or understanding risk factors or pathophysiology data are listed in Table 5.3.

Secondary prevention

A **screening intervention** enables the discovery of a disorder in its asymptomatic stage. To be effective against any targeted disease, the screening intervention should satisfy all the following conditions:

1. The disorder is relatively prevalent.

2. The test is reasonably safe, inexpensive, and acceptable to the patient.

3. The test recognizes the majority of patients with the disorder (high sensitivity) while mislabeling few patients as having the disorder (high specificity).

4. Follow-up confirmation tests are safe and, ideally, noninvasive and affordable.

5. Treatment of the disorder in its asymptomatic stage will improve the patient's prognosis compared with those patients who have a similar disorder and are treated only when the disease becomes symptomatic.

TABLE 5.3	Potential Opportunities for Disease Prevention Through Modifications in Lifestyle/Understanding of Risk Factors

Home
Teach firearm safety.
Advise against smoking in bed.
Use smoke detectors.
Monitor hot water temperature (elderly and toddlers).
Prevent falls (elderly).

Outdoors
Use seat belts while driving.
Use bicycle and motorcycle helmets.
Advocate regular physical activity.
Prevent melanoma through sun protection.

General
Advise regarding:
   practice of safe sex
   use of contraceptives
   preventive dental care
   use and abuse of stimulants, including alcohol, caffeine, tobacco, illicit drugs
Ensure immunizations.
Preventive eye care including glaucoma screening.
Evaluate hearing in individuals at high risk for hearing loss.
Provide regular health maintenance.

Work environment
Review safety precautions commensurate with type of occupation.

Nutrition
Educate regarding:
   balanced diet
   fiber content
   vitamin supplements
   calcium supplements
Help manage stress

6. The ultimate outcome of the disorder has grave consequences for the well-being of patients, regarding morbidity and/or mortality.

Of these characteristics, the two that are most difficult to evaluate and quantify are the sensitivity/specificity and the efficacy of the available interventions for disease diagnosed in its asymptomatic stage.

Examples of screening interventions that have not been shown to benefit patient outcome include yearly chest x-ray for the screening of lung cancer, carcinoembryonic antigen (CEA) for colo-rectal cancer screening, the use of a battery of blood tests in asymptomatic individuals, complete routine urinalysis in nonpregnant/nondiabetic patients, and the use of electrocardiograms in otherwise healthy individuals. Strategies currently undergoing investigation as potentially useful screening strategies include the prostate-specific antigen (PSA) alone and in combination with transrectal ultrasound for the early diagnosis of prostatic cancer, fecal occult blood testing for colorectal cancer screening, and serum markers for ovarian cancer (CA-125) alone or in combination with transvaginal ultrasound.

A major application of screening interventions in adults involves the early detection of cancer. While proponents argue that earlier detection of cancer will lead to its cure, opponents argue that cancer has its natural growth rate and finite prognosis, that the overall prognosis is unaffected regardless of the time of detection, and that the improvement in mortality is merely a reflection of the cancer being detected early (lead-time bias). Nevertheless, the physician's obligation to detect cancers early, if possible, is indisputable. A detailed list of screening recommendations for many neoplasms is shown in Table 5.4.

Breast cancer screening combines monthly breast self-examination at midmenstrual cycle with an annual exam by a physician, supplemented by yearly mammography, depending on the patient's age (see Table 5.4). The initiation of the screening is influenced by a family history of breast cancer. Cervical cancer, a prime example of the usefulness of screening, is detected early by regular Pap smears of the cervix, the process beginning from the time sexual activity starts. The frequency depends on the age and the results of previous tests.

Complete skin inspection for detection of skin cancer entails examination of the entire skin in patients at high risk for skin cancer or those with precursor lesions. As with breast cancer, the role of self-examination cannot be overemphasized.

TABLE 5.4 Cancer Screening: Recommendations for Screening and Its Overall Effectiveness in Changing the Natural History of the Disease

Neoplasm	General Recommendations	Recommendations by Special Societies/Panel of Experts
Breast cancer[a]	Breast examination by a physician every 1 to 2 yrs. from age 40. Yearly mammography, from age 50. Screening may be stopped by age 75. If family history of breast cancer is present, start yearly mammography at age 35. Monthly breast self-examination at midcycle.	ACOG: annual or biannual mammography and annual breast examination by a physician starting at age 40.
Colorectal cancer[a]	Flexible sigmoidoscopy every 3 to 5 years starting at age 50. Usefulness of fecal occult blood testing (FOBT) is being determined.	USPTF: screening only for those at high risk for colorectal cancer (positive family history) starting at age 50. ACS: yearly FOBT starting at age 40, and flexible sigmoidoscopy for 2 consecutive years at age 50 and every 3 years thereafter, if the initial flexible sigmoidoscopic examinations are normal.
Cervical cancer[a]	Pap smears every 1 to 3 years, from commencement of sexual activity. Screening can be stopped by age 65 if the examinations are consistently normal.	Screening to begin at age 18 or beginning of sexual activity, with annual tests for 3 years and thereafter, every 3 years, if the three prior Pap smears were normal.
Prostate cancer[b]	Yearly rectal examinations after age 40.	USPTF: Digital rectal examination, serum markers, or transrectal ultrasound not recommended in asymptomatic men. ACS: yearly rectal examination starting at age 40. See text for the BPH guideline panel recommendations.
Skin cancer[a]	Complete skin inspection only for patients at high risk, family or personal history of skin cancer, or precursor lesion (i.e., dysplastic nevi).	AAD: annual complete examination for all patients as well as monthly self-examination.
Ovarian cancer[b]	Careful examination of the uterine adnexa during pelvic examination. Role of serum markers and/or transvaginal ultrasound still under investigation. If history of ovarian cancer or breast cancer in first degree relatives: serum markers and transvaginal ultrasound done sequentially may be beneficial.	
Testicular cancer	Routine examination only in high-risk patients: those with testicular atrophy, cryptorchidism, or orchiopexy.	ACS: testicular exam as part of the periodic health examination and monthly self-examination in post-pubertal man.

[a]Interventions are effective in changing natural history.
[b]Effectiveness of interventions unknown in changing natural history.
AAD: American Academy of Dermatology; ACOG: American College of Obstetricians and Gynecologists; ACS: American Cancer Society; BPH: Benign prostatic hypertrophy; USPTF: United States Preventive Task Force.

ALTERNATIVE MEDICINE

■ Definition

Alternative medicine defies definition because the term encompasses a broad spectrum of practices and beliefs. Many are well-known, others are exotic or mysterious, and some are unquestionably dangerous. Perhaps a reasonable definition is medical practices that do not conform to the standards of the traditional Western medical community and are not taught widely at U.S. medical schools or generally available at U.S. hospitals.

■ Types of Alternative Therapies

At one time, **osteopathy** was considered an alternative therapy; it is now integrated with modern Western medicine because the curriculum taught in osteopathic schools is comparable with that in the allopathic (traditional) medical schools. Some of the better-known alternative therapies are described in the following.

Chiropractic

In this therapeutic system, diseases are regarded as the result of an irritation of the spinal cord due to subluxation of the spine and that manipulation of the spine can lead to cure.

Acupuncture

In the ancient Chinese practice of acupuncture, insertion of needles into specific points on the body's surface supposedly improves the flow of the energy around the body. Acupuncture is believed to relieve pain, induce surgical anesthesia, and heal several disorders.

Homeopathy

In this German system of therapeutics founded by Samuel Hahnemann (1755–1843), all disease symptoms are believed to originate from the body's attempts at healing. Accordingly, the patient is treated with small doses of a drug that, in large doses, would mimic the symptoms of the patient's disease. Most homeopathic medications are said to be harmless and are given individually rather than in the "dangerous mixtures" that were customary during Hahnemann's time.

Massage therapy

Massage therapists manipulate soft tissue with their hands using unperfumed or perfumed oil. This reduces friction and, thus, relieves musculoskeletal pain while supposedly curing many other illnesses.

Reflexology

Also known as zone therapy, reflexology is manipulation and massage of the feet to locate and treat disease or dysfunction elsewhere in the body.

Transcendental meditation

Transcendental meditation (TM) is a technique for obtaining a state of physical relaxation and psychological calm by implementing the regular practice of a relaxation procedure that entails the repetition of a selected word or mantra.

Imagery

Imagery is based on the belief that pleasant thoughts—for example, imagining that the body is healing itself, reading literature, or watching humorous videos—can cause a healing effect.

Herbal medicine

Plant products of various kinds such as minced palmetto berries, chopped valerian root, and others, including some with pharmacologic properties, are administered orally or through enemas to cure various disorders.

Holistic medicine

Holistic medicine—which encompasses a "whole body" approach to health, as opposed to a focus on individual organs— has gained respectability in recent years. This therapeutic modality includes meditation, exercise, dieting, and abstinence from smoking, alcohol, and other addictive substances.

Ayurvedic medicine

This ancient East Indian mode of therapy relies on the use of various herbs to treat illness and maintain health. Ayurvedic medicine emphasizes the interaction of medications with diet and/or activities. By the repeated distillation and processing of herbal agents, as well as by avoidance of interacting diet (e.g., milk, certain vegetables) and/or activities (e.g, physical activity for several hours after taking medication), this mode of therapy also aims to minimize or eliminate side effects from medication.

Naturopathy

Naturopathy emphasizes a drug-free system of therapy, making use of physical forces such as air, light, water, heat, and massage for healing.

TABLE 6.1	The 10 Most Frequent Conditions and Alternative Therapies Used
Condition	**Therapies**
Back problems	Chiropractic, massage
Allergies	Spiritual healing, lifestyle diets
Arthritis	Chiropractic, relaxation techniques
Insomnia	Relaxation techniques, imagery
Sprains or strains	Massage, relaxation techniques
Headache	Relaxation techniques, chiropractic
High blood pressure	Relaxation techniques, homeopathy
Digestive problems	Relaxation techniques, megavitamins
Anxiety	Relaxation techniques, imagery
Depression	Relaxation techniques, self-help groups

Self-help groups

With the increasing use of electronic communication, more and more people are relying on other patients and advice from nontraditional healers.

■ Use of Alternative Medicine

Americans often use unconventional therapy upon the failure of, or in conjunction with, traditional therapy for various indications. According to a 1990 study, as many as 34% of the public used at least one unconventional therapy in the previous year. The 10 most frequent medical conditions for which the public uses alternative medicine are listed in Table 6.1.

The highest use of unconventional therapy is re-ported among North Americans aged 25–49 years who have higher-than-average education and income. The majority use unconventional therapy for chronic, non-life-threatening, medical conditions. Among those who use unconventional therapy for serious medical conditions, 72% did not inform their medical doctors that they had done so. According to one estimate in 1990, Americans made 425 million visits to providers of unconventional therapy compared with 388 million visits to all U.S. primary care physicians. The expenditures associated with the use of unconventional therapy were estimated to be $13.7 billion, three-quarters of which was paid out-of-pocket, compared with $12.8 billion spent out-of-pocket annually for all hospitalizations in the United States.

■ Role of Physicians

Physicians should learn more about alternative therapies, understand what they are, and apply scientific methods to test them. They should promote open communication with patients who seek help from these methods, and they should always ask patients about their use of unconventional therapy when obtaining medical histories. According to Relman, no such thing as alternative medicine exists—only medicine that has been proven to work and medicine that has not. Unconventional medicine may work, but we will never know without better evidence. In today's frantic and increasingly impersonal world, many patients seek simplicity, clarity, attention, and a human touch from their doctors. Physicians should welcome this demand from their patients and spend more time with them. In the era of managed care, this may seem unrealistic, but physicians must remain their patients' advocates and make time for their patients.

<hr/>

CHAPTER 7 MEDICAL ETHICS

The medical profession has long subscribed to a body of ethical statements developed primarily for the benefit of the patient. The American Medical Association (AMA) has summarized these principles, which define the essentials of honorable behavior and expected standards of conduct among physicians (Table 7.1). As medical historian Lester King said, "Members of a profession thus found themselves in a position of authority that rested on trust." This dual relationship imposed on the members of a profession a particular moral obligation, which was made explicit by a code of ethics.

■ Physician and the Profession

Ethically, clinicians are responsible for reaching a decision that is not only clinically and technically sound but also morally appropriate—one that is suitable for the specific problems of the particular patients they are treating.

Medicine has no solitary goal. In the encounter between patient and clinician, many appropriate goals are pursued simultaneously. These are summarized in Table 7.2. Essential to sound decision making is a realistic understanding of the goals of treatment by both the

TABLE 7.1	American Medical Association Principles of Medical Ethics

I. A physician shall be dedicated to providing competent medical service with compassion and respect for human dignity.

II. A physician shall deal honestly with patients and colleagues, and strive to expose those physicians deficient in character or competence, or who engage in fraud or deception.

III. A physician shall respect the law and also recognize a responsibility to seek changes in those requirements which are contrary to the best interests of the patient.

IV. A physician shall respect the rights of patients, of colleagues, and of other health professionals, and shall safeguard patient confidences within the constraints of the law.

V. A physician shall continue to study, apply, and advance scientific knowledge, make relevant information available to patients, colleagues, and the public, obtain consultation, and use the talents of other health professionals when indicated.

VI. A physician shall, in the provision of appropriate patient care except in emergencies, be free to choose whom to serve, with whom to associate, and the environment in which to provide medical services.

VII. A physician shall recognize a responsibility to participate in activities contributing to an improved community.

TABLE 7.2	Goals for Physicians in Patient Encounters

Always
Avoidance of harm to the patient in the course of care (*primum non nocere*).
Palliation (relief of pain and suffering) and comfort care *in all situations.*

Before disease is established
Prevention of disease and untimely death.

When disease is established
Cure of disease and restoration of health, *when possible.*
Improvement or maintenance of functional status *when cure is not possible.*
Education and counseling regarding the condition and its prognosis.

physician and the patient. The physician's task is to inform the patient about which goals are attainable. In defining the goals of the encounter, according to Jonsen, Siegler, and Winslade, the clinician should consider the following issues: the nature of the disease; the preferences of the patient; and social, cultural, political, and economic realities.

Nature of the disease

In determining the nature of a patient's disease and how to manage it, the physician must ask the following questions: What is the current medical status, diagnosis, and prognosis? What is the recommended treatment? What are the reasonable alternative treatments and what would be the effect of no treatment? What goals are attainable for this particular patient with this specific condition? What trade-offs must be made among the possible goals—for example, between relief of suffering and maximal preservation of function? Of course, any such determination in medicine must be expressed in probabilities rather than in certainties.

Preferences of the patient

What are the patient's personal goals in this encounter? Is the patient fully informed and has the patient had time to consider the reasonable options? Will the probable outcomes of the suggested course of action be consistent with the patient's value system and life plan? Although usually the same as the clinician's, the patient's goals will occasionally differ from those of the clinician for personal or psychological reasons, and some accommodations must be made.

Social, cultural, political, and economic realities

Any goals sought by clinicians and patients must be pursued within the context of religious, social, cultural, political, and economic realities. Access to scarce resources, the mandates of the current health care system, the wealth or poverty of individuals and communities, religious and cultural beliefs, and family pressures will facilitate the attainment of some goals and render the achievement of others unlikely.

■ Basic Concepts in Medical Ethics

Informed consent

Informed consent is rooted in the English common law on battery, which forbids harmful or offensive nonconsensual touching. No special exceptions were made for medical care, except in emergency situations. The modern American judicial expression of consent is that of Justice Cardozo in 1914: "Every human being of adult years and sound mind has a right to determine what shall be done with his [or her] own body; and a surgeon who performs an operation without his [or her] patient's consent commits an assault for which he [or she] is liable for damages." In the latter half of this century, the courts began merging the physician's traditional duty to secure consent with an obligation of disclosure, perhaps best understood as a duty to warn patients of potential side effects or consequences of medical treatment, resulting in the legal concept of "informed consent."

The purpose of informed consent is to provide the patient with the information necessary to allow a reasonable person to make a prudent treatment choice. According to the President's Commission, adequate informed consent involves more than just a signature on the bottom of a list of possible complications; it requires effort on the part of the physician to ensure the patient's comprehension: "Such recitations can be so overwhelming that patients are unable to distinguish truly significant information and to make sound decisions." Rather, informed consent attempts to foster a conversational partnership between doctor and patient in the clinical setting.

The elements incorporated into the current doctrine of informed consent require the physician to ensure that the patient has a clear understanding of the following:

- the disease process (diagnosis in understandable terms),
- the prognosis (probable course of this patient's specific disease),
- the benefits and burdens of the recommended treatment,
- the benefits and burdens of reasonable alternative treatments, and
- the probable effect of no treatment (this is always an option).

The consent that follows this disclosure entails the patient's voluntary, autonomous authorization to proceed with the proposed intervention.

Patient's right to refuse treatment

Adult patients of sound mind have the right to refuse any treatment on their own behalf, and courts have increasingly granted surrogate decision makers the right to withdraw treatment as well. This right even extends to the withdrawal of treatment from patients who are not judged to be terminal. The *Bartling* decision in California states that "competent adult patients with serious illnesses which are probably incurable but have not been diagnosed as terminal have the right over the objections of their physicians and the hospital to have life support equipment disconnected, despite the fact that withdrawal of such devices will surely hasten death."

Since the *Bartling* decision, there have been no legal cases challenging to the right of the "decisional patient" (i.e., one who is capable of making a decision) to refuse any treatment, including fluid and nutrition.

Confidentiality and the patient's right to privacy

The basis for the principle of confidentiality is respect for an individual's privacy and the special relationship of trust in the doctor–patient encounter. Because confidentiality is considered necessary for the good of society and to prevent harm to the patient, it is not to be breached without a compelling reason.

Legal exceptions exist to the patient's right to confidentiality. Physicians may breach confidentiality to testify in court; to report communicable disease; to report child, spouse, or elder abuse; and to report gunshot or suspicious wounds if a reasonable cause to believe that the wound occurred as the result of a crime exists. Aside from these specific situations, breach of confidentiality can rarely be justified ethically; such breach can be justified only when all of a few specific conditions are met. These are listed in Table 7.3.

Decision-making capacity

"Competence" and "incompetence" are legal terms. Technically, a patient remains competent until a court decides otherwise; however, the determination of decision-making capacity can be made by medical personnel and does not require a court hearing.

The assessment of a patient's ability to make autonomous judgments requires the evaluation of the following three distinct aspects of decision-making capacity:

Understanding. The ability to comprehend the given information about diagnosis and treatment and to appreciate the impact of the disease and its consequences.

Evaluating. The ability to deliberate in accordance with one's own values, to manipulate information rationally, and to compare the risks and benefits of the options.

Communicating. The ability to communicate choices to persons providing medical care.

TABLE 7.3	Breach of Patient Confidentiality by the Physician

Breach of privacy is permissible when all of the following conditions are met:
—A high probability exists of serious physical harm to an identifiable, specific person.
—A benefit will result from breaking the confidence (i.e., the harm can be prevented).
—The breach is a last resort; persuasion and other approaches have failed.
—The breach is generalizable; it would be reasonable for doctors, in general, to breach such confidence.

Incapacitated (nondecisional) patients

When a surrogate acts for an incapacitated patient, the basis for his or her decision is either "substituted judgment" or the "best interests" standard. Substituted judgment is the guideline the surrogate uses if the patient has expressed a preference before becoming incapacitated or if the surrogate knows the patient well enough to determine what the patient would choose if he or she were still decisional.

The best interests standard is what the surrogate must use when he or she is unsure of what the patient might choose or if the patient has never been decisional. It is what a reasonable person might choose in the same context and is based on what is ultimately best for the particular patient in his or her particular circumstances. When a patient has a legal guardian, this individual has the right to make decisions, including the refusal of life-sustaining treatment, based on the patient's best interests considering the diagnosis, prognosis, and medical goals of treatment.

■ Specific Issues in Medical Ethics

"Do-not-resuscitate" orders

The issue of cardiopulmonary resuscitation (CPR) should be addressed early in the treatment course of a seriously ill patient in whom cardiac or pulmonary arrest might likely occur. The subject should be approached sensitively as part of the overall therapeutic plan. The comfort and therapeutic measures that will remain in effect should be discussed first. The legal authority for the decision to write a do-not-resuscitate (DNR) order may emanate from the specific request of a decisional patient, from the dictates of an advance directive, or from the judgment of a guardian.

In some states, surrogate laws establish a hierarchy of decision-making authority for the nondecisional patient; in others, moral authority but no legal authority exists for the following order: spouse, adult children, parents, siblings. If no relatives or friends are available for consultation, the decision should be based on medical indications, taking into consideration whether CPR would further the reasonable personal medical goals of the patient in his or her current particular circumstances.

Ordinarily, DNR simply means no CPR. A DNR order may have no other significance and may be compatible with all other modalities of treatment including intensive care. On the other hand, a DNR order may be the first step in the withdrawal of other treatment; thus, specific orders detailing what may remain in use must be written to avoid misunderstandings. The rationale and specific orders need to be discussed fully with the nursing staff and the patient's other caregivers so no uncertainties about care plans remain. Sometimes, patients or their families fear abandonment by health care professionals when a DNR order is written; therefore, physicians and nurses alike should be more attentive and aware of comfort measures. The patient and family must know from the outset that "no code" does not mean "no care."

Withdrawal versus withholding of treatment

Psychologically, for the physician, refraining from starting a treatment is easier than discontinuing it. A moment's reflection demonstrates that this is illogical; the decision to omit treatment is just as much a willful judgment as the decision to withdraw it. The decision to withhold a specific treatment may create an "up-front" barrier—denying up-front a treatment that might be effective. Thus, a decision to withhold treatment must actually have more substantial reasons than a decision to discontinue, or withdraw, treatment that has clearly failed. When the effectiveness of a treatment is uncertain, the bias clearly must be in favor of a time-limited trial. If the treatment proves to be ineffective for a particular patient in a given circumstance, it can be stopped. Through the use of this model, the patient has a reasonable chance of attaining the goals of the specific therapy.

Futility

Occasionally, patients will demand or request treatment modalities that the physician believes to be ineffective or even contraindicated medically because they are futile. Futility has been defined as any effort to achieve a result that is possible but that experience suggests is highly improbable. Some consider futility to be a disproportionate burden including treatment that will not serve any useful purpose, that may cause needless pain and suffering, and that will not achieve the goal of restoring the patient to an acceptable quality of life (as defined by that patient).

Professional integrity requires that the ethical physician refuse requests for futile interventions. The President's Commission stated the following: "The well-being principle circumscribes the range of alternatives offered to patients: informed consent does not mean that patients can insist upon anything they might want. Rather, it is a choice among medically accepted and available options, all of which are believed to have some possibility of promoting the patient's welfare." And the Council on Ethical and Judicial Affairs of the AMA stated that "the right of the patient to choose does not imply the right to demand care beyond appropriate options based on medical judgment and accepted standards of care, nor are physicians required to provide care in ways that in their personal judgment violate the principles of medical ethics."

Resolution of this sort of impasse requires a dialogue

with the patient to elicit the reasons behind the request for a medically futile intervention. Often, such a conversation will solve the dilemma; if not, the physician may need to transfer the patient to the care of another. Many physicians unreasonably fear liability for not "doing everything" such as using every available technology if the patient requests it, but the law rarely dictates the particulars of clinical practice and does not require that physicians do everything requested by a patient, agent, or guardian.

Acquired Immune Deficency Syndrome (AIDS)

Ethical issues concerning AIDS include maintaining medical compassion, determining medical futility, caring for the nondecisional patient, and alleviating physician stress and anxiety. The physician may need to overcome homophobia and attempt to understand patients from different social backgrounds. A gap between doctor and patient will make having ethical discussions regarding medical indications, patient preferences, and allocation of resources (CPR and intensive care) more difficult. Because AIDS is a relatively new disease and therapies evolve so rapidly, additional unique issues exist relating to medical uncertainty in diagnosis, prognosis, and the withdrawal of treatment when it becomes futile.

Another problem posed by AIDS is the risk to health professionals. The risk of occupational transmission is minimal, but despite good infection control measures, it is not nonexistent. The thoughts, feelings, and fears of caregivers who provide bedside care need to be addressed using credible scientific information and psychological support, but the ethical responsibility for the care of AIDS patients is clear. The AMA Council on Ethical and Judicial Affairs has stated, "A physician may not ethically refuse to treat a patient whose condition is within the physician's current realm of competence solely because the patient is sero-positive. Persons who are sero-positive should not be subjected to discrimination based on fear or prejudice."

Pain control

Recent national initiatives and the medical literature reflect the lack of optimal pain control in both adults and children. Fear that pain control may be inadequate is widespread and may be responsible, in part, for the increasing interest in euthanasia and assisted suicide.

Several reasons exist concerning the problem of substandard pain control. The drug of choice may be poor; for example, meperidine is clearly inferior to morphine for controlling the severe pain of bony metastases. The dose of the chosen drug may be inadequate or the dosing interval too long. Fear of causing addiction in chronic pain or terminal situations in which large doses must be continued for long periods is another reason for withholding adequate analgesics. Underdosing of a narcotic in terminal situations for fear of producing respiratory depression is another common mistake.

Studies have shown that addiction is rare in patients who receive opioids for pain, even if the drug must be continued for protracted periods. If the patient is receiving morphine for the pain of terminal malignancy, the question of addiction is irrelevant. The experiences of hospices and oncology services show that respiratory depression is uncommon in patients who are receiving opioids for pain control. The physician must balance the issue of pain control with the rare, undesired effect of respiratory depression.

One ethics panel has addressed the issue as follows: "In the patient whose dying process is irreversible, the balance between minimizing pain and suffering and potentially hastening death should be struck clearly in favor of pain relief. Narcotics and other pain medications should be given in whatever dose and by whatever route is necessary for relief." Most ethicists would agree that it is morally permissible to "increase the dose of narcotics to whatever dose is needed" although the medication may contribute to the depression of respiration or blood pressure, the dulling of consciousness, or even death—providing the primary goal of the physician is to relieve suffering. The proper dose of pain medication is the dose that is sufficient to relieve pain and suffering—even if it causes unconsciousness.

Advance directives

Medical advances have widened the range of options a patient has for the treatment of many diseases, but also have resulted in increased patient concerns about invasive, expensive, and unwanted treatment. An advance directive (AD) provides valuable written evidence of an individual patient's desires to physician and family alike. An AD is a statement a patient makes while still capable of making decisions concerning how treatment decisions should be made at some future time if he or she loses the capacity to make such decisions. Two types of ADs, the Living Will (LW) and the Power of Attorney for Health Care (PAHC), exist.

Most statutory forms of LW are documents stating the desire of the signer to die a natural death and not to be kept alive by medical treatment and machines. In many states, the principal may also stipulate that fluid and nutrition are to be discontinued in the event that the signer is left in a persistent vegetative state. Usually, the LW becomes effective on the determination of a "terminal" illness or "imminent" death (death expected within 6 months) or when two physicians make the diagnosis of a persistent, vegetative state. Usually, there is no provision for adding a personal statement with specific instructions.

Power of Attorney for Health Care documents provide a way for the signer to appoint a person to act as health care agent, or proxy, to make health care decisions in the event that the signer becomes nondecisional. The PAHC allows the principal to add specific directions; often, the agent may be given authority to have feeding tubes withheld or withdrawn (even in the absence of a persistent vegetative state). The PAHC typically becomes effective when two physicians determine that the principal is no longer decisional.

Patients may ask for advice about advance directives. The statutory form of PAHC has the advantage of allowing all the options of an LW plus the advantage of allowing for the insertion of specific instructions and, most important, of providing an agent—someone who knows the principal well and can take an active role in the decision-making process on the patient's behalf. Filling out both forms is not advantageous. Because the specific laws regarding LW and PAHC vary from state to state, checking the provisions and activating clauses in your own jurisdiction is wise.

Ethics consultation

Advances in medicine have resulted in increased ethical dilemmas. Questions now concern not only what can be done for this patient but what should be done. In most hospitals today, ethics consultation is available to physicians and patients to help resolve the vexing problems that sometimes arise in patient care. Institutional ethics committees (ECs) have many different configurations. Many are standing committees comprised of members of the professional staff that report to the medical executive committees or governing staff of the hospital. Most meet monthly or more frequently, as occasion demands. Typically, ECs have three tasks: 1) education, of committee members first and of staff and community later; 2) formulation of policy at the request of the medical staff or institutional administration (ordinarily the EC is not a policy-making body); and 3) specific case consultation on request.

An ethics consultation might be considered by the attending physician for some of the following reasons: 1) to clarify issues regarding decisional capacity, informed consent, or advance directives; 2) to provide counsel on the ethical aspects of withdrawal of treatment in specific cases; and 3) to help resolve conflicts regarding ethical issues that might arise between patients and caregivers, or between family and caregivers, or among staff members.

In case consultation, no single ethical principle suffices. Cases vary too much to allow for such generalizations. The consultant usually allows the details of the case to frame the issues; the consultation process allows the patient, family, and others to identify the important factors and values at stake. This medical casuistry—solving issues by considering the clinical circumstances that surround and affect the cases instead of applying a set of rules or principles to them—characterizes the consultant's ethical analysis.

After analysis of the issues, the EC or the ethics consultant, acting on behalf of the EC, must ensure that the information is complete and that the ethical problem is delineated clearly. In clarifying the possible options, the EC must ensure that the patient will have as much autonomy as possible. The recommendations should be consistent with the patient's preferences or best interests and with ethical and, if possible, with legal principles. Recommendations should be made as recommendations only; the attending physician and the patient must decide whether to take or reject them, as is true of all consultations.

Euthanasia and assisted suicide

The important aspect of agency marks the difference between euthanasia and assisted suicide. Euthanasia, in which the physician is the agent, is an intentional act to cause the immediate death of a person with a terminal, incurable, or painful disease by the medical administration of a lethal drug. In assisted suicide, the physician provides the lethal drug with instructions for its use, but the patient is the agent who decides when and if to use the drug.

Euthanasia is illegal in all states. Suicide is not illegal, but all states now have some sort of legal prohibition against assisted suicide. Thirty-one states have a specific law against assisting a suicide; in the remaining states, prosecution is possible under other existing statutes.

Official medical organizations are uniform in their stance that these actions are unethical. The American College of Physicians Ethics Manual states, "Although a patient may refuse a medical intervention and the physician may comply with this refusal, the physician must never intentionally and directly cause death or assist a patient to commit suicide."

In several recent surveys, the majority of the public has expressed support for some form of physician-assisted death under some circumstances. In 1994 the voters of Oregon authorized controlled physician-assisted suicide. Court challenges delayed implementation until October 1997. In November 1997, another vote failed to repeal the 1994 initiative; thus, Oregon is the only state in which physician-assisted suicide is legal under stipulated safeguards. The "Laboratory of the States" will test this issue.

Analyzing the stimulus for these initiatives that have such widespread public support and attempting to change those factors that are amenable to change is the responsibility of physicians. Prominent among the fears

tinction between withholding and withdrawing treatment are true, EXCEPT:

A. There is no legal or ethical difference between withholding and withdrawing a specific treatment regimen.

B. Once treatment begins, it cannot be discontinued; therefore, withholding treatment becomes an important consideration in many cases.

C. The difference between these is not based on any logic.

D. In case of uncertainty, one should not withhold a time-limited treatment trial, which can be stopped if it later proves to be ineffective.

Refer to items A through I below for questions 17 and 18:

A. Fear of addiction

B. The patient's ability to understand the information given

C. Ability to evaluate given information in personal terms

D. Principle of informed consent

E. The patient's mental competence

F. Fear of respiratory depression

G. Communication skills and ability

H. PRN rather than a regular schedule

I. Inadequate agent and/or dose

17. Select any THREE items to consider in determining a patient's decisional capacity.

18. Select any FOUR items to consider when administering pain control in terminal malignancy.

■ Answers

1. A	2. D	3. C	4. D	5. A
6. D	7. D	8. D	9. E	10. D
11. C	12. C	13. A	14. D	15. D
16. B	17. B, C, G		18. A, F, H, I	

SUGGESTED READING

General

Books and Monographs

Bennett JC, Plum F (eds.). Cecil Textbook of Medicine. 20th ed. Philadelphia: W. B. Saunders, 1996.

Isselbacher KJ, Braunwald E, Petersdorf RG, et al. (eds.). Harrison's Principles of Internal Medicine. 14th ed. New York: McGraw-Hill, 1998.

Orland M, Saltman R (eds.). Manual of Medical Therapeutics. 29th ed. Boston: Little, Brown & Co., 1997.

Stein, JH (ed.). Internal Medicine. 4th ed. St. Louis: Mosby, 1994.

Articles

Frisse ME, Florence V. A library for internists IX. Recommended by the American College of Physicians. Ann Intern Med 1997;120:836–846.

Bedside Techniques

Books and Monographs

Bates B, Hoekelman RA. A Guide to Physical Examination. 6th ed. Philadelphia: J. B. Lippincott, 1995.

DeGowin, RL. DeGowin & DeGowin's Bedside Diagnostic Examination. 6th ed. Revised by RL DeGowin. Jochimsen PR, Theilen Eo (contributors). New York: McGraw-Hill, 1994.

Swash M, Mason S. Hutchinson's Clinical Methods. 19th ed. Philadelphia: W. B. Saunders, 1989.

Articles

Eddy DM, Clanton CH. The art of diagnosis. N Engl J Med 1982;306:1263–1268.

Prevention and Screening

Catalona WJ, Smith DS, Ratliff TL, et al. Measurement of prostate-specific antigen in serum as a screening test for prostate cancer. N Engl J Med 1991;324:1156–1161.

Eddy, DM. Screening for breast cancer. Ann Intern Med 1989;111:858–859.

Eddy DM. Screening for cervical cancer. Ann Intern Med 1990; 113:214–226.

Eddy DM. Screening for colorectal cancer. Ann Intern Med 1990; 113:373–384.

Guide for Adult Immunization/ACP Task Force on Adult Immunization and Infectious Diseases Society of America. 3rd ed. Philadelphia: American College of Physicians, 1994.

Hayward RS, Steinberg EP, Ford DE, et al. Preventive care guidelines. Ann Intern Med 1991;114:758–783.

Mandel JS, Bond JH, Church TR, et al. Reducing mortality from colorectal cancer by screening for fecal occult blood. N Engl J Med 1993;328:1365–1371.

Shapiro ED, Berg AT, Austrian R, et al. The protective efficacy of polyvalent pneumococcal polysaccharide vaccine. N Engl J Med 1991;325:1453–1460.

Alternative Medicine

Delbanco DL. Herbs: Mainstream magic and menace. Ann Int Med 1994;121:803–804.

Eisenberg DM, Kessler RC, Foster C, et al. Unconventional medicine in the United States. N Engl J Med 1993;328:246–252.

Relman AS. Alternative medicine: A shot in the dark. The Wall Street Journal, July 12, 1995.

Medical Ethics

Books and Monographs

Jonsen AR, Siegler M, Winslade WJ. Clinical Ethics. 2nd ed. New York: Macmillan, 1986:15–16.

La Puma J, Schiedermayer D. Ethics Consultation—A Practical Guide. Boston: Jones and Bartlett, 1994:20.

President's Commission for the Study of Ethical Problems in Medicine and Biomedical and Behavioral Research. Washington, DC, 1982.

President's Commission for the Study of Ethical Problems in Medicine and Biomedical and Behavioral Research. Washington, DC. 1982:42–44.

Articles

AMA Council on Ethical and Judicial Affairs. Ethical issues involved in the growing AIDS crisis. JAMA 1988;259:1360–1361.

AMA Council on Ethical and Judicial Affairs. Guidelines for CPR—Ethical considerations in resuscitation. JAMA 1992; 268:2282–2288.

American College of Physicians Ethics Manual 4th ed. Ann Int Med (In press).

Bartling vs. Superior Court 163 Cal.App3d 186, 1984.

King LS. Medicine—trade or profession. JAMA 1985;253: 2709–2710.

Schloendorff vs. Society of New York Hospital, 211 NY 125,105 NE 92,95 (1914).

Wanzer SH, Federman DD, Adelstein SJ, et al. The physician's responsibility toward hopelessly ill patients—a second look. N Engl J Med 1989;320:844–849.

PART II

Robert H. Fisher

ALLERGY AND CLINICAL IMMUNOLOGY

CHAPTER 8

BASIC MECHANISMS

The immune system plays a critical role in the body's defense against pathogens. Both defects and over-activity (generally termed **hypersensitivity**) of the immune response can cause disease. Hypersensitivity results in symptoms via inflammatory mediators, antibodies, complement, and cells. The term **allergy,** derived from the Greek words *allo* and *ergo*, implies "other" or "bad" work by the body's immune system.

Lymphocytes and **macrophages** are the key cells in immune defense. The lymphocytes may be derived from the thymus (**T cells**) or bone marrow (**B cells**). T cells, which may be helper or suppressor types, provide cellular immunity, and B cells produce antibodies. As shown in Figure 8.1, the macrophage can serve as an antigen-processing cell (APC). Foreign antigens from pathogens are first internalized and then presented as peptides on the APC's surface. The peptides are bound to other surface proteins called histocompatibility proteins, which provide cell markers called major histocompatibility complex (MHC). Aside from enabling T cells to determine whether cells are foreign, MHC also serves as binding sites for T cells. T suppressor cells (TS cells) can recognize and bind the MHC complex, termed MHC I, which is present on nearly all cells in the body. T helper cells (TH cells) recognize a separate MHC protein, called MHC II, which is generally limited to cells that are APCs. The protein on the T cell that binds to MHC II is called CD4 (cluster of differentiation antigen 4). These interactions cause the macrophage to produce interleukin (IL)-1, which stimulates the T cell and helps uncommitted T helper cells to differentiate into TH_1 or TH_2 cells. TH_1 cells promote cell-mediated defenses against viruses, fungi, and bacteria; TH_2 cells defend against parasites and produce additional IL-4 and IL-5, which activate the eosinophils. Most individuals produce predominantly TH_1 cells. Allergic patients usually have an overabundance of TH_2 cells.

The proteins that TH_2 cells secrete (called cytokines) promote the clinical expression of allergies. IL-4 and IL-5 result in increased amounts of immunoglobulin E (IgE) and tissue eosinophilia, respectively. Eosinophils release toxic substances such as major basic protein (MBP) that can exacerbate asthma. IL-4 may also promote inflammation by increasing expression of adhesion proteins on blood vessels to which eosinophils bind, thus allowing egress into tissues. Cytokines produced by TH_1 and TH_2 cells are summarized in Table 8.1. To counteract the allergic response, the macrophage produces IL-12. Interferon-gamma is also produced by pre-existing TH_1 cells. Both of these help uncommitted T helper (T_0) cells differentiate into TH_1. Interferon-gamma (IFN-γ) also inhibits the ability of TH_2 cells to produce IL-4.

An immature form of antibody (IgM) is found on B-cell surfaces. IgM serves as an antigen receptor. Following antigen-binding by the IgM, the B cells initially produce and secrete additional IgM, followed later by production of other antibody classes such as IgG, IgA, or IgE. Antibody production is enhanced by the binding of B cells to T cells, which express a protein called the CD40 ligand. Lack of T-cell help or abnormal CD40 binding can impair antibody production or the switch from IgM to IgG. If TH_2 cells predominate, IgM is replaced by IgE, allowing the increased likelihood of a later immediate-type allergy.

During T-cell development, those cells that recognize self-antigens are destroyed in the thymus, and those with receptors that recognize foreign antigens survive. However, the depletion of self-reactive cells is thwarted if infection or other toxic effects cause self-antigens to mimic foreign antigens. In such situations, macrophages may produce increased amounts of interleukin-1 (IL-1). In excess, IL-1 can cause fever, leukocytosis, thrombocytosis, and an elevated sedimentation rate—all signs of inflammation. Some autoimmune reactions may occur when TH_1 cells mistake the body's own cells as foreign. Gel and Coombs have classified hypersensitivity reactions into four types (Table 8.2), providing a framework for understanding these reactions.

Type I Reactions

Type I (**immediate hypersensitivity**) reactions have a rapid onset, appearing within minutes. **Anaphylaxis** (a serious, life-threatening allergic reaction with rapid onset) following a bee sting or penicillin injection is one such example. These reactions involve inflammatory mediator release from tissue mast cells or blood basophils (Figure 8.2). Macrophages, platelets, and eosinophils may also be activated by allergens or pathogens. IgE antibodies made by B cells bind to receptors on mast cells and basophils. When the IgE on these cells comes in contact with allergen, intracellular signals are triggered. Basophils and mast cells then release preformed

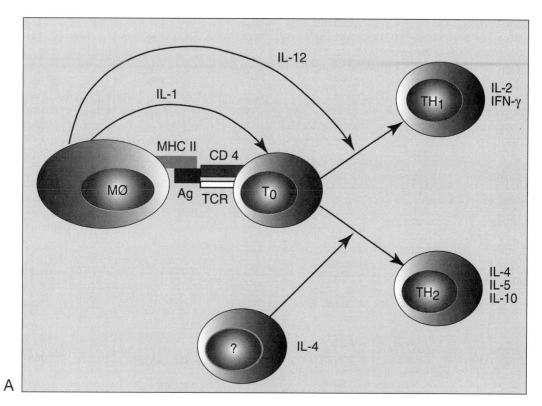

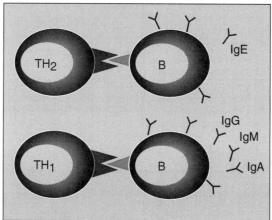

FIGURE 8.1. A. Macrophage (MØ) processes foreign antigens and presents them as peptides on its surface in association with the major histocompatibility complex (MHC). T helper cells recognize these peptides by the T-cell receptor (TCR) owing to interactions with the T cell's CD4 antigen. Suppressor/cytotoxic T cells recognize MHC class I antigens because of interactions with CD8. The MØ then produces interleukin (IL)-1, which stimulates the T cell, and IL-8 (not shown), which activates neutrophils. T_0 cells then differentiate into TH_1 cells, which promote cell-mediated defenses against viruses, fungi, and bacteria, or TH_2 cells, which promote defense against parasites. IL-12 from the MØ, and IFN-γ from pre-existing TH_1 cells, help T_2 cells differentiate into TH_2, and IL-4 locally helps differentiation into TH_2 cells. The cytokines from TH_2 cells are associated with atopic conditions including asthma. B. When TH_2 cells interact with B lymphocytes, the B cells preferentially produce IgE antibodies. TH_1 interactions promote the production of some IgG subclasses, IgM, and IgA.

mediators, such as histamine, from their granules. They also produce de novo (newly formed) mediators when phospholipase A_2 acts on the membrane lipids, releasing arachidonic acid.

■ Preformed Mediators

Histamine, a preformed mediator, stored almost entirely in mast cells and basophils, is rapidly released

TABLE 8.1.	TH₁ and TH₂ Cytokines and Their Actions	
Group	**Cytokine**	**Actions**
TH₁	IL-2	Promotes clonal proliferation of T cells.
	IFN-γ	Antiviral, up-regulates antigen-presenting cells and down-regulates TH₂ cells.
TH₂	IL-4	Promotes switching to IgE and up-regulates VCAM* expression on endothelium. Promotes differentiation of TH₁ cells to TH₂.
	IL-5	Chemotactic for eosinophils, also activates them and prolongs their survival.
	IL-10	Down-regulates antigen-presenting cells and TH₁ cells.
	IL-13	Acts like IL-4, promotes TH₂ differentiation.
Shared	IL-3	Growth factor especially for mast cells and basophils; primes basophils to respond to stimuli.
	GM-CSF	Growth factor, also promotes eosinophil growth.

*VCAM = vascular cell adhesion molecule.

after cellular activation and causes vascular leak and venodilation. Following local release in the skin, erythema, itching, and wheal formation occur. Thus, itching is predictive of mast cell or basophil activation. On a larger scale, histamine can evoke vasopermeability with resultant loss of vascular fluid into tissues—a process termed third spacing of fluid—leading to hypotension, abdominal pain, and **urticaria** (hives; see chapter 13). Nasal vasodilatation causes nasal congestion. Type I reactions lead to pruritus and sneezing because histamine binds to type 1 receptors (H_1) which are also present on afferent nerves. Histamine binding to type 2 (H_2) receptors causes flushing, hypotension, and headache because H_2 receptors are located on blood vessels. Pulmonary symptoms include chest tightness and wheezing.

Although elevated blood histamine level is a good indication of a type I reaction, the rapid metabolism of histamine makes this test impractical. Given the stability of mast cell–derived tryptase in the blood for several hours, serum tryptase levels can retrospectively confirm a type I reaction.

■ *De Novo* Mediators

De novo mediators—leukotrienes, prostaglandin D_2 (PGD_2), and platelet-activating factor (PAF)— which are derived from cell membrane phospholipids of mast cells or basophils, cause bronchoconstriction and stimulate mucus secretion (Figure 8.3). Corticosteroids can inhibit the production of these agents by inhibiting phospholipase A_2. Nonsteroidal anti-inflammatory drugs (NSAIDs)—aspirin, for example—may shunt more arachidonic acid into the lipoxygenase pathway and cause more leukotriene synthesis in susceptible individuals. Drugs that block binding of leukotrienes to their receptors (e.g., zafirlukast) and those that block produc-

TABLE 8.2.	Classification of Hypersensitivity Reactions			
Type	**Synonym**	**Time/Course**	**Antibody Role**	**Cellular Role**
I	Immediate	Minutes	IgE triggers basophils and mast cells.	Basophils and mast cells release mediators.
II	Cytotoxic	<1 hour	Antibody binds to cells or tissues, fixes complement, and causes damage.	Cells are targets.
III	Serum sickness; immune complex	7–14 days	Antibody forms complexes with antigen; complex fixes complement and settles into blood vessels.	Neutrophils are attracted by complex in blood vessel and cause further damage.
IV	Delayed	2–3 days	—	Macrophage produces IL-1 and IL-12, promoting TH₁ response. TH₁ produces IL-2 and IFN-γ, resulting in cellular infiltrate.

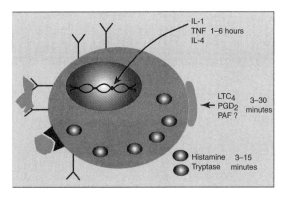

FIGURE 8.2. Mast cells (and basophils) express the high-affinity IgE receptor on their surface, to which allergen-induced IgE binds. A mast cell activates when two IgE molecules are cross-linked. Histamine and tryptase stored in granules are then rapidly released. Arachidonic acid is generated by the effect of phospholipase A$_2$ on cell membrane; production of leukotriene C$_4$ (LTC$_4$), prostaglandin D$_2$ (PGD$_2$), and platelet activating factor follows. IL-1 and tumor necrosis factor (TNF) stored in granules may also be released, but additional amounts are later generated due to gene transcription.

tion of leukotrienes (e.g., Zileuton, a lipoxygenase inhibitor) can benefit some asthmatics.

■ Cytokines and the Late-Phase Reaction

Release of preformed and de novo mediators is rapid. Mast cells and basophils also begin to produce new protein cytokines several hours after IgE-mediated stimulation. Gene regulatory factors migrate from the cytoplasm to the nuclei of mast cells and basophils and enhance gene transcription of cytokines such as tumor necrosis factor (TNF) and IL-4 (Figure 8.4). The local release of IL-4 will selectively enhance the migration of eosinophils and basophils to sites of allergic inflammation. After migration into the tissues, basophils can release additional IL-4, leukotrienes and histamine. It is now known that "immediate" type I reactions often evoke a late-phase reaction (LPR) within 4–8 hours, probably due to cellular inflammation and tissue damage by chemotactic and pro-adhesive cytokines. Corticosteroids and drugs capable of stabilizing mast cells (such as sodium cromolyn or nedocromil) inhibit the LPR.

■ Anaphylactoid Reactions

These reactions, which mimic a type I reaction, follow non–IgE-dependent degranulation of mast cells or basophils and are often induced by certain drugs (morphine and codeine), contrast dye, bacterial peptides, and anaphylatoxins of the complement system (C3a, C5a). These systemic reactions mimic anaphylaxis but

are termed **anaphylactoid** to indicate that they bypass the usual IgE-dependent mechanism.

■ Diagnosis of Type I Reactions

The clinical identification of a specific sensitivity to an allergen enables avoidance of that allergen, verification of a type I allergy diagnosis, and initiation of immunotherapy or desensitization. Immunotherapy increases the level of blocking IgG antibodies, blunts seasonal changes in IgE, depresses basophil histamine release, and shifts T-helper-cell profiles from TH$_2$ to TH$_1$ by raising IFN-γ levels. An elevated total IgE level is rarely helpful clinically. Allergen testing relies on the presence of specific IgE antibodies either in serum or on skin mast cells or basophils. The most common, accurate, and least expensive test is skin testing for allergens.

Skin testing

The most commonly performed skin test for allergens is the **epicutaneous** or **prick test,** which involves pricking the skin with a small needle or lancet having a drop of stock allergen on it. Such testing correlates well with actual nasal or lung challenge with allergen and is 90% sensitive and 95% specific for identifying allergens. Only the prick test should be performed for diagnosing food allergies, and because it is safer, it should always

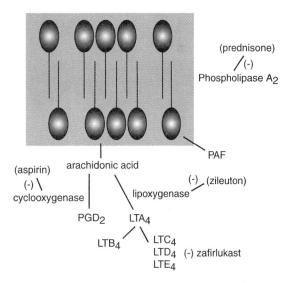

FIGURE 8.3. Phospholipase A$_2$ acts on membrane phospholipids to produce arachidonic acid and PAF; prostaglandins and leukotrienes are produced from arachidonic acid. Cyclooxygenase inhibitors (aspirin) block prostaglandin production, but may also cause increased leukotriene production. Lipoxygenase inhibitors (zileuton) inhibit leukotriene synthesis. Phospholipase A$_2$ is inhibited by corticosteroids, which can inhibit production of inflammatory mediators at all levels.

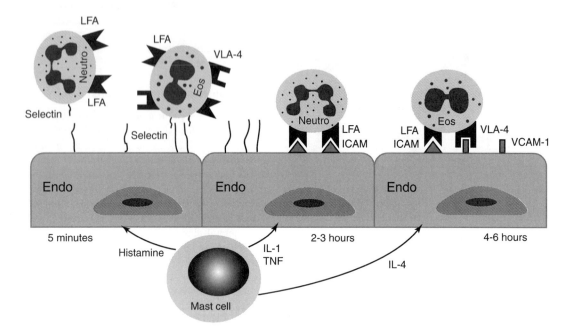

FIGURE 8.4. Tissue mast cells resting near vascular endothelium (endo)-release histamine and cytokines. Histamine promotes weak attachment and rolling of leukocytes along the endothelium. Both neutrophils (neutro) and eosinophils (eos) interact with endothelium. Subsequent release of IL-1 and TNF by the mast cell causes increased expression of intercellular adhesion molecules (ICAM) by the endothelial cells, and neutrophils and eosinophils are anchored to the endothelium. IL-4 produced during the late phase by mast cells causes selective enhancement (up-regulation) of vascular cell adhesion molecule-1 (VCAM-1) on the endothelium. VCAM-1 is recognized by very late antigen-4 (VLA-4), which is present on eosinophils and basophils but not on neutrophils, resulting in selective recruitment of these cells.

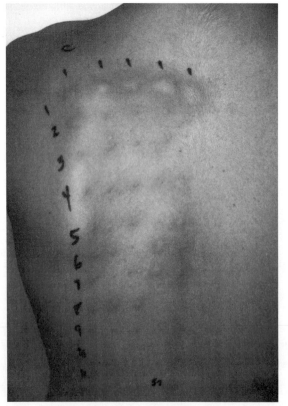

FIGURE 8.5. Results of a prick test on an allergic patient. The patient has strongly positive wheal and flare reactions to several grass allergens (row 1) but not to other allergens (such as trees, row 9). A saline control is also found to be negative.

precede intradermal skin testing in the evaluation of other allergies. The **intradermal test** involves an injection of 0.02–0.03 ml of diluted allergen (usually about 1:100–1:500) through a 27-gauge needle, which raises an intradermal wheal. By introducing nearly 1000 times more allergen than the prick test, it is more sensitive (95–98%) but less specific (85%). Both the prick test and the intradermal test can be read within 15 minutes (Figure 8.5) of testing. A positive control using histamine and a negative saline control are always performed concurrently. Antihistamines must be stopped (generally 3–5 half lives of the agent) prior to skin testing.

Radioallergosorbent test

The **radioallergosorbent test (RAST)** measures specific serum IgE. The allergen is linked to a disk in a test tube or microtiter well and incubated in the patient's serum. If IgE is present against that allergen, it will adhere and remain attached to the disk. The disk is then washed and incubated with an antibody against human IgE (such as goat antihuman IgE). The second antibody is linked to radioactive iodine. After rewashing the disk, the amount of bound IgE is noted by the amount of radioactivity in the tube or well. The RAST is almost as sensitive as the prick test for most common allergens but has several limitations, such as poor binding by some allergens, false-positives with high total IgE levels (>500 ng/ml), and its limited availability (only via special laboratories). When severe eczema, dermatographism, or the use of tricyclic antidepressants preclude skin testing (1–3% of patients), alternate diagnostic tests such as RAST are useful. However, because skin tests are more sensitive than RASTs, skin tests should always be used to detect potentially life-threatening allergens such as Hymenoptera venom (bee stings) or type I penicillin allergy.

Type II Reactions

Also known as **cytotoxic reactions,** type II reactions are mediated by antibodies directed against cells and can use complement to help **cell lysis** or rupture cells**.** The ABO mismatch-type transfusion reaction best exemplifies them. Because complement fixation is common, IgG and IgM antibodies, which have the ability to bind complement, are the most important. The antigen recognized as foreign can truly be foreign (e.g., transfusion or early rapid graft rejections) or may be neo-antigens on a host's own cells. Alpha-methyldopa (Aldomet), an antihypertensive, can cause **hemolysis** by inducing the cells to express neo-antigens on their surface. A cell can also be lysed as an "innocent bystander" when a drug (penicillin or quinidine) binds to its surface. Hemolytic antibody on cells can be detected using the **Coombs test.**

Type II reactions can also occur owing to chronic pathologic antibody production. Autoantibody production occurs in systemic lupus erythematosus (SLE) and is directed against nuclear material. Autoantibodies can cause illness without cellular damage. Long-acting thyroid-stimulating antibodies (LATS) can cause hyperthyroidism; antibodies against C1 esterase inhibitor (C1 INH) can accelerate clearance of C1 INH, precipitating **angioedema** (see chapter 13).

Type III Reactions

In a type III reaction—also called **serum sickness**—a foreign antigen is bound by the patient's own antibodies, forming immune complexes that subsequently fix complement. Immune complexes may enhance IL-1 production, resulting in fever. Complexes, depending on the ratios of antigen and antibody, could settle into blood vessels, leading to **vasculitis** (vascular inflammation). Vasculitis causes leukocyte infiltration, nuclear damage of the endothelial cells, and extravasation of red blood cells. Cutaneous vasculitis can sometimes present as an atypical **urticaria** (see chapter 13) or palpable purpura. Vasculitis elsewhere is associated with respective organ dysfunction. Typical characteristics of type III reactions are fever, joint pains, proteinuria, lymphadenopathy, consumption of complement factor 4, eosinophilia, and a high sedimentation rate, occurring 7–14 days after exposure. Antinuclear antibodies (ANA) and anti–double-stranded DNA antibodies are seen in drug-induced lupus.

Type IV Reactions

In type IV reactions, an antigen triggers macrophages to produce cytokines, which in turn activate local lymphocytes. Macrophage IL-1 and IL-8 enhance leukocyte infiltration. Local IFN-γ production of T cells increases MHC II expression on APCs and enhances defense against viruses, mycobacteria, and intracellular bacteria.

Type IV responses can be inhibited by corticosteroids. They are also known as **delayed hypersensitivity** since the clinical onset is delayed by 24–72 hours. The tuberculin skin test embodies a type IV reaction.

 # RHINITIS, SINUSITIS, AND CONJUNCTIVITIS

Rhinitis

■ Definition and Etiology

Rhinitis, or nasal inflammation, may be allergic or nonallergic; the cause must be determined by the history, physical examination, and selected studies. Allergic rhinitis can be perennial or seasonal. Commonly, **acute rhinitis** is viral and **chronic rhinitis** is allergic.

■ Epidemiology

Rhinitis is a leading problem in primary care, with an estimated 15% incidence in the U.S. population younger than age 30. Like other atopic diseases (e.g., asthma), allergic rhinitis also has a genetic basis, with almost two-thirds of subjects having an affected first-degree relative. Since IgE levels peak around age 11, allergic rhinitis—especially perennial—is more prevalent in children and young adults. Seasonal symptoms (brought on, for example, by ragweed in the early fall, mold in the late fall, tree pollens in the spring, and grasses in the summer) suggest an allergic component. However, some allergens are perennial (such as dust mites, indoor pets, and certain molds). Worldwide, the most common allergen is the *Dermatophagoides* mite species. Because human dander is the food source for these mites, they accumulate in bedding, carpeting, and feather pillows, harboring the main allergenic protein in their feces. Aeroallergies most often result from wind-driven pollen grains. Because some viral infections may be seasonal, nonallergic rhinitis may also be seasonal.

■ Pathophysiology

When the nose fails to warm and humidify air, bronchospasm can result, and failure to filter (mouth breathing) results in a predisposition to lower respiratory tract infections. The nasal turbinates, being covered with ciliated epithelium, increase the epithelial surface area for warming, humidifying, and filtering. Excess airflow over these areas can lead to **mucosal hypertrophy,** which, if pronounced, presents as nasal congestion. In **septal deviation,** this effect may arise from shunting airflow to the unobstructed nostril or by breathing air with very low humidity. Similarly, conditions that cause increased blood volume (e.g., pregnancy) or vasodilatation (medications) will produce congestion.

In allergic rhinitis, the allergen activates mucosal mast cells and triggers mediator release (see chapter 8). A cholinergic reflex causes additional rhinorrhea with mucus secretion. Histamine appears to play a role in sneezing as newer, selective H1 antagonists effectively treat this symptom. Late-phase reactions mediated by cytokines may explain the chronicity of rhinitis symptoms. Edema around the eustachian tube opening can cause partial obstruction and concomitant dysfunction.

■ Clinical Features

Patients with rhinitis report a variable degree of nasal congestion, rhinorrhea, postnasal drainage, and sneezing. Sneezing is very common in *seasonal* allergic rhinitis and, when absent, should suggest nonallergic causes. In *perennial* allergic rhinitis, nasal congestion and thick secretions are reported with less prominent sneezing. In all forms of rhinitis, increased mouth breathing of relatively cool, dry air can exacerbate associated asthma. Nasal congestion can provoke **sleep-disordered breathing** and cause chronic fatigue. Eye and throat itching and irritation are common. "Ear popping" and serous otitis follow eustachian tube dysfunction. The nasal mucosa is often pale and edematous (versus reddened in nonallergic rhinitis), and "allergic shiners" (dark circles under the eyes) are frequent. A lumpy appearance of the pharyngeal mucosa (**posterior pharyngeal lymphoid hyperplasia)** and **anterior cervical adenopathy** are other findings. In children, the "allergic salute" (rubbing or wiping the nose with the back of the hands to allay pruritus) along with nasal creases are striking. With eustachian tube dysfunction, the tympanic membrane may be retracted.

■ Diagnosis

Figure 9.1 illustrates the differential diagnosis of rhinitis. The patient's history is critical and should include information about exposure to potential allergens at home and work, drug use, and family history. In the common cold, the most frequent form of nonallergic rhinitis, constitutional symptoms are common, and nasal

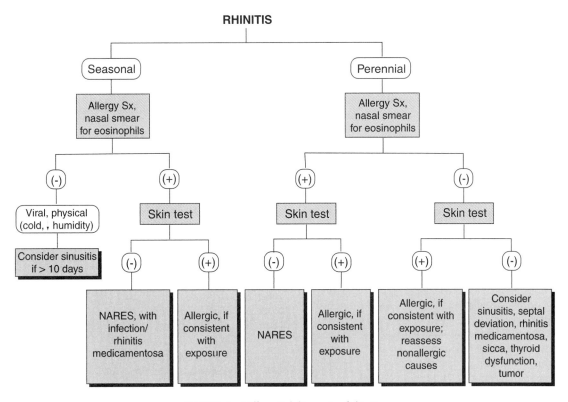

FIGURE 9.1. Differential diagnosis of rhinitis.
Sx= symptoms; (+) = positive; (−) = negative; NARES = nonallergic rhinitis with eosinophilia.

smear shows no eosinophils. Nonallergic rhinitis with eosinophilia (NARES) features perennial nasal congestion, nasal polyps, and slight pruritus, but skin testing demonstrates no allergies. Aside from being associated with nonallergic asthma, polyps may also block sinus drainage, causing recurrent sinusitis. Nonsteroidal anti-inflammatory drugs (NSAIDs) should be avoided in asthmatics with nasal polyps because such medications may induce asthmatic attacks.

Rhinitis medicamentosa is inflammation of the nasal mucosa caused by excessive use of medication such as vasoconstrictor nasal sprays, which temporarily reduce nasal congestion but cause rebound congestion. Rhinitis often follows habitual cocaine snorting; septal ulcers and perforation may also be noted. A subset of patients with nonallergic rhinitis have **vasomotor rhinitis,** with an abnormal cholinergic reflex response to physical stimuli (bright lights; cooling of the skin; and warm, moist air). Often middle-aged or older, these patients may have a history of rhinorrhea and sneezing when walking barefoot on a cold floor or when eating certain foods—for example, soup (gustatory rhinitis).

Other conditions can mimic rhinitis by causing congestion or apparent rhinorrhea. Normal blood flow to the nostrils cycles periodically, with a mild unilateral increase in resistance, especially on recumbency. This may worsen with high cardiac output (stress), increased blood volume (pregnancy), vasodilatation (ß-blockers and central α-agonists), or hormonal changes (birth control pills, hypothyroidism). Anatomic obstruction (polyps, septal deviation, intranasal malignancy) may cause constant congestion that responds poorly to therapy. Unilateral obstruction with infection in a child may be caused by a foreign body; when a nasal polyp is the cause, cystic fibrosis should be considered. Profuse rhinorrhea after head trauma or surgery may be caused by cerebrospinal fluid leakage, which can be quickly confirmed using a glucose dipstick (value over 40 mg/dl is nearly diagnostic). With excessive mucosal dryness (**Sjögren's syndrome),** patients often report nasal congestion and associated sinus discomfort. In both allergic rhinitis and NARES, the nasal smear shows eosinophils. Although this implies allergies, skin testing or RAST to show specific IgE is necessary for diagnosis. Chronic nasal congestion without positive skin tests or eosinophilia could suggest the need for a workup to rule out chronic sinusitis and should direct attention to other nonallergic causes for congestion (listed previously in this chapter).

■ Management

Table 9.1 outlines the management of rhinitis. For allergic rhinitis, avoidance of allergens is the first choice (Table 9.2); however, it is difficult to avoid outdoor aeroallergens. Medical management routinely includes the use of nasal saline washes (to reduce inflammatory cells and mediators), anti-inflammatory nasal sprays (corticosteroid sprays and sodium cromolyn), and oral antihistamine-decongestants. The steroid sprays are used once or twice a day, and cromolyn is used several times a day. Both corticosteroids and cromolyn should be used regularly and prophylactically; the clinical response may take several days. For patients with nasal polyps or severe allergic rhinitis, a course of oral steroids may reduce polyp size and lessen symptoms; topical steroid sprays can be used afterward. Besides cessation of topical decongestant, rhinitis medicamentosa often requires concurrent topical steroids, oral antihistamine-decongestants, and brief oral corticosteroid therapy. Ipratropium bromide nasal spray is effective in treating vasomotor rhinitis.

Several classes of first-generation antihistamines have variable anticholinergic and antiserotoninergic properties, which are sometimes desirable (to "dry up" secretions or provide mild sedation). Besides being effective H1 antagonists, the newer generation of antihistamines cause very little sedation and possess relatively little anticholinergic activity. Unmetabolized terfenadine and astemizole, in clinical states of impaired hepatic metabolism (from cirrhosis or concomitant use of macrolide antibiotics or azole antifungals), can prolong the QT interval in the ECG, with rare instances of conduction abnormalities and arrhythmias, including the torsade de pointes form of ventricular tachycardia.

Patients with hypertension should be monitored for worsening symptoms while receiving oral decongestants (e.g., pseudoephedrine or phenylephrine). Topical decongestants are occasionally useful, especially with underlying sinusitis. However, because they can cause rebound nasal congestion, they should be given for no more than three consecutive days. Immunotherapy with allergen extracts is quite effective for controlling allergic rhinitis symptoms if the allergens are clearly identified and adequate doses can be tolerated. Immunotherapy may be effective because it can 1) blunt basophil histamine release, 2) inhibit seasonal rises in specific IgE, and 3) produce blocking IgG antibodies. Indicated for patients with symptoms present at least 6 months per year, immunotherapy is also effective for patients with seasonal symptoms who respond poorly to drugs. Upon its cessation, approximately one-third of patients will continue to benefit from immunotherapy, one-third will gradually worsen over the years, and the remainder will relapse more quickly. Given the rare fatalities, such therapy should be initiated only by trained allergists. Because of the increased risk for life-threatening anaphylaxis, immunotherapy is contraindicated in patients using ß-blockers.

■ Complications and Prognosis

Although rhinitis is not lethal, it does add to the morbidity and perhaps mortality of other illnesses. It increases the likelihood of developing sinusitis due to obstruction of the sinus ostia and exacerbates pre-existing asthma. The use of first-generation antihistamines by patients with rhinitis can impair work performance and/or driving ability. Most patients with rhinitis, especially allergic rhinitis, have an excellent prognosis with a regimen of allergen or irritant avoidance, topical corticosteroids, or oral antihistamines.

Sinusitis

■ Definition

Although sinusitis is most commonly viral, the term often implies documented bacterial or fungal overgrowth in the sinuses with greater than 10,000 infectious units/ml. Diagnosed clinically and/or radiographically, sinusitis may be acute (<30 days), subacute (1–2 months), or chronic (>2 months).

■ Epidemiology

Almost one in eight adults will experience chronic sinusitis. **Maxillary sinusitis** accounts for 90% of all cases of sinusitis, followed by **ethmoidal sinusitis** in 5–10% of the cases. Thus, maxillary sinusitis is used as a prototype for this discussion. **Acute sinusitis** is very common in children, with 5–10% of upper respiratory infections becoming complicated by acute sinusitis. Although this rate appears to be lower among adults, exact figures are unavailable. Typical bacterial isolates are *Streptococcus pneumoniae, Haemophilus influenzae,* and *Moraxella (Branhamella) catarrhalis.* Groups A and C streptococci and *Streptococcus viridans* are less frequent. Anaerobic grampositive organisms such as Peptococcus and Peptostreptococcus can be found in cases of chronic sinusitis along with Bacteroides species. ß-lactamase-producing bacteria, resistant to ampicillin and amoxicillin, are present 20% of the time.

TABLE 9.1. Medical Management of Rhinitis

Therapeutic	Examples	Frequency[a]	Useful for[b]				Comments	Cost/Day
			S/I	C	PRN	NA		
Avoidance	pillow, mattress cover, air filters	—	S	+	—	—	Usually reduces but does not eliminate symptoms. Only an adjunct to management.	20–30¢
1st-generation antihistamine	diphenhydramine, clemastine, chlorpheniramine, hydroxyzine	BID TID	++	+/-	++	+/-	Fairly rapid onset; drying effect sometimes useful. Can be sedating and can cause urinary retention in men.	$1
2nd-generation antihistamine	fexofenadine, astemizole, loratadine, cetirizine	QD BID	++	+/-	+	—	Usually nonsedating and little tachyphylaxis. Do not give astemizole with erythromycin.	$2–3
Decongestant	pseudoephedrine, phenylpropanolamine	BID TID	—	+	+	+/-	Nonsedating but can cause agitation and insomnia, and may worsen hypertension. Often given with an antihistamine.	20–30¢
Cromolyn	Nasalcrom™	TID	+	+	—	—	Given as topical spray, relatively free of systemic effects.	$2–3
Topical corticosteroid	beclomethasone, triamcinolone, budesonide, fluticasone	QD BID	+	++	—	+	Topical spray, few systemic effects. Rarely causes nose bleed. Can be effective for NARES, vasomotor.[c]	$2–3
Saline	Ocean™, Ayre™	TID QID	+/-	+	+/-	+/-	Safe. Often an adjunct to medications.	5–10¢
Immunotherapy	—	Q wk	++	+	—	—	Must determine allergens and correlate with symptoms. Effective but takes months to year to begin; occasional reaction. Can work when medications fail.	$1–2

[a]BID = twice a day; Q wk = once a week; QD = once a day; QID = 4 times a day; TID = three times a day.
[b]C = congestion; NA = nonallergic; PRN = as needed; S/I = sneeze/itch.
[c]NARES = nonallergic rhinitis with eosinophilia.

TABLE 9.2.	Methods for Reducing Allergen Exposure
Allergen Type	**Methods**
Outdoor allergens	Close windows, use central air conditioning or window unit. Wear face mask (trees, grasses, molds) when exposed to cut grass or moldy areas such as compost piles.
Indoor allergens	
Mite	Provide adequate ventilation.
	Remove feather pillows, down comforters.
	Cover pillow, mattress, and box spring with airtight covering.
	No carpeting in bedrooms or use only machine-washable area rugs.
	Wash bedding in hot water (>140°F) every 2 weeks.
	Maintain humidity <50% and temperature <70°F.
	Use acaricide (tannic and benzoic acid) on carpet and stuffed furniture every 2–4 months.
	Minimize knickknacks; frequently dust with damp cloth.
	Vacuum rugs, mattress, and drapes using multilayered collection bag every 2 weeks.
	Replace dust filters in furnace/central air conditioning unit regularly.
	Place cheese cloth across forced air vents.
Molds	Maintain humidity <40%.
	Treat areas containing mildew and bathroom tiles with mold-killing cleansers.
	Add mold inhibitors to wall and ceiling paint.
	Empty water pans (e.g., from under refrigerator).
	Store firewood outside.
Animals	Minimize exposure, or at least keep pets out of bedroom and off furniture.
	Bathe cat or dog weekly.
	Wash hands thoroughly after touching all animals.

■ Pathophysiology

Among the four paranasal sinuses (maxillary, ethmoid, sphenoid, and frontal), the first two develop soon after birth; development of the others may lag until age 3–6. The posterior ethmoid cells and sphenoid sinuses drain by gravity into the superior meatus between the superior and middle turbinates, and the anterior ethmoid cells and maxillary sinuses drain into the middle meatus (Figure 9.2). This region, the **osteomeatal complex,** is readily obstructed by mucosal edema or polyps. Bacteria can enter the sinuses through the ostia, or by contiguous spread, as in a dental abscess. The pathogenesis is summarized in Figure 9.3.

The cross-sectional areas of the sinus ostia largely determine gas exchange and mucus clearance, and thus, even modest obstruction, as in rhinitis, will increase the risk for sinusitis. A low PaO_2 also causes vasodilatation, leading to transudation and mucosal congestion. Because the maxillary ostia are located high on the medial wall, ciliary action is required to clear the secretions against gravity. Thus, increased mucus viscosity (cystic fibrosis), reduced ciliary function (smoking, ciliary dyskinesia, viruses, hypoxia), or low PaO_2 (smoking) increase the likelihood of maxillary sinusitis.

■ Clinical Features

Acute sinusitis often follows upper-respiratory viral infections. Its features are persistent symptoms of viral rhinitis lasting more than 10 days: pain in the cheeks radiating into the incisor teeth, fever, bad breath, purulent rhinorrhea, nasal congestion, or, occasionally, a nocturnal cough from postnasal drip of sinus secretions. Untreated sinusitis can lead to more serious complications, including cavernous sinus thrombosis, intracranial abscess, or subperiosteal abscess of the orbit. Eye swelling, exophthalmos, or focal neurologic changes after an unresolved upper respiratory infection suggest such a sequence.

Chronic sinusitis, which follows prolonged osteomeatal obstruction, manifests with chronic rhinorrhea, nasal congestion, decreased sense of smell, chronic cough from postnasal drip, or headaches. Asthmatics often report worsening asthma symptoms when a sinus infection develops; the majority of these patients report improved control of asthma following treatment of the sinusitis. **Allergic fungal sinusitis** is rare, caused most frequently by *Aspergillus* and occurring in highly allergic patients.

■ Diagnosis

The history and a clinical suspicion are key to diagnosing sinusitis. In acute sinusitis, sinus tenderness may be demonstrable, and the nasal smear often shows numerous neutrophils. Incisor toothache, poor response to decongestants or antihistamines, or discolored nasal discharge seen by the patient or on physical examination increase the likelihood of bacterial sinusitis twofold to threefold. These factors, combined with the overall clinical impression by the primary care

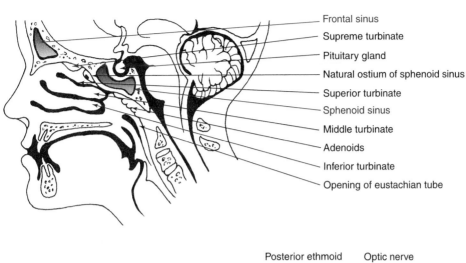

Frontal sinus
Supreme turbinate
Pituitary gland
Natural ostium of sphenoid sinus
Superior turbinate
Sphenoid sinus
Middle turbinate
Adenoids
Inferior turbinate
Opening of eustachian tube

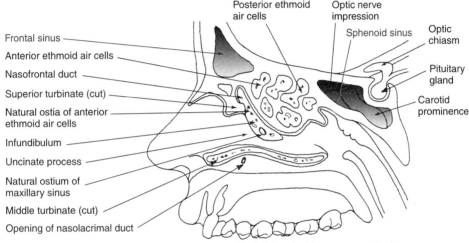

Posterior ethmoid air cells
Optic nerve impression
Sphenoid sinus
Optic chiasm
Pituitary gland
Carotid prominence

Frontal sinus
Anterior ethmoid air cells
Nasofrontal duct
Superior turbinate (cut)
Natural ostia of anterior ethmoid air cells
Infundibulum
Uncinate process
Natural ostium of maxillary sinus
Middle turbinate (cut)
Opening of nasolacrimal duct

Medial view (turbinates removed)

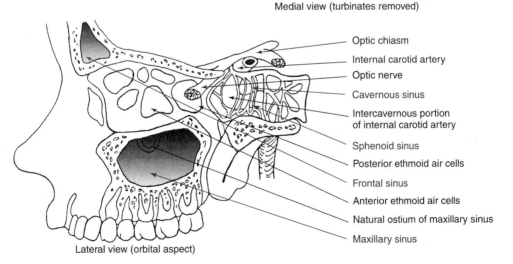

Optic chiasm
Internal carotid artery
Optic nerve
Cavernous sinus
Intercavernous portion of internal carotid artery
Sphenoid sinus
Posterior ethmoid air cells
Frontal sinus
Anterior ethmoid air cells
Natural ostium of maxillary sinus
Maxillary sinus

Lateral view (orbital aspect)

FIGURE 9.2. Anatomy of the nasal cavity and the sinuses showing the osteomeatal complex.

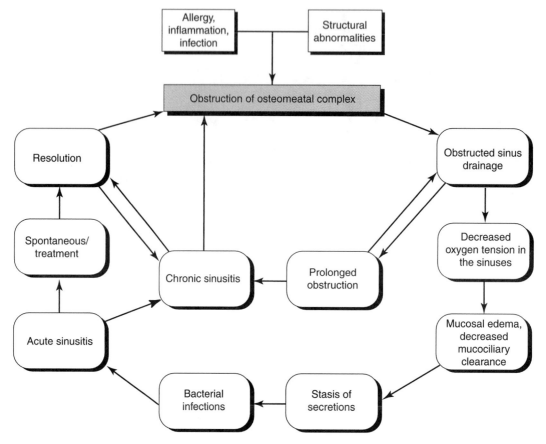

FIGURE 9.3. The pathogenesis of acute and chronic sinusitis.

physician, can effectively stratify patients into high or low risk for sinusitis.

Although some studies suggest that transillumination may be useful in diagnosis, others dispute its diagnostic value as an isolated test. The vast majority of patients (>85% of children) with 10 consecutive days of symptoms will have radiographic evidence for sinusitis. Computed tomography (CT) scans are more sensitive than standard radiographs in demonstrating sinusitis; given the ready availability of CT, the cost for limited cuts of the sinuses compares favorably with that for conventional sinus films, making CT the first study of choice. In allergic sinusitis due to *Aspergillus*, a mass effect can be seen in sinus CT. Flexible rhinoscopy in skilled hands also aids diagnosis when a purulent discharge can be visualized below the middle turbinate in the area of the maxillary ostium. Sinus aspiration is generally reserved for those patients who do not respond to a full course (greater than 4 weeks) of appropriate management including antibiotics, or for those with a rapidly progressive course while taking antibiotics.

■ **Management**

Promoting drainage and treating the bacterial infection are the dual goals in treating sinusitis. Because most children and adults with recurrent sinusitis have allergies, allergy treatment is also critical.

The bacteriology of sinusitis is discussed in chapter 147. Anaerobic bacteria more often play a role in chronic sinusitis. Treatment options are listed in Table 9.3. Some sinus infections resolve spontaneously. Oral and short courses of topical decongestants may be helpful. Oral steroids and topical steroid sprays may reduce osteomeatal complex obstruction, especially when polyps are present. Appropriate antibiotics (amoxicillin, 500 mg three times a day being the most common agent used) should be given for at least 3 weeks. If the response is not adequate in 10–14 days, ß-lactamase-resistant drugs should be used. The initial choice of a ß-lactamase-resistant drug such as clarithromycin (500 mg twice daily) or amoxicillin/clavulanate (500 mg/125 mg) three times a day is appropriate for smokers and childcare workers because they are more likely to harbor ß-lactamase-producing *Haemophilus influenzae.* In ß–lactam allergy, erythromycin or trimethoprim-sulfamethoxazole can also be used as a first-line therapy.

Documented anatomic obstruction or failure of sinusitis to resolve after 2–3 months of therapy with a course of oral steroids and antibiotics against *H. influenzae* and anaerobic bacteria warrant surgical drainage. Endoscopic sinus surgery, designed to improve osteomeatal drainage, is also highly successful (80% of cases).

IgG subclasses, immunoglobulin responses to encapsulated bacteria, and ciliary function should be evaluated in patients with recurrent episodes (3 or more in 6 months or 4 in 1 year) who have been appropriately treated (see chapter 14).

■ Complications and Prognosis

Sinusitis can exacerbate asthma. If untreated, the infection can spread to adjacent bone and vascular structures, causing osteomyelitis or thrombosis, and into the intracranial cavity, resulting in meningitis. With appropriate antibiotic therapy, the prognosis is excellent for most patients. Those with recurrent sinusitis and an underlying immunodeficiency generally respond well to prophylactic antibiotics, but they may require immunoglobulin replacement. Anatomical obstruction of the sinus ostia generally responds to surgical intervention.

Conjunctivitis

Allergic conjunctivitis often complicates allergic rhinitis and may be the most bothersome symptom for some patients. Ocular allergy commonly manifests with seasonal allergic conjunctivitis characterized by a mild conjunctivitis with photophobia, moderate itching, gritty sensation in the eyes, tearing, a slight discharge, and mild conjunctival injection. Oral antihistamines and topical agents such as antihistamines (naphazoline, levocabastine), NSAIDs (ketorolac), mast cell stabilizers (lodoxamide, tromethamine), and artificial tears are all helpful.

Other conditions encountered in atopic individuals include atopic keratoconjunctivitis, vernal conjunctivitis, and giant papillary conjunctivitis. Atopic keratoconjunctivitis coexists with atopic dermatitis. Vernal conjunctivitis is usually seasonal, causing conjunctival interstitial inflammation and flat-topped papules. The patient, usually a child, reports extreme ocular pruritus with mucus strands. Giant papillary conjunctivitis, with giant papillae under the lids and corneal abrasions related to friction of the papillae on the cornea, may follow the use of gas-permeable contact lenses. Frequent lens cleaning can sometimes reduce symptoms.

TABLE 9.3.	Treatment Options in Sinusitis		
Treatment	**Frequency**	**Cost**	**Comments**
Steam	BID–TID	+/–	May relieve symptoms.
Oral decongestant	BID–TID	+	May improve drainage.
Topical decongestant	QD–BID	+	May improve drainage but risk of rebound. Usually avoided.
Topical corticosteroid	QD–BID	++	May shorten clinical course and improve drainage.
Oral corticosteroid	QD	+	Can improve symptoms when severe and improve drainage. Limit to 4–7 d taper (start at 0.5–1 mg/kg).
Antibiotics			
1st line			(All courses for 3 weeks)
Amoxicillin	TID	+	Usually effective at 500 mg/dose. 15–20% β lactamase resistance.
Erythromycin	TID–4/xd	+	Suitable in penicillin allergy at 1–1.5 g/day.
TMP/SMX	BID	+	Suitable in penicillin allergy at 160/800 mg/dose.
2nd line			
Amoxicillin/clavulanate	TID	+++	Effective at 500 mg/dose × 3 wks.
Cephalosporin	BID–TID	++	Cefuroxime 250 mg 2x/d × 3 wks or cefaclor 500 mg 3x/day.
Macrolide	QD–BID	++	Clarithromycin 500 mg 2x/d × 2–3 weeks

TMP/SMX = Trimethoprim/sulfamethoxazole.
+/– = trivial.

CHAPTER 10

BRONCHIAL ASTHMA

■ Definition

Bronchial asthma (commonly termed "asthma") is a common disease, characterized by reversible bronchial obstruction and nonspecific **bronchial hyperresponsiveness.** Airway inflammation, another hallmark, correlates with the severity of chronic symptoms. Asthma is sometimes subcategorized into *extrinsic*—when allergens trigger an allergic response—and *intrinsic*—when no allergic trigger can be identified.

■ Epidemiology and Pathogenesis

Asthma affects 5% of the population (i.e., 12 million Americans) and is the prime cause of absenteeism from school and a frequent cause of work absences. During the 1980s, yearly deaths from asthma doubled from 2000 to approximately 4000. The overall mortality rate now is 1 in every 3,000 patients, but this rate is at least five times higher for African Americans. Lack of access to medical care and inappropriate medication use both contribute significantly to the rising morbidity and mortality of asthma.

Most asthmatics have allergies. Seasonal or perennial rhinitis coexists with asthma in about 75% of children and 50–60% of adults. In these persons, asthma exacerbations frequently follow allergen exposure. Occupational exposure to allergens and sensitizing agents can cause **occupational asthma.** Occupational exposure generally involves isocyanates (in urethane foam) and organic acids (for electronic solders) or chemicals and proteins, which induce IgE responses—such as acid anhydrides (used as plasticizers), nickel salts, and cereal proteins. These agents may cause epithelial damage with only modest obstruction early in the disease. Exposure may evoke immediate symptoms, but commonly symptoms are delayed for several hours. Continued exposure progressively worsens bronchial hyperresponsiveness (BHR) and asthma, both of which can become severe and irreversible if the affected person does not leave the offending environment. In **reactive airways dysfunction syndrome** (RADS), a subset of occupational asthma, patients develop BHR and symptoms after a toxic exposure. Prior asthma is absent; only lymphocytic infiltrates and relatively little inflammation are seen histologically.

Asthma attacks may also follow drug use or preservative exposure. Metabisulfites, used as preservatives in salad bars, beers, sauerkraut, and many other foods may cause severe symptoms in some asthmatics. Aspirin, which causes asthma attacks in 10% of patients,

similarly affects one-third of asthmatics with nasal polyps.

A subset of asthma is **exercise-induced asthma** (EIA). Patients with EIA generally develop bronchoconstriction during the cool-down period following strenuous exercise in a cool, dry environment. A high level of ventilation during exercise and the temperature and relative humidity of the ambient air are critical to its genesis.

Respiratory tract inflammation can exacerbate asthma. Viruses, most commonly rhinovirus, influenza, and the respiratory syncytial virus (RSV), impede ciliary clearance of mucus and may promote adhesion molecule expression and mediator release. Therapy of sinusitis improves asthma symptoms in many asthmatics; thus, bacterial sinusitis seems to play a role in asthma. In a small subset of highly allergic asthmatics, type I reactions may follow fungal colonization of the bronchi by *Aspergillus* (allergic bronchopulmonary aspergillosis; see chapter 217).

■ Pathophysiology

Despite the overlapping aspects in their clinical expression, the key features of asthma are bronchial obstruction, bronchial hyperresponsiveness, and inflammation.

Bronchial obstruction

Bronchial obstruction is clinically measured indirectly by assessing airflow. Because airflow resistance is proportionate to the fourth power of the airway radius, even small changes in the lumen can cause major airflow changes. Reversible bronchial obstruction can follow smooth muscle contraction, mucosal edema, or intraluminal debris such as mucus. Collectively, the contribution of each determines the rate of reversibility. Smooth muscle contraction can be induced by cold, dry air (exercise), histamine, prostaglandin D_2 (PGD_2), and leukotriene C_4 (LTC_4), as well as vagally by acetylcholine release. Bronchoconstriction thus produced is transient and frequently resolves spontaneously or after bronchodilator use.

Bronchial hyperresponsiveness

Nonspecific BHR, determined through bronchoprovocation testing (chapter 211), is an important criterion for asthma. Asthmatics are many times more sensitive to irritants such as smoke, cold air, and air pollution than those without asthma, and the degree of

BHR roughly correlates with asthma severity. Although the mechanism of BHR in asthma is still undefined, it is believed that epithelial damage affords the allergens or irritants greater access to afferent nerve endings. The degree of BHR correlates with eosinophilic inflammation. Baseline obstruction due to inflammation may also evoke BHR by causing uneven deposition of inhaled irritants throughout the lung, resulting in proximal deposition of more concentrated solutions.

Inflammation

Most if not all asthmatics manifest airway inflammation, including basement membrane thickening, epithelial damage, cellular infiltrates, and excess mucus production. These changes not only limit bronchodilator responsiveness, but also take days or weeks to reverse. Eosinophils play a very important role in asthmatic inflammation, and their toxic granule contents probably cause much of the epithelial damage observed in asthma. Pathologists refer to the disease as **chronic desquamative eosinophilic bronchitis.**

After exposure to stimuli (e.g., an allergen), asthmatics can have an isolated "early" bronchial obstruction, with largely bronchospasm and edema, which generally occurs within 10–15 minutes and resolves in 1 hour. Nearly half of those displaying such an early response also show a late response, occurring spontaneously 4–8 hours after exposure and resolving in a day or two. This late phase, believed to be caused by inflammation, is relatively refractory to bronchodilators compared with the early phase. Development of late-phase reactions contributes to BHR. The cellular events in early-phase and late-phase inflammation are depicted in Figure 10.1. Drugs that inhibit mast cell activation (e.g., cromolyn or nedocromil) and drugs that block cytokine production (e.g., corticosteroids) can block the late phase.

Airflow obstruction produces disturbances in gas exchange. With worsening airflow obstruction, the ventilation-perfusion mismatch worsens, and progressive **hypoxemia** (a low PaO_2) results. Respiratory muscles work and their oxygen demand (**work of breathing**) increase as well, which necessitates diversion of an increasing proportion of the cardiac output to the respiratory muscles, a process that seriously imperils the cerebral and coronary blood flow. Declining perfusion of these vital organs, in the face of deteriorating systemic oxygenation, predisposes them to cellular hypoxia and subsequent dysfunction (see chapter 248). Hyperventilation during acute attacks leads to a low $PaCO_2$ (**hypocapnia**) and a high pH (respiratory alkalosis). With worsening obstruction, the 1-second forced expiratory volume ($FEV_{1.0}$) progressively decreases and the $PaCO_2$ drops linearly with the $FEV_{1.0}$. When the $FEV_{1.0}$ decreases to 20–30% of normal (<1.0L), the $PaCO_2$

begins to rise (**hypercapnia**), which generally follows an $FEV_{1.0}$ lesser than 0.75L.

■ Clinical Features

Asthma is a chronic illness with episodic exacerbations and a wide spectrum of clinical severity. At one extreme is **episodic asthma,** characterized by very infrequent attacks of bronchospasm with interspersed normal periods; on the other extreme is **chronic asthma,** characterized by persistent airflow obstruction that paroxysmally worsens. The intensity of airflow obstruction in the individual episode determines the severity of the acute event, and the frequency and severity of exacerbations—and the severity of airflow obstruction between episodes—determine the severity of chronic asthma. Chronic asthma can be mild, moderate, or severe (Table 10.1). Most patients have mild to moderate illness, and between attacks many patients function normally with minimal or no symptoms. However, during acute exacerbations, even patients with otherwise mild disease can experience moderate to severe symptoms.

Asthmatics commonly report shortness of breath, wheezing, and chest tightness. Nearly all asthmatics have at least some symptoms (dyspnea, wheezing, and/or cough) when exercising in cool, dry air. Almost all chronic asthmatics, irrespective of daytime symptoms, experience nocturnal symptoms, highlighting the need for the treating physician to inquire regarding both daytime and nocturnal symptoms. A mild form of asthma may present with only a recurrent cough (**cough-variant asthma).**

Classically, asthmatic attacks occur in paroxysms, in which the patient swiftly exhibits an intense sense of air hunger. Acute episodes feature **tachypnea** and **tachycardia.** Fever is absent unless infection is associated. Wheezing, the sine qua non of asthma, manifests as a high-pitched, expiratory, continuous, musical sound, best heard at the mouth and without using a stethoscope. Chest-wall movements may be diminished, and chest percussion generally reveals increased resonance. Breath sounds may be decreased and, aside from the wheeze, some middle to late inspiratory crackles may be heard; confusion with heart failure (**cardiac asthma**) is then possible. As the attack becomes more severe, inability to recline, accessory muscle use, pulsus paradoxus, diaphoresis, and impaired mentation and judgment follow. The attack may terminate spontaneously or after the use of a bronchodilator.

The degree of airflow obstruction roughly correlates with the severity of asthma symptoms and many of the associated physical findings. While wheezing may be noted on examination, symptoms of airflow limitation are

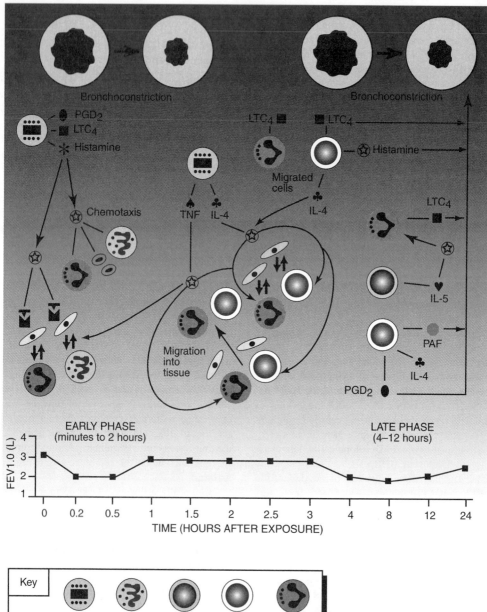

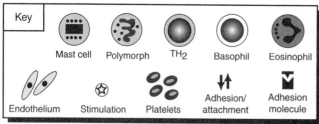

FIGURE **10.1.** Early-phase and late-phase reaction in asthma.

not generally apparent until the peak expiratory flow rate (PEFR) or the $FEV_{1.0}$ declines to less than 60% of the predicted values (predicted values are obtained from nomograms). Most patients have acute symptoms as the PEFR falls below 60%, with wheezing and a prolonged expiration being universal beyond this point.

As the PEFR decreases to less than 50% of predicted, symptoms become severe, especially in those whose illness is normally mild. In addition to chest tightness and dyspnea at rest, patients may report generalized fatigue from the extra work required to breathe. A severe asthmatic attack nearly always causes inability to recline, and this finding in a diaphoretic patient unequivocally indicates very severe airflow obstruction. Conversation consists of short or fragmented sentences ("shortened word-strings"). The hallmarks of a severe degree of airflow obstruction are accessory muscle use and pulsus paradoxus (see Tables 10.2 and 10.3). With further reductions in airflow, wheezing disappears, and in conjunction with the generalized decrease in breath sounds, causes the so-called **silent chest.** Accessory muscle use becomes evident when the $FEV_{1.0}$ has fallen to about 1.25L. Pulsus paradoxus, (>12 mm Hg decrease in systolic BP on inspiration) appears when the FEV_1 decreases to less than 1.0–0.75L. A PEFR of 30–40% of predicted is a harbinger of impending respiratory muscle fatigue and respiratory arrest. **Status asthmaticus—** which is largely preventable—is a clinical state of acute, severe asthma for which this threat looms large. Although this state of severe obstruction evolves over a few days in most patients, in a minority, an explosive start rapidly progresses to severe obstruction with a high risk of death **(acute asphyctic asthma** or **acute explosive asthma).** As the cerebral and/or coronary blood flow diminish, impaired mentation, confusion, tachycardia, ventricular irritability, and lethal arrhythmias follow.

Oximetry or arterial blood gases are often obtained when the PEFR is less than 40%. Because oximetry reflects only oxygenation and not $PaCO_2$, exclusive reliance on oximetry should be avoided. As the asthma attack worsens, the PaO_2 and $PaCO_2$ decrease; with worsening airflow obstruction, $PaCO_2$ normalizes first and then rises. An asthmatic with a normal $PaCO_2$ during an acute attack is in serious trouble.

■ Differential Diagnosis

Accurate diagnosis requires history and physical examination, supplemented by spirometric evidence of reversible obstruction or BHR. Spirometry between attacks may be normal or may show airflow obstruction (see chapter 211). Airflow obstruction in itself does not prove asthma. Because asthmatics also have BHR, response to histamine or methacholine can assist diagnosis. Although the illness is typical in most patients (history, findings, and spirometry), a few with relatively normal spirometry may manifest only cough or episodic chest tightness. Although bronchoprovocation testing can be useful in this setting (see chapter 211), it is superfluous in patients who demonstrate airflow obstruction and not indicated when the $FEV_{1.0}$ is less than 70% of predicted.

Asthma, emphysema, and bronchitis all share the feature of airflow obstruction, and it can be difficult to distinguish between them, especially when a history of smoking is present. Airflow obstruction in the asthmatic shows reversibility, which may be seen on treatment (especially in chronic asthma after initiating corticosteroid therapy), or more commonly, on spirometry, as an improvement in $FEV_{1.0}$ by 15–20% over baseline following inhalation of a ß agonist. Extra-thoracic airway obstruction (tumor or granuloma) may present with wheezing. Careful auscultation over the area of the trachea and flow-volume loop (chapter 224) may be useful. Peribronchial tumors and foreign bodies, other causes of obstruction, may be suggested by localized wheezing and confirmed by imaging.

TABLE 10.1.	Chronic Asthma: A Suggested Severity Classification		
Measure	**Mild (green zone)**	**Moderate (yellow zone)**	**Severe (red zone)**
PEFR			
%pred/PB	≥80%	60–80%	≤60%
Variability/day[a]	<20%	20–30%	>30%
BDR[b]	≤80%	≥80%	Chronically ≤80%
Nocturnal episodes	≤2/mo	>2/mo	Almost daily
prn β agonist use	≤3/wk	>3/wk	Daily
Clinical			
Symptoms	±/0	Almost daily	Continuous
Activity limitation	None	Almost none	Limited despite optimal medication
Hospitalizations	—	—	(+) in the preceding year
Prior life-threatening episodes	—	—	+

Note: Zones refer to peak expiratory flow rate (PEFR) monitoring system. Yellow and red zones generally correlate with a PEFR of 60–80% and <80% of personal best, respectively. Otherwise, clinical correlates are similar.
[a]Variability of PEFR throughout the day.
[b]BDR = Restoration of PEFR to predicted after bronchodilator application; PB = post-bronchodilator.

TABLE 10.2. Clinical Pharmacology of Commonly Used Agents in Asthma

Class	Agent	Effect	Mechanism of Action	Use	Route	Side Effects/Comments
β-2 agonists	Albuterol, metaproterenol, pirbuterol, terbutaline	↓ vascular permeability, bronchodilation.	↑ c-AMP, inhibits histamine release from basophils.	Isolated early phase reactions, EIA, for immediate relief of bronchospasm.	Oral/MDI/nebulizer; use as needed only.	Tachycardia, tremor, nervousness, ?may increase mortality with excessive use.
β-2 selective	Salmeterol	Same as above.	Same as above, but lipophilic, thus longer half-life.	May be used to reduce frequency of use of β agonists.	MDI	Same as above. Not effective for acute attacks.
Phosphodiesterase inhibitor	Theophylline	Acts as a bronchodilator.	Inhibits histamine release from basophils.	As a secondary agent in asthma.	Oral/IV	Narrow therapeutic index; drug levels vulnerable to many factors; GI side effects, agitation, potassium wasting, seizures. Slow onset of action.
Mediator release inhibitor	Cromolyn/nedocromil	Affects early and late phase response; ↓ BHR.	Stabilizes mast cells; inhibits neuropeptide release; ↓ eosinophil chemotaxis.	EIA; allergic asthma, especially cat-induced asthma; prophylactic use.	MDI (Cromolyn and Nedocromil) MDI and nebulizer (cromolyn only)	
Corticosteroids (oral/IV)	Prednisone and methylprednisolone	Prevents latephase response; ↓ BHR; potentiates action of β-2 agents.	Down-regulates TH2 cytokines in lung, inhibits adhesion molecule expression.	Antiinflammatory agent; pivotal in acute asthma to produce clinical improvement and prevent relapse.	IV/Oral	May alter mental status, cause fluid retention, potassium wasting, hyperglycemia, and hypertension. Long-term use may lead to osteoporosis, aseptic necrosis, and cataracts.
Corticosteroids (inhaled)	Beclomethasone, flunisolide; fluticasone, triamcinolone, budesonide	Same as above.	Same as above.	Prophylactic use in chronic asthma.	MDI or dry powder	Variable absorption from tracheobronchial tree; long-term effects on pituitary-adrenal function unknown; may cause oral thrush.
Leukotriene blocker/inhibitor	Zileuton, zafirlukast	Prevents bronchospasm.	Inhibits leukotriene synthesis/blocks leukotriene receptor.	Prophylactic use in chronic asthma.	Oral	Diarrhea, headache, liver function impairment. Zafirlukast is cleared through hepatic P450CYP3A4 system.

↓ = decreases/reduces. ↑ = increases/raises. EIA = exercise-induced asthma.

Congestive heart failure, cystic fibrosis, pulmonary embolism, carcinoid syndrome, mastocytosis, and mycoplasma infection can also mimic asthma. Angina or esophageal spasm may present with chest tightness. Vocal cord dysfunction (intentional or unconscious apposition of the vocal cords during inspiration) can mimic severe asthma. In these patients, wheezing is loudest over the larynx, and diagnosis is made by laryngoscopy. Counseling and speech therapy can be beneficial. Some drugs (ß blockers and NSAIDs) can precipitate asthma, and angiotensin-converting enzyme inhibitors can cause coughing. Cough without wheezing or tightness can be due to rhinitis, sinusitis, gastroesophageal reflux, or cough-variant asthma.

Management

Management of the ambulatory asthmatic

The therapy for asthma depends on its type, attack frequency, and severity. Allergic or occupational asthma is best treated by avoidance of the causative agent. Air filtration units with high-energy particulate air (HEPA) filters may help supplement dust-avoidance measures. Because many asthmatics (75% of children, 50% of adults) have an allergic component to their illness, a screening allergy evaluation is prudent, particularly for those younger than 40. Identification and avoidance of potential allergens and allergy immunotherapy can reduce BHR and the frequency of exacerbations. A careful history of home and work exposures is also important—especially in asthma of new onset in an adult.

Objective follow-up of an asthmatic's progress is best conducted using a peak flow meter because the perception of symptoms is highly variable. The patient should monitor the PEFR regularly over a course of time to determine his or her best levels ("personal best"), which may then be used as a guide for management. Medication adjustment is required if the PEFR values consistently decrease from the personal best by 20%. Patients should see their physician if ß-agonist inhalation fails to improve the PEFR to above 80% of their personal best or if their pretreatment PEFR decreases to 50%

below the personal best. Frequent interruption of sleep by asthmatic attacks calls for medication adjustment, with a prime goal of therapy being minimization—if not complete elimination of—the nocturnal attacks. Adequate control of asthma implies a normal lifestyle during day and night.

Exercise-induced asthma is treated prophylactically with inhaled cromolyn, nedocromil, or ß agonists. If no other symptoms exist, this will usually suffice. If episodic asthma symptoms occur at rest, the attacks may be terminated by use of inhaled ß agonist. However, if episodes (especially if nocturnal) occur more than two to three times per week, a prophylactic anti-inflammatory drug should be used.

Patients who continue to have symptoms should be treated with a stepwise approach (Figure 10.2): 1) maximization of an inhaled anti-inflammatory agent, 2) as-needed (PRN) ß agonists, 3) addition of a long-acting theophylline, and 4) PRN use of oral corticosteroids. Steroid-sparing approaches (e.g., use of methotrexate) are as yet somewhat controversial. When patients routinely require a ß agonist more frequently than twice a day, the addition of a long-acting selective ß agonist such as salmeterol should be considered. However, both salmeterol's delayed onset of action and the need to carry a more rapid-acting agent for acute attacks should be emphasized to the patient.

Pharmacologic therapy

The clinical pharmacology of commonly used agents in ambulatory asthma is shown in Table 10.2. ß-2 agonists offer immediate relief from bronchospasm; many physicians now endorse only their as-needed use, instructing patients to contact their physicians when they are used more than four times a day. Aside from concerns that the regular use of ß-2 agonists increases risk of mortality, some believe they may offset the effects of topical corticosteroids on BHR. Inhaled steroids are safe but can occasionally cause oral candidiasis or hoarseness, which is preventable by gargling after use and by use of a spacer. Allergy shots reduce the late-phase response and BHR when allergens are properly identified, but may take

TABLE 10.3.	Acute Asthma: Evaluating the Severity						
Severity Category	PEFR L/min	Wheeze	Accessory Muscle Use	Chest Wall Retraction	PaCO$_2$	Pulsus Paradoxus	Mentation
Mild	>200	±	None	None	↓	Absent	Normal
Moderate	100–200	+	Present	None	↓	±	Normal
Severe	80–100	++	++	±	Normal	++	Normal
Very severe	<80	May be absent	+++	Present	↑	++	Confusion, loss of judgment

↓ = decreased; ↑ = increased; ± = may or may not be present.

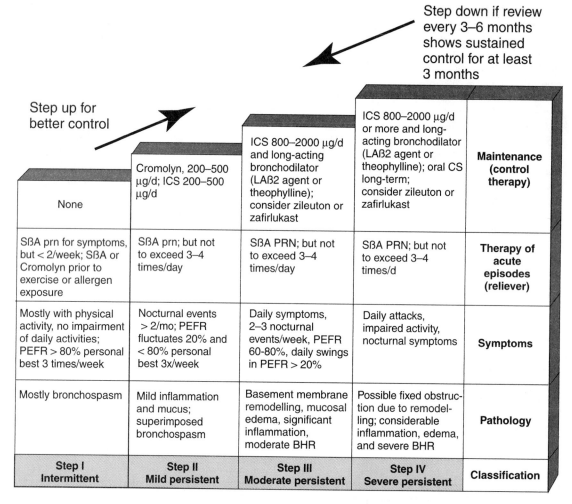

Step down if review every 3–6 months shows sustained control for at least 3 months

Step up for better control

Step I Intermittent	Step II Mild persistent	Step III Moderate persistent	Step IV Severe persistent	Classification
None	Cromolyn, 200–500 µg/d; ICS 200–500 µg/d	ICS 800–2000 µg/d and long-acting bronchodilator (LAß2 agent or theophylline); consider zileuton or zafirlukast	ICS 800–2000 µg/d or more and long-acting bronchodilator (LAß2 agent or theophylline); oral CS long-term; consider zileuton or zafirlukast	Maintenance (control therapy)
SßA prn for symptoms, but < 2/week; SßA or Cromolyn prior to exercise or allergen exposure	SßA prn; but not to exceed 3–4 times/day	SßA PRN; but not to exceed 3–4 times/day	SßA PRN; but not to exceed 3–4 times/d	Therapy of acute episodes (reliever)
Mostly with physical activity, no impairment of daily activities; PEFR > 80% personal best 3 times/week	Nocturnal events > 2/mo; PEFR fluctuates 20% and < 80% personal best 3x/week	Daily symptoms, 2–3 nocturnal events/week, PEFR 60-80%, daily swings in PEFR > 20%	Daily attacks, impaired activity, nocturnal symptoms	Symptoms
Mostly bronchospasm	Mild inflammation and mucus; superimposed bronchospasm	Basement membrane remodelling, mucosal edema, significant inflammation, moderate BHR	Possible fixed obstruction due to remodelling; considerable inflammation, edema, and severe BHR	Pathology

FIGURE 10.2. Stepwise care in asthma.
BHR = bronchial hyperreactivity; CS = corticosteroid; ICS = inhaled corticosteroid; LAβ₂ = long-acting β₂ agent; PRN = as needed; SβA = short-acting β₂ agent.

months to work. They may improve BHR and symptom scores and reduce the need for medication.

Delivery devices

Metered dose inhalers (MDIs) are effective and generally preferable to oral medications because the drug is delivered to the lung, causing minimal systemic effects. However, only 10–20% of the drug actually enters the lung when using typical MDIs. Much of the spray impacts the tongue and throat and is swallowed. Many patients, particularly children, the elderly, and those with arthritis, have trouble coordinating inspiration with actuation of the MDI. Spacer devices, which differ in their mechanism of operation, may address these problems. Because MDIs currently use fluorocarbon propellants, inhalers are also being developed that deliver powder driven by the patient's inspiratory flow to the lungs.

Nebulizers are more convenient to use in young children. Clinically, many patients with bronchospasm respond better to nebulized ß-agonist solutions than to MDIs administered with spacers. Better distribution of the drug was considered the cause, but the greater dispersion of drug may be likely. Thus, if 10–20 puffs from an MDI with spacer are used, a comparable response might occur.

Scope of therapy

With proper, well-supervised medical care, most asthmatics can avoid emergency department (ED) visits (emergent care) or hospitalizations. However, a heavy allergen burden or infection may precipitate rapid deterioration in asthmatics, necessitating emergent care. The cost of such care relative to careful outpatient management is much greater. The annual medical cost of asthma care can be reduced substantially by enrolling patients in programs that provide asthma education, routine outpatient visits, and 24-hour telephone access to physicians. The need for emergent care can be further reduced by regular use of inhaled corticosteroids and early initiation of oral corticosteroids as needed. Corticosteroids given to those who are discharged after emergent care can reduce the need for later hospitalization.

Guidelines for outpatient asthma management established by an international consensus are outlined in Table 10.3. Patients should contact their physicians 1) if their asthma symptoms worsen, 2) if the PEFR decreases by 20% from their "personal best," or 3) if the PEFR diurnal variation is 20% or more (a drop from the "green zone" to the "yellow zone"). They are evaluated for exposures and infection(s), are advised to increase the frequency of use of ß agonist (PRN) or alter its delivery, or are given an additional medication (such as theophylline). Those who fail to respond acutely to ß-agonist aerosol, who continue to be symptomatic for several days, or who drop into the "red zone" with greater than 40% reduction in PEFR should be evaluated for infection and, unless contraindicated, started on oral prednisone (0.5–0.75 mg/kg for the first 2 days followed by a taper over the next several days by about 20% less each day; an average course for an adult is 40 mg, 40 mg, 30 mg, 20 mg, 10 mg, and stop). Those with more severe asthma who require frequent steroid intervention may benefit from a slightly higher initial dose and longer taper. A single morning dose is often adequate. Divided doses may provide better relief of nocturnal symptoms, but they can also evoke more severe adrenal suppression.

Management of acute asthma

In treating acute asthma, ß-2 agonists are of prime importance, the objectives being rapid symptom relief and prevention of status asthmaticus (Figure 10.3). Albuterol is administered as an aerosol. Patients whose PEFR is less than 50% of their personal best or those with severe obstruction (PEFR <100L/min) who fail to readily respond by 10% or more to nebulized ß agonists in the outpatient setting require emergency care.

In emergency management of asthma, supplemental oxygen is started first, to maintain the O_2 saturation greater than 90%. Rapid evaluation can then follow, and PEFR is measured. If the history and examination support a diagnosis of asthma, nebulized albuterol is administered, with 2.5 mg (0.5 ml) in 2.5 ml of saline. This dose is repeated at 20-minute intervals for three doses and hourly thereafter until side effects (tremor and tachycardia) appear or the attack begins to subside. Deceptively enough, tachycardia is often due to the airflow obstruction in the acutely ill asthmatic. If patients are unable to participate with nebulization

or if the exacerbation is part of a systemic allergic reaction, 0.3 ml of 1:1000 epinephrine can be given subcutaneously. Use of parenteral epinephrine must be weighed against the potential for cardiac side effects in patients with risk factors for coronary disease and in those older than 50. A common mistake is failure to administer epinephrine in critically ill patients, given concerns about hypertension or coronary artery disease. Routine use of aerosolized anticholinergic agents confers no additional benefits in acute, severe asthma.

Those with mild or moderate attacks could be observed after administration of a ß-2 agent. Those who attain a posttreatment PEFR greater than 70% of predicted can be discharged from the ED, on a tapering regimen of corticosteroids. Given their high likelihood of relapse, those who attain a posttreatment PEFR of only 40–70% of predicted require observation prior to discharge. Some EDs with appropriate facilities might elect to observe these patients for several hours as improvement often occurs within that time.

All patients presenting to an ED with severe asthma or who are at risk for complications (Table 10.4) should receive corticosteroids initially (prednisone at 30–40 mg every 6 hours). A severe asthmatic attack that has an explosive onset accompanied by respiratory arrest, inability to speak, confusion, complications (pneumothorax, pneumonia, pneumomediastinum), angina, myocardial infarction, or serious arrhythmias should be managed in the intensive care unit after therapy with oxygen, ß-agonist, and IV corticosteroids is initiated in the ED. Others with a severe episode can be observed in the ED after receiving the same therapy. PEFR is measured before administering treatment and 30 minutes thereafter. Patients who worsen despite therapy or improve only partially and those with persistent, severe asthma after treatment should be admitted for observation. If significant improvement ensues, they could be observed further and then discharged on an appropriate regimen of bronchodilators, close follow-up with a primary physician, and a tapering course of corticosteroids.

Management of the patient hospitalized for asthma

Hospitalized patients should have a complete blood count (CBC), differential count, electrolyte measurement, an ECG (for patients older than 40 or at high risk for coronary disease), and arterial blood-gas study if the initial PEFR is less than 40% of predicted. Chest x-rays contribute little in the absence of *a priori* suspicion of pneumonia or barotrauma (pneumothorax or pneumomediastinum). Abundant eosinophils in the sputum Gram's stain may help confirm allergic exacerbation; excess neutrophils may suggest infection.

CLINICAL ASSESSMENT

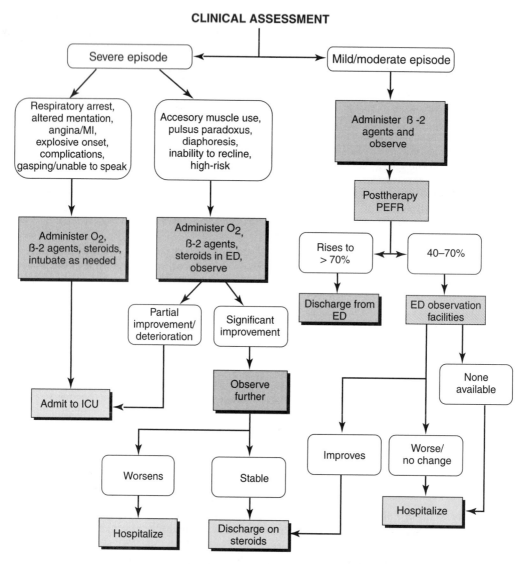

FIGURE 10.3. Management of acute asthma.

Pharmacologic management of the asthmatic hospitalized for acute, severe asthma (status asthmaticus), as summarized in Table 10.5, consists of oxygen, nebulized bronchodilators (given either hourly or by continuous nebulization until bronchospasm begins to abate or side effects emerge), and corticosteroids (at first IV and later PO, as soon as stability is attained). Corticosteroids are gradually tapered as the patient improves. Concomitant use of an H2 blocker may reduce the occurrence of steroid-related gastric stress ulcers; however, cimetidine reduces theophylline clearance, thereby raising the serum theophylline level.

Another potentially useful measure includes theo-

phylline. Monitoring the serum levels of theophylline is critical as it is potentially toxic. In the spontaneously breathing patient, sedation must be avoided. Because the illness often evolves over many days and may involve compromised fluid intake, rehydration is important. However, overhydration to "liquefy tenacious mucus" is without merit.

Endotracheal intubation and mechanical ventilation may become necessary because of worsening asthma, with the usual indications being respiratory arrest, unconsciousness, progressive fatigue, development and/or progression of hypercapnia, and significant mental obtundation or progressive confusion. In general, the asthmatic requires these measures when 1) the possibility of maintaining spontaneous ventilation until achieving an effective bronchodilator/corticosteroid regimen is dubious, or 2) when the patient's general appearance and the course, despite comprehensive therapy, attests to progressive respiratory failure (worsening inability to recline, combativeness, confusion, dull sensorium, escalating tachypnea, and compromised accessory muscle use). Hy-

TABLE 10.4. Recommended Guidelines for Outpatient Management of Chronic Asthma					
Asthma Severity	Inhaled β-2 Agonist	Cromolyn Sodium	Nedocromil	Inhaled Corticosteroid	Others[a]
Mild	PRN, no more than 3x/wk[b]	Before exercise or before antigen exposure[c]	Before exercise or before antigen exposure		
Moderate without nocturnal symptoms with nocturnal symptoms (e.g., ≥ weekly)	prn ≤3–4 x/day Salmeterol; Albuterol ≤3–4 x/day	Daily	Daily	200–500 μg/day 800–1,000 μg/day[d]	ThSR++, βA++
Severe[e]	Same as moderate with nocturnal symptoms				OCS QD[f]

Note: Patient should be evaluated for possible allergy component and follow avoidance. If indicated, undergo immunotherapy for improved symptomatic control.
[a]OCS = oral corticosteroid; βA = oral β$_2$ agonist; ThSR = sustained release theophylline.
[b]Use either β-agonist or cromolyn or nedocromil.
[c]Use either cromolyn or nedocromil.
[d]Use inhaled corticosteroid with Theophylline SR or oral β-2 agonist or long-acting β-agonist. Daily dose above 1000 μg requires specialist supervision.
[e]Evaluate and treat underlying illness such as sinusitis.
[f]QD = single daily dose.
++ = useful; generally necessary.

TABLE 10.5. Evaluating Acute Asthma: Harbingers of Trouble

History
1. Prior hospitalization for asthma.
2. Prior endotracheal intubation and mechanical ventilation for asthma.
3. Chronic steroid dependence.
4. Prior explosive or near-fatal asthma.
5. Noncompliance with medications.
6. Extremes in evolution of current illness: an extremely short one and a very protracted course.
7. Absence of perception of dyspnea in the face of severe airflow obstruction.
8. Associated systemic illnesses, e.g., diabetes mellitus, coronary artery disease, etc.

Physical findings
1. Confusion, lethargy, and/or altered mental status.
2. Accessory muscle use and retraction.
3. Inability to recline, diaphoresis.
4. Ability to recline in the face of very severe obstruction.
5. Respiratory rate >30; heart rate >120; pulsus paradoxus (>12 mm Hg).
6. Silent chest.
7. PEFR ("peak flow") <100 L/min (or <40% of predicted).
8. Hypercapnia.

Response to therapy
1. PEFR <70% of predicted at the end of 2 hours, following bronchodilator treatment.
2. Untoward progression of the following findings: posture, diaphoresis, accessory muscle use, breath sounds, PEFR.

percapnia alone should not be a reason for intubation. A regimen of noninvasive ventilation with a tight-fitting face mask, continuous positive airway pressure (CPAP), and IV bicarbonate where required to offset acidosis, offers an alternative to be used in selected situations when the need to intubate is less urgent.

Preventing relapse

Early intervention using corticosteroid therapy is pivotal to prevent relapse, and both the patient and the physician must be properly educated regarding this therapy (Table 10.6). Careful management of chronic asthma—with an emphasis on anti-inflammatory agents—is key to preventing relapses and status asthmaticus (Table 10.7). The physician should remember the

adage that "the time to treat status asthmaticus is three days before it happens."

■ Complications and Prognosis

Many physicians believe that untreated asthma can progress to an obstructive form of the illness with only partial reversibility. Patients with poorly controlled asthma who are undergoing surgery are also at greater risk for postoperative complications and complications due to radiocontrast study. Without adequate *and* timely treatment, the mortality rate is several times higher than the previously mentioned 1 for 3000 cases. Although asthma is a chronic illness, most patients should be able to lead normal lives, especially if they receive proper care.

TABLE 10.6.	Medications in the Treatment of Acute Severe Asthma		
Agent	**Dose**	**Route**	**Comments**
Albuterol	2.5 mg in 2.5 ml saline	Nebulizer, initially for three doses at 20-minute intervals, then hourly. May also be given by continuous nebulization.	May cause tachycardia, tremor, and nervousness.
Methylprednisolone	40–125 mg q 6h	IV	Start treatment in ED; higher doses do not show any additional benefit, but lower doses may not be as effective.
Prednisone	40–60 mg q 6h	Oral administration.	
Epinephrine	0.3 ml (1:1000 solution)	Subcutaneous administration. A suspension in oil available for pediatric use, for sustained local absorption.	May cause angina with prior CAD. Drug of choice for asthma with anaphylaxis. Patients with a history of explosive asthma should carry preloaded epinephrine syringe (EpiPen™) to use when such attacks recur.
Ipratropium bromide	0.5 mg	Nebulizer, given every hr for 3–4 doses.	Not a standard regimen in acute asthma, but may be useful when the response to β-2 agents and steroids is suboptimal.
Theophylline	5–6 mg/kg (Loading dose) 0.5–0.7 mg/kg/hr maintenance	IV infusion in about 20 min for loading. IV infusion	Toxicity generally related to serum level. Therapeutic level 10–20 µg/ml, but a level of 9–12 µg/ml may be safer.
Magnesium sulfate	2.0 g (total dose)	Two doses of 1.0 g each, infused IV in 20 min, given 20 min apart.	Not a standard regimen. If serum levels are low, correct the deficiency.

TABLE 10.7.	Status Asthmaticus: Keys to Preventing Relapse	
Patient Education		**Physician Education**
Identify triggers of attacks.		Intervene early and decisively when disease is out of control.
Control and avoid triggers.		Give antiinflammatory therapy.
Know when to call the physician.		Use reliable methods to monitor control of disease.
Recognize early warning signs of loss of disease control.		Overcome fear of using corticosteroids.
Be compliant with medications.		
Control the environment.		
Learn side effects of medications.		

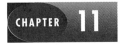

ANAPHYLAXIS

■ Definition

It has long been known that "protective" immunizations with toxins could unexpectedly produce severe and often fatal reactions upon re-exposure. Anaphylaxis is a constellation of allergic responses with features dependent on organ involvement and dose and route of exposure. Symptoms can range from mild, generalized urticaria (see chapter 13) to respiratory and circulatory collapse. Anaphylactic reactions are mediated through IgE; anaphylactoid reactions, which resemble anaphylaxis, do not require IgE recognition.

■ Etiology and Epidemiology

The annual incidence of anaphylaxis in the general population is 3 per 100,000, accounting for 500–700 deaths yearly in the United States. Seen once for every 3000 inpatient admissions, anaphylaxis is most commonly caused by drug allergy, followed by Hymenoptera (bee) stings and food allergies. First reported in 1979, latex allergy became an important cause of anaphylaxis during the 1990s, and several fatalities have occurred. Three high-risk groups are known for latex allergy: spina bifida patients, employees of rubber manufacturers, and health care workers. Latex allergy seems to develop either from occupational exposure or by recurrent intraoperative contact. In adults, most anaphylaxis deaths are caused by a combination of hypoxia, cardiac arrhythmias, and laryngeal edema. Anaphylactoid reactions also cause more than 500 deaths each year, with the majority caused by radiocontrast media.

■ Pathogenesis

Several mechanisms have been proposed for anaphylaxis. A type I IgE-dependent reaction is a common mechanism and is typically seen with reactions to proteins (e.g., venoms, insulin, foods) and smaller-weight haptens (penicillin, sulfa). These reactions involve vascular leak, vasodilatation, and bronchospasm owing to the release of platelet-activating factor (PAF), histamine, leukotriene C_4, and prostaglandin D. Released by mast cells, tryptase can be measured in serum 1–8 hours after the onset of anaphylaxis. Mast cells may also produce nitric oxide, which acts as a vasodilator and could prolong hypotension.

At least two well-described anaphylactoid reactions do not require IgE. One such mechanism is immune complex-anaphylatoxin–induced mast cell degranulation. Patients reacting to some drug infusions form IgG complexes that activate complement, which, in turn, activates mast cells and basophils. In patients undergoing hemodialysis, anaphylatoxin can be directly produced by reaction with the dialysis membrane. Direct cell activation is a third type of reaction, but it is poorly understood. Agents such as morphine, codeine, and contrast media cause mediator release from the cells of certain individuals. Ironically, atopic individuals are at no greater risk for IgE-mediated reactions, but they are four to five times more likely to have an adverse response to direct degranulation reactions. It is believed that their cells are relatively unstable—perhaps owing to unique features of the bound IgE.

Regardless of the mechanism, patients with a prior anaphylactic reaction are at increased risk of its repetition on re-exposure. Penicillin, the most frequent cause of anaphylaxis, causes mild reactions in 0.5–1% of persons. Repeat exposure will cause a recurrent reaction in about 10–20% of these patients. Similar rates of recurrence are seen for other hapten drugs. In the U.S. population, 20% of persons produce IgE against Hymenoptera venoms, but reactions are seen in only 0.5%. However, patients with a prior systemic reaction have a 40–50% risk of another systemic reaction when re-stung. Because IgE levels gradually wane over time, the severity and likelihood of repeat reaction depends partly on the duration since the last exposure. Non–IgE-dependent reactions are also highly recurrent (30–40% risk for radiocontrast), but whether avoidance influences this rate is uncertain.

Other forms of anaphylaxis may be idiopathic or may be induced by NSAIDs or exercise. Although NSAIDs inhibit cyclo-oxygenase and may shunt arachidonic acid into the leukotriene pathway, whether they activate mast cells or basophils is not known. The rate of NSAID anaphylaxis, 1:1000 in the general population, is higher among asthmatics with nasal polyps.

■ Clinical Features

The presentation varies in severity and with organ system. Often, patients report a vague sense of impending doom as a **prodrome.** Manifestations may be cutaneous (pruritus, flushing, urticaria, and angioedema), upper respiratory with laryngeal edema (stridor, dysphagia, and respiratory distress), respiratory (sneezing, congestion, or initial ocular itch with later bronchospasm), gastrointestinal (nausea, vomiting, diarrhea, and cramping), and cardiovascular (vasodilatation causing skin flushing and vascular leak with associated hypotension and compensatory tachycardia). Histamine-induced coronary artery spasm may cause ischemia in patients with previous coronary artery disease. Patients receiving ß blockers are especially prone to severe cardiovascular compromise because they are unable to develop tachycardia and are relatively resistant to epinephrine. Uterine contraction during anaphylaxis could cause miscarriage.

Anaphylaxis owing to percutaneous allergen challenge (e.g., injection or insect sting) has a rapid onset (within minutes) and is complete in 30 minutes. Life-threatening anaphylaxis after allergy injections almost always follows within 20 minutes. Owing to its slower absorption rate, oral allergen exposure evokes less severe, delayed symptoms (less than 1 hour). However, reactions to peanuts and eggs can be rapid and lethal.

■ Differential Diagnosis

When evaluating a patient with possible anaphylaxis, rapid decision making and initiation of life-saving therapy are essential. Further evaluation can follow stabilization. When anaphylaxis cannot be excluded in the acute setting, assuming this diagnosis is generally the safest course of action. A brief history and physical examination are helpful. If a patient is known to be allergic to certain medications, Hymenoptera, or foods, a presumptive diagnosis is easy if exposure has occurred. Prior history of asthma, cardiovascular disease, MedicAlert™ bracelets proclaiming anaphylaxis,

ß-blocker use, or 'reactions to needles' should be noted. At least some of the following typical signs and symptoms should be present: urticaria, rhinorrhea, wheeze, abdominal cramps, or hypotension. Unless there has been ß-blocker use, tachycardia is usual. Elevated plasma tryptase with attacks can confirm anaphylaxis. By definition, the diagnosis of idiopathic anaphylaxis is one of exclusion.

The differential diagnosis includes anaphylactoid reactions (such as contrast, transfusion, and dialysis reactions)—which are treated as anaphylaxis—and asthma and urticaria. Vasovagal episodes and anxiety are other imitators, usually elicited by a fear of procedures. Patients with vasovagal episodes can experience hypotension and nausea, as in anaphylaxis, but have bradycardia and are usually pale (not flushed), diaphoretic, and without wheezing or urticaria. Patients with anxiety may have a rapid pulse, paraesthesias, and light-headedness but no other signs of anaphylaxis.

Side effects such as hypotension (overdose or increased sensitivity to an antihypertensive) or flushing (rapid infusion of vancomycin) from medications can mimic anaphylaxis. Carcinoid syndrome, aspiration of a foreign body, pulmonary embolism, myocardial infarction, and adrenal insufficiency may also occasionally be confused with anaphylaxis. A lack of precipitators and atypical features help determine the diagnosis. When in doubt, measurement of serum tryptase 1–4 hours after the onset of an attack will help establish or exclude anaphylaxis.

■ Management

Acute intervention (Table 11.1) must be quick and decisive, including the use of epinephrine. Adverse outcomes including fatality are more likely caused by slow recognition and undertreatment than complications from therapy. Early subcutaneous administration of epinephrine may head off more severe reactions. If anaphylaxis is caused by a sting or injection in an extremity, a tourniquet should be applied proximally and epinephrine can be injected directly into the sting site (if on an arm or leg) to delay absorption. For severe cardiovascular collapse unresponsive to subcutaneous injection, some physicians advocate a slow IV infusion of epinephrine. IV epinephrine infusion may induce myocardial damage in adults with risk factors for coronary disease and should thus be reserved for patients in extremis.

A team approach to address *airway, breathing,* and *circulation* is helpful. A patent airway must be maintained by repositioning the head, endotracheal intubation, or emergency cricothyroidotomy, if necessary. Give supplemental oxygen to maintain oxygen saturation above 90%. Endotracheal intubation may be necessary

TABLE 11.1. Treatment of Anaphylaxis		
Medication	**Route**	**Dose**
Epinephrine	SubQ	0.3 ml of 1:1000 every 10–20 min
Albuterol	Nebulized	0.5–1.0 ml of 0.5% nebulized every 20 min up to three times
Oxygen	Nasal/Mask	40–100% to maintain PaO2 >60 mm Hg, SaO2 >90%
H1 antihistamine	IM	25–50 mg of hydroxyzine or diphenhydramine q 6–8h
H2 antihistamine	IV	Cimetidine 300 mg IV q 6 h
Corticosteroid	IV	250 mg hydrocortisone or 50 mg methylprednisolone q 6 h × 2–4 doses
Aminophylline	IV	For persistent bronchospasm, and if not currently using the drug, load with 5–6 mg/kg over 30 min, then maintenance of 0.3–0.5 mg/kg hr
For cardiovascular collapse		
Saline	IV	Infuse rapidly 1–2 liters over 20–30 min until systolic BP is ≥80 mm Hg, then use sufficient fluid to maintain BP
Epinephrine	IV[a]	After the initial dose, continuously infuse a 4 µg/ml solution starting at 1 µg/min under careful cardiac monitoring, to keep systolic BP ≥80 mm Hg
Dopamine	IV	200 mg in 500 ml D5W (0.4 mg/ml) starting at 5 µg/kg/min, increase rate by 5–10 µg/kg/min as necessary up to a rate of 20–50 µg/kg/min
Levarterenol	IV	4–8 mg in 1 liter of D5W or saline, to infuse at a maximal rate of 2 ml/min
Glucagon	IV	1 mg in 1 liter D5W 5–15 ml/min for refractory hypotension

[a]If no contraindication.

for respiratory failure that is refractory to the measures in Table 11.1. Circulation is assessed by pulse rate, blood pressure, and capillary filling of the nail beds. The patient is placed in the Trendelenburg position. A large-bore IV (16–18 g) should be used to establish access for fluids. Hypotension is treated by rapid infusion of normal saline, followed, if necessary, by an infusion of dopamine or levarterenol bitartrate. Corticosteroids should be infused as soon as IV access has been achieved. Patients who use ß blockers and are refractory to these interventions may benefit from glucagon infusion. Intravenous diphenhydramine will reduce cutaneous manifestations but not respiratory, gastrointestinal, or cardiovascular complications. Some physicians find IV cimetidine, which blocks H2 effects of histamine, useful for treating hypotension and flushing.

■ Prevention

Although anaphylaxis is not always avoidable, its frequency and severity can be reduced for most patients. Many common-sense measures are often overlooked (Table 11.2). Patients with venom sensitivity should adopt additional measures such as avoiding wearing clothes with light-colored floral patterns and staying away from trash cans and open soda and juice containers when outdoors to reduce the likelihood of stings. Patients with a suspected food allergy should undergo skin testing by an allergist to confirm the diagnosis. They should carry a preloaded epinephrine syringe when dining out and carefully read the ingredients on all food labels.

Premedication regimens are available for patients at risk for anaphylactoid reactions to radiocontrast dyes.

TABLE 11.2. A Strategy for Preventing Anaphylaxis
• Wear MedicAlert bracelet to indicate prior adverse reactions.
• Document prior adverse drug reactions in the medical record.
• Patients should wait in office 30 minutes after parenteral drug administration.
• Avoid causative or cross-reacting medications (e.g., cephalosporins with penicillin allergy; an NSAID when drug reactions to another have occurred).
• Use lower ionic contrast media and premedicate when a history of prior reaction exists.
• Substitute ß blockers with other antihypertensives for patients at risk.
• Patients with prior anaphylaxis should undergo desensitization to Hymenoptera venom.
• Appropriate patients at risk should carry injectable epinephrine.
• If reaction has formed due to sting or injection in extremity, place tourniquet proximal to sting.

Use of low ionic strength agents reduces the risk, as does premedication with prednisone (50 mg or 1 mg/kg every 6 hours for 3 doses) and diphenhydramine (1.5 mg/kg, up to 50 mg) IM 30–60 minutes before study. Ephedrine (25 mg), which has also been added to this regimen, is not recommended for patients at high risk for heart disease. Finally, in a patient known to be allergic to a drug (e.g., a ß lactam antibiotic) that is essential for his or her care, desensitization before administering a therapeutic dose greatly diminishes the risk of anaphylaxis.

CHAPTER 12

DRUG ALLERGY

■ Definition

Drug allergy is an adverse reaction based on immune recognition, expressed as a hypersensitivity reaction (Table 12.1). Although allergic reactions form a minority (10%) of adverse reactions to drugs, they are often severe. Prior exposure to the drug is usually required to develop immune recognition; however, the reaction is often unforeseen because the prior exposure may have been uneventful, the patient might have been exposed to a cross-reacting drug, or the exposure might have been occult or forgotten. Type II–IV reactions have delayed onset compared with most expected toxic or metabolic drug side effects.

■ Etiology and Epidemiology

The high frequency of all adverse drug reactions parallels the frequent use of medications, particularly in the elderly. The average outpatient will consume three over-the-counter medications containing nine active ingredients per month. Drug reactions cause 5% of hospitalizations in the elderly (Table 12.2). A serious drug reaction occurs in 5% of patients hospitalized for 6 days or less but in 40% hospitalized more than 2 weeks.

Nonallergic reactions may be predictable or unpredictable (Table 12.3). Rather than memorizing long lists of medications and their possible adverse effects and interactions, the physician should do the following:

1) review the profile of each drug in the *Physician's Desk Reference* (PDR) or similar guide before prescribing, 2) use available software for drug interactions (e.g., the HyperCard-based Drug Interaction Software program published by *The Medical Letter*), and 3) be familiar with several broad categories of agents. A small group of seven drug types (aspirin, digoxin, anticoagulants, antibiotics, diuretics, steroids, and hypoglycemic agents) cause most drug reactions. Antibiotics are the group most likely to cause unpredictable allergic reactions.

Despite overlaps and exceptions, classifying allergic reactions along the type I–IV hypersensitivity scheme is helpful. Because immune recognition is involved, clues for the diagnosis of drug allergy include the following: 1) no reaction on prior exposure, 2) reaction after several days (for types II–IV), 3) reactions after exposure to doses well below the therapeutic norm, 4) a small proportion of the population affected, and 5) unusual presentation with recognized allergic syndromes. It is worth remembering that some patients are prone to multiple drug allergies. A patient with a proven allergy to penicillin is 10 times more likely to experience an IgE-mediated allergic reaction to another antibiotic. A familial trait for increased drug allergy may exist. Allergy to penicillin (and its derivatives) is the most common drug allergy; because penicillin can cause any of the type I–IV reactions, it is a prototype for the pathophysiology and presentations described in the following.

Type I Reactions

A type I reaction involves mast cell or basophil activation. Classic, IgE-dependent mediator release is seen with complete antigens such as proteins (serum, insulin) or haptens such as penicillin or sulfa drugs bound to proteins. Pseudoallergic reactions cause mediator release without immune recognition by IgE. This form of release can be seen 1) with agents that directly degranulate mast cells such as morphine, codeine, and radiocon-

TABLE 12.1.	Types of Allergic Reactions	
Reaction Type	**Common Causative Agents**	**Clinical Presentations**
Type I		
Anaphylactic	Penicillin, chymopapain, insulin, sulfonamides	Urticaria, anaphylaxis
Anaphylactoid	Contrast media, morphine, codeine	Urticaria, hypotension
Type II	Transfusion reaction, quinidine, methicillin	Hemolysis, thrombocytopenia, nephritis
Type III	Penicillin, hydralazine, procainamide, antithymocyte globulin, sulfonamides	Serum sickness (fever, arthralgias, purpuric rash, proteinuria) hypersensitivity angiitis
Type IV	Parabens, nitrofurantoin, neomycin, topical antihistamines, ethylenediamine, sulfonamides	Contact dermatitis, pulmonary fibrosis, photosensitivity, toxic epidermal necrolysis

trast; 2) as a result of bacterial contamination, which activates cells directly or indirectly by generating anaphylatoxins; and 3) when immune complexes plus complement are generated, which then activate mast cells. This last case may be a mechanism for protamine-induced reactions.

The most common type I reaction arises from penicillin and its derivatives. IgE antibodies are usually directed against the ß lactam ring, which is shared with the cephalosporins (Figure 12.1). Occasionally, IgE is directed against the side chains, but such IgE antibodies are less clinically important. Reactive metabolites of penicillin can bind proteins and thus cross-link IgE on cells. Penicilloyl and penicilloate are two prominent metabolites. Penicilloyl is the "major determinant" because 85% of patients with type I penicillin allergy make IgE antibodies to it. Penicilloate and penilloate are "minor determinants." However, these terms are misleading because they do not correlate with the severity of reactions caused by these metabolites. Corresponding cephalosporin metabolites are less stable, perhaps accounting for the lower allergenicity of cephalosporins.

Although patients with rhinitis and asthma are no more likely to have IgE-mediated drug reactions than the general population, they are more likely to have anaphylactoid reactions to contrast dyes, and these reactions are more severe.

Some drug reactions resemble type I reactions, but the mechanism is not clear. Local anesthetics evoke wheal and flare reactions in susceptible persons. Aspirin-sensitive patients, especially those with the aspirin triad (nasal polyps and asthma), can experience asthma attacks, urticaria, or nasal/ocular symptoms. Almost 10% of asthmatics experience worsening airflow after aspirin ingestion, but when asthma is associated with nasal polyps, this incidence increases.

■ Clinical Features of Type I Reactions

Reactions can be subdivided by onset as immediate, accelerated, and delayed. *Immediate reactions* (e.g., anaphylaxis or isolated hives) usually occur within 30 minutes. *Accelerated reactions* (usually pruritus only, with or without hives and erythema) occur between 2 hours and 3 days. *Delayed reactions*, which simulate a **morbilliform** (measles-like) **rash,** typically present after 5–10 days of drug use and may not involve IgE antibodies.

The route, rate of administration, and dose play an important role in the clinical presentation. Oral medications are more slowly absorbed than parenteral ones and thus are less likely to elicit serious type I reactions. Minute doses (<1μg) cause partial degranulation with mild to minimal symptoms. This is the principle underlying drug desensitization regimens. Greater exposure may lead to localized hives, pruritus, or cough, usually within minutes. This can be followed by hypotension, gastrointestinal symptoms, and respiratory compromise. Many patients report an eerie sense of impending doom prior to the reactions. Although anaphylactoid reactions also cause symptoms within minutes, warmth or flushing commonly precedes them.

■ Diagnosis of Type I Reactions

Drugs that cause allergic reactions are listed in Table 12.4. Diagnosing drug allergy is often a process of deduction when the patient is using multiple medications.

TABLE 12.2.	Determinants/Causes of Drug Reaction(s) in Hospitalized Patients

Drug allergy
Idiosyncrasy
Drug interactions
Wrong dose
Wrong dosing interval
Wrong patient
Polypharmacy (multiple drugs)
Length of stay

TABLE 12.3.	Examples of Predictable and Unpredictable Drug Reactions

Forms	Examples
Predictable forms	
Toxic side effects	Drowsiness from antihistamines.
Toxic supratherapeutic	Heart block from digoxin; CNS dysfunction from lidocaine.
Drug interactions	Theophylline toxicity when a macrolide antibiotic is added.
Unpredictable forms	
Drug intolerance	Hypotension at low dose of antihypertensive; hyponatremia on starting dose of diuretic.
Secondary effects	Fever and chills due to Jarisch-Herxheimer reaction when treating syphilis.
Idiosyncratic	Hemolysis in glucose-6-phosphate dehydrogenase deficiency; anaphylaxis in response to penicillin; aspirin-induced bronchospasm.

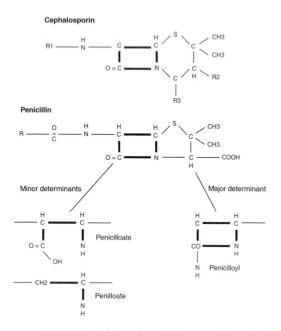

FIGURE 12.1. Penicillin and cephalosporins share the ß lactam ring (in bold). Penicillin determinants include penicilloyl (major determinant), penicilloate, and penilloate (minor determinants). Most patients allergic to penicillin react to major determinant although the most severe reactions are usually against the minor determinants.

Almost any drug can cause almost any form of reaction, and reactions may occur days, weeks, or even months after initiating use. Skin testing, when available, is the preferred method for diagnosing type I reactions. Ideally, patients with true type I reactions to drugs should be amenable to testing for IgE antibody through skin tests or RAST. Unfortunately, this is often not true for small molecular-weight drugs. Proteins, such as insulin, being large enough to cross-link IgE, can be used for skin tests. Reagents for penicillin skin testing are available, but not for most other drugs. Skin tests for other agents are also not as reliable as that for penicillin—a possible exception being skin testing for topical anesthetics. Because contrast agents directly degranulate cells, they lack any test; avoidance or premedication are the only ways to reduce the risk of reactions to them. Without reliable skin testing, a presumptive diagnosis is made by history, clinical presentation, onset of reaction, and established knowledge that the suspected drug has evoked allergic reactions. Other clues are prior reactivity to a similar or cross-reacting medication (e.g., sulfonamide-allergic patients using a thiazide diuretic), discontinuation followed by re-exposure to a drug, and rapid improvement when a drug is discontinued.

Pre-Pen™ is commercially available for penicillin testing. This will detect patients with IgE directed against the major determinant but will miss those (about 10%) who are allergic only to the minor determinants—an unfortunate omission because patients who make IgE to minor determinant more often have severe anaphylactic reactions to penicillin. The likelihood of missing minor-determinant sensitivity can be minimized by prick testing with 100,000 units/ml penicillin G and intradermal tests with 1000 units/ml. However, testing with preparations of minor determinant mixes, which are usually available at referral centers, is preferable. Patients without prior histories of penicillin reaction have a 1–2% chance of a systemic IgE-mediated reaction, which rises to 5–20% in those with prior histories and 40% in those with prior histories of severe anaphylaxis. When a skin test is performed using both Pre-Pen™ and minor determinant, the result is positive in 2% of patients without positive histories. Those with negative skin tests and positive histories have only a 2% risk of an IgE-mediated reaction, and usually such reactions are mild (pruritus with or without urticaria). However, a positive skin test and positive history increase the risk of a serious reaction to 50–70%.

Most reactions to topical anesthetics are vasovagal, toxic, or trauma-related. Group I local anesthetics are p-amino benzoic derivatives and include procaine benzocaine. IgE against these can cross-react with paraben preservatives, which are commonly found in lotions and some injectable medications. Group II includes lidocaine and mepivacaine. Cross-reactivity is rare between groups I and II. Skin testing is conducted with anesthetics lacking preservatives or epinephrine to provide a less ambiguous study. When a positive skin test is found, patients frequently have a negative test for an appropriate substitute.

■ Management of Type I Reactions

Mild to moderate reactions (pruritus with or without urticaria) can be treated symptomatically with antihistamines such as hydroxyzine, 25 mg, every 8 hours or doxepin, 10 mg, every 12 hours. When possible, the

TABLE 12.4.	Common and Uncommon Causes of Allergic Drug Reactions	
Common (>1%)	**Uncommon (<.1%)**
Amoxicillin	Potassium chloride
Trimethoprim-sulfamethoxazole	Diazepam
Ampicillin	Furosemide
Whole blood	Tetracycline
Cephalosporins	Digoxin
Penicillin	Allopurinol
Quinidine	Anticoagulants

drug should be discontinued. The patient is watched closely for development of **erythema multiforme major** (Stevens-Johnson syndrome) or serum sickness. More serious anaphylactoid or anaphylactic reactions should be treated as outlined in chapter 11.

Avoidance is the best therapy. In most cases of infection, other classes of antibiotics can be used. Patients with penicillin sensitivity are much more likely than the general population to have a reaction to cephalosporins; thus, cephalosporins should be avoided as a substitute for penicillin. Aztreonam, a monobactam, reportedly has little or no cross-reactivity with penicillin. When penicillin or a related ß lactam antibiotic is clearly indicated in an allergic patient (e.g., endocarditis, syphilis with pregnancy, or listeria meningitis), skin testing should precede administration of the drug. Patients with positive histamine tests and negative penicillin tests are able to use ß lactam antibiotics although many physicians will first administer a test dose of 1/1000th the therapeutic dose to confirm safety. If pruritus or mild urticaria

develops, an antihistamine such as diphenhydramine or hydroxyzine can be given. Patients with positive skin testing to penicillin require desensitization, but only if, after reconsideration, the need to give the drug still clearly outweighs the risk. Desensitization should be performed in an intensive care unit with careful monitoring and epinephrine at bedside. Similar desensitizations can be carried out for other drugs such as sulfa drugs or insulin.

Insulin allergy, although fairly common, is almost always mild and transient. Immune responses to insulin can include IgE-mediated local reactions with swelling and itching or more severe generalized pruritus and urticaria. Patients sensitized to beef or pork insulin can also display cross-reactive IgE to recombinant human insulin. Desensitization is not useful for contrast media. These patients have a 30% risk for recurrent reactions. When diagnostic procedures with these agents are necessary, the risk for reaction can be reduced by using newer nonionic agents and premedicating patients.

Type II Reactions

The classic type II reaction is an ABO transfusion mismatch. Small molecular-weight drugs may also evoke such reactions, and depending on the location where the drug settles, cause hemolysis or organ damage. Penicillin can coat red cells or platelets, and **thrombocytopenia** or hemolysis results when IgG or IgM antipenicillin antibodies attach to cells with fixation of complement. Type II hematologic reactions may also result from phenacetin, quinidine, heparin, and sulfonamides. Methyldopa may

induce red cells to express new antigens that bind cytotoxic antibody and cause hemolysis. Interstitial nephritis may follow nafcillin and phenytoin-induced linear antibody and complement deposition on the renal tubular basement membrane. History and evidence of antibody deposition on red cells (direct Coombs test) or in affected organs are key to diagnosing these reactions. Stopping the drug is essential; corticosteroids are not always beneficial.

Type III Reactions

A type III reaction (also called serum sickness) involves immune complex deposition, complement fixation, and vasculitis. Such reactions may follow use of antithymocyte globulin, penicillin, and hydralazine. Cutaneous symptoms often begin with erythema around the sides of the fingers, palms, and feet. Drug-induced hypersensitivity angiitis, most often caused by sulfonamides, can also affect the kidneys and lungs. Propylthiouracil can induce vasculitis initially involving the face and ear

lobes. Biopsy of affected skin shows fibrinoid necrosis of small, dermal vessels with polymorphonuclear infiltration and C3 and IgM deposition on direct immunofluorescent staining.

Pruritus generally responds to antihistamines, which may, theoretically, reduce vascular changes and immune complex deposition. Gradual spontaneous improvement occurs over 7–14 days although corticosteroids may hasten recovery.

Type IV Reactions

Type IV reactions follow the topical use of drugs such as topical anesthetics or co-ingredients such as methylparaben and ethylenediamine. Oral medications rarely cause a diffuse eczematoid response. A photosensitive

cutaneous rash, which characteristically occurs in sun-exposed areas, may follow oral or parenteral use of tetracyclines. A fibrotic lung reaction may follow nitrofurantoin. A component of type IV hypersensitivity has been alleged in some cases of drug-induced interstitial nephritis or hepatitis. In **fixed drug eruption,** a probable example of type IV sensitivity, a delayed, localized pruritic rash occurs in the same location on the skin each time certain drugs are systemically used.

These rashes usually abate spontaneously with the cessation of the drug or the offending agent. Antihistamines may allay pruritus. Topical corticosteroids may ease symptoms, but application over a large area requires care.

CHAPTER 13   URTICARIA AND ANGIOEDEMA

Urticaria

■ Definition

Urticaria (hives), a symptom complex arising from a variety of causes, consists of raised, usually pruritic cutaneous lesions that vary in size from several millimeters to several centimeters. The term is from the *Urtica urens* nettle, which causes stinging and itching. Key categories of urticaria are listed in Table 13.1.

■ Epidemiology and Etiology

Urticaria can occur at any age, but is most frequent in young adults. Nearly 15% of the general population has had at least one bout of urticaria at some time, and on any given day, 1 of every 1000 people experience it. Patients can have isolated urticaria or urticaria with coexisting angioedema (see the second portions of this chapter). Urticaria will spontaneously resolve within 6 months in most patients. Causes of urticaria are listed in Table 13.1. Because urticaria usually occurs within 30–90 minutes of exposure, many patients are able to associate the onset of urticaria with these exposures and thus limit the duration of the urticaria. Use of a food-and-activity diary is sometimes helpful in determining when the urticaria is delayed in onset. Chronic urticaria is more of a diagnostic challenge, and in 80% of patients, the cause is never clearly established.

■ Pathology

Approximately 2–3% of patients will have evidence for leukocytoclastic vasculitis in biopsy specimens, including immunoglobulin and complement deposition in vascular walls. Rarely, in physical urticaria (e.g., delayed pressure urticaria), a polymorphonuclear infiltrate can be seen. Mast cell degranulation is considered central to most urticarias. Histamine release has been demonstrated both in locally draining veins in several forms of urticaria and in biopsy specimens of cold urticaria (urticaria brought on by exposure to cold). Some afferent nerve fibers in the skin release substance P, a neuropeptide that can degranulate mast cells. Histamine from mast cells activates these afferent fibers, causing the release of additional substance P in a feed-forward amplification reaction.

Mediators not associated with mast cell activation also are important in urticaria. Many antihistamines can act as serotonin antagonists, and those most useful for cold urticaria are potent serotonin antagonists. Patients with cholinergic urticaria (prickly heat) may have an abnormality of acetylcholine release from nerves in the skin. Intradermal injection of methacholine causes abnormal wheal responses in one-third to one-half of these patients. Interestingly, many of the effective antihistamines also have anticholinergic activity.

Some patients with chronic urticaria produce autoantibodies against the IgE high-affinity receptor. Excess cutaneous blood flow or vascular leakage might exacerbate urticaria in these patients, thus explaining how vasodilators such as alcohol and heat or factors that increase cardiac output such as hyperthyroidism and stress occasionally precipitate urticaria. The C1q complement component has amino acid homology with collagen, and in some patients with collagen vascular disease and autoantibodies against C1q, hypocomplementemic urticarial vasculitis may develop.

■ Clinical Features

The clinical presentation (Table 13.2) depends on the form of urticaria and its cause. Although it has many alleged precipitants, it is frequently spontaneous. *Typical urticaria* is one to several centimeters in size, circular, and pruritic. The lesions blanch and resolve within 6 hours. Lesions that do not blanch and take more than a day to resolve, or that leave bruising, should be considered atypical and make an underlying vasculitis suspect. *Cholinergic urticaria* consists of 2–3-mm red papules that coalesce into large areas and follows warming of the corresponding body area. If the core body temperature is raised 1°C, more generalized constitu-

TABLE 13.1.	Key Categories of Urticaria
Type	**Clinical Considerations**
Acute (<6 weeks)	
Etiology known	Bacterial or viral infections.
	Ingestion of foods or drugs.
	Topical exposure (soaps, shampoos, detergents, and lotions).
	Occasionally aeroallergens.
Etiology unknown	Idiopathic.
Chronic (>6 weeks)	
Nonphysical	
Underlying disease	E.g., bacterial infection, thyroid disease, parasitic infestation, hepatitis, autoimmune—usually typical hives, but persist >24 hours with autoimmune.
Contact urticaria	Due to contact with IgE-mediated allergen (e.g., cat saliva).
Cholinergic	Coalescing papular due to cholinergic nerve activation with heating.
Adrenergic	Papular-like cholinergic, but with white zones around wheal, provoked with stress.
Physical	
Dermatographism	Streaks of wheal and flare due to mechanical trauma, often excoriated.
Pressure urticaria	Immediate, <30 minutes, or delayed; burning wheals for immediate; induration for delayed at sites of pressure.
Cold	Induration at cold exposed sites.
Vibratory	Urticaria (or angioedema in hands or feet) due to vibratory stimuli.
Aquagenic	Due to tepid water exposure.
Solar	Sun-exposed areas, depends on wave length.

TABLE 13.2.	Clinical Diagnosis and Treatment of Common Chronic Urticarias	
Classification	**Diagnosis**	**First-line Treatment**
Nonphysical		
Bacterial infection	CBC and differential, sedimentation rate, chest x-ray, sinus x-rays as appropriate.	Appropriate antibiotic.
Contact urticaria	Prick skin test to confirm IgE antibodies.	Avoidance, careful washing after contact, possibly allergy immunotherapy.
Cholinergic	Typical rash, occurs with body warming, methacholine skin test positive in <50% of cases.	Antihistamines with anticholinergic properties (e.g., doxepin 10 mg 1–3 times per day); gradual warm-up and cool-down with exercise.
Physical		
Dermatographism	Lightly stroke with broken tongue blade to produce linear wheals.	Daily antihistamine (e.g., loratadine, astemizole, fexofenadine, or cetirizine).
Pressure	Apply 15 pounds to 1 square inch area for 10–15 minutes.	Prophylactic antihistamine for immediate type; colchicine or nonsteroidal anti-inflammatory agents for delayed type.
Cold	Apply plastic-wrapped ice cube to skin for 5 minutes, remove and observe for induration for 10 minutes.	Warm garments, cyproheptadine, or doxepin prior to exposure.
Vibratory	Place extremity on vortexer or reproduce exposure for 5–10 minutes.	Avoidance, antihistamine prior to exposure.

tional symptoms such as hypotension and wheezing can occur. Physical urticarias are fairly rare and can be brought on by exposure to vibration, pressure, or certain ultraviolet wavelengths. For some of these forms,

urticaria is a misnomer because the lesions swell and burn, and rarely can fever and arthralgias coexist.

Urticarias caused by an underlying primary disorder reflect the symptoms of the primary condition, such as weight loss and fatigue (hyperthyroidism); weight loss, fatigue, and fever (malignancies or infection); hair loss, Raynaud's phenomenon, and arthralgias (systemic lupus erythematosus, SLE); or anorexia and high-colored (dark) urine (hepatitis).

■ Diagnosis

The history and physical findings are the most helpful elements of the workup and are usually sufficient for diagnosis. Extensive laboratory studies are not helpful. If chronic urticaria is not easily controlled with nonsedating antihistamines, a CBC, differential count, and sedimentation rate are appropriate. In suspected vasculitis—particularly with constitutional symptoms such as arthralgias or fatigue—ANAs, urinalysis, C3, C4, and CH50 are warranted. Poor response to therapy or abnormal laboratory tests suggest the need for skin biopsy to check for **urticarial vasculitis.** Exercise anaphylaxis occurs only with exercise, in contrast to cholinergic urticaria. Given the occasional association of urticaria with hyperthyroidism, the thyroid-stimulating hormone (TSH) level should be checked. In women with postpartum urticaria, postpartum hyperthyroidism should be excluded. Recent travel or gastrointestinal symptoms should prompt stool examination for ova and parasites. Chest x-ray, stool for occult blood, cryoglobulin, and cryofibrinogen tests are occasionally helpful.

Several illnesses may mimic urticaria. *Erythema chronicum migrans* in Lyme disease may be mistaken for urticaria. In systemic mastocytosis, urticaria may be associated with hypotension, gastrointestinal symptoms, stomach ulcers, and flushing. In *urticaria pigmentosa*, the skin often has hyperpigmented lesions, and stroking it causes **Darier's sign**—linear wheals with larger beady hives. In *dermatographism,* a benign condition, figures can be drawn (urticaria with whealing) on the skin by lightly stroking with a sharp object. Patients often have linear wheals with flare owing to scratching. Although pruritic, these lesions usually do not occur spontaneously. *Papular urticaria* consists of crops of small pruritic papules, usually near the ankles and wrists and caused by local reactions to insect bites, especially fleas. *Erythema multiforme* is often associated with bacterial or viral infections and can present with mucus membrane lesions and cutaneous "iris" lesions. These have pale centers with erythematous rims.

■ Management

Urticaria is typically episodic and mostly self-limited. Although uncomfortable, urticaria without associated angioedema is rarely life-threatening. A stepwise treatment plan with the fewest adverse reactions should be adopted (Figure 13.1). In cases in which a stimulus can be identified, avoidance is the first choice. Drugs that immunologically cross-react with offending agents (such as cephalosporins in ß lactam allergy) or ones with similar mechanisms of action (such as NSAIDs) should be avoided. Physical urticarias can be improved by prudent measures such as using sun block and wearing protective clothes for solar urticaria, gradual warming oneself with tepid showers or mild warm-up sessions for cholinergic urticaria, avoiding sudden cold exposure or ice-cold foods and liquids for cold urticaria, and so on. Patients with cold urticaria should be warned not to jump into cool lakes or swimming pools; they also need special premedication when undergoing surgery for coronary artery bypass grafts as ice-cold saline is used to produce cardioplegia.

The mainstay of drug therapy for the urticarias has been antihistamines. Those with significant anticholinergic or antiserotoninergic effects often have worked best in the past. The newer, nonsedating antihistamines such as cetirizine and fexofenadine work well in mild, uncomplicated urticaria or dermatographism. Some studies suggest that a combination of hydroxyzine plus cyproheptadine is more effective than either drug alone, but cyproheptadine can be very sedating and promotes weight gain. Occasionally, a combination of an H1 antagonist plus an H2 blocker such as cimetidine, 300 mg twice daily, will work better than H1 inhibition alone. One of the most potent antihistamines is doxepin, which is a tricyclic antidepressant with antiserotoninergic, anticholinergic, and H2 blocking effects. Since its H1 inhibition is 1000 times that of diphenhydramine (Benadryl), relatively low starting doses of 10 mg at bedtime or twice a day can be used.

Although most patients respond well to antihistamines, 10–20% may not. Frequently, a short course of oral corticosteroids will help break the cycle of recurrent hives, and antihistamines will then often suffice to maintain the patients symptom-free. When urticaria persists, the physician must weigh the morbidity of the urticaria against potential side effects of corticosteroids. If corticosteroid maintenance is required, the lowest possible dose should be given. Corticosteroid-dependent patients may be able to taper or stop the steroid dose when stanozolol (an anabolic steroid with potential androgenergic side effects) is added. Anecdotally, colchicine, calcium channel blockers, and oral β-adrenergic agonists are occasionally successful.

Aside from avoidance, the physical urticarias are treated similarly to common urticaria. All urticaria patients should be advised to contact their physicians if they experience angioedema.

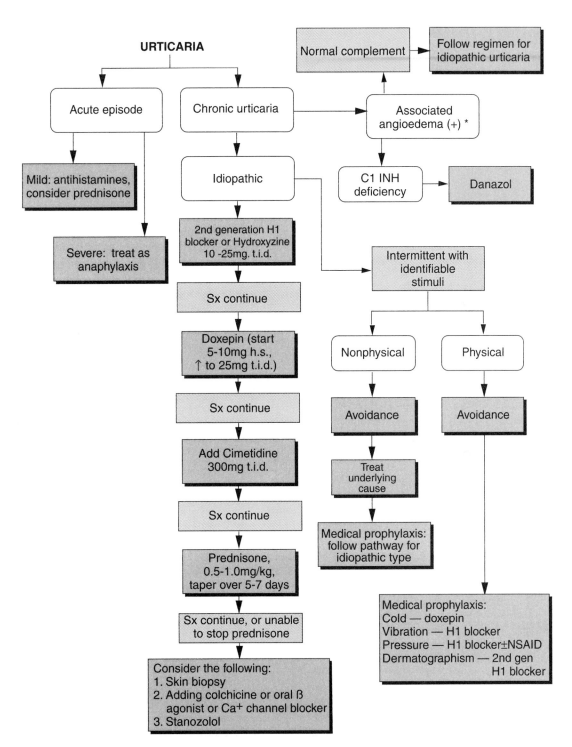

FIGURE 13.1. Treatment of urticaria. For mild episodes less frequent than once a week, treatment may be given as needed; for more frequent episodes, preventive treatment is needed.

* = Patients with associated angioedema should also be evaluated for a complement disorder and treated more aggressively with prophylactic medications outlined in the idiopathic column.

Angioedema

Angioedema presents as indurated areas of swelling that often feel numb or burn. Occurring most often in areas of loose tissue such as the lips and eyelids, angioedema histologically resembles typical urticaria, but the edema and vasodilatation occur deeper in the subcutaneous tissue where few afferent nerve endings exist. Urticaria may be associated in about 80–90% of cases. The cause may mimic that of urticaria, but several other causes should be considered for isolated angioedema. Angiotensin-converting enzyme (ACE) inhibitors can cause angioedema alone, and this can occur months after starting the drug. ACE inhibitors may permit activation of the bradykinin system.

Life-threatening, isolated angioedema can also be due to C1 esterase inhibitor (C1 INH) deficiency, which can be genetic or acquired. The genetic form, also termed **hereditary angioneurotic edema,** presents during the teen years but can occur at any age. A history of trauma may be present. Most patients have low levels of C1 INH, usually owing to reduced transcription of the gene, but in 15% the levels are normal and consists of poorly functioning protein. The acquired form is associated with malignancies or autoimmune diseases. These patients make autoantibodies, which can either accelerate the breakdown of C1 INH or directly bind to it and cause its removal. Both the genetic and acquired forms have low functional amounts of C1 INH and low C4 levels, but patients with the acquired form also have low serum C1 levels.

Angioedema in the gastrointestinal tract or larynx evokes nausea, cramping, or throat tightness. Its potential for laryngeal involvement makes it a more serious issue than isolated urticaria. Although nearly all the fatalities occurred in patients with isolated angioedema from C1 INH deficiency, all urticaria patients should be questioned carefully for any history of tongue or lip swelling, throat discomfort, or gastrointestinal symptoms. If such symptoms are present, the patient should be instructed in self-administration of epinephrine and provided with a self-administration kit (EpiPen™ or Anakit). These patients may also be more aggressively treated with potent antihistamines such as doxepin. Patients with C1 INH deficiency are successfully treated with danazol or stanozolol. Virilization (severe masculine somatic characteristics) is a problem with stanozolol.

During acute attacks, especially with impending respiratory compromise, adults should be given 0.3 ml of 1:1000 epinephrine subcutaneously and sent immediately by ambulance to the nearest emergency facility. Injection can be repeated after 15 minutes. The protective effects of epinephrine can wear off in 15–20 minutes; a tapering course of corticosteroids and an additional dose of antihistamine should be started within this time. Epinephrine is not always effective in C1 INH deficiency. Fresh frozen plasma to replace the C1 INH may be used, but it also supplies substrate for activated complement and bradykinins. These patients may require intubation or tracheostomy for respiratory impairment.

CHAPTER 14 — IMMUNODEFICIENCY

Host defenses against microbes and the various deficiencies thereof that predispose to infection are discussed in chapter 141. This chapter discusses the adult immunodeficiency disorders other than the acquired immune deficiency syndrome (AIDS). Despite their relative rarity in adults, these other immunodeficiencies deserve attention because appropriate intervention can limit the potentially serious infectious complications.

Although the immune system can be divided into the *humoral* (antibodies and complement) and *cellular* (T cells, natural killer cells, macrophages, and neutrophils) components, interplay between these two groups (as in T-cell cytokine production to promote B-cell antibody production). Patients with humoral deficiencies suffer recurrent infections with encapsulated bacteria and occasionally enteric viruses and Giardia, whereas with T-cell defects and normal humoral immunity, recurrent infections with *Pneumocystis carinii*, fungi, viruses, and mycobacteria predominate. (See Tables 14.1 and Table 14.2.)

■ Humoral Defects

Defects in humoral response can occur owing to lack of production or inadequate production of antibodies and antibody consumption.

Lack of antibody production

This was first described in **X-linked hypogamma-globulinemia.** The immature B cells in affected boys produce only very small quantities of all the immuno-

TABLE 14.1.	Representative Features of Cellular and Humoral Immunodeficiency	
Type	**Clinical Features**	**Initial Diagnostic Tests**
Cellular		
Neutrophils	Recurrent pyodermic cutaneous infections, especially staphylococcus.	CBC with differential, nitroblue tetrazolium reduction.
T-lymphocytes	Opportunistic infections (mycobacterial, fungal, pneumocystis).	Delayed hypersensitivity skin tests (mumps, Candida, trichophyton), lymphocyte count, possibly helper/suppressor (CD4/CD8) enumeration by flow cytometry.
Humoral		
B cell/ Immunoglobulin	Recurrent infections with encapsulated bacterial organisms resulting in pneumonia, sinusitis, otitis. May have chronic diarrhea due to *Giardia lamblia*.	Lymphocyte count, quantitative IgG, IgA, and IgM and pre-existing antibody titers to tetanus, rubella, *H. influenzae*. If normal but high suspicion, check IgG subclasses and response to pneumococcal and *H. influenzae* immunization.
Complement	Infections with encapsulated bacteria, especially Neisseria. Possible collagen-vascular symptoms.	CH50, C3, C4
Secondary	May be due to underlying illness such as diabetes mellitus, nephrotic syndrome, drug effect, or absent spleen.	Appropriate screening test such as glucose, urine for protein.

TABLE 14.2.	Immunodeficiency Treatment
Deficiency	**Treatment**
General	Maintain good nutrition; treat any underlying illness; avoid live virus vaccines; treat acute infections rapidly with appropriate antibiotic.
Chronic granulomatous disease	Possible prophylaxis with antistaphylococcal antibiotic. Interferon-gamma-1b (Actimmune™) may be beneficial.
T lymphocytes	If due to genetic defect, may be appropriate for transplantation; patients with adenosine deaminase (ADA) deficiency may benefit from ADA-polyethylene glycol replacement, gene therapy, or bone marrow transplant.
Complement	Immunize against *H. influenzae* and pneumococci to boost antibody protection; may require daily prophylactic antibiotic on rotating schedule (such as alternating sulfonamide, clarithromycin, amoxicillin-clavulanate every 2 months).
Immunoglobulin	For subclass deficiency, prophylactic antibiotic such as for complement may suffice; for common variable, may require intravenous immunoglobulin (IVIG) replacement; start at 300–400 mg/kg/month, adjust dose subsequently to maintain 4-week trough at ≥400 mg/day.

globulins. Resistance to fungi, mycobacteria, most viruses, and parasites is generally adequate, but enteroviral and Giardia infections can occur. Although all classes of immunoglobulins are lacking in **common variable immunodeficiency** (CVI), an idiopathic disorder, the infectious complications are not as severe as in X-linked hypogammaglobulinemia. In CVI, antibody production is normal in childhood, but the disease manifests in adults of either gender. Usual initial features are recurrent sinusitis and respiratory infections. Because antibody deficiency impairs the ability to fight encapsulated

bacteria (pneumococcus and *Haemophilus influenzae*), it should be suspected in any adult with two or more proven pneumonias in a year. Chronic diarrhea is common, caused by *Giardia lamblia,* Campylobacter, or nodular lymphoid hyperplasia with features that mimic sprue. Pernicious anemia, hypothyroidism, and hemolytic anemia may coexist.

Most patients with CVI have normal peripheral B-cell numbers but no plasma cells in their bone marrow. B cells or T cells may, however, be defective. In some, B cells do not respond to T-cell cytokines; in others, B cells produce but cannot secrete antibody. Defective T-helper-cell activity may create vulnerability to mycobacterial and fungal infections. The risk for gastrointestinal malignancies and lymphoma is greatly (100x) enhanced, necessitating close follow-up of these patients.

Inadequate antibody production

Among the four subclasses of IgG antibodies, IgG_1 is the most plentiful; failure to produce IgG_1 leads to a low total IgG level. However, patients with isolated IgG_2 or IgG_3 deficiencies may have low–normal total IgG. IgG_1 and IgG_3 preferentially bind proteins, and IgG_2 and IgG_4 recognize carbohydrate antigens. IgG_4 levels are naturally quite low, and its value in host resistance is unclear. Although an abnormally low IgG subclass level may cause recurrent infection, immunodeficiency should be confirmed by measuring a patient's response to immunization. Thus, baseline titers to *Haemophilus influenzae* B, pneumococci, and tetanus toxoid should be measured and retested several weeks after immunization.

IgA deficiency (<5 mg/dl) is fairly common (1:500–600 adults), but it does not always cause disease. Phenytoin, carbamazepine, D-penicillamine, sulfasalazine, and chloroquine can induce reversible IgA deficiency. Some patients with recurrent respiratory infections have coexisting IgG subclass deficiencies or poor IgG antibody response to immunization.

Antibody consumption

Patients with protein-losing enteropathies or the nephrotic syndrome can lose antibody in sufficient amounts to impair immunity. Typically presenting with edema and low-serum albumin, these patients can develop recurrent respiratory infections with pyogenic organisms.

■ Complement Deficiency

The complement system amplifies immune response by helping lyse antibody-bound bacteria, or by coating pathogens (opsonization), allowing their clearance by phagocytic cells and the reticuloendothelial system. Resistance to some bacteria, particularly encapsulated ones, is defective in complement deficiency. Susceptibility to **Neisserial infections** (e.g., meningococci) is especially enhanced in terminal complement component deficiency. Although the CH50 can screen for complement dysfunction, C3 and C4 measurement can indicate affected pathways.

■ Cellular Responses

Immune dysfunction can follow altered activity of any of the cell types (T cell, macrophage, neutrophil, or natural killer) that provide cellular protection, although the most common natural abnormalities are associated with T-cell dysfunction. **Natural killer** (NK) cells have a low-affinity IgG receptor that allows them to bind antibody-coated cells and participate in antibody-directed cytotoxicity. They may also provide natural resistance to virally infected cells. Altered NK activity may predispose persons to recurrent herpes virus infections. The T cell is critical in amplifying immune surveillance. T-cell defects are frequently associated with other abnormalities and defective antibody responses. T helper cells (CD4+) recognize antigen presented by APCs and subsequently secrete cytokines in the proximity of B cells that have bound this antigen to positively select those cells and magnify the immune response. TH_1 cells further augment the immune response against viruses by producing IFN-γ. T suppressor cells (CD8+) carry out antibody-directed lysis of virally infected cells and tumor cells and also suppress abnormal autoimmune responses. Infants lack functional T cells owing to absent thymic precursor tissue in **DiGeorge's syndrome;** they suffer recurrent *Candida* and viral infections.

The macrophage, with its receptors for immunoglobulin and complement, is important for clearing antibody-coated or complement-coated pathogens. Alcoholics with cirrhosis have defective macrophage IgG receptor processing, and life-threatening bacterial infections are most likely to occur in those with the most severely impaired immunoglobulin handling. Defects or loss of the macrophage could impair one's ability to recognize foreign pathogens and mount a response. Asplenic patients (surgical splenectomy or autosplenectomy from sickle cell disease) also lack activated macrophages and are prone to sepsis from encapsulated bacteria.

The neutrophil is usually the first cell to migrate to a site of pathogen invasion. Neutrophils accumulate in response to local trauma and on a true immunologic basis. Once neutrophils arrive at sites of infection, they provide protection by phagocytosis and killing by the production of hydrogen peroxide in their granules. If neutrophils have defective phagocytosis or lack the ability to produce hydrogen peroxide, affected individuals experience chronic granulomatous disease manifested by recurrent infections with gram-positive and gram-negative bacteria, usually involving skin, mucous membranes, and the respiratory tract.

■ Diagnosis

The more severe immunodeficiency states (e.g., severe combined, Wiskott-Aldrich, Hyper-IgE syndrome) are diagnosed in infancy or early childhood. In others, a high index of suspicion and thorough past medical history are very important. Chronic diarrhea, recurrent sinusitis or pneumonia, recurrent infections, and failure to clear infections readily despite appropriate therapy for opportunistic infections should raise a suspicion of immunodeficiency. Recurrent infections can also be due to diabetes mellitus, renal failure, and alcoholism; control of these conditions may improve the immune status.

Patients with humoral defects will typically experience recurrent infections (sinusitis, otitis, or meningitis) with encapsulated organisms. Laboratory studies should include a WBC count and differential, flow cytometry (only if infected), quantitative immunoglobulin levels, and, if this is normal, IgG subclasses and antibody titers to tetanus toxoid and encapsulated organisms. Low titers should be reassessed by titers 3–5 weeks after immunization. Determination of isohemagglutinin titers to measure IgM antibody function and CH50 should be performed. Delayed hypersensitivity skin tests for mumps, *Candida*, and trichophyton can help determine whether the cellular arm of immunity is functional.

Patients with atypical viral or mycobacterial infections or chronic fungal infections should be investigated for cellular immunity. A good initial screening test for macrophage and T-cell function is skin testing for delayed hypersensitivity. Constitutional symptoms should suggest tuberculosis, thymoma, or lymphoma. Flow cytometry for elucidating helper, suppressor, and killer cells is useful. When patients have adequate T-cell numbers but questionable function, T-cell response to mitogens (phytohemagglutinin) should be studied. In patients with cutaneous abscesses, the pus should be examined for neutrophils, and neutrophil studies should include nitro blue tetrazolium dye reduction.

■ Management

Treatment varies according to the underlying cause of the immunodeficiency (Table 14.2). Use of prophylactic antibiotics directed against causative bacteria is used for many immunodeficiencies. Patients with complement or splenic dysfunction may respond to immunization. If patients with documented immunoglobulin deficiencies continue to experience recurrent infections despite antibiotic prophylaxis, IV immunoglobulin (IVIG) replacement can be given. However, patients with associated IgA deficiency must be treated carefully with IgA-depleted IVIG preparations to prevent anaphylactic reactions. Patients with immunodeficiency should not be exposed to live attenuated viral vaccines because disseminated disease can follow.

■ Questions

Instructions: For each question below, select only **one** lettered answer that is the **best** for that question.

1. A 50-year-old gardener is stung by a wasp. Within 10 minutes, generalized urticaria and hypotension develop. In the emergency department, obtundation, hypotension, and hypoxemia are found. Aside from the history of bee sting, no other history is available. She is intubated and treated for shock. Which of the following laboratory studies is the best to confirm the diagnosis?
   A. A serum total IgE level
   B. A serum IFN-g level
   C. A serum tryptase level
   D. A serum total IgG level

2. Mary K, a 19-year-old woman, has had 2 years of increasing perennial nasal congestion and rhinorrhea, with sneezing, itching, and ear popping, especially when indoors. Among these, which symptom most suggests an allergic etiology?
   A. Nasal congestion
   B. Rhinorrhea
   C. Ear popping
   D. Sneezing and itching

3. Mary K's nasal smear shows numerous eosinophils. This finding is consistent with which of the following?
   A. NARES
   B. Rhinitis medicamentosa
   C. Allergic rhinitis
   D. Vasomotor rhinitis
   E. NARES and allergic rhinitis
   F. Rhinitis medicamentosa and vasomotor rhinitis

4. Because Mary K's symptoms are perennial, to which of the following allergens can she be expected to be predictably allergic?
   A. Ragweed
   B. Dermatophagoides mite
   C. Oak pollen
   D. Dog dander

5. Mary K requests a remedy that will most rapidly control her nasal pruritus and rhinorrhea so that she can attend a wedding the next day. Which of the following would you prescribe?
   A. Topical nasal steroids
   B. Oral decongestants
   C. Topical decongestants
   D. Oral antihistamines
   E. Avoidance of allergens

6. A 26-year-old man with asthma missed 11 days of work last year. He uses an inhaled ß agonist 2 to 3 times a day and wakes up three nights a week with his asthma. All of the following are true EXCEPT:
   A. Asthma is the most common cause of absenteeism from school.

B. Most patients with asthma have allergies.

C. The risk for asthma mortality is five times greater for African Americans than the general population.

D. Adequate asthma control is defined as a partial or complete response to his ß agonist.

E. Occupational exposure may account for as many as 20% of asthma cases.

7. A 31-year-old woman has daily chest tightness and shortness of breath, which predictably occur with exercise, but also at rest, 4 to 5 times per week. Spirometry confirms reversible airflow obstruction. Which one of the following is most appropriate to prescribe now?

A. Sustained-release theophylline, 300 mg q 12 h

B. Sustained-release ß-2 agent (salmeterol), 2 puffs twice a day

C. Beclomethasone MDI, 2 puffs 2 times/day; and albuterol MDI, 2 puffs PRN for episodes of bronchospasm

D. Cromolyn sodium MDI, 2 puffs 4 times/day

E. Cromolyn sodium MDI, 2 puffs 4 times/day; and albuterol MDI, 2 puffs PRN for episodes of bronchospasm

F. Cromolyn sodium MDI, 2 puffs 4 times/day; sustained release theophylline, 300 mg q 12 h; and albuterol MDI, 2 puffs PRN for episodes of bronchospasm

8. Ron, a 48-year-old business executive, went jogging in a nearby park 2 hours after lunch. Twenty minutes into his run he developed lightheadedness, abdominal cramping, and shortness of breath. In the emergency department he was found to be hypotensive, with generalized urticaria. ECG is normal except for sinus tachycardia at 118 beats per minute. The chest x-ray is normal. Your best initial diagnosis is:

A. Pulmonary embolism

B. Myocardial infarction

C. Exercise-induced anaphylaxis

D. Gastrointestinal bleeding

9. Which of the following can be measured in serum 3 hours after the episode described in question 8 to verify the diagnosis?

A. Tryptase

B. Histamine

C. Creatinine kinase

D. Nitric oxide

E. Complete blood count

F. Serum troponin

10. A patient with syphilis experiences fever and chills several hours after being treated with penicillin. Which of the following is most likely?

A. A toxic reaction

B. A secondary drug effect

C. A drug interaction

D. An allergic reaction

E. An idiosyncratic reaction

11. The onset of a reaction characterized by a purpuric rash, fever, and joint pains is most likely to occur:

A. 1 hour after starting a drug

B. 12 hours after starting a drug

C. 2 days after starting a drug

D. 10 days after starting a drug

12. A 55-year-old man has had four sinus infections during the past 14 months and two documented cases of pneumococcal pneumonia in the last 2 years. He has no cutaneous infections, thrush, or risk factors for HIV. His chest x-ray last week was normal. Which of the following laboratory studies would be most useful?

A. A serum total IgE level

B. Determination of the CD4/CD8 ratio

C. Quantitative immunoglobulin levels including IgG subclasses

D. Neutrophil reduction capacity

■ **Answers**

1. C	2. D	3. E	4. B	5. D
6. D	7. C	8. C	9. A	10. B
11. D	12. C			

SUGGESTED READING

Textbooks and Monographs

Baker JR Jr., Zylke JW. Primer on allergic and immunologic Diseases. JAMA 1997;278:1799–2034.

Bierman CW, Pearlman D, Shapiro G, et al. Allergy, Asthma and Immunology from Infancy to Adulthood. 3rd ed. Philadelphia: WB Saunders Co., 1996.

Busse W, Holgate S. Asthma and Rhinitis. Oxford: Blackwell Scientific, 1994.

Expert Panel Report 2. Guidelines for the Diagnosis and Management of Asthma. Publication No. 97-4051. Bethesda, MD: National Asthma Education Program, Office of Prevention, Education and Control, National Heart, Lung and Blood Institute, National Institutes of Health, April 1997.

International Consensus Report on Diagnosis and Management of Asthma. Publication No. 92-3091. Bethesda, MD: U.S. Department of Health and Human Services, National Heart, Lung and Blood Institute, National Institutes of Health, 1991.

Patterson R, Grammer L, Greenberger P. Allergic Diseases: Diagnosis and Management. 5th ed. New York: Lippincott-Raven, 1997.

Articles

Basic Mechanisms

Costa JJ, Weller PF, Galli SJ. The cells of the allergic response. JAMA 1997;278:1815–1822.

Fleisher TA, Tomar RH. Introduction to diagnostic laboratory immunology. JAMA 1997;278:1823–1834.

Huston DP. The biology of the immune system. JAMA 1997;278:1804–1814.

Smith T. Allergy testing in clinical practice. Annals Allergy 1992;68:293–301.

Varney VA, Holgate ST. Allergy testing in respiratory medicine. Br J Hosp Med 1996;56:406–408.

Rhinitis, Sinusitis, and Conjunctivitis

Bertolini J, Pelucio M. The red eye. Emerg Med Clin North Am 1995;13(3):561-79.

Ferguson BJ. Allergic rhinitis. Recognizing signs, symptoms, and triggering allergens. Postgrad Med 1997;101:110–116.

Low DE, Desrosiers M, McSherry J, et al. A practical guide for the diagnosis and treatment of acute sinusitis. CMAJ 1997;156 Suppl 6:S1–S14.

Naclerio R, Solomon W. Rhinitis and inhalant allergens. JAMA 1997;278:1842–1848.

Senior BA, Kennedy DW. Management of sinusitis in the asthmatic patient. Ann Allergy Asthma Immunol 1996;77:6–15.

Williams JW, Simel DLT. The rational clinical examination: Does this patient have sinusitis? JAMA 1993;270:1242–1246.

Bronchial Asthma

Abramson MJ, Puy RM, Weiner JM. Is allergen immunotherapy effective in asthma? Am J Resp Crit Care Med 1995;151:969–974.

Bernstein D. Occupational asthma. Med Clin North Am 1992;76:917–934.

Corbridge TC, Hall JT. The assessment and management of adults with status asthmaticus. Am J Resp Crit Care Med 1995;151:1296–1316.

McFadden ER, Gilbert I. Asthma. N Engl J Med 1992;327:1928–1937.

McFadden ER, Gilbert I. Exercise-induced asthma. N Engl J Med 1994;330:1362–1367.

Anaphylaxis

Greenberger P, Patterson R. The prevention of immediate generalized reaction to radiocontrast media in high-risk patients. J Allergy Clin Immunol 1991;87:867–872.

Heffner D. Anaphylaxis. Lippincotts Prim Care Pract 1997;1:220–223.

Kam PC, Lee MS, Thompson JF. Latex allergy: an emerging clinical and occupational health problem. Anaesthesia 1997;52:570–575.

Melton AL. Managing latex allergy in patients and health care workers. Cleve Clin J Med 1997;64:76–82.

Drug Allergy

Adkinson NF. Grand rounds at the Johns Hopkins Hospital: Drug allergy. JAMA 1992;268:771–773.

deShazo RD, Kemp SF. Allergic reactions to drugs and biologic agents. JAMA 1997;278:1895–1906.

Urticaria and Angioedema

Maher J. Urticaria and angioedema. A simple approach to a complex problem. Lippincotts Prim Care Pract 1997;1:172–182.

Volcheck GW, Li JT. Exercise-induced urticaria and anaphylaxis. Mayo Clin Proc 1997;72:140–147.

Immunodeficiency

Puck JM. Primary immunodeficiency diseases. JAMA 1997;278:1835–1841.

PART III

Rebekah Wang-Cheng
Albert Liebman

BEHAVIORAL MEDICINE

■ Physician-Patient Encounter

A well-conducted interview is crucial not only for establishing a diagnosis but also for dealing with emotions and building a trusting, open relationship with the patient. The physician may use a variety of cognitive, affective, behavioral, and social strategies to enhance the process (Table 15.1).

The interview has special importance in psychiatry because physical signs are sparse and many syndromes lack laboratory or neuroimaging abnormalities. Disorders such as psychosis, delirium, and dementia necessitate history taking from both the patient and other observers. Table 15.2. summarizes key areas to explore in the psychiatric interview.

Careful observation of the patient may disclose nonverbal behaviors that reflect learned and unconscious patterns in the context of social situations. Recognizing such inner distress may provide significant clues to diagnosis and can facilitate communication with the patient (Table 15.3).

TABLE 15.1.	Therapeutic Strategies in the Physician-Patient Encounter

Cognitive
Negotiation of priorities and expectations
Explanation of illness
Suggestion for treatment
Patient education

Affective
Empathy
Encouragement of emotional expression
Encouragement and hope
Reassurance

Behavioral
Encouragement of patient to take an active role in his or her own recovery
Praise of desired behaviors
Attention to compliance issues

Social
Use of family and social supports
Use of community agencies or other health care providers

Adapted with permission from Novack J. Gen Intern Med 1987; 2:346–355.

TABLE 15.2.	Key Areas to be Explored in the Psychiatric Interview

1. What symptoms prompted the patient to seek medical care?

2. What is the patient's present life situation? Seeking psychiatric attention generally presupposes a life predicament.

3. What is the developmental life history (childhood, school, occupational, marriage, and relationship history, and salient life events)?

4. Have there been any past episodes of mental distress? If so, what was the treatment?

5. Is there a family history of any mental illness, alcoholism, or drug abuse? What are family members' personalities, and their adaptation, particularly in education, occupation, marriage, parenthood, and relationships?

6. Is there any history of past interventions? What are current medications?

7. What are the current stresses and the support system of the patient? What is the patient's ability to function in the current situation and the patient's past display of "hardiness"?

■ Imaging Techniques in Psychiatry

Neuroimaging techniques, which consist of anatomic and functional modalities, increasingly contribute to our understanding of brain activity and its relationship to specific psychiatric disorders. Anatomic scans, including computed tomography (CT) and magnetic resonance imaging (MRI), have demonstrated structural changes in certain psychiatric disorders such as schizophrenia and Alzheimer's dementia. These tests may also disclose mass lesions such as subdural hematomas or tumors that may mimic psychiatric illnesses.

Functional imaging techniques—positive emission tomography (PET), single photon emission computed tomography (SPECT), functional MRI, and electroencephalography (EEG)—may reveal brain activity that correlates with clinical psychiatric syndromes, such as obsessive-compulsive disorder, Alzheimer's disease, and

TABLE 15.3.	Nonverbal Behavior to Observe in the Psychiatric Interview

1. Dress and demeanor.

2. Posture and carriage.

3. Body movements, including presence of unusual posturing.

4. Gaze, particularly unusual staring or averted gaze.

5. Facial display of happiness, sadness, surprise, fear, anger, interest, disgust.

6. Vocal quality can reflect mood as well as the pattern of engaging others.

7. Nonverbal utterances such as screams, cries, and laughter.

8. Tears, which are not an unusual display and may represent anger as well as sadness.

Huntington's chorea. More targeted pharmacologic treatments for psychiatric disorders have developed as a result of these technologies.

■ Role of the Psychiatrist in Medical Care

The neurobiology of the brain as an organ of the body and a person's conscious activity, manifested as behavior, is expressed by the terms "brain" and "mind." Advances in neurochemistry and brain imaging techniques have identified correlations of "brain" changes with dysfunctional behavior patterns, or psychiatric disorders.

In determining as accurate a diagnosis as possible, the psychiatrist follows the nomenclature of the *Diagnostic and Statistical Manual of Mental Disorders*, currently in its 4th edition, and known as DSM-IV), published by the American Psychiatric Association. The classification includes five axes (Table 15.4).

The need for a psychiatric consultation depends on the severity and complexity of the problem and the primary care physician's (or psychologist's) degree of expertise in dealing with these problems. Prompt diagnosis and treatment by the psychiatrist may reduce the patient's overall morbidity and shorten the hospital stay. In recent years, psychiatric consultative services have developed in medical outpatient settings. The psychiatrist may assist other physicians in the medical care of outpatients suffering from drug abuse, alcoholism, high-risk sexual behavior, and violent behavior by identifying co-

existing treatable psychiatric disorders and by aiding in the recognition of intractable, maladaptive behavioral problems in their patients. Specific community resources can then be targeted for patients as needed.

■ Psychiatric Emergencies

An acute change in behavior may present as a psychiatric emergency (delirium, psychoses, etc.). The physician must quickly perform a clinical evaluation and assess the degree and immediacy of threat to the individual and/or others. In addition to the crucial mental status examination, the physician should obtain and monitor vital signs and perform a physical examination if feasible and appropriate.

The physician needs to ask the following questions in the differential diagnoses of the acute behavioral change:

- Does the patient have an acute medical illness? Could the patient have suffered a head injury?
- Has there been acute use or withdrawal of a drug (or drugs) and/or alcohol?
- Has the patient been taking any prescription or over-the-counter drugs?
- Does the patient have a history of previous psychiatric treatment; if so, what was the diagnosis?
- Has there been an immediate personal or social crisis in the person's life, such as a divorce or death?

The treatment process usually requires two stages— the indicated immediate treatment at the time of presen-

TABLE 15.4.	Multiaxial Classification of the *Diagnostic and Statistical Manual of Mental Disorders-IV* (DSM-IV)

Axis I
Clinical disorders
Other conditions that may be a focus of clinical attention

Axis II
Personality disorders
Mental retardation

Axis III
General medical conditions

Axis IV
Psychosocial and environmental problems ("stressors")

Axis V
Global assessment of functioning

tation, followed by the determination of the optimal site for further definitive treatment and care. Some situations may require a civil commitment process, if a danger to the patient or others exists and the patient refuses

hospitalization. A follow-up plan is always necessary in the management of the psychiatric emergency, and a team approach, which includes internists, psychiatrists, social workers, and so forth, is essential.

<table><tr><td>CHAPTER</td><td>16</td></tr></table> # SOMATIC DISTRESS DISORDERS

S omatic distress (somatoform) disorders constitute an umbrella term that includes somatization disorders (SD), hypochondriasis, and conversion disorder. The diagnosis of somatization disorder requires fulfillment of all three criteria listed in Table 16.1. Usually, the patient is disinterested in the physi-

cian's efforts to link the psychologic experience to the illness. Most seek out more specialists and tests; some eventually choose other forms of therapy (alternative medicine), and some may become reclusive, ostensibly to minimize their suffering.

Somatization Disorder

The individual with somatization disorder (SD) experiences anxiety as a somatic, or physiological, phenomenon rather than a medical one. No generally accepted theory exists regarding the psychologic causation of these disorders. However, these patients have a higher incidence of major depression and anxiety compared with the general population. SD differs from malingering, in which patients consciously feign sickness for secondary gain.

The estimated prevalence rate of SD is 3–4% among primary care patients. The care of SD patients entails higher costs (nine times the U.S. per capita cost) than for the average patient and increased frequency of hospitalizations and outpatient visits.

■ Pathophysiology and Clinical Features

SD often begins in adolescence and usually prior to age 30. Table 16.1 lists the complete diagnostic criteria.

TABLE 16.1.	Criteria for Somatization Disorder

1. Usual onset before age 30.
2. Multiple unexplained physical complaints.
3. Symptoms must include the following:
   — Pain in four different sites (e.g., head, joints, chest, abdomen).
   — Two GI symptoms without pain (e.g., constipation, bloating).
   — One sexual symptom without pain (e.g., anorgasmia, decreased libido).
   — One pseudoneurological symptom without pain (e.g., paresthesias, syncope).

Adapted from DSM-IV.

Its chronic course with remissions and exacerbations significantly impairs daily functioning. These patients report multiple symptoms, described in meticulous detail, often supported by lists or daily logs. Many of the patients that physicians consider the most frustrating and challenging suffer from SD. As many as two-thirds of these patients may have a concomitant personality disorder. As the patient's frustration with physicians and the "system" increases, and each new physician is confronted with this "difficult" patient, a vicious cycle is created.

Approximately 80% of patients with SD are women, and many were raised in dysfunctional families. Commonly, a parent or other family member also suffered from somatizing behavior or from chronic illness. SD is strongly associated with childhood sexual and physical abuse. Sexually abused women had significantly more medical problems, greater levels of somatization, and more risky health behaviors compared with nonabused women; fewer than 2% of them had ever discussed the abuse with a physician. This underscores the importance of taking a sexual history.

■ Management

The cornerstone of treatment is a supportive, ongoing doctor-patient relationship, in which the physician takes the patient seriously and is genuinely interested in relieving the patient's suffering. The physician should be cognizant of the patient's perceived sense of powerlessness.

Frequent, short visits of 15–20 minutes, scheduled every 4–6 weeks, may reassure the patient while also reducing patients' phone calls and requests for extra appointments. When appropriate, the physician should help the patient to understand how psychosocial factors affect physical health. Rather than extensively counseling, the physician can simply discuss the association of job or marital stress to the symptom (e.g., headache). If

done appropriately in the context of a trusting relationship, the patient will learn some different coping skills.

Psychiatric consultation can help define more clearly the patient's malady and identify comorbid treatable disorders such as panic disorder and depression.

Hypochondriasis

Hypochondriacs have a recurring, persistent belief that they are, or will become, afflicted with a serious disease. The patient has a focus of somatic distress in a particular location that serves as the nidus for the hypochondriacal fears. Serious organic disease should be excluded first. The DSM-IV criteria for the diagnosis requires that symptoms have lasted for six months.

The belief that one is suffering from a serious disease is common to all the somatic distress syndromes, but it can also be a part of a depressive disorder and is commonly seen in patients with panic disorder or other anxiety states. This preoccupation with the body can also be expressed in delusional form in schizophrenia. Patients with medical entities of obscure etiology (e.g.,

fibromyalgia, irritable bowel syndrome) that lack definitive treatment often have hypochondriacal-like states of mind.

The patients in this category tax the therapeutic ingenuity of the primary care physician because of the lack of specific curative measures. The frequent association with treatable psychiatric syndromes dictates careful psychiatric evaluation. Uncontrolled pharmacologic studies using imipramine and fluoxetine to treat monosymptomatic hypochondriasis (illness phobia) have yielded encouraging results with moderate improvement. The lethal potential of imipramine overdose must be considered. Cognitive therapy measures can also be considered.

Conversion Disorder

Conversion disorder, formerly known as **hysteria,** presents with symptoms that simulate a neurologic disorder, such as anesthetic limbs, loss of motor function, aphonia, visual disturbance including blindness, and behavior suggesting seizures. The onset is usually sudden and dramatic. The term "conversion" means displacement of psychic energy as a result of repression of unacceptable impulses and drives.

A medical or neurological condition should be excluded before the diagnosis of conversion disorder can be made.

Treatment calls for a collaboration of psychiatry with medicine and neurology. Comorbid personality disorder, dissociative reaction symptoms, and somatization disorder may be present. The pseudoneurologic symptoms usually remit in a relatively short period of time with appropriate diagnosis. Pharmacologic treatment of accompanying syndromes such as anxiety disorders and depressive disorders is important.

Factitious Disorders

Factitious disorders are the intentional feigning of physical and/or psychological symptoms. The full-blown form is known as **Munchhausen's syndrome.** The confusing nature of these patients' symptoms leads to emergency department (ED) visits, hospitalizations, and even exploratory surgery. The motivations behind such behavior are not always obvious. An underlying severe personality disorder exists and often is a borderline personality disorder. Many of these patients may be associated with the health care field and are adept at simulating illnesses (e.g., hypoglycemia as a result of

surreptitious insulin use). However, the patient universally assumes a sick role, ostensibly to resolve internal distress. In Munchhausen's "by proxy," a parent repeatedly presents a child for medical care. Genuine illness is absent; the child unwittingly collaborates with the parent in assuming the role of someone who is sick.

These patients should be directly confronted before further harm occurs. Obviously, the patient will resist the diagnosis; thus, this requires careful and sensitive management. Psychiatric consultation is essential very soon after the diagnosis is suspected.

Pain Disorders

Persistent pain, unresponsive to medical treatment and not reasonably explained by demonstrable illness, is an increasingly frequent and costly medical problem. Chronic pain greatly affects the patient's personal and work life, often with attendant economic consequences.

The exact role of psychologic factors in this disorder is unknown. Psychosocial measures fail to distinguish between pain patients and the general population. Clearly, the consequences of a pain disorder that may result in economic hardship, social limitations, and damaged self-esteem can profoundly affect the cognitive and affective spheres. In many of these patients, the disorder occurs after a medical disorder, often an injury.

Chronic pain involves several stages of pain processing (Table 16.2). The first stage reflects nociceptive processing dependent on tissue injury, with subsequent stimulation of peripheral nerves, involvement of the spinothalamic tracts, and subsequent stimulation of the brain. The second stage of pain processing involves an emotional response of the organism to potentially damaging stimuli. Animal studies implicate the cingulate gyrus. In the third stage, one cognitively interprets pain sensations. Although pain usually creates anxiety, in this stage of pain processing, depression, anger, and fear are common reactions. In the final stage, the individual takes steps to mitigate the pain. In the last two stages of the pain experience, when chronicity has occurred, therapeutic strategies such as biofeedback, relaxation training, graduated exercise programs, medications for anxiety and depression, and counseling psychotherapy can prove useful.

Prolonged **postsensory stimulus disturbance** (including continuing pain) following noxious skin stimuli–producing injury may be caused by a change in the central nervous system and at the site of injury. Thus, studies suggest that "pain may beget pain." Pain in acute injury should be optimally treated to decrease the possible sensitization of neural structures, which sets the stage for a chronic pain process.

Patients with a chronic pain disorder are often referred to a pain clinic. Such a clinic usually operates as a multidisciplinary team with a multimodal therapeutic approach. Each patient presents with a unique situation that requires an individual assessment of biologic, psychologic, and sociological factors. The emphasis in the pain clinic is to improve the patient's ability to function rather than to eliminate the pain.

Although opiates do not completely relieve pain, opiate addiction is common among these patients. Weaning from opiates is a frequent task in the pain clinic. The use of less addicting pain medications along with carefully selected psychotropic drugs may relieve symptoms.

The psychiatrist has a dual role in the treatment of the chronic pain patient. The first is to identify clear-cut psychiatric syndromes responsive to specific pharmacologic interventions. The second is to render a comprehensive view of the patient's premorbid style of coping so as to identify opportunities for successful interventions.

TABLE 16.2.	Stages of Pain Processing
Acute	
Stage 1: Injury and nociceptive response in the CNS	
Stage 2: Emotional response to pain stimuli	
Chronic	
Stage 3: Cognitive processing of the continuing pain experience	
Stage 4: Behavioral adaptations to the chronic pain	

CHAPTER **17** ANXIETY DISORDERS

The anxiety disorders are a group of clinical syndromes in which the subjective experience of anxiety is the salient feature. Each syndrome, however, presents with a unique set of manifestations. In individual patients, symptoms of anxiety need to be distinguished from the reactions of fear and worry over life's ordinary concerns. In general, "fear" is the way one responds to a physical threat, but "anxiety" is more of a threat to one's sense of mental control; it has no distinguishable stimulus, external or internal. Furthermore, because no threat is immediately identifiable, anxiety lacks a time definition.

Panic Disorder

Panic disorder is characterized by sudden, recurrent attacks of intense anxiety occurring without warning and causing a terrifying sense of imminent disaster. In the United States, its prevalence rate is 1% with a lifetime incidence of 2–3%. Onset is usually in adolescence and young adulthood. The long-term course is highly variable and characterized by remissions and exacerbations. Association with major depression is noteworthy, and substance abuse (especially alcohol) and personality disorders may complicate treatment and outcomes.

Panic disorder seemingly has a biologic basis. Lactate infusion and yohimbine administration provoke symptoms of panic in predisposed individuals. Growth hormone response to clonidine, an alpha-2 adrenergic agonist, is blunted in patients with panic disorder. Brain perfusion abnormalities in the hippocampal regions have also been noted (PET and SPECT studies) in these patients.

■ Clinical Features

Panic attacks usually have an abrupt onset of intense somatic symptoms (Table 17.1) that often result in visits to hospital emergency departments. Frequently, the disease is first diagnosed by a perceptive ED physician. Even those with an established diagnosis may still visit the ED during an attack, driven by the severity of symptoms and accompanying fear. Without prompt and effective treatment, **agoraphobia** (a fear of leaving the home or venturing into the open) may develop in the

TABLE 17.1.	Common Features of Panic Disorder

Somatic symptoms
Palpitations and rapid heart rate
Trembling and shaking
Chest pain
Difficulty breathing
Sensation of choking
Hyperventilation
Dizziness and feeling of faintness
Sensation of heat and sweating
Paresthesias, particularly of the face
Interpretations of imminent disasters (examples)
Having a heart attack
Sense of suffocation
Losing control of oneself
Going crazy

patient who begins to anticipate the return of a panic attack in a public place.

■ Management

Therapy begins with a clear presentation of the diagnosis to the patient because such a patient has usually formed erroneous concepts regarding the symptoms prior to an accurate diagnosis. Benzodiazepines (which are addictive), tricyclic antidepressants, and monoamine oxidase inhibitors (MAOIs) and selective serotonin re-uptake inhibitors (SSRIs) are all effective in preventing panic attacks. Because of more frequent side effects and inconvenient dietary restrictions, the MAOIs are usually reserved for patients for whom treatment has failed.

Of the benzodiazepines, alprazolam (Xanax) is the most widely studied and used and is clearly the most effective in reducing anticipatory anxiety and preventing panic attacks. One should use the lowest effective dosage because this drug is very potent and addicting. The principal side effects of sedation, ataxia, and incoordination may limit the dosage. The dosages and half-lives of anxiolytic drugs are shown in Table 17.2 lists. Given the multitude of available agents, physicians should become familiar with a few anxiolytics that they find most efficacious. Withdrawal symptoms (restlessness, nervous feelings, tremor, insomnia, and, in extreme situations, convulsions) can occur with benzodiazepine therapy, commensurate with dosage and length of treatment. They can be avoided by dose tapering; a dose reduction of alprazolam to 0.5–1.0 mg/week is appropriate.

Tricyclic antidepressants are also effective (imipramine, 25–50 mg/day). Theoretically, they act by down-regulating beta-adrenergic receptors. By using a combination of imipramine and alprazolam, one might use lower dosages of each to minimize side effects.

Alprazolam is rapidly effective in preventing panic attacks, whereas imipramine takes longer (2–4 weeks). Drug tolerance and the need for increased daily doses over time have not been noted with alprazolam and imipramine. Because of its more tolerable side-effect profile, alprazolam has better patient acceptance than imipramine.

The selective serotonin re-uptake inhibitors (SSRIs) are also effective and have been approved by the FDA for use in panic disorder. Treatment may be initiated in low doses to avoid adverse effects that may be triggered in panic patients who are very sensitive to body sensations and can be titrated up as necessary. Their long-term efficacy in panic disorder remains to be clarified.

Behavior therapy (consisting of graded exposure to situations that have assumed a phobic nature for

TABLE 17.2.	Dosages and Half-Lives of Anxiolytic Drugs	
Drug	**Daily Dosage Range (mg)**	**Half-Life**
Benzodiazepines		
Alprazolam	0.75–4.0 (anxiety)	Short-intermediate
	1.5–12 mg (panic)	
Chlordiazepoxide	15–100 mg	Long[a]
Clorazepate	15–60 mg	Long[a]
Diazepam	6–40 mg	Long[a]
Halazepam	60–160 mg	Long[a]
Lorazepam	1.5–6 mg	Short-intermediate
Oxazepam	30–120 mg	Short
Prazepam	20–60 mg	Long[a]
Azaperone		
Buspirone	15–60 mg	Short (delayed onset of action over days)

[a]Benzodiazepines with long half-lives have active metabolites.

the patient) can be a useful supplement to pharmacologic treatment in selected patients. This approach can be especially useful in treating agoraphobic symptoms.

Generalized Anxiety Disorder

In 1894, Freud described two forms of anxiety: 1) generalized anxiety disorder (GAD), a chronic form of generalized or free-floating anxiety that can coexist with or occur separately from 2) panic disorder, a pattern of acute anxiety attacks that can erupt suddenly into consciousness without being precipitated by any thoughts. This delineation of generalized anxiety disorder from panic disorder remains valid to this day.

The following disorders need to be differentiated from GAD: schizophrenia, bipolar disorder, somatization disorder, borderline personality, obsessive-compulsive disorder, phobic disorders, and medical illnesses such as hyperthyroidism and pheochromocytoma. Alcohol withdrawal syndrome, particularly if the patient conceals his or her alcohol consumption from the physician, and psychoactive drugs, especially amphetamines, can simulate a primary anxiety state.

As a result of the increasing refinement in the diagnosis of psychiatric disorders (social phobia, "anger attack syndrome," acute stress reactions, and post-traumatic stress disorders), the diagnosis of GAD has become less and less appropriate.

■ Clinical Features

Common symptoms of generalized anxiety disorder include a feeling of inner tension; difficulty concentrat-

ing, often with a feeling of one's mind going "blank"; difficulty falling asleep and maintaining sleep; fatigue; muscle tension; and often autonomic symptoms such as palpitations, trembling, and breathlessness. Social and occupational functioning and interpersonal relations are significantly disrupted.

■ Management

Because treatment of GAD is symptomatic, every effort should be made to delineate other psychiatric disorders from GAD that may yield more definitive resolution. The benzodiazepines and buspirone are the current drugs most effective in treating GAD. The benzodiazepines are anxiolytic and sedating; they interact with the benzodiazepine GABA complex. Buspirone—the only currently available azaperone—is anxiolytic but not sedating; it modulates serotoninergic neurotransmission via the 5 HT-1A receptor (Table 17.3).

Because of their addictive potential, benzodiazepines should be used at the lowest effective dose with dose adjustments depending on clinical response. Periodic tapering and attempts at discontinuation are appropriate. Even with gradual tapering, however, prolonged therapy is often needed.

Post-traumatic Stress Disorder

Post-traumatic stress disorder (PTSD), which is brought on by a threat to one's life or personal integrity, has been recognized as a formal psychiatric diagnosis since 1980. The onset may be acute (occurring immediately or within days of the event) or delayed. Often the acute form resolves, only to be followed by subsequent symptoms, which then assume the form of a characteristic PTSD.

Extreme situations such as war, violent crime, and natural disasters are the most common causative factors. Observation of Vietnam War veterans resulted in the complete characterization and description of PTSD. A prevalence rate of 15% in Vietnam veterans has been noted, with an incidence of 2% approximately 20 years after wartime service.

■ Clinical Features

Symptoms occurring in acute stress reactions range from a sensation of being in a "daze," to feeling a sense of detachment and depersonalization, to various conversion symptoms. Amnesia for the event, prominent agitation and restlessness, hyperarousal symptoms of vigilance, increased scanning, irritability, sleeplessness, and difficulty concentrating are varying manifestations.

A re-experiencing of the traumatic event(s) by thought, images, and intense affect is the most prominent symptom. Flashback episodes may vary in intensity and evolve to dissociative experiences. The patient attempts to avoid situations that might evoke the intense symptoms. Significantly impaired social and occupational functioning and disruption of marital and other interpersonal relationships are common. Depression and anhedonia (loss of pleasure in one's normal pursuits) may be prominent. Impulse control is impaired; thus, alcoholism and drug abuse are frequent. Chronic PTSD has led to significant morbidity and mortality in many patients, as exemplified by Vietnam veterans.

■ Management

Pharmacologic treatment is usually combined with a variety of psychologic techniques including behavioral conditioning, support groups, and other behavioral approaches. Pharmacologic therapy has been better studied in the chronic PTSD than in the acute stress forms. Nevertheless, treatment used in the chronic disorder may be effective in the acute form.

Pharmacologic therapy is usually prolonged. For prominent depressive symptoms, a trial of antidepressants, including serotonin re-uptake inhibitors and tricyclic antidepressants, may be effective. Neuromodulators, such as carbamazepine, and beta-blocking agents may be useful. Benzodiazepines have not been systematically studied and their short-term use in selected acute forms of the disorder may be logical. Buspirone and trazodone, because of some antiaggressive and anti-irritability features without addiction potential, may have a unique place in long-term treatment. When suicidal hazard is present or severe symptoms prevail, inpatient psychiatric care may be necessary.

TABLE 17.3.	**Advantages and Disadvantages of Benzodiazepines and Buspirone**	
Characteristics	**Benzodiazepines**	**Buspirone**
Advantages	Sedation (can be controlled by dosage)	No sedation
	Rapid effect	No withdrawal symptoms
	Few subjective side effects	No interaction with alcohol
	Safe in overdose as single agent	No impaired cognition
	Diminishes autonomic symptoms	Safe in overdose
Disadvantages	Sedation when unwanted	Slow onset of action (several weeks)
	Cognitive impairment, primarily memory	Poor clinical response in patients previously on benzodiazepines
	Interaction with CNS depressants including alcohol	Frequent side effects (dizziness, lightheadedness, nausea, headaches)
	Psychomotor impairment (dose-related)	
	Withdrawal syndrome	
	Abuse risk in addiction-prone persons	

Obsessive-Compulsive Disorders

Community surveys estimate a 1.5–2.1% incidence of obsessive-compulsive disorder (OCD) in the U.S. population. The presence of intrusive, compelling thoughts, images, or ideas involving impulsive acts constitute the **obsessions.** Their theme, although variable in different individuals, is repetitive and remarkably constant in any one individual. The themes usually involve harm to oneself or to others resulting from some act on the part of the afflicted. The **compulsions** consist of repetitive actions designed to ward off some dreaded consequence. Lady Macbeth's hand-washing is the obvious famous example for compulsive behavior. The obsessive thoughts are regarded by the patient as alien, and this insight distinguishes this disorder from psychosis.

Despite the established association between obsessions and compulsions in **Tourette's syndrome,** it has only recently become obvious that patients with either OCD or Tourette's syndrome have a significant number of family members with the other disorder. Thus, a common gene may exist, containing a phenotype of either OCD or Tourette's syndrome.

Effective drug therapy is through agents that affect primarily the serotoninergic neurotransmitter system (Table 17.4). Clomipramine and fluoxetine are currently the drugs of choice; both are apparently equally effective. Clomipramine is a tricyclic compound, but it possesses a specific inhibitory effect on serotonin re-uptake into presynaptic terminals. It may decrease libido and the ability to achieve orgasm. Fluoxetine is a serotonin re-uptake inhibitor that may cause anxiety, restlessness, insomnia, and inhibition of orgasm. Duration of treatment is uncertain but may be prolonged. Behavioral therapy may be useful.

TABLE 17.4.	**Drugs for the Treatment of Obsessive-Compulsive Disorder**		
Drug	**Initial Dose**	**Maintenance**	**Half-Life**
Clomipramine	25 mg	100–250 mg	32 hrs
Fluoxetine	10 mg	20–80 mg	160 hrs
Fluvoxamine	50 mg	100–300 mg	16 hrs

Specific Phobias

A specific phobia is a persistent, invariable, inappropriate fear reaction to a specific object, creature, activity, or situation. Symptoms include shakiness, trembling, palpitations, dry mouth, breathlessness, lightheadedness (which can progress to a vasovagal faint), and sometimes a choking sensation. Some provocateurs are certain animals or insects, heights, enclosed spaces such as elevators, airplane flight, bridges, and, in medical situations, a fear of needles and blood. Cognitive-behavioral therapy involving exposure can be an appropriate measure. Alprazolam and clonazepam can be effective in blocking symptom response.

Agoraphobia is a phobic reaction to open spaces. Agoraphobia almost always occurs in patients with a history of panic disorder and commonly begins shortly after the initial panic attack. These individuals fear that the panic attack will recur in a public place from which they cannot exit quickly or easily (e.g., freeways, shopping malls, bridges, and movie theaters, where a hasty exit could be embarrassing or dangerous). The prompt and effective treatment of the accompanying panic disorder is the key to successful management. Intensive cognitive-behavioral therapy is indicated for the impaired agoraphobic patient.

Also known as **social anxiety disorder,** social phobia is characterized by a conditioned fear of and, consequently, avoidance of social situations in which the person would be exposed to the possible scorn of others and thereby suffer intolerable humiliation. The anticipation of such an event provokes the characteristic somatic accompaniments of anxiety as previously described. The severity of the disorder is highly variable, but shy children (behaviorally inhibited at age 21–31 months) are at increased risk to develop this disorder. The peak age of onset is between 11 and 15 years, and it usually is chronic. Relatives of social phobics have a higher incidence of the disorder than relatives of normal controls.

This disorder is often the hidden cause for school dropout and other social and occupational failures. Social phobics also might discover the calming effect of alcohol as well as the ability of alcohol to help them overcome inhibitions. The high prevalence rate of social phobia among alcoholics may stem from this reason.

Pharmacotherapy has shown great promise in many clinical trials. Clonazepam (0.75–3 mg daily) produces clinically significant improvement in 80% of patients;

alprazolam (1–10 mg daily, averaging 3 mg per day) is effective in 67%. Fluoxetine has shown promise in preliminary trials. Cognitive-behavioral approaches may be useful.

CHAPTER 18

DEPRESSIVE DISORDERS

Characterized by a significant, often profound change in an individual wherein the person becomes distressed and despondent, a depressive disorder may begin at any age from childhood to late life. The average age of onset, however, is the late 20s. Onset may be fairly acute or the depression may have been present for years in a low-grade form.

This variability in course and severity has led to a classification of the depressive disorders into the current categories of major depressive disorder, dysthymic disorder, and depressive disorder not otherwise specified. Recently the term **subsyndromal symptomatic depression** has been proposed as another clinical syndrome of depression. Indeed, a spectrum of depressive manifestations exists, and the awareness of this helps the physician recognize and treat depressed patients—even those whose manifestations are not typical.

Major Depressive Disorder

The 12-month prevalence of major depressive disorder is 10%, with a lifetime prevalence of 17%. For women, the lifetime prevalence is 20–25%, compared with 7–12% for men. The patient with a depressive disorder becomes dysfunctional in family, social, and occupational roles. The economic burden is also profound, with direct and indirect costs exceeding $40 billion in 1990.

Primary care physicians currently treat only two-thirds of patients with depression, owing to lack of insurance coverage, a perceived stigma on the part of patients in consulting a psychiatrist, and a shortage of mental health professionals. Nevertheless, depression remains both underdiagnosed by some primary care physicians and overdiagnosed by others.

■ Pathophysiology

The cause of depression is unclear, but a dysregulation of neurotransmitter function has been postulated. Impaired availability of norepinephrine and/or serotonin at synapses is a possible biochemical mechanism. Although some depressed patients show changes in brain function or functional brain imaging, these changes are not consistent enough for diagnostic use. Individuals with a first-degree blood relative with a mood disorder are at increased risk to develop clinical depression. A family history or prior episode doubles the personal risk for a depressive episode. The familial risk appears to be even higher in bipolar patients. Other risk factors for depression include feminine gender, postpartum state, and stressful life events.

■ Clinical Features

These patients describe their mood as "depressed," "blue," or "down in the dumps" and often report feeling hopeless. They have lost interest in their usual pursuits (**anhedonia**) and are unable to feel pleasure in life. Depressed mood and anhedonia are the two major features of depression, one of which must be present to diagnose definitively. (See Table 18.1 for other criteria.)

Often cognitive function is affected, resulting in poor concentration, slower mental processes, and a decreased ability to perform complex mental tasks. Psychotic manifestations are present in some patients (see chapter 19). A common manifestation is unusual irritability, which may be most striking in adolescents and the elderly and is evident to family members but often unnoticed by the patient.

Aside from mood and thought processes, physical well-being is also affected, causing decreased energy, fatigue and lethargy, and a loss of usual motivations. Psychomotor agitation or retardation and apathy may exist. Anorexia and weight loss are common. Sleep is characteristically disturbed, usually with a middle (inability to maintain sleep) or terminal (early morning awakening) insomnia. Terminal insomnia is often immediately accompanied by anxiety and, later, some decrease in symptoms by evening, thus constituting a diurnal variation in mood. Patients suffering from major depression often become preoccupied with thoughts of death, and suicide is a serious risk. As many as 15% of severely

TABLE 18.1.	Diagnostic Criteria for Depression

A. Five (or more) symptoms for at least 2 weeks
  • Depressed mood[a]
  • Anhedonia[a]
  • Weight change
  • Sleep disturbance
  • Psychomotor agitation or retardation
  • Fatigue
  • Feelings of worthlessness/guilt
  • Poor concentration
  • Recurrent thoughts of death or suicide

B. Symptoms cause significant functional impairment.

C. Symptoms not accounted for by the following:
  • Substance abuse
  • Medical condition
  • Bereavement

[a]Must include at least one of these.
Adapted from DSM-IV.

depressed patients commit suicide; 60% of all suicides result from depression. Overdose with drugs is the most common method, but hanging or shooting are also used. Risk factors for suicide are listed in Table 18.2. All patients with suspected depression should be directly questioned about previous suicidal attempts and current thoughts ("Have you considered ending your life?"). Any expressed wish, threat, or gesture should be taken very seriously. One should specifically ask if any definite plans are being considered. Most patients are relieved to express such thoughts. Ascertaining what the precipitant might be for considering suicide is imperative. If the situation is not resolved, the suicidal ideation will likely persist. Psychiatric evaluation should be obtained as soon as suicidal intent is expressed. The patient should be hospitalized for close observation, if the safety of the patient is in question.

■ **Diagnosis**

A number of scales are available to assess depression. The **Beck, Zung, and Hamilton General Health Questionnaire,** filled out by the patient, is one of these; the **PRIME-MD** (Primary Care Evaluation of Mental Disorders) is another (Figure 18.1), developed especially for use by primary care physicians. Based on the patient's answers, further directed inquiry can ensue.

No biologic or imaging tests are available to confirm the clinical diagnosis of a depressive disorder. An associated dysregulation of the hypothalamic-pituitary-adrenal axis has been postulated, and some depressed patients show elevated cortisol levels that are not suppressed by dexamethasone. In most studies, a dexamethasone suppression test shows a sensitivity of 40–50% and a specificity of 70–90% for detecting depression. Pharmacologic treatment that results in a clinical remission will often show a reversal of the hypercortisolism. Persistent nonsuppression of cortisol after dexamethasone following therapy of depression indicates a high risk of early relapse and poor outcome, which might reflect insufficient treatment or the patient's lack of response to the treatment.

Depression may be related to medication (beta-blockers, reserpine, and corticosteroids) or to substance abuse. Strokes (especially left-hemispheric), Parkinson's disease, endocrine and autoimmune disorders, and certain cancers may contribute to depression. Adjustment reactions and seasonal affective disorder (discussed in the following) usually cause less functional impairment and are of shorter duration. Dysthymia causes milder symptoms that persist for two years or longer. Bipolar affective disorder (chapter 19) is suggested by a strong family history, prior episodes of hypomania, and onset in one's 20s.

■ **Management**

Antidepressant therapy

Drug therapy is the primary treatment of depressive disorders (Table 18.3). Initial antidepressant therapy, in appropriately diagnosed cases, leads to a remission rate of approximately 80%. The three classes of antidepressant drugs are **tricyclic antidepressants** (TCAs), **monoamine oxidase inhibitors** (MAOIs), and **selective serotonin re-uptake inhibitors** (SSRIs). Other antidepressants, loosely termed **heterocyclics,** are useful when any of the agents from the three classes above have led

TABLE 18.2.	Factors Associated with Suicide

Caucasian
Masculine gender
Advanced age
Previous attempts
Detailed plan
Hopelessness
Living alone
General medical illness
Substance abuse
Psychosis
Depression
Personality disorder
Family history of suicide

PATIENT QUESTIONNAIRE

Updated for DSM-IV™

NAME: _____   **AGE:** _____

SEX: ☐ Male ☐ Female   **TODAY'S DATE:** _____

INSTRUCTIONS: This questionnaire will help in understanding problems that you may have. It may be necessary to ask you more questions about some of these items. Please make sure to check a box for <u>every</u> item.

*During the **PAST MONTH,** have you been bothered **A LOT** by...*				*During the **PAST MONTH...***	
	YES **No**		**YES** **No**		**YES** **No**
1. stomach pain	☐ ☐	12. constipation, loose bowels, or diarrhea	☐ ☐	21. have you had an anxiety attack (suddenly feeling fear or panic)	☐ ☐
2. back pain	☐ ☐	13. nausea, gas, or indigestion	☐ ☐	22. have you thought you should cut down on your drinking of alcohol	☐ ☐
3. pain in your arms, legs, or joints (knees, hips, etc)	☐ ☐	14. feeling tired or having low energy	☐ ☐		
4. menstrual pain or problems	☐ ☐	15. trouble sleeping	☐ ☐	23. has anyone complained about your drinking	☐ ☐
5. pain or problems during sexual intercourse	☐ ☐	16. your eating being out of control	☐ ☐	24. have you felt guilty or upset about your drinking	☐ ☐
6. headaches	☐ ☐	17. little interest or pleasure in doing things	☐ ☐	25. was there ever a single day in which you had five or more drinks of beer, wine, or liquor	☐ ☐
7. chest pain	☐ ☐				
8. dizziness	☐ ☐	18. feeling down, depressed, or hopeless	☐ ☐		
9. fainting spells	☐ ☐				
10. feeling your heart pound or race	☐ ☐	19. "nerves" or feeling anxious or on edge	☐ ☐	Overall, would you say your health is: Excellent ☐ Very good ☐ Good ☐ Fair ☐ Poor ☐	
11. shortness of breath	☐ ☐	20. worrying about a lot of different things	☐ ☐		

FIGURE 18.1. PRIME-MD.
(© Pfizer Inc., all rights reserved. PRIME-MD is a trademark of Pfizer Inc. Used with permission.)

TABLE 18.3.   Principles of Antidepressant Therapy

1. Early, close monitoring for side effects and clinical response
2. Titration to appropriate dosage
3. Adequate trial of 3–10 weeks to reach clinical efficacy
4. Monitoring of drug-drug interactions (e.g., cytochrome P-450 induction)
5. Treatment for minimum of 4–6 months after complete remission
6. Drug change if lack of response
7. Maintenance treatment required for recurrent episodes
8. Supportive physician contact essential

to an inadequate response or to side effect(s). A special indication may be patients who experience sexual dysfunction while on SSRIs.

Tricyclic antidepressants

A major limiting factor in the use of TCAs is their side effects, which result from their actions on a number of neurochemical receptors: histamine H-1, muscarinic, and alpha-1 adrenergic receptors (Table 18.4). Many psychiatrists prefer nortriptyline and desipramine to the other compounds because of a better side-effect profile. An adequate therapeutic trial of TCAs requires a full dosage for at least 4–8 weeks. Poor therapeutic results are mostly due to inadequate dosage. (See Table 18.5 for therapeutic ranges.) Serum levels afford an accurate gauge for adequate TCA dosing.

Selective serotonin re-uptake inhibitors (SSRIs)

SSRIs have become first-line treatment for mild to moderate depression, owing to a fairly even efficacy in outpatient therapy, a lower incidence of limiting side effects, a narrow therapeutic range, and less need for dose titration.

Monoamine oxidase inhibitors

Patients receiving MAOIs need to avoid tyramine-containing foods and sympathomimetic agents because the diet-drug or drug-drug interaction can produce a hypertensive crisis. Other adverse effects are orthostatic hypotension, weight gain, edema, insomnia, and sexual dysfunction. Patients should be instructed to discontinue the drug 2 weeks before a surgical or dental procedure or use another drug because of the risk of drug interactions. These toxic possibilities make these drugs a secondary treatment choice.

Side effects of antidepressants

Mild side effects occur in approximately 50% of patients taking antidepressants, but usually less than

10% will need to discontinue therapy as a result. In general, the side effects of TCAs continue throughout the course of treatment, and the consequent dropout rate in trials is considerable. In contrast, the side effects of the SSRIs occur at the onset of treatment and, if significant, one may try another compound in the same group since "cross-reactivity" may not occur. Table 18.6 compares the side effect profiles of some of the newer agents.

TABLE 18.4.   Physiologic Effects of Tricyclic Antidepressants

Histamine H-1 receptor blockade
  Sedation
  Weight gain
  Hypotension
  Potentiation of central depressant drugs

Muscarinic receptor blockade
  Blurred vision
  Constipation
  Urinary retention
  Dry mouth
  Sinus tachycardia

Alpha-1 adrenergic receptor blockade
  Dizziness
  Postural hypotension
  Reflex tachycardia
  Potentiation of antihypertensive medications (alpha-1 blockers)

TABLE 18.5.   Therapeutic Dosages of Commonly Used Antidepressants

Drug	Trade Name	Dose Range (mg/day)
Tricyclics		
Amitriptyline	Elavil	75–300
Doxepin	Sinequan	75–300
Desipramine	Norpramin	75–300
Nortriptyline	Pamelor	40–200
Heterocyclics		
Trazodone	Desyrel	150–600
Bupropion	Wellbutrin	225–450
Venlafaxine	Effexor	75–375
Nefazodone	Serzone	100–600
SSRIs		
Fluoxetine	Prozac	10–40
Paroxetine	Paxil	20–50
Sertraline	Zoloft	50–150

TABLE 18.6.	Side Effects of Newer Antidepressants				
Side Effect	Fluoxetine	Paroxetine	Sertraline	Venlafaxine	Nefazodone
Half-life (hrs)	168	24	24	5	4
Activating	+++	+	++	++	+
GI distress	+	+	+++	++	+
Loss of orgasm	Yes	Yes	Yes	Yes	Yes

+ mild
++ moderate
+++ pronounced

Duration of treatment

Three phases of treatment exist: *acute,* which lasts 6–12 weeks until symptom abatement or remission; *continuation,* which usually lasts 6 months, to prevent relapses; and *maintenance therapy,* to prevent recurrence, which is frequent in depression. Fifty percent of patients have a relapse after one episode, 70% after two, and 90% after three. Long-term treatment has been recommended for patients who have had recurrent episodes. Such therapy for 2–3 years has yielded favorable results and is indicated for patients who have had three major episodes, onset before age 20, a life-threatening episode in the past 3 years, recurrence within 1 year after medication was discontinued, or two episodes plus a first-degree relative with depression. For those with a bipolar disorder who are at risk for frequent recurrence, therapy may be life-long.

Psychotherapy

Some patients benefit from referral to a mental health professional for psychotherapy in addition to medication. The role of psychotherapy alone in the treatment of depression is somewhat controversial. In general, medication alone is more effective, with a response rate of approximately 70%, whereas the response to psychotherapy alone is approximately 50%. A combination of medication and psychotherapy, however, does not improve the response rate above that of medication alone.

Short-term cognitive, interpersonal, or behavioral therapy has shown good results in patients who have mild or moderate depression. Patients with a contraindication to antidepressants or who have an inadequate drug response are also candidates. Other indications might be a prior positive response to psychotherapy and recent or chronic stressful life events.

Seasonal Affective Disorder

Seasonal affective disorder (SAD) is a recently described clinical syndrome that occurs in the autumn and winter seasons and is characterized by depressed mood, lack of energy, and a tendency to sleep excessively, overeat, and crave carbohydrates. Surveys conducted in East Coast cities of the United States suggest a 16–20% incidence. The syndrome appears to be most common in women and young adults. To be diagnostic, the symptoms must occur yearly during the same time period. The application of bright-light therapy has achieved a good response in approximately 70% of patients. Improvement is seen 4–5 days after initiation of light therapy. A daily exposure for one hour to a light intensity of 10,000 Lux is required.

CHAPTER **19** ## PSYCHOTIC DISORDERS

Psychosis is characterized by bizarre subjective mental experience and behavior that deviates grossly from the ordinary. The DSM-IV notes that "the narrowest definition of psychosis is restricted to delusions or prominent hallucinations with the hallucinations occurring in the absence of insight into their pathologic nature." Clearly, neurobiologic processes are altered in patients with psychoses, with attendant disrup-

TABLE 19.1.	The Psychotic Disorders			
Disorder	**Age of Onset**	**External Precipitant**	**Chronicity**	**Need for Maintenance Treatment**
Schizophrenia	Late teens, 20s	No	Yes	Yes
Bipolar-manic	20s–40s	First episode	Yes	Yes
Bipolar-depressed	20s–30s	First episode	Yes	Often
Delirium	>60	Yes	No	No
Psychosis in dementia	>60	Sometimes	Yes	Often
Substance abuse	Teens–35	Yes	No	No
Medication-induced	Any age	Yes	No	No
Brief reactive	Teens–35	Yes	No	No

tion in cognitive processes, leading to gross impairment of coherence and intention.

Neural systems have been postulated to become "heated up," and then each neuron behaves in a more random fashion—that is, the neurons become less precise in responding to the excitatory and inhibitory inputs from the other neurons in the system. Given the multitude of conditions that can provoke psychosis, this theory would suggest a common mechanism of neural network perturbations leading to the attendant disturbed mental experience and psychotic behavior. A variety of pathologic processes, infectious agents and toxins, medical illness, and other unknown processes can produce a psychotic state. Common psychotic disorders are listed in Table 19.1.

Schizophrenia

Schizophrenia is regarded as the quintessential psychotic disorder, in which the patient presents with florid, bizarre manifestations. Reported worldwide, schizophrenia has a life-time morbidity risk of approximately 8 per 1000. The onset is most often abrupt, beginning during adolescence and in the early 20s in men but allegedly later in women, though still usually by the third decade of life.

■ Pathophysiology

Epidemiologic, cytoarchitectural, and immunocytochemistry brain studies led to a neurodevelopmental hypothesis of the cause of schizophrenia. This theory contends that schizophrenics harbor brain lesions that originated very early in life, in the intrauterine period, perhaps due to infection (viral), perinatal trauma, or abnormal patterns of neural migration. A genetic defect may render the fetal brain susceptible to early viral infection or associated immune response mechanisms or both. This immature neural circuitry is exposed by synaptic pruning, a process that continues into late adolescence. A theoretical model hypothesizes an "overpruning" of axonal-dendritic connections, especially in the hippocampus, parahippocampal gyrus, and cingulate and prefrontal cortices during the normal course of postnatal cortical development. This overpruning is thought to lead to the onset of symptoms.

■ Clinical Features

Schizophrenia presents as an acute psychosis with a dramatic onset. Usually, someone notices the patient's inappropriate behavior. The patient experiences hallucinations, either auditory or visual, which may be very frightening for the patient. Memories appear de novo without relation to real events and evolve into delusions, which are impervious to modification by persuasion and are thought to be imposed by some external force (paranoia). Delusions have varying content and may be somatic ("I know I have brain cancer"), persecutory ("My father is trying to poison me"), or grandiose ("I control the universe").

■ Management

The patient is highly excitable, and because a psychosis precludes insight, the patient usually does not believe treatment is necessary and, more often than not, resists it. Hospitalization is required in the acute initial psychotic episode because of the hazards of self-harm and aggressive behavior. A commitment process is sometimes required in order to obtain treatment for the patient.

Neuroleptics

The treatment of schizophrenia and, indeed, all psychoses was dramatically changed by the introduction of chlorpromazine in the 1950s. It was the first in a series of drugs called neuroleptics (antipsychotic drugs), whose main efficacy is in the treatment of psychotic disorders. Neuroleptics were presumed to exert their therapeutic effect by blocking dopamine postsynaptic receptors. This led to the hyperdopaminergic theory of schizophrenia. The action of the new antipsychotic drugs that do not exert their principal effect on the dopaminergic system questions this unitary theory of neurotransmitter dysfunction in schizophrenia. Most of the neuroleptics cause extrapyramidal side effects to one degree or another that can be disconcerting for the patient. Antipsychotic agents are listed by class along with dosages and side effects in Table 19.2.

The neuroleptics exert two principal beneficial roles in the treatment of psychoses. The first and the most immediate is a calming or tranquilizing effect that relieves the agitation of the patient and, thus, prevents aggressive acts. The patient can then be more agreeable to treatment. This action is an immediate one and dependent on careful dose titration. This goal is best accomplished by the concomitant parenteral administration of an anxiolytic drug, such as lorazepam. The second clinical effect is to reduce the intensity of and perhaps eliminate the florid psychotic symptoms of hallucinations, delusions, thought disorder, and distressed mood. This effect has its onset by 1–2 weeks after optimum dosage is reached and must be reckoned with in discharge planning.

The efficacy of antipsychotic drugs in the acute phase is well established. The successful treatment of the chronic phase is more difficult. Approximately 40% of patients presumed to be under adequate therapy and two-thirds of patients not receiving treatment will suffer a psychotic relapse within 1 year. The intramuscular depot form of neuroleptics, given in 1–3-week intervals, is being used increasingly. Optimum dosing of neuroleptics is a difficult problem because the drugs have the potential liability of extrapyramidal symptoms including **akathisia** (inability to remain in a sitting posture, with motor restlessness), aggravation of the negative symptoms of schizophrenia by producing lethargy and sedation, and the long-term hazard of **tardive dyskinesia** (involuntary movement of the facial muscles and tongue). The long-term course of schizophrenia is usually a difficult one for the patient, the family, and the health care system. Follow-up studies after discharge from care for an acute psychotic episode reveal that, in many cases, recurrent and/or persistent problems remain. Unemployment, social difficulties, and a restricted lifestyle are common. In fact, a complete recovery with resumption of a productive, normal lifestyle should occasion the physician to question the very diagnosis of schizophrenia.

TABLE 19.2. Dosages and Side Effects of Antipsychotic Drugs

Drug	Dose (mg)	Anticholinergic	Sedation	Hypotension	Extrapyramidal
Phenothiazines					
Chlorpromazine	100	++++	+++	+++++	++
Thioridazine	90–100	++++	+++	+++++	+
Fluphenazine	2	++	+	++	++++
Perphenazine	10	++	+	++	+++
Trifluoperazine	5	++	+	++	++++
Thioxanthenes					
Thiothixene	3–5	++	++	++	++++
Dibenzapines					
Loxapine	10–15	+++	++	+	+++
Clozapine	150	+++	+++	+++	+
Indoles					
Molindone	8–10	+++	+	++	+++
Butyrophenones					
Haloperidol	2–3	+	++	+	+++++
Diphenylbutylpiperidines					
Pimozide	2–3		++	+	+++++
Risperidone	4–6	+	+++	++	+

+ mild; ++ moderate; +++ pronounced; ++++ +++++ severe

First-Generation Antipsychotics

Haloperidol

The most commonly used neuroleptic for treatement of psychosis is haloperidol. Parenteral administration is required because of the need for prompt symptom control, in a usual initial dose of 2–5 mg, followed by hourly dosing. Concurrent administration of lorazepam, parenterally in clinically titrated doses of 1–2 mg, has markedly decreased haloperidol requirements in the acute phase. The most common side effect of haloperidol in acute phase treatment is acute dystonic reactions with muscle spasms and involuntary postures, which can be treated with 25 mg diphenhydramine IV.

Second-Generation Antipsychotics

Clozapine, risperidone, olanzapine, and quetiapine

Clozapine has a low affinity for dopamine 2 (D2) receptors, but a strong affinity for 5-HT2 receptors.

It has demonstrated efficacy in schizophrenic patients resistant to the older antipsychotics. **Agranulocytosis** (an acute condition characterized by pronounced leukopenia) has been reported in patients receiving clozapine; thus, WBC counts should be routinely monitored in these patients. At present, clozapine is recommended in patients not responding adequately or those who develop intolerable side effects from therapeutic doses of the usual neuroleptics. Risperidone, like clozapine, also has a lower propensity for extrapyramidal effects. Its most significant neurotransmitter system effect is still in question, but it has a high affinity for 5-HT2 receptors and D2 receptors. The optimum dosage is approximately 6 mg/day. Its complete side effect profile and place in treatment of the psychoses remains indeterminate. The other second-generation antipsychotic drugs listed appear to cause less extra pyramidal side effects and offer the promise of a beneficial effect on the negative and disability symptoms of schizophrenia.

Manic Psychosis

Manic psychosis is characterized by gross disturbance in mood, behavior, and thought. **Primary manic psychosis** is usually a part of a bipolar disorder, in which recurrent manic episodes are its hallmark. More than 90% of individuals who have a primary manic episode will suffer future episodes. Major depressive episodes may alternate with manic episodes. The illness most commonly begins in early life with a peak onset in the 20s. However, onset in adolescence, middle age, or late life is not uncommon.

Secondary manic psychosis is caused by medications, infections, metabolic derangements, and neurologic disorders. Although less frequent than primary manic psychosis, it should be considered, particularly in hospitalized patients, when the symptoms resemble a delirium (see the following).

■ Clinical Features

The most prominent feature is a disturbance in mood, which is euphoric and grandiose with a heightened vision of one's capacities. Associated irritability may occur, especially if the person senses he or she will be thwarted. Euphoria usually leads to unrealistic behavior in the occupational, interpersonal, and sexual spheres. Excessive buying and attempts at inappropriate business deals are common. The patient manifests little need for sleep and may be awake for days at a time in the manic state. Insight is remiss and family members usually must intervene to obtain treatment for the patient. Physical overactivity and a thought pattern of rapid, loose

associations prompting pressured speech are manifestations. The psychosis may be severe with persecutory delusional states as well as auditory hallucinations. Despite the euphoria and mania, suicide risk is quite high. Comorbid substance abuse, particularly of alcohol, is not uncommon in bipolar disorders.

■ Management

The first manic episode almost always requires hospitalization. Lithium carbonate is the mainstay in the treatment of acute manic episodes and the prophylactic management of the bipolar patient. However, in the acute manic phase, neuroleptics are also often necessary for the immediate treatment of agitation, albeit at lower doses than in the acute treatment of schizophrenia. Lorazepam, intramuscularly, can also decrease restlessness and hyperactivity. Usual lithium doses are 900–1500 mg/day. Serum levels can help gauge the dose; acutely manic patients often require doses toward the high end of the therapeutic range (0.5–1.5 mEq/L serum levels). Lithium therapy, which can have significant medical complications (Table 19.3), requires close monitoring. Bipolar disorders respond variably to lithium, somewhat dependent on the type of symptom expression. Approximately 60–80% of classic bipolar patients will respond adequately to the drug. Divalproex sodium (valproate compounds) is effective in manic patients, including treatment of the acute phase; however, its role in the long-term treatment of manic psychosis is unknown.

TABLE 19.3.	Medical Complications of Lithium Therapy
Complication	**Comment**
Leukocytosis (14,000–18,000/mm^3 range)	Requires no intervention.
Goiter and/or hypothyroidism	Lithium interferes with iodine trapping. More common in women than men. Does not necessitate stopping lithium.
ECG changes	T-wave depression, sinoatrial block.
Glucose intolerance	Could be problematic in diabetics.
Drug interactions leading to increased lithium toxicity	Tetracycline, NSAIDs, carbamazepine, thiazide.
Skin toxicity	Acne or worsening of prior psoriasis.
Nephrogenic diabetes insipidus	Reversible with dose reduction or cessation.
Interstitial nephritis or nephrotic syndrome	Necessitates permanent cessation of lithium therapy.
Lower extremity edema	May respond to a diuretic.
Weight gain	Usually minimal.
Neuropsychiatric problems	Confusion may occur in the elderly. Drowsiness, delirium, blurred vision, tinnitus, ataxia, and slurred speech (with toxic levels).

Major Depressive Disorder with Psychosis

Psychotic symptoms may occur in some patients with a depressive illness. Most common after age 45, this delusional depression can be seen in younger patients as well. The diagnosis is particularly difficult in the elderly, who may have cognitive deficits secondary to dementia. Agitation accompanied by somatic, persecutory, or paranoid delusions and marked withdrawal are the features. Auditory hallucinations occur in 20% and visual hallucinations in 7% of these patients. Delusions are characteristic and involve a preoccupation with one's guilt, a need for self-punishment, and suicidal ideation. The psychotic, depressed patient, particularly a man living alone, is at great risk of suicide.

Given the high suicide risk, difficulty in treatment, and profound self-neglect of the delusional patient, hospitalization is usually needed. Approximately 30–40% of these patients will respond to tricyclic antidepressants alone; the response rate increases to 60–70% with the addition of a neuroleptic. The second-generation antidepressants, including SSRIs and atypical antidepressants (bupropion and venlafaxine), are equally effective with fewer side effects than the tricyclics in this situation.

In most cases, electroconvulsive treatment (ECT) produces a faster clinical response than drug therapy. The severity of illness demands urgent treatment in some; ECT is appropriate initial therapy in these cases. Relapse after remission is not infrequent, necessitating follow-up ECT with medication and/or maintenance ECT.

Psychosis in the Course of Medical Illness

Psychosis in the course of a medical illness is manifested as delirium, an acute disorder of brain function characterized by acute onset with the predominant symptoms of fluctuating consciousness, disorientation, perceptual distortions, profound restlessness and agitation, disturbance of the sleep-wake cycle, and visual hallucinations. Both recent and remote memory are impaired and distorted. The delirious patient requires hospitalization for safety reasons because of associated combativeness. Emotional lability accompanies fluctuations during a 24-hour period. Autonomic nervous system dysregulation is present with sweating, tachycardia, and often a flushed appearance; speech is often fragmented, rambling, and incoherent. Elderly hospitalized patients are particularly prone to delirium, often caused by infections, particularly with sepsis, organ failure, metabolic derangements (dehydration at the time of admission is a risk factor), neurologic events including stroke, postoperative states, and medications. The more severe the illness, the greater is the risk of delirium. Determining the cause is of primary importance because recovery from the delirium depends on treatment of the underlying illness. Delirium is lethal in one-fifth of elderly patients.

Delirium must be differentiated from other psycho-ses, particularly alcohol and drug withdrawal, psychosis due to hallucinogenic drugs, manic psychosis, and agitation in a demented patient.

Treatment requires attention to the environment, limiting stimulation as much as possible. Nursing attention is crucial and so are safety measures. Neuroleptics can effectively control the agitation and decrease the severity of the thought disturbance, delusions, and hallucinations. Haloperidol is the most frequently prescribed neuroleptic, given parenterally in a dose of 1–5 mg initially (depending on the age and status of the patient). Doses of 0.5–2.0 mg can be repeated hourly with careful monitoring of the patient's response. The frequency of dosing is decreased as response occurs. Lorazepam (1–2 mg parenterally or orally) can also be used to augment tranquilization and to decrease the neuroleptic requirements. Neuroleptic overdosing can cause excess sedation, stupor, and severe extrapyramidal symptoms. The course of recovery varies, but persistent delirium requires further diagnostic evaluation.

Psychosis of Dementing Diseases

Deficits in memory, **aphasia** (deterioration of language function), **agnosias** (impaired ability to recognize various sensory stimuli), and **apraxia** (impaired performance of skilled or purposeful movements), which then result in global intellectual impairment, are characteristic of **dementia.** Psychosis can occur in the course of dementing diseases. Delusions (frequently of theft and infidelity) complicate Alzheimer's disease in as many as 30% of patients. These delusions may sometimes precede far advanced cognitive symptoms, and families often bear the brunt of accusatory behavior on the part of the patient. Hallucinations, most often visual, have been reported in approximately 25% of patients. Patients with Alzheimer's disease often display irritability, agitation, and aggressive behavior. Psychosis should be suspected when such symptoms develop or behavior changes suddenly in the course of dementia.

Anxiolytic medications may be beneficial to demented patients, but severe behavioral problems from psychosis often require neuroleptics, given in small doses and for short periods. Long-term neuroleptic therapy can be avoided by carefully watching for the appearance of psychotic symptoms, providing good nursing care, and using anxiolytics (e.g., lorazepam, buspirone).

Psychosis Caused by Pharmacologic Agents

Many commonly used drugs may cause psychosis, often from an idiosyncratic reaction, a toxic overdose, or withdrawal. The differential diagnosis usually involves the exclusion of direct brain involvement by the disease process, a delirium, or a manic state. Hallucinations, paranoid delusions, and agitation are common. The list of drugs that reportedly produce psychotic states is long. High-dose steroids are a common cause. Treatment consists of withdrawal of the drug (psychosis usually remits promptly after this) and treatment with a neuroleptic for acute symptoms. At times, the administration of lorazepam alone may suffice for moderate symptoms.

Psychosis Caused by Psychoactive Substance Abuse

Cocaine and amphetamines may produce acute toxic states with psychotic manifestations. Amphetamines trigger a release of catecholamines from storage sites in the central and peripheral nervous systems. The action of cocaine is somewhat similar to amphetamines as it inhibits the re-uptake of catecholamines both peripherally and centrally. Accordingly, in the acute toxic phase, the patient manifests evidence of sympathetic system overactivity as well as a variety of psychiatric and neurologic symptoms and signs. Bizarre behavior, agitation, panic, tachycardia, hypertension, and hyperthermia may be seen. The toxic psychosis of chronic amphetamine or cocaine use is manifested by visual, auditory, and, sometimes, tactile hallucinations. Paranoid ideation with panic is characteristic. The presentation to the emergency department of a young person with sudden, recent onset of a psychosis should arouse suspicion of substance abuse.

The administration of diazepam or lorazepam IV is an appropriate measure in treating acute psychosis. Propranolol, parenterally, may be useful in blocking peripheral sympathetic effects. Treatment of the psycho-

sis may also require the short-term use of a neuroleptic. The hallucinogens, lysergic acid diethylamide (LSD) and methylenedioxymethamphetamine (MDMA), can also provoke psychotic episodes. The effects of these agents are believed to be mediated via 5-HT receptors in the brain. The most constant effect of these agents is to produce visual hallucinations and perceptual distortions. The effects on mood are variable, ranging from euphoria to panic and depression and, sometimes, to suicidal ideation and action. Rage reactions and paranoid delusions may also occur. Sympathomimetic effects may be manifest with hypertension, tachycardia, tremor, and sweating. The best acute treatment of toxic psychosis is to provide a protective, tranquil environment and to administer benzodiazepines, either diazepam or lorazepam, parenterally, at least initially.

Brief Reactive Psychosis

The criteria for diagnosing this disorder, also termed **brief psychotic disorder,** include the following: the appearance of the psychotic symptoms shortly after, and apparently in response to, a traumatic event that would be markedly stressful to anyone in the culture; confusion and rapid shifts of intense affects; and delusions or hallucinations accompanied by disorganized thought processes and behavior. The duration of the psychosis is

usually a matter of days but no longer than 2–4 weeks, and full recovery with no residual effects should occur. Other types of psychotic disorders should be excluded. Treatment with a neuroleptic and/or anxiolytic for a short period of time may be required. After the patient recovers from the psychosis, vulnerability factors can be determined.

Neuroleptic Malignant Syndrome

This rare syndrome may occur at any time during the use of antipsychotic drugs but most commonly in the acute phase of psychosis. Postulated to be the result of dopamine depletion—particularly in the basal ganglia and hypothalamus—neuroleptic malignant syndrome is reported most frequently in the course of treatment with haloperidol, thiothixene, and the piperazine phenothiazines, but is not limited to these drugs. Concomitant use of other psychotropic drugs such as lithium, antidepressants, and benzodiazepines is present in more than 50% of reported cases.

Fever, tachycardia, labile blood pressure, generalized

muscular rigidity leading to rhabdomyolysis, tremors, and fluctuating consciousness are clinical features of the disorder. As it is lethal in nearly 20% of the cases, the syndrome constitutes a medical emergency. Leukocytosis is also common, and the illness may at first be mistakenly assumed to be infectious. Fatalities have occurred as late as 30 days later owing to renal failure, arrhythmias, pulmonary emboli, and aspiration pneumonia.

Treatment is supportive and involves prompt discontinuation of psychotropic drugs and the use of bromocriptine, a dopamine agonist. Dantrolene is employed to counteract muscular spasm and rigidity.

CHAPTER 20 EATING DISORDERS

The manifestations of eating disorders vary from severe restriction of food intake and emaciation in anorexia nervosa to compulsive overeating and obesity, but an underlying theme is a preoccupation with external appearance. Although anorexia nervosa, bulimia nervosa, and compulsive overeating are identified as discrete disorders, they exist on a continuum and share some common features.

The vast majority (>90%) of eating disorders in the United States occur in women, with women between the ages 14 and 40 having the highest incidence. A history of sexual abuse prior to age 18 is a common thread in as many as 50% of women with eating disorders. Many of these women also suffer from depression. Estimates of prevalence rates in the United States range from 1% to 19%, but the overall prevalence is probably 1%.

Although public awareness about eating disorders has become more widespread, the disorder remains somewhat hidden. Diagnosis may be delayed until serious medical complications arise because the patient conceals the problem even from close family members. Because most of these young women are seen initially by a gynecologist or primary care physician, these physicians must be aware of clues to early diagnosis.

Anorexia Nervosa

Anorexia nervosa usually has its onset in adolescence and is characterized by extreme weight loss, an intense fear of gaining weight, and a distorted body-image concept. The DSM-IV criteria are listed in Table 20.1. The typical patient is a teenage girl, with an average or above-average intelligence from a white, middle-class family, in which parental overcontrol or perfectionism may exist. Commonly, the girl is involved in athletic pursuits such as gymnastics or ballet. Obsessive-compulsive personality features may be present. A break-up with a boyfriend or remarks about her weight by other family members or peers may be cited as a precipitant for the weight loss. The weight loss arises from severe restriction of food intake and/or compulsive exercise; it is not unusual for these girls to exercise for 2 or 3 hours per day. They maintain energy by drinking large amounts of caffeinated diet soda. Besides weight loss, the other major symptom is secondary amenorrhea or, in the case of the prepubertal patient, primary amenorrhea. Cold intolerance, lightheadedness, palpitations, or peripheral edema may be noted.

The most obvious physical sign is **cachexia** (general weight loss and wasting). The skin may be dry, and **lanugo hair**—a fine growth that is normally present in newborn babies—may be noted on the face or upper extremities. Bradycardia, with pulse rates

TABLE 20.2.	Medical Complications of Anorexia Nervosa
Hematologic	Bone marrow hypoplasia with leukopenia and anemia
Cardiac	Bradycardia, hypotension, arrhythmias, rarely cardiomyopathy
Metabolic	Volume depletion, hypochloremic metabolic alkalosis, increased serum carotene
Endocrine	Low or normal thyroxine (T_4) levels, osteoporosis
Gynecologic	Amenorrhea, low LH, FSH, and estrogen levels

as low as 30 or 40 beats per minute, and hypotension, with systolic pressures less than 90 mm Hg, are fairly common. In anorexia nervosa, medical complications can arise in many systems, as listed in Table 20.2.

■ Laboratory Studies

Blood tests may be within normal limits. Electrolytes should be obtained because potassium, sodium, and magnesium may be decreased. Marrow hypoplasia may result from malnutrition and be reflected in anemia, leukopenia, and thrombocytopenia. Thyroid function studies may show a low T_4 but the TSH is normal (euthyroid sick pattern). Estrogen, LH, and FSH are at low pubertal levels, which results in the amenorrhea. Liver function tests may be abnormal. Serum carotene is usually elevated and may even cause a yellowish-orange tint to the skin in some patients.

An ECG should be obtained in every patient. Sinus bradycardia, T-wave inversion, ST depression, and QT prolongation may be noted. QT prolongation may be ominous as it has been associated with sudden death.

TABLE 20.1.	Diagnostic Criteria for Anorexia Nervosa

1. Failure to maintain body weight at 85% of normal for age and height.
2. Intense fear of gaining weight or becoming fat.
3. Distorted body concept and undue influence of weight on self-evaluation.
4. Amenorrhea as defined by the absence of at least three consecutive menstrual cycles.

Adapted from DSM-IV.

Management

Medical and psychiatric care of anorexia nervosa is a challenge. The physician needs to be aware of potential complications because the long-term mortality rate is between 5% and 15%. Early referral to a mental health professional with experience in treating eating disorders, regular counseling with a dietitian to evaluate and monitor nutritional intake, and family therapy are all critical. Outpatient care is preferable, but hospitalization is indicated when body weight is extremely low, metabolic abnormalities or dehydration are present, or psychosis is evident.

Because no medication consistently induces weight gain or prevents further loss, cognitive-behavior therapy remains the mainstay of treatment. This usually involves 10–20 sessions over 3–6 months in which cognitive restructuring of the patient's extreme concerns about shape and weight takes place. In addition, education of the patient in the use of self-control measures and the introduction of regular patterns of eating are essential.

This approach has been more effective than treatment with antidepressant drugs.

Drug treatment may be helpful if concurrent depression exists. The tricyclic antidepressants are somewhat effective. Because of their potential for cardiac side effects and the underlying bradycardia and QT prolongation often seen in anorexia nervosa, they must be used with caution. More recently, fluoxetine, an SSRI, has been used with some success. However, because fluoxetine might suppress appetite, food intake must be carefully monitored. Cyproheptadine, an antihistamine that stimulates appetite, has been helpful in severe cases of anorexia resistant to previous treatment. Because some patients have delayed gastric emptying or a sensation of bloating, metoclopramide may be of benefit.

Given the prolonged, extremely low estrogen levels, the risk of osteoporosis is high. Adequate calcium intake or supplementation may help preserve bone density. Vitamin and protein supplementation may also be indicated for many patients.

Bulimia Nervosa

Patients with bulimia nervosa engage in recurrent episodes of binge eating followed by purging through vomiting, laxative use, diuretics, or enemas (Table 20.3). The average binge consists of 4000 calories, eaten rapidly, followed by quick vomiting. The patient has no self-control over the eating binge and usually feels very guilty afterward.

Anorexia nervosa and bulimia overlap considerably. Bulimia occurs predominantly in older (20–40 years) white women. (See Table 20.4.) Bulimic persons are usually of normal weight or obese. They tend to be very well groomed and concerned with external appearance. Although "binging and purging" are the primary characteristics, bulimic persons also might restrict their food

TABLE 20.4.	Physical Findings in Bulimia Nervosa
Face	Bilateral painless parotid enlargement
Teeth	Loss of enamel, many cavities (from contact with gastric acid)
Throat	Petechial hemorrhages from vomiting
Abdomen	Bloating, distention, hyperactive bowel sounds
Fingers	Callus on dorsal surface from inducing vomiting (Russell's sign)

intake, go on periodic diets, and compulsively exercise. Low self-esteem and depression are very common. Substance abuse, particularly with alcohol, occurs in approximately one-third. Shoplifting and sexual promiscuity are also common. Anxiety and personality disorders (especially borderline personality) may be present.

Usual symptoms are nonspecific symptoms such as weakness; edema of the hands and feet; fainting spells; gastrointestinal symptoms such as abdominal bloating, pain, or constipation; and menstrual irregularities. Persons with bulimia are even more secretive than those with anorexia. Since cachexia is uncommon, the disorder may escape detection for years.

Laboratory Studies

Blood counts and protein levels are usually normal. Even in cases of recent, active purging, electrolyte ab-

TABLE 20.3.	Diagnostic Criteria for Bulimia Nervosa

1. Recurrent episodes of binge eating of a large amount of food within a 2-hour period characterized by a lack of control.
2. Recurrent inappropriate behavior to prevent weight gain such as vomiting, laxatives, diuretics, enemas, fasting, or excessive exercise.
3. These behaviors occur at least twice a week for 3 months.
4. Self-evaluation is unduly influenced by body shape and weight.

Adapted from DSM-IV.

normalities are rare. Cardiac examination is normal; an ECG is necessary to detect any abnormalities such as prolonged QT interval or flattened T waves. Aspiration pneumonia, a Mallory-Weiss tear, or even gastric rupture can follow the vomiting, and pancreatitis has also been reported. Chronic use of syrup of ipecac can lead to a cardiomyopathy or skeletal myopathies.

■ Management

Bulimia nervosa is a chronic disorder with frequent remissions and relapses. Relapses are common (50–60% after 1 year), especially at stressful times throughout the person's life. A multidisciplinary approach is important because of the medical, psychiatric, and underlying personality disorders. Collaboration with a mental health professional is usually very helpful. Treatment options include individual psychotherapy, group therapy, family therapy, behavioral therapy, electroconvulsive treatments, and pharmacotherapy. The relapse rate remains high regardless of which method is used.

Tricyclic antidepressants, especially imipramine and desipramine, have had approximately a 50–75% response rate. More recently, encouraging results have been noted with the use of trazodone and fluoxetine. Anticonvulsants such as phenytoin and carbamazepine, MAOIs, and lithium have also been used, but their high potential for adverse side effects makes them less desirable.

| CHAPTER **21** | **SUBSTANCE ABUSE** |

Alcohol is the most commonly abused substance in the United States, but addiction also occurs with prescription drugs such as barbiturates, benzodiazepines, and narcotics, and illicit drugs such as amphetamines, marijuana, opiates, and cocaine. Direct treatment costs and indirect losses to society from substance abuse are billions of dollars every year.

Many people who drink or take drugs on occasion do not become addicted. Predicting who will eventually develop dependence is not possible because many factors, such as family influences, genetics, personality, psychiatric disorders, and the addictive properties of the substance, determine the development of addiction. Abuse is characterized by a pathologic use of the substance that has personal and social consequences in a 12-month period (Table 21.1). Three specific features are essential in dependence: tolerance, withdrawal, and compulsive use (Table 21.2).

| TABLE **21.1.** | **Criteria for Substance Abuse** |

Recurrent substance use (only one or more of the following needs to occur within a 12-month period)[a]
- resulting in a failure to fulfill major role obligations at home, work, or school
- in situations in which it is physically hazardous (e.g., driving an automobile)
- causing recurrent related legal problems
- despite persistent social/interpersonal problems

Adapted from DSM-IV.
[a]Criteria can apply to any substance such as alcohol, cocaine, narcotics.

| TABLE **21.2.** | **Criteria for Substance Dependence** |

Presence of three or more of the following at any time in a 12-month period:

1. Tolerance: *either* need for markedly increased (≥50%) amounts of substance to achieve effect *or* markedly diminished effect with same amounts of substance.

2. Withdrawal: *either* at least two characteristic symptoms within hours to days after reduction/cessation of substance *or* substance taken often to relieve or avoid symptoms.

3. Substance taken in larger amounts over a longer period than person intended.

4. Desire but unsuccessful efforts to cut down intake.

5. A great deal of time is spent in obtaining and using substance and recovering from its effects.

6. Important activities are reduced or given up because of substance use.

7. Continued use despite persistent or recurrent problems likely caused by the substance.

Adapted from DSM-IV.

Substance abuse is a chronic relapsing condition. Abusers repeatedly attempt to quit before they are successful. Six stages of behavior change have been identified: precontemplation, contemplation, preparation, action, maintenance, and termination (Table 21.3). Understanding where the patient is can facilitate successful change by identifying the particular issues at that stage.

■ **Role of the Family**

To accommodate a chemically dependent member, most families develop coping strategies that are often unhealthy and may even perpetuate the dependence. Such family members are termed **codependent.** Because of this dysfunctional family process, family treatment must be integral to rehabilitation. Children in these homes may need specialized counseling and peer-support groups (e.g., Children of Alcoholics [COA] groups). When patients lack family support, options include referral to a halfway house or transitional living arrangements to enable the development of new social structures that promote sobriety.

■ **Role of the Self-Help Group**

Nonprofessional, twelve-step support programs modeled after Alcoholics Anonymous (AA) are available virtually everywhere. The only requirement for membership is the contemplation (Table 21.3). Groups exist for almost any behavior: Narcotics Anonymous, Overeaters Anonymous, Gamblers Anonymous, and so on. If the dependent person is not contemplative, family members may find 12-step groups for significant others helpful, such as AlAnon, NarAnon, and Alateen.

■ **Prevention**

The individual physician can do much to prevent alcohol and chemical dependency by identifying high-risk individuals, such as children of alcoholics. In every clinical encounter, physicians should promote healthful lifestyle changes (regarding diet, exercise, and work habits) and alternative coping strategies

TABLE 21.3. Stages of Behavior Change in Addicted Personalities

Stage	Behavior
Precontemplation	No intention of changing and denies problem, lacks information, intends to remain ignorant.
Contemplation	Acknowledges the problem; serious thoughts about solving it.
Preparation	Committed to action, but not necessarily ready; needs to plan detailed action scheme.
Action	Expends most time and energy (of all stages) modifying behavior and surroundings.
Maintenance	Can be in this stage for a few months or a lifetime; is at risk for relapse if not committed.
Termination	Has confidence that addiction no longer presents a threat without any continuing effort.

(e.g., exercise, stress reduction, relaxation therapy, biofeedback, and meditation) for dealing with anxiety, depression, and general stress. Early referral to appropriate counseling settings is also a responsibility of the primary care physician. Physicians should involve themselves in general public health initiatives and educational measures for children, discouraging the use of mood-altering drugs, alcohol, and tobacco.

Tobacco Abuse

Despite widespread use of tobacco, the overall smoking rate in the United States has declined dramatically from 42% of the population in 1965 to 26% in 1991. Nearly 90% of lung cancer deaths and 20% of all U.S. deaths are caused by tobacco abuse. Smoking is heavily implicated in deaths from arteriosclerotic cardiovascular disease, chronic obstructive pulmonary disease, and cancers of the head, neck, and pancreas. Smoking is also the most important modifiable cause of poor pregnancy outcome.

Environmental tobacco smoke (ETS) may cause lung cancer in nonsmoking adults, respiratory infections and asthma in children, and may be a risk factor for sudden infant death syndrome (SIDS).

The Fagerstrom scale helps indicate the degree of nicotine dependence (Table 21.4).

Two basic types of treatment are available: self-help and assisted strategies. Approximately 90% of successful quitters have used self-help techniques, such as quitting "cold turkey." Assisted methods include clinics, hypnosis, acupuncture, and nicotine adjuncts, e.g., nicotine chewing gum, transdermal patches, or nasal spray. The patches are available in several dosage strengths, thus enabling gradual nicotine withdrawal. Smoking while wearing the nicotine patch can cause cardiac ischemia or even lethal myocardial infarction. The patch is most effective if used in conjunction with

TABLE 21.4.	Fagerstrom Scale of Nicotine Tolerance			
Question	**Points**	**Question**	**Points**

Question	Points	Question	Points
1. When do you smoke your first cigarette?		6. Do you smoke when you are so ill you must remain in bed?	
a. Less than 30 minutes after awakening	1	a. Yes	1
b. More than 30 minutes after awakening	0	b. No	0
2. Do you find it difficult not to smoke in places where it is forbidden?		7. What is the nicotine content of your brand?	
a. Yes	1	a. 0.9 mg or less	0
b. No	0	b. 1.0–1.2 mg	1
		c. 1.3 mg or more	2
3. Which cigarette is most satisfying?			
a. First one of the day	1	8. How often do you inhale?	
		a. Never	0
4. How many cigarettes a day do you smoke?		b. Sometimes	1
a. 1–15	0	c. Always	2
b. 16–25	1		
c. 26 or more	2	Maximum total score: 11	
d. Any other	0		
5. Do you smoke more in the morning?		Highly dependent: Score of 7 or more	
a. Yes	1		
b. No	0		

Adapted with permission from Fagerstrom KO, Schneider NG. Behav Med 1988; 12:159–182.

a formal counseling program. Many employers have on-site smoking cessation programs or pay for employees to participate in outside programs. Free group programs, sponsored by local voluntary agencies and Mormon or Seventh-day Adventist churches, exist in many areas. Programs are also offered by state branches of the American Lung Association and American Cancer Society. Quit rates range from 15–40% at 1-year follow-up. Recidivism is high, but exact data are not available.

Bupropion, an atypical antidepressant, was approved in 1997 for use in smoking cessation. Given as a sustained-release preparation, it may be used in daily doses of 150–300 mg, either alone or in conjunction with the nicotine patch or gum.

Physician counseling is an important factor in smoking cessation and does not have to be lengthy or involved. The physician should provide advice, encourage the patient to set a quit date, refer to formal programs, and prescribe adjunctive medication, if indicated. Physicians must be especially attentive to high-risk groups, such as adolescents and pregnant women, but counseling about smoking cessation should be a part of routine practice.

Alcohol Abuse

Three out of four U.S. adults use alcohol, and 5–10% of these are alcoholics. Although alcohol consumption declined slightly when the legal drinking age was raised to 21, alcohol remains the most costly substance of abuse with an annual cost to society of $100 billion. Over 100,000 yearly deaths are related to alcohol. People dying from alcohol-related causes, such as cirrhosis, lose an average of 26 years from their life expectancy.

The American Medical Association defines alcoholism as "an illness characterized by significant impairment that is directly associated with persistent and excessive use of alcohol. Impairment may involve physiological, psychological or social dysfunction."

Simply stated, alcoholism is present when a person experiences repeated harm from drinking.

Alcoholism is regularly underdiagnosed in medical practices, with detection rates as low as 50% in one study. Psychiatrists are correct more often than their medical and surgical colleagues. The diagnosis is less likely to be made in patients with higher income, higher education, and private insurance, but in reality only approximately 5% of alcoholics fit the "skid row" stereotype.

Alcoholism is a complex disorder in which genetic, environmental, and personality factors interact. Male gender and a family history appear to be the two major risk factors for alcoholism. No biologic marker has yet been identified, but the risk among sons of alcoholic fathers may be as much as 25%. Other possible risk factors include tobacco use, history of hyperactivity, unemployment, being reared in a broken home, or being of Irish, Scandinavian, or American-Indian descent.

■ Clinical Features and Diagnosis

Medical history taking should routinely include inquiries about alcohol use. Questions such as: "How often do you use alcohol?" or "When was your last drink?" asked in a matter-of-fact, nonjudgmental way are not offensive and are more likely to elicit an honest response than questions regarding quantity of alcohol consumed. Use of a short screening questionnaire such as the CAGE test (Table 21.5) is another aid to diagnosis. A positive response to any question implies that the person is at risk for alcoholism.

Any of the following behavioral clues should arouse concern: emotional lability, loss of friends, difficulty with work, divorce or other family problems, sleep disturbance, self-medication, history of trauma (especially unexplained rib fractures), defensiveness or evasiveness when asked about alcohol, and driving while intoxicated or having other clashes with the law. Obviously, symptoms of liver disease, pancreatitis, or gastritis should alert one to surreptitious alcohol abuse. Other clues are insomnia, anxiety, depression, dyspepsia, headache, palpitations, or recurring minor trauma.

In early alcoholism, abnormal physical findings are sparse. Odor of alcohol on the breath or excessive use of mouthwash may be warning signs. Hypertension, tachycardia, or other cardiac arrhythmias are occasionally related to alcoholism. A plethoric face and bilateral parotid enlargement may be seen, on occasion.

No diagnostic laboratory markers exist. With heavy alcohol consumption, gamma-glutamyl transferase (GGT) levels rise and return to normal after weeks of abstinence. Obesity, medications (e.g., anticonvulsants), and liver disease not related to alcohol use can also elevate GGT. Macrocytosis with an MCV above 90 is another finding. Alkaline phosphatase, aspartate aminotransferase (AST), uric acid, cholesterol, and triglycerides may be elevated as well.

TABLE 21.5.	CAGE Screening Test for Alcoholism
Have you ever . . .	
• felt a need to	**C**ut down on drinking?
• felt	**A**nnoyed by criticism of your drinking?
• felt	**G**uilty about drinking?
• taken an	**E**ye-opener?

To diagnose alcoholism, at least one of the following criteria must be present: dependence, continued drinking, major alcohol-related illness (e.g., hepatitis, cirrhosis), or alcohol tolerance. Tolerance can be defined as a blood alcohol level >0.10 mg% on any office or emergency department visit, a level usually attained after three to four servings of alcohol. Alternative criteria for tolerance are a blood alcohol level of 0.15 mg% without signs of intoxication, or 0.30 mg% at any time.

One of the biggest obstacles in treating the alcoholic patient is overcoming the denial. It may take persistence over several encounters with the patient to make the diagnosis. Arguing with the patient serves no useful purpose and engenders more defensiveness and denial. The physician should continue to maintain a positive relationship with the patient without participating in the denial, explaining firmly but sympathetically why an alcohol problem might be present. Adverse medical effects already noted should be shared with the patient in a straightforward manner without using scare tactics or threats. The physician should show concern, convey a clear message of hope, and spend time educating the patient about the disease process and the long course of recovery.

■ Medical Complications

Medical complications as a result of alcohol abuse are varied and diffuse. Gastrointestinal problems include decreased salivary production with resultant dental problems; gastritis and upper gastrointestinal (GI) bleeding; and acute pancreatitis, eventually leading to chronic pancreatitis with malabsorption, diarrhea, and even secondary diabetes mellitus. Ninety percent of alcoholics have fatty liver; alcoholic hepatitis and eventual cirrhosis develops in as many as 30%.

Malnutrition and vitamin deficiencies are frequent in alcoholics, causing neurological problems such as peripheral neuropathy. Other neurological problems of alcoholism include Wernicke-Korsakoff syndrome, cerebellar degeneration, alcoholic dementia, and alcohol-related seizures. Miscellaneous complications include hypertension, arrhythmias, hypothermia, hypogonadism, increased susceptibility to pulmonary infections, and increased risk for cancer of the GI tract, urinary tract, bladder, and liver. Alcohol is directly toxic to bone marrow, causing thrombocytopenia, leukopenia, anemia, and macrocytosis.

■ Management

Managing acute alcohol withdrawal

Withdrawal/detoxification from alcohol is the first step. Hospitalization is recommended for metabolic or nutritional interventions, detoxification from other drugs, and for comorbid medical conditions. The severity of the withdrawal symptoms varies depending on the duration and amount of alcohol intake. Symptoms, which usually peak in approximately 24–72 hours, are of three main types: autonomic hyperactivity, neuronal excitation, and sensory distortion. Tremulousness, diaphoresis, tachycardia, and hypertension result from autonomic hyperactivity. Seizures occur within the first 48 hours after abstinence and are usually generalized, tonic-clonic, and limited to one or two episodes. The patient may have general clouding of the sensorium and perceptual disturbances, such as **formication** (tactile hallucination, as if small insects are creeping under the skin) or auditory or visual hallucinations.

Since the advent of benzodiazepines for treatment of withdrawal, full-blown **delirium tremens** (DTs) is uncommon. DTs usually occur 70–80 hours after cessation of alcohol consumption and are associated with more severe hyperadrenergic symptoms; disorientation and hallucinations are associated.

Benzodiazepines (Table 21.6) are the pharmacologic agent of choice and are effective in both inpatient and outpatient settings. With benzodiazepine therapy, symptoms are relieved sooner and complications (e.g., seizures and arrhythmias) lessened. Administering chlordiazepoxide in response to symptoms rather than on a fixed schedule has reduced the total drug dose and duration of therapy. Mild to moderate symptoms of alcohol withdrawal can be treated with benzodiazepines on an outpatient basis. Given the risk of cross-addiction, benzodiazepines should be stopped when withdrawal is completed.

Clonidine, an alpha-2 adrenergic agonist, has shown control of autonomic hyperactivity in alcohol withdrawal, probably by reducing catecholamine levels. Because it does not prevent seizures, clonidine should not be used alone. Similarly, ß-blockers (e.g., atenolol), given with benzodiazepines, decrease symptoms and reduce benzodiazepine requirements.

Long-term management of alcoholism

The optimal treatment program for rehabilitation and recovery from alcoholism is still unclear. Athough even brief interventions by the physician encouraging a patient to abstain from alcohol can be effective, pharmacologic treatment for alcohol abuse with disulfiram is of limited use. Disulfiram is an aversive drug that interacts with ingested alcohol to cause severe headache, flushing, and hypotension. Consistently favorable results do not exist, and disulfiram may cause hepatotoxicity, neuropathy, and cardiotoxicity. Patients should be made aware of alcohol-disulfiram reactions and cautioned to avoid alcohol—even in mouthwashes and cooking wines.

Naltrexone, an opioid-receptor antagonist approved for the treatment of alcoholism, has reduced craving in abstinent patients and prevented relapse. Naltrexone is not habit-forming and its side effects include nausea, headache, dizziness, and arthralgia. The usual dose is 50 mg per day. Because studies to date have only been of short duration, long-term (>3–6 months) naltrexone therapy is not recommended. For relapse prevention, psychological intervention should occur for those taking naltrexone.

Because inpatient programs lack proven superiority and their cost-effectiveness is of concern, residential programs are probably not essential in all instances. Those who have failed outpatient programs, those with serious medical or psychiatric problems, or those with cross-addictions to cocaine, narcotics, or benzodiazepines may benefit from residential programs.

Alcoholics Anonymous groups have existed for 50 years, and consistent attendance at meetings correlates with abstinence. These groups offer support, help participants resist the compulsions, and provide strategies to deal with the pressures that prompt the return to drinking. AA is also excellent for eliminating the denial of the alcoholic patient.

TABLE **21.6.**   **Management of Alcohol Withdrawal**

General
Thiamine 100 mg IM or IV stat and PO daily[a]
Hydration usually not necessary unless vomiting or poor intake
Folic acid and multivitamins
Magnesium sulfate 2.0 g IV q 6 h if hypomagnesemia and normal renal function

Withdrawal symptoms
Benzodiazepines (oral route preferred; if IV, should be given slowly over 2–3 minutes)
- Lorazepam 2–4 mg PO/IM/IV q 6 h
  OR
- Chlordiazepoxide 50–100 mg PO or 12.5 mg IV q 2–4 h
  OR
- Diazepam 10–20 mg PO/or 5–10 mg slow IV q 2–4 h
Beta blockers
- Atenolol (preferred for fewer side effects) 50–100 mg PO qd
Alpha-2 receptor agonist
- Clonidine 0.2 mg PO TID

Delirium/Hallucinations
Haloperidol 0.5–5.0 mg IM or 5–10 mg PO q 2 h until controlled

Seizures
Phenytoin (therapeutic value is uncertain)
- Loading dose: 10 mg/kg IV at 50 mg/min
- Maintenance dose: 100 mg PO q 8 h

[a]Deficiency in 30–80% of alcoholics.

Both inpatient and outpatient programs have approximately a 6-month efficacy rate of 80%, but recidivism is high, with only approximately 50% of alcoholics remaining abstinent one year after completing treatment. Early intervention is most likely to be effective; health complications can also be thus prevented.

Sedative-Hypnotics

Abuse of sedative-hypnotics, which are prescription drugs, often begins as an iatrogenic problem. These drugs exert alcohol-like effects on mood and consciousness and reduce anxiety and inhibitions.

Use does not necessarily correlate with abuse, but the potential for inducing tolerance and escalating drug use is constant. Dependence can occur even with appropriate therapeutic doses. As the daily dose and duration of treatment increase, the probability of physical dependence rises. The potential for misuse and addiction is greatest in patients with a history of alcohol abuse. The rapid-acting lipophilic drugs—secobarbital, pentobarbital, ethchlorvynol (Placidyl), glutethimide (Doriden), methaqualone (Quaalude), diazepam (Valium), and lorazepam (Ativan)—probably have the highest abuse potential.

■ Clinical Features

The person with acute intoxication may exhibit slurred speech, unsteady gait, general slowing of mental functions, drowsiness, and impaired judgment. Given the inhibitory effect on the arousal and respiratory centers of the brain stem, higher doses produce stupor, coma, and respiratory depression. Psychomotor testing will demonstrate a slowing of performance, reaction time, and coordination. Anterograde amnesia is also a consequence, which results in a partial or complete failure to acquire or store information after taking the drug. Ethchlorvynol in large doses may cause pulmonary edema.

■ Management of Withdrawal Syndrome

Anxiety, fearfulness, and insomnia may follow discontinuation of these drugs. Usually, the withdrawal syndrome is self-limited, and recovery is complete several days or weeks after the drug is eliminated. Abrupt discontinuation of benzodiazepines with short half-lives (oxazepam, lorazepam, alprazolam, etc.) and barbiturates carries a significant potential for seizures, delirium, and hallucinosis. Tremors, diaphoresis, and restlessness similar to alcohol withdrawal may develop. Even long-acting drugs such as chlordiazepoxide and diazepam can produce a significant abstinence syndrome.

Besides delirium, hallucinations, and disorientation, barbiturate withdrawal may be associated with fever, usually within 36 to 72 hours after barbiturate termination. Withdrawal from barbiturates should be very gradual, and phenobarbital is ideal for detoxification because of its wider safety range. Tolerance can be determined by pentobarbital loading with 200 mg. If after 1 hour, withdrawal symptoms are not controlled, 100 mg is given PO hourly until the point of toxicity or a total of 800 milligrams is reached. The total pentobarbital dose is converted to phenobarbital equivalents (100 mg pentobarbital = 30 mg phenobarbital), which is given in divided doses three or four times a day, tapering by 5–10% daily. Consultation with an individual who is experienced in barbiturate detoxification is recommended.

Opioids

Because most opiate abuse is parenteral, many patients present with medical complications, including skin infections, endocarditis, nephropathy, hepatitis, overdose, and, most recently, acquired immunodeficiency syndrome (AIDS), which is the fastest growing cause of all illicit drug–related deaths. Many of these complications are related to the sharing and use of contaminated needles. Heroin or cocaine is involved in two-thirds of all drug deaths. Nearly 40% of illicit drug deaths occur in the 30–39-year-old age group. Rates are increasing, particularly for men, and even more so for African-American men.

Opiates cause euphoria or dysphoria, drowsiness, diaphoresis, constipation, pruritus, miosis, pulmonary edema, and respiratory depression. Physical dependence develops quite rapidly, especially with intravenous (IV) use, because of the unpleasant withdrawal symptoms. To treat patients for whom opiates have had an acutely toxic effect with respiratory depression, naloxone, an opiate antagonist, should be administered IV (0.4 mg) every 3 to 5 minutes up to three doses. However, this may precipitate acute withdrawal symptoms.

Intense drug craving, abdominal and muscle cramps, nausea, vomiting, diarrhea, lacrimation, and frequent yawning characterize opiate abstinence symptoms. Mild to moderate autonomic hyperactivity is seen with tremor, restlessness, rhinorrhea, mydriasis, and piloerection or "goose-flesh," seen commonly on the chest. Because this syndrome is not life-threatening, patients do not always require medical detoxification.

Methadone, 5 mg, is given orally initially; if objective signs of withdrawal do not improve, the dose may be increased, usually by no more than 5 mg per dose, every 4–6 hours. In general, 20–40 mg of methadone in four divided daily doses is adequate for most patients; later, a single daily dose may suffice. The dose should be tapered by 5–20% per day, depending on the severity of the habit. Opiate withdrawal via high-dose methadone (75–100 mg/day), which carries a high failure rate, should be conducted only by experts in this area.

Detoxification may be followed by highly structured, behaviorally oriented, residential treatment programs, lasting from 6 to 24 months. Those who are strongly pressured (either legally or socially) to remain in treatment do best. In highly motivated patients, naltrexone may be instituted in a monitored program. Methadone maintenance should be reserved for those who have failed or refused such programs or for those with very severe psychopathology.

All high-risk patients should be screened for HIV, counseled on reducing their risks of acquiring HIV, and educated about "safe sex" and the risks of using contaminated drug paraphernalia. Needle and syringe exchange programs and education regarding safer injection practices are part of a "harm reduction" approach.

Cocaine and Other Stimulants

"Stimulants" include decongestants (e.g., phenylpropanolamine and ephedrine); anorectics (e.g., phentermine, phenmetrazine, and fenfluramine); methylphenidate (Ritalin) used for attention deficit disorder (ADD) and narcolepsy; agents such as d-1 amphetamine (Benzedrine), d-amphetamine (Dexedrine), methamphetamine (Desoxyn); and cocaine. Among these, cocaine is presently the most widely abused. Toxic reactions to all of these drugs are similar.

■ Pathophysiology

Cocaine and amphetamines share similar neurochemical and clinical effects. They act by blocking re-uptake of norepinephrine, dopamine, and serotonin at synaptic junctions, which results in increased energy, a sense of well-being, and decreased appetite. Cocaine has a shorter plasma half-life (90 min; amphetamines, 6–12 hrs). With both agents, euphoria rapidly declines despite the presence of the stimulant in the plasma.

■ Clinical Features

Abusers engage in intensive binges alternating with a few days of abstinence, compared with alcoholic or opiate abusers, who use daily. Impaired judgment, impulsiveness, hypersexuality, compulsively repeated actions, and hyperactivity may occur with acute intoxication, along with euphoria. Anxiety bordering on panic, paranoia, and delusions may occur—even in persons with no premorbid psychiatric conditions. The most common acute presentations (Table 21.7) are psychiatric (altered mental state or behavior), cardiac

(chest pain, palpitations, or syncope), or neurologic (seizures) symptoms.

TABLE 21.7. Common Presentations/Complications of Cocaine Abuse

General
Sudden death
Malnutrition (Vit B, C deficiencies)
Rhabdomyolysis with acute renal failure

Head and neck
Perforated nasal septum
Chronic rhinitis

Cardiac
Chest pain
Myocardial infarction
Ventricular arrhythmias
Cardiomyopathy

Pulmonary
Pulmonary edema
"Crack lung"
Pneumothorax
Pneumomediastinum

Psychiatric
Depression/suicide
Psychosis
Anxiety

Neurologic
Seizures
Headaches
Cerebral hemorrhage/infarctions

■ Withdrawal Syndrome

Abstinence from stimulants has three sequential phases: crash, withdrawal, and extinction. The crash immediately follows a binge and may last a day or a week. Features are depression, agitation, and insomnia followed by a craving for sleep. Withdrawal symptoms are decreased energy and anhedonia that fluctuate with near-normal moods, lasting for 6–18 weeks. Periods of intense craving for the drug occur within this time. The extinction phase lasts indefinitely, but craving for the drug may be induced by conditioned cues.

■ Management

Treatment of cocaine abuse is often modeled after alcohol programs. Inpatient treatment was pre-viously considered necessary for cocaine withdrawal but, because of the expense and lack of controlled studies demonstrating the superiority of the approach, daily outpatient programs are being used more. Long-term treatment often involves a twelve-step group, such as Cocaine Anonymous. Such treatment is imperative because the risk of relapse may persist for years. Success rates of treatment range from 30–70%.

Pharmacologic therapies reduce cocaine craving, but the effects are often temporary and side effects limit their use. Long-term courses of desipramine have yielded some of the best treatment results.

Marijuana

Men are twice as likely as women to be frequent users of marijuana. Smoking or ingestion create a sense of euphoria, and both stimulation and, later, sedation may occur. The sense of passage of time is slowed, appetite is stimulated, and the user's sense of humor may be heightened or inappropriate. Paranoid ideation, depersonalization reactions, and, rarely, a toxic psychosis may occur. Reassurance is usually effective in mild cases; sometimes a low dose of benzodiazepine is useful, and a neuroleptic may rarely be required.

Chronic use may cause **"amotivational" syndromes** with apathy, social withdrawal, and school or work dysfunction. Bronchitis and other pulmonary effects may also occur in heavy users.

Hallucinogens

Lysergic acid diethylamide and similar drugs may cause transient psychotic episodes, the management of which is similar to marijuana. Organic hallucinogens (Jimson weed, mescaline, psilocybin) and similar plant alkaloids (belladonna) may cause anticholinergic toxicity. The most important hallucinogen is phencyclidine (PCP), known as "angel dust," which may result in toxic psychosis, coma, myoclonic seizures, rhabdomyolysis, and renal failure. Although intoxications with most other hallucinogens only require reassurance or mild sedation, phencyclidine can cause violent outbursts requiring restraints and neuroleptics (e.g., haloperidol).

Anabolic Steroids

As many as 5–10% of high school boys use anabolic steroids at some time, and their use is most prevalent among football players. Another one-third of the users simply use them to increase muscle bulk. Anabolic steroids are considered a class III controlled substance. Adverse effects include increased secondary sex characteristics, risk for infectious disease if used IV, increased aggressive behavior, and dependency.

Impaired Health Professionals

Physicians, dentists, podiatrists, nurses, pharmacists, and veterinarians all have increased access to medicinal mood-altering drugs and the ability to self-prescribe without easily being detected. The level of denial, rationalization, and manipulative behavior is high, and the drug use may be overlooked by colleagues. "Impaired professional" programs, where confidentiality is preserved, make it easier for the impaired colleague to receive help.

Physicians have a responsibility to each other and to society to be alert to the signs of functional impairment in their peers caused by substance abuse or other disorders. Clinicians who suspect that a colleague is impaired should seek the guidance of a local expert to effect appropriate referral and therapy. Individual and group counseling and randomized urine drug screens for at least 2 years are usually part of such a program. Success rates of 70–90% are common.

<table>
<tr><td>CHAPTER</td><td>22</td><td>CLINICAL TOXICOLOGY</td></tr>
</table>

A ccidental or intentional overdoses are medical emergencies comprising approximately 10–15% of all emergency department visits. Almost any substance may be ingested including household poisons, prescribed drugs, over-the-counter preparations, and illicit drugs. Any unexplained or unusual illness, especially involving changes of consciousness, should prompt suspicion of toxic ingestion.

■ Basic Management

Initial stabilization

The ABCs of resuscitation—**a**irway, **b**reathing, and **c**irculation— are the most urgent considerations. An open airway is established and supplemental oxygen begun. If a gag reflex is absent, an endotracheal tube must be inserted to protect the airway. Cardiopulmonary resuscitation should commence if spontaneous respiration or pulse is absent. Intravenous access is gained with a large bore (18 gauge or larger) peripheral or central catheter. If blood pressure is low (<90 mm Hg systolic) or if perfusion is compromised, the patient is placed in the **Trendelenburg position** and appropriate amounts of intravenous crystalloid infused. Care must be taken to avoid fluid overload. Central monitoring may be warranted, especially if no response to fluid resuscitation occurs. Electrocardiographic monitoring is particularly important with tricyclic antidepressants and cocaine.

All unconscious patients should be given dextrose (50 ml of 50% glucose IV over 3–4 minutes), naloxone (2.0 mg IV and repeated three or four times, if narcotic overdose is suspected), and oxygen. Lower doses of naloxone (0.2–0.4 mg) may be necessary to avoid precipitating withdrawal in a suspected narcotic addict. Thiamine (100 mg IV or IM) should precede glucose in all alcoholics to prevent precipitation of **Wernicke's encephalopathy.**

Specific antidotes

Antidotes are available for a few poisonings (Table 22.1). The correct use of antidotes requires knowledge of the pharmacology of both the poison and the antidote. Antidotes could be harmful, and in an asymptomatic patient, supportive, watchful care may avoid iatrogenic toxic complications.

■ General Principles of Evaluation

After basic management (ABCs), the clinician should consider several key questions in a suspected toxic emergency. Does the patient's current presentation or history indicate any offending substance? What are specific physical findings? Do the clinical features and laboratory tests support one diagnosis? Is a unique therapy available that will make a difference?

History

A complete history of recent medication use, both prescription and over-the-counter; intake of alcohol and other drugs; and occupational or other exposures is

TABLE 22.1.	Common Antidotes for Poisonings	
Poison	**Antidote**	**Dose/Comment**
Acetaminophen	Acetylcysteine	140 mg/kg load, then 70 mg/kg q 4 h × 17 doses
Anticholinergics	Physostigmine	1–2 mg IV over 5 min
Benzodiazepines	Flumazenil	0.2 mg IV, then 0.3–0.5 mg q 1 min to 3.0 mg total
Beta-blockers	Glucagon	5–10 mg IV. Titrate 2–10 mg/hr until response
Ca++ channel blockers	Calcium	1 g calcium chloride over 5 min IV with cardiac monitoring
Carbon monoxide	Oxygen	100% by mask
Digoxin	Digoxin fab	mg ingested divided by 0.6 = vials required; if unknown, 10–20 vials IV
Ethylene glycol and methanol	Ethanol	10% IV: 7.5 ml/kg load, then 1 ml/kg/hr maintenance
Opiates	Naloxone	2–4 mg IV

important. If the patient is unable to give a reliable history, efforts should be made to contact friends, family, co-workers, or neighbors. One should inquire if any pill bottles or drug paraphernalia were found at the scene where the patient was found. Prior medical and psychiatric history (prior ingestions or overdose or underlying depression) should be ascertained. Although a complete history is helpful, diagnostic and therapeutic efforts may have to be initiated without it.

Key physical findings

Vital signs should be obtained when the patient arrives in the emergency department and, if unstable, should be stabilized and frequently monitored. Hypertension may follow use of amphetamines, cocaine, and anticholinergic drugs. Hypotension may indicate poisoning with sedative-hypnotics, antihypertensives, narcotics, or tricyclic antidepressants. Hyperpnea could be from salicylates or other drugs causing metabolic acidosis.

During the initial examination, the physician should concentrate on assessing the level of consciousness; almost half of all cases of coma are due to toxins. In comatose patients, physicians should check for head and neck trauma and stabilize the neck prior to moving the patient. A focused neurological examination should ensue. Muscle tone will be increased with amphetamines, phencyclidine, and antipsychotics, and decreased with sedative-hypnotics and narcotics. Fasciculations may indicate lithium or organophosphorus toxicity. Tremor is common with lithium or amphetamine overdose and withdrawal from alcohol or sedative-hypnotics. Seizures may occur from the use of alcohol, theophylline, tricyclic antidepressants, cocaine, and phencyclidine. The skin should be inspected carefully for cyanosis, flushing, rash, injury, or signs of skin popping or IV drug use. Breath odors can also provide diagnostic clues. Some odors, such as ethanol, ammonia, and glue, may be obvious. Cyanide can produce a bitter almond odor; methyl salicylate, a wintergreen smell. The eyes should be carefully inspected for miosis (narcotics, phenothiazines, and organophosphorus), mydriasis (anticholinergics, amphetamines, and cocaine), nystagmus (phenytoin, phencyclidine, and many sedative-hypnotics), and optic neuritis (methanol). Cardiopulmonary and abdominal examination should be performed as the diagnostic studies and treatment progress.

General diagnostic tests are listed in Table 22.2. In most cases, because toxicology data may be delayed, treatment should begin based on the clinical impression. Negative toxicology screens are falsely reassuring, and excessive reliance on quantitative data can be dangerous. The history, physical examination, and routine laboratory tests will lead to the correct diagnosis in most cases. Contact with a local poison control center is quite useful.

TABLE 22.2.	Diagnostic Studies in Suspected Poisonings
Blood tests
Glucose
Electrolytes, BUN, creatinine
Calculate osmolality and anion gap; measure osmolality in selected cases
Complete blood count, including platelets and differential
Liver function, calcium, phosphate
Coagulation studies
Arterial blood gas analysis, especially if obtundation or respiratory embarrassment is present
Electrocardiogram for QRS or QT prolongation, arrhythmias, ischemia
Radiographs
Chest x-ray
Abdominal x-ray to look for radiopaque drugs/toxins
Cross-table cervical spine x-ray if trauma suspected
Toxicology screens
Save 30 ml of serum, 60 ml of urine, 60 ml of gastric aspirate for analysis
Quantitative assays for specific drugs (e.g., acetaminophen, phenytoin, phenobarbital, aspirin)

■ Removal of the Offending Substance

Topical decontamination

Some toxins, such as organophosphorus insecticides, may cause intoxication via cutaneous absorption. Skin-to-skin contact with patients should be avoided; if it occurs, the skin should be flushed immediately with copious amounts of water and dilute soap solution. In patients with skin contamination, the clothing should be decontaminated or destroyed.

If the eyes are involved, they must be irrigated immediately with plain water or normal saline for at least 30 minutes, facilitated by a local anesthetic, such as 0.5% tetracaine. Long-term use of the anesthetic should only be with ophthalmological consultation. For acidic/basic contaminants, pH paper may be used to ensure that all toxic material was removed by washing. Early referral to an eye specialist is urged.

Methods of enhanced drug removal

Besides lack of demonstrated usefulness in most cases, forced diuresis is potentially hazardous. Usually, small amounts of drugs are removed and both pulmonary and cerebral edema may occur. Toxin removal may be enhanced by a variety of methods. Catharsis with mannitol or sorbitol (0.5 to 2.0 gm/kg) or saline cathartics ($MgSO_4$, magnesium citrate, or disodium phosphate) can remove unabsorbed orally ingested toxins. Hemodialysis is effective for water-soluble substances that are not highly protein-bound and is recommended in severe poisonings with salicylate, ethylene glycol, methanol, bromide, lithium, or isopropyl alcohol. In hemoperfusion, toxin is removed from the blood by direct contact with an adsorbent resin such as charcoal and then the blood is returned to the body. Selected instances of possible benefit from hemoperfusion/dialysis are listed in Table 22.3.

TABLE 22.3.	Methods for Enhanced Toxin Removal in Severe Cases of Poisonings
Method	**Indication**
Hemodialysis	Lithium, salicylate, methanol, ethylene-glycol
Hemoperfusion	Paraquat, theophylline, phenobarbital, salicylate
Peritoneal dialysis	Same indications, much less efficient than hemodialysis

Aspirin

Both intentional and accidental aspirin overdose is common as it is present in many medications. Salicylate poisoning affects the central nervous system and Krebs cycle enzymes, and uncouples oxidative phosphorylation. Because aspirin is a weak acid, acidemia increases its penetration into the CNS. The minimum acute toxic dose is usually 150 mg/kg; severe toxicity occurs at doses greater than 300 mg/kg. Levels must be interpreted with an estimate of the time elapsed since ingestion (Figure 22.1). Levels of more than 50 mg/dl usually require treatment. With concomitant acidosis, toxicity occurs at lower blood levels.

Early symptoms are nausea, vomiting, tinnitus, and hyperventilation. Initial respiratory alkalosis is followed by severe metabolic acidosis. Increased agitation and irritability may progress to seizures and coma. Hypoglycemia and pulmonary edema may also be present. Serum salicylate level should be obtained rapidly and repeated every 4–6 hours, especially if a sustained-release or enteric preparation was the culprit.

Emesis or lavage, as well as the administration of activated charcoal, will help reduce the amount of salicylate load. Forced alkaline diuresis is used with sodium bicarbonate (1 mEq/kg/h) to promote urinary excretion and combat acidosis. A urine pH of at least 7 should be attained, and deficits of fluid, glucose, and potassium should be corrected. In severe cases

with persistent seizures or acidosis, hemodialysis is recommended, especially with serum levels more than 100 mg/dl.

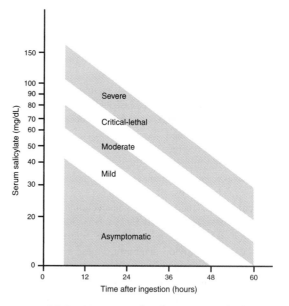

FIGURE 22.1. Nomogram for determining salicylate intoxication.
(Adapted with permission from: Done AK. Pediatrics 1960;26:800.)

Acetaminophen

With ingestion of large amounts of acetaminophen, an intermediate metabolite accumulates, which, by rapid glutathione depletion, causes oxidative liver injury (see Figure 102.1 and chapter 102). Acute tubular necrosis may also occur. Doses exceeding 7.5 grams may be toxic, but usually 15 grams or more must be ingested at one time to produce liver toxicity.

■ Clinical Features

Untreated patients progress through four clinical stages. In the stage 1 (12–24 hours), mild gastrointestinal symptoms occur. A transient improvement (stage 2) occurs 24–48 hours after ingestion; the patient feels well, but liver enzymes begin to rise. Stage 3 occurs three to four days postingestion, with jaundice, coagulopathy, and signs of hepatic encephalopathy. Stage 4 is the recovery period, which begins approximately five days postingestion, when normalization of liver function tests begins. Although most treated patients suffer no residual liver damage, mortality exceeds 75% in untreated cases.

Serial acetaminophen levels can predict toxicity from the **Rumack-Matthew nomogram** (Figure 22.2). In general, levels of 200 μg/ml at 4 hours after ingestion, or 50 μg/ml at 12 hours, indicate the likelihood of hepatotoxicity. Prolongation of acetaminophen half-life from the normal 2 hours to 4 hours, hyperbilirubinemia, and prolongation of prothrombin time are all indicators of serious liver injury.

■ Management

Patients presenting within 4–6 hours of ingestion should receive syrup of ipecac. Acetaminophen is rapidly absorbed; induced emesis or lavage is not likely to be effective several hours after ingestion. Activated charcoal probably should not be administered because it adsorbs the antidote, N-acetylcysteine.

Acetylcysteine, a glutathione precursor that prevents accumulation of the toxic intermediary, is the treatment of choice. In acetaminophen overdose of at least 7.5 gm in adults, acetylcysteine therapy should be initiated within 15–24 hours of ingestion. (Otherwise, only supportive measures are indicated.) Since the taste of acetylcysteine is poorly tolerated, it is best given mixed with cola or fruit juice or by nasogastric tube. A loading dose

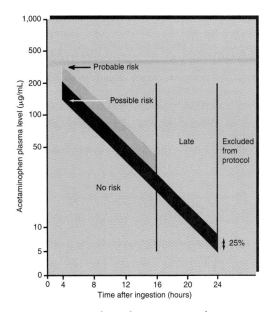

FIGURE 22.2. Rumack-Matthew nomogram for acetaminophen poisoning.
(Adapted with permission from: Hall AH, Rumack BH. American Family Physician 1986;33:109, figure 3.)

of 140 mg/kg is given initially, followed by 70 mg/kg every 4 hours for 17 doses. With prompt treatment, the outcome is very favorable. Once hepatic toxicity has occurred, exchange transfusions and resin hemoperfusion may be tried.

Nonsteroidal Anti-inflammatory Drugs

Nonsteroidal anti-inflammatory drugs (NSAIDs) can be divided by chemical structure into two major classes, **carboxylic acids** and **enolic acids.** Both classes have similar pharmacologic properties, but overdose with

TABLE 22.4.	Complications of Overdose with Nonsteroidal Antiinflammatory Agents
Gastrointestinal	Nausea, vomiting, ulceration
Neurologic	Drowsiness, disorientation, coma, convulsions
Renal	Metabolic acidosis, acute renal failure (especially in elderly)
Respiratory	Apnea, cyanosis
Allergic	Bronchospasm, urticaria in sensitive patients, anaphylactic shock (sulindac, tolmetin)
Cardiovascular	Hypotension, bradycardia, tachycardia
Hepatic	Hepatitis (sulindac), necrosis (phenylbutazone)
Hematologic	Aplastic anemia, hemolytic anemia

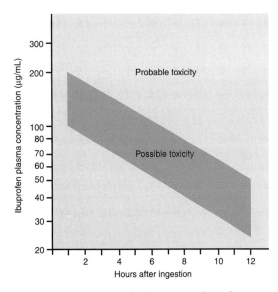

FIGURE 22.3. Nomogram for determining ibuprofen toxicity in ibuprofen overdose.
(Adapted with permission from: Hall AH, et al. Ann Emerg Med 1986;15:1309.)

enolic acid derivatives (e.g., phenylbutazone, piroxi-cam) may be more serious than with carboxylic acid overdoses. The major symptoms seen in overdose greater than 100 mg/kg are mild CNS depression and gastrointestinal upset, which usually respond to sup-portive care. More serious effects have been reported but are rare (Table 22.4) and usually follow ingestions of more than 400 mg/kg. Figure 22.3 shows the correlation of plasma ibuprofen levels with symptomatic toxicity. The nomogram may help identify those patients who are initially asymptomatic but later develop com-plications.

Vomiting should be induced if the patient presents soon after ingestion. Activated charcoal and a cathartic will help decrease absorption. Treatment is usually supportive with airway control, fluid therapy and cor-rection of acidosis, hypotension, or bradycardia, if needed. Because of high protein binding, hemodialysis or hemoperfusion are not effective. No antidotes are available.

Tricyclic Antidepressants

Tricyclic antidepressant overdose is probably the most common life-threatening ingestion. Mortality has been estimated to range from 0–15%, primarily owing to cardiovascular complications. The majority of deaths occur within the first 6 hours of admission. TCAs have a narrow therapeutic index: ingestion of 10 mg/kg may be toxic and more than 20 mg/kg may be le-thal. All of the tricyclic compounds and the tetracyclic maprotiline have virtually identical toxicity. The newer heterocyclic compounds and the selective se-rotonin re-uptake inhibitors are considerably less toxic.

■ Clinical Features

Symptoms and signs, primarily of the nervous and cardiovascular systems, usually appear within a few hours of overdose. Mild symptoms are anticholinergic effects, which include blurred vision, dry mouth, urinary and stool retention, and dizziness. Some cases may rapidly progress to delirium, hallucinations, seizures, and coma. Hyperthermia may be initially present; later in the course, hypothermia may be severe. Respiratory depres-sion may be severe, and aspiration pneumonia and the adult respiratory distress syndrome may occur.

Hypertension or hypotension may be present. The QRS complex usually exceeds 100 msec, and the QT interval is prolonged. Sinus tachycardia reflects the anticholinergic effect and does not, by itself, indicate serious cardiac abnormality. TCAs, through a quinidine-like direct membrane effect, produce conduction distur-bances and a ventricular tachycardia, often of torsades-de-pointes type.

Initial hypertension may give way to sudden hy-potension because TCAs inhibit sodium-potassium–activated ATPase, directly inhibit cardiac contractility, and produce peripheral alpha blockade and vasodilation. Hypotension is a harbinger of cardiac arrest. Serum

TABLE 22.5.	Summary of Treatment of Tricyclic Overdose	
Symptom/Sign	**Treatment[a]**
Convulsions	Diazepam 0.1 mg/kg IV per dose as needed Alkalinization Phenytoin, 15 mg/kg IV over 30 min
Coma	Airway support
Hypotension	Crystalloid infusion Alkalinization Vasopressors: norepinephrine[d] Inotropic agents: dobutamine[d]
Ventricular arrhythmias[b]	Alkalinization Lidocaine Phenytoin, 15 mg/kg IV over 30 min
Prolonged QRS (≥0.10 sec)	Alkalinization Phenytoin, 15 mg/kg IV over 30 min
Bradyarrhythmia/ heart block[c]	Isoproterenol Pacemaker

[a]Basic and advanced cardiac support is initiated first, when indicated.
[b]Any arrhythmia that compromises hemodynamic status should be treated by cardioversion. Quinidine, procainamide, and disopyramide are contraindicated for any tricyclic overdose.
[c]Mobitz II second-degree or third-degree heart block.
[d]Preferred agents.
(Reprinted with permission from: Frommer DA, Kulig RW, Marx JA, et al. JAMA 1987; 257(4):525.)

levels, which usually require a long time to test for, are unreliable indicators of the severity of the intoxication or of prognosis.

■ Management

A summary of treatment options in tricyclic overdose is provided in Table 22.5. When the patient arrives in the emergency department, basic management should be initiated. Gastric lavage and cathartics are essential. Syrup of ipecac should be avoided because of the rapid fluctuation in level of consciousness and, thus, the risk of aspiration as drowsiness occurs. Charcoal, 50 to 100 gm, very effectively binds TCAs. Because enterohepatic circulation occurs, repeated use of charcoal and cathartics is indicated.

In several large tests, survival in antidepressant overdose was approximately 95% with conservative treatment alone. Physostigmine, once considered an antidote, is now rarely used because of serious complications. Neurologic toxicity includes coma and seizures. Coma, which usually resolves in 24 hours, is treated with respi-ratory support and meticulous medical management. Seizures may precede cardiac arrest and should be aggressively treated with IV diazepam or lorazepam. Hypotension is treated with fluids, usually normal saline and bicarbonate. If the patient remains hypotensive after volume loading, hemodynamic monitoring and pressors should be initiated. Norepinephrine and phenylephrine are preferred. Alkalinization, either by hyperventilation or sodium bicarbonate, may significantly reduce cardiotoxicity by decreasing QRS widening, correcting hypotension, and reducing arrhythmias. Serum pH should be maintained above 7.45 to increase protein binding. Cardiac conduction delays are common and QRS prolongation exceeding 120 msec occurs in 25% of TCA overdoses. Phenytoin improves conduction through the His-Purkinje system and may be the drug of choice to correct conduction delays and control ventricular arrhythmias. Supraventricular tachycardias may be cautiously treated with beta blockers. Isoproterenol can be used for significant bradyarrhythmias and torsades de pointes until overdrive pacing can be established.

Benzodiazepines

Benzodiazepines are the most popular class of sedative-hypnotics in the United States. They are commonly prescribed for insomnia, anxiety and panic disorders, perioperative sedation, muscle strain, and seizure disorders (see Table 17.2 for dosages and half-lives). Because of their wide therapeutic index, serious toxic reactions seldom occur; nonetheless, they are often implicated in intentional or iatrogenic overdose.

■ Clinical Features

Mild manifestations of toxicity include disinhibition, slurred speech, ataxia, and sedation. These can progress to respiratory depression, stupor, and coma, which predispose the patient to pulmonary aspiration of gastric contents. In particular, if other drugs such as alcohol, narcotics, or TCAs have been ingested, hypoventilation may occur.

■ Management

Until recently, treatment of benzodiazepine overdosage was limited to supportive management. The usual measures of lavage, charcoal, cathartics, and mechanical ventilation, if necessary, were successful in the majority of cases. However, flumazenil (Mazicon), the first specific benzodiazepine antagonist, can be used for both diagnosis and treatment of benzodiazepine overdose. An initial bolus of 0.2 mg of flumazenil is given IV over 30 seconds. Within 1–2 minutes, sedation and respiratory depression are usually reversed. A dose of 0.3–0.5 mg may be repeated after 3–5 minutes, if an adequate response is not noted. Most patients will respond to cumulative doses of 0.2–1.0 mg; however, in severe overdose, as much as 5.0 mg may be required. Because the half-life of flumazenil is short (approximately 50 minutes), patients must be observed closely for recurrence of sedation or hypoventilation.

Nausea, dizziness, agitation, hot flushes, headache, and sweating are among the adverse effects of flumazenil. Seizures may occur if the patient has been taking benzodiazepines for seizure control or if the patient has ingested both a benzodiazepine and a TCA. If the seizure warrants pharmacologic control, a nonbenzodiazepine anticonvulsant, such as phenytoin, should be used.

Miscellaneous Drugs

All medicinal agents can be taken in overdose, either deliberately or accidentally, and treatment is usually supportive. Treatment advances in the management of poisoning occur regularly. If the clinician is not familiar with the treatment of a specific substance, prescribing information, a poison control center, and the Poisindex should be consulted.

■ Questions

Instructions: For each question below, select only **one** lettered answer that is the **best** for that question.

1. A 55-year-old man who was brought to the emergency department with a suspected imipramine overdose developed seizures shortly afterward. Which of the following statements concerning seizures due to TCA overdose is incorrect?
   A. They may be either grand mal or myoclonic.
   B. They are treated initially with IV diazepam.
   C. Seizure may respond to alkalinization with sodium bicarbonate.
   D. Physostigmine treatment may exacerbate them.
   E. Seizures indicate concomitant stimulant drug ingestion as well.

2. Tom J. knows that he has a drinking problem. He has thought seriously about seeking help, but is not committed to action. Which of the following describes his stage of behavior change?
   A. Precontemplation
   B. Contemplation
   C. Preparation
   D. Action
   E. Maintenance

3. A 52-year-old man is admitted for alcohol withdrawal. He is tremulous and diaphoretic and his heart rate is 110. What is the most appropriate initial treatment?
   A. Naltrexone
   B. Lorazepam
   C. Haloperidol
   D. Phenytoin

4. A 30-year-old man is brought to the emergency department by his roommate. He complains of chest pain and appears somewhat agitated. His roommate suspects that he is using drugs. Which of the following drugs is most likely?
   A. Alcohol
   B. Heroin
   C. Cocaine
   D. Marijuana

5. An unconscious young woman is brought to the emergency department. After establishment of an airway, she should receive all of the following EXCEPT:
   A. Oxygen
   B. Lorazepam

C. Dextrose
D. Naloxone

6. Upon physical examination in a suspected overdose, nystagmus is noted. Which of the following drugs is the likely possibility?
   A. Amitriptyline
   B. Thorazine
   C. Phenytoin
   D. Theophylline

7. To prevent liver damage with acetaminophen overdose, the treatment of choice is which of the following?
   A. exchange transfusions
   B. hemodialysis
   C. activated charcoal
   D. N-acetylcysteine

8. A psychiatric consultation is requested on an elderly hospitalized man with diabetes who presents with delirium. Under which axis will the diabetes fall in the *Diagnostic and Statistical Manual on Mental Disorders* classification?
   A. Axis I
   B. Axis II
   C. Axis III
   D. Axis IV
   E. Axis V

9. In a normal-weight, 20-year-old college student, which of the following physical signs would be most suggestive of bulimia?
   A. Bilateral parotid enlargement
   B. Cheilosis
   C. Abdominal bloating
   D. Lower extremity edema

■ Answers

1. E	2. B	3. B	4. C	5. B
6. C	7. D	8. C	9. A	

SUGGESTED READING

Books and Monographs

American Psychiatric Association. Diagnostic and Statistical Manual of Mental Disorders. 4th ed. Washington, DC: American Psychiatric Association 1994.

Articles

Biopsychosocial Approach

Engel GL. The need for a new medical model: a challenge for biomedicine. Science 1977;196:129–135.

George MS, Ketter TA, Post RM. SPECT and PET imaging in mood disorders. J Clin Psych 1993;54:6–13.

Leon AC, Olfson M, Broadhead WE. Prevalence of mental disorders in primary care. Arch Fam Med 1995;4:857–61.

Novack DH. Therapeutic aspects of the clinical encounter. J Gen Int Med 1987;2:346–355.

Somatic Distress Disorders

Gamsa A. The role of psychological factors in chronic pain. 1. A half century of study. Pain 1994;57:5.

Noyes R, Kathol RG, Fisher MM, et al. Psychiatric comorbidity among patients with hypochondriasis. Gen Hosp Psychiatr 1994;16:78–87.

Smith GR. The course of somatization and its effects on utilization of health care resources. Psychosomatics 1994;35:263–267.

Anxiety Disorders

Fierman EJ, Hunt MF, Pratt LA, et al. Trauma and post-traumatic stress disorder in subjects with anxiety disorders. Am J Psychiatry 1993;150:1872–1874.

Fleet RP, Dupuis G, Marchand A, et al. Panic disorder in emergency department chest pain patients: prevalence, comorbidity, suicidal ideation, and physician recognition. Am J Med 1996;101:371–380.

Mannuzza S, Chneier FR, Chapman TF, et al. Generalized social phobia: reliability and validity. Arch Gen Psychiatry 1995;52:230–237.

Shader RI, Greenblatt DJ. Use of benzodiazepines in anxiety disorders. N Engl J Med 1993;328:1398–1405.

The Depressive Disorders

Brown C, Schulberg HC, Madonia MJ, et al. Treatment outcomes for primary care patients with major depression and lifetime anxiety disorders. Am J Psychiatry 1996;153:1293–1300.

Christiansen PE, Behnke K, Black CH, et al. Paroxetine and amitriptyline in the treatment of depression in general practice. Acta Psychiatr Scand 1996;93:158–163.

Guscott R, Taylor L. Lithium prophylaxis in recurrent affective illness: efficacy, effectiveness, and efficiency. Br J Psych 1994;164:741–746.

Richelson E. Pharmacology of antidepressants: characteristics of the ideal drug. Mayo Clin Proc 1994;69:1069–1081.

Rosenthal NE. Diagnosis and treatment of seasonal affective disorder. JAMA 1993;270:2717–2720.

Psychotic Disorders

Fujii DE, Ahmed I, Jokumsen M, et al. The effects of clozapine on cognitive functioning in treatment-resistant schizophrenic patients. J Neropsychiatry Clin Neurosci 1997;9:240–245.

Rosenheck R, Cramer J, Xu W, et al. A comparison of clozapine and haloperidol in hospitalized patients with refractory schizophrenia. N Engl J Med 1997:337;809–815.

Tueth MJ. Emergencies caused by side effects of psychiatric medications. Amer J Emerg Med 1994;23:212–216.

Eating Disorders

Jimerson DC, Wolfe BE, Brotman AW, et al. Medications in the treatment of eating disorders. Psychiatr Clin North Am 1996;19:739–754.

Warren MP. Anorexia, bulimia, and exercise-induced amenorrhea: medical approach. Curr Ther Endocrinol Metab 1997;6:13–17.

Substance Abuse

Cherubin CE, Sapiera JD. The medical complications of drug addiction and the medical assessment of the intravenous drug user: 25 years later. Ann Intern Med 1993;119:1017–1028.

Hurt RD, Sachs DP, Glover ED, et al. A comparison of sustained-release bupropion and placebo for smoking cessation. N Engl J Med 1997;337:1995–2202.

Lieber CS. Medical disorders of alcoholism. N Engl J Med 1995;333:1058–1065.

Saitz R, Mayo-Smith MF, Roberts MS, et al. Individualized treatment for alcohol withdrawal. A randomized double-blind controlled trial. JAMA 1994;272:519–523.

Wadler GI. Drug use update. Med Clin North Am 1994;2:439–455.

Clinical Toxicology

Dec GW, Stern TA. Tricyclic antidepressants in the intensive care unit. J Intensive Care Med 1990;5:69–81.

Done AK. Salicylate intoxication. Significance of measurement of salicylate in blood in cases of acute ingestion. Pediatrics 1960;26:800.

Kruse JA. Methanol poisoning. Intensive Care Med 1992;18:391–397.

Kulig K. Initial management of ingestions of toxic substances. N Engl J Med 1992;326:1677–1681.

McClain CJ, Holtzman J, Allen J, et al. Clinical features of acetaminophen toxicity. J Clin Gastroenterol 1988;10:76–80.

Mendelson JH, Mello NK. Management of cocaine abuse and dependence. N Engl J Med 1996;334: 965–972.

Schwartz JL. Methods of smoking cessation. Med Clin North Am 1992;76:451–476.

Vernon DD, Gleich MC. Poisoning and drug overdose. Crit Care Clin 1997;13:647–67.

Whitwam JG, Amrein R. Pharmacology of flumazenil. Acta Anaesthesiol Scand Suppl 1995;108:3–14.

Wadler GI. Drug use update. Med Clin North Am 1994;2:439–455.

Clinical Toxicology

Done AK. Salicylate intoxication. Significance of measurement of salicylate in blood in cases of acute ingestion. Pediatrics 1960;26:800.

Kruse JA. Methanol poisoning. Intensive Care Med 1992;18:391–397.

Kulig K. Initial management of ingestions of toxic substances. N Engl J Med 1992;326:1677–1681.

McClain CJ, Holtzman J, Allen J, et al. Clinical features of acetaminophen toxicity. J Clin Gastroenterol 1988;10:76–80.

PART **IV**

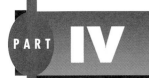

Virinderjit S. Bamrah
John C. Wynsen
James L. Sebastian

CARDIOVASCULAR DISEASES

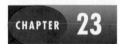 **COMMON PRESENTATIONS OF HEART DISEASE IN ADULTS**

Chest Pain/Discomfort

Chest pain or discomfort, an exceedingly common symptom, should be fully characterized by asking the appropriate questions, which may be recalled with the mnemonic PQRST (Table 23.1). The history is the most useful tool for elucidating its cause (Table 23.2).

Dyspnea

Dyspnea, or shortness of breath, in patients with chronic heart failure results from pulmonary venous hypertension. Mild heart failure may cause dyspnea only on exertion. With progressive heart failure, the threshold for dyspnea decreases, and patients may report orthopnea, paroxysmal nocturnal dyspnea, or episodic acute pulmonary edema.

Orthopnea is dyspnea occurring in recumbency and is promptly relieved by sitting the patient up or elevating his or her head. When caused by cardiac disease, orthopnea signifies a high left ventricular (LV) filling pressure owing to enhanced venous return. It may also occur in patients with asthma, chronic obstructive lung disease (COPD), massive ascites, or bilateral diaphragmatic paralysis. **Paroxysmal nocturnal dyspnea** (PND) is slightly more specific for left heart failure, but it also occurs in patients with chronic obstructive pulmonary disease and asthma. Usually, the patient awakens gasping for breath and feeling suffocated 2–5 hours after falling asleep. Dyspnea and the associated cough and wheezing ("cardiac asthma") abate in 15–30 minutes, usually by sitting up, walking, or opening a window. PND in COPD is relieved by coughing up mucus.

Edema

Peripheral edema develops when fluid volume expands by about 5 L (a 10-lb weight gain) caused by sodium and water retention. Edema owing to heart disease reflects **right heart failure;** it is gravity-dependent and, thus, is first noted in the feet and ankles of ambulatory persons. Right heart failure and edema usually develop late in heart disease.

Fatigue

Commonly reported by patients with heart disease, fatigue is subjective and nonspecific and is often due to noncardiac causes. When seen in patients with heart failure, fatigue signifies a low cardiac output. Sometimes, it is iatrogenic—following use of β-blockers or excessive use of diuretics.

Palpitations

Palpitations can be described as experiencing an unpleasant awareness of one's heartbeat, often caused by changes in cardiac rhythm or contraction force. Palpitations do not necessarily indicate the presence of heart disease or arrhythmia; normal persons may report them under conditions such as exercise, acute anxiety, or excessive use of caffeine or other stimulants.

Palpitations may also be caused by arrhythmias, particularly extrasystoles. The patient often senses the forceful beat after the extrasystole occurs, not the extrasystole itself.

All forms of tachycardia, hyperkinetic or high cardiac output states, and volume overload of the heart may evoke palpitations. The onset of rapid heart action (whether it starts and ends suddenly or gradually) and its regularity should be determined.

Other Symptoms

Many other symptoms may occur in patients with heart disease and should be inquired about and recorded. For example, **hemoptysis,** or bloody expectoration, may be seen in mitral stenosis, pulmonary infarction, or pulmonary hypertension or with an aortic aneurysm eroding the tracheobronchial tree. A dry, nonproductive **cough,** often worse when supine, is seen in pulmonary congestion caused by heart failure. **Nocturia**—large volumes of urine at night rather than simply increased frequency—is common in patients with heart failure. Anorexia, abdominal fullness, and weight loss (cardiac cachexia) may occur in patients with advanced heart

TABLE 23.1.	Important Chest Pain Characteristics
P	— Provocative (what activities precipitate pain?) Palliative (what alleviates pain?)
Q	— Quality (describe pain and any associated symptoms)
R	— Region (describe location of pain) Radiation (does pain radiate and, if so, where?)
S	— Severity (describe intensity of pain)
T	— Timing (describe usual duration of each episode) Time (how long since episodes first began?)

TABLE 23.2.	Frequent Causes of Chest Pain and Their Characteristics				
Condition	Provocative Factors (P)	Palliative Factors (P)	Quality (Q)	Region (R)	Timing (T)
Stable angina	Emotion, exercise, meals, cold	Rest, nitroglycerin	Pressure, tightness, ache, heaviness	Variable—see text	<10 min
Unstable angina	Same as stable angina, but may be present at rest	Nitroglycerin, sometimes	Same as stable angina	Same as stable angina	>10 min
Myocardial infarction	—	Relief of coronary obstruction	Same as stable angina	Same as stable angina	>30 min
Pericarditis	Breathing, supine position	Sitting upright	Sharp, pleuritic	Left precordial	Hours/days
Dissecting aortic aneurysm	—	None	Severe, tearing	Substernal, interscapular	Abrupt onset, hours
Anxiety	Emotion	Removal of stimulus	Sharp, stabbing	Left breast, pinpoint area	Variable
Pneumonia, pulmonary embolism/infarction	Deep inspiration	Analgesics	Generally sharp	Substernal, site of pulmonary infarction	Abrupt onset minutes/hours
Chest wall pain	Chest wall movement, palpation	Rest, salicylates	Sharp	Variable	Seconds/hours
Esophageal reflux	Supine position, empty stomach	Antacids, meals	Burning	Substernal, epigastric	<1 hour

TABLE 23.3.	Functional Classification of Heart Disease: A Comparison of New York Heart Association (NYHA) and the Canadian Cardiovascular Society (CCS) Criteria	
Class	NYHA	CCS
	Evaluates overall functional capacity.	Evaluates functional capacity in angina.
I	No limitation of physical activity.	No limitation of activity. Angina does not follow ordinary physical activity.
II	Slight limitation of physical activity. Ordinary physical activity results in fatigue, palpitations, dyspnea, or anginal pain.	Slight limitation of ordinary activity. Angina may be provoked by walking >2 blocks on level ground or climbing >1 flight of stairs at a normal pace and under normal conditions.
III	Marked limitation of physical activity. Ordinary physical activity causes fatigue, palpitations, dyspnea, or anginal pain.	Marked limitation of ordinary activity. Angina provoked by walking 1–2 blocks on ground or climbing 1 flight of stairs under normal conditions.
IV	Unable to carry on any physical activity without discomfort. Symptoms of cardiac insufficiency or angina may be present even at rest and increase with any physical activity.	Severe limitation of activity. Inability to carry on any physical activity without angina. Angina may occur at rest.

failure; fever and chills in infective endocarditis; epistaxis in hypertension; and recurrent pneumonias in large left-to-right shunts. Syncope is another manifestation of heart disease and may signify aortic stenosis, neurocardiogenic syncope, or arrhythmias.

■ Functional Classification of Heart Disease

Functional capacity is an important prognostic indicator in heart disease. The most widely used method is the New York Heart Association (NYHA) Functional Classification, which measures disability in heart failure (see chapter 30, Table 30.5). This system is a fairly subjective measure of disability but more realistically estimates a patient's functional improvement or decline over time and also the effects of therapy. A similar system, the Canadian Cardiovascular Society Criteria, rates disability from angina (Table 23.3).

CHAPTER 24

CARDIOVASCULAR EXAMINATION

■ Arterial Pulse

Arterial pulse (Figure 24.1) is best evaluated by palpating the brachial or, less preferably, the radial artery to determine the rate and rhythm. All accessible arterial pulses should be felt and compared bilaterally; normal arterial pulses are symmetric. As the closest accessible arteries to the aortic valve, the carotids should be palpated, one at a time, for assessing pulse volume and contour, which accurately reflect LV ejection velocity, stroke volume, and aortic valve function. The normal carotid, felt as a gentle tap, has a rapid upstroke. Distal pulses, with their greater amplitude and velocity of flow, can mask diagnostic clues.

A **high-volume (amplitude) pulse,** or bounding pulse, corresponds to increased pulse pressure (systolic minus diastolic pressure) that follows rapid ejection of a large stroke volume into the aorta against a low systemic vascular resistance. It occurs in hyperkinetic states (anxiety, fever, thyrotoxicosis, anemia), aortic regurgitation, patent ductus arteriosus, arteriovenous fistula, bradycardia, and arteriosclerosis. A **small-volume pulse** corresponds to decreased pulse pressure that follows slow ejection of a normal or low stroke volume; it also may occur when the systemic vascular resistance is high. The pulse is weak and thready in left heart failure and shock. In severe aortic valvular stenosis, the pulse is typically low volume, with a slowly rising upstroke and a delayed peak (*pulsus parvus et tardus*; *parvus* means "slow rising" and *tardus* means "late"). In the elderly with aortic valve stenosis and hypertension or arteriosclerosis, these features may be absent.

In **pulsus bisferiens** (*bis* means "twice" and *feriens* means "beating"), the pulse has two strong systolic peaks; the percussion and tidal waves occur before the dicrotic notch. Pulsus bisferiens is seen in severe aortic regurgitation, aortic regurgitation with stenosis, and hypertrophic obstructive cardiomyopathy.

In a **dicrotic pulse,** the second palpable peak occurs in diastole and is an exaggerated dicrotic wave following the dicrotic notch (aortic valve closure). Associated with a low cardiac output and low peripheral resistance, dicrotic pulse is typically seen in heart failure, hypovolemic shock, and young patients with fever. It is **rare** in patients older than 45 years.

Pulsus alternans indicates alternately strong and weak pulses, occurring at regular intervals or sometimes detected in the brachial or radial pulses by palpation, it usually requires a blood pressure cuff for detection (manifesting as a sudden doubling of rate as the blood pressure cuff is slowly deflated). Pulsus alternans is produced when high and low stroke volumes are ejected alternately from larger and smaller end-diastolic volumes of the LV. Its presence always indicates severe LV dysfunction.

Pulsus paradoxus is an excessive drop (>10 mm Hg) in systolic pressure during inspiration. In normal subjects, systolic pressure (measured with a blood pressure

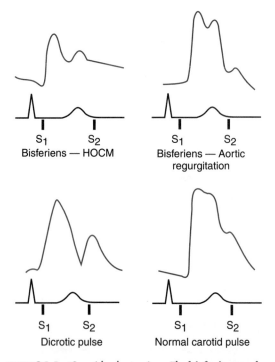

FIGURE 24.1. Carotid pulse tracings. The **bisferiens pulse** contains two systolic peaks that occur in conditions with rapid ejection of blood through the aortic valve. In the **dicrotic pulse,** the second palpable wave is diastolic and is due to an exaggerated dicrotic wave following the dicrotic notch (aortic valve closure). A normal carotid pulse is shown for comparison. HOCM = hypertrophic (obstructive) cardiomyopathy.

cuff) falls 3–10 mm Hg during inspiration. When the paradox exceeds 20 mm Hg, it is usually specific for cardiac tamponade due to pericardial effusion. In pericardial tamponade, right ventricular (RV) filling increases during inspiration, causing a larger RV volume and a raised intrapericardial pressure; this lowers inspiratory LV filling and leads to a diminished inspiratory LV stroke volume and pulse amplitude. Pulsus paradoxus may be noted in other conditions such as acute severe asthma, severe cardiomegaly, marked obesity, and massive pulmonary embolism.

■ Venous (Jugular) Pulse

Bedside evaluation

Bedside examination of the jugular venous pulse allows evaluation of the right atrial pressure and the morphology of the venous pulse waveforms. Examining the right internal jugular vein is preferred to the external jugular vein for pulse wave analysis because the right vein is in a direct line with the superior vena cava and, thus, better reflects right atrial events.

The patient should rest quietly in bed with his or her neck muscles relaxed and trunk elevated to a sufficient angle—usually 30–45 degrees—to allow the venous pulse to be visible in the sternal angle above the manubrium. Venous pulses are often best seen with tangential lighting. To estimate jugular venous pressure, the vertical distance from the sternal angle to the top of the oscillating venous column is measured (Figure 24.2). This distance is ordinarily less than 3 cm. Because the sternal angle is approximately 5 cm above the mid-right atrium, regardless of body position, the jugular venous pressure would equal 5 cm plus 3 cm (the height of the oscillating venous column), or 8 cm H_2O. This value can be converted to mm Hg by dividing it by 1.3 (1 mm Hg = 1.3 cm of blood); thus, the upper limit of normal jugular venous pressure is 6 mm Hg.

Jugular venous pressure reflects the mean right atrial or central venous pressure. The most common cause of an elevated right atrial pressure is **RV failure.** Other causes include tricuspid regurgitation and abnormalities of RV filling (pericardial tamponade, constrictive pericarditis, or rarely, tricuspid stenosis) (Figure 24.3). The normal jugular venous pressure decreases with inspiration and increases with expiration. In superior vena cava obstruction, the venous pressure is elevated but the venous waves and respiratory fluctuation are absent.

Hepatojugular reflux

In incipient or early right heart failure when the venous pressure is normal, a positive **hepatojugular reflux** may be elicited. When steady pressure is applied to the abdomen (liver) for 15–20 seconds (ensuring that

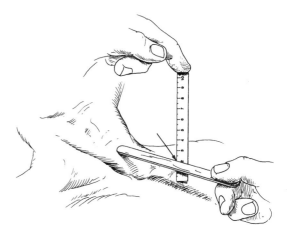

FIGURE 24.2. Measuring the jugular venous pressure.
(From: Adair OV, Havranck EP (eds.). Cardiology Secrets. Philadelphia: Henley & Belfus, Inc., 1995, p. 17. Used with permission.)

the patient does not perform a Valsalva maneuver) in normal individuals, the venous column rises transiently but returns to normal, despite continued abdominal compression. If the venous column increases more than 1 cm and remains high throughout the period of compression and gradually declines only after compression is relieved, this indicates positive hepatojugular reflux. The hepatojugular reflux occurs as the abnormal RV is unable to handle the increased venous return during abdominal compression.

Jugular venous pulse waves

The normal jugular venous pulse has two visible peaks (the a and v waves) and two troughs (the x and y descents) (see Figure 24.3). Another positive deflection after the a wave, the c wave, is not palpable but can be recorded; however, it is of little clinical importance.

- The **a wave** is produced by retrograde blood flow in the jugular veins caused by right atrial contraction. The a wave immediately precedes the carotid upstroke and the first heart sound, S_1.
- The **x descent** reflects a fall in right atrial pressure that occurs with right atrial relaxation and the downward movement of the tricuspid valve ring owing to RV systole. The x descent is often the most easily detected motion in the jugular pulse; it occurs during systole and ends just prior to S_2.
- The **v wave** results from venous inflow to the right atrium during ventricular systole while the tricuspid valve is closed. It occurs roughly coincident with the carotid pulse and the S_2.
- The **y descent** results from the fall in atrial pressure that occurs as the tricuspid valve opens.

Normally, the *a* wave is more visible than the *v* wave, and the *x* descent is more prominent than the *y* descent. In fact, the *v* wave and *y* descent are often not visible in healthy adults owing to the very compliant normal right atrium.

Abnormalities of jugular venous pulse waves

The ***a* wave** is increased in RV hypertrophy, tricuspid or pulmonic stenosis, or contraction of the atrium against a closed tricuspid valve (so-called cannon *a* wave, Figure 24.3). Cannon waves occur regularly in junctional rhythm and irregularly in atrioventricular dissociation. The normal *a* wave is absent and the *x* descent less prominent in atrial fibrillation.

The ***x* descent** becomes deeper in pericardial tamponade and constrictive pericarditis. It is attenuated or disappears with tricuspid regurgitation (being replaced by a *cv* wave) and is attenuated in atrial fibrillation.

The classic cause of an enlarged *v* wave is tricuspid regurgitation. An enlarged ***v* wave** may also be seen in mitral regurgitation, but only when left atrial pressure recordings are made from a wedged pulmonary artery catheter.

A rapid, deep ***y* descent** is seen in tricuspid regurgitation, constrictive pericarditis, and severe right heart failure. The *y* descent becomes dominant in atrial fibrillation. A slow *y* descent suggests impeded RV filling and may be seen in tricuspid stenosis or pericardial tamponade.

■ Cyanosis

Cyanosis is a bluish discoloration of the skin and mucous membranes. It is conventionally divided into central and peripheral types. **Central cyanosis** reflects arterial desaturation and is recognized as a blue tinge of the tongue, conjunctivae, lips, nose, ears, and nail beds. It occurs in lung diseases, and congenital heart diseases with right-to-left shunt. In **peripheral cyanosis** the arterial oxygenation is normal; however, an increased extraction of oxygen peripherally by the tissues, due to sluggish blood flow, leads to an excess of reduced hemoglobin. Seen in the ears, nose, lips, nails, and fingertips but not in the tongue or conjunctivae, peripheral cyanosis occurs with low cardiac output states, exposure to cold, and arterial and venous obstruction.

The absolute requirement for cyanosis is only the presence of at least 5 g/dl of reduced hemoglobin in the capillary blood. Thus, in a person with a hemoglobin of 15 g/dl, it reflects an oxygen saturation of 66% or less. For the same reasons, cyanosis may appear even with slightly lesser levels of desaturation in polycythemic states; however, cyanosis in an anemic patient indicates severe desaturation of hemoglobin (e.g., 50% in a patient with a hemoglobin of 10 g/dl). Smaller concentrations of

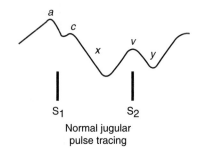

Normal jugular
pulse tracing

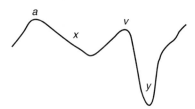

Constrictive pericarditis

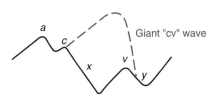

Severe tricuspid regurgitation

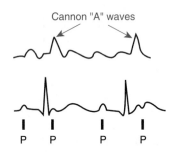

FIGURE   24.3. Jugular venous pulse tracings. **Normal jugular venous pressure**—The *a* wave and *x* descent are normally more prominent than the *v* wave and *y* descent. The *c* wave may be recorded but is not palpable on examination. **Constrictive pericarditis**—The steep *y* descent (diastolic ventricular filling) results from elevated venous pressures and rapid early diastolic filling. As the rigid pericardium suddenly limits further inflow, the pressure rapidly rises. **Severe tricuspid regurgitation**—A giant *cv* wave of tricuspid regurgitation is shown. **Cannon a waves** in complete heart block—Note the large *a* waves in the venous pulse, which occur due to atrial contraction against a closed tricuspid valve during ventricular systole.

methemoglobin and sulfmethemoglobin (1.5 and 0.5 g/dL, respectively) may also cause central cyanosis.

■ Palpation of the Precordium

The **apical impulse** is located normally in the fourth or fifth left intercostal space, at or inside the midclavicular line. It can best be felt with the fingertips and is normally produced by the left ventricle. The apical impulse occupies a maximal area of 2–3 cm and should be located no more than 10 cm to the left of the midsternal line. If the apical impulse is not felt with the patient supine (which is common in patients older than 50), the left lateral position should be used.

Besides location, one should note the duration, force, and contour of the apical impulse (Table 24.1). Normally, the apical impulse is felt as a brief, gentle tapping motion that ends before midsystole.

Simultaneous auscultation of S_1 and S_2 during precordial palpation allows one to estimate the duration of the apical impulse (Figure 24.4). A **sustained** apical impulse is one that maintains its peak into the second half of systole. It is caused by LV hypertrophy.

TABLE 24.1.	Causes of Abnormal Apical Impulse	
Hyperkinetic	**Sustained**
Hyperdynamic states	Normal location (suggests
Exercise	normal LVEF)
Excitement	Hypertension
Thyrotoxicosis	Aortic stenosis
Severe anemia	HOCM
Volume overload	Lateral displacement
Aortic regurgitation	Chronic volume overload
Mitral regurgitation	states
Ventricular septal defect	LV dilation with
	decreased LVEF

LV = left ventricle; LVEF = left ventricular ejection fraction; HOCM = hypertrophic cardiomyopathy.

The force of the apical impulse, although subjective, should be determined. A normal impulse is felt as a gentle tap whereas a **hyperkinetic** impulse (exaggeration of the normal contour) may be found in volume overload and other hyperdynamic states.

Other palpable cardiovascular events and structures may be found on examination. Rapid LV distension during early and late diastole may produce distinctly visible and palpable impulses—corresponding in timing to ventricular (S_3) and atrial (S_4) gallops, respectively. A systolic bulge, medial to the apical impulse, can be produced by an LV aneurysm. An apical tap in mitral stenosis is a palpable first heart sound. A palpable S_2 in the second left interspace may occur in pulmonary hypertension. **Thrills** are merely murmurs loud enough to be palpable; these are usually low-frequency murmurs. A left parasternal pansystolic impulse (lift) indicates RV dilation and/or hypertrophy. Severe mitral regurgitation may be associated with a late systolic parasternal lift owing to expansion of the left atrium beneath the RV.

■ Cardiac Auscultation

Examination and auscultation are usually best done from the patient's right side and ideally in quiet surroundings. A good-quality stethoscope, having both a diaphragm and bell, is essential. The diaphragm detects higher frequency sounds (>300 Hz) and is applied with moderate pressure. The bell detects lower frequency sounds (30–150 Hz) and is applied with the least pressure necessary to create a skin seal; excess pressure lessens the transmission of low-frequency sounds.

Auscultation should be done with the patient supine, but also when the patient is sitting and lying on the left side. At times, other positions (e.g., standing and squatting) and maneuvers (e.g., isometric exercise or Valsalva maneuver) that alter loading conditions may provide additional diagnostic information.

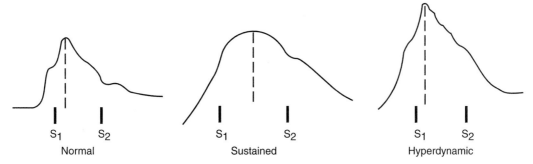

FIGURE 24.4. Major types of apical impulses. The **normal** apical impulse is felt as a brief tapping sensation, which clearly peaks before mid-systole (simultaneous auscultation of S_1 and S_2 is required). A **hyperdynamic** apical impulse is an exaggerated form of a normal impulse contour; it is not sustained or late-peaking but simply more forceful. A **sustained** apical impulse is prolonged and late-peaking; the peak of the impulse may still be felt in the latter half of systole.

Four primary precordial areas for cardiac auscultation are as follows:

- Aortic area—the 2nd right and 3rd left intercostal spaces (ICS)
- Pulmonic area—the 2nd left ICS
- Tricuspid area—the 4th and 5th left ICS adjacent to the left sternal border
- Mitral area—the cardiac apex

Each physician should adopt a systematic method of listening, but it is imperative to focus attention on one auscultatory event in the cardiac cycle at a time. Many cardiac and noncardiac variables can affect the intensity of heart sounds and murmurs (Table 24.2).

First heart sound (S₁)

The first heart sound, S_1, signals the beginning of ventricular systole and is generated by mitral and tricuspid valve closure (Figure 24.5). Although audible over the entire precordium, it is loudest over the apex and left lower sternal border. Its pitch, although relatively high, is lower than S_2; therefore, it is heard best by using the diaphragm of the stethoscope.

The intensity of S_1 is determined primarily by valve mobility, force of ventricular contraction, and most important, the velocity of valve closure (Table 24.3). S_1 is louder when atrioventricular valves are widely separated at the onset of ventricular contraction, such as in mitral stenosis with pliable leaflets, a short PR interval, tachycardias, and increased diastolic flow rates. Alternatively, a soft S_1 occurs when the atrioventricular valves are partially closed at the onset of ventricular contraction, as with a long PR interval, acute aortic regurgitation, and decreased flow rates (low cardiac output). Finally, the S_1 may vary in intensity from beat to beat in atrial fibrillation, reflecting variable ventricular filling and thus contractility.

Second heart sound (S₂)

Evaluation of S_2 is a key component of the cardiac physical examination. S_2 is best heard over the base of the heart, especially at the left upper sternal border. The closure of the aortic (A_2) and pulmonic (P_2) valves at end-systole generates S_2 (see Figure 24.5). Abnormalities of S_2 relate primarily to alterations in intensity or timing (Table 24.4).

A_2 is the louder component and is audible at all locations on the chest wall. In normal subjects, P_2 is heard

TABLE 24.2.	Conditions Affecting Intensity of Heart Sounds and Murmurs	
	Noncardiac Conditions	**Cardiac Conditions**
Decreased intensity	Emphysema Obesity Muscular chest wall Pericardial fibrosis Pericardial effusion	Low cardiac output
Increased intensity	Thin chest Anemia	Hyperdynamic states

FIGURE **24.5.** The cardiac cycle and related hemodynamic events. The relationship of intracardiac pressures to the timing and sequence of heart sounds is shown. S_4 is a late diastolic event occurring after atrial contraction, and S_3 is an early diastolic event occurring during the rapid-filling phase of the left ventricular volume curve. Ao = aortic pressure; LV = left ventricular pressure; LA = left atrial pressure.

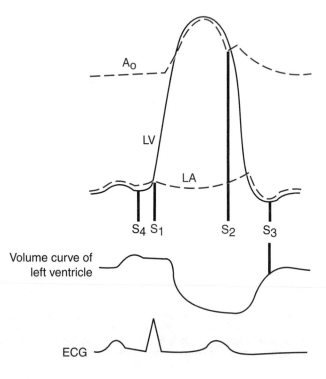

TABLE 24.3.	Factors Affecting Intensity of First and Second Heart Sounds		
			S_2
	S_1	A_2	P_2
Increased	PR <160 ms Mitral stenosis with pliable valve Hyperdynamic states Holosystolic MVP Rapid heart rates	Systemic HTN Hyperdynamic states Aortic dilation	Pulmonary HTN Atrial septal defect
Decreased	PR >200 ms Poor LV systolic function Mitral stenosis with rigid valve LBBB Acute aortic regurgitation	Calcific aortic stenosis Aortic regurgitation	Pulmonic stenosis

A_2 = aortic component of second heart sound; HTN = hypertension; LBBB = left bundle branch block; LV = left ventricle; MVP = mitral valve prolapse; PR = PR interval; P_2 = pulmonic component of second heart sound.

TABLE 24.4.	Alterations in the Second Heart Sound and Their Causes		
Single S_2	Fixed Splitting	Paradoxical Splitting	Wide Splitting
Aging	ASD	Complete LBBB	Complete RBBB
Severe AS	Right heart failure	RV pacing	Atrial septal defect
Pulmonic stenosis	VSD + pulmonary HTN	Ischemic heart disease	Pulmonary HTN with right heart failure
Any cause of delayed A_2		Aortic stenosis	LV pacing
		HCM	Pulmonic stenosis
			Severe MR
			VSD

AS = aortic stenosis; ASD = atrial septal defect; HCM = hypertrophic cardiomyopathy; HTN = hypertension; LBBB = left bundle branch block; LV = left ventricular; MR = mitral regurgitation; RBBB = right bundle branch block; RV = right ventricular; VSD = ventricular septal defect.

only at the upper left sternal border and is always less audible than A_2 at this location. An audible P_2 at the apex is an abnormal finding and strongly suggests pulmonary hypertension or atrial septal defect (apical impulse is caused by an enlarged RV).

A **single** S_2 results from attenuation of either A_2 or P_2. A single S_2, a common finding in older adults, arises from an inaudible P_2 caused by increased anteroposterior chest diameter.

The timing, or **splitting**, of S_2 varies with the phases of respiration. Normally, the split widens during inspiration and narrows during expiration. Slow, regular respirations are best for auscultating S_2.

- Wide splitting of S_2 during expiration with further widening during inspiration, i.e., a widely split S_2 having normal respiratory variation occurs when P_2 is delayed (e.g., right bundle branch block) or with early A_2 (e.g., mitral regurgitation).
- Fixed splitting of S_2 occurs when the RV cannot augment its stroke volume (e.g., in right heart failure) or when respiration-induced changes in filling, and hence stroke volumes, are similar in both ventricles (e.g., in atrial septal defect).

- Paradoxical splitting of S_2 occurs typically in conditions that delay the onset of LV depolarization and, thus, LV ejection (e.g., in left bundle branch block) or those that delay aortic valve closure (e.g., in severe aortic stenosis). In paradoxical splitting of S_2, A_2 follows P_2 during expiration and coincides with P_2 during inspiration.

Diastolic sounds

A **ventricular gallop** (S_3) sound occurs in early diastole, 140–160 ms after S_2 as the active ventricular relaxation ends. It corresponds to the end of the rapid filling phase on the LV volume curve (Figure 24.5). It is a low-frequency sound, best heard with the bell of the stethoscope lightly applied to the apex (LV S_3) or left lower sternal border (RV S_3). Often, gallops are heard only in the left lateral position.

The S_3 is caused by an interplay between ventricular filling and ventricular compliance (Table 24.5). An S_3 will be intensified by maneuvers that enhance ventricular filling and lessened by maneuvers that diminish venous return. Although an S_3 occurs in many conditions, most commonly, a nonphysiologic S_3 is associated with

TABLE 24.5.	Causes of Left Ventricular S_3 and S_4 Gallops	
	S_3	**S_4**
Physiological	Children and young adults Common during pregnancy Hyperkinetic states Rarely present after age 40	Rarely a normal finding
Pathological	High diastolic flow states Mitral regurgitation Ventricular septal defect Patent ductus arteriosus Aortic regurgitation Systolic dysfunction Diastolic dysfunction Hypertrophic cardiomyopathy Restrictive cardiomyopathy Constrictive pericarditis (pericardial knock)	Coronary artery disease Hypertension Aortic stenosis Hypertrophic cardiomyopathy Acute mitral regurgitation Dilated cardiomyopathy Hyperkinetic states

abnormally high LV filling pressures, low cardiac output, and a dilated, poorly contractile LV. An S_3 is not heard when significant mitral stenosis is present. A "pericardial knock," a higher pitched diastolic sound that occurs earlier (closer to A_2) than the usual S_3, is heard in patients with constrictive pericarditis.

Atrial gallop (S_4) is a dull, low-frequency sound that precedes S_1 and is best heard over the apical impulse (left-sided S_4) or left lower sternal border (right-sided S_4). The techniques used to elicit an S_3 sound also apply for the S_4. The S_4 is attributed to forceful atrial contraction to fill a noncompliant or stiff ventricle (Table 24.5). An S_4, although abnormal, is quite common in older adults. It implies a less serious alteration of overall LV function and better prognosis than a pathologic S_3. The S_4 disappears in atrial fibrillation.

A **summation** gallop occurs in the presence of tachycardia in a patient who has both an S_3 and an S_4. During tachycardia, the shortened diastole forces the S_4 and S_3 into a loud, single diastolic sound.

Mitral **opening snap** (OS) is a sharp, high-frequency sound heard best over the left lower sternal border in patients with mitral valve stenosis. It is attributed to the sudden arrest of a rapidly opening mitral valve that is stenotic but pliable. Immobility or calcification of the mitral leaflets causes softening or disappearance of the OS. The A_2-OS interval correlates inversely with the severity of the mitral stenosis; because left atrial pressure increases with the progression of severe mitral stenosis, the OS occurs earlier, resulting in a narrow A_2-OS interval.

Systolic sounds

Ejection click (EC) is a sharp, high-frequency sound audible immediately after S_1. ECs occur in aortic and pulmonary valvular stenoses as well as in dilation of the ascending aorta and pulmonary artery. An aortic EC is audible over the entire precordium and varies little with respiration. A pulmonary EC is most audible along the left upper sternal border, becoming louder during expiration and less audible or absent during inspiration. ECs occur owing to abrupt cessation of the systolic motion of the dome-shaped, stenotic aortic and pulmonary valves. As the valves become stiff and calcified in aortic and pulmonary valvular stenosis, the EC disappears.

Nonejection clicks are associated with mitral valve prolapse. They are high-frequency sharp clicks occurring over the apex or left lower sternal border. These may occur as isolated findings or be followed by late systolic murmurs. Maneuvers such as squatting and gripping one's hand move a midsystolic click toward S_2 whereas standing and performing the Valsalva maneuver move the click toward S_1. A midsystolic click arises from the sudden tension on the chordae tendineae or from the sudden halt of the prolapsing mitral valve leaflet during ventricular systole.

Prosthetic valve sounds

A ball-in-cage prosthesis (Starr-Edwards) has loud, metallic opening and closing sounds. Disc valves produce distinct closing sounds but usually no audible opening sounds. Porcine valves in the aortic position usually generate no abnormal sounds, but when placed in the mitral position, they may produce an opening snap followed by a diastolic rumble.

A pressure gradient exists across all prosthetic valves because the valve area of a prosthesis is typically smaller than that of a normal native valve. This causes a barely audible systolic murmur across prosthetic aortic valves and a soft diastolic rumble across prosthetic mitral valves.

Heart murmurs

A prolonged series of audible vibrations constitute a heart murmur. Heart murmurs are traditionally classified as systolic, diastolic, or continuous (Table 24.6). During auscultation of a murmur, its timing in the cardiac cycle in relation to S_1 and S_2, intensity, quality (e.g., blowing, harsh, rumbling), duration, and radiation (e.g., to the neck, axilla, or back) should be defined. Additionally, if a patient with a systolic murmur has a coexistent arrhythmia, the effect of varying diastolic filling periods on the intensity of the murmur should be noted. Commonly, the intensity of outflow murmurs (e.g., aortic sclerosis or stenosis) will clearly increase in intensity in the beat following a longer diastole whereas murmurs owing to mitral regurgitation will remain unchanged.

The grading system for murmur intensity is described in Table 24.7. Most innocent murmurs are grades I or II. With a grade III murmur, one should initiate a search for pathology. Grade IV to VI murmurs are uncommon to rare. Whereas some systolic murmurs may be innocent, all diastolic and continuous murmurs are abnormal and pathological.

Systolic murmurs

Systolic murmurs are categorized according to their duration and relationship to S_1 and S_2. The most

TABLE 24.7.	Grading System for Murmur Intensity
Grade	**Description**
I/VI	Very faint; barely audible
II/VI	Soft but readily audible
III/VI	Moderately loud; no thrill
IV/VI	Very loud; thrill present
V/VI	Louder; thrill present; still requires a stethoscope on the chest to be heard
VI/VI	Audible with stethoscope close to, but not touching, chest; thrill present

important point to ascertain is whether the systolic murmur extends to S_2. Ejection murmurs usually are crescendo-decrescendo in shape and end prior to S_2. Regurgitant or pansystolic murmurs are usually of more uniform intensity and extend to or even through S_2.

A midsystolic **ejection** murmur occupies only the ejection portion of systole. Ejection (and thus the murmur) begins at the time of semilunar valve opening, following S_1. Because the pressure gradient and blood flow markedly diminish before semilunar valve closure (S_2), these murmurs usually end prior to S_2. These murmurs are classically diamond-shaped (crescendo-decrescendo). However, determining whether a systolic murmur extends to S_2 is more important than determining its shape.

The most common type of midsystolic ejection murmur is the flow murmur, which arises owing to the normal turbulence of aortic blood flow during systolic ejection. Most pathologic midsystolic ejection murmurs originate at the semilunar valve; the classic example is aortic stenosis (Figure 24.6).

Regurgitant or **pansystolic** murmurs begin with S_1 and extend to S_2. A truly pansystolic murmur implies a large and continuous pressure differential between two chambers, causing a high-velocity stream of flow throughout systole. The resulting murmur is classically high-frequency, blowing in quality (not harsh), and relatively uniform in intensity (Figure 24.7). All pansystolic murmurs are pathologic.

Late systolic murmurs occur in the latter part of systole, well after S_1 and end in or after A_2. If caused by mitral valve prolapse, a midsystolic click may precede the murmur. All late systolic murmurs are pathologic.

Diastolic murmurs

Early diastolic regurgitant murmurs are heard with aortic and pulmonic regurgitation. Because the pressure difference and thus regurgitant flow between the aorta and left ventricle (or pulmonary artery and right ventricle) decrease throughout diastole, these murmurs are classically decrescendo (Figure 24.8). Unless it is specifically sought, the murmur of aortic regurgitation can be easily missed on auscultation. It is best heard with

TABLE 24.6.	Classification and Causes of Heart Murmurs

INNOCENT MURMURS
SYSTOLIC MURMURS
  Ejection (midsystolic; crescendo–decrescendo)
    Subvalvular, valvular, and supravalvular aortic or pulmonic stenosis
    Malformed but nonstenotic aortic valve (aortic sclerosis)
    Dilation of aortic or pulmonary artery
    Increased systolic flow—e.g., aortic regurgitation, atrial septal defect
  Regurgitant (pansystolic; constant amplitude)
    Mitral and tricuspid regurgitation
    Ventricular septal defect
  Late systolic (onset well after S_1; end in A_2)
    Mitral regurgitation—papillary muscle dysfunction or mitral valve prolapse
DIASTOLIC MURMURS
  EARLY (onset with A_2 or P_2; decrescendo; high-pitched)
    Aortic and pulmonic regurgitation
  MID-DIASTOLIC (begin after S_2; low-pitched rumble)
    Mitral or tricuspid stenosis
    Increased atrioventricular valve flow without stenosis—mitral and tricuspid regurgitation, atrial and ventricular septal defects, aortic regurgitation (Austin Flint)
CONTINUOUS MURMURS (systolic/early diastolic; peak late systole)
  Patent ductus arteriosus
  Ruptured aneurysm of sinus of Valsalva
  Coronary arteriovenous fistula

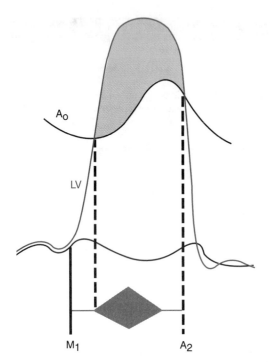

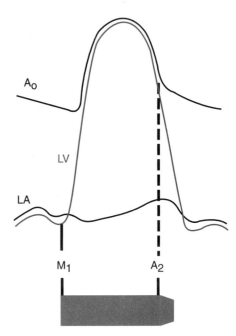

FIGURE 24.6. Midsystolic murmur in aortic stenosis. Left ventricular (LV) and aortic (Ao) pressure tracings are shown. The hatched area is the LV-Ao pressure gradient across the stenosis. The diamond-shaped midsystolic murmur begins after the mitral component of the first heart sound (M_1), as the aortic valve is not yet open. The murmur ends before aortic valve closure (A_2).

FIGURE 24.7. Pansystolic murmur in mitral regurgitation. Left ventricular (LV), aortic (Ao), and left atrial (LA) pressure tracings in typical mitral regurgitation are shown. The classic holosystolic murmur of mitral regurgitation begins with and may replace the first heart sound (M_1). The murmur continues up to and even through the second heart sound (A_2) since, at that time, left ventricular pressure still exceeds left atrial pressure and thus the pressure gradient causing the regurgitant flow continues to exist.

FIGURE 24.8. Early diastolic murmur in chronic aortic regurgitation. Left ventricular (LV) and aortic (Ao) pressure curves in chronic aortic regurgitation are shown. Note the low aortic diastolic pressure. The hatched area is the LV-Ao diastolic pressure gradient driving the AR flow. The murmur of aortic regurgitation begins with the second heart sound (A_2). Since the gradient between the aorta and LV is maximal almost instantaneously and then slowly decreases, the murmur has a high-pitched, slow-decrescendo character.

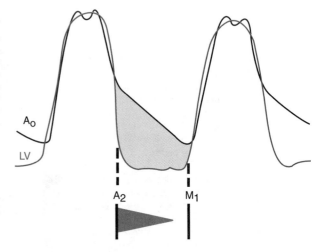

the patient sitting up and leaning forward, with breath held in expiration. The murmur of pulmonary regurgitation owing to pulmonary hypertension is termed a Graham Steell murmur.

Mid-diastolic murmurs are caused by increased diastolic flow across normal mitral and tricuspid valves or normal diastolic flow across stenosed or distorted mitral and tricuspid valves. Classically, the murmur of mitral stenosis follows the opening snap of the mitral valve and then diminishes in intensity, only to increase again at the end of diastole (presystolic accentuation, Figure 24.9). These murmurs are of low frequency, heard best with the bell of the stethoscope with the patient in the left lateral position. They too can be easily missed unless carefully sought.

A diastolic rumbling murmur may also be heard in patients with severe aortic regurgitation (Austin Flint murmur). This murmur has been ascribed to vibrations of

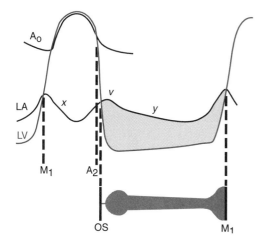

FIGURE 24.9. Mid-diastolic murmur in mitral stenosis. Left ventricular (LV), left atrial (LA), and aortic (Ao) pressure curves in mitral stenosis are shown. Note the elevated LA pressure. The pink-shaded area represents the LA-LV diastolic pressure gradient, showing the late diastolic rise in gradient associated with atrial contraction. The low-pitched diastolic rumble of mitral stenosis is immediately preceded by the high-pitched mitral opening snap (OS).

the anterior mitral leaflet sandwiched between the aortic regurgitant stream on one side and blood across the mitral orifice on the other.

Continuous murmurs

Continuous murmurs occur when a large and persistent pressure difference throughout the cardiac cycle exists. This may occur between two communicating chambers or vessels with no intervening valve or across a severely stenosed segment of an artery. Typically, a continuous murmur begins in systole and continues without interruption or change into diastole. These murmurs usually peak at S_2.

Pericardial friction rub

A pericardial friction rub is a superficial scratching sound heard over the precordium in acute pericarditis. Faint rubs are best heard with the patient sitting up and leaning forward; they are notorious for their evanescence. Friction rubs may be triphasic with systolic, diastolic, and presystolic components. The systolic component is loudest and virtually always present. All three components are present in only about 50% of cases.

Effects of physical maneuvers on murmurs

Certain physical maneuvers can profoundly affect murmur intensity by acutely changing loading conditions (Table 24.8). These maneuvers can augment the intensity of soft murmurs or gallops and aid in the differential diagnosis of various murmurs.

TABLE 24.8.	Effects of Physical Maneuvers on Heart Sounds and Murmurs		
Maneuver	**Technique**	**Pathophysiology**	**Effect**
Valsalva	Place hand on patient's abdomen and exert downward pressure as patient exerts outward pressure	During strain phase: ↓ venous return/cardiac output; ↓ LV chamber size	↓ Most heart sounds and murmurs except: • ↑ in HCM • MVP, earlier click and/or murmur
Rapid standing	Abrupt assumption of upright posture	Abrupt ↓ in venous return	Augments in HCM and MVP ↓ in aortic stenosis, mitral and tricuspid insufficiency
Respiration	Normal respiration	Inspiration: ↑ venous return	Inspiration ↑ right heart murmurs and gallops
Isometric handgrip	Sustained handgrip for 20–30 sec	↑ systemic resistance and arterial pressure	Augments aortic and mitral insufficiency, ventricular septal defect Decreases HCM and MVP
Post PVC or prolonged RR interval	Auscultate murmur in beat following a longer RR interval	↑ ventricular filling ↑ contractility	Augments aortic stenosis; No change in mitral insufficiency

HCM = hypertrophic cardiomyopathy; LV = left ventricle; MVP = mitral valve prolapse; PVC = premature ventricular contraction.

| CHAPTER **25** | ELECTROCARDIOGRAPHY |

■ Anatomy of the Conduction System

The **sinus node** is located in the right atrium near its junction with the superior vena cava, and the **atrioventricular (AV) node** is located in the right atrium between the opening of the coronary sinus and attachment of the septal leaflet of the tricuspid valve. The AV node is continuous with the **His bundle** that is present on the right side of the membranous ventricular septum. As it reaches the muscular portion of the ventricular septum, the His bundle continues as a slender **right bundle** on the right side of the ventricular septum to the apex of the RV and then enters the moderator band. Numerous branches from the His bundle penetrate the membranous ventricular septum below the aortic ring to enter the LV, where they are grouped into anterior and posterior fascicles of the **left bundle.** All three fascicles, i.e., the right-bundle and the anterior and posterior left-bundle branches, break into numerous Purkinje fibers that spread over the endocardial surfaces of the two ventricles.

■ Basic Electrophysiology

In the resting or polarized state, there is a 20-fold greater concentration of K^+ intracellularly than extracellularly, making the inside of the myocardial cell electrically negative by −90 mV as compared to the outside (Figure 25.1). On **depolarization** (phase 0), a sudden influx of Na^+ into the cell through specific Na^+ channels (fast channels) in the cell membrane causes the inside of the cell to become rapidly positive (+20 mV). Phase 1 **(initial repolarization)** ensues, during which the potential falls from +20 to 0 mV. In turn, this phase is followed by phase 2, or the **plateau** phase, which indicates slow repolarization caused predominantly by Ca^{++} influx. In phase 3, **rapid repolarization** occurs owing to the efflux of K^+ from the cell, enabling the membrane potential to return to the resting level. During phase 4, the Na^+ efflux and K^+ influx maintain the cell in its **resting,** or polarized, state.

Cells that can spontaneously generate an electrical impulse are present in the sinus node and AV junction. These pacemaker cells show a spontaneous diastolic depolarization; i.e., the resting membrane potential drifts slowly upward during phase 4 until the threshold is reached, and then another action potential results. The normal cardiac impulse arises in the sinus node and travels through the anterior, middle, and posterior internodal tracts to the AV node. Upon reaching the AV node, the impulse suddenly slows (decremental conduction, 50 mm/sec) and, after about 60–100 ms, enters the His-Purkinje system. From the AV node, the impulse travels rapidly (2000–3000 mm/sec) over the His-Purkinje system. Thereafter, conduction from the endocardium to the epicardium is relatively slow (200–500 mm/sec).

The midportion of the ventricular septum is activated from left to right, followed sequentially by the lower septum, RV apex, RV free wall, LV free wall, and bases of both ventricles. The RV outflow tract, or crista supraventricularis, is activated last. Repolarization follows the same pathway as depolarization, with the exception of the ventricular wall, which repolarizes from the epicardium to the endocardium.

The normal rate of impulse formation in the sinus node is 60–100 beats per minute. The sinus node is controlled by the sympathetic and parasympathetic nervous system. If the sinus node fails, the AV junction depolarizes the heart at a rate of 40–60 beats per minute. If both the sinus node and AV junction fail, the His-Purkinje system will drive the heart at 20–40 beats per minute.

■ Electrocardiographic Leads

A graphic recording of changes in cardiac electrical potential as detected by an electrocardiograph is called an electrocardiogram (ECG) (Figure 25.2). Three standard bipolar ECG leads are commonly placed on the extremities. Lead I records the potential difference between the left arm and right arm; lead II, between the left leg and right arm; and lead III, between the left leg and left arm. The positive and negative sides of all leads are configured to record upright complexes in all three leads in normal persons. Three additional leads are placed on the extremities (the augmented leads aVR, aVL, and aVF) and, together with the three standard limb leads, make a hexaxial system that provides frontal plane representation on the ECG. The six precordial leads, V_1 through V_6, provide a horizontal (transverse) representation on the ECG.

The direction and spatial orientation of the electrical force profoundly affect the ECG waveform configuration in a given lead. By convention, a lead records an electrical force coming toward it as positive and one directed away from it as negative. If the electrical force is parallel to the lead, the recorded wave will show maximal amplitude whereas an electrical force

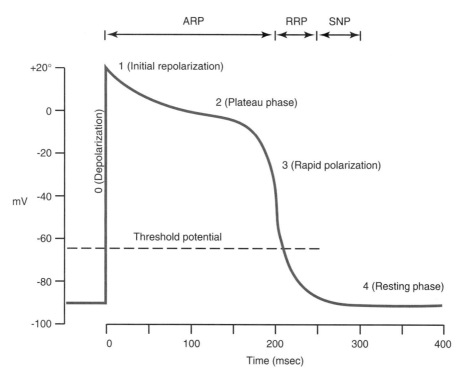

FIGURE 25.1. Action potential of the normal myocardial cell. The myocardial cell has a resting transmembrane potential (phase 4) of -90 mV. On excitation, the transmembrane potential is lowered to threshold potential, causing depolarization (phase 0), followed by three phases of repolarization, which return the cell to resting transmembrane potential (phase 4). During phases 1,2, and early phase 3, the cell is completely inexcitable (ARP, absolute refractory period). During the late phase 3, the cell is excitable by a strong stimulus (RRP, relative refractory period). During the last portion of phase 3, even a subthreshold stimulus can excite the cell. SNP = supernormal period.

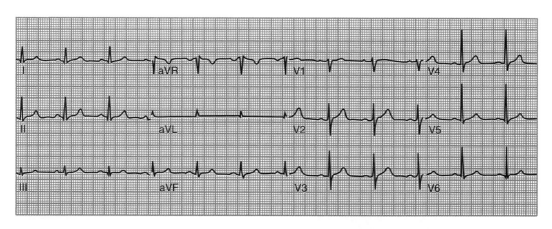

FIGURE 25.2. Normal ECG. A normal ECG shows, in sequence, P, QRS and T waves. It is recorded on graph paper for rapid measurement of time intervals and amplitudes. At a standard speed of 25 mm/s, the interval between vertical thin lines is 0.04 s. At standard calibration, a 1-mm height equals 0.1 mV.

perpendicular to the lead may show little voltage deflection.

■ Normal Electrocardiogram

Electrical axis on the ECG

The ECG is recorded on graph paper for rapid measurements of time intervals and amplitudes. At a standard speed of 25 mm/sec, the interval between vertical thin lines is 0.04 second. At standard calibration, a 1 mm height equals 0.1 mV. A normal ECG shows, in sequence, P, QRS, and T waves (Figure 25.2). The surface ECG records only the net resultant electrical force. Given the depolarization of the entire heart in sequence, the direction (axis) of depolarization changes from moment to moment. The mean axis of the total depolarization of atria (mean P axis), ventricles (mean QRS axis), and ventricular repolarization (mean T axis) in the frontal plane can be calculated from the six limb leads, i.e., I, II, III, aVR, aVL, and aVF. In clinical practice, the mean QRS axis is more important than the other two axes (Figure 25.3).

In normal persons, the mean QRS axis is between −30° and +110° (Figure 25.3). An axis in the −30° to −90° range is abnormally deviated to the left, and an axis between +110° and 180° is abnormally deviated to the right; the axis in the right upper quadrant (−90° to +180°) could be an abnormal right or left axis deviation. A left axis deviation occurs in patients with inferior wall myocardial infarction and left anterior hemiblock. A right axis deviation is found in patients with RV hypertrophy, lateral wall infarction, and left posterior hemiblock. In infancy, the mean QRS axis is usually between +90° and +150° but shifts leftward with age.

P wave

Depolarization of the atria results in a P wave. As the impulse from the sinus node travels inferiorly and leftward, limb leads I, II, III, aVL, and aVF usually record an upright P wave, and aVR records a negative P wave because the impulse is traveling away from this lead. All precordial leads show a positive P wave, except V_1, which may show a positive, negative, or biphasic P wave.

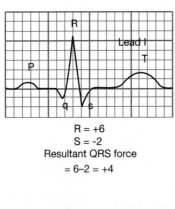

R = +6
S = -2
Resultant QRS force
= 6−2 = +4

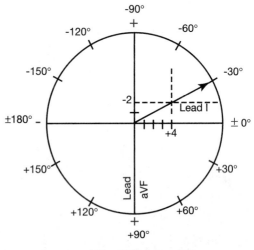

Mean QRS axis = -30°

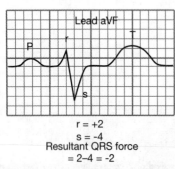

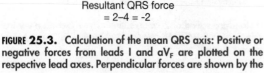

r = +2
s = -4
Resultant QRS force
= 2−4 = -2

FIGURE 25.3. Calculation of the mean QRS axis: Positive or negative forces from leads I and aV_F are plotted on the respective lead axes. Perpendicular forces are shown by the dotted lines. The line connecting the center with the point of intersection of perpendiculars represents the mean QRS axis.

A normal P wave is less than 2.5 mm high and less than 0.10 sec wide. Its initial portion represents right atrial depolarization and the terminal portion reflects left atrial depolarization.

P-R interval

The P-R interval, measured from the start of the P wave to the beginning of the QRS complex, indicates the time from the start of atrial depolarization to the beginning of ventricular activation. Normally 0.12 to 0.20 sec, this interval is inversely related to the heart rate. Most of the conduction delay occurs in the AV node.

QRS complex

The Q wave is the first negative wave and the R wave the first positive wave after a P wave. The S wave is the first negative wave after the R wave. The QRS complex reflects depolarization of the ventricles. The initial **Q wave,** an electrical force directed to the right and anteriorly, reflects depolarization of the left midseptum and is recorded as a small r (<5 mm) in lead V_1 and a small q (<2 mm) in leads I, aVL, V_5, and V6. The main QRS represents depolarization of the free ventricular walls. Because the LV muscle mass exceeds the RV muscle mass, the main depolarization force, which is oriented leftward and posteriorly, appears as an **R wave** in leads I, aVL, V_5, and V_6, and as an S in aVR, V_1, and V_2. The terminal **S wave** reflects activation of the base of the heart and RV outflow tract.

The QRS duration, normally 0.06 to 0.10 second, is the time period between initiation and completion of ventricular depolarization. Ventricular activation time (intrinsicoid deflection), measured from the onset of QRS to the peak of R, is the amount of time the electrical force takes to travel from the endocardium to the epicardium (normally <0.035 sec in V_1 or V_2 and <0.045 sec in V_5 or V_6).

ST segment

The ST segment is the isoelectric portion between the S and T waves. This segment denotes the time that the ventricles are partially repolarized, corresponding to phase 2 of the action potential.

T and U waves

The T wave reflects rapid repolarization of the ventricles. After the T wave, another positive wave, U, is sometimes seen, especially in the midprecordial leads. This wave is usually attributed to repolarization of the papillary muscles. The atrial repolarization produces a negative T wave that is difficult to identify because it is hidden by the QRS complex.

◼ ECG Changes in Specific Diseases

Myocardial ischemia, injury, and infarction

With severe and prolonged hypoperfusion, the affected myocardium progresses from a stage of reversible **ischemia,** to a stage of reversible **injury,** and finally to irreversible **infarction.** As ischemia persists, the area most deprived of blood supply—usually the subendocardial region—becomes necrotic. This necrotic region is surrounded by injured tissue that in turn is surrounded by ischemic tissue.

In **Q-wave infarction** (previously termed transmural infarction), the earliest ECG change is a tall and spiked T wave, followed by ST-segment elevation in leads facing the infarcted region and reciprocal ST-segment depression in the opposite leads. ST-segment elevation becomes isoelectric within the first few days. This regression unmasks a symmetrically inverted T wave, reflecting transmural ischemia. A few hours to a few days after the onset of ST-segment elevation, a pathologic Q wave appears in the same leads, which persists for months, years, or indefinitely and serves as an ECG sign of an old scar. Thus, the only ECG sign of acute myocardial injury is ST-segment elevation, which along with a new Q wave, indicates an acute Q-wave infarction (Figure 25.4). During the first few hours of an infarction, the ECG may be entirely normal.

Non–Q-wave infarction (previously termed subendocardial infarction) produces ST-segment depression and T-wave inversion without pathologic Q waves.

In some young, healthy subjects, a normal variant of repolarization occurs (Figure 25.5) with ST-segment elevation, primarily in leads I, aVL, and V_4 through V_6. The ST segment is concave upward and starts from the descending limb of the R wave before it reaches the baseline. No T-wave abnormalities are noted. This pattern may occasionally be confused for an infarct. An elevated ST segment in myocardial injury tends to be convex upward.

Cardiac hypertrophy

In **left atrial enlargement** (P-mitrale), the P wave is wider (>2.5 mm) and double-peaked, with the second peak representing left atrial depolarization. Since the P axis shifts leftward (−30° to +45°), the double-peaked P wave is best seen in leads I, II, aVL, and V_4 through V_6. In V_1, the P wave is biphasic and the terminal negative component is deep and wide (>0.04 sec). Left atrial enlargement is commonly seen in aortic stenosis, cardiomyopathy, hypertension, coronary artery disease, and mitral valve disease.

With **right atrial enlargement** (P-pulmonale), the P waves are tall (>2.5 mm) and spiked, usually in leads II, III, aVF, and V_1. The P axis shifts to the right (>+75°).

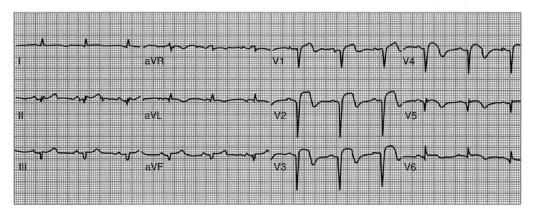

FIGURE 25.4. ECG changes in extensive, acute anterior myocardial infarction. ST-segment elevation, T-wave inversions, and Q waves can be seen in leads V_1 through V_6. The Q waves in leads II, III and aV_F are the residua of an old inferior wall myocardial infarction.

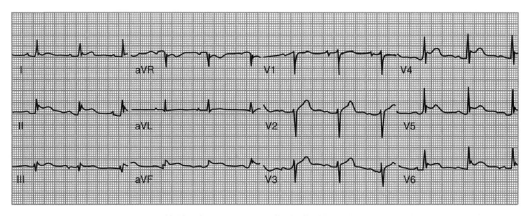

FIGURE 25.5. ECG showing early repolarization. ST-segment elevation with upward concavity is seen in leads I, II, aV_F, and V_3 through V_6. Persistence of this pattern over months and years is highly suggestive of early repolarization.

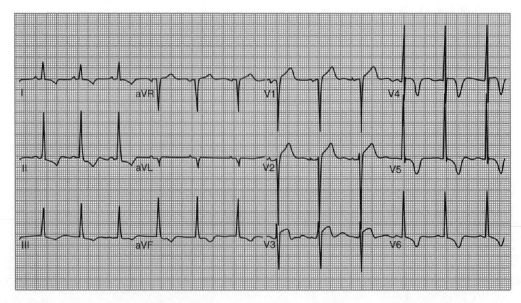

FIGURE 25.6. ECG changes in left ventricular hypertrophy. Note increased QRS voltage and secondary ST-T changes.

Right atrial enlargement occurs in pulmonary stenosis, pulmonary hypertension, cor pulmonale, and tricuspid stenosis.

Increased LV mass results in greater amplitude of QRS (Figure 25.6). Because voltage criteria alone may falsely suggest **LV hypertrophy,** especially in thin-chested individuals, the point scoring system described by Estes is more specific for diagnosis (Table 25.1). Similar diagnostic criteria are used for **RV hypertrophy** (Table 25.2, Figure 25.7).

Acute pericarditis

In acute pericarditis, virtually all the leads except aVR and V_1 record ST-segment elevation, indicating diffuse injury. As the inflammation subsides several days later, the ST segments become gradually isoelectric, and the T waves then become inverted.

Electrolyte disturbances and drug effects

In **hyperkalemia,** the T waves become tall and spiked (Figure 25.8). With an increasing degree of hyperkalemia, the P waves become less distinct and may totally disappear, the QRS complex widens, and ultimately, QRS-T assumes a sine-wave configuration. **Hypokalemia** produces ST-segment depression, T-wave flattening, and prominence of U and P waves. A progressively less distinct T wave merges into the U wave, causing prolongation of the Q-T (actually Q-U) interval. In severe hypokalemia, the QRS also widens. **Hypocalcemia** prolongs the ST segment, and **hypercalcemia** shortens the ST segment.

Digitalis produces a sagging or "hammock-shaped" ST depression, flat or inverted T waves, and shortened Q-T interval. These changes may follow even a therapeutic dose and, thus, constitute the "digitalis effect." Procainamide and quinidine prolong the Q-T interval, flatten or invert T waves, and widen the QRS.

TABLE 25.1.	Estes Criteria for Left Ventricular Hypertrophy (LVH)	
Criteria		**Points**

1. Voltage
   R and/or S >20 mm in any one or more
   of the six limb leads, OR
   S >25 mm in V_1, V_2 or V_3, OR
   R >25 mm in V_4, V_5 or V_6
		3

2. ST-segment deviation opposite to the main
   QRS complex
   In the absence of digitalis therapy
   In the presence of digitalis therapy
		3
		1

3. Left axis deviation (QRS axis to the left of −15°)		2
4. QRS duration >0.09 s		1
5. Ventricular activation time >0.04 s		1

A sum of 4 points indicates probable LVH and ≥5 points indicates definite LVH.

TABLE 25.2.	Diagnostic Criteria for Right Ventricular Hypertrophy
Right axis deviation (QRS axis to the right of +110°) R/S ratio in lead V_1 >1, provided R in V_1 is >5 mm R in V_2 >7 mm R in V_1 + S in V_5 or V_6 >10.5 mm Secondary ST-segment depression and T-wave inversion in leads V_1 and V_2 Persistence of prominent S wave in leads V_4 through V_6	

Neurologic conditions

In neurologic conditions such as head trauma and subarachnoid hemorrhage, an ECG may show bizarre, wide and tall, or deeply inverted T waves with Q-T prolongation.

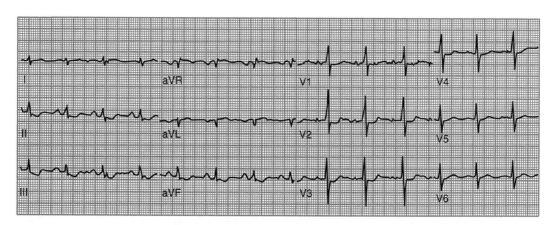

FIGURE 25.7. ECG changes in right ventricular hypertrophy. Note the rightward mean QRS axis, prominent R wave in V_1 with R/S ratio of >1, and persistence of S waves in leads V_5 and V_6.

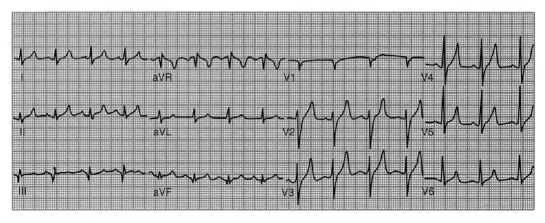

FIGURE 25.8. ECG changes in hyperkalemia. Note the tall and spiky T waves in most leads, especially V$_2$ through V$_6$.

CHAPTER 26   NONINVASIVE CARDIAC IMAGING

■ Roentgenography

Chest radiography permits an assessment of the size and configuration of the heart and great vessels, the pulmonary vascularity, and calcification of cardiac valves and other structures.

Cardiac silhouette

The **cardiothoracic ratio,** which is an index of cardiac size (normal is <0.5), can be determined on standard chest radiographs by dividing the maximal transverse width of the heart by the maximal internal width of the thorax above the diaphragm. On posteroanterior (PA) and special oblique views, chest radiograph is useful in screening for enlargement of specific heart chambers; however, this technique is only moderately reliable, and echocardiography is the preferred method of assessing chamber sizes.

Great vessels

A dilated **pulmonary artery** accentuates the shadow of the pulmonary artery segment seen on the left heart border and occurs in conditions of increased pulmonary blood flow (e.g., left-to-right shunts), pulmonary arterial hypertension, and poststenotic dilatation in pulmonary valvular stenosis. An attenuated pulmonary artery segment occurs in the tetralogy of Fallot, tricuspid atresia, and Ebstein's anomaly.

In a PA projection, dilatation of the **ascending aorta** (as in aortic valvular stenosis and aneurysms of the ascending aorta) causes a prominent convexity of the right upper cardiac shadow. Dilatation, elongation, and

tortuosity of the **aortic arch** cause a prominent aortic knob. Hypertension, arteriosclerosis, and aortic insufficiency produce aortic dilatation.

Pulmonary vascularity

A careful examination of the lung fields in a chest radiograph discloses the pulmonary vascularity. Differentiating pulmonary arteries from veins on chest radiographs is difficult; it is, however, easier in the right lung field. In general, upper lobe veins are vertical and remain lateral to the corresponding arteries. The lower lobe veins are more horizontal, remain medial to the arteries, and are usually more prominent than those in the upper lung fields.

In left heart failure and mitral stenosis, as pulmonary venous pressure increases, the veins in the upper lung fields become more prominent than those in the lower lung fields (redistribution of the pulmonary blood flow). When the pulmonary wedge pressure approaches 25–30 mm Hg, it exceeds the capillary oncotic pressure and fluid accumulates in the lung interstitium. The lung fields appear hazy and the small pulmonary vessels indistinct. **Kerley's B lines,** attributed to thickened interlobular septa owing to edema, appear as 1-2-cm horizontal lines in the lower lung fields near the costophrenic angles (Figure 26.1). Worsening of heart disease prompts further fluid transudation into the alveoli, causing **pulmonary edema** (which appears on chest radiographs as confluent opacities in the central lung fields resembling butterfly or bat wings) or interlobar and/or **pleural effusions.**

Pulmonary arteries gradually taper as they proceed peripherally. Enlarged central pulmonary arteries that abruptly taper peripherally indicate pulmonary arterial hypertension (cor pulmonale, Eisenmenger's syndrome, or primary pulmonary hypertension). In severe pulmonary hypertension that follows left heart disease, both pulmonary veins and arteries become prominent. In large left-to-right shunts, the central and peripheral arteries also become enlarged without any sudden peripheral tapering.

Calcification

Calcification of various cardiac structures is visible on PA chest radiographs but is more easily detected using fluoroscopy. Mitral valvular calcification indicates prior rheumatic disease. A congenitally bicuspid aortic valve, the pericardium in constrictive pericarditis, atrial myxomas, ventricular aneurysms, intracardiac blood clots, and the coronary artery walls may all undergo calcification.

■ Echocardiography

Echocardiography uses ultrasound, generated by a piezoelectric crystal held against the chest wall, to image cardiac structures. It is used in three types of studies. **Motion mode (M-mode) tracings,** which show motion within a single beam of sound, lack spatial orientation, but the resulting high-resolution record of the cardiac cycle helps to *time* events and measure chamber diameters easily.

Two-dimensional (2D) echocardiography provides a two-dimensional image by steering the sound beam 30 times/sec through an arc of up to 90°. The images obtained from several transducer positions on the chest wall or upper abdomen (transthoracic 2D echo) provide

superior *spatial* resolution, allowing assessment of structural movement in real time. **Transesophageal echocardiography,** obtained by placing a transducer in the esophagus, provides excellent two-dimensional images of the posterior cardiac chambers and aorta.

Doppler **echocardiography** can provide information on blood flow within the heart. The sound reflected by red cells moving within the heart changes frequency (Doppler shift) in proportion to the cells' velocity, allowing one to measure the direction and velocity of blood flow through the cardiac valves and to detect abnormal flow patterns.

Echocardiography is useful in imaging structural abnormalities that underlie numerous heart diseases. It can detect mitral valve prolapse, mitral and aortic stenosis, valvular vegetations, congenital diseases, and intracardiac tumors. Transesophageal echocardiography is superior to transthoracic echo for evaluating the function of prosthetic valves; investigating atrial masses, atrial septal defects, and aortic dissection; and monitoring ventricular function during cardiac surgery. In addition to determining blood-flow velocity across stenotic valves, Doppler echocardiography can be used to calculate transvalvular pressure gradient and to detect and quantify regurgitant lesions. Echocardiography is the test of choice for detecting, quantifying, and locating pericardial effusion and tamponade.

Echocardiography, in conjunction with exercise or pharmacologic stress (**stress echocardiography**), is also useful in detecting coronary artery disease. Echocardiography allows evaluation of LV function, detecting abnormal LV segmental wall motion and the compli-

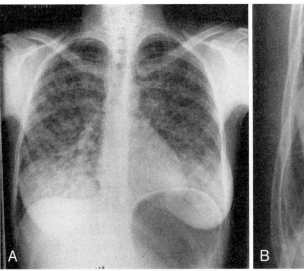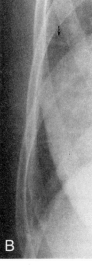

FIGURE 26.1. Chest radiograph showing left heart failure with diffuse lung infiltration (**panel A**). Kerley B lines, seen in the periphery of the right lung, are better seen in the magnified view (**panel B**).
(Courtesy, Radiology Museum, St. Joseph's Hospital, Milwaukee, Wisconsin.)

cations of myocardial infarction. With two-dimensional echocardiography, LV volumes and ejection fraction can be measured, and cardiac output can be measured on a beat-by-beat basis using Doppler echocardiography.

■ Radionuclide Imaging

Three types of radionuclide imaging procedures are clinically useful in cardiac diagnosis: radionuclide angiocardiography, myocardial perfusion imaging, and infarct imaging.

Angiocardiography

The most commonly used radionuclide for cardiac angiography is **technetium 99m** (^{99m}Tc), which is tagged to the patient's own red blood cells. This technique helps determine systolic and diastolic ventricular function and intracardiac shunts.

In the **first-pass method,** a scintillation camera records the activity of a peripherally injected radionuclide bolus as it travels for the first time through the cardiac chambers and blood vessels. In the **equilibrium method** (multigated acquisition, MUGA), images of the heart are recorded over several hundred cardiac cycles for several minutes after the radionuclide has equilibrated throughout the vasculature. A computer generates a single, composite cycle. The resulting ventricular images, displayed in a cine format throughout the cardiac cycle, greatly facilitate the detection of segmental wall motion abnormalities.

With either method, the ejection fraction and absolute end-diastolic and end-systolic volumes of the ventricles can be calculated. Radionuclide angiocardiography has many clinical applications (Table 26.1).

Myocardial perfusion imaging

The imaging stress test enhances the accuracy of the standard electrocardiographic treadmill stress test by nearly 10–20% in detecting coronary artery disease.

Thallium-201(^{201}Tl) and ^{99m}Tc-Sesta MIBI are the most suitable radionuclides for myocardial perfusion imaging. As a biological substitute for ionic K^+, ^{201}Tl is rapidly extracted from the bloodstream by normally functioning myocardial cells. Ischemic or infarcted areas accumulate little ^{201}Tl and appear "cold." Following initial uptake by myocardial cells, ^{201}Tl undergoes exchange with the systemic pool and gradual equilibration so that transiently ischemic areas show reversible defects (i.e., perfusion defects in the initial scans return to near-normal perfusion in the delayed images) (Figure 26.2). However, infarcted areas show fixed defects. In

TABLE 26.1.	Clinical Applications of Radionuclide Angiocardiography	
Objective	Setting	Comments
Determine/monitor LV function	Chest pain and abnormal baseline ECG, or Asymptomatic patients with a positive exercise ECG.	May detect coronary artery disease, which can be confirmed by coronary angiography
	Recent myocardial infarction	Significant reduction in LVEF (≤40%) indicates poor prognosis
	During or following therapy with cardiotoxic drugs (e.g., doxorubicin)	May detect myocardial damage from drugs
	Aortic regurgitation	May help determine optimal timing for intervention
	Congestive heart failure	May detect an etiology (LV aneurysm or global LV dysfunction)
Detect RV dysfunction	Acute inferior wall myocardial infarction	RV dysfunction may cause a low output state in inferior wall myocardial infarction
Detect RV and LV dysfunction	Chronic obstructive lung disease	Long term oxygen therapy may be needed with RV dysfunction; overall management may be altered by LV dysfunction
Detect and quantitate intracardiac shunts	Unexplained hypoxemia and/or erythrocytosis	—

LV = left ventricular; ECG = electrocardiography; LVEF = left ventricular ejection fraction; RV = right ventricular.

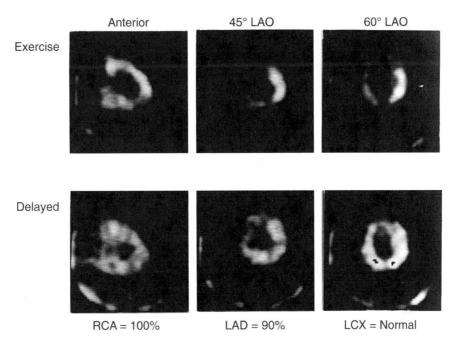

Exercise   Anterior   45° LAO   60° LAO

Delayed

RCA = 100%   LAD = 90%   LCX = Normal

FIGURE 26.2. Exercise thallium-201 perfusion imaging. **Exercise images** *(top panels)* show perfusion immediately after exercise in anterior, 45° left anterior oblique (LAO), and 60° LAO views. Perfusion defects are evident in the septal and inferior segments. **Delayed images** *(bottom panels),* repeated 4 hours after exercise, show that the perfusion defects have "filled in," indicating reversible myocardial ischemia in the septal and inferior segments. Coronary angiography (not shown) revealed total occlusion of the right coronary artery (RCA), 90% stenosis of left anterior descending (LAD) artery, and normal left circumflex (LCX) artery.

severe coronary disease owing to exercise-induced left ventricular (LV) failure, initial images may show LV dilatation and increased lung uptake of ^{201}Tl.

Intravenous dipyridamole or adenosine may be used in patients unable to exercise **(pharmacologic stress).** These agents greatly augment blood flow through the normal—but not stenotic—coronary vessels resulting in heterogeneity of blood flow among different myocardial regions. The accuracy of pharmacologic stress tests is similar to that of exercise imaging tests.

Myocardial perfusion imaging is clinically useful in patients with resting abnormal ECGs in whom an exercise ECG would be unreliable and in patients who cannot achieve near-maximal heart rates during exercise stress tests. Current clinical applications are summarized in Table 26.2.

Infarct imaging

Technetium-99m stannous pyrophosphate (^{99m}Tc-PYP) binds to calcium and organic macromolecules in the acutely damaged myocardium and appears as a "hot spot" on perfusion imaging. Unlike the fixed defects of ^{201}Tl imaging, which cannot distinguish acute from old

TABLE 26.2. **Clinical Applications of Myocardial Perfusion Imaging**

Diagnosis of coronary artery disease
  Patients with an intermediate pre-test likelihood of disease
  Asymptomatic patients with positive exercise ECG test
  Non-anginal chest pain in middle-aged or elderly men
  Non-anginal chest pain in patients with positive or inconclusive exercise ECG test
  Patients with atypical angina
  Typical angina in men <40 years and in women <60 years
  Typical angina in patients with negative exercise ECG test.
Evaluation for multi-vessel disease
  Perfusion defects in multivessel territories
  Exercise-induced LV dilatation
  Increased lung uptake of ^{201}Tl
Assess myocardial viability in hypokinetic areas of LV
Assessment of efficacy of angioplasty/detection of restenosis
  Serial ^{201}Tl imaging before and after coronary angioplasty

infarctions, ^{99m}Tc-PYP delineates only the acutely infarcted myocardium. ^{99m}Tc-PYP imaging becomes positive 48 hours after acute myocardial infarction and remains positive for 6 days. The sensitivity and specificity are excellent for Q-wave infarction but less accurate for non–Q-wave infarction.

The main clinical use of ^{99m}Tc-PYP imaging is to confirm, localize, and evaluate the size of an acute myocardial infarction in patients in whom serial ECGs are inconclusive or difficult to interpret. False-positive results occur in some cases of unstable angina, myocardial contusion, ventricular aneurysms, and calcified heart valves and also after electrical defibrillation.

<table><tr><td>CHAPTER</td><td>27</td></tr></table>

CARDIAC CATHETERIZATION

Cardiac catheterization is a powerful diagnostic tool that provides precise assessment of anatomic and physiologic changes in many cardiovascular diseases. Because this technique provides direct and definitive information, it is considered the gold standard against which various noninvasive tests are judged. In general, this technique permits measurements of the following:

1. Pressures in various cardiac chambers and blood vessels

2. Pressure gradients across stenotic cardiac valves

3. Cardiac output

4. Systemic and pulmonary vascular resistances

5. Hemodynamic changes during stress (e.g., supine exercise)

6. Shunts between systemic and pulmonary vessels

Selective injection of contrast material during catheterization helps define the coronary anatomy, quantify valvular regurgitation, calculate the chamber volume (particularly the LV end-diastolic and end-systolic volumes and ejection fraction). This technique permits cardiac pacing and electrophysiologic studies. In addition, several therapeutic modalities, such as coronary angioplasty, atherectomy, stent placement, and selective administration of thrombolytic agents, can be performed during the procedure (chapters 31 and 32).

■ Measurement of Intravascular Pressures

A fluid-filled catheter is routinely introduced into the vascular system to record pressure curves from the cardiac chambers and great vessels. Phasic and mean (electronically measured) pressures are usually recorded from the right atrium, pulmonary artery, pulmonary capillary wedge position, and aorta, but only phasic

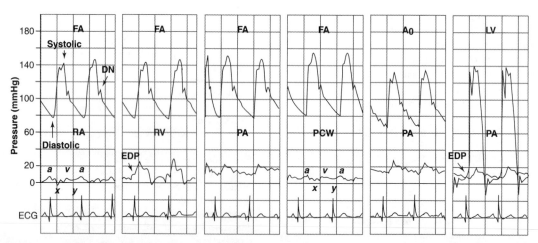

FIGURE 27.1. Phasic pressure curves obtained from different cardiac chambers and vessels during right and left heart catheterization. FA = femoral artery; Ao = aorta; LV = left ventricle; RA = right atrium; RV = right ventricle; PA = pulmonary artery; PCW = pulmonary capillary wedge; DN = dicrotic notch; EDP = end-diastolic pressure.

TABLE 27.1.	Normal Values for Intravascular Pressure Measurements				
Site	Systolic Pressure (mm Hg)	End-Diastolic Pressure (mm Hg)	a wave (mm Hg)	v wave (mm Hg)	Mean Pressure (mm Hg)
Right atrium	—	—	2.5–9	2–7	1–5
Right ventricle	15–30	0–8	—	—	—
Pulmonary artery	15–30	3–12	—	—	9–20
Pulmonary capillary wedge	—	—	4–6	6–20	3–12
Left ventricle	90–140	4–14	—	—	—
Aorta	90–140	60–90	—	—	70–105

pressures are recorded from the right and left ventricles (Figure 27.1). The mean pressure is calculated as the diastolic pressure plus one-third of the pulse pressure. Tables 27.1 and 27.2 list the normal values for various hemodynamic measurements obtained by cardiac catheterization.

Normally, the pulmonary artery diastolic, mean pulmonary capillary wedge, mean left atrial, and LV diastolic pressures *prior to atrial contraction* are similar. Thus, pulmonary artery diastolic or pulmonary artery wedge pressure accurately reflects the LV filling pressure and can be readily monitored at bedside by a *pulmonary artery* (Swan-Ganz) catheter.

■ Measurement of Cardiac Output

Cardiac output (systemic blood flow) is usually expressed as the cardiac index (L/min/m^2) after correction for body surface area. It can be measured by three methods:

- In the **Fick** method, cardiac output is calculated by dividing the oxygen consumption (VO$_2$, in ml/min) by the arteriovenous oxygen difference (in ml/L).
- In the **indicator-dilution** method, a bolus of indocyanine green dye is injected into the pulmonary artery, and its concentration in the systemic circulation (LV, aorta, or peripheral artery) is continuously recorded; cardiac output is calculated from the time-concentration curve.
- In the **thermodilution** method, a bolus of cold saline is injected into the right atrium through a multilumen catheter. The thermistor at the catheter tip, positioned in the pulmonary artery, senses an initial decrease in temperature followed by a progressive rise, and the time-temperature curve thus obtained helps compute the cardiac output.

■ Other Studies

Vascular resistance, or resistance to blood flow, is calculated separately for the systemic and pulmonary

TABLE 27.2.	Normal Values for Hemodynamic and Flow Measurements
Measurement	Normal Values
Cardiac index	2.5–4.2 L/min/m^2
Stroke index	40–70 ml/m^2
Stroke work index	40–80 g·m/m^2
Pulmonary vascular resistance	0.2–3 Wood units
Systemic vascular resistance	10–20 Wood units
Oxygen consumption	110–150 ml/min/m^2
Arterio-venous oxygen difference	30–50 ml/L blood
LV end-diastolic volume	50–90 ml/m^2
LV end-systolic volume	14–34 ml/m^2
LV ejection fraction	50–75%

LV = left ventricular.

$$\text{Wood units} = \frac{\text{Pressure difference (mm Hg)}}{\text{Flow (L/min)}}$$

circulations. The functional **orifice area** of stenotic valves can be calculated by measuring the pressure gradient and blood flow across the valve. The angiographic stroke volume minus the Fick stroke volume indicates the amount of blood regurgitating across the incompetent valve.

The presence of an abnormal communication between the systemic and pulmonary circulations allows **shunting** of blood from one to the other without traversing the capillary bed. The magnitude of the shunts can be calculated by oximetry or the indicator-dilution method. Cineangiocardiography, following selective injection of contrast material, is helpful in localizing the shunt.

■ Indications for Cardiac Catheterization

The primary role of cardiac catheterization is to provide precise anatomic and physiologic information about cardiac abnormality in patients in whom surgical intervention is being contemplated. The recent

TABLE 27.3.	Indications for Bedside Pulmonary Artery Catheterization
Acute myocardial infarction complicated by: 　Moderate or severe heart failure 　Hypotension not easily corrected by volume infusion 　Suspected right ventricular infarction 　Mechanical complications 　　Ventricular septal rupture 　　Papillary muscle rupture 　　Ventricular free wall rupture with cardiac tamponade Intractable postinfarction ischemia	Intractable heart failure, before inotropic and vasodilator 　therapy Confirmation and management of cardiac tamponade Differentiation between cardiogenic and noncardiogenic 　pulmonary edema Perioperative monitoring in high-risk cardiac patients Management of sepsis and/or multisystem organ 　dysfunction

availability of pulmonary artery catheters has made bedside hemodynamic monitoring practical and extended its use to coronary and intensive care units (Table 27.3).

The incidence of complications of cardiac catheterization relates to the underlying heart disease and experience of the operator. Right heart catheterization is associated with minimal morbidity and no mortality in adults. In most cardiac catheterization laboratories and with experienced operators, the risk of death with coronary catheterization is less than 0.1% and the incidence of arterial complications is 1.0% or less.

CHAPTER 28 DISORDERS OF CARDIAC RHYTHM AND CONDUCTION

■ **Basic Electrophysiologic Principles and Applied Pharmacology of Antiarrhythmic Agents**

The cardiac transmembrane potential, as explained in chapter 25, consists of five phases resulting from ion fluxes (see Figure 25.1). In the myocardium, there are "fast" and "slow" response cell types, which differ in the ions to which they respond and in other electrophysiologic respects. **Fast-response** cell types are found in atrial and ventricular myocardium and the His-Purkinje system. **Slow-response** cell types occur in the sinoatrial (SA) and atrioventricular (AV) nodes. Phase 0 is caused by the rapid influx of either sodium (fast-response cell types) or calcium (slow-response cell types). Phase 2 is mediated by slow calcium influx, and phase 3, by potassium efflux.

As would be expected from the respective ions involved, inhibitors of fast-response cell types (Na^+-dependent tissue) are the local anesthetics and related antiarrhythmic agents, such as sodium channel blockers. Conversely, inhibitors of slow-response cell types (Ca^{++}-dependent tissue) include the calcium-channel-blocking agents.

Terms

Automaticity refers to the initiation of cardiac impulses as a result of spontaneous depolarization during phase 4. When this diastolic depolarization reaches a threshold, a spontaneous action potential results. Cells in the SA node, distal AV node, some atrial tissue, and the His-Purkinje system normally possess this property of automaticity and can initiate a spontaneous action potential. Owing to its inherently higher discharge rate, the sinus node suppresses these other potential automatic foci and thus masterminds the cardiac rhythm.

Conduction is the propagation of a cardiac impulse and is most closely related to phase 0 of the action potential. Interventions that affect phase 0 will affect conduction.

The (absolute) **refractory period** is defined as the minimum interval between two propagating impulses. The refractory period is most closely linked to the action potential duration (length of phase 3) in most cardiac cells. Agents that lengthen phase 3 will lengthen the refractory period, prolonging the period of time during which a cell is unable to initiate an action potential following completion of an earlier action potential.

Nervous system stimulation

The **autonomic nervous system** has little direct effect on fast-response cell types but significantly alters conduction velocity and the rate of automaticity in slow-response cell types. **Sympathetic** stimulation causes enhanced calcium influx, which leads to an increase in both conduction velocity and the slope of phase 4 diastolic depolarization in slow-response cell types, thus increasing the rate of firing. **Parasympathetic** stimulation causes enhanced potassium efflux, causing cell hyperpolarization and a decrease in the slope of phase 4 diastolic depolarization with a reduction in cell firing rate. Parasympathetic stimulation also provokes a reduction in conduction velocity of AV nodal cells.

Mechanisms of cardiac arrhythmias

Cardiac arrhythmias can be broadly divided according to their mechanisms into abnormalities of impulse formation (automaticity), impulse conduction, or both. Although the precise mechanism of most clinical arrhythmias cannot yet be identified, contending that a given arrhythmia is most likely caused by one electrophysiological mechanism or another is possible. Additionally, many variables can precipitate or exacerbate arrhythmias, including myocardial ischemia, hypoxia, congestive heart failure, electrolyte abnormalities, scarred myocardium, drug toxicity, or antiarrhythmic drug use.

Abnormalities of automaticity

Abnormalities of automaticity include **inappropriate rates of discharge** of the sinus node, which is the normal cardiac pacemaker (e.g., inappropriate sinus bradycardia or tachycardia), or of an ectopic pacemaker, which gains control of the atrial or ventricular rhythm (e.g., paroxysmal atrial tachycardia, accelerated idioventricular rhythm, accelerated junctional rhythm, and nonparoxysmal junctional tachycardia).

A second category of abnormalities of automaticity includes **triggered activity.** Triggered activity is caused by **afterdepolarizations,** which are abnormal action potentials arising as a consequence of an earlier action potential. They cannot arise *de novo* but are entirely dependent on a preceding impulse (the "trigger") for their generation. Afterdepolarizations may occur singly or trigger other afterdepolarizations. **Torsades de pointes,** a unique type of polymorphic ventricular tachycardia, is one such example.

Abnormalities of conduction

Abnormalities of impulse conduction include **conduction delay** or **block** with or without **reentry.** A bradyarrhythmia may occur in the absence of reentry (e.g., AV block, bundle-branch blocks). In the presence of reentry, tachyarrhythmias may occur if reentry causes a self-perpetuating tachycardia. Most forms of ventricular tachycardia and many atrial tachycardias occur on the basis of a reentrant mechanism.

Mechanisms of reentry

Reentry can occur in all portions of the cardiac electrical system. Reentry requires 1) an area of depressed conduction with unidirectional block (i.e., retrograde but not antegrade conduction occurs at the depressed site) and 2) slow impulse propagation in the retrograde direction at the depressed site (Figure 28.1). As mentioned, reentry in the ventricular muscle may prompt ventricular tachycardia. Other reentrant loops may involve atrial muscle fibers (atrial fibrillation and flutter), the AV node (AV nodal reentrant tachycardia),

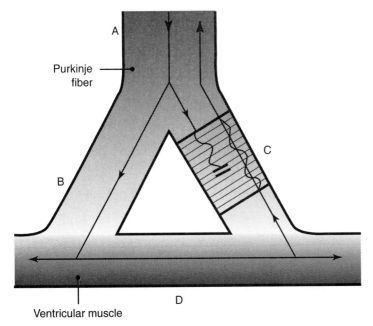

FIGURE 28.1. Mechanism of reentry in a branched terminal of the Purkinje system contacting ventricular muscle. An impulse traveling antegrade in Purkinje fiber *A* is blocked by a unidirectional block in Purkinje fiber *C*. However, the initial impulse from fiber *A* is able to conduct normally through Purkinje fiber *B* to ventricular muscle *D*. This impulse then travels retrograde to the distal branch of fiber *C* (which has not yet been depolarized) and through the site of the unidirectional block to again reach fiber *A*. If retrograde conduction through the site of unidirectional block is slow enough for the cells of fiber *A* to have regained excitability, then a self-perpetuating circuit or reentrant loop is formed. In this example, ventricular tachycardia would result.

Purkinje fiber

Ventricular muscle

and large reentrant loops comprised of the atria and ventricles linked not only by the AV node but also by specialized conducting tissue known as **accessory pathways** (Wolff-Parkinson-White syndrome).

Any factor that leads to a local alteration of conduction and/or refractoriness may lead to a reentrant rhythm. Examples include localized myocardial fibrosis, premature stimuli (such as premature atrial or ventricular complexes), or acute myocardial ischemia.

Halting reentrant rhythms

Reentrant arrhythmias can be interrupted by interventions that disrupt the reentrant circuit. This disruption may be accomplished through mechanical intervention, such as catheter-based radio-frequency ablation (destruction) of accessory pathways, or through pharmacologic means with antiarrhythmic agents. Antiarrhythmic agents prevent tachyarrhythmias in multiple ways. They may disrupt a reentrant circuit by either producing bidirectional block at the former site of unidirectional block in

a Purkinje fiber or by prolonging the refractory period of tissue in the region proximal to the site of unidirectional block, making this tissue unexcitable (Figure 28.2). These agents may also preempt reentrant rhythms by preventing the formation of premature stimuli.

Proarrhythmia

Antiarrhythmic agents, in particular those in Class I and Class III (see Table 28.1), have proarrhythmic potential. These agents, because of their ability to alter conduction and/or refractoriness, can lead to the development or exacerbation of ventricular arrhythmias in 2–10% of patients, especially those with decreased LV systolic function.

Antiarrhythmic agents

Antiarrhythmic agents are commonly grouped in classes according to the Vaughan Williams classification scheme (Table 28.1). Although this scheme has many

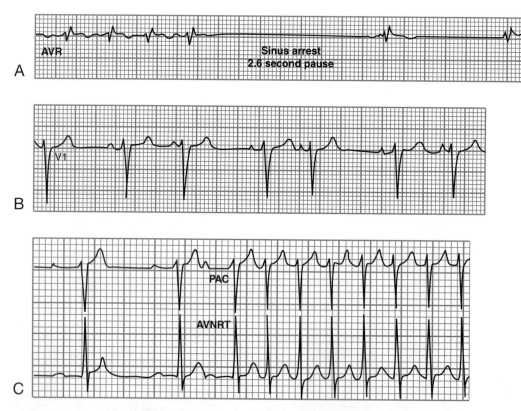

FIGURE 28.2. A. Sinus arrest. Following a run of supraventricular tachycardia at a rate of 110 beats/min, sinus arrest occurs, resulting in a 2.6-sec pause, followed by a slow junctional escape rhythm at a rate of 30 beats/min. This type of alteration, between a tachyarrhythmia and a bradyarrhythmia, is characteristic of the sick-sinus syndrome.

B. **Premature atrial complexes.** In this strip, PACs are conducted without aberration. C. **AV nodal reentrant tachycardia (AVNRT).** A PAC is found to initiate a run of AVNRT at a rate of 170 beats/min. No P waves are evident because they are obscured in the QRS complex.

TABLE 28.1.	Vaughan Williams Classification of Antiarrhythmic Drugs				
Class	**Category**	**Subclass**	**Agent(s)**	**Primary Electrophysiological Effect**	
I	Sodium-channel blockers	A	Procainamide Disopyramide Quinidine	Moderate inhibition of phase 0 depolarization Slows conduction Prolongs action potential duration, and thus refractory period	
		B	Lidocaine Tocainide Mexiletine	Mild/moderate inhibition of phase 0 depolarization, Minimal effect on conduction Shortens action potential duration and thus refractory period	
		C	Flecainide Propafenone	Marked inhibition of phase 0 depolarization Marked slowing of conduction Little effect on action potential duration	
II	β-adrenergic receptor blockers		Propranolol Atenolol Metoprolol Others	In absence of catecholamines, no electrophysiological effect In presence of catecholamines, slows SA nodal discharge rate and slows conduction through AV node	
III	Potassium-channel blockers		Amiodarone Bretylium Sotalol	Prolongs repolarization	
IV	Calcium-channel blockers		Verapamil Diltiazem	Active in slow-response cells Slows SA nodal discharge rate Slows conduction and increases refractory period of AV node	

limitations, and although agents within a given class may differ significantly in their electrophysiologic, hemodynamic, or myocardial depressant effects, the scheme nonetheless enhances communication concerning these agents. The safe use of any antiarrhythmic drug depends on a thorough knowledge of its pharmacology, dose range, metabolism, drug interactions, and side-effect profile (Table 28.2).

Specific Arrhythmias

Normal sinus rhythm arises from the sinus node. In adults, the normal discharge rate is between 60 and 100 beats per minute. The P wave is normally upright in leads I, II, and aVF and inverted in lead aVR.

Sinus Nodal and Atrial Rhythm Disturbances

■ Sinus Tachycardia

Sinus rhythm with a heart rate exceeding 100 beats per minute is termed **sinus tachycardia.** The sinus node responds to sympathetic or parasympathetic stimulation with either an increase or decrease, respectively, in the rate of phase 4 diastolic depolarization, which in turn leads to an increase or decrease in the sinus node discharge rate. Numerous stresses may cause sinus tachycardia, including anxiety or excitement, fever, congestive heart failure, and sympathomimetic (e.g., albuterol) and vagolytic drugs (e.g., atropine).

■ Sinus Bradycardia

Sinus bradycardia is sinus rhythm at a rate less than 60 beats/min. Physiologic **sinus bradycardia** occurs in well-conditioned athletes with enhanced vagal tone and in the elderly. Pharmacologic agents (e.g., digoxin, β-blockers, diltiazem, verapamil), maneuvers (e.g., eyeball manipulation, carotid sinus massage), and various disease states (e.g., hypothyroidism, sick sinus syndrome) may prompt sinus bradycardia. Usually, augmented stroke volume compensates for the slower heart rate; thus, cardiac output remains adequate. The only current long-term solution to symptomatic sinus bradycardia is electrical pacing.

TABLE 28.2. An Overview of Antiarrhythmic Drugs

Drug	Direct Electrophysiological Actions	Effect on ECG	Clinical Indications	Dose	Major Route of Elimination	Adverse Effects/Drug Interactions
Class I A Quinidine	Reduces conduction velocity and prolongs refractoriness in most cardiac tissues. Suppresses automaticity from ectopic sites. Mild alpha-blocker and vagolytic agent, thus may enhance AV conduction.	Prolongs the QT interval; mildly prolongs QRS complex.	SV/Ventr arrhythmias. Slows the intrinsic (atrial) rate of atrial arrhythmias, but may raise ventr. rate by vagolytic effect. Administer other rate-slowing drugs (digitalis, β-blockers etc.) before quinidine for SV arrhythmias.	P.O: 300–600 mg q 6 hr.	Liver	Cause drug discontinuation in 30% of patients. Cardiac: proarrhythmia, including torsades de pointes; GI: diarrhea, nausea, vomiting, anorexia; CNS: cinchonism (tinnitus, visual changes, hearing loss, confusion); Blood-thrombo cytopenia. Increases serum digoxin levels 2-fold.
Procainamide	Same as quinidine. Insignificant vagolytic properties.	Same as quinidine.	SV/Ventr arrhythmias, same as for quinidine.	P.O: 2–6 g/d; q 3–4 h doses (procainamide) and q 6 h doses for sustained-release form. IV: 100 mg q 5 min until arrhythmia control or up to a total of 1 g, then infuse at 2–6 mg/min.	Kidneys Metabolites: N-acetylprocainamide (NAPA), which has Class III actions. Therapeutic Levels: 8–20 µg/ml (including NAPA).	Limit long-term use. Cardiac:same as quinidine. Other: systemic lupus-like syndrome (15–20% of patients). GI: nausea, vomiting.
Disopyramide	Same as quinidine; prominent vagolytic effects.	Same as quinidine.	SV and ventr arrhythmias.	P.O: 100–400 mg q 6–8 h.	Kidneys	Cardiac: same as quinidine; also may cause/worsen CHF. Other: blurred vision, urinary retention, closed-angle glaucoma, dry mouth.
Class I B Lidocaine Mexiletine Tocainide	Weak Na++-channel blockers. Shorten phase 3 and action potential duration at normal heart rates and in normally polarized tissue. Minimally affect conduction velocity and reduce refractory period.	May shorten QT interval.	Ventr arrhythmias.	Lidocaine: load with 1–2 mg/kg IV; repeat 50 mg bolus in 10 min; then infuse 1–4 mg/min. Therapeutic levels 2–4 µg/ml. Tocainide: 400–600 mg q8h. P.O. Mexiletine: P.O. 200–300 mg q8 h.	Liver	Cardiac: proarrhythmia (all agents). Lidocaine: Primary toxicity: CNS, with confusion, coma, seizures. Mexiletine: GI: anorexia, nausea, vomiting; CNS: tremor, dysarthria, nystagmus. Tocainide: same as Mexiletine (GI and CNS); agranulocytosis (0.2%) and pulmonary fibrosis.
Moricizine	Does not neatly fit into the classification schema. Similar Na++-channel-blocking properties as class IA drugs but mildly shortens phase 3.	Usually no change.	SV and ventr arrhythmias.	P.O: 100–400 mg q8h.	? Liver	Cardiac: proarrhythmia. GI: nausea, vomiting, diarrhea. CNS: dizziness, headache.

Drug	Action	ECG effects	Indications	Dose/Route	Metabolism	Toxicity/Side effects
Class I C Flecainide	Potent Na^{++} channel blockade but minimal effect on action potential duration. Markedly depresses conduction in all cardiac fibers. Mildly prolongs refractory period.	Decreases sinus rate. Moderately prolongs QRS interval. May increase PR interval.	SV arrhythmias without organic heart disease. Avoid in patients with ventr. arrhythmias (especially sustained) and poor systolic function (high risk of proarrhythmia).	P.O: 100–200 mg q12 h.	Liver	Cardiac: proarrhythmia in certain subgroups; heart block; may cause/worsen CHF.
Propafenone	Similar to flecainide except for mild β-blocking properties.	Same as flecainide.	SV and ventr. arrhythmias. May have proarrhythmic potential.(use with caution).	P.O: 150–300 mg q8–12 h.	Liver	Cardiac: proarrhythmia and heart block; may cause/worsen CHF. Other: bronchospasm, dizziness, taste disturbance.
Class II Propranolol	Prototypical β-blocker. Primarily affects slow-channel dependent tissue (SN and AV nodes). Decreases SN firing rate and prolongs AV nodal conduction.	Decreases sinus rate. Prolongs PR interval.	Slowing ventr. rate in SV arrhythmias. Prevention of exercise-induced arrhythmias. Prevent sudden death in post-MI patients.	P.O: 10–200 mg q6–8h. IV: 0.25–0.5 mg, q 5 min for ≤0.15 to 0.20 mg/kg	Liver	Cardiac: severe bradycardia, heart block; may cause/worsen CHF. Other: bronchospasm, lethargy, impotence.
Class III Amiodarone	Lengthens repolarization by blocking outward K^+ currents. Prolongs action potential duration and refractoriness of all cardiac tissues. Blocks Na^{++}-channels Slows conduction by reducing phase 0 upstroke velocity. Blocks the slow-Ca^{++} channels (reducing SN discharge rates and prolonging AV conduction) and noncompetitively inhibits β-receptors.	Prolongs QRS, PR and QT. Slows sinus rate.	SV and ventr. arrhythmias. Limited by its potential for severe toxicity.	P.O: loading: 800–1600 mg qd for 1–3 wks; Maintenance: 200–400 mg qd Therapeutic drug level: 1–2.5 µg/ml	Liver Concentrated in lung, liver, heart and fatty tissue. Half-life: 50 d.	Cardiac: proarrhythmia, severe bradycardia, heart block. Other: pulmonary fibrosis, hepatitis, hyper- and hypothyroidism, peripheral neuropathy, skin photosensitivity and discoloration. Increases digoxin levels and potentiates warfarin effect.
Bretylium	Causes initial release but then prevents further release of norepinephrine from adrenergic nerve terminals.	Prolongs QT interval.	Life-threatening ventr. arrhythmias not responsive to other drugs (e.g., lidocaine or procainamide)	IV only: loading: 5–10 mg/kg at 1–2 mg/kg/min; Maintenance: 0.5–2 mg/min.	Liver	Cardiac-proarrhythmia, orthostatic hypotension.

AVNRT = AV nodal reentrant tachycardia; CHF = congestive heart failure; CNS = central nervous system; GI = gastrointestinal; RBC = red blood cells; SN = sinus node; SV = supraventricular; ventr = ventricular; VT = ventricular tachycardia.

TABLE 28.2. *(continued)* An Overview of Antiarrhythmic Drugs

Drug	Direct Electrophysiological Actions	Effect on ECG	Clinical Indications	Dose	Major Route of Elimination	Adverse Effects/Drug Interactions
Sotalol	Nonselective β-blocker; blocks outward potassium current. Does not block sodium channels.	Decreases sinus rate, prolongs PR and QT intervals.	SV and ventr arrhythmias	P.O: 80–240 mg q12 h.	Kidneys	Cardiac: proarrhythmia including torsades de pointes, severe bradycardia, heart block, may cause/worsen CHF; Other: fatigue.
Class IV Verapamil	Antagonizes Ca^{++} influx in slow-channel dependent tissue. Does not block Na^{++} channels. Reduces firing rate by decreasing the slope of phase 4 depolarization in SN. Decreases the maximum upstroke velocity of phase 0 depolarization and prolongs AV nodal conduction time and refractory period	Decreases sinus rate and prolongs PR interval.	Rate slowing/termination of SV arrhythmias. Do not use acutely in patients with sustained VT (causes severe hypotension). Not useful for recurrent VT.	P.O: 80–120 mg q6–8 h. IV: 10 mg over 1–2 min.		Cardiac: hypotension, severe bradycardia, heart block, may cause/worsen CHF. Other: elevated liver enzymes, peripheral edema.
Other Adenosine	Increases outward K^+ conductance similar to acetylcholine. Produces marked, brief slowing of AV node conduction and SN discharge rate.	AVNRT or AV reentrant tachycardia utilizing an accessory pathway.	IV: 6 mg bolus. Use 12 mg IV if ineffective.	Metabolized by RBC and vascular endothelium; effects potentiated by dipyridamole and competitively antagonized by methylxanthines. Half-life <10 sec.		Fleeting dyspnea, flushing and chest pain.

AVNRT = AV nodal reentrant tachycardia; CHF = congestive heart failure; CNS = central nervous system; GI = gastrointestinal; RBC = red blood cells; SN = sinus node; SV = supraventricular; ventr = ventricular; VT = ventricular tachycardia.

Sinus Arrhythmia

Sinus arrhythmia is a common, normal event. Sinus rhythm in most individuals is characterized by varying P-P intervals. When the difference between the longest and shortest P-P intervals exceeds 0.12 seconds, it is referred to as sinus arrhythmia. Neither the P-wave morphology nor P-R interval changes. Sinus arrhythmia is termed **phasic** when the rate is faster during inspiration or **nonphasic** when the rate change is not affected by the respiratory cycle.

Sinus Arrest

Sinus arrest is defined as a pause of variable duration caused by the failure of the sinus node to initiate an impulse. Usually, the pause is terminated promptly by a secondary pacemaker site in the heart, and symptoms are absent. In a patient who is experiencing symptoms, permanent pacing may be required. Sinus arrest is seen in sick sinus syndrome, ischemic syndromes, digitalis toxicity, or conditions of excess vagal tone (Figure 28.2A).

Wandering Atrial Pacemaker

Wandering atrial pacemaker involves transient shifts in location of the dominant pacemaker. Locations may vary among different portions of the SA node, atria, or the AV junction. A continual change in the P-wave morphology occurs with varying P-R and R-R intervals. Treatment is rarely necessary.

Premature Atrial Complexes

A premature atrial complex (PAC) is manifested on the ECG by a premature, morphologically abnormal P wave. Depending on the degree of prematurity, the PAC may be nonconducted (no subsequent QRS complex), aberrantly conducted (widened QRS complex), or normally conducted. The P-R interval of a PAC lengthens with increasing degrees of prematurity: the more premature the PAC, the longer the P-R; the later the PAC, the more normal the P-R.

Common, benign events, PACs may be produced by use of tobacco, caffeine, or alcohol; emotional stress; or by myocardial ischemia, atrial distension, or hypoxia. They usually cause no symptoms but may cause palpitations or trigger other atrial or AV-nodal reentrant tachycardias (Figure 28.2 B,C).

Atrial Flutter

Atrial flutter is a common arrhythmia, thought to be owing to a reentrant mechanism (Figure 28.3A, B), that occurs either in a short-lived, paroxysmal form or a sustained, chronic form. Brief episodes of atrial flutter may occur in many acute illnesses (e.g., thyrotoxicosis, acute pulmonary embolism, alcohol intoxication) and are especially common soon after open-heart surgery. In a few patients, no organic heart disease is evident. Atrial flutter commonly occurs in ischemic heart disease but is not usually caused by acute myocardial ischemia.

The **ECG** in atrial flutter demonstrates "saw-tooth" flutter (F) waves occurring regularly at 250–350 beats/min. The undulating F waves are best appreciated in leads II, III, and aVF, with an absence of isoelectric baseline between the F waves. Most commonly, a 2:1 AV block exists, resulting in a ventricular rate of 125–175 beats/min, although higher-grade, variable AV blocks may occur. With 2:1 AV block, the alternate flutter waves may be obscured by the QRS or T waves. In these instances, carotid sinus massage or intravenous adenosine may help by increasing the degree of AV block, thereby unmasking the otherwise obscured F waves (Figure 28.3 B).

The **treatment** of atrial flutter is directed at its conversion into sinus rhythm. Treating the underlying cause (e.g., congestive heart failure) often results in the spontaneous resumption of sinus rhythm. Cardioversion at low energies (25–50 joules) usually restores sinus rhythm and is the method of choice when spontaneous reversion does not occur or when hemodynamic instability or acute myocardial ischemia exists. Rapid atrial pacing may also be attempted, especially after open heart surgery when epicardial pacing leads are already in place. Simple rate control can be achieved with a variety of drugs, including verapamil, β-blockers, or digitalis. Rate control is important to achieve before instituting Type IA agents such as quinidine, procainamide, or disopyramide because these drugs slow the atrial rate but enhance AV conduction, thus increasing ventricular response.

Atrial Fibrillation

In atrial fibrillation, there is complete disorganization of atrial electrical activity. The atria, if viewed directly, display only a writhing motion with total loss of effective contraction.

The **ECG manifestations** include 1) fibrillatory (f) waves that are variable in amplitude, causing random oscillations of the baseline, and 2) an irregular ventricular response, usually between 100 and 160 beats/min in the untreated patient (Figure 28.3 C). QRS complexes are usually normal but may be widened owing to aberrancy **(Ashman's phenomenon)**. This aberrancy is suggested by a relatively long RR cycle immediately preceding a relatively short RR cycle, which is terminated by the aberrant QRS complex resembling right bundle branch block. These aberrant beats may occur singly or in multiples and thus may mimic ventricular tachycardia (Figure 28.3 D).

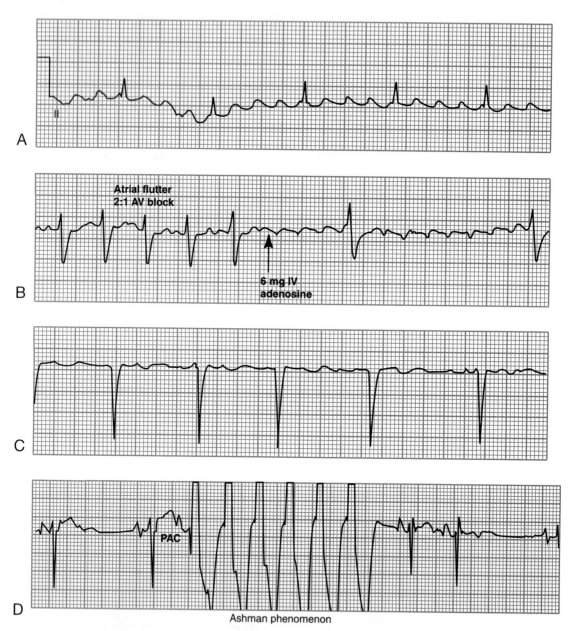

A

B

Atrial flutter
2:1 AV block

6 mg IV
adenosine

C

D

PAC

Ashman phenomenon

FIGURE 28.3. A. **Atrial flutter** with 4:1 AV block. The atrial deflections consist of rapid, sawtooth-shaped regular undulations (F waves). B. **Atrial flutter** with 2:1 AV block. The diagnosis of atrial flutter may be missed in 2:1 AV block. The F waves may be made more obvious by briefly increasing the degree of AV block (in this case, with IV adenosine). C. **Atrial fibrillation**. The P waves are replaced by fine, undulating fibrillatory waves (f waves). In the absence of complete AV block, the R-R intervals are irregular. D. **Ashman's phenomenon**. Aberrant conduction occurs when a premature atrial impulse(s) occurs after a long preceding cycle length. In this example, the premature impulses consist of a six-beat run of atrial tachycardia, beginning with the premature P wave labeled PAC. Thus, aberrant conduction of supraventricular impulses may mimic ventricular tachycardia.

Clinical manifestations

As with atrial flutter, atrial fibrillation may occur in paroxysmal or sustained forms. Usually found in patients with hypertension, ischemic heart disease, mitral valvular disease, or chronic lung disease, atrial fibrillation may also occur in many other conditions, for example, pericarditis, thyrotoxicosis, pulmonary embolism, or alcohol intoxication. It uncommonly can occur in structurally normal hearts and, in this instance, is termed **lone atrial fibrillation.**

Acutely, atrial fibrillation may cause **adverse consequences** owing to a rapid ventricular rate, loss of the atrial contribution ("atrial kick") to ventricular filling, or peripheral emboli. The onset of atrial fibrillation is particularly poorly tolerated in patients with noncompliant LV chambers such as those with aortic stenosis or hypertrophic cardiomyopathies and in patients who poorly tolerate tachycardias such as those with mitral stenosis.

Management

As with all arrhythmias, the correction of the underlying cause is paramount. The main objectives of treatment are to control the ventricular rate, restore sinus rhythm, and prevent systemic emboli. A rapid ventricular rate is traditionally controlled with digitalis. Other agents such as β-blockers and rate-limiting calcium channel blockers (verapamil, diltiazem) may be required. A goal is to achieve a resting heart rate of 70–80 beats/min and a rate below 110–120 beats/min after mild exertion.

Atrial fibrillation rarely reverts spontaneously to sinus rhythm, and thus, it requires either chemical or electrical **cardioversion.** If atrial fibrillation is associated with hemodynamic compromise, then immediate synchronized DC cardioversion is warranted (100–200 joules). Electrical cardioversion is associated with a 1–3% risk of systemic embolism; thus, full **anticoagulation** with warfarin is warranted in all patients who have had atrial fibrillation for longer than 2 days. Anticoagulation should be maintained for 3 weeks before and 2–4 weeks after cardioversion. Heparin should be used followed by warfarin if immediate cardioversion is required. No anticoagulation is needed for atrial fibrillation less than 2 days' duration.

Type IA antiarrhythmic agents, as well as the class III agent sotalol, may be used in an attempt to convert atrial fibrillation to sinus rhythm, but the success rate is typically low. More often, these agents are used to prevent recurrences following electrical cardioversion. Amiodarone is the most efficacious agent for maintaining sinus rhythm following cardioversion but has significant toxicity.

All antiarrhythmic agents can themselves induce arrhythmias (proarrhythmia), and their potential adverse effects also need to be considered. Despite continued antiarrhythmic therapy in patients successfully converted from atrial fibrillation, the **recurrence rate** after 1 year is high—20–40%.

Prophylactic anticoagulation

Chronic atrial fibrillation carries a substantial risk of embolization causing 15% of all ischemic strokes.

Furthermore, more than one-third of affected patients will experience an ischemic stroke within their lifetime. Long-term anticoagulation with warfarin to maintain an International Normalized Ratio (INR) between 2.0–3.0 reduces thromboembolic risk by 50–75%. Aspirin is far less efficacious and confers only a small reduction in risk of stroke. Patients in chronic atrial fibrillation who have mitral stenosis, a prior history of thromboembolism, recent (prior 3 months) history of congestive heart failure, or history of hypertension (with no contraindications for full anticoagulation) are candidates for chronic warfarin therapy. Patients younger than age 65 years with none of these risk factors are considered to be at low risk for thromboembolism and can be treated with aspirin alone.

■ Multifocal Atrial Tachycardia

Multifocal atrial tachycardia is characterized by an atrial rate higher than 100 beats/min; at least three different P-wave morphologies in any one lead; and variable P-P, P-R, and R-R intervals (Figure 28.4A). Caused by enhanced automaticity in the atria, multifocal atrial tachycardia is usually found in the elderly, particularly those with severe obstructive lung disease, coronary artery disease, or diabetes mellitus. Verapamil, which reduces abnormal atrial automaticity, may prove effective as treatment. Vigorous efforts also should be aimed at improving the underlying cardiac or pulmonary status.

■ Paroxysmal Atrial Tachycardia with AV Block

Paroxysmal atrial tachycardia (PAT) results from enhanced atrial automaticity combined with evidence of conduction (AV) block. Digitalis toxicity is responsible for most cases (Figure 28.4 B). The ECG demonstrates abnormal P waves with an atrial rate from 150–250 beats/min; the ventricular rate depends on the degree of AV block.

In a patient receiving digitalis, it should be assumed that PAT is caused by digitalis toxicity, and potassium supplements should be given instead of digitalis. In a patient not receiving digitalis, digitalis can be given to slow the ventricular response; if PAT remains, then class IA, IC, or III drugs may be added to restore sinus rhythm.

Atrioventricular Junctional Rhythm Disturbances

■ Premature Junctional Beats

Premature junctional beats arise in the AV junction and are transmitted in an antegrade fashion to the

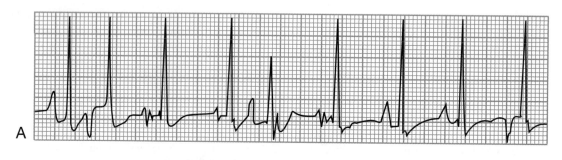

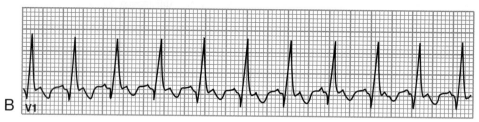

FIGURE 28.4. A. **Multifocal atrial tachycardia.** At least three different P-wave morphologies and varying P-R and R-R intervals are evident in this tracing. B. **Paroxysmal atrial tachycardia** with 2:1 AV block. The P waves occur regularly at 250/min, resulting in a regular ventricular rate of 125 beats/min. PAT with AV block is often caused by digitalis intoxication. This patient had a preexisting complete right bundle branch block.

ventricles, producing a premature, but normal-appearing, QRS complex. The impulse also conducts to the atria in a retrograde fashion, producing a retrograde P wave that may occur before, during, or after the QRS complex. Treatment is usually not necessary.

■ AV Junctional Escape Beats and Junctional Rhythm

If suprajunctional pacemaker sites fail to discharge, then latent pacemaker cells of the AV junction will discharge at a rate of 40–60 beats/min to prevent ventricular asystole. These **escape beats** may occur singly; however, if the normally dominant pacemaker (usually the SA node) continues to fail to discharge, then the escape beats can occur sequentially, termed a **junctional escape rhythm** (Figure 28.5A). The escape interval is greater than the basic P-P interval. Retrograde P waves may be present, but the QRS is normal.

Therapy is directed at increasing the discharge rate of the normal suprajunctional pacemaker. Occasionally, a pacemaker may be required.

■ Nonparoxysmal AV Junctional Tachycardia

In nonparoxysmal AV junctional tachycardia, the AV junction, rather than remaining the default pacemaker, wrests control from the SA node owing to its enhanced automaticity and usually discharges at a rate of 70–130 beats/min (a rate of 70 represents a "tachycardia" for

the normally slow-discharging AV junction). Retrograde P waves may be present, but AV dissociation may also occur.

Digitalis toxicity is most often responsible; however, acute myocardial infarction and myocarditis are other causes. Treatment is directed at the underlying cause (Figure 28.5 B).

■ Paroxysmal Supraventricular Tachycardia

An abrupt onset and termination are characteristic of the paroxysmal supraventricular tachycardias (PSVTs). Approximately 60% of PSVTs are owing to reentry involving the AV node, 30% are caused by a concealed accessory pathway, and the remainder are due to sinus node reentry, intra-atrial reentry, or an ectopic atrial focus (paroxysmal atrial tachycardia).

AV nodal reentry tachycardia

AV nodal reentry tachycardia (AVNRT) is characterized by a regular, narrow-complex tachycardia at a rate of 150–250 beats/min. Dual parallel AV nodal pathways—α and β pathways— exist in patients with AVNRT. The α pathway is slower conducting and has a shorter refractory period than the faster-conducting, longer-refractory β pathway. Premature atrial impulses are blocked in the slow-to-recover β pathway but are conducted slowly down the α pathway; thus, the β pathway is able to conduct them retrogradely. This "slow antegrade–fast retrograde" reentrant circuit, termed the **type I variety,** accounts for 90% of AVNRT cases. Because of the fast retrograde conduction to the atria, the P wave is most often buried in the QRS complex and not seen. When seen, it distorts the terminal portion of the R wave in lead V1.

In the uncommon **type II variety** of AVNRT, the slow α pathway has the longer refractory period, and the premature impulse travels down the fast β pathway and retrograde up the slow α pathway. In this instance, inverted P waves appear shortly before each ensuing QRS.

Concealed accessory pathway tachycardia

A concealed bypass tract, consisting of specialized conduction tissue linking the atrium and ventricle, may provide the necessary substrate for a reentrant tachycardia (e.g., Wolff-Parkinson-White syndrome). Most commonly, the reentrant circuit consists of normal antegrade conduction through the AV node (resulting in a normal-appearing QRS complex) and retrograde conduction from the ventricle to the atria via the accessory pathway (orthodromic tachycardia). In this instance, the retrograde P wave usually distorts the ST segment (Figure 28.6A).

Frequently, PSVT occurs in young patients with normal hearts. The symptoms caused by these PSVTs depend on the rate of the tachycardia and the underlying heart disease.

Management

With reentrant forms of PSVT, termination of the tachycardia is accomplished by blocking one of the limbs of the circuits. Vagal maneuvers, such as carotid sinus massage, gagging, or Valsalva maneuver, may terminate the attack and should be tried initially. If these maneuvers fail, adenosine (6–12 mg by rapid IV bolus) is 95% successful in restoring sinus rhythm. Verapamil (5 to 10 mg IV) may also be used. If the arrhythmia is associated with hemodynamic compromise, then synchronized DC cardioversion is necessary.

For chronic drug therapy, digoxin, β-blockers, verapamil, or diltiazem are initially given, with class IA antiarrhythmic agents being reserved for recalcitrant cases. Recently, catheter ablation has become the preferred therapy for both AVNRT and concealed accessory pathway tachycardias, obviating long-term drug therapy.

■ Preexcitation Syndromes

Preexcitation syndromes include the **Wolff-Parkinson-White (WPW) syndrome** and its variants. On the ECG, features of the WPW pattern consist of a short P-R interval (<0.12 sec), prolonged QRS duration

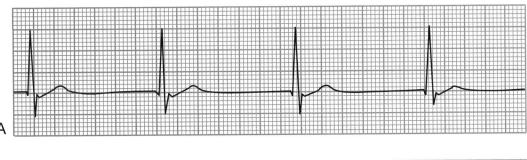

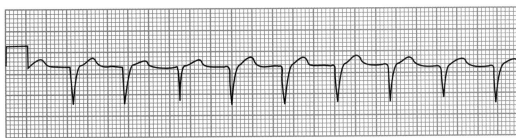

FIGURE 28.5. **A. Junctional rhythm.** There is a regular, narrow-complex rhythm at a rate of 52 beats/min. No P waves are visible. In this instance, the junctional rhythm serves as a passive escape mechanism. **B. Nonparoxysmal junctional tachycardia.** There is a regular, narrow-complex rhythm at a rate of 125 beats/min. No P waves are visible. This rhythm results from abnormal enhancement of impulse formation at the AV junction, commonly from digitalis toxicity.

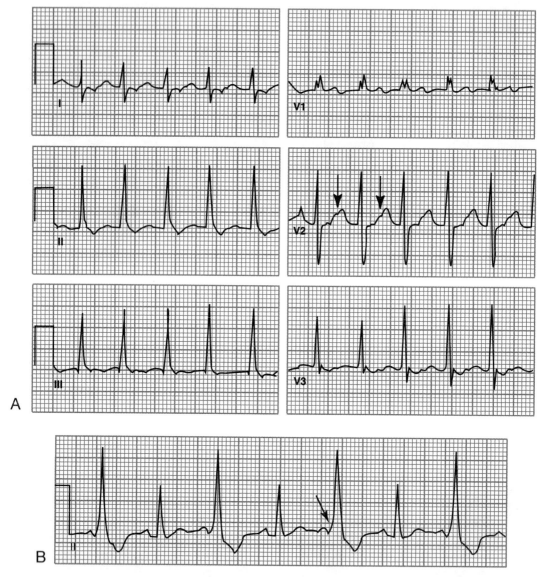

FIGURE 28.6. A. Wolff-Parkinson-White syndrome **with orthodromic conduction.** This six-lead strip shows a tachycardia at 135 beats /min in which the supraventricular impulses conduct antegrade down the AV node and retrograde to the atrium via the accessory pathway. In lead V₂, the arrows point to retrograde P waves deforming the upslope of the T waves. Each P wave is causally related to the prior QRS. The QRS complex is narrow because the ventricles are activated via the normal conduction pathway (AV node and His-Purkinje system). B. **WPW with antidromic conduction.** This strip demonstrates intermittent preexcitation. The arrow points to a "preexcited" ventricular complex. Note the short PR interval (100 ms) and the slurred QRS upstroke (the delta wave, *arrow*). The preexcited complexes are a result of antegrade conduction down the accessory pathway.

(>0.11 sec, owing to the addition of a delta wave), and secondary ST-T wave changes (Figure 28.6 B).

In these patients, the existence of anomalous or accessory fibers bridging the AV groove has been demonstrated. The impulse from the sinus node conducts rapidly through the accessory pathway and activates a portion of the ventricle, resulting in a delta wave. The remainder of the sinus impulse travels normally through the AV node and depolarizes the remaining portion of the ventricles. Thus, the QRS complex in the WPW pattern represents a fusion complex owing to near-simultaneous activation of the ventricles through two different pathways.

Clinical manifestations

The prevalence of WPW syndrome in the general population is about 0.15%, with a 2:1 preponderance for men. This anomaly is considered to be congenital and is probably inherited, and it may be associated with other cardiac anomalies (e.g., Ebstein's anomaly, mitral valve prolapse).

Approximately 10–40% of patients develop tachyarrhythmias, with the most common variety being paroxysmal supraventricular tachycardia that occurs on a reentrant basis. Usually, the impulse transmits antegrade through the AV node in the usual fashion and retrogradely through the accessory pathway back to the atria (**orthodromic tachycardia**) (Figure 28.6A). Less commonly, the impulse conducts antegrade through the accessory pathway and retrogradely through the His bundle and AV node (**antidromic tachycardia**) (Figure 28.6B).

Because the accessory pathway may have the potential to conduct impulses rapidly, patients with WPW are at risk for developing very fast ventricular rates, if atrial arrhythmias, such as atrial fibrillation or flutter were to occur. In general, rapid ventricular rates faster than 200 beats/min during atrial fibrillation are characteristic of WPW syndrome. Patients may develop chest pain, heart failure, or syncope during these rapid tachycardias. However, the long-term prognosis for WPW is usually good, and the incidence of sudden death is low.

Management

Treatment is not necessary for patients with WPW who have no history of tachycardias or for patients with a history of infrequent, asymptomatic tachycardias. In patients with symptomatic tachycardias, treatment options consist of 1) lifelong drug therapy with agents that delay conduction in the AV node, accessory pathway, or both, or 2) destruction of the accessory pathway by surgery or catheter (radiofrequency) ablation. Because it offers a permanent cure and obviates the need for drug therapy, catheter ablation is becoming the prefered treatment. Patients with hemodynamic compromise require immediate, synchronized DC cardioversion.

In patients with anterograde conduction over the AV node (orthodromic tachycardia), acute drug treatment is similar to that of AV nodal reentrant rhythms (e.g., IV adenosine or verapamil). In patients with atrial fibrillation or flutter and antegrade conduction over the accessory pathway (antidromic tachycardia), IV procainamide or electrical cardioversion should be the initial treatment. Intravenous digitalis, adenosine, or verapamil are contraindicated because they may increase the ventricular response by blocking the AV node and lead to ventricular fibrillation.

Diagnosis of narrow-complex tachycardia

Narrow QRS tachycardias arise from supraventricular structures, i.e., sinus node, atria, and AV junction. By definition, they imply fast heart rate with normal width and configuration of the QRS complex. Narrow QRS complexes occur in a range of tachycardias (Table 28.3). The general approach to these entities is summarized in Figure 28.7, Table 28.4, and Table 28.5. Some key considerations are summarized as follows:

1. 12-lead ECG tracings, rather than recordings of a single-lead, are preferable for the analysis of an arrhythmia.

2. The location of the P wave relative to the QRS complex (before, within, or after) should be determined, and the presence of 1:1 AV conduction should be noted. The presence of AV block would terminate AV-dependent rhythms and so exclude conditions such as AV nodal reentrant tachycardias or AV reciprocating tachycardias using an accessory pathway. If AV block is present, the differential diagnosis is that of an atrial arrhythmia—either an ectopic atrial focus or reentry in the SA node or atrial tissue.

3. In the presence of 1:1 AV conduction, the relative timing of atrial and ventricular activation—the R-P and P-R intervals—should be assessed. The R-P interval is the duration between the start of the QRS and the following P wave. The P-R interval is the duration between the onset of the P wave and the start of the QRS. If a P wave is identifiable, determining whether the R-P exceeds P-R or the P-R exceeds R-P can suggest other differential diagnoses (Table 28.4).

4. The morphology of the P wave should be determined.

5. Esophageal ECG can be helpful in demonstrating atrial activity when P waves are not apparent on the surface ECG; however, this technique requires the intraesophageal placement of an electrode to record atrial activity.

6. Carotid sinus massage can help in the differential diagnosis of tachyarrhythmias. By increasing vagal tone, carotid sinus massage causes 1) a slight transient decrease of sinus tachycardia rate; 2) no effect or abrupt termination of AV nodal reentrant tachycardia or supraventricular tachycardia using an accessory pathway, or 3) AV block with continuation (at a slower ventricular rate) of atrial flutter, or atrial fibrillation. Carotid massage should be avoided in patients with known carotid disease, carotid bruits, or prior stroke.

7. Adenosine can be used to produce brief, high-grade block of the AV node, which will terminate supraven-

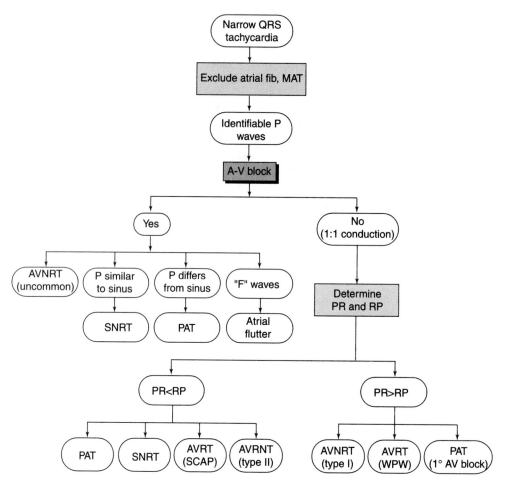

FIGURE 28.7. Differential diagnosis of tachycardia with a narrow QRS. This schema excludes atrial fibrillation, multifocal atrial tachycardia, and nonparoxysmal atrial tachycardia and assumes an identifiable P wave is present. It should be noted that AVNRT is most commonly not associated with an identifiable P wave but, rather, the P wave is "obscured" in the QRS. A fib = Atrial fibrillation; AVNRT = AV nodal reentrant tachycardia; AVRT = AV nodal reciprocating tachycardia; MAT = multifocal atrial tachycardia; PAT = paroxysmal atrial tachycardia; SCAP = slow-conducting accessory pathway; SNRT = sinus node reentrant tachycardia; WPW = Wolff-Parkinson-White syndrome.

tricular tachycardias such as AV node reentry or those using accessory pathways. By producing transient AV nodal block, adenosine may aid in the diagnosis of atrial fibrillation, atrial flutter, and other atrial tachycardias, as well as wide QRS tachycardias. Adenosine only rarely terminates ventricular tachycardia. Caution must be exercised when antegrade conduction over an accessory pathway exists, because adenosine may favor conduction over the accessory pathway (by blocking the AV node) and thus increase the ventricular rate.

Ventricular Arrhythmias

■ Premature Ventricular Complexes

Premature ventricular complexes (PVCs) are the most common ventricular rhythm disturbance. On the ECG, PVCs produce a wide-complex QRS owing to their abnormal ventricular origin and anomalous conduction pattern. The T wave is oriented opposite to the major QRS deflection. Commonly, the atria and sinus node are not depolarized in a retrograde fashion. Therefore, a

---

TABLE 28.3. Narrow QRS Tachycardias

Reentrant
　SA nodal reentry
　AV nodal reentrant tachycardia
　　Type I (slow-fast)
　　Type II (fast-slow)
　AV reciprocating tachycardia (WPW)
　　Orthodromic
　　Antidromic
　Atrial flutter
Automatic
　Paroxysmal atrial tachycardia
　Multifocal atrial tachycardia
　Nonparoxysmal AV junctional tachycardia
　Sinus tachycardia
Other
　Atrial fibrillation

TABLE 28.4. Differential Diagnosis of Tachycardias Based on Timing of RP and PR Intervals

RP > PR (short PR):
PAT—This is the most likely diagnosis.
Sinus node reentry—P wave resembles sinus P wave.
Type II AVNRT—In this unusual form of AVNRT, there is antegrade conduction down the fast pathway and retrograde conduction up the slow pathway. The P wave in front of each QRS is causally related to the prior QRS (retrograde P-wave).
WPW—(with antegrade conduction down the AV node and slow conduction up a retrograde pathway) The P wave in front of each QRS is causally related to the prior QRS (retrograde P-wave).
PR > RP (long PR)
Type I AVNRT—In this more common form of AVNRT, where there is antegrade conduction down the slow pathway and retrograde conduction up the fast pathway. Normally, no P wave is seen, as it is obscured in the QRS. However, when the P wave is seen it usually distorts the terminal R wave of the QRS (e.g., in lead V_1 R' [R prime]).
WPW—This is the most likely diagnosis. When a retrograde P wave is seen in this arrhythmia, it is often found distorting the ST segment.
PAT with 1st degree AV block—P wave differs from sinus.

AVNRT = AV nodal reentrant tachycardia; PAT = paroxysmal atrial tachycardia; WPW = Wolff-Parkinson-White syndrome.

compensatory pause exists—that is, the R-R interval containing the PVC is twice the duration of the preexisting basic R-R interval. If a compensatory pause does not exist, then the PVC is termed **interpolated.**

PVCs arising from the same focus usually maintain a fixed coupling interval to the preceding QRS complex. The fixed interval suggests that the PVC's existence depends on the preceding impulse and thus a reentrant mechanism. If the coupling interval varies by more than 0.08 sec, then **ventricular parasystole** should be considered. In ventricular parasystole, an ectopic ventricular focus, presumably with increased automaticity, activates the ventricles concurrently with, but independent of, the impulse of the basic rhythm.

Two successive PVCs are termed a **couplet,** and three successive PVCs, at a rate of 100 beats/min or greater, are termed **ventricular tachycardia.** PVCs of similar morphology are termed **unifocal,** but if the morphology varies in the same lead, they are termed **multifocal** or **polymorphic.** If PVCs successively alternate with a sinus beat, the rhythm is termed **bigeminy** (Figure 28.8).

PVCs may be associated with structurally normal hearts and, in the absence of significant symptoms, do not require treatment. PVCs may become manifest or exacerbated with excess caffeine, alcohol, emotional stress, sympathomimetic agents, hypoxia, or other conditions, including any type of heart disease. Their prognostic importance depends on the type and severity of the underlying heart disease. In the presence of coronary artery disease and, particularly, poor LV systolic function, PVCs signify an increased risk of cardiac death.

Nevertheless, eradication of PVCs with antiarrhythmic therapy has not been proven to improve outcome (except for β-blockers in patients following myocardial infarction), and it may in fact increase mortality owing to proarrhythmic mechanisms. Thus, in patients with PVCs, reversible factors should be sought and corrected when

---

TABLE 28.5. Clues to Differentiating Narrow QRS Tachycardias (with AV Block)*

Type of Tachycardia	Clue (s)
AVNRT	AVNRT and AV block are an uncommon combination
SNRT	P similar to sinus P
PAT	P wave differs from sinus
Atrial flutter	Saw tooth flutter waves without intervening isoelectric baseline

*The above schema excludes atrial fibrillation, multifocal atrial tachycardia, and nonparoxysmal atrial tachycardia and assumes an identifiable P wave is present. AVNRT is most commonly not associated with an identifiable P wave, but rather, the P wave is "obscured" in the QRS.
AVNRT = AV nodal reentrant tachycardia; AVRT = AV nodal reciprocating tachycardia; F waves = saw-tooth flutter waves without intervening isoelectric baseline; PAT = paroxysmal atrial tachycardia.

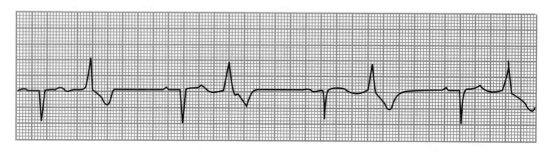

FIGURE 28.8. **Bigeminy.** Every other QRS represents a premature ventricular complex (PVC).

possible. If drug treatment is instituted, β-blockers should be tried first. Other antiarrhythmic agents should be used with great caution and preferably under guidance of electrophysiologic testing.

■ Ventricular Tachycardia

Ventricular tachycardia (VT) arises from impulses generated from the His-Purkinje system, ventricular myocardium, or both, and can arise from abnormalities of impulse formation (automaticity, triggered activity), or conduction, (e.g., reentry). Most episodes are owing to reentry.

In VT, the QRS complex exceeds 0.12 sec in duration, with T-wave vectors directed opposite to the main QRS deflection. The R-R intervals are usually regular. Because the atria are controlled by the sinus node, AV dissociation is usually present (Figure 28.9A); however, retrograde activation of the atria from the ventricles (ventriculoatrial association) may occur. If in the same lead the QRS complexes do not vary in contour, VT is termed **monomorphic** (Figure 28.9 B); if contours vary, VT is **polymorphic** (Figure 28.10). VT is further subdivided into two types: **sustained** (>30 sec duration or associated with hemodynamic compromise) and **nonsustained** (>3 consecutive beats lasting <30 sec) (Figure 28.9C).

The spectrum of manifestations of VT ranges from none to hemodynamic collapse. VT almost always implies a diseased heart. Occuring in all forms of ischemic heart disease, cardiomyopathies, and valvular disease, VT may result from proarrhythmia caused by many drugs and in patients with long Q-T intervals.

The main differential diagnosis of a wide QRS complex tachycardia is between VT and supraventricular tachycardia (SVT) with aberrancy. Certain historical, clinical, and ECG variables, as described in Table 28.6, may help differentiate between these two conditions. VT is much more common than SVT with aberrancy, and any wide QRS complex tachycardia should be considered VT until proven otherwise. In the presence of known structural heart disease—particularly a prior myocardial

infarction—a diagnosis of VT is very likely. Also, VT usually has more profound hemodynamic effects than SVT, but normal hemodynamics do not rule out VT. Intravenous verapamil must be avoided in these patients unless the diagnosis of SVT with aberrancy is an absolute certainty, because verapamil may cause profound hypotension in a patient with VT.

Management of VT

Steps in the management of VT consist of terminating the VT, identifying underlying causes, and eliminating reversible factors (e.g., hypokalemia, ischemia, bradycardia, fluid overload), thus preventing recurrence. VT associated with hemodynamic compromise requires urgent synchronized DC cardioversion.

For acute treatment, IV lidocaine is usually the initial agent of choice, followed by procainamide or bretylium. Bretylium is reserved for patients with refractory, sustained VT. Patients having recurrent sustained VT or symptomatic nonsustained VT require chronic treatment. Those with hemodynamically significant VT should undergo electrophysiologic testing, and many will require both chronic antiarrhythmic therapy and an implantable cardioverter-defibrillator (ICD). In others, endocardial resection, aneurysmectomy, or catheter ablation techniques may be successful.

The treatment of patients with asymptomatic nonsustained VT (a common clinical problem) is controversial. β-adrenergic-blocking agents may be administered empirically. Empiric amiodarone or drug therapy selected on the basis of electrophysiologic testing are alternative approaches. As with PVCs, it is not clear whether eradication of asymptomatic nonsustained ventricular arrhythmias actually improves prognosis, and treatment with class I drugs may, in fact, be harmful. There is an increasing emphasis on implantation of ICDs, especially in patients with coexistent LV dysfunction.

Torsades de pointes

Torsades de pointes (twisting of points) refers to a type of polymorphic VT occurring in the presence of a

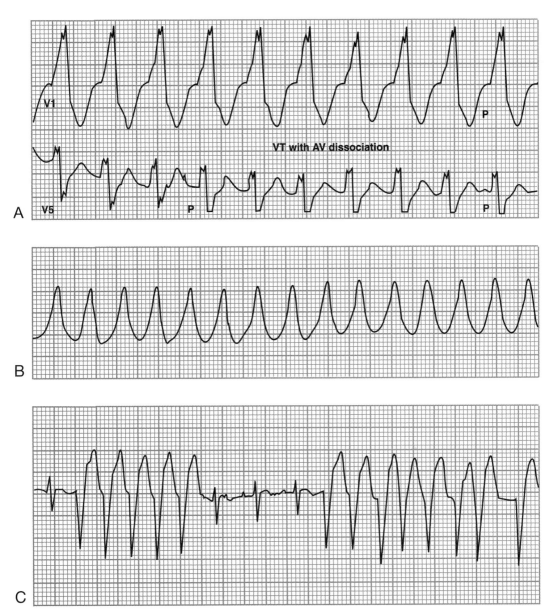

FIGURE 28.9. Ventricular **tachycardias** (VT). A. **VT with AV dissociation**. This strip demonstrates VT at 130 beats/min with evidence of dissociated P waves (P). AV dissociation during a wide QRS tachycardia is strong evidence that the tachycardia is of ventricular origin. B. **Monomorphic VT.** The monotony of each complex contrast with the pattern of polymorphic VT (see Fig. 28.10). C, **Nonsustained VT.** Five- and eight-beat runs of nonsustained VT are demonstrated. In this strip, the eight-beat run is irregular, demonstrating that VT need not be absolutely regular.

long Q-T interval. Morphologically, this VT is characterized by the gradual oscillation, around the baseline, of the peaks of successive QRS complexes (Figure 28.10). Torsades de pointes occurs at a rapid rate in clusters and is self-terminating. Patients present with recurrent dizziness and syncope, and ventricular fibrillation and sudden death are common. Early after-depolarizations, rather than re-entry, are thought to be the mechanism for this arrhythmia.

The syndrome may be congenital or acquired. The acquired form may be caused by antiarrhythmic agents that prolong repolarization (e.g., class IA agents or

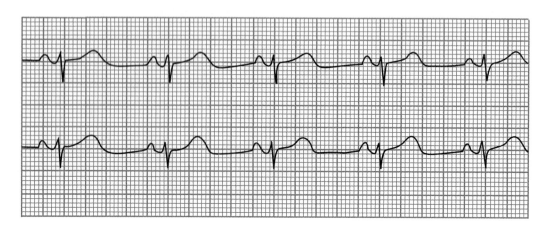

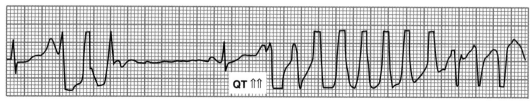

Torsades de pointes

FIGURE 28.10. Torsades de pointes. The *upper strip* demonstrates sinus bradycardia with a mildly prolonged Q-T interval (480 msec, corrected). The *lower strip*, recorded minutes later, demonstrates an episode of torsades de pointes with marked prolongation of the Q-T interval (>600 msec). The prolonged Q-T interval resulted from the long pause immediately preceding the VT.

TABLE 28.6.	Differential Diagnosis of Wide-QRS-Complex Tachycardia on the 12-Lead ECG	
	Ventricular Tachycardia	**Supraventricular Tachycardia**
AV dissociation	Present	Absent
QRS duration	>140 msec if RBBB	<140 msec if RBBB
	>160 msec if LBBB	<160 msec if LBBB
Axis deviation	−90 to ±180°	All other axes
QRS configuration		
RBBB		
Lead V1	Mono or biphasic	Triphasic (rSR′)
Lead V6	R/S <1	R/S >1
LBBB		
Lead V₁†	Slurred S wave (Q-S [nadir] >70 ms)	Absence of same (Q-S [nadir] <70 ms)
Precordial Leads		
(+) concordance*	present	absent
(−) concordance	present	absent
If baseline bundle-branch block present	QRS morphology different	QRS morphology same

LBBB = left bundle branch block; RBBB = right bundle branch block;
* (+) concordance indicates that QRS complexes in leads V1-V6 are all upright; (−) concordance indicates that QRS complexes in leads V1–V6 are all inverted; † QS nadir refers to duration of QRS onset to S wave nadir.

sotalol), potassium and magnesium depletion, certain psychotropic drugs, bradyarrhythmias, and liquid protein diets.

Treatment of this arrhythmia involves removing the causative drug, if present, and vigorously correcting electrolyte deficiencies. Any agent that may prolong the Q–T interval is contraindicated. Intravenous magnesium (regardless of actual serum magnesium levels) may terminate the arrhythmia. Alternative acute therapies include overdrive atrial or ventricular pacing and isoproterenol administration. Chronic treatment may involve oral β-blockers at maximally tolerated doses. If the arrhythmia recurs despite drug therapy, left-sided cervicothoracic sympathetic ganglionectomy has proven helpful, as has permanent pacing. Select patients with congenital long QT syndrome and recurrent syncope may require ICD implantation.

Ventricular escape beats

If the SA node and AV junction fail or conduction defects block the impulses from reaching the ventricles, then the ventricular Purkinje network will activate the ventricles and prevent ventricular asystole. These beats may occur singly or in succession. This escape usually occurs at a rate of 20–40 beats/min.

Accelerated idioventricular rhythm

Three or more ventricular complexes occurring at a rate of 60–100 beats/min comprise an accelerated idioventricular rhythm (AIVR), and this arrhythmia characteristically begins with a ventricular escape com-

plex (Figure 28.11A). Enhanced automaticity of ventricular tissue causes AIVR. This arrhythmia is commonly observed in acute myocardial infarction and only rarely leads to ventricular fibrillation. Because episodes of AIVR are brief and commonly asymptomatic, treatment is not needed. If symptoms occur, atropine or pacing may be required.

■ Ventricular Fibrillation

Ventricular fibrillation (VF) is characterized electrocardiographically by baseline undulations with variable amplitude and periodicity (Figure 28.11B). No QRS complexes or T waves are evident. Because no effective cardiac contraction occurs, VF is a catastrophic event in which pulse and blood pressure are absent. Loss of consciousness ensues, followed by death within 3–5 minutes unless resuscitation is promptly instituted. The most common causes of VF include acute myocardial infarction, advanced coronary disease with LV systolic dysfunction, marked electrolyte disturbances (e.g., hypokalemia), drug toxicity or proarrhythmia, hypothermia, and electrocution.

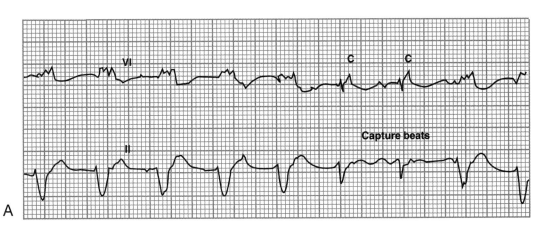

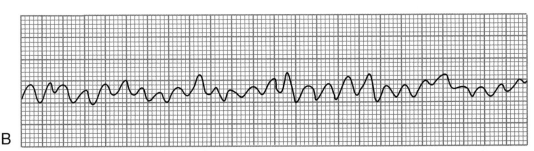

FIGURE 28.11. **A. Accelerated idioventricular rhythm** (AIVR) with capture beats. The basic rhythm is ventricular tachycardia at a rate of 95 beats/min. Capture beats *(C)* result from capture of the ventricles by sinus impulses. (This patient had an underlying right bundle branch block, and thus the capture beats are conducted accordingly.) The presence of capture beats provides strong evidence that the prevailing rhythm is of ventricular origin. **B. Ventricular fibrillation.** Broad complexes are seen occurring rapidly and at irregular intervals. There are no discrete QRS complexes.

Conduction Disorders

■ Heart Block

Optimal cardiac performance depends on an orderly sequence of events occurring in the cardiac conduction system: pacemaker impulses arising in the SA node initially depolarize the atrial myocardium, propagate slowly through the AV node, and finally spread through the His-Purkinje network to the ventricular myocardium. Failure of conduction can occur anywhere in this electrophysiological chain but is most readily recognized in the AV node, His bundle, and bundle branches.

First-degree AV block

First-degree AV block is defined as a delay in conduction from the sinus node to the ventricles with a resultant P-R interval longer than 0.20 sec (Figure 28.12A). It is most commonly caused by abnormally slow conduction through the AV node although all impulses are conducted.

Second-degree AV block

Second-degree AV block is characterized by intermittent failure of the AV conduction.

Type I second-degree AV block (also termed **Mobitz type I** or **Wenckebach**) is the more common type. Characterized by a progressive lengthening of the P-R interval and shortening of the R-R interval until a P wave fails to conduct, second-degree AV block causes an increased R-R interval (Figure 28.12 B). Typically, the beat following the nonconducted P wave has the shortest P-R interval.

The most common site of type I second-degree AV block is the AV node. In such patients, the QRS complex is narrow and the prognosis is benign. Type I block may occur in normal individuals as a manifestation of enhanced vagal tone, but it also occurs in a wide variety of medical conditions, such as acute inferior-wall myocardial infarction and congenital or acquired diseases of the AV node, or with medications that slow AV conduction. Less commonly, type I AV block is caused by conduction disease below the AV node—in the His bundle or its branches. In these patients, the QRS is usually widened.

In most cases, type I AV block does not require specific treatment. However, in patients who develop type I block in the absence of an identifiable acute process, particularly the elderly with severe coronary artery disease or calcific aortic disease, electrophysiologic testing should be considered to identify the site of the block. If the block is within or below the His bundle, particularly if the patient has had prior dizziness or syncope, then permanent pacing is indicated.

Type II second-degree AV block (also termed **Mobitz type II** AV block) differs from type I block in that abrupt failure of AV conduction occurs without the preceding gradual P-R prolongation (Figure 28.12C). The location of the type II block is always within or below the His bundle.

Most patients with type II block have broad QRS complexes indicative of conduction system disease, and symptoms (dizziness or syncope) are common. Causes include sclerodegenerative diseases of the conduction system, anterior wall myocardial infarction, calcific aortic valve disease, hypertensive heart disease, and cardiomyopathy. Permanent pacing is indicated in all symptomatic patients with type II block and should be strongly considered even in asymptomatic patients.

In a third type of second-degree AV block, the ratio of P waves to QRS complexes is 2:1 or higher. These cases ("high-degree blocks") cannot always be accurately categorized as either type I or type II. If the QRS is narrow, the block is likely in the AV node; but if the QRS is wide, then the block may be in the AV node or His-Purkinje system.

Complete AV block

Complete or **third-degree AV block** is characterized by total independence of the atria and ventricles owing to the complete failure of atrial impulses to be conducted to the ventricles. In the presence of sinus rhythm, third-degree AV block is characterized by total dissociation between P waves and QRS complexes, with the ventricles being controlled by a subsidiary pacemaker site (Figure 28.12D). The site of the conduction defect may be at the AV node or infranodal (within or below the His bundle).

The site of the block has prognostic value. If the QRS complexes are narrow and the ventricular rate exceeds 50 beats/min, then the block is likely at the AV node, and the prognosis is usually favorable. These patients are usually asymptomatic, and their heart rate is able to increase with exercise. Causes include congenital complete heart block, in which the block is permanent, as well as acute myocardial infarction, drug intoxication, or myocarditis, in which the block is transient.

If the QRS complexes are wide and the ventricular rate is 30–40 beats/min, then the site of the block is likely infranodal. Infranodal blocks account for the vast majority of episodes of complete heart block, causing slow heart rates that are unresponsive to autonomic influence. Symptoms are frequent. Reversible causes are infrequent, and permanent pacing is usually indicated.

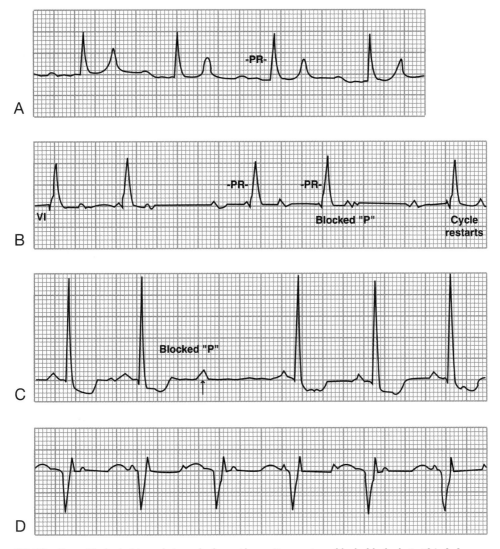

FIGURE 28.12. Heart block. A. Normal sinus rhythm with **first-degree AV block.** The P-R interval is 360 msec. B. **Type I second-degree AV block.** There is progressive prolongation of the P-R interval until a P wave is blocked, following which the cycle restarts. C. **Type-II second-degree AV block.** P-R intervals are constant until the third P wave is suddenly blocked. D. **Third-degree or complete AV block.** Regularly occurring P waves at a rate of 115 /min and regularly occurring QRS complexes at a rate of 80/min are evident. There is no relationship between the P waves and the QRS complexes.

Atrioventricular dissociation

AV dissociation is defined as activation of the atria and ventricles by two independent foci (Figure 28.13). Conduction block may or may not exist.

AV dissociation is usually owing to one of three general causes:

1. With failure of the normal dominant pacemaker (as in sinus bradycardia), normally latent pacemaker cells in the AV junction gain control of the cardiac rhythm. The atria are under the abnormally slow control of the SA node, and the ventricles are under the control of the AV junction. In this type of AV dissociation, the ventricular rate is faster than the atrial rate, and heart block is not present.

2. Latent pacemakers may gain control, not through failure of higher pacemakers, but rather through abnormal acceleration of their normally slow discharge rate. These pathologic latent pacemakers

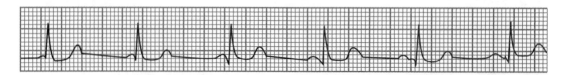

FIGURE 28.13. Atrioventricular dissociation. There are regular atrial and ventricular rates of 65 beats/min, but no relationship between P waves and QRS complexes. In this instance, there is a slow sinus rhythm and junctional rhythm in competition with one another. The junctional impulses fail to be conducted retrogradely to "capture" the atria. Thus, the sinus node and AV junction discharge at similar rates but independent of one another. This strip is an example of isorhythmic AV dissociation.

actively take over from a normally functioning SA node. An example is accelerated junctional or ventricular tachycardia. Again, the ventricular rate exceeds the atrial rate, and heart block is not present.

3. In conduction block, the ventricles are under the control of a slower discharging, normally latent pacemaker (e.g., complete heart block with a ventricular escape rhythm). In this third cause of AV dissociation, the ventricular rate is slower than the atrial rate, and conduction block is present.

Bundle branch blocks

Conduction of an impulse may be slowed or totally interrupted in the right bundle, main left bundle, or anterior and posterior fascicles of the left bundle.

Right bundle branch block

Right bundle branch block (RBBB) is characterized by a delayed RV activation. On auscultation, S_2 is widely split owing to delayed closure of the pulmonic valve but maintains its respiratory variation. RBBB occurs in sclerodegenerative disease of the conduction system, acute pulmonary embolism, chronic coronary disease, septal trauma (such as during right heart catheterization), and occasionally in otherwise healthy persons.

The clinical significance of RBBB depends on the type and severity of underlying heart disease, if any. As an isolated finding, it is usually harmless, and progression of RBBB to complete AV block is rare. Delayed RV activation generates a secondary R wave (R′) in the right precordial leads (rsR′) and wide S waves in leads I, V_5, and V_6. The QRS duration exceeds 0.12 sec in complete RBBB, and the T wave is directed opposite to the terminal portion of the QRS. Because RBBB does not affect the initial portion of the QRS, Q waves retain their usual significance.

Left bundle branch block

Left bundle branch block (LBBB) results from slow conduction in the main left bundle or, rarely, simultaneous slow conduction in its anterior and posterior fascicles. On auscultation, delayed closure of the aortic valve results in a reversed or paradoxical splitting of S_2. LBBB occurs in sclerodegenerative disease of conduction tissue, cardiomyopathies, calcific aortic valve disease, and hypertensive or coronary heart disease. LV hypertrophy is commonly found in patients with LBBB. As opposed to RBBB, LBBB is rarely seen in patients without other demonstrable evidence of heart disease, and the prognosis depends on the associated heart disease.

The ECG in LBBB demonstrates a broad monophasic R wave in leads I, V_5, and V_6, which is usually notched or slurred; deep S waves in V_1 and V_2; absence of the normal small septal Q waves in leads I, V_5, and V_6; and secondary T wave changes. LBBB is considered **complete** when the QRS width exceeds 0.12 sec and **incomplete** when it is less than 0.12 sec. By affecting the initial portion of ventricular activation, LBBB interferes with the ECG diagnosis of myocardial infarction.

Left anterior hemiblock

Left anterior hemiblock (LAH) is the most common variety of conduction abnormality. Impaired conduction in the anterior fascicle delays activation of the anterosuperior portion of the LV and produces the following ECG features: a left axis deviation exceeding 30°; qR pattern in leads I and aVL; rS pattern in leads II, III, and aVF; and only negligible prolongation of the QRS. LAH may also result in persistence of S waves in leads V_5 and V_6 and the presence of a qrS pattern in leads V_1 and V_2, which may mimic an anterior myocardial infarction.

Left posterior hemiblock

Impaired conduction in the posterior fascicle delays activation of the posteroinferior portion of the LV. ECG features consist of right axis deviation that exceeds +110°; presence of a qR pattern in leads II, III, and aVF; and presence of rS pattern in leads I and aVL. Other conditions that cause right axis deviation, such as lateral infarction, RV hypertrophy, and vertical heart, must be excluded. Because it implicates the broadest fascicle with a dual blood supply, isolated left posterior hemiblock is rare.

Bifascicular blocks

Impairment of conduction can develop simultaneously in any two of the three fascicles; the impulse then propagates to the ventricles through the remaining fascicle. RBBB, in combination with LAH, is the most common type of bifascicular block. It is characterized by a mean QRS axis above 30°; rS' in leads V₁ and V₂; and deep S waves in V₅ and V₆. Approximately 5% of patients with RBBB plus LAH develop second-degree or third-degree AV block. RBBB plus left posterior hemiblock is characterized by EC changes of RBBB and right axis deviation of exceeding +110°. It progresses to advanced AV block in 5–10% of cases. Simultaneous block in the left anterior and posterior fascicles manifests as LBBB.

Trifascicular block

Simultaneous block in all three fascicles manifests as complete AV block. Incomplete trifascicular block indicates bifascicular block plus a prolonged P-R interval, indicating slow conduction in the third fascicle. In most patients, a prolonged P-R interval results from a delayed impulse at the AV node rather than in the third fascicle. Patients with fascicular blocks can develop advanced AV block that may result in dizziness and syncope, at which time permanent pacemaker insertion is indicated.

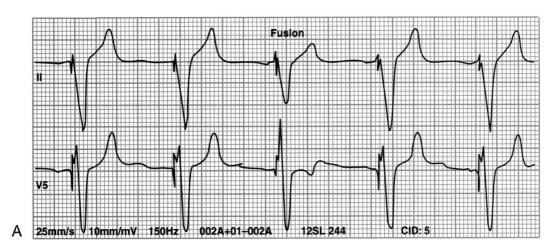

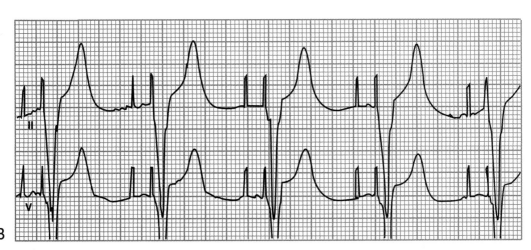

FIGURE 28.14. Artificially paced rhythms. **A. Ventricular pacing.** This strip demonstrates an electronic ventricular pacemaker maintaining a rate of 60 beats/min. Note the pacemaker "spike" preceding each QRS complex. The third complex in each lead represents a fusion beat, which occurs when the ventricles are excited simultaneously from both supraventricular and ventricular foci. The resultant complex appears to be a mixture of a supraventricular and ventricular complex. **B. AV sequential pacemaker.** With leads in both the atrium and ventricle, the first spike causes the atria to depolarize. The 200-msec delay that follows represents the programmed P-R interval. Ventricular depolarization then follows as the next spike.

Asymptomatic patients need only periodic clinical follow-up.

Sick Sinus Syndrome

Sick sinus syndrome implies sinus node disease leading to a variety of cardiac arrhythmias, including 1) sinus bradycardia unrelated to medications or excessive vagal tone, 2) sinus arrest or SA block, and 3) alternating episodes of tachyarrhythmia and bradycardia. Most patients also show some evidence of abnormal AV conduction.

The underlying cause of the syndrome consists of a degenerative process that destroys sinus nodal and surrounding atrial tissue. The AV node and His bundle may also be involved. A significant number of patients also have coronary artery disease, hypertension, or cardiomyopathy. The most common symptoms are palpitations, dizziness, lightheadedness, and syncope. Ambulatory ECG monitoring is often helpful in documenting the ECG manifestations of sinus node dysfunction.

Asymptomatic individuals with sick sinus syndrome require no treatment. In patients with symptoms that are believed to arise from a conduction defect, permanent pacing is employed. In addition, antiarrhythmic drugs may be used to prevent or slow coexisting atrial tachyarrhythmias.

Permanent Pacemakers

A permanent pacemaker consists of an electrode lead and a pulse generator or battery. In the most common type, the electrode lead is inserted transvenously into the RV apex or, less often, surgically implanted into the LV wall (epicardium). The generator is inserted into a subcutaneous pocket below the clavicle or in the abdominal wall. The power source consists of lithium cells with a life expectancy of 5–10 years.

A letter code has been devised as a shorthand

TABLE 28.7.   North American Society of Pacing and Electrophysiology Pacemaker Code

I	II	III	IV
Chamber Paced	Chamber Sensed	Response to Sensing	Rate Modulation
0 = None	0 = None	0 = None	R = Rate modulation
A = Atrium	A = Atrium	T = Triggers pacing	
V = Ventricle	V = Ventricle	I = Inhibits pacing	
D = Dual (A + V)	D = Dual (A + V)	D = Triggers and inhibits pacing	

TABLE 28.8.   Indications For Permanent Pacing

1. Acquired AV block
   Complete AV block permanent or intermittent, symptomatic or asymptomatic
   Mobitz type II AV block, symptomatic or asymptomatic
   Type I (Wenckebach) AV block, symptomatic
   Atrial fibrillation with complete AV block or advanced AV block and symptomatic bradycardia
2. Acquired AV block associated with myocardial infarction
   Newly acquired bundle-branch block and transient advanced AV block
   Type II second-degree AV block
   Complete AV block
3. Chronic bifascicular and trifascicular block
   Bifascicular block with intermittent symptomatic complete heart block
   Bifascicular or trifascicular block with type II second-degree AV block, symptomatic or asymptomatic
   Bifascicular or trifascicular block with syncope when other causes are not identifiable
4. Sinus node dysfunction
   Sinus node dysfunction with documented symptomatic bradycardia (the bradycardia may be spontaneous or due to concomitant drug therapy)
   Sinus bradycardia with bradycardia-dependent ventricular or supraventricular arrhythmias
5. Hypersensitive carotid sinus
   Recurrent syncope or dizziness in a patient with easily-induced asystole (>3 sec) upon light carotid stimulation in the absence of drugs which depress SA or AV node; symptoms should be clearly related to carotid stimulation

notation to describe the complex function of pacemakers (Table 28.7). The first letter indicates the chamber paced; the second letter, the sensed chamber; the third, the mode of pacemaker response to a spontaneous cardiac impulse; and the fourth letter, recently added, indicates that the pacemaker has the property of rate modulation (i.e., the unit can increase its pacing rate in response to increased physiological need).

Most patients in need of a permanent pacemaker should be considered for dual-chamber pacing (Table 28.8). Pacer systems that include atrial pacing (as opposed to a simple VVI system, which paces and senses only the ventricle [Figure 28.14]) have the advantage of maintaining AV synchrony, reducing the incidence of congestive heart failure, the incidence of future atrial fibrillation (and thereby the risk of embolization), and overall mortality. Contraindications for dual-chamber pacing include 1) fixed atrial fibril- lation or flutter or any intractable supraventricular arrhythmia and 2) patients with terminal disease or extreme debility in whom simple ventricular pacing would suffice. Simple VVI pacing may be appropriate in those occasional patients with infrequent, symptom- atic bradycardia.

Complications of permanent pacing include infection and erosion at the site of battery implantation, failure to capture (pace) the ventricular or atrial myocardium, and failure to appropriately sense (owing to undersensing or oversensing).

Patients with permanent pacemakers should be monitored periodically to check the function and trouble- shooting these complicated devices. The need for battery replacement is often heralded by a spontaneous, auto- matic slowing of the pacing rate—a property built into the pacemaker to alert the physician to the need for battery replacement.

<table><tr><td>CHAPTER</td><td>29</td><td>SYNCOPE</td></tr></table>

Syncope is a sudden, and usually self-limited, transient loss of consciousness that is typically associated with a loss of postural tone. Episodes are recurrent in about one-third of patients.

■ **Etiology**

The underlying theme of syncope is a tran- sient, global decrease in cerebral perfusion lasting from 5–10 sec. Causes are legion, ranging from benign to life-threatening, and are not uncommonly elusive (Figure 29.1). In elderly patients, cardiac causes pre- dominate, whereas among younger patients, noncardiac diagnoses such as vasodepressor syncope, orthostatic hypotension, or emotional conditions are more likely causes.

Cardiac causes

Syncope may be caused by structural heart disease, cardiac arrhythmias, or both. **Structural heart disease** causing syncope commonly involves LV or RV outflow obstruction, such as aortic stenosis or some variants of hypertrophic cardiomyopathy. Syncope in aortic stenosis is exertional, since stroke volume fails to increase in tandem with exercise-induced peripheral vasodilation. Peripheral vasodilatation may also be reflexly induced in response to stimulation of LV mechanoreceptors by marked increase in LV systolic pressure during exercise. In mitral stenosis, syncope follows rapid tachycardias or atrial fibrillation. Effort syncope and chest pain also occur in pulmonary hypertension.

Cardiac arrhythmias are often responsible for syn- cope, especially in the elderly. The arrhythmias may be rapid or slow and supraventricular or ventricular. **Brady- arrhythmias** may follow sick sinus syndrome or admin- istration of digitalis, β-blockers, and Ca^{++} channel blockers with negative chronotropic effects. In high- degree AV block, the site of the block and the adequacy of ventricular escape rhythm determine the onset of syncope, with a more distal block and slow escape rhythm often evoking syncope.

TABLE 29.1.	Important Elements of History-Taking in a Patient with Syncope

What was patient doing just before blacking out?
Were there any apparent precipitating events?
Was there any prodrome?
What was the time course of events? If there were other symptoms, what were their onset and progression?
Was there any injury related to the syncopal episode?
Was there any bowel or bladder incontinence?
What does the patient remember about "coming to"?
How long was the patient "out"?
Are there any persistent symptoms?
What medications is the patient taking now?
Did anyone (observer) witness this event?
Have there been any previous similar episodes?

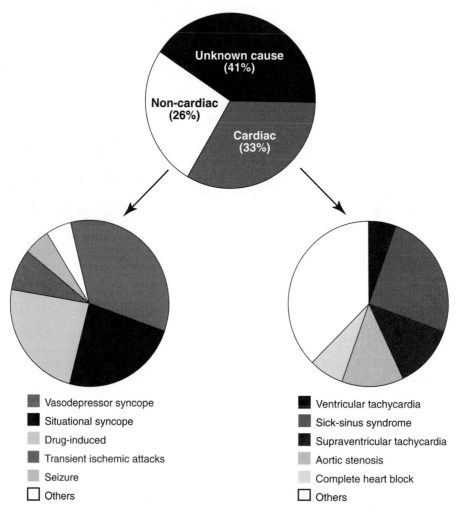

Vasodepressor syncope
Situational syncope
Drug-induced
Transient ischemic attacks
Seizure
☐ Others

Ventricular tachycardia
Sick-sinus syndrome
Supraventricular tachycardia
Aortic stenosis
Complete heart block
☐ Others

FIGURE 29.1. Relative frequency of some common causes of syncope. Among a total of 433 cases a cardiac etiology was seen in 110; non-cardiac causes in 144 and an unknown mechanism in 179 cases. The most frequent non-cardiac condition causing syncope is orthostatic hypotension ($n = 43$) followed by vasodepressor syncope ($n = 35$); the most frequent cardiac cause is ventricular tachycardia ($n = 49$), followed by sick sinus syndrome ($n = 15$).
(Data from: Kapoor WN. Medicine 1990;69:160–175. Used with permission.)

A **supraventricular tachycardia** may cause syncope even with normal ventricular and valvular function. Not uncommonly, a paroxysmal supraventricular tachycardia causes the elderly to develop hypotension, cerebral hypoperfusion, and a feeling of faintness. Supraventricular arrhythmias complicating an accessory pathway that facilitates accelerated conduction are particularly liable to cause syncope.

Ventricular tachycardia, owing to structural heart disease, or **antiarrhythmic drugs,** especially class IA agents, may cause hypotension and syncope (e.g., torsades de pointes, see Figure 28.10). Syncope in **pacemaker** patients may be due to pacemaker malfunction (loss of capture or under-sensing).

Noncardiac causes

The noncardiac causes of syncope can be recalled with the mnemonic "SVNCOPE"—*s*ituational, *v*asodepressor, *n*eurologic, *c*arotid sinus hypersensitivity, *o*rthostatic hypotension, *p*sychiatric/emotional, and *e*xtra.

Situational syncope

Situational syncope may be mechanical (decreased venous return that occurs on a Valsalva maneuver) or reflex (vagal stimulation or vasodepressor responses that cause sinus bradycardia, sinus arrest, or high-degree AV block). Examples include cough syncope (high intrathoracic pressure with low venous return), postmicturition syncope (rapid decrease in peripheral vascular resistance owing to drainage of distended urinary bladder), and defecation syncope (prolonged Valsalva maneuver). Elderly persons with hypertension—especially those receiving vasodilators—may suffer postprandial hypotension causing dizziness, syncope, and falls.

Vasodepressor syncope

The Bezold-Jarisch reflex is critical to the pathogenesis of vasodepressor syncope (Figure 29.2). Upright posture, vasodilation, and increased venous pooling decrease ventricular filling. This decrease in "preload" and systolic blood pressure causes catecholamine release, which causes vigorous contraction of the (small) ventricle. The Bezold-Jarisch reflex is activated via intracardiac vagal mechanoreceptors. Increased neural input to the brainstem via synapses with vagal efferents causes both bradycardia and hypotension; syncope ensues. Hypotension results from peripheral vasodilation. β-blockers, by short-circuiting the Bezold-Jarisch reflex, prevent bradycardia, hypotension, and syncope.

This type of syncope is a common sequel to emotional stress, threat of physical injury, sudden pain or discomfort, or the sight of blood or needles. Fatigue, hunger, fever, heat, and prolonged standing or recumbency are predisposing factors in susceptible persons. Patients often report a prodrome of a "queasy" feeling, nausea, sweating, lightheadedness, weakness, blurred vision, and tinnitus.

Neurologic diseases

A minority of syncope cases may be caused by seizures, which may be difficult to diagnose without a bystander account and without the patient's recollection of the events preceding the event. Syncope occasionally causes brief spells of tonic-clonic activity or irregular muscle twitching that are falsely interpreted as seizures. Patients with transient ischemic attacks, strokes, or cerebral emboli present with focal neurologic deficits rather than syncope; nonetheless, vertebrobasilar insufficiency may cause syncope.

Carotid sinus hypersensitivity

The normal response to carotid sinus massage includes brief slowing of the sinus rate and slowing of AV nodal conduction. Carotid sinus hypersensitivity may be suggested by syncope that follows turning of the head, shaving, or wearing a tight collar. The immediate responses may be cardioinhibitory (bradycardia), vasodepressor (a drop in systolic BP of ≥ 50 mm Hg), or a mixed-type with elements of both responses.

Orthostatic hypotension

When a person assumes an upright posture, normal homeostatic mechanisms (arteriolar and venous constriction, enhanced heart rate, and lower-extremity muscle tone) prevent a significant decrease in systolic blood pressure. Patients with orthostatic hypotension may have inadequate responses or impaired reflexes that cause postural symptoms. Symptomatic orthostatic hypotension may be related to inadequate volume, autonomic impairment (either primary or secondary, such as diabetes), or medications. Diuretics, vasodilators, tricyclic antidepressants, antihypertensives, phenothiazines, and long-acting nitrates commonly cause postural changes in blood pressure, particularly in the elderly.

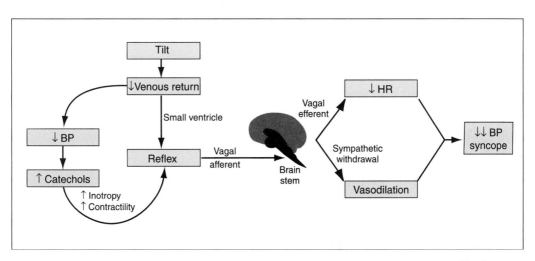

FIGURE 29.2. Bezold-Jarisch reflex. The Bezold-Jarisch reflex is critical to the pathogenesis of vasodepressor syncope. The reflex is activated via intracardiac vagal mechanoreceptors. Increased neural input to the brainstem via synapses with vagal efferents causes both bradycardia and hypotension, with syncope ensuing. BP = blood pressure; HR = heart rate.
(Redrawn from: Abi-Samra F, et al. PACE 1988;11:1201–1214 and Linzer M. Am J Med 1991;90:1–5. Used with permission.)

Psychogenic/emotional causes

Emotional abnormalities are an important cause of syncope and should be suspected in young patients with recurrent syncope and no cardiac disease. Patients with generalized anxiety disorders, panic attacks, and somatization disorders may present with syncope.

■ Diagnosis

The approach to evaluating syncope, as outlined in Figure 29.3, focuses on determining the presence of underlying heart disease because syncope of cardiac origin is more lethal than that of noncardiac or unknown cause. A detailed and accurate history, preferably corroborated by a bystander account, is critical (Table 29.1). Syncope must be distinguished from vague symptoms and syndromes not associated with loss of consciousness, such as vertigo, dizziness, faintness,

drop attacks, and dysequilibrium (a sensation of imbalance). Medications should be thoroughly reviewed, including prescription, over-the-counter, and illicit drugs (Table 29.2).

Supine and upright heart rate and blood pressure should be checked. The pulse rate normally increases by at least 10 beats/min with an orthostatic systolic blood pressure drop of >10 mm Hg and a diastolic drop of >5 mm Hg. Failure of the pulse to rise may indicate autonomic impairment or medication effects. The neck should be inspected for jugular venous distention, and the carotid pulse wave and its amplitude. Cardiac auscultation can detect aortic stenosis, mitral stenosis, pulmonic stenosis, and hypertrophic cardiomyopathy with obstruction. If no carotid bruits exist and carotid sinus hypersensitivity is a diagnostic possibility, then carotid sinus massage should be performed while the patient's heart rate and BP are being monitored.

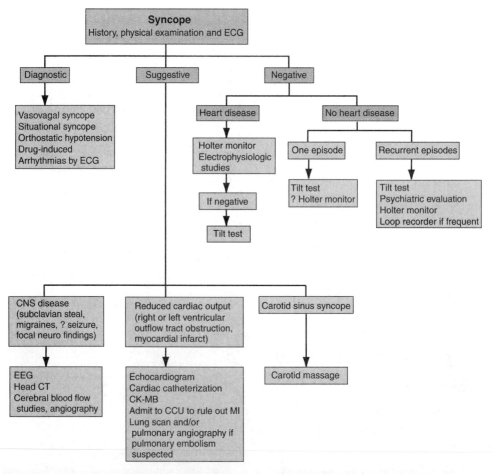

FIGURE 29.3. Approach to the evaluation of syncope. TIA, transient ischemic attack; EEG, electroencephalogram; CT, computed tomography; CK-MB, creatine kinase -MB fraction; CCU, cardiac care unit; MI, myocardial infarction. (Adapted from: Kapoor WN. Am J Med 1991;90:91–106.)

TABLE 29.2. Common Drugs Causing Syncope

Diuretics	Vasodilators
Beta blockers	Calcium channel blockers
Digitalis	Nitrates
Antiarrhythmics	Antidepressants
Phenothiazines	Hypoglycemics (Including Insulin)
CNS depressants	Alcohol
	Cocaine

(From: Kapoor WN. Am J Med 1991; 90: 91–106. Used with permission.)

Ancillary studies

Electroencephalograms (EEG) and computed tomography of the head are not indicated unless the history strongly suggests seizures or the physical examination shows a focal neurologic deficit. **ECG** may detect ischemic heart disease, prior myocardial infarction, chamber hypertrophy, conduction delays, a short P-R interval (accessory pathway), or a long Q-T interval. **Transthoracic and Doppler echocardiography** may confirm valvular heart lesions and quantify LV function; transesophageal echocardiography provides little additional information.

Ambulatory (Holter) monitoring may uncover significant tachyarrhythmias or bradyarrhythmias or intermittent high-degree AV block. For those with infrequent symptoms or spells, cardiobeepers and memory loop recorders (transtelephonic continuous loops) may provide useful diagnostic information.

Signal-averaged ECG (SAECG) amplifies and filters high-frequency late potentials in the terminal part of the QRS and is most useful when underlying ischemic heart disease is causing ventricular tachycardia. A normal SAECG excludes lethal ventricular arrhythmias as the cause of syncope, but such a test has a low positive predictive value when used in unselected patients.

Electrophysiologic testing and tilt-table testing

The major indication for electrophysiologic testing (EPT) is the inability to confirm noninvasively an arrhythmia as the cause of syncope in patients with underlying heart disease. When positive, EPT will show ventricular tachycardia in 46%, bradycardia from SA or AV nodal disease in 30%, and supraventricular tachycardias in 23% of patients. Predictors of positive EPT are conduction system disease (left bundle branch block), LV dysfunction (ejection fraction <40%), and effort syncope. Predictors of a negative EPT are recurrent syncope, lack of injury during episodes, no underlying heart disease, normal baseline ECG, and normal Holter monitoring. A nondiagnostic EPT in syncope confers a low risk of sudden death (about 2%).

Indications for tilt-table testing are summarized in Table 29.3. Vasodepressor syncope may be unmasked with tilt-table testing. A positive study is the induction of syncope or near-syncope associated with bradycardia, hypotension, or both.

■ Management
Cardiac syncope

A precise diagnosis is crucial to the rational management of cardiac syncope. Valvular disease that obstructs ventricular inflow or outflow may require surgery. With symptomatic bradyarrhythmias, offending drugs (e.g., β-blockers, digoxin) should be discontinued, if possible, before placement of a permanent pacemaker. Patients with documented sick sinus syndrome may need a permanent pacemaker. Paroxysmal supraventricular tachycardia owing to AV nodal reentry or an accessory pathway may be treated with drugs or catheter ablation.

Arrhythmias accompanied by hemodynamic compromise should be managed acutely. With symptomatic ventricular arrhythmias, precipitating factors (such as ischemia, hypoxia, or drugs) should be corrected. If ischemia is documented, antianginal regimens and possibly revascularization are appropriate treatments. Electrophysiologic testing should guide drug selection or placement of an automatic implantable cardioverter-defibrillator in those presumed to be symptomatic from ventricular arrhythmias; empiric antiarrhythmic drug therapy has no proven benefit.

Noncardiac syncope

Patients with situational syncope should be educated about appropriate strategies to avoid recurrences. Treatment of recurrent vasodepressor syncope includes β-blockers or disopyramide (both negative inotropes), transdermal scopolamine (anticholinergic), or hydrofluorocortisone (a mineralocorticoid to promote salt retention and volume expansion).

TABLE 29.3. Indications for Tilt-Table Testing

- Suspected neurally mediated syncope
- Recurrent idiopathic syncope with or without prodrome
- To differentiate convulsive syncope from seizure disorder
- Evaluate recurrent dizziness/vertigo if associated with syncope or presyncope
- Diagnosis of psychogenic syncope

Patients with autonomic insufficiency should be distinguished from those with volume-mediated or drug-induced orthostasis. In addition to maintaining an optimal circulating volume, avoiding excessive diuretic use, and discontinuing or adjusting doses of potentially offending drugs, patients may use mechanical measures, such as compression hose or body stockings. Beneficial drugs are ephedrine, hydrofluo-rocortisone, or prostaglandin synthesis inhibitors (indomethacin).

Patients with carotid sinus hypersensitivity may benefit from placement of a permanent pacemaker if a cardioinhibitory response is documented with carotid sinus massage. Patients with vasodepressor or mixed responses may benefit from denervation and/or local irradiation.

CHAPTER 30 CONGESTIVE HEART FAILURE

ongestive heart failure (CHF) is defined clinically as a constellation of symptoms and signs denoting congestion of the systemic and/or pulmonary venous beds and low cardiac output owing to the inability of the cardiac chambers to discharge their contents adequately. In this condition, despite adequate filling of the ventricles, cardiac output is inadequate to meet the metabolic demands of the body. The impaired ventricular function is associated with diminished exercise capacity, a high incidence of ventricular arrhythmias, and reduced life expectancy. Several terms are used relative to CHF, as defined in Table 30.1.

Congestive heart failure is a common syndrome, afflicting approximately 1% of the U.S. population (approximately 3 million people) and contributing to approximately 270,000 deaths annually.

TABLE 30.1.	Various Forms of Congestive Heart Failure
Left heart failure	— Pulmonary venous congestion
Right heart failure	— Systemic venous congestion
Acute heart failure	— Typified by acute pulmonary edema
Chronic heart failure	— Typified by congestive cardiomyopathy
High-output failure	— Higher than normal cardiac output that is still inadequate to meet vastly increased metabolic demands, (e.g., thyrotoxic heart disease)
Low-output failure	— Heart failure with lower-than-normal cardiac output

■ Pathophysiology

Normal circulation

The pump function of the heart is dependent on the load placed on the heart during systole and diastole and myocardial contractility.

Preload

Ventricular end-diastolic volume represents preload. The relationship between preload and stroke volume is defined by **Starling's law,** which states that up to a limit, the stroke volume (or stroke work) is directly proportional to the end-diastolic volume of the ventricle (Figure 30.1). Factors such as total intravascular volume, venous return, and atrial function influence the end-diastolic volume. Normal LV end-diastolic volume is attained at an end-diastolic pressure of up to 14 mm Hg. However, if the LV becomes more rigid (less compliant), as in LV hypertrophy, a higher end-diastolic pressure is required to distend the ventricle to a normal end-diastolic volume (Figure 30.2). Because measurement of LV volume is difficult in vivo, **LV filling pressure** (pulmonary capillary wedge, pulmonary artery diastolic, or LV end-diastolic pressure) is used as an indicator of preload.

Afterload

Afterload is the stress acting on contractile fibers in the ventricular wall after the onset of shortening. According to **Laplace's law,** afterload (wall stress) is directly proportional to ventricular pressure and ventricular radius and indirectly proportional to wall thickness. Aortic input impedance, systemic vascular resistance (SVR), and mean aortic pressure are indirect indicators of afterload. SVR can be calculated as follows:

$$SVR\ (Wood\ units) = \frac{Mean\ aortic\ pressure\ (mm\ Hg) - Mean\ right\ atrial\ pressure\ (mm\ Hg)}{Cardiac\ output\ (L/min)}$$

With a given preload and contractility, LV stroke volume and afterload show an indirect relationship.

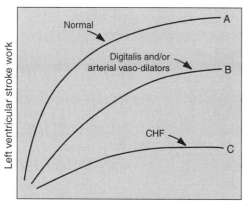

FIGURE **30.1.** Ventricular function (Starling's) curves: In the normal individual (*line A*), a slight increase in left ventricular (LV) filling pressure should result in a large increase in LV stroke work. With the markedly depressed ventricular function of CHF (*line C*), even a large increase in LV filling pressure results in only a small increase of LV stroke work. Treatment with digitalis enhances contractility and treatment with arterial vasodilators decreases afterload in patients with CHF, shifting the ventricular function curve from C to B.

Although a normal ventricle can adjust to changing afterload and deliver a normal stroke volume by using an intrinsic homeometric mechanism, a diseased ventricle loses this ability, and its systolic performance becomes profoundly afterload-dependent (Figure 30.1).

Myocardial contractility

Myocardial contractility (inotropic state) indicates the intrinsic capacity of myocardial fibers to shorten independent of their preload and afterload. The maximum velocity of contraction (V_{max}) is an index of contractility. Sympathomimetic amines, digitalis, glucagon, and tachycardias enhance myocardial contractility, and β-adrenergic-blocking agents reduce it. As shown in Figure 30.1, at a given preload and afterload, an upward and leftward shift of the ventricular function curve indicates increased contractility; a downward and rightward shift indicates decreased contractility.

Systemic circulation

Cardiac output is distributed to various organs depending on their metabolic needs. Blood pressure is the product of cardiac output and systemic vascular resistance. Autonomically mediated vasomotor tone plays a vital role in matching the perfusion of a particular organ to its demands.

Circulatory reserve

Increased oxygen demands during exercise are met by two mechanisms: augmented cardiac output and increased oxygen extraction by the tissues. Increased sympathetic activity on exercise augments both heart rate and myocardial contractility, thus raising cardiac output. Starling's law also becomes operational at high levels of exercise.

Compensatory mechanisms in heart failure

Although either systolic or diastolic dysfunction can cause CHF, in approximately two-thirds of patients, the primary hemodynamic abnormality is systolic dysfunction (i.e., impaired myocardial contractility and inability of the heart to discharge normally). Several compensatory factors evolve to restore normal cardiac output (Figure 30.3). However, as these mechanisms are expended to maintain the resting cardiac output, the cardiac reserve becomes eroded. Moreover, several deleterious effects are associated with these compensatory mechanisms (Table 30.2).

Ventricular hypertrophy and dilatation

Impaired contractility and pressure overload stimulate myocardial **hypertrophy.** The hypertrophied ventricle can generate greater force to overcome the increased afterload. In contrast, conditions associated with volume overloading, such as aortic regurgitation, cause ventricular **dilatation** to compensate for increased volume. An enlarged chamber can generate a greater stroke volume. However, as the ventricle enlarges, wall stress also increases, raising the myocardial oxygen demand. In both ventricular hypertrophy and dilatation, beyond a certain stage, myocardial O_2 demand exceeds the supply, resulting in diffuse myocardial fibrosis and further reducing the contractile function.

After a large anterior wall infarction, the LV may

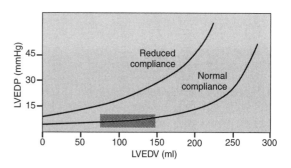

FIGURE **30.2.** Diastolic pressure-volume (compliance) curves. The initial portion of the normal curve is fairly flat; consequently, a significant increase in left ventricular end-diastolic volume (LVEDV) results in only a small increase in left ventricular end-diastolic pressure (LVEDP). With increasing LVEDV beyond a certain limit, small increases in LVEDV cause rapid increases of LVEDP. With reduced compliance, the curve is shifted upward and to the left, indicating that even normal LVEDV is associated with high LVEDP. The shaded area indicates the normal range for LVEDV and LVEDP.

FIGURE **30.3.** Pathogenesis of congestive heart failure and the influence of various compensatory factors that become active in an attempt to maintain normal pump function. (CAD, coronary artery disease.)

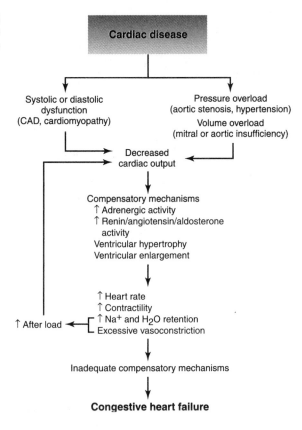

TABLE 30.2. Compensatory Mechanisms in Congestive Heart Failure

Mechanism	Salutary Effects	Deleterious Effects
Ventricular hypertrophy	↑ Force of contraction, ↑ Wall stress	↑ O_2 demand, ↓O_2 supply ↓ Diastolic compliance
Ventricular dilatation (increased preload, Starling's law)	↑ Stroke volume	↑ O_2 demand, ↑ wall stress, ↑ pulmonary congestion, ↑ systemic congestion
↑ Sympathetic activity	↑ Contractility, ↑ heart rate, ↑ Venous tone (preload)	↑ O_2 demand, ↑ systemic arterial tone (afterload) causing ↓ stroke volume
↑ Renin-angiotensin-aldosterone system	↑ Salt and water retention; ↑ venous return and preload	↑ Pulmonary congestion, ↑ systemic congestion, ↑ vasoconstriction (↑ afterload)
↑ O_2 extraction	↑ O_2 delivery	—

enlarge and assume a spherical configuration (ventricular remodeling). Although this adaptive change maintains stroke volume, the remodeling process has deleterious long-term effects on global LV function and prognosis.

Starling's law

The ventricular function curve becomes progressively depressed (downward shift) with increasing se-

verity of heart failure as large changes in preload result in only small changes in stroke volume (Figure 30.1). In CHF, renal blood flow is markedly reduced, which activates the renin-angiotensin-aldosterone system, causing retention of sodium and water and expansion of the intravascular volume. Expanded central blood volume, by increasing the preload, activates the Starling's mechanism and increases the stroke volume. However, the deleterious effects of this mechanism include increased myocardial oxygen demands and pulmonary and/or systemic venous congestion manifested by dyspnea, edema, and hepatomegaly.

Neurohormonal activity

CHF is associated with increased levels of several neurohormones: norepinephrine, renin-angiotensin, antidiuretic hormone, atrial natriuretic neuropeptide, and prostaglandins.

Increased sympathetic discharge is beneficial in maintaining the normal circulatory status in heart failure through several different mechanisms, e.g., tachycardia, stimulation of contractility, arteriolar constriction, and venoconstriction. Despite the increased blood catecholamine level, the norepinephrine content of the failing myocardium decreases.

Increased activity of the systemic and tissue renin-angiotensin system in CHF has been well documented. A decrease in renal blood flow and reduced concentration of renal tubular Na^+ and Cl^- ions as well as activation of atrial mechanoreceptors stimulate the renin-angiotensin system. A potent vasoconstrictor and stimulator of sympathetic nervous system, angiotensin II also contributes to cell growth and cardiac remodeling. It also stimulates secretion of aldosterone and vasopressin, which in turn promote sodium and water retention and loss of potassium and magnesium.

Plasma levels of arginine vasopressin (antidiuretic hormone) may be elevated in CHF. This hormone is also a potent vasoconstrictor, and its release is stimulated by angiotensin II. Increased levels of atrial natriuretic peptide also are present in CHF. This compound is generated in the atrial tissue and promotes diuresis, natriuresis, and vasodilation. It inhibits the renin-angiotensin-aldosterone system as well as vasopressin.

The primary disadvantage of generalized arteriolar constriction is that it augments afterload, with increased resistance to LV ejection and a reduced stroke volume. This establishes a vicious cycle of reduced cardiac output, increased sympathetic activity, increased arteriolar constriction, and further reduction of cardiac output. A high level of circulating catecholamines indicates a poor long-term prognosis.

Increased oxygen extraction

Normally, peripheral tissues extract 3.5–5.0 ml of O_2 from each 100 ml of arterial blood. In low-output states, tissues extract greater amounts of oxygen, causing widening of the arteriovenous O_2 difference.

■ Etiology

Several disease states affecting predominantly the left and/or right side of the heart account for CHF (Table 30.3). Despite some overlaps, heart failure may be caused by predominantly systolic or predominantly diastolic dysfunction.

Predominantly systolic dysfunction

Abnormal loading conditions

A **pressure overload,** or increased afterload, is imposed on the LV by conditions such as aortic stenosis, coarctation of the aorta, and systemic hypertension. Pulmonary stenosis and pulmonary hypertension place a pressure overload on the RV. Ventricular hypertrophy subsequently develops to overcome the increased outflow resistance. A hypertrophied ventricular wall is more stiff, causing end-diastolic pressure to rise. Progressive contractile failure follows several years of ventricular hypertrophy, culminating in ventricular dilatation and failure.

TABLE 30.3. Etiology of Congestive Heart Failure

Predominantly Systolic Dysfunction	Predominantly Diastolic Dysfunction
Conditions causing pressure overload:	Marked left ventricular hypertrophy
Hypertension	Hypertrophic cardiomyopathy
Aortic stenosis	Hypertension
Coarctation of aorta	Severe myocardial ischemia
Pulmonary hypertension	Mitral stenosis
Pulmonary thromboembolic disease	Left atrial myxoma
Conditions causing volume overload:	Infiltrative cardiomyopathies (amyloidosis, hemochromatosis)
Aortic incompetence	Pericardial constriction
Mitral incompetence	Cardiac tamponade
Ventricular septal defect	
Atrial septal defect	
Myocardial contractile failure:	
Myocardial infarction	
Dilated cardiomyopathies	

A **volume overload** is placed on the LV by conditions such as aortic or mitral regurgitation, patent ductus arteriosus, and ventricular septal defect. Tricuspid regurgitation, pulmonary regurgitation, and atrial septal defect impose a volume overload on the RV. To accommodate the increased volume, ventricular dilatation occurs relatively early, and over several years, ventricular hypertrophy ensues. The heart tolerates volume overload better than pressure overload.

Myocardial contractile failure (intrinsic myocardial failure)

In myocardial infarction, maintenance of cardiac output depends on the infarct size: whereas the residual normal muscle can compensate and maintain normal output in small infarcts, such compensatory mechanisms fail in large infarcts, resulting in heart failure and/or cardiogenic shock. In cardiomyopathies, myocardial contractility is reduced diffusely, resulting in global ventricular dysfunction and heart failure.

Predominantly diastolic dysfunction

Diastolic dysfunction implies impaired ventricular filling; however, systolic function is preserved. LV hypertrophy—as in hypertrophic cardiomyopathy, aortic stenosis, or hypertension (especially in combination with diabetes mellitus)—reduces LV compliance. Filling such a stiff ventricle requires a powerful left atrial contraction. Left atrial pressure rises, which affects the pulmonary circulation, causing congestion and dyspnea (Figure 30.2). If atrial fibrillation develops in this setting, the resulting loss of atrial kick as well as reduced diastolic time for ventricular filling by tachycardia further aggravate the CHF. Intense myocardial ischemia can also reduce LV compliance and cause pulmonary edema.

Mitral stenosis and left atrial myxoma cause CHF by mechanically obstructing the mitral orifice, restricting LV filling, impeding left atrial emptying, and in turn, causing pulmonary vascular congestion. Similarly, systemic venous congestion develops in tricuspid stenosis, tricuspid atresia, and right atrial myxoma. In these conditions, ventricular filling is impeded by the mechanical obstruction, but the ventricle itself is normal.

■ Clinical Features

The manifestations of heart failure can be attributed to three main hemodynamic changes: 1) decreased cardiac output causing inadequate perfusion of various organ systems, 2) left atrial hypertension with pulmonary venous congestion, and 3) right atrial hypertension with systemic venous congestion. Depending on the underlying mechanism, these features may be present in varying combinations (Table 30.4).

Signs and symptoms increase as CHF worsens, causing a progressive loss of functional capacity. The New York Heart Association (NYHA) Functional Classification is a widely used measure of disability in heart failure and provides important prognostic information (Table 30.5).

Left Heart Failure

Symptoms

Dyspnea, the cardinal symptom of left heart failure, implies awareness of breathing or shortness of breath. It is usually attributed to decreased compliance

TABLE 30.4.	Clinical Manifestations of Congestive Heart Failure
Left Heart Failure	**Right Heart Failure**
Symptoms	
Dyspnea	Edema
Orthopnea	Dyspnea
Paroxysmal nocturnal dyspnea	Abdominal distension and discomfort
Acute pulmonary edema	Anorexia, nausea
Hemoptysis	Weight loss
Nocturia	Weakness
Fatigue	Anxiety
Signs	
Cardiomegaly	Positive hepatojugular reflux
Left ventricular S_3	Jugular venous distension
Loud P_2	Liver enlargement
Functional mitral incompetence	Splenic enlargement
Pulsus alternans	Dependent edema
Pulmonary crackles	Ascites
Cheyne-Stokes breathing	Cyanosis
Pleural effusion	Cardiomegaly
	Right ventricular S_3
	Functional tricuspid incompetence
	Cardiac cachexia

TABLE 30.5.	New York Heart Association Functional Classification of Congestive Heart Failure

Class	Description
I	No symptoms on ordinary activity
II	Symptoms* occur on ordinary activity
III	Symptoms occur on less than ordinary activity
IV	Symptoms present at rest

*Symptoms include dyspnea, fatigue, and/or angina.

of the lungs owing to pulmonary venous congestion and edema. With mild heart failure, dyspnea occurs only on exertion, but as CHF progresses, the activity threshold declines.

Orthopnea indicates dyspnea during recumbency, with relief on sitting up. Relief in an upright posture presumably occurs due to an increase of intrathoracic space and reduction of pulmonary venous congestion, as the blood pools in the lower extremities.

In **paroxysmal nocturnal dyspnea** (PND), the patient typically sleeps 1–4 hours and then awakens acutely short of breath, feeling suffocated. The patient may sit upright and gasp for breath, walk for a few minutes, or open a window to obtain some fresh air. Sweating, pallor, cyanosis, cold extremities, and cough may be associated signs. The episode subsides in approximately 10–30 minutes, and the patient sleeps comfortably for the rest of the night. Wheezing may be present during PND ("cardiac asthma").

Acute **pulmonary edema** is a consequence of sudden, severe decompensation of the LV or severe mitral stenosis. The patient notes abrupt, agonizing dyspnea and persistent cough productive of white or pink, frothy sputum. Use of accessory muscles of respiration and an extreme degree of anxiety are accompaniments. The skin is cold, pale, and gray with profuse sweating. The attack subsides spontaneously or with treatment, usually after a few minutes to a few hours. However, severe pulmonary edema can be lethal.

Cheyne-Stokes breathing is defined as periods of apnea alternating with hyperpnea (rapid breathing). Usually occurring in elderly patients with left heart failure who have concomitant central nervous system disease, it is ascribed to a disturbance of feedback control of the respiratory center owing to prolongation of circulation time, cerebrovascular disease, or sedation.

Expectoration of blood, or **hemoptysis,** may occur in severe left heart failure or pulmonary edema, varying from rusty-colored or pink, frothy sputum to frank blood. Hemoptysis also may arise from pulmonary thromboembolism, to which patients with heart failure are predisposed.

Patients frequently note **fatigue** on mild exertion. Low cardiac output causing decreased O_2 delivery to skeletal muscle, electrolyte depletion (hypokalemia), and physical deconditioning are possible causes.

Many patients report **dizziness,** weakness, and lack of balance. Most of these episodes are brief and occur when the patient is in an upright posture. Dizziness in patients with cardiac disease is due to low cardiac output resulting in poor perfusion to the brain. **Angina decubitus,** or nocturnal angina, may be another manifestation of left heart failure.

Physical signs

A small-volume pulse is caused by low stroke volume. **Pulsus alternans** refers to a strong pulse alternating with a weak one, despite equal duration of the cardiac cycles. It implies severe myocardial failure. Tachycardia, pallor, cyanosis, and cold and clammy extremities indicate a hyperadrenergic state.

Tachypnea, or rapid, shallow breathing, is attributed to pulmonary venous congestion and decreased lung compliance. An audible **ventricular gallop** (S_3) over the cardiac apex is an early sign of left heart failure and indicates an enlarged and poorly contracting LV.

Functional ("secondary") **mitral regurgitation** may develop with LV enlargement and improper coaptation of the mitral valve leaflets. As the LV shrinks in response to therapy, this type of mitral incompetence may disappear (see chapter 34).

Pulmonary findings in left heart failure consist of **bibasilar rales (crackles),** diminished breath sounds over the bases, and, occasionally, bilateral rhonchi. Transudation of fluid into the alveoli and bronchiolar narrowing explain these findings.

Ancillary studies

Chest radiography is a valuable tool for diagnosis and follow-up of left heart failure. Although the heart may or may not be enlarged, its silhouette may suggest LV enlargement. Lung fields show vascular redistribution and Kerley B lines (Figure 26.1). In frank pulmonary edema, confluent opacities appear in the central lung fields bilaterally near the hila, producing a "bat's wing" appearance (Figure 30.4) In persistent left heart failure, pleural effusion(s) may develop either on the right side or bilaterally. Pleural effusions, however, are more common in biventricular failure and usually occur when pulmonary capillary wedge pressure is significantly elevated.

In early left heart failure, pulmonary function tests show premature closure of peripheral airways at low lung volumes, causing maldistribution of intrapulmonary air. Lung compliance is decreased.

Echocardiography and **radionuclide ventriculography** demonstrate an enlarged and poorly contractile LV. **Cardiac catheterization** shows high pulmonary capillary wedge and LV end-diastolic pressures, an abnormally wide arteriovenous oxygen difference, and decreased ejection fraction. However, severity of symptoms correlate poorly with the LV ejection fraction.

Arrhythmias such as atrial flutter, atrial fibrillation, premature ventricular complexes, and bouts of nonsustained ventricular tachycardia are common in chronic CHF and indicate a poor prognosis. Ventricular tachycardia or ventricular fibrillation are frequent terminal events.

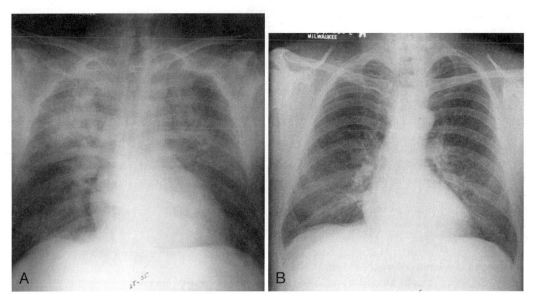

FIGURE 30.4.   Chest radiograph in acute cardiogenic pulmonary edema showing bilateral confluent opacities ("bat wing"). (B) Follow-up x-ray a few days later, showing significant clearing, although some mild congestive changes remain.
(Courtesy of the Radiology Museum, St. Joseph's Hospital, Milwaukee, Wisconsin.)

Right Heart Failure

The symptoms and signs of right heart failure are caused by two primary factors: systemic venous congestion and RV dilatation. Systemic venous pressure increases as a result of an increased blood volume in the systemic veins secondary to inadequate RV emptying during systole. Generalized venoconstriction in response to sympathetic overactivity also causes such an increase. In the vast majority of patients, LV failure or mitral valve disease is the principal cause of right heart failure. Other causes include pulmonary emboli, chronic obstructive pulmonary disease, and pulmonary hypertension.

With left heart failure and/or pulmonary venous hypertension, passive pulmonary arterial hypertension develops to maintain forward flow. Once the pulmonary arterial pressure attains a certain level, pulmonary arterioles actively constrict by a reflex mechanism that worsens the pulmonary hypertension. This places a pressure overload on the RV, which subsequently fails as the compensatory mechanisms become ineffective in maintaining the forward output.

With progressive decrease of RV stroke volume, the signs and symptoms of pulmonary venous congestion (e.g., pulmonary vascular redistribution, dyspnea) become less marked. It is not uncommon for a patient with severe mitral stenosis to be free of orthopnea despite advanced right heart failure.

Symptoms

Patients usually note **edema** of the ankles and feet initially, which later spreads to the legs and abdomen. The edema is bilateral and pitting. In bedridden patients, edema may first develop over the sacrum. In its advanced stage, edema becomes widespread (anasarca), with ascites and edema of the external genitalia.

Right-upper-quadrant **abdominal pain** occurs owing to liver enlargement. **Anorexia** and **nausea** develop secondary to congestion of the gastrointestinal tract. Absorption of nutrients is impaired, and in persistent systemic venous congestion as seen in patients with constrictive pericarditis, significant protein loss may result (protein-losing gastroenteropathy). All these factors cause gradual **weight loss** and, ultimately, **cardiac cachexia.** Other symptoms include fatigue, daytime oliguria, and nocturia.

Physical signs

Jugular venous distention and jugular venous pressure (JVP) exceeding 3 cm above the sternal angle are indicative of right heart failure. The neck veins fill from below. A **positive hepatojugular reflux**—i.e., persistent elevation of the JVP during sustained pressure in the right upper abdomen—is an early sign of right heart failure. On close examination of the venous pulse, a sharp y descent is frequently found. RV gallop (S_3) is audible over the left lower sternal border and indicates increased RV end-diastolic volume.

Hepatomegaly and, occasionally, **splenomegaly** occur in right heart failure. An enlarged liver is tender to light pressure. After prolonged or recurrent episodes of right heart failure, widespread patchy necrosis, which is followed by fibrosis, develops in the liver owing to ischemic injury of the liver cells. Ultimately, cardiac cirrhosis follows.

Functional tricuspid incompetence, manifested by a pansystolic murmur over the left lower sternal border, prominent v waves in the neck veins, and a pulsatile liver, develops as the RV dilates. Because the tricuspid valve no longer protects the systemic veins from RV systolic pressure, systemic venous congestion worsens. As the tissues extract more oxygen owing to poor tissue perfusion and the capillary deoxyhemoglobin exceeds 5 g/dl, **peripheral cyanosis** becomes evident.

Ancillary studies

The chest radiograph shows dilatation of the superior and inferior vena cava, right atrium, RV, and main pulmonary trunks. Associated pleural effusion indicates coexistent left heart failure.

The **echocardiogram** may reveal dilatation of the RV and paradoxical septal motion indicating RV volume overload, especially when functional tricuspid incompetence develops. **Cardiac catheterization** reveals high central venous, right atrial, and RV end-diastolic pressures and pulmonary arterial hypertension. The pulmonary capillary wedge pressure is elevated when right-sided failure is associated with LV failure or mitral stenosis; however, it is normal when right heart failure arises from obstructive lung disease or pulmonary emboli.

Liver function tests become abnormal in advanced cases. Urinalysis commonly shows slight proteinuria and high specific gravity. Blood urea nitrogen may rise owing to poor renal perfusion (prerenal failure).

■ Prognosis

The overall 1-year survival in CHF varies from 10–60%. Milder degrees and initial episodes of CHF are easily controllable and have a better prognosis than chronic, severe CHF. Correctable diseases, such as valve lesions, hypertension, and some congenital lesions, when treated early, have a much better prognosis than untreatable diseases. Poor prognostic factors include LV dysfunction, poor exercise tolerance, presence of coronary artery disease, S_3 gallop, ventricular arrhythmias, atrial flutter or fibrillation, and increased neurohormonal factors.

■ Management

Management should alleviate symptoms, treat the primary or underlying cardiac disease to prevent recurrence of CHF, and thus improve survival.

General measures

Depending on the severity of heart failure, complete bedrest or frequent rest periods should be advised to reduce the cardiac workload and promote diuresis. Use of elastic stockings, passive leg exercises, and low-dose heparin therapy are useful to prevent thromboembolic complications. Careful exercise training should be encouraged to prevent physical deconditioning.

The head of the patient's bed should be elevated to decrease ventricular preload by pooling the blood in the legs. Caloric intake should be restricted in overweight patients. Supplemental O_2 is helpful in severe CHF. Factors that precipitate episodes of CHF should be identified and treated (Table 30.6).

Increasing myocardial contractility

Because depressed myocardial contractility is the underlying cause in most cases of heart failure, enhancement of myocardial contractility would be expected to improve cardiac performance. Of the various positive inotropic agents, digitalis preparations are the most useful clinically. They enhance myocardial contractility by promoting the availability of Ca^{++} to actin and myosin. Enhanced contractility improves ventricular ejection fraction, stroke volume, and exercise tolerance.

TABLE 30.6.	Factors Contributing to Decompensation in CHF

Cardiac
  Recurrent myocardial ischemia
  Acute myocardial infarction
  Tachyarrhythmias
  Infective endocarditis
Noncardiac
  Systemic infections
  Heavy alcohol consumption
  Thyrotoxicosis
  Excessive salt intake
  Excessive fluid ingestion
  Pulmonary embolism
  Increased physical or emotional stress
Drugs
  Poor compliance with medications
  Use of negative inotropic agents (β-blockers)
  Use of prostaglandin inhibitors (NSAIDs) causing fluid
    retention

Even though digitalis is a direct vasoconstrictor, as the CHF improves and adrenergic tone is withdrawn, the net effect is vasodilation. In contrast to catecholamines, digitalis increases the myocardial contractility without concomitant tachycardia or systemic arterial constriction. It is particularly useful in patients with cardiomegaly, severe symptoms, reduced ejection fraction and ventricular gallop.

Digitalis

The most commonly used digitalis preparations are digoxin and digitoxin. **Digoxin** is available as 0.125-mg, 0.25-mg, and 0.5-mg tablets as well as for IV use. Slightly more than three-fourths of the oral dose is absorbed. Effects start within 1–2 hours and reach a peak level 2–3 hours after ingestion. The half-life of digoxin is 1.6 days. It is excreted unchanged, predominantly by the kidneys.

Therapy is usually begun with 0.75 mg of digoxin in divided doses during the first 24 hours, and then maintained at 0.125–0.5 mg daily. In patients with renal insufficiency, the dose should be reduced to 0.125 mg daily or administered on alternate days. The therapeutic serum level of digoxin is usually 1–2 ng/ml, with digitalis toxicity usually developing at serum levels exceeding 2 ng/ml. However, the diagnosis of digitalis toxicity is made by clinical and ECG findings because a wide range of digitalis levels can create a toxic state in patients.

Digitoxin has a long half-life of approximately 7 days and is used primarily for long-term maintenance in 0.1-mg/day doses. Because digitoxin is metabolized predominantly in the liver, it is perhaps more useful as long-term therapy in patients with chronic renal insufficiency.

Digitalis in therapeutic doses produces ST-segment depression and Q-T interval shortening. With toxic amounts, a variety of arrhythmias may occur, such as multifocal premature ventricular contractions; bigeminy; atrial tachycardia with block; nonparoxysmal junctional tachycardia; atrioventricular dissociation and first, second, or third degree AV blocks. Nausea, anorexia, vomiting, and altered vision (seeing as if through a green or yellow filter) may also be reported. Hypokalemia, hypomagnesemia, hypoxia, and hypercalcemia may precipitate digitalis toxicity. Patients with acute myocardial infarction, myocarditis, and cor pulmonale are more sensitive to digitalis.

Treatment of digitalis toxicity consists of discontinuing the drug and administering a potassium supplement (if hypokalemia is present). In more severe toxicity, antiarrhythmic agents, such as lidocaine, procainamide, propranolol, or phenytoin, are necessary to control the tachyarrhythmias. A temporary pacemaker may be required when complete AV block develops with slow ventricular rate resistant to atropine. For severe digoxin toxicity causing life-threatening arrhythmias, digoxin immune Fab (free digoxin binding antibody fragments) is the treatment of choice.

Other inotropic agents

Dopamine and **dobutamine** are sympathetic agonists with potent positive inotropic effects and without significant chronotropic effect. In addition, dobutamine lowers systemic vascular resistance. Neither dopamine in small doses nor dobutamine affects blood pressure significantly. These agents are available only for intravenous use. They are useful on a short-term basis, in patients with refractory CHF. Some patients with refractory CHF exhibit sustained improvement in response to intermittent, short-term dobutamine infusions.

Recently, a new class of positive inotropic agents with vasodilating properties, the bipyridine compounds, (e.g., **amrinone** and **milrinone**) have become available. They reduce systemic vascular resistance and preload, augment cardiac output, and reduce symptoms. Their mode of action at the cellular level differs from that of digitalis and catecholamines: they inhibit cellular phosphodiesterase, resulting in an increase in the cyclic AMP level. Both agents are available in intravenous form for short-term use in patients with refractory heart failure. Although these agents improve hemodynamics and symptoms acutely, they have not been shown to improve survival. Vesnarinone and pimobendan have recently been shown to be useful in CHF. These agents enhance sensitivity of contractile elements to calcium and thus augment contractility.

Lowering ventricular preload

Expanded intravascular volume owing to abnormal salt and water retention by the kidneys as well as elevated ventricular filling pressure are responsible for the pulmonary vascular congestion that results in dyspnea, orthopnea, and paroxysmal nocturnal dyspnea and for the systemic vascular congestion causing edema, hepatomegaly, distended neck veins, and ascites. One way to reduce this expanded intravascular volume is to limit salt intake to 1–2 g/day (17–34 mEq Na^+). A sitting or semi-sitting posture also reduces the ventricular preload by pooling blood in the periphery.

The most effective way to reduce the preload is by the judicious use of **diuretics** (Table 30.7). These agents reduce the reabsorption of Na^+ in the renal tubules, causing natriuresis and diuresis. As the pulmonary congestion is relieved, oxygenation of blood and exercise tolerance improve. Because the ventricles are operating at the flat portion of Starling's curve, cardiac output is only slightly changed, despite a reduction of the preload

TABLE 30.7. Commonly Used Diuretics

Drug	Dose	Route	Onset of Action (min)	Peak Effect (h)	Duration of effect (h)	Class Site of Action	Class Adverse Effects
A. *Thiazides*							
Chlorthalidone	25–50 mg qd	PO	120	2–6	24–72	Distal convoluted tubule (Metolazone acts in proximal convoluted tubule also)	Hypokalemia, hyponatremia, hypochloremic alkalosis, glucose intolerance, increased cholesterol, nausea, skin rash
Hydrochlorothiazide	25–50 mg qd	PO	120	4–6	6–12		
Indapamide	2.5–5 mg qd	PO	60–120	2	36		
Metolazone	2.5–10 mg qd	PO	60	2	12–24		
B. *Loop Diuretics*							
Furosemide	20–200 mg	IV	5	0.5	2	Ascending limb of loop of Henle	Hypokalemia, hypomagnesemia, hypocalcemia, hyponatremia, hypochloremic alkalosis, increased cholesterol, hearing loss
	20–240 mg qd or bid	PO	30	1–2	6–8		
Bumetanide	0.5–1 mg (max 10 mg)	IV	5	0.5–0.75	2		
	0.5–2 mg (max 10 mg)	PO	30–60	1–2	4–6		
C. *Potassium-Sparing*							
Spironolactone	25–200 mg qd	PO	(3 days)	1–2	48–72	Late distal convoluted tubule	Hyperkalemia, hyponatremia, hyperchloremic acidosis, gynecomastia and hirsutism
Triamterene	50–100 mg qd or bid	PO	(2–4 days)	2–4	7–9	Collecting ducts	Hyperkalemia, hyponatremia
Amiloride	5–10 mg qd (max 40 mg)	PO	120	3–4	24		

(Figure 30.1). However, overzealous use of diuretics, which causes excessive contraction of intravascular volume, can reduce the cardiac output and also promote thromboembolic complications.

The aim of diuretic therapy is relieving symptoms of pulmonary and systemic venous congestion while not compromising the cardiac output. The optimal dose of diuretics can be determined by performing serial clinical examinations, measurement of body weight, blood pressure measurements in the supine and standing positions (to detect postural hypotension), and blood urea nitrogen determinations.

The second major class of pharmacologic agents used to decrease the ventricular preload are the **venodilators** such as nitrates. By pooling blood in the periphery, they decrease venous return, reducing the filling pressures of both ventricles. (They are discussed with afterload reduction in the next section.)

Reducing left ventricular afterload

In CHF, aortic input impedance and ventricular afterload are inappropriately elevated, which tends to lower the stroke volume and increase myocardial O_2 demand. Arteriolar **vasodilators** break this cycle; they reduce aortic impedance, which facilitates systolic emptying of the LV, thus increasing cardiac output and decreasing myocardial O_2 demand (Table 30.8). The arteriolar vasodilators (Table 30.8) are particularly useful in treating patients with left heart failure caused by acute mitral or aortic regurgitation because these drugs promote forward ejection into the aorta and reduce regurgitation into the left atrium and LV, respectively. On the other hand, in heart failure due to valvular stenosis, vasodilators may evoke hypotension because the stenotic valves do not allow increase in cardiac output to compensate for arterial dilatation.

Patients with heart failure frequently show venoconstriction that augments pulmonary blood volume and contributes to pulmonary congestion. Venodilators (e.g., nitrates) reduce pulmonary blood volume, preload, and pulmonary congestion, thus relieving dyspnea and enhancing exercise tolerance.

Because of its potency and rapid onset of action, IV **sodium nitroprusside** is an ideal agent for short-term use in patients with refractory CHF. Pulmonary wedge pressure (left heart filling pressure), peripheral blood pressure, cardiac output, heart rate, and urine output should be monitored during sodium nitroprusside therapy.

Angiotensin-converting enzyme (ACE) inhibitors have a balanced effect on the arterial and venous beds. Both the ACE inhibitor and a combination of nitrates and hydralazine improve hemodynamic status, exercise capacity, and survival. ACE inhibitors minimize the loss of serum K^+ and blunt the stimulation of the renin-angiotensin system by diuretics.

β-blockers

β-blockers are negative inotropic agents and, therefore, are usually contraindicated in CHF. However, recent studies in idiopathic dilated cardiomyopathy have shown that judicious use of **metoprolol** can actually improve symptoms and cardiac function and prevent clinical deterioration. Recent studies using **carvedilol** have shown beneficial effects in CHF. The mechanism of these favorable effects is not clear, and the role of β-blockers is not yet established in the treatment of CHF.

Drainage of effusions and ascites

Persistent hydrothorax and ascites, by encroaching on the chest cavity, worsen dyspnea. If unresponsive to diuretic therapy, thoracentesis and paracentesis, respectively, may be required.

TABLE 30.8.	**Commonly Used Vasodilators**						
Drug	Mechanism of Action	Venodilation	Arteriolar Dilation	Dose	Route	Duration	Adverse Effects
NITRATES							
Nitroprusside	Direct	Major	Major	5–150 µg/min	IV	Minutes	Hypotension, thiocyanate toxicity
Nitroglycerin	Direct	Major	Minimal	10–100 µg/min	IV	Minutes	Hypotension, dizziness, syncope,
				0.3–0.6 mg	SL	Minutes	headache, nausea
				0.5–2 in. q 4–6 h	Topical	Hours	
				0.2–0.6 mg/h	Topical	Hours	
Isosorbide dinitrate	Direct	Major	Minimal	2.5–10 mg q2–3h;	SL	Hours	
				10–40 mg q 3–6h	PO	Hours	
HYDRALAZINE	Direct	None	Major	10–75 mg q 6 h	PO	Hours	Tachycardia, headache, nausea, drug-induced lupus
ACE INHIBITORS							
Captopril	ACEI	Major	Moderate	6.25–25 mg TID	PO	Hours	Hypotension, hyperkalemia,
Enalapril	ACEI	Major	Moderate	2.5–10 mg BID	PO	Hours	cough, proteinuria, azotemia,
Lisinopril	ACEI	Major	Moderate	5–20 mg BID	PO	Hours	angioedema, agranulocytosis

ACEI = angiotensin converting enzyme inhibition; PO = oral; SL = sublingual.

◼ Treatment of CHF Due to Diastolic Dysfunction

Treatment is based on interventions that reduce LV diastolic pressure and, at the same time, augment diastolic filling. Restriction of salt intake and careful use of diuretics as well as vasodilators (nitrates) decreases LV end-diastolic volume and pressure, reduces pulmonary congestion, and relieves dyspnea. Control of tachycardia improves ventricular filling by increasing the diastolic filling period. Because a forceful atrial contraction can account for 35–40% of ventricular filling in the presence of a stiff, hypertrophied ventricle, restoration of normal sinus rhythm in atrial fibrillation will greatly enhance ventricular filling. Calcium channel-blockers may favorably influence the compliance characteristics of the ventricular myocardium (lusitropic function). Because the systolic function is mostly normal in these patients, positive inotropic agents (digitalis) and arterial vasodilators (hydralazine, ACE inhibitors) may not be useful.

Treatment of acute pulmonary edema

Pulmonary edema develops when the influx of fluid into the interstitial space or the alveoli from the intravascular space exceeds its efflux via the pulmonary lymphatics (see chapter 225). It may be cardiogenic (high-pressure form), when pulmonary capillary wedge pressure exceeds the plasma colloid osmotic pressure, or noncardiogenic (low-pressure form), when the pulmonary vascular permeability increases. Chest radiographs are very helpful in diagnosis of pulmonary edema, but cannot differentiate between high-pressure and low-pressure forms.

Acute pulmonary edema is a medical emergency and can be fatal unless promptly treated. The goals of treatment are to maintain systemic arterial oxygenation and rapidly relieve pulmonary congestion (Table 30.9).

Treatment of arrhythmias

Frequent premature ventricular complexes and bouts of nonsustained ventricular tachycardia are common in CHF. Structural changes in the myocardium, myocardial ischemia, electrolyte disturbances, and neurohormonal factors contribute to these arrhythmias. These arrhythmias increase the risk for sudden death. Conventional antiarrhythmic agents do not reduce this risk, and ironically, promote arrhythmogenesis through proarrhythmic effects.

Current recommendations for managing these arrhythmias include optimizing therapy for CHF (especially with ACE inhibitors), maintaining serum potassium and magnesium levels in the high-normal range, and correcting ongoing myocardial ischemia. Ventricular arrhythmias associated with significant symptoms, such as presyncope and syncope, require evaluation with electrophysiologic studies and aggressive management with antiarrhythmic agents (e.g., amiodarone) and automatic implantable cardioverter-defibrillator.

Refractory CHF

With CHF refractory to standard treatment with diuretics, digoxin, and vasodilators, patients should be hospitalized, evaluated, and treated for any precipitating factors (Table 30.6). Patients with severe, persistent CHF should be considered for individualized therapy under invasive monitoring with a pulmonary artery catheter. After the baseline hemodynamic status is evaluated, therapy with diuretics, vasodilators (IV sodium nitroprusside), digoxin, and/or sympathomimetic amines (dopamine or dobutamine) is initiated. The goal is to achieve the optimal hemodynamic values (mean pulmonary capillary wedge pressure <15 mm Hg, systemic vascular resistance <1200 dynes/sec/cm^5, mean right atrial pressure <8 mm Hg, and mean systemic blood pressure >80 mm Hg). Patients are subsequently switched to oral medications and counseled regarding salt restriction, exercise, and flexible diuretic regimen. In patients refractory to intensive medical treatment, LV assist devices may be considered as a temporary bridge to heart transplantation.

Heart transplantation

Heart transplantation is reserved for patients with intractable functional Class III-IV CHF who have little likelihood of survival during the next 6–12 months. The ideal patients are relatively young (<60 years) who do not have multiorgan disease. In such patients, the chances of improved quality of life and return to employment are high. Significant pulmonary hypertension (pulmonary vascular resistance >6 Wood units), collagen vascular disease, HIV positivity, and severe, complicated diabetes mellitus are the major contraindications.

These patients are prone to acute and chronic rejection of the allograft. However, with the long-term use of immunosuppressant agents, 1- and 5-year survivals are 90% and 70%, respectively. The complications of heart transplantation include episodes of rejection, nephrotoxicity, bone marrow suppression, opportunistic infections, accelerated coronary atherosclerosis, and neoplasia.

◼ Prevention of Heart Failure

Controlling various risk factors for atherosclerosis and treating hypertension go a long way in preventing the initial LV dysfunction that eventually results in CHF.

TABLE 30.9. Management of Acute Cardiogenic Pulmonary Edema		
Drug/Maneuver	**Dose**	**Comments**
Upright or semi-upright posture	—	Decreases venous return (preload); Increases lung volumes; decreases work of breathing.
Oxygen therapy	100% by mask or 6–8 L/min by nasal prongs; if ineffective, proceed to endotracheal intubation	Optimal oxygenation dilates pulmonary vasculature.
Continuous positive pressure breathing		Improves gas exchange, reduces respiratory work and reduces preload.
Morphine sulfate	2–5 mg IV, repeat every 20 min (total <15 mg)	Relieves anxiety, reduces preload by venodilation.
Loop Diuretics		Reduce preload by vasodilation and rapid diuresis.
Furosemide	20–120 mg IV	
Bumetanide	1 mg IV	
Vasodilators		
Nitroglycerin	0.4 mg SL,	
or	5–200 µg/min IV (inf)	Reduces preload and afterload.
Sodium nitroprusside	5–10 µg/min (inf)	
Digoxin	0.25–0.5 mg IV	Reduces ventricular rate if patient has atrial fibrillation, and also enhances contractility.
Bronchodilator		
Aminophylline	5 mg/kg IV over 15 min, then 0.5–0.9 mg/kg/hr (inf)	Relieves bronchospasm, vasodilator and positive inotropic agent.
Rotating tourniquets	Apply BP cuffs to three limbs, raise pressure up to 10 mmHg below diastolic BP, release pressure every 15 min and rotate to different limbs	Reduces preload.
Correct	Tachy-arrhythmias or brady-arrhythmias and AV asynchrony	
Dopamine or dobutamine	2–5 µg/kg/min	Positive inotropic agents, useful especially if hypotension present.
Intra-aortic balloon counterpulsation		Reduces afterload and improves myocardial blood flow, useful if hypotension is present.
Determine etiology		Establish and correct the cause as rapidly as possible.
Treat diastolic dysfunction		If etiology is predominantly diastolic dysfunction and systolic function is normal, use diuretics and nitrates cautiously; avoid digoxin and direct acting vasodilators; β-blockers and calcium channel-blockers may be required to control hypertension and/or ischemia, heart rate.
Ultrafiltration		Removes excess water.

inf = infusion; SL = sublingual.

Once LV dysfunction begins, stimulation of neurohormones, vasoconstriction, LV remodeling, and salt retention, all interrelated processes, worsen LV dysfunction and convert asymptomatic LV dysfunction into symptomatic CHF. It is now well established that early ACE inhibitors at the stage of asymptomatic LV dysfunction can slow the progression of symptomatic CHF and enhance survival.

CHAPTER **31** # CORONARY ARTERY DISEASE

The clinical manifestations of coronary artery disease (CAD)—angina, myocardial infarction, sudden death, arrhythmias, and ischemic cardiomyopathy—arise from impairment of coronary blood flow that results from narrowing of the coronary arterial lumen by atheromatous plaques.

Atherosclerosis

▪ Pathogenesis

Atherosclerosis, the process of hardening and thickening of medium and large arteries, begins in childhood and adolescence, and slowly progresses over decades to become clinically manifest during mid and late adulthood. The earliest lesions ("fatty streaks") are eccentric, yellowish, flat intimal lesions. These consist of foam cells (macrophages and smooth muscle cells filled with cholesterol esters) and T–lymphocytes, and they may progress to fibrous plaques during the second decade of life. Covered by pearly-gray, dense connective tissue matrix, fibrous plaques can protrude into the vessel lumen and restrict blood flow. They become complicated when the fibrous cap fissures or cracks, allowing platelet and fibrin mural clots to form. Calcification and bleeding also occur within these lesions.

These atheromas are mostly located in the epicardial segments of the coronary arteries, especially at branch points (bifurcations) and usually spare intramural segments. Smaller vessels may be involved in smokers and diabetics.

While the precise mechanism of atherosclerosis is elusive, it is usually believed to follow endothelial injury brought about by shear forces, risk factors (oxidized low density lipoprotein particles), and viral or immunologic factors, thus rendering the endothelium more permeable and thrombogenic. The release of several vasoactive, chemotactic, and growth factors leads to proliferative lesions.

▪ Risk Factors

Being water-insoluble, lipids are transported in blood as lipoprotein particles, of which there are five types: **chylomicrons**, **very–low-density** (VLDL), **intermediate-density** (IDL), **low-density** (LDL), and **high-density** (HDL) lipoproteins. LDL and IDL are the most atherogenic. HDL participates in reverse transportation of cholesterol from tissues to the liver and thus exerts a strong protective role from CAD.

Excess dietary saturated fat and cholesterol, obesity, hypothyroidism, nephrotic syndrome, and inherited conditions (e.g., primary hypercholesterolemia) lead to high levels of total cholesterol and LDL-cholesterol. Feminine gender, physical activity, and moderate alcohol intake correlate with high HDL levels; obesity, diabetes, smoking, and physical inactivity correlate with low HDL levels (Table 31.1).

The prevalence of CAD increases with advancing age. In women, its prevalence is low prior to menopause but then rapidly increases. Three primary risk factors, however, are associated with most of the risk for CAD:

- Increasing one's **total cholesterol level** from 200 to 240 mg/dl increases the risk of CAD fivefold.
- **Smoking** one pack of cigarettes per day increases the risk of CAD three- to fivefold. The risk increases with heavier and prolonged use but declines by 50% within a few years of smoking cessation and to the level of nonsmokers in 5 years. Nicotine, an adrenergic agonist and a coronary vasoconstrictor, adversely affects clotting factors and serum lipids.
- Even a moderate degree of **hypertension** increases the incidence of CAD fivefold.

TABLE 31.1.	Risk Factors for Coronary Atherosclerosis	
Modifiable	**Nonmodifiable**
Hypercholesterolemia	Age (men, ≥45 yrs; women, ≥55 yrs)
Cigarette smoking	Family history (men, <55 yrs; women, <65 yrs)
Hypertension	
Physical inactivity	
Low HDL-cholesterol (<35 mg/dl)	
Diabetes mellitus	
Truncal obesity	

Strong epidemiologic evidence (e.g., the Framingham study) shows that the coexistence of multiple risk factors amplifies the adverse impact. Thus, the risk of CAD increases tenfold in patients with all three risk factors when compared to subjects without these risk factors (14.6/1000 vs 1.6/1000).

■ Clinical Syndromes

Stable Angina Pectoris

Classic angina pectoris (Heberden's angina) is a discomfort in the substernal area precipitated by exercise or emotion and relieved by rest. **Stable angina** implies that the pattern of angina—i.e., the activity threshold of developing angina and its intensity, duration, and relief with rest and/or nitroglycerin—is unchanged for months and years and is fairly predictable. The angina is termed **typical** when three features are present: 1) substernal discomfort, 2) precipitation by activity or emotional stress, and 3) relief with rest and/or nitroglycerin. When only two of three features are present, the episodes are described as **atypical** angina.

Coronary arteriography shows significant CAD in approximately 90% of patients with typical angina and 50% of patients with atypical angina. CAD is demonstrable in fewer than 10% of cases with only one or none of the features of angina (nonanginal chest pain).

Etiology

Atherosclerotic obstruction of one or more coronary arteries (>50% reduction in diameter) is the major cause of angina pectoris in about 90% of patients. Transient spasm of normal or atherosclerotic coronary arteries causes angina in some. In the few with typical angina pectoris and entirely normal coronary arteries (syndrome X), ischemia is attributed to small-vessel disease.

Angina commonly accompanies aortic valve disease, especially aortic stenosis. Marked RV hypertrophy may lead to angina occasionally. Systemic lupus erythematosus and polyarteritis nodosa, which affect small coronary vessels, are rare causes of angina.

Pathophysiology

Angina results from an inadequate oxygen supply relative to the myocardial O_2 demand (Figure 31.1). Increased heart rate, contractility, LV chamber size, and/or systolic blood pressure increase the myocardial O_2 needs. Even under basal conditions, the myocardium extracts oxygen nearly maximally from coronary arterial blood, leading to a wide coronary arteriovenous O_2 difference. Thus, the only means of increasing the myocardial O_2 supply is to increase the coronary blood flow, which in turn is dependent on coronary vascular

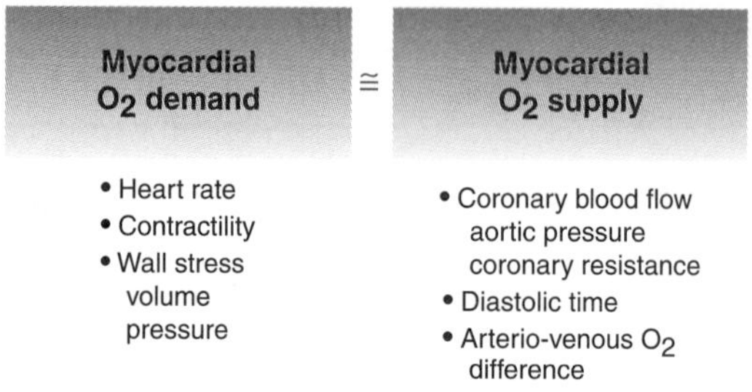

FIGURE 31.1. Factors determining myocardial oxygen demand and supply. Myocardial O_2 demand depends on heart rate, contractility, and left ventricular wall stress. Wall stress depends on the left ventricular diameter and systolic pressure. Normally, under physiological stress such as exercise, the myocardial O_2 supply can increase with the increase in demand. In coronary artery stenosis, the supply is inadequate relative to the demand, leading to myocardial ischemia.

resistance and perfusion pressure (aortic diastolic pressure – LV end-diastolic pressure).

Coronary arteriolar dilatation is the primary means of enhancing coronary blood flow. With mild to moderately severe (50-90%) stenotic lesions, arterioles distal to the obstruction dilate and tend to maintain normal blood flow at rest (but not during exercise). In severe (>90%) coronary stenosis, even maximal arteriolar dilatation cannot keep up normal resting coronary blood flow, resulting in ischemia at rest. Enlargement of dormant collateral vessels is another compensatory mechanism to maintain coronary blood flow. Although it is inadequate to meet the myocardial O_2 demands, particularly during stress, collateral flow may prevent or limit the size of a myocardial infarction in the distribution of a slowly occluding coronary artery.

Minor atherosclerotic plaques may also inhibit the production of endogenous vasodilator and platelet inhibitors (e.g., endothelium-dependent relaxing factor and prostacyclin), thereby permitting platelet clumping with release of the vasoconstrictor thromboxane A_2, causing coronary vasospasm. An imbalance of vascular autonomic tone and activation of serotonin receptors may also evoke vasospasm.

Thus, the spectrum of angina seen in patients consists of **exertional angina** (owing to a fixed obstruction), **rest angina** (due to vasospasm or a very severe, fixed obstruction), and **mixed angina** which has a varying activity threshold (owing to obstruction and vasospasm). As ischemia develops, the earliest change consists of diastolic dysfunction followed by systolic dysfunction, ECG changes, and angina (Figure 31.2).

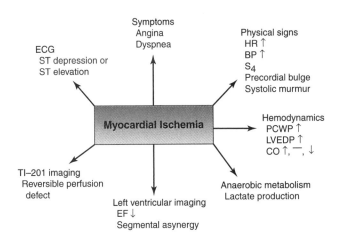

FIGURE 31.2. Manifestations of myocardial ischemia. HR = heart rate; BP = blood pressure; S_4 = fourth heart sound; PCWP = pulmonary capillary wedge pressure; LVEDP = left ventricular end-diastolic pressure; CO = cardiac output; EF = ejection fraction.

Clinical features

Angina pectoris is episodic chest discomfort, precipitated by physical activity. The discomfort frequently rises to a crescendo, forcing the patient to rest. Less often, it builds up to a tolerable intensity, enduring until activity is discontinued. Angina is usually more common during the morning hours. Rarely, angina abates itself during continued activity, enabling the patient to exercise even more vigorously without interruption ("walk-through" or "second-wind" angina). The Canadian Functional Classification of stable angina is shown in Table 23.3.

Angina is a deep, aching, visceral pain, poorly localized and usually described as a tightness, heaviness, or burning or choking sensation in the chest. Occasionally, it is described as indigestion. Angina may be accompanied by acute anxiety, nausea, sweating, and dyspnea. The pain is most commonly felt substernally or across the anterior chest (or occasionally precordially) and may radiate to the inner aspect of the left arm, right arm, shoulders, neck, jaw, upper abdomen, and interscapular area. Pain in the region of the cardiac apex is not typical. The pain intensity may vary. Most episodes last 3–5 minutes, but severe attacks may last up to 30 minutes.

Physical examination during an episode of angina may reveal tachycardia, hypertension, abnormal precordial pulsation, and an atrial gallop (S_4) or mitral insufficiency murmur secondary to papillary muscle dysfunction. These cardiovascular findings are usually absent between episodes.

Ancillary studies

Electrocardiography

In one-half to two-thirds of patients with stable angina, a standard 12-lead ECG is normal. In the remaining, evidence of old myocardial infarction or

TABLE 31.2. Indications for Exercise Stress Testing
CAD
A. Diagnosis
Men with atypical angina
Women with typical or atypical angina
Asymptomatic men:
– in special occupations (e.g., pilots, firemen, bus drivers, railroad engineers)
– 2 or more risk factors for atherosclerosis
– before entering exercise training programs
B. Prognosis (risk stratification) with established CAD
Stable angina
Post-myocardial infarction
Annual follow-up
C. Assessing treatment efficacy
Medical
Revascularization procedures (angioplasty, surgery)
Non-CAD
A. Evaluation and treatment efficacy of exercise-induced arrhythmias
B. Functional evaluation of valvular heart disease
C. Functional evaluation in heart failure

repolarization changes (ST-T abnormalities) may be seen. During spontaneous angina, most patients show an abnormal ST-segment depression (horizontal or downsloping ST depression of >0.1 mV), indicating subendocardial ischemia.

Exercise stress test

Exercise stress tests help in evaluating patients with suspected CAD because most patients with stable angina have a normal resting ECG (Table 31.2). A focused history and clinical examination and a control 12-lead ECG are essential before the stress test to exclude the

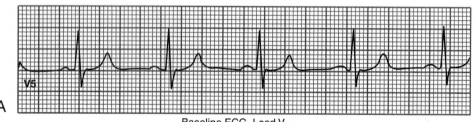

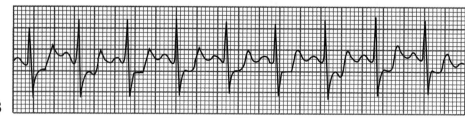

FIGURE 31.3. ECG changes in angina. A. Baseline ECG, with lead V$_5$ showing an isoelectric ST segment. B. During peak exercise, lead V$_5$ shows 2.5-mm horizontal ST-segment depression, indicating marked myocardial ischemia. HR = heart rate; BP = blood pressure.

TABLE 31.3.	Contraindications to Exercise Stress Testing

A. Cardiovascular
   Acute myocardial infarction
   Recent change in resting ECG
   Unstable angina
   Arrhythmias/conduction defects
      Uncontrolled life-threatening arrhythmias
      Second- or third-degree AV block
      Fixed-rate pacemaker
   Decompensated heart failure
   Critical aortic stenosis
   Severe obstructive hypertrophic cardiomyopathy
   Acute myocarditis, pericarditis or endocarditis
   Uncontrolled hypertension (BP >200/105 mm Hg)
B. Non-cardiac
   Severe pulmonary hypertension
   Acute pulmonary embolism or infarction
   Any acute, systemic illness

possibility of unstable angina or recent myocardial infarction (Table 31.3). The patient should be fasting for about 4–6 hours, and digitalis, diuretics, β-blockers, and nitrates should be withheld before the test. Exercise is performed on a treadmill or upright bicycle and the ECG is monitored continuously while the following variables are observed: the extent of ST depression or elevation, the level of activity that produces it, the duration that it persists after exercise, arrhythmias, R-wave amplitude, blood pressure, atrial and/or ventricular gallop, and apical systolic murmur.

- A positive stress test is indicated by a horizontal or down-sloping ST depression greater than 1 mm for 60–80 msec, using the P–R segment as the reference (Figure 31.3). ST depression indicates subendocardial myocardial ischemia.
- ST-segment elevation in leads showing Q waves usually indicates underlying LV aneurysm, and that in leads without Q waves, transmural ischemia.
- T-wave abnormalities, conduction defects, and arrhythmias are not specific signs of myocardial ischemia.
- A significant fall of systolic blood pressure (>10 mm Hg) indicates LV dysfunction.

The overall sensitivity and specificity of stress test for detecting CAD are 60% and 70% respectively. False-positive tests occur significantly more often in women.

The predictive value of exercise ECG test is highly dependent on the **pretest likelihood** of disease. For example, in a middle-aged man with several risk factors and typical angina (very high pretest likelihood of CAD), a positive exercise ECG does not add much to the diagnosis of CAD and a negative test is probably false-negative. Similarly, in a young, premenopausal woman with atypical angina (low pretest probability of CAD), a positive exercise ECG is probably false-positive and a negative test does not add much diagnostic information. Conditions that frequently interfere with the interpretation of exercise ECG tests include left bundle branch block, LV hypertrophy, atrial flutter or fibrillation, and ST–T changes and/or Q waves in most leads on baseline ECG. Exercise testing using nuclear imaging is discussed in chapter 26.

Coronary arteriography

Using selective **coronary arteriography,** one can visualize the coronary vessels, estimate the site and severity of narrowing, assess the status of the vessel distal to the lesion, determine the status of collaterals to the obstructed artery, and determine the number of diseased coronary arteries (Table 31.4). Coronary arteriography, however, yields little information about coronary blood flow. This procedure carries a 0.1% mortality. Rarely, myocardial infarction, coronary artery dissection, embolic stroke, hypotension, arrhythmias, or thromboembolism occur, usually in patients with left main CAD or severe LV dysfunction.

Left ventriculography is routinely done in conjunction with coronary arteriography to assess global and regional LV function and to determine the existence of mitral insufficiency. During on-going ischemia, segmental asynergy and low global ejection fraction are usually noted if a large area of myocardium is ischemic.

Natural history

Stable angina may progress to several outcomes. Patients may exhibit continued stability without change, develop unstable angina followed by a myocardial infarction, die suddenly, sustain multiple myocardial infarctions that lead to ischemic cardiomyopathy, or, rarely, extinguish the angina, (presumably by infarction in the ischemic region or development of adequate collateral vessels).

The number of obstructed coronary vessels and the status of LV function are the key long-term prognostic indicators. **Long-term prognosis** is excellent in patients with angina and normal coronary arteries. Single-, double-, and triple-vessel disease carry a yearly mortality of 2%, 6%, and 10%, respectively. Left anterior descending coronary artery stenosis has a yearly mortality of 4%, while that of the left main coronary artery carries the worst prognosis; one-half of these patients die by the fifth year and 80% by the 10th year. Severe LV dysfunction with CAD has a mortality of 50% at 1 year and 85% at 5 years.

The following ECG criteria from a symptom-limited stress test indicate a poor prognosis: marked downsloping ST depression (>2 mm) at low levels of stress (stage 1 of Bruce's protocol or heart rate <120 beats/min), persistent ST depression for greater than 5 minutes after cessation of exercise, or systolic hypotension during exercise and ventricular ectopy along with ST depression. Heart failure, prior myocardial infarction or hypertension, abnormal resting ECG, and angina at rest or with minimal effort also carry a poor prognosis.

Differential diagnosis

Angina pectoris is diagnosed from the patient history. Until proven otherwise, all chest discomfort induced by exertion and/or emotion, relieved with rest and/or nitroglycerin, is angina. Several common conditions must be distinguished from angina (see Table 23.2). The pain of pulmonary hypertension is spontaneous, substernal, often prolonged, and accompanied by dyspnea. Diffuse esophageal spasm may be induced by cold liquids. Peptic ulcer pain is epigastric, related to food intake rather than exertion, relieved by antacids, and accompanied by epigastric tenderness. Pain from gallstones or biliary disease is spontaneous or postprandial, waxes and wanes, is epigastric or in the right upper quadrant, and remits on its own in a few hours or following spasmolytics and analgesics. Local tenderness and relationship to movement of the trunk are the main features of musculoskeletal pain. Cervical radiculopathy causes neck and upper chest pain, radiating into the arms.

Management

Management strategies in angina (Figure 31.4) incorporate the following principles: 1) relieving acute episodes, 2) preventing future episodes, 3) retarding the progression of atherosclerosis (through exercise and

TABLE 31.4.	Indications for Coronary Arteriography
Indication	**Purpose**
Patients with disabling angina pectoris despite adequate medical therapy	To delineate coronary anatomy for potential revascularization
Patients with angina and a strongly positive exercise stress test at a low level of stress (<5 METS or heart rate <120 beats/min),	To assess the severity of CAD
Patients with chest pain of unclear origin	As a diagnostic measure
Patients who redevelop disabling angina after coronary artery bypass grafting	To differentiate graft occlusion from native CAD

FIGURE **31.4.** Management strategies for patients with chronic, stable angina.

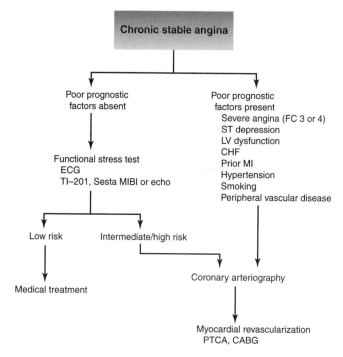

diet), and 4) enhancing survival by revascularization procedures in high-risk patients.

Antianginal drug therapy

Angina follows an imbalance of myocardial O_2 demand and supply, and drugs that improve this imbalance are useful in treating angina (Table 31.5).

Nitrates

Nitrates are well established in both the acute relief and prophylaxis of angina. They interact with guanylate cyclase in vascular smooth muscle cells, oxidize sulfhydryl groups, and are converted into S—nitrosothiols, which augment cyclic GMP, which in turn causes smooth muscle cell relaxation.

Glyceryl trinitrate **(nitroglycerin),** the drug of choice for immediate relief of angina, reverses myocardial ischemia by several mechanisms:

- It causes dilatation of the venous bed, thus reducing LV preload. As a result, the LV chamber becomes smaller, and the myocardial O_2 demand is reduced.
- By reducing the LV end-diastolic pressure, it increases the blood supply to the subendocardial region.
- It dilates the collateral coronary vessels, resulting in enhanced perfusion to ischemic myocardium.
- It also dilates stenotic segments of coronary arteries, thereby enhancing blood flow.

Nitrates are also spasmolytics, relieving any spasm of the

major coronary arteries. Commonly used nitrate preparations are listed in Table 31.6. The long-acting nitrates are indicated for angina prophylaxis. Nitroglycerin may also be used prophylactically before performing activities likely to cause angina. Patients should avoid using nitroglycerin while standing up. If three tablets of nitroglycerin taken at 5-minute intervals do not relieve angina, the patient should be advised to go to the nearest hospital.

Nitrates may cause throbbing headache, hypotension, dizziness, and lightheadedness. Continuous use of nitrates over a 24-hour period induces tolerance, presumably from depletion of sulfhydryl groups, and so, a 12-hour nitrate-free interval during each 24-hour period is recommended to maintain responsiveness.

β-Adrenergic blocking agents (β-blockers)

β-blockers exert their antianginal effect primarily by lowering myocardial O_2 demand. Effective doses vary widely among patients and are determined by the abolition of angina, resting heart rate of about 50 beats/min, or the development of serious side effects (Tables 31.7 and 31.8). β-blockers are often combined with nitrates in preventing angina. β-blockers counteract nitrate-induced tachycardia and increased contractility, and nitrates prevent β-blocker-induced LV enlargement.

β-blocker therapy should not be abruptly halted, because of the possibility of rebound angina or myocardial infarction from exposure of β-receptors to endogenous catecholamines.

Calcium antagonists

Verapamil, diltiazem, nifedipine, and amlodipine are the calcium channel blockers available for use, and all are potent vasodilators. Nifedipine and amlodipine are the most potent vasodilators, and verapamil and diltiazem also have mild negative inotropic effects. Diltiazem and verapamil have a depressant effect on the SA and AV nodes, whereas nifedipine and amlodipine lack any effect on the conduction system. Because of their negative inotropic effects, verapamil and β-blockers should not be combined in patients with LV dysfunction, as frank congestive heart failure may result. However, nifedipine instead may be safely combined with β-blockers.

Aspirin

Use of low-dose aspirin (80–325 mg/day) in chronic stable angina may reduce the incidence of acute myocardial infarction and unstable angina.

Percutaneous transluminal coronary angioplasty

Approximately 40% of patients with CAD and angina have discrete single-vessel or multivessel disease, making them amenable to treatment with percutaneous transluminal coronary angioplasty (PTCA). In this procedure, a balloon catheter is advanced into the stenotic artery, positioned across the lesion, and inflated for 30 seconds to a few minutes. A larger-diameter lumen results due to compression and disruption of atherosclerotic plaque and disruption of internal elastic lamina and, sometimes, the media of the artery.

PTCA is successful in dilating the stenosis and relieving angina in 85–90% of suitable patients. It is associated with a 1% mortality rate. The target vessel may abruptly occlude from dissection or clotting in approximately 4–5% of patients, resulting in uncontrolled ischemia and necessitating emergency bypass surgery. Following successful PTCA, approximately 40% of arteries restenose within 6 months. While aspirin helps prevent early reocclusion of a dilated vessel, no agent has so far successfully reduced long-term restenosis rate.

PTCA is less invasive and less expensive than bypass surgery and should be strongly considered in patients with disabling angina, suitable coronary anatomy, and objective signs of ischemia. Standard PTCA is more likely to be complicated by abrupt closure and/or high restenosis rate when performed for severe eccentric lesions, long lesions, lesions at branch points and calcified lesions. Newer techniques such as rotational or directional atherectomy (atheromatous material is pul-

TABLE 31.5.	Effects of Antianginal Agents on the Determinants of Myocardial O₂ Demand and Supply		
	Nitrates	**β-Blockers**	**Ca++ Blockers‡**
Demand:			
LV wall stress	↓↓	↑	↓
Volume	↓↓	↑	↓
Pressure	↓	↓	↓
Contractility	↑	↓↓	↓
Heart rate	↑	↓↓	↓
Net change	↓	↓	↓
Supply:			
Perfusion pressure*	↑	↓	↓
Coronary resistance	↓	↑	↓↓
Diastolic period	0, ↓	↑↑	↑
Collateral flow	↑	0	0, ↑
Net change	↑	↑	↑

↑ = increase, ↓ = decrease, 0 = no change; ↑↑ = significant increase, ↓↓ = significant decrease.
*Perfusion pressure = (aortic diastolic pressure) − (LV diastolic pressure).
‡Changes associated with verapamil and diltiazem; nifedipine causes reflex increase in heart rate and contractility.

TABLE 31.6.	Commonly Used Nitrate Preparations				
Preparation	Route	Dose		Onset (min)	Duration (hr)
Nitroglycerin	Spray	0.4 mg		2–5	<0.5
Nitroglycerin	SL	0.3–0.6 mg		2–5	<0.5
Isosorbide dinitrate	SL	2.5–10 mg		3–5	1–2
Nitroglycerin	PO	2.5–9 mg		30–45	2–8
Isosorbide dinitrate	PO	5–30 mg		15–30	3–6
Isosorbide dinitrate (SR)	PO	40 mg		30–60	6–10
Isosorbide mononitrate	PO	20–40 mg		30	6–8
Nitroglycerin paste (2%)	Topical	0.5–2 in		20–60	3–8
Nitroglycerin patches	Topical	0.2–0.6 mg/hr		30–60	8–14
Nitroglycerin	IV	10–200 µg/min		Immediate	Minutes

IV = intravenous; PO = oral; SL = sub-lingual; SR = sustained release.

TABLE 31.7. Commonly Used Beta-Blockers

Drug	Route	Dose	Half-Life (hrs)	Cardioselective*	ISA
Propranolol	Oral	10–120 mg QID	4–6	—	—
Propranolol LA	Oral	40–160 mg BID	4–0	—	—
Metoprolol	Oral	50–100 mg BID	3–4	+	—
Nadolol	Oral	40–160 mg QD	14–25	—	—
Atenolol	Oral	50–100 mg QD	6–9	+	—
Betaxolol	Oral	15–20 mg QD		+	—
Timolol	Oral	10–20 mg BID	3–4	—	—
Pindolol	Oral	10–30 mg BID	3–4	—	+
Acebutolol	Oral	200–800 mg QD	3–4	+	+
Labetalol	Oral	100–400 mg BID	6 (α & β blocker)	High	—
Propranolol	IV	1 mg at 3–5 min intervals (max 0.1–0.15 mg/kg)	—	Low	—
Esmolol	IV	Loading, 500 µg/kg/min × 1 min Maintenance, 50–200 µg/kg/min	+	Moderate	—
Metoprolol	IV	5 mg at 5 min × 3	+	Moderate	—

*Noncardioselective agents block β-1 receptors in the heart and β-2 receptors in the bronchial tree and peripheral circulation.
+ = present; — = absent; ISA = Intrinsic sympathomimetic activity; BID = Twice daily; QD = Once daily.

TABLE 31.8. Adverse Effects of Beta-Blockers

Due to β-blockade	Unrelated to β-blockade
Bradycardia	Lethargy
Hypotension	Depression
Heart failure	Confusion
Cold extremities	Hallucinations
Bronchospasm	Nausea
Inhibition of metabolic and circulatory adjustments to hypoglycemia	Constipation
	Impotence

TABLE 31.9. Coronary Artery Bypass Surgery

Effectiveness:
  More effectively prevents unstable angina than medical therapy
  Improves left ventricular function, especially during exercise
  Improves the long-term survival in the following high-risk subsets:
    Left main coronary artery stenosis
    3-vessel CAD with LV dysfunction
    2-vessel CAD when one of the vessels is LAD, with LV dysfunction
    Proximal LAD and LV dysfunction
  No advantage over medical therapy in one-vessel CAD
Indications:
  Disabling angina, poorly controlled
  Poorly tolerated medical therapy and unsuitable anatomy for PTCA
  High-risk CAD (see above)

LAD = Left anterior descending; LV = left ventricular; PTCA = percutaneous transluminal coronary angioplasty.

verized or actually removed) are more suitable for such lesions. Availability of stainless steel stents has greatly helped in the treatment of abrupt closure or threatened closure after standard PTCA. Furthermore, the use of stents rather than standard PTCA has reduced the restenosis rate to about 20%.

Coronary artery bypass surgery

Direct myocardial revascularization, or coronary artery bypass grafting (CABG), involves an aortocoronary bypass using short segments of the saphenous vein or internal mammary artery to anastomose the aorta to the coronary arteries distal to the obstruction(s). The revascularization increases the amount of blood flow to the ischemic myocardium, thereby totally relieving angina in almost 60% of cases and markedly reducing it in another 20%. Almost 85% of the vein bypasses are patent and functional 1 year after the operation. While only 50% of the vein grafts are patent 10 years after bypass, 90% of mammary artery grafts are patent at 10 years.

The effectiveness of and indications for surgical therapy are outlined in Table 31.9. Important considerations in choosing CABG over medical therapy or PTCA include the extent and severity of CAD, LV function, severity of angina, response of angina to medical therapy, results of the exercise stress test, and age, occupation, and general condition of the patient. The procedure has a hospital mortality of 1–2%, and a perioperative myocardial infarction rate of 5–10% in patients with adequate LV function.

Unstable Angina

Unstable angina is very common and falls between brief, exercise–induced anginal episodes and the intense and prolonged pain of myocardial infarction. When extracardiac factors, such as anemia, tachyarrhythmias, hypertension, increased physical or emotional stress, and thyrotoxicosis are excluded as contributing to the unstable condition, this syndrome suggests increasing severity of coronary stenosis with a higher risk for myocardial infarction and sudden death than stable angina. The pathogenesis of unstable angina is shown in Figure 31.5.

TABLE **31.10.** Patterns of Unstable Angina
1. New onset of severe angina (Class III or IV) within the previous 2 months
2. Worsening of previous stable angina to Class III or IV angina within the previous 2 months
3. Rest angina (usually prolonged ≥20 min) within the past 1 week
4. Post-myocardial infarction angina (>24 hours)
5. Variant angina

Diagnosis

The history or evolution of symptoms is crucial to the diagnosis of unstable angina (Table 31.10). A history of new onset of angina within the previous 2 months; recent worsening of previously stable angina in terms of frequency, activity threshold, intensity, duration and radiation of pain, poor response of pain to nitroglycerin; and prolonged episodes of rest pain (≥20 min) indicate a diagnosis of unstable angina. Physical examination generally discloses little information. An atrial gallop and apical systolic murmur of mitral insufficiency may be audible during an episode of acute ischemia. The ECG may show ST-segment depression or elevation and T-wave flattening or inversion. Generally, these ST-T changes accompany the episodes of chest pain and may normalize as pain is relieved.

Coronary angiography generally reveals multivessel CAD, with left main stenosis being found in 10% of patients. The angiographic appearances commonly suggest ruptured coronary plaques with associated thrombi. Coronary arteries are normal in 5–20% of cases, and in a significant number of these, vasospasm may be responsible.

The ejection fraction and segmental wall motion may be entirely normal if active ischemia is absent during left ventriculography. If critical stenoses compromise resting coronary flow (hibernating myocardium), segmental wall motion abnormalities are usually present, which may improve upon repeating the ventriculogram after nitroglycerin administration.

Natural history

Adverse prognostic factors with an enhanced risk of myocardial infarction or sudden death are summarized in Table 31.11. The overall incidence of death and myocardial infarction during hospitalization is 1–2% and 5–15%, respectively. Over a 30-month follow-up,

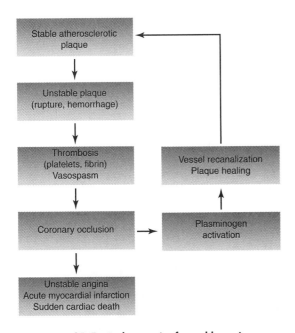

FIGURE 31.5. Pathogenesis of unstable angina.

TABLE 31.11.	Adverse Prognostic Factors in Unstable Angina*
History	Age >65 years
	Recurrent prolonged (>20 min) rest angina
	Poor response to nitroglycerin
	Previous myocardial infarction
Physical examination	Hypotension
	Cardiomegaly
	New mitral regurgitation murmur
	Heart failure (pulmonary edema, S_3, rales)
Ancillary studies	ST-T changes in ECG
	Low EF on echocardiogram
Cardiac catheterization	Critical multivessel or left main disease
	Abnormal LVEDP
	↓ Cardiac output
	↓ EF

*Short-term risk of death or nonfatal myocardial infarction.
LVEDP = left ventricular end-diastolic pressure; EF = ejection fraction.

a mortality rate of 10% and myocardial infarction rate of 19% are noted. The acute phase of unstable angina usually lasts 3–4 months before attaining stability.

Management

The choice, timing, and aggressiveness of management of unstable angina are determined by 1) the certainty of diagnosis and severity of underlying CAD, 2) severity of symptoms, 3) hemodynamic status, 4) history of prior revascularization procedures and drug therapy, and 5) the presence of coexistent medical conditions (Figure 31.6). Conditions that enhance the risk of acute myocardial infarction and/or sudden death are summarized in Table 31.11.

Patients with a normal or unchanged ECG; the absence of severe, prolonged (>20 min), or rest angina within the preceding 2 weeks; or the absence of new-onset angina for over 2 weeks are at a low risk of new coronary events. They can be managed on an ambulatory basis and further evaluated within 72 hours with repeat ECGs, evaluation for extracardiac conditions causing instability of symptoms, and a noninvasive stress test.

High-risk patients should be admitted to an intensive care unit and promptly started on therapy consisting of supplemental O_2; IV heparin; aspirin (160–325 mg daily); IV nitroglycerin (10–200 µg/min) to relieve chest pain or to reduce systolic blood pressure by 10%; IV β-blockers to achieve a heart rate of 50–60 beats/min; assessment of LV function by echocardiography or nuclear scanning during the next 24 hours; and evaluation for myocardial infarct by daily ECGs and measurement

of cardiac enzymes. Patients with an intermediate risk can be given medications orally.

In most patients, ischemic symptoms are controlled within 30 minutes of intensive medical treatment. If they remain symptom-free and hemodynamically stable during the next 24 hours, they can be moved from the intensive care unit. Patients with prior revascularization procedures, LV ejection fraction below 0.5, heart failure, hypotension, malignant ventricular arrhythmias or severe AV block, recurrent angina or ST-T changes, and new mitral regurgitation murmur, should undergo a cardiac catheterization and coronary arteriography. The remaining patients, after the second stable 24-hour period, can

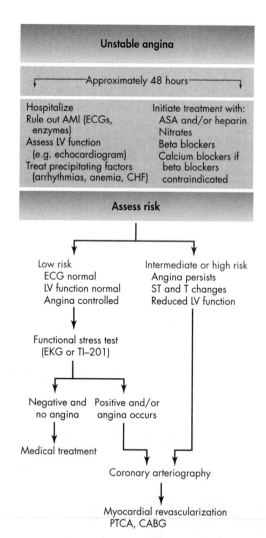

FIGURE 31.6. Management strategies in unstable angina. AMI = acute myocardial infarction; ASA = aspirin; CHF = congestive heart failure.

undergo functional stress test including pharmacologic stress test, if the patient is unable to exercise. Cardiac catheterization and coronary angiography should be performed in patients with ischemic response on functional testing or those with inconclusive results.

In patients in whom the initial chest pain does not respond within 30 minutes, other entities (e.g., evolving acute myocardial infarction, aortic dissection, pulmonary embolism) should be ruled out. If intractable myocardial ischemia is still the most likely possibility, the patient should undergo an urgent cardiac catheterization and coronary angiography, preferably in conjunction with intraaortic balloon counterpulsation.

Coronary artery bypass surgery should be recommended for high-risk patients (Tables 31.9 and 31.11). Other patients should be considered for coronary angioplasty or continuation of medical therapy, depending on the coronary anatomy. Severity of symptoms, hemodynamic status, and response to medical therapy should dictate the timing of revascularization procedures.

Prinzmetal's (Variant) Angina

Some episodes of angina occur at rest and are accompanied by ST-segment elevation and ventricular ectopy or heart block. These episodes may be precipitated by cocaine, or tobacco smoking or may occur spontaneously. The attacks tend to occur at similar times of the day. Angina and ST-segment elevation disappear following sublingual nitroglycerin. ST-segment elevation indicates transmural rather than subendocardial ischemia.

Vasospasm, either in atherosclerotic or normal coronary arteries, is the usual causative mechanism. Coronary angiography demonstrates severe, fixed, atherosclerotic lesions in the proximal region of one or more major coronary arteries in most patients with Prinzmetal's angina. Coronary vasospasm can be angiographically demonstrated during a spontaneous attack of variant angina or after induction with IV ergonovine maleate.

A significant number of patients (18%) develop myocardial infarction or die suddenly within 3 months of diagnosis of variant angina. The active phase of disease lasts 3–6 months, following which some patients go into a long remission when coronary vasospasm cannot be induced, even with ergonovine.

Because therapy depends on the presence or absence of fixed coronary stenosis, coronary angiography should be the first step in the management. In patients with severe, fixed stenosis, PTCA or CABG is generally very effective in relieving angina. Drug therapy with aspirin, calcium channel blockers, and nitrates also should be implemented. In patients with absent or mild CAD, calcium antagonists and nitrates are the mainstay of treatment.

Silent (Painless) Ischemia

Most patients with CAD experience both painful and painless episodes of myocardial ischemia. However, some patients with CAD have only asymptomatic (silent) ischemic episodes. Despite being silent, these episodes adversely impact the prognosis. There is no agreement regarding the strategies to detect or treat such entirely asymptomatic patients. Obviously, when a severe ischemic response is detected, coronary arteriography should be considered to define the severity of CAD.

CHAPTER 32 ACUTE MYOCARDIAL INFARCTION

Defined as necrosis of the myocardium, myocardial infarction (MI) is characterized by severe and prolonged chest pain, progressive ECG changes, and a transient rise of cardiac enzymes. Of the nearly 1.5 million cases of MI that occur yearly in the United States, roughly 30% are lethal; more than half of these deaths occur before the person arrives at the hospital.

■ Etiology

Myocardial infarction typically follows the sudden occlusion of a major coronary artery, usually caused by formation of a platelet and fibrin thrombus over the site of a disrupted atheromatous plaque. With slowly evolving obstruction, collateral channels may develop, which can limit or prevent infarction. Patients with multiple risk factors, unstable angina, and variant angina are more prone to develop acute MI. Hypercoagulability, collagen vascular disease, and cocaine abuse are other major risk factors for acute MI.

Generally, occlusion of the left anterior descending artery can be demonstrated in an anterior wall MI. Occlusion of the right or circumflex artery occurs in an inferior, inferolateral or posterior MI. Rarely, MI occurs with normal coronary arteries, where coronary embolism or vasospasm has been incriminated.

■ Pathology and Pathophysiology

The pathologic changes of acute MI consist of coagulation necrosis followed by fibrosis. The earliest histologically recognizable changes begin 6–12 hours after the onset of MI and include an eosinophilic appearance of myocardial fibers, with indistinct and fuzzy appearance of their cross striations. Neutrophilic infiltration begins in 18–24 hours. By 48 hours, the infarct zone appears pale, with interspersed hemorrhagic and healthy areas. Fibrosis starts after the third week, and scar formation is complete in 6–8 weeks. Interruption of coronary blood flow causing hypoxia and accumulation of injurious metabolites, such as potassium, calcium, lipids, and oxygen-free radicals, impair LV function, leading to ventricular arrhythmias.

■ Clinical Features

Although acute MI can occur at anytime of the day, it most commonly occurs within a few hours of awakening. The usual symptom is **substernal pain** radiating along one or both arms and the neck, lasting from 30 minutes to several hours (usually <24 hours), with associated nausea, vomiting, sweating, weakness, and anxiety. The pain does not respond to nitroglycerin. Prior to the MI, most patients report either new-onset angina or a change in the pattern of angina. Pain may be absent during acute MI in the elderly and some diabetic patients, presenting instead as arrhythmia, new or worsening heart failure, cerebrovascular accident, confusion, or severe weakness. In some patients, MI is totally asymptomatic and is detected on a routine ECG.

During the initial few hours of acute MI, the patient is in pain, with acute anxiety, pallor, and cold clammy skin. Bradycardia and hypotension, signs of parasympathetic overactivity, are frequent, especially in inferior wall MI. Tachycardia and hypertension (signs of sympathetic overactivity) may be noted with anterior wall MI. As the pain is relieved, the blood pressure usually returns to the preinfarction level. In anteroapical MI, an abnormal precordial systolic bulge, representing the dyskinetic anteroapical segment, may be visible and palpable. A soft S_1 due to reduced myocardial contractility and an apical atrial gallop (S_4) are common. A

pericardial friction rub may arise on the second or third day and last for 1–2 days. Slight fever may also occur early in the first week.

Killip has suggested the following clinical classification of acute MI based on these signs:
- Class I—uncomplicated
- Class II—mild LV failure (S_3, pulmonary rales)
- Class III—acute pulmonary edema
- Class IV—cardiogenic shock

■ Ancillary Studies

Electrocardiography

As a **Q-wave MI** evolves, the earliest ECG change is hyperacute (tall and spiked) **T waves** in the leads facing the infarct, ascribable to subendocardial myocardial ischemia. This early change is followed by elevation and reciprocal depression of ST segments in the leads facing and opposite to the infarct, respectively. The **ST elevation,** attributed to an electrical gradient that develops in the subepicardial layers between the injured and adjoining healthy cells, usually obscures the T waves.

ST elevation, the only ECG sign of acute myocardial injury, is transient, becoming isoelectric by 2 weeks at most. However, during its early course, a pathologic **Q wave** appears in the leads facing the infarct. Since the infarct segment is electrically inert, the initial QRS vector is directed away from it and is recorded as a negative wave (Q). The Q wave lasts months, years, or indefinitely and is the ECG sign of an old scar. A **symmetrically inverted T wave** appears as the ST-segment regresses, reflecting transmural ischemia; this also persists for months to years (see Figure 25.4).

Very early in MI, an ECG may show no changes, and thus it should be repeated daily for at least 3 days to facilitate their detection when MI is suspected. The standard 12-lead ECG can approximately localize MI (Figure 25.4): Q waves in leads V_1 and V_2, anteroseptal; V_3 and V_4, midanterior; I and aVL, anterolateral; V_1–V_6, extensive anterior, and Q in II, III, and aVF, inferior (diaphragmatic). In true posterior MI, V_1 and V_2 show tall, broad R and upright T waves, given the separation of these leads from the infarct by the healthy anterior wall. A non–Q wave (subendocardial) infarct leads to ST depression and T-wave inversion.

The ECG has several limitations in diagnosing MI. Associated conduction defects (left bundle branch block), Wolff-Parkinson-White syndrome, multiple prior infarcts, infarction of the LV apex or high lateral wall, or a small myocardial infarct anywhere may not show the typical ECG changes.

Laboratory tests and imaging studies

Slight leukocytosis and a left shift usually occur on the second day after MI and last for 3–7 days. The erythrocyte sedimentation rate also rises during the second or third day and may persist for 1–2 weeks.

With myocardial cell death, the enzymes **creatine kinase** (CK) and **lactate dehydrogenase** (LDH) leak into the blood, and their serum levels serve diagnostic and prognostic purposes in acute MI. The serum CK level rises within 8 hours, peaks in 24 hours, and becomes normal within 72–96 hours. Serum LDH concentration rises in 24–48 hours, peaks at 48–72 hours, and becomes normal in 7–10 days. Elevations of these enzymes, however, are not specific for acute MI. CK, being present in skeletal muscle and brain, rises after IM injections and surgery, in skeletal myopathies, hypothyroidism, electrical cardioversion, trauma, convulsions and central nervous system diseases. LDH, being present in the RBC, liver, kidneys, and lungs, rises in hemolysis, leukemia, liver disease, cancer and lung or renal infarction.

Isoenzymes of CK and LDH are more specific for detecting acute MI, and a high **CK-MB fraction** is most specific for myocardial injury. CK-MB usually peaks at 24 hours after the onset of acute MI, and so, it should be measured on admission and every 12–24 hours until MI is excluded. With reperfusion, CK-MB peaks at 12 hours. The fast-moving fraction of LDH, **LDH1,** rises in acute MI and several other diseases, but an elevated LDH1/LDH2 ratio exceeding 1 is highly suggestive of acute MI. Subforms of MB-CK and cardiac **troponin I** or **T** are very sensitive and specific for the diagnosis of acute MI.

Serial chest radiographs in acute MI are helpful for detecting left heart failure, but bedside films do not reliably reflect cardiac size.

^{99m}Tc-stannous pyrophosphate (PYP) binds to Ca^{++} and organic macromolecules in the acutely necrotic myocardium, causing a "hot spot" during myocardial imaging. Scans become positive at 48 hours after the onset of acute MI and remain so for up to 7 days. The sensitivity and specificity of PYP are excellent for detecting Q-wave MI, but not non–Q-wave MI. PYP imaging is mainly used to confirm and localize MI when ECG and serum enzyme tests are equivocal and to monitor the size of the MI.

On ^{201}Tl or ^{99m}Tc-Sesta-Mibi myocardial imaging, the infarct appears as a cold spot because the isotope does not accumulate in the infarct zone. Unlike PYP imaging, these become positive immediately after the onset of MI. However, they cannot separate old MI from new or distinguish between an MI and severe ischemia.

Radionuclide angiography and **echocardiography** can reliably estimate the LV ejection fraction (global function) as well as segmental wall motion abnormalities (regional function). Akinetic or dyskinetic segments correspond to old and new infarcts, and the ejection fraction helps determine the long-term prognosis following MI. Echocardiography can reliably detect and localize the segmental wall motion abnormalities which develop almost instantly following MI. It can also identify ventricular aneurysms, intraventricular mural blood clots, pericardial effusion, mitral regurgitation due to a ruptured papillary muscle, ventricular septal rupture and right ventricular (RV) infarction.

Hemodynamic monitoring and coronary angiography

Because physical signs do not always mirror the underlying hemodynamic changes, and clinical and radiographic changes of heart failure lag behind intracardiac pressure changes, hemodynamic variables sometimes need to be measured directly (Table 32.1). The right atrial pressure does not reliably reflect the status of the LV following infarction, but the pulmonary capillary wedge pressure (PCWP) accurately mirrors the LV filling pressure.

A balloon-tipped, flow-directed (Swan-Ganz) catheter is used to measure right atrial and pulmonary artery pressures as well as cardiac output and PCWP and thereby stratify patients with acute MI (Table 32.2). Using serial measurements of PCWP, cardiac output, systemic vascular resistance, and blood pressure, one can

TABLE 32.1. Indications for Hemodynamic Monitoring

Significant hypotension and hypoperfusion not easily corrected by fluids
Moderate to severe heart failure
Suspected mechanical complications, such as:
  Mitral insufficiency due to papillary muscle dysfunction
  Ventricular septal rupture with left-to-right shunt
Persistent ischemic pain
Refractory arrhythmias
Persistent sinus tachycardia, hypoxia, or acidosis

TABLE 32.2. Hemodynamic Subsets of Patients With Acute MI

Subset	Systemic BP (mm Hg)	PCWP (mm Hg)	CI (L/min/m²)
Normal	N	≤12	2.7 ± 0.5
Hyperdynamic state	↑	<12	>3.0
Heart failure	N or ↓	>18	≤2.5
Hypotension			
Hypovolemia	↓	<9	<2.2
Cardiogenic shock	↓	>18	<1.8
RV infarction	↓	≤18	<1.8

BP = blood pressure; CI = cardiac index; N = normal; PCWP = pulmonary capillary wedge pressure; RV = right ventricular.
(Modified from: Forrester JS et al. N Engl J Med 1976; 295:1404.)

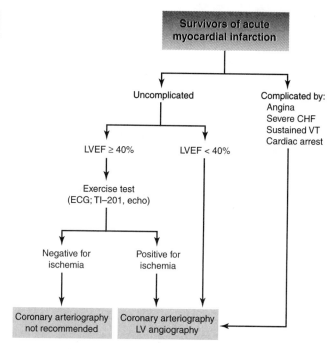

FIGURE 32.1. Indications for cardiac catheterization and arteriography in survivors of acute myocardial infarction. CHF = congestive heart failure; LVEF = left ventricular ejection fraction; VT = ventricular tachycardia.

rationally manage heart failure and cardiogenic shock and, by comparing the O_2 content of blood samples from various right heart chambers, discern a ventricular septal rupture from acute mitral regurgitation due to papillary muscle rupture.

Coronary angiography, while not routinely done during the acute phase of MI, is indicated in severe heart failure due to mechanical complications (e.g., papillary muscle rupture), post-MI angina, or ischemia unresponsive to aggressive medical therapy (Figure 32.1).

▪ Differential Diagnosis

The initial presentation of acute MI can be confused with several acute conditions, including acute pulmonary embolism, aortic dissection, acute pericarditis, acute pancreatitis, biliary colic, and ruptured peptic ulcer. When characteristic evolutionary ECG changes and typical rising serum enzymes are seen, the diagnosis of acute MI is obvious.

▪ Natural History and Prognosis

Most deaths from acute MI occur during the first 24 hours, and two-thirds of these occur during the first hour. Over 50% of all acute MI deaths occur before the patients reach a hospital, with ventricular fibrillation causing most fatalities. For patients admitted to a coronary care unit, the hospital mortality is 8–10%, mostly during the first 48 hours. The in-hospital mortality

declines progressively, and later deaths depend on patient age, total myocardium lost from the current and prior MI, and coexisting diseases (Table 32.3).

▪ Management

The major objectives of management are: a) to relieve the symptoms, b) to reduce mortality by promptly detecting, treating and, where possible, preventing ventricular fibrillation and limiting infarct size, c) to rehabilitate patients for return to a normal life and d) to prevent progression of underlying atherosclerosis.

Resuscitation promptly undertaken by trained bystanders or rescue personnel can reduce the prehospital mortality from MI. Trained paramedics also can administer lidocaine and defibrillation for ventricular arrhythmias, atropine for bradyarrhythmias, and morphine for pain. The initial management of suspected MI after patients arrive at the emergency department is outlined in Table 32.4. Caring for patients in the coronary care units (CCUs) with continuous ECG monitoring helps identify and treat arrhythmias, thus reducing arrhythmia-related hospital deaths.

LV dysfunction, caused mainly by myocardial damage from MI, is the major cause of in-hospital morbidity and mortality. Irreversible ischemic myocardial damage is nearly complete in 4–6 hours after the onset of the symptoms of acute MI. However, in the early hours, a sizable amount of myocardium within the threatened area is still viable, with the potential for either recovery or necrosis, depending on the O_2 supply/demand balance. Pharmacologic agents (nitrates, β-blockers) can lower O_2 demands but their ability to save myocardium is limited. Because coronary thrombosis is the imme-

diate cause of most acute MIs, recent therapeutic interventions have aimed at opening the infarct-related artery. The benefit is greatest if reperfusion is established within the first hour of acute MI, and so early reperfusion has become the mainstay of treatment for acute MI.

Reperfusion therapy

Thrombolytic agents

With successful reperfusion, chest pain, ST-segment elevation, and reperfusion arrhythmias resolve and the total CK and CK-MB levels peak much earlier (about 12 hours). Large-scale trials of thrombolytic agents have shown improvement in early and late mortality as well as preservation of LV function (Table 32.5). Also, patients with sustained patency of an infarct-related artery show less ventricular remodeling, infarct expansion, aneurysm formation, and late potentials on signal-averaged ECG.

The indications and contraindications to thrombolytic therapy are listed in Tables 32.6 and 32.7. Aspirin (160–325 mg/d), given concurrently, enhances the benefits of all three thrombolytic agents. Also, heparin, given in conjunction with tissue plasminogen activator (tPA) for 3–5 days, reduces the rate of reocclusion of infarct-related artery.

Patients should be followed closely, with a 12-lead ECG about 90 minutes after starting thrombolytic therapy. In high-risk patients (Table 32.8) not responding to thrombolytic agents (continuing chest pain, persistent ST elevation), emergent coronary arteriography and rescue angioplasty should be considered. Others, who can

TABLE 32.3.	Indicators of Adverse Outcome in Acute MI

Age >70 years
Heart failure (S_3 gallop, sinus tachycardia, rales, cardiomegaly, radiographic evidence of pulmonary congestion)
History of prior angina
Hypotension
History of prior MI
High enzyme rise
LV ejection fraction <40%
Persistent occlusion or reocclusion of infarct-related artery
Silent ischemia
Recurrent angina
ECG signs
    Anterior location of infarct
    Complex ventricular arrhythmias
    Bundle branch block
    Second- or third-degree AV block
    Number of leads with ST elevation
    Abnormal signal-averaged ECG
Associated diseases
    Diabetes mellitus
    Hypertension
    Pulmonary disease

TABLE 32.4.	Initial Management of Suspected Acute MI in the Emergency Department*

1. Establish the diagnosis
    Concise history and examination
    12-lead ECG and enzymes
2. Assess hemodynamic status (BP, rhythm, organ perfusion)
3. If ST elevation is present, administer 0.4 mg nitroglycerin sublingually, ×3 doses 5 min apart; repeat 12-lead ECG (avoid nitroglycerin if there is hypotension)
4. Obtain IV access
5. Start continuous ECG monitoring
6. Administer soluble aspirin, 325 mg po†
7. Start supplemental O_2, 4–6 L/min by nasal cannula
8. Initiate IV thrombolytic treatment as soon as acute MI is diagnosed (ST elevation and no contraindications)
9. Administer morphine sulfate for pain relief
10. Administer metoprolol if there is no contraindication
11. Admit to Coronary Care Unit
12. Emergency cardiology consult for possible direct coronary angioplasty/intraaortic balloon counter pulsation (if hemodynamically unstable, severe heart failure, cardiogenic shock)

*These steps should be undertaken promptly and nearly simultaneously.
†Aspirin alone reduces early mortality by 21%.

TABLE 32.5. Comparison of Various Thrombolytic Agents	SK	APSAC	rt-PA
Dose (IV)	1.5 MU in 1 hr	30 mg in 5 min	15-mg bolus; 0.75 mg/kg over next 30 min; then 0.5 mg/kg over next 60 min.
Recanalization	50%	60%	75%
Hypotension	5%	None	None
Half-life	18 min	95 min	4 min
Allergic reaction(s)	Yes	Yes	No
Fibrinogen depletion	Severe	Severe	Moderate
Intracranial bleeding	0.4%	0.4%	0.5%
Cost per dose	$100	$1,500	$2,500

APSAC = Anisoylated plasminogen streptokinase activated complex; rt-PA = recombinant tissue plasminogen activator; SK = streptokinase.

TABLE 32.6. Indications for Use of Thrombolytic Agents
• Typical chest pain lasting ≥30 min, suggestive of acute MI
• 2 mm ST segment elevation in at least 2 contiguous precordial ECG leads (≥1 mm in standard leads) and within 6 hrs of onset of chest pain (6–12 hrs if anterior wall MI or the pain remains persistent)

be followed conservatively, should undergo cardiac catheterization only if angina or other evidence of myocardial ischemia recurs. Thrombolytic agents may cause hypotension, bleeding, and intracranial hemorrhage. They may cause a hemorrhagic stroke in 0.4–0.5% of patients.

Primary percutaneous transluminal coronary angioplasty

Direct (primary) percutaneous transluminal coronary angioplasty (PTCA) is highly successful in opening infarct-related arteries, preserving LV function, and reducing mortality. Its indications are shown in Table 32.8.

Routine care of patients in cardiac care units

Patients with acute MI require complete physical and mental rest, to lower their heart rate and blood pressure and thus myocardial O_2 demand. After an initial 24 hours of confinement to bed, patients with uncomplicated MI can sit on the bedside or be assisted to a chair. Sitting lowers cardiac work slightly, facilitates urination, and reduces the perils of bedrest, such as venous thromboembolism and physical deconditioning. Because mild arterial hypoxemia is common, supplemental oxygen (2–4 L/min by nasal prongs or mask) is appropriate. An IV access is started and kept open by slowly infusing 5% dextrose in 0.45% saline. Most cases of uncompli-

cated MI require 1–3 days of care in CCU and 6–7 days in the hospital.

A liquid diet (1000 calories) is given for 24–48 hrs, following which a soft, easily digestible diet can be prescribed; a regular diet may be given after 5 days. The daily Na^+ intake should not exceed 4 g and calories must be restricted if the patient is overweight. Patient education regarding the disease and risk factor modification should begin in the CCU. Smoking and alcohol are forbidden. A stool softener (dioctyl calcium sulfosuccinate), bisacodyl, or milk of magnesia is routinely given to avoid straining at stool. Urinary bladder catheterization should be avoided unless voiding is severely difficult.

Drug therapy in the CCU

Drug therapy consists mainly of analgesics, antithrombotic agents, β-blockers, nitrates, and angiotensin-converting enzyme (ACE) inhibitors.

Unless contraindicated, **aspirin,** 160–325 mg/day, is highly recommended at first patient contact and should be continued indefinitely. Given early in acute MI, aspirin reduces hospital mortality by 21%. Even when given later, it reduces the long-term risk of MI recurrence or cardiac death.

For pain relief, **morphine sulfate** is given, 2–4 mg IV every 5 minutes until pain is fully relieved or a total of 20 mg is given. Morphine, being vagotonic and sympatholytic, may cause hypotension, bradycardia, respiratory depression, nausea, and vomiting in excessive doses. Because persistent pain may denote ongoing myocardial ischemia, nitroglycerin (sublingually followed by IV) and β-blockers may also be given to relieve pain; however, hypotension *must* be avoided.

Bedrest predisposes to venous thromboembolism, and systemic embolism can follow the formation of a LV mural thrombus. Passive leg movements, early ambulation, and anticoagulants can prevent these complications.

Full-dose **heparin** is given, maintaining an activated partial thromboplastin time (aPTT) at 1.5–2.0 times control, especially in high-risk patients with prior thromboembolism, large anterior or apical MIs, heart failure, shock, atrial fibrillation, cardiomegaly, obesity, LV mural thrombi or when prolonged bed-rest is anticipated. Heparin is followed by warfarin for at least 3 months, maintaining an INR at 2.0–3.0. Long-term warfarin significantly reduces rates of reinfarction and cardiac death. In patients not receiving full anticoagulation, low-dose heparin is given (7500 U every 12 hrs, subcutaneously) until fully ambulatory.

β-blockers improve the myocardial O_2 supply/demand ratio, relieve ischemic pain, limit infarct size, and prevent arrhythmias. In early MI, IV metoprolol is started at 5 mg every 5 minutes for 3 doses, followed by 50–100 mg orally twice daily. β-blockers without intrinsic sympathomimetic activity reduce sudden cardiac death and reinfarction rates (Table 31.6). Therefore, unless contraindicated, long-term β-blockers are strongly advocated in all MI survivors, especially high-risk cases with ventricular arrhythmias, recurrent angina, and impaired LV function.

Unless there is hypotension, **nitroglycerin** infusion can be started at 5 μg/min and gradually increased to reduce systolic blood pressure by approximately 10% from the baseline. Early nitrate therapy reduces the degree of LV remodeling as well as relieves pain by controlling and preventing myocardial ischemia.

ACE inhibitors prevent LV remodeling, heart failure, and reinfarction in patients with an LV ejection fraction less than 40%. Unless there is hypotension, captopril is started at 6.25 mg three times daily and increased up to 50 mg three times daily.

■ **Complications**

Postinfarction angina and infarct extension

Recurrent ischemic pain after relief of initial MI pain is termed unstable angina. It may be either ischemia in a vascular territory distant from the infarct ("ischemia-at-a-distance") or peri-infarction ischemia (in the same vascular territory as the infarct). ST-T changes during angina in leads without Q waves suggest ischemia at a distance, indicating high risk. Urgent coronary angiography and suitable myocardial revascularization are indicated in all patients with recurrent post-MI angina, as such patients are at high risk for reinfarction and sudden death.

Extension indicates occurrence of another MI within 3 weeks of the preceding one. Generally, ECG changes occur in the same leads as the previous MI. Extension should be treated as a new acute MI.

Cardiac arrhythmias

Atrial arrhythmias can result from sinus node ischemia, increased vagal tone, or due to LV failure.

Sinus bradycardia is common in early acute inferior-wall MI. When associated with hypotension, premature ventricular contractions or accelerated junctional or idioventricular rhythm, atropine (0.4–1.0 mg IV, repeated in 2 hours if necessary) is given, and if there is no response, a temporary pacemaker is placed. **Sinus**

TABLE 32.8.	Indications for Direct PTCA

1. Thrombolytic agents contraindicated
2. Patients with acute MI in high-risk subsets:
   Cardiogenic shock
   Heart failure
   Large anterior wall MI
3. Inferior wall MI complicated by:
   Posterior extension
   Right ventricular infarction
   Third-degree AV block

AV = atrioventricular; MI = myocardial infarction; PTCA = Percutaneous transluminal coronary angioplasty.

TABLE 32.7.	Contraindications to Thrombolytic Therapy	
Absolute		**Relative**
Active internal bleeding		Peptic ulcer disease
History of major GI or GU bleeding		Significant liver disease
Recent stroke (<8 wks)		Remote stroke >8 weeks
Major bleeding diathesis		Chronic renal failure
History of cerebral hemorrhage		Uncontrolled hypertension (>180/110 mmHg)
Intracranial tumor		Recent (<2 wks) biopsy, lumbar puncture, thoracentesis, paracentesis
Major surgery, trauma, head injury within 8 wks		Major arterial puncture, dental extraction
Prolonged or traumatic CPR within 2 weeks		Left heart thrombus
Diabetic or other hemorrhagic retinopathy		Oral anticoagulants
Acute pericarditis		Infective endocarditis

tachycardia is often due to heart failure, pulmonary embolism, pericarditis, or anemia.

Atrial tachycardia, atrial flutter, and **atrial fibrillation** are due to LV failure or atrial ischemia. These arrhythmias cause very rapid ventricular rates and hemodynamic impairment or angina and should be treated by electric countershock. The ventricular rate may be controlled in asymptomatic or mildly symptomatic patients by β-blockers, digoxin, or calcium channel blockers.

Premature ventricular complexes (PVCs) and other ventricular arrhythmias occur in almost 90% of patients with acute MI, but only symptomatic or sustained arrhythmias are treated. In these patients, serum potassium and magnesium levels should be maintained in the high-normal range. β-Blockers also may help reduce the frequency of ventricular arrhythmias. Ventricular fibrillation occurs in 15–20% of patients with acute MI.

Primary **ventricular tachycardia** and **ventricular fibrillation** (due to acute ischemia) occur within the first 48 hours of MI and usually do not recur. Secondary ventricular tachycardia and fibrillation, which occur in the presence of predisposing factors (e.g., heart failure, shock, bundle branch block, or LV aneurysm) occur later than 48 h after MI, tend to be recurrent, carry poor prognosis, and require electrophysiologic testing for definitive therapy. Either situation requires immediate treatment.

When PVCs or ventricular tachycardia develop, IV lidocaine is the drug of choice; if it fails, IV procainamide or bretylium is generally effective. Ventricular tachycardia with stable hemodynamics should be treated with drugs first, and if refractory to drug therapy or associated with hemodynamic impairment, it should be treated by electric countershock (100 W-sec). Prophylactic lidocaine, although controversial, may be considered in patients <70 years old who are admitted during the first 6 hours of MI, because the frequency of ventricular tachycardia or ventricular fibrillation is higher in early MI.

Conduction disturbances

Nodal and infranodal atrioventricular (AV) blocks may complicate acute MI. Because the right coronary artery supplies the inferior LV wall, AV node, and His bundle, these structures usually sustain ischemia in **acute inferior-wall MI,** leading to **first-degree, second-degree,** or **third-degree AV block.** The block is located in the AV node, and therefore with third-degree (complete) AV block, an escape rhythm usually arises from the His bundle, with a stable rate of 50–60 beats/min. These blocks are generally transient, lasting 2–3 days. Atropine or a temporary pacemaker is advisable if the escape rate is unusually slow and accompanied by hypotension or ventricular arrhythmias. Acute inferior-wall MI with

third-degree AV block carries a mortality of 25–40%.

Occlusion of the left anterior descending artery leads to **anterior-wall MI,** which affects the right bundle and left anterior fascicle of the left bundle. These bundle-branch blocks (usually bifascicular, with left axis and right bundle branch block) may progress to Mobitz type II and third-degree AV block. Complete heart block in acute anterior-wall MI invokes a slow and unstable escape rhythm from the distal bundle branches or Purkinje fibers, which often degenerates into ventricular fibrillation. Given the much greater myocardial damage in anterior MI, complete heart block in this setting is lethal in 70% of patients. A temporary pacemaker, while advisable when complete heart block or right bundle branch block (with or without left hemiblock) complicates the early course of anterior MI, does not reduce the high mortality of acute anterior MI because a large amount of myocardium is lost; however, in a few cases, it may help. Complete heart block in acute MI may last up to 2 weeks, but bundle-branch blocks may persist for longer periods of time, indicating a higher risk of recurrent complete heart block and sudden death during the ensuing year. Permanent pacemakers may be of benefit, particularly in patients with anterior wall MI who had transient high-grade atrioventricular block and continue to show bifascicular bundle branch block.

Heart failure

High LV filling pressures, due to either decreased compliance or heart failure, usually accompany acute MI. Large MIs (myocardial loss >28%) evoke a process of initial infarct expansion and later enlargement of normal myocardial regions, termed **ventricular remodeling,** which causes heart failure. The degree of remodeling and severity of heart failure correlate with the amount of myocardium lost.

Oral or IV furosemide usually adequately controls symptoms of mild heart failure. In severe cases or pulmonary edema, furosemide or bumetanide is given IV, and if the blood pressure is normal, nitroglycerin or IV sodium nitroprusside may be considered. Blood pressure, heart rhythm, urine flow, hemodynamics, blood urea nitrogen, creatinine, electrolytes, and serial chest radiographs are monitored. Unless there are atrial arrhythmias, digitalis is not very useful. Coexisting severe heart failure and cardiogenic shock call for dopamine or dobutamine (inotropic support). Ventricular septal or papillary muscle rupture should be detected early (see Mechanical Complications below).

Right ventricular infarction

Approximately 35% of patients with inferior or posterior LV infarction also sustain a RV infarction. In patients with inferior-wall MI, an ST elevation in right-sided lead V_4 is highly suggestive of this entity. Its distinct hemodynamic pattern includes hypotension, markedly elevated right atrial and systemic venous pressures (jugular venous distention), equalization of diastolic pressures, and low cardiac output. Pulmonary capillary wedge pressure may be normal or moderately high. In most cases, hypotension improves on volume expansion; inotropic agents and AV sequential pacemaker may rarely be needed.

Mechanical complications

Ventricular septal rupture occurs in 3% of cases of acute MI, usually in the first week after infarction. This catastrophe leads to a sudden, loud pansystolic murmur over the left lower parasternal area and severe congestive heart failure and/or cardiogenic shock. The differential diagnosis is from acute mitral regurgitation (MR) due to a ruptured papillary muscle (Table 32.9). Complete rupture of the body of the papillary muscle causes shock and rapid death. When the tip of one of the heads of the papillary muscle ruptures, acute MR follows with heart failure and/or cardiogenic shock; death may occur several days or weeks later.

In MR and septal rupture, the circulation should be rapidly stabilized with IV nitroprusside and intra-aortic balloon counterpulsation, followed by urgent coronary arteriography and left ventriculography and then urgent surgical repair of the septal defect or valve. Coronary bypass surgery is also often required.

Rupture of the **LV free wall** causes 10% of all deaths in acute MI. More common in elderly, hypertensive women, it sometimes follows severe cough or straining at stool. Most patients die suddenly, and others, having perhaps only a slow oozing of blood, may survive for a few hours or days. Most patients report ongoing or recurrent chest pain from myocardial ischemia or pericarditis. A pericardial friction rub may be heard. The peripheral pulses may be thready, and neck veins grossly distended from cardiac tamponade. Electromechanical

dissociation is common (see below). Hemopericardium evokes intense vagotonia with sinus bradycardia and AV junctional rhythm. When suspected, immediate pericardiocentesis, saline, and isoproterenol infusion, followed by emergency repair of the rupture, could be life-saving.

Cardiogenic shock

A detailed discussion of cardiogenic shock follows in chapter 40.

Electromechanical dissociation

In electromechanical dissociation (pulseless electrical activity), the force of ventricular contraction is severely impaired, despite regular electrical activity. This usually fatal condition occurs in acute mitral regurgitation due to ruptured body of the papillary muscle, massive pulmonary embolism, massive hemopericardium due to LV free wall rupture, after prolonged cardiopulmonary bypass, and in severe three-vessel coronary disease.

Pericarditis

Pericarditis often complicates acute MI, usually within the first 4 days, and is characterized by dull, achy precordial pain, which is worsened by stooping, bending, or breathing (pericardial-type chest pain), and atrial arrhythmias. The pericardial friction rub is usually evanescent. ECG may show diffuse ST-T changes. Salicylates, indomethacin, or a short course of corticosteroids promptly resolve various features of pericarditis. Anticoagulants are contraindicated.

Thromboembolic complications

A mural thrombus may form at the site of endocardial injury due to infarction and is seen much more often in anterior-wall MI (33%) than inferior-wall MI (2%). Systemic embolism may follow in a few days to weeks in high-risk cases (large anterior MI, congestive heart failure, or shock). While high-risk cases

TABLE 32.9. Differential Diagnosis of a Systolic Murmur Developing During the Course of a Myocardial Infarction	
Ruptured Ventricular Septum	**Mitral Regurgitation (MR)**
More common after anterior wall MI	More common after inferior wall MI
Presents with severe congestive heart failure and shock	Involves papillary muscle (dysfunction or rupture)
Systolic murmur/thrill	Murmur generally audible in dysfunction, but may not be heard at all in rupture; rupture causes acute left heart failure, pulmonary edema and hypotension
Doppler echocardiogram may be very useful	Echocardiogram shows MR
Prominent v wave in LA pressure tracings	↑LA pressure and v wave in pressure tracings
Step up in SaO_2 on moving catheter from RA into RV	No step-up in SaO_2 from RA into RV

LA = left atrium; RA = right atrium; RV = right ventricle; SaO_2 = O_2 saturation.

require full-dose heparin followed by short-term oral anticoagulation, all patients with acute MI should receive prophylaxis against venous thromboembolism from the legs and pelvis.

Dressler's syndrome (postmyocardial infarction syndrome)

Presumed to be an immunologic reaction to necrotic myocardium, Dressler's syndrome complicates about 3% of all cases of acute MI. Beginning most often 2 weeks to several months after an MI, its features are recurrent fever, pericardial-type chest pain, pericardial friction rub, atrial arrhythmias, leukocytosis, and bloody pericardial and/or pleural fluid. Despite the recurrences, constrictive pericarditis is unlikely. Acute attacks are treated with aspirin, indomethacin, or steroids.

True and false aneurysms of the left ventricle

LV true aneurysm following Q-wave MI usually involves the anterolateral or apical segments and,

when large, can cause congestive heart failure, systemic emboli from a mural thrombus, and/or ventricular arrhythmias. Large aneurysms produce abnormal chest wall pulsations. Chest radiographs may show a bulge on the left heart border and, occasionally, calcification in the aneurysm wall or mural thrombus. On ECG, persistent ST-segment elevation may be seen in leads showing Q waves. LV aneurysms carry an unfavorable long-term prognosis. Aneurysmectomy is indicated in cases of intractable heart failure and ventricular tachycardia despite medical therapy or in recurrent systemic emboli despite anticoagulation, but it is possible only if the remaining LV has a normal wall motion.

Rarely, the LV free wall ruptures, but the blood leakage into the pericardium is slow and contained by pericardial-epicardial adhesions. Such **pseudoaneurysms,** whose walls have only pericardium, enlarge over time and may rupture fatally. Therefore, they should be corrected surgically.

Non–Q-Wave Myocardial Infarction

Traditionally, MIs were classified as **transmural,** if the ECG showed Q-waves, or **nontransmural** (subendocardial), if the ECG showed only ST-T-wave changes. Because it is difficult to predict from the ECG whether a given MI is transmural (full ventricular wall thickness) or only subendocardial, MIs are presently categorized simply as **Q-wave MI** or **non–Q-wave MI,** each having different patho-anatomy and prognosis (Table 32.10). In non–Q-wave MI, the early mortality is lower, myocardial damage relatively less, and LV function is preserved. The infarct-related artery is usually open, albeit severely stenosed; if it is totally occluded, collateral flow is usually present. Given the relatively large amount of viable but threatened myocardium,

these patients may suffer repeated episodes of angina and reinfarction. The long-term prognosis approaches that of Q-wave MI.

Besides the routine treatment of acute MI, patients with non–Q-wave MI should be given diltiazem (unless heart failure is present) and aspirin, as both agents reduce the mortality and reinfarction rate. Thrombolytic agents have not been shown to be beneficial and β-blockers are not cardioprotective in non–Q-wave MI. All patients with poor prognostic factors (Table 32.11) should undergo prompt coronary arteriography, followed by myocardial revascularization. Stress tests (noninvasive) can be used to judge the need for coronary angiography in others.

■ Predischarge Evaluation

The average 1-year mortality after hospital discharge is 10–15%. The risk for recurrent angina and reinfarction varies widely in post-MI patients, but most patients likely to develop these complications do so within the first 3 months after hospital discharge.

Before discharge, patients without clinical heart failure, LV dysfunction, or post-MI angina and arrhythmias should undergo a low-level exercise stress test, which is safe and helps to classify patients based on risk. Patients with a positive test (ST depression >1 mm, angina, systolic hypotension) should have coronary arteriography, and those with a clearly negative test can be safely managed on medical therapy.

TABLE 32.10.	**Important Differences Between Q-Wave MI and Non-Q-Wave MI**	
	Non-Q-wave MI	Q-wave MI
Patency of infarct-related artery	High	Low
Amount of myocardial damage	Small	Large
Incidence of recurrent angina and reinfarction	High	Low
In-hospital mortality	2–5%	5–10%
One-year mortality	29%	10–20%

TABLE 32.11.	Factors Indicating a Poor Prognosis in Non-Q-Wave MI

Recurrent angina and/or reinfarction
Left ventricular dysfunction, heart failure
Complex ventricular arrhythmias
ECG signs
   Anterior ST-T changes
   Persistent ST depression
   Left ventricular hypertrophy
^{201}Tl perfusion imaging
   Perfusion defects in >1 vascular territory
   Large size of perfusion defect
   Reversible perfusion defect
   Left ventricular dilation
   Increased lung uptake
Multi-vessel coronary artery disease

Posthospitalization Period

The goal in the posthospitalization period is to rehabilitate the patient physically and emotionally to return to work at the end of 8–12 weeks. Minor chores are allowed, but not isometric exercise. The level of activity achieved later during the hospitalization should be maintained, and the pace and duration of exercise slowly increased. The development of angina, dyspnea, or undue fatigue generally implies that the exercise level should be reduced.

Office visits are scheduled at 1 and 2 months after discharge before returning to work. A symptom-limited exercise stress test during the second visit can establish safe limits of activity and determine the level of exercise for body-conditioning programs. Achieving cardiovascular training requires 30 minutes of dynamic exercise (preferably involving both arms and legs, including warm-up and cool-down periods) 3 times weekly on alternate days, which attains 70% of a safely attained maximal heart rate during a symptom-limited stress test. Besides enabling extended work with a smaller rise in pulse and blood pressure, these long-term training programs enhance the patient's sense of well-being. Uncontrolled hypertension, heart failure, arrhythmias, and disabling angina are contraindications to exercise training and should be controlled before a high-intensity training program is begun.

Secondary Prevention

Long-term use of β-blockers clearly reduces reinfarction and sudden death rates significantly (26–34%) in post-MI patients. Most cardiologists now recommend prophylactic β-blockers (unless contraindicated) for all intermediate-risk and high-risk patients following MI. Aspirin and oral anticoagulants provide long-term cardioprotection. Risk/benefit considerations, however, will dictate continuing aspirin indefinitely. ACE inhibitors can prevent heart failure and recurrent MI in patients with reduced LV function. Patients who continue cigarette smoking following MI increase their mortality by 25–50%. Besides modifying diet to achieve ideal body weight and reduce serum cholesterol levels, drug therapy should be undertaken to control hypertension and hyperlipidemia.

Sudden Death

Sudden death is defined as unexpected death occurring instantly or within 1 hour after the onset of symptoms. It is more common in men and most frequently (about 80%) caused by atherosclerotic CAD. Nearly 50–60% of all deaths due to CAD are sudden.

The risk for sudden death is higher with heavy cigarette smoking, hypertension, LV hypertrophy or intraventricular block on ECG, complex ventricular arrhythmias, cardiomegaly, excessive obesity, and stressful lifestyle. About 25% of sudden death patients experience angina, palpitations, undue fatigue, or dyspnea on the day of death.

Ventricular fibrillation is often the immediate mechanism and is often associated with several underlying conditions (Table 32.12). About one-third of the survivors reveal an acute MI. Pathologically, the coronary arteries show severe multivessel disease in most patients and fresh thrombosis over old plaques in about one-third.

Cardiopulmonary resuscitation (CPR) instituted within 3–4 minutes of the onset of ventricular fibrillation can save some lives. Following CPR, patients should be admitted to a CCU for further observation, given the very high recurrence rate of ventricular fibrillation. Coronary angiography is indicated, followed by coronary revascularization or aggressive antiischemic medical therapy. For preventing recurrent cardiac arrest, implantation of cardioverter-defibrillator is the most effective treatment.

Ischemic Cardiomyopathy

In some patients, atherosclerotic CAD causes multiple LV infarcts leading to dilated cardiomyopathy. Angina may or may not be reported. This entity is differentiated from the usual nonischemic congestive cardiomyopathy by coronary arteriography. The prognosis is poor.

TABLE 32.12.	**Conditions Associated With Sudden Cardiac Death**

Coronary artery disease
  Atherosclerosis
    Acute myocardial ischemia
    Previous MI
  Congenital anomalies
  Miscellaneous: spasm, embolism, trauma, dissection,
    arteritis
Myocardial diseases
  Hypertropic or dilated cardiomyopathies
  Infiltrative cardiomyopathies, e.g., sarcoid, tumor,
    infection, dysplasia
  Arrhythmogenic right ventricular dysplasia
  Congenital heart diseases, e.g., tetralogy of Fallot
	Valvular heart diseases, e.g., aortic stenosis, mitral valve
	  prolapse
	Electrophysiologic disorders
	  Long QT syndromes
	  Pre-excitation syndromes
	  Conduction system disorders
	Miscellaneous
	  Acute, massive pulmonary embolism
	  Primary pulmonary hypertension
	  Aortic dissection
	  Severe cardiac tamponade

Besides controlling heart failure, treatment may include coronary revascularization and heart transplantation as appropriate.

In some patients with normal systolic function, diastolic dysfunction from severe myocardial ischemia may cause acute left heart failure and pulmonary edema. Angina may be absent; the ECG shows only ischemia but no prior MI. Because revascularization may benefit most of these patients, coronary angiography should be performed.

CHAPTER 33   CONGENITAL HEART DISEASES

Congenital heart disease occurs in 0.5 to 1.0% of all live births and, overall, shows a masculine predisposition. Maternal viral illnesses (e.g., rubella) and use of drugs (e.g., thalidomide) in early pregnancy are recognized causes, as well as certain chromosomal anomalies and single gene mutations. Children of affected parents also show a 2-fold to 4-fold rise in prevalence. A classification of these disorders is shown in Table 33.1. The clinical features, natural history and complications of the more common congenital heart diseases are listed in Table 33.2; various diagnostic studies and therapy of these conditions are summarized in Table 33.3.

Atrial Septal Defect

Atrial septal defects (ASD) are classified into several types by their location in the atrial septum. **Sinus venosus defect** is an upper defect, where the superior vena cava opens into both the right and left atria. **Ostium secundum defect,** the most common congenital heart disease in adolescents and adults, is 2–3 times more common in women and may be familial. The defect, 1–3 cm in size, occurs in the midportion (fossa ovalis region) of the atrial septum. **Endocardial cushion defects,** including septum primum or atrioventricular (AV) canal defects, are low defects, involving the mitral and tricuspid valves or upper ventricular septum. They may be incomplete (ostium primum defect) or complete. In **ostium primum,** the upper margin of the defect is crescentic, and the lower margin is the mitral and tricuspid valve tissue. In most cases, the anterior mitral valve leaflet has a cleft and abnormal chordal attach-ments. A **complete AV canal defect** has a high ventricular septal defect in addition to a low ASD and cleft mitral and tricuspid valves. The ostium primum defect is 2–3 times more common in women, but a complete AV canal defect has no gender predilection.

The normal fetal shunt is right to left through the foramen ovale. Soon after birth, pulmonary arterioles rapidly involute; the thicker and less compliant RV turns relatively thin and more compliant. As the inflow resistances of the two ventricles change, the left-sided filling pressure rises and right-sided filling pressure abates, and the foramen ovale closes functionally. A persistent, abnormal interatrial opening initiates a left-to-right shunt, owing to the gradually decreasing RV inflow resistance (compared to the LV). The extent of the shunt depends on the size of the defect, the relative resistance in the two circulations, and the relative RV and LV

| **TABLE 33.1.** | **Classification of Congenital Heart Diseases** |

Abnormal pulmonic-systemic communications
  Left-to-right shunt (acyanotic)
    Atrial septal defect
    Ventricular septal defect
    Patent ductus arteriosus
  Right-to-left shunt (cyanotic)
    Decreased pulmonary vascularity
      Cyanotic type of tetralogy of Fallot
      Complete transposition of great vessels with severe
        pulmonic stenosis
    Increased pulmonary vascularity
      Complete transposition of great vessels
      Truncus arteriosus
Vascular and valvular abnormalities
  Coarctation of the aorta
  Aortic stenosis
  Mitral valve incompetence
  Pulmonic stenosis
  Cor triatriatum
    Ebstein's anomaly
Cardiac malpositions (e.g., dextrocardia)

*Not a complete list of all congenital heart diseases.

compliance. Whereas large defects equalize the atrial pressures, hypertension and coronary disease lower LV compliance and increase the shunt. As age increases, rising pulmonary vascular resistance evokes pulmonary hypertension and RV hypertrophy, which raise the RV inflow resistance and reverse the shunt (**Eisenmenger's syndrome**).

In endocardial cushion defects, many derangements may occur: left-to-right shunt through the ostium primum defect, left-to-right shunt via a ventricular septal defect, shunt from the LV to right atrium, and mitral or tricuspid incompetence through cleft mitral or tricuspid valves. The relative resistances in the pulmonary and systemic circuits determine the direction of the shunt. Both ventricles face an increased volume work that leads to biventricular failure.

Excess RV stroke volume prolongs RV ejection time, delaying pulmonic valve closure, while a smaller LV stroke volume shortens the LV ejection time, hastening aortic valve closure. The ensuing widely split S_2 from the early A_2 and late P_2 varies little with respiration (fixed split), because venous return to the atria during phases of respiration is equalized across the ASD.

Ventricular Septal Defect

In adults, ventricular septal defects (VSD) constitute 10% of all congenital abnormalities, being equally frequent in men and women. Nearly 80% of the defects occupy the outflow region of the ventricular septum, between the pulmonary valve and septal tricuspid valve leaflet. The remainder occupy the inflow region (muscular portion) of the septum.

The extent and direction of the shunt depend on the size of the VSD and the relative resistances in the systemic and pulmonary circulations. A large VSD, with a cross-sectional area equal to that of the aortic valve, leads to equal systolic pressures in the LV, aorta, RV, and pulmonary artery and permits unfettered

blood flow from the LV to the RV. Thus, in a large VSD, pulmonary hypertension is severe. With the pulmonary vascular resistance well below the systemic levels, a large left-to-right shunt evolves. Volume overload causes the LV to distend and fail. A medium-sized VSD, being more restrictive, raises the RV and pulmonary artery systolic pressures only moderately, whereas in a small VSD, these remain normal. Over the years, large left-to-right shunts and pulmonary hypertension foster obliterative pulmonary vascular disease, raise pulmonary vascular resistance, and ultimately reverse the left-to-right shunt (Eisenmenger's syndrome).

Patent Ductus Arteriosus

Patent ductus arteriosus (PDA) is the third most common congenital heart disease in adults, being 2–3 times more common in women. Maternal rubella (German measles) during intrauterine life of the fetus is an etiologic factor. The pulmonary orifice of the ductus is located immediately distal to the bifurcation of the main pulmonary trunk, and the aortic orifice of the ductus lies distal to the origin of the left subclavian artery. In addition to pulmonic stenosis, PDA may occur with aortic coarctation and VSD.

During fetal life, oxygenated maternal blood bypasses the lungs and reaches the aorta via the ductus arteriosus, which closes functionally within several hours to 1 week and anatomically within a few days to several weeks after birth. The functional closure follows an increase in PaO_2 and changes in prostaglandins. However, a ductus remaining patent after birth shunts blood from the aorta to the pulmonary artery during both systole and diastole, causing LV volume overload. The caliber of the ductus and level of

TABLE 33.2.   Clinical Features, Natural History and Complications of Congenital Heart Diseases

Lesion	Clinical Features	Natural History	Complications
Atrial septal defect (ASD), ostium secundum type	No symptoms in most; fatigue and dyspnea. Atrial arrhythmias and heart failure after age 40. Thin and frail, usually child or adolescent; Pulse N or ↓ volume; equal a and v waves; HDN LPA; S_1 N; S_2 wide, fixed split; SEM from flow into pulmonary artery; MDM from flow across tricuspid; S_3.	Eisenmenger's syndrome in 20%, mostly with advancing age; PH lowers longevity; 1st, 4th and 6th decade mortality of 0.6%, 4.5% and 7.5% respectively.	Eisenmenger's syndrome, PH, Heart failure, atrial arrhythmias. Very low risk of infective endocarditis.
Atrial septal defect (ASD), ostium primum type	Heart failure, failure to thrive, and respiratory infections begin in late childhood or adolescence. Atrial fibrillation or flutter initiates heart failure. Symptoms develop during infancy in complete a-v canal defects; Down's syndrome in almost 50%. Cyanosis, poor physical development; JVD if right heart failure; large a wave (from MR or TR or both); precordial bulge and Harrison's groove; holosystolic MR murmur and findings of MR; VSD and MR murmur superimposed.	Primum-type defect and mild MR: same as ostium secundum ASD. If MR more severe, early heart failure. Complete a-v canal defects: heart failure during infancy and early death.	Eisenmenger's syndrome; associated mitral regurgitation enhances the risk of infective endocarditis.
Ventricular septal defect (VSD)	No symptoms with small VSD. Dyspnea, fatigue, effort intolerance respiratory infections, failure to thrive. Arterial pulse N or brisk. No JVD; precordial bulge and Harrison's groove (±) HDN apical impulse with large shunts. S_1 usually covered by the holosystolic murmur, S_2 widely split, S_3 with ≥2:1 shunt; brief mid-diastolic murmur; holosystolic murmur in LP area most important sign, murmur only early systolic in very small VSD.	Defect commonly decreases in size and may disappear. Eisenmenger's syndrome rare in children but most frequent in young adults.	Eisenmenger's syndrome, Infective endocarditis, paradoxical embolism.
Patent ductus arteriosus (PDA)	No symptoms with small PDA. Heart failure during the third and fourth decades with large L-R shunts. Infective arteritis. Poor development and CHF. Harrison's groove, pigeon chest, and wide pulse pressure with large PDA. Continuous thrill with systolic accentuation in the 1st and 2nd left intercostal spaces; typical rough, continuous (systole-diastole) murmur over the left upper sternal border. S_3 and mid-diastolic flow apical murmur from excess diastolic blood flow across the mitral valve. These suggest at least 2:1 L-R shunt.	Small PDA does not affect the cardiovascular system nor shortens longevity. Potential site for infective arteritis.	Eisenmenger's syndrome, PDA aneurysm; infective endarteritis, CHF, frequent respiratory infections and retarded growth.
Eisenmenger's syndrome	Symptoms more frequent in large VSD and PDA; onset often during infancy or childhood; in most ASD cases, onset in adulthood; fatigue, exertional dyspnea, angina, syncope, hemoptysis, and right heart failure; squatting (knee/chest position) uncommon. Patients with PDA tolerate it better since the head and neck blood flow maintained; with worsening disease, hemoptysis, predisposition to brain abscess, and strokes. Central cyanosis; in PDA, toenails cyanotic, with pink fingernails (differential cyanosis); clubbing; low volume or normal pulse, "a" wave in neck veins and v wave with TR; RV heave, right-sided S_4, pulmonary ejection click, upper left parasternal SEM; pulmonary valvular incompetence from severe PH (early diastolic [Graham-Steell] murmur); loud P_2; S_2 narrowly split or absent; signs of right heart failure; tricuspid incompetence; arterial hypoxia, polycythemia, hyperuricemia.	Average survival into the mid thirties; death most commonly from hemoptysis, cardiovascular collapse, and heart failure; pregnancy carries a very high risk of maternal and infant mortality.	Cerebral thrombosis, cerebral abscess, paradoxical embolism and infective endocarditis.

	Clinical Features	Prognosis	Complications
Tetralogy of Fallot	Cyanosis early after birth; dyspnea relieved by squatting; syncope, physical underdevelopment. Clubbing (fingers and toes), arterial and jugular venous pulses, N. S_1 N; soft and delayed or totally absent P_2, loud A_2; aortic ejection click due to a dilated aorta; SEM over the mid-left sternal border (pulmonary stenosis); murmur intensity inversely related to the stenosis severity; continuous murmur of bronchial collaterals over chest wall in severe Fallot's.		Infective endocarditis of pulmonary valve, paradoxical embolism, cerebral abscess and cerebral thrombosis.
Transposition of great arteries	More common among men and offspring of diabetic mothers; dyspnea, cyanosis, heart failure, and growth retardation. Anteriorly located aorta causes very loud A_2. Associated VSD, PDA, or PS determine type of murmur.	Prognosis depends on the magnitude of the R-to-L shunt. Survival into adulthood possible, and survival into the sixties not rare.	
Corrected transposition	Symptoms depend on the nature of associated anomalies (such as tricuspid [left-sided] incompetence, VSD, pulmonary stenosis, and complete heart block). Anteriorly located aortic valve causes a very loud A_2.	Untreated, nearly 75% die by 6 months of age, and the rest rarely survive adolescence; patients with large ASD or VSD and significant PS may survive infancy.	
Coarctation of aorta	No symptoms in many; headaches, nosebleeds, cold feet, chest pain and claudication. Modest hypertension in the arms; absent, ↓, or delayed leg pulses; right arm to leg systolic pressure gradient >30 mm Hg; hypertensive retinopathy unusual; thrills and continuous murmurs over the scapular areas and ribs from enlarged collateral (intercostal) arteries; LV heave and S_4 due to LVH. S_1 N; loud A_2; aortic ejection click from dilated ascending aorta; SEM over right upper sternal edge; EDM due to aortic insufficiency; continuous murmur over left interscapular area from the coarcted segment.		Infective endocarditis, aortic rupture, heart failure, stroke due to rupture of cerebral aneurysm, mycotic aneurysm of the poststenotic dilated segment of aorta, myelopathy due to thrombosis of anterior spinal arteries, or CAD.
Pulmonic stenosis (PS)	Mild or moderate PS may be asymptomatic; fatigue, dyspnea, right heart failure and syncope with severe stenosis. Prominent "a" wave in neck veins; palpable RV heave; S_1 N; soft and delayed or absent P_2; pulmonic ejection click; right-sided S_4; murmur length correlates with severity of PS; functional tricuspid incompetence and R-to-L shunt via a patent foramen ovale with onset of right heart failure.	Survival into adulthood in 25%; the remaining die from complications. Only 10% live beyond 6th decade.	
Ebstein's anomaly	Symptoms most often develop in neonatal life or infancy and occasionally in adulthood with exertional dyspnea, fatigue, paroxysmal arrhythmias. Cyanosis, atrial arrhythmias, tall "v" waves, pulsatile liver, systolic murmur with inspiratory accentuation, with or without Wolff-Parkinson-White syndrome; widely split S_1 and S_2; S_3 and S_4 frequent.	Many patients survive only into the third or fourth decade.	Infective endocarditis.

CAD = Coronary artery disease; EDM = early diastolic murmur; HDN = hyperdynamic; LPA = Left parasternal area; LV = Left ventricle; LVH = Left ventricular hypertrophy; MDM = mid-diastolic murmur; MR = mitral regurgitation; N = normal; PH = Pulmonary hypertension; RV = Right ventricle; SEM = systolic ejection murmur; TR = tricuspid regurgitation; ± = may be present.

TABLE 33.3.   Diagnostic Studies in and Therapy of Congenital Heart Diseases

Lesion	ECG and Chest X-ray (CXR)	Echocardiography	Cardiac Catheterization	Therapy
Atrial septal defect (ASD), ostium secundum type	ECG: NSR in young, AF in old; Axis N or rightward; rSR′ or RSR′ in right chest leads. CXR: Heart N or increased size; RA and RV enlarged; PA enlarged; may be aneurysmal.	RV volume overload; ASD directly seen in subcostal, parasternal or apical views; Color-flow Doppler or contrast study can show the shunt.	Locates the ASD, excludes associated anomalies, measures PA pressures; can diagnose any associated CAD.	Surgical closure if shunt is ^{3}1.5: 1.0, ideally between 3–6 years of age, closure in adolescents and adults if shunt is still left to right. No surgery if Eisenmenger's syndrome present.
Atrial septal defect (ASD), ostium primum type	ECG: Left axis, p mitrale, p pulmonale, 1 st° or higher a-v blocks, atrial arrhythmias; rSR′ in right chest leads. LVH (MR) RVH (PH). CXR: same as secundum ASD; chamber enlargement variable; pulmonary plethora.	RV volume overload; anterior mitral leaflet lies in close proximity to the ventricular septum in systole and diastole; cleft in the anterior mitral leaflet on 2-D echo.	Step-up of SaO$_2$ at the right atrial level; left ventriculogram: gooseneck deformity of the LV outflow tract (sine qua non), MR and a LV-right atrial shunt.	Prevent infective endocarditis, treat heart failure and pulmonary infections. Surgical correction between 5–6 yrs or earlier. Marked MR: replace valve, operate at a later age. Total correction of complete a–v canal before 2 yrs of age may prevent Eisenmenger's syndrome.
Ventricular septal defect (VSD)	ECG: LVH, and/or RVH, left atrial hypertrophy, qRS pattern in left chest leads indicates LV volume overload. CXR: cardiomegaly, LV, RV, LA enlargement; enlarged PA and branches; pulmonary plethora.	2-D and Doppler echo locate and quantitate VSD, assess the size of L-R shunt, and estimate RV and PA pressure.	Determines the extent of shunt, locates site of VSD, and detects any additional malformations. PA pressure depends on the size of the VSD.	Infective endocarditis prophylaxis and treatment of heart failure. Surgical closure before the child enters school for medium-sized VSDs with left-to-right shunt (>1.5:1).
Patent ductus arteriosus (PDA)	ECG: LVH with medium-sized or large PDA. CXR: cardiomegaly, enlarged LV, LA, Aorta and its arch and pulmonary artery and its branches; pulmonary plethora, ductus calcification in older persons.	PDA only occasionally seen directly on 2-D echo. LA, LV enlargement. Color-flow Doppler echo detects L-R shunt and extent of pulmonary hypertension.	Confirms diagnosis and identifies other anomalies. Step-up in the SaO$_2$ in the main PA above the RV. PA pressure either normal or high. Aortography precisely locates the PDA and measures its size.	Infective endarteritis prophylaxis. Surgical division of the ductus. Medical therapy for CHF in inoperable patients; Eisenmenger's syndrome contraindicates surgery. Risk of surgery exceeds the risk for infective endarteritis in asymptomatic middle-aged and elderly with a small ductus.
Eisenmenger's syndrome	ECG: Right axis deviation, RVH with strain and right atrial hypertrophy. CXR: marked enlargement of PA and major branches, marked attenuation of distal pulmonary arteries peripherally. Central pulmonary arteries enlarge most in Eisenmenger's due to ASD; enlarged RV and right atrium.	2-D echo shows the intracardiac anatomy and RA, RV and PA enlargement. Doppler echo detects valvular regurgitation and estimates PA pressure.	PA and RV systolic pressures = systemic levels. Elevated right atrial pressure; large "a" wave; PA wedge pressure = N. Markedly high pulmonary vascular resistance (>10 Wood units). Moderate to marked arterial desaturation. Shunts may be right-to-left, bidirectional, or absent. Selective angiocardiography can locate the shunt. Can assess pulmonary vascular reactivity at baseline and after inhalation of 100% O$_2$ or administration of vasoactive agents.	Management of heart failure and various hematologic abnormalities; long-term anticoagulants for thromboembolic complications; nifedipine, prostacyclin and alpha-adrenergic blockade may be helpful. Single lung transplantation with repair of intra-cardiac defects promising.

Tetralogy of Fallot	ECG: Moderate right axis deviation, moderate RVH, tall monophasic R in V_1, and rS in V_2-V_6; biventricular hypertrophy in the acyanotic type CXR: absent pulmonary artery segment and enlarged aorta; aortic arch right-sided (25%); normal/slightly increased heart size, boot-shaped heart shadow ("coeur en sabot"); oligemic lung fields in cyanotic type and prominent or increased lung vessels in acyanotic type	VSD in a membranous septum and biventricular origin of dilated aorta; preserved continuity between posterior aortic wall and anterior mitral leaflet; narrowed subpulmonic RV outflow tract in the short-axis view.	Required to estimate the site and size of VSD, degree of pulmonary stenosis, and to detect other anomalies; selective angiocardiography for delineating RV outflow tract anatomy	Infective endocarditis prophylaxis, treatment of anemia and excessive erythrocytosis; propranolol to prevent anoxic spells. Total correction indicated whenever possible. Surgical mortality 2.5–3.0%; ventricular arrhythmias, complete heart block, right bundle branch block, RV aneurysm and aortic regurgitation postoperatively. Blalock-Taussig operation or a Waterson operation are temporary procedures
Transposition of great arteries	ECG: Right atrial enlargement, right axis deviation and RVH; LVH with PS CXR: Cardiomegaly and narrow mediastinum ("egg-shaped heart"); pulmonary plethora	2-D echo: aorta located anteriorly; runs parallel to the pulmonary artery	SaO_2 much lower in aorta than in the PA. Sequential sampling can locate level of shunt. Angiocardiography can establish the diagnosis and define the precise anatomy	Treat heart failure; palliative procedures (atrial septostomy, PA banding, or systemic-pulmonary anastomosis may be needed in infants. Mustard's operation (rearranging the venous in-flow) and Rastelli's operation (correcting the ventricular outflow) may be successful
Corrected transposition			Diagnosis established by angiocardiography	Surgical correction of associated abnormalities
Coarctation of aorta	ECG: LVH with strain. CXR: Heart size N or ↑; enlarged ascending aorta and aortic knuckle; enlarged left subclavian artery, concave coarcted region and poststenotic dilatation cause a figure-3 configuration of the left margin of the aorta at the coarcted area ("3" sign); notching of lower rib margins from enlarged intercostal vessels (Figure 33.1, Dock's sign).	2-D echo, align with Doppler can identify the site and length of coarctation and assess pressure gradient across it.	Can measure pressure gradient across coarctation and detect associated anomalies (coronary artery disease in adults and bicuspid aortic valve). Aortography extremely important to define the degree and extent of coarctation.	Corrective surgery when systolic pressure gradient is ≥50 mm Hg, ideally between 8-16 years; surgical mortality <5%. In most cases, BP normalizes within several weeks after surgery; balloon angioplasty is an alternative; infective endarteritis prophylaxis and treatment of heart failure and high BP. β-blockers and ACE-inhibitors ideal for BP control.
Pulmonic stenosis (PS)	ECG: Right atrial enlargement, right axis deviation, and RVH with strain; height of R in V_1, correlates with the degree of PS. CXR: prominent poststenotic dilatation; pulmonary oligemia; right atrial and RV enlargement	2-D echo and Doppler visualizes the valve morphology and determines pressure gradient.	Can localize the obstruction and estimate its severity (mold = systolic gradient across the pulmonic valve, <50 mm Hg; moderate, 50 to 80 mm Hg; severe, >80 mm Hg) and exclude associated abnormalities	Direct surgical relief of PS with low risk; percutaneous balloon valvuloplasty quite effective for severe or moderately severe PS.
Ebstein's anomaly	ECG: P pulmonale, right bundle-branch block, and prolonged P-R CXR: marked right atrial enlargement, small RV, and normal or oligemic lungs.	Tricuspid valve closure delayed; downward displacement of its septal leaflet.	On careful pullback of the electrode catheter from the RV apex a chamber is observed (between the right atrium and RV below) with pressure curve characteristic of right atrium but electrogram characteristic of RV.	Control of heart failure and, in a few, surgical replacement of the tricuspid valve. Radiofrequency ablation of the bypass tracts to abolish atrial arrhythmias

2-D = 2-dimensional; AF = Atrial fibrillation; CAD = Coronary artery disease; LV = left ventricle; LVH = Left ventricular hypertrophy; N = normal; NSR = normal sinus rhythm; PA = Pulmonary artery; PH = Pulmonary hypertension; RA = right atrium; RV = right ventricle; RVH = Right ventricular hypertrophy; SaO_2 = Arterial hemoglobin saturation.

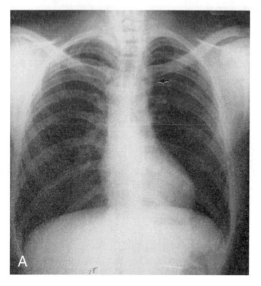

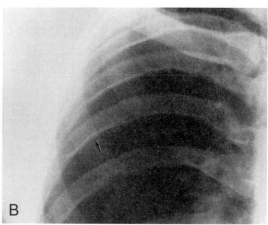

FIGURE 33.1. **A. Chest x-ray of a patient with coarctation of the aorta. Note the bulge above and lateral to the aortic arch, probably due to an enlarged subclavian artery (*arrow*).**

B. Magnified view of the ribs showing notching in their lower borders.
(Courtesy of the Radiology Museum, St. Joseph's Hospital, Milwaukee, Wisconsin.)

pulmonary vascular resistance determine the magnitude of the left-to-right shunt.

Other conditions causing a continuous precordial murmur include aortopulmonary septal defect, ruptured aneurysm of the sinus of Valsalva into the right heart chambers, combined aortic regurgitation and VSD, coronary or pulmonary arteriovenous fistula, and cervical venous hum.

Eisenmenger's Syndrome

Eisenmenger's syndrome represents a reversed or bidirectional shunt through systemic-pulmonary communications, such as VSD, ASD, and PDA, which originally allowed a large left-to-right shunt. In these large left-to-right shunts, pulmonary vascular resistance gradually rises relative to the systemic resistance, thus effacing the left-to-right shunt. When resistances in the two vascular beds equalize, the shunt disappears or becomes bidirectional. If the pulmonary vascular resistance surpasses the systemic, a right-to-left shunt evolves. Pulmonary arterial pressure approaching systemic level imposes a pressure overload on the RV. The pulmonary blood flow decreases and is lower than the systemic, which remains normal.

Tetralogy of Fallot

In adults, Fallot's tetralogy, or the combination of VSD with pulmonary stenosis, is the most common cyanotic congenital heart disease. It has a wide clinical and physiologic spectrum. At one extreme, pulmonary stenosis is mild to moderate, permitting a left-to-right shunt through the VSD (acyanotic type of tetralogy of Fallot). At the other extreme there is pulmonary atresia leading to right-to-left shunt, and the bronchial collaterals supply the pulmonary circuit. Most cases constitute a cyanotic type of tetralogy of Fallot, with severe pulmonary stenosis causing a right-to-left shunt. In addition to VSD and pulmonary stenosis, RV hyper-trophy and a variable degree of overriding of the aorta complete the original tetrad. Pulmonary stenosis is often infundibular and occasionally valvular. Since pulmonary stenosis is progressive, acyanotic tetralogy of Fallot may progress to a cyanotic type.

The degrees of pulmonary valvular obstruction and systemic vascular resistance determine the hemodynamics. As the RV communicates with both the aorta (via its overriding origin) and LV (via VSD), its systolic pressure is always at a systemic level. When the resistance from pulmonary stenosis is low relative to systemic vascular resistance, the shunt is predominantly left to right. As resistance to ejection into the pulmonary artery increases due to progressive pulmonic stenosis, the left-to-right shunt decreases; when the pulmonary resistance exceeds the systemic resistance, the shunt is entirely right to left.

Transposition of the Great Arteries

In transposition of the great arteries, the septum dividing the aorta from the pulmonary artery develops abnormally, and thus, the aorta arises from the RV, and the pulmonary artery arises from the LV. The aorta is anterior and parallel to a posteriorly located pulmonary artery.

Transposition in its pure form is incompatible with life; survival depends on mixing of blood between the right and left circulations through ASD, VSD, or PDA. Also, because the pulmonary and systemic circulations operate in parallel, rather than in series, the shunt has to be bidirectional. In **corrected transposition of the great arteries,** another congenital heart disease, inversion of the ventricles along with transposition of the great arteries results in physiologic correction of circulation. Systemic venous blood flows into the right atrium, across the mitral valve (bicuspid), into a ventricle having the anatomic characteristics of the LV (fine trabeculation and no infundibulum), and is ejected into the pulmonary artery. Oxygenated blood from pulmonary veins flows into the left atrium, across the tricuspid valve into a ventricle with RV characteristics (coarse trabeculation and an infundibulum), and is ejected into the aorta.

Coarctation of the Aorta

Coarctation of the aorta occurs in 1 of every 2000 persons and is more common in men. Anatomically, there is a curtain-like infolding of the media that obstructs the blood flow. In the more common adult-type, the obstruction occurs just distal to the origins of the left subclavian artery and ligamentum arteriosum. Coarctation may coexist with bicuspid aortic valve, VSD, mitral regurgitation, endocardial fibroelastosis, cerebral aneurysms, and Turner's syndrome (in 20% of cases). Hypertension, the main feature of coarctation, is due to as-yet unknown mechanisms, but a lack of pulsatile renal blood flow, stimulating the renin-angiotensin system, seems to play a major role. Pseudocoarctation of the aorta (kinking and tortuosity without obstruction) and saddle embolism in the descending aorta should be considered in the differential diagnosis of coarctation of the aorta.

Pulmonary Stenosis

A valvular type of pulmonary stenosis is the most common type of obstructive disease in the RV outflow tract; supravalvular and subvalvular obstruction is less common. RV hypertrophy follows the RV pressure overload.

Ebstein's Anomaly

In Ebstein's anomaly, the tricuspid valve tissue is redundant and dysplastic, and the septal and posterior valve leaflets are attached lower than normal. Thus, the upper RV becomes a portion of the right atrium. The tricuspid valve is frequently incompetent, the RV is hypoplastic, and the foramen ovale is patent with a right-to-left shunt.

Malpositions of the Heart

Normally, the cardiac apex is located on the left side of the midline and is described as levocardia. When the cardiac apex lies on the right side of the midline, it is termed **dextrocardia,** and when it is located in the midline, it is termed **mesocardia.** Generally, no serious abnormality of the heart exists when dextrocardia is a part of **situs inversus** (i.e., mirror-image reversal of all body organs). However, serious congenital heart malformations occur in patients with isolated dextrocardia or in levocardia with situs inversus.

CHAPTER 34

VALVULAR HEART DISEASE

Mitral Regurgitation

Mitral regurgitation (MR) is the abnormal ejection of a portion of LV stroke volume from the high-pressure LV to the low-pressure left atrium during all or part of systole. This regurgitation is caused by abnormalities or dysfunction in any of the supporting structures of the mitral valve (anterior and posterior mitral leaflets, mitral annulus, chordae tendineae, papillary muscles, or regional LV segments).

■ Pathophysiology

The pathophysiology of MR depends on its acuteness and severity and the degree to which compensatory mechanisms adapt to the regurgitant volume (Table 34.1). **Acute MR** is poorly tolerated since the left atrium cannot accommodate the sudden volume excess; thus the left atrial, pulmonary venous, and pulmonary capillary wedge pressures rise severely, and pulmonary congestion follows. The contractility of the volume-primed LV increases via the Starling mechanism, evoking a supernormal ejection fraction.

In **chronic MR**, left atrial hypertrophy, dilation, and distensibility determine the left atrial and pulmonary venous pressures. An enlarging left atrium dampens the rise in these pressures. LV chamber hypertrophy and initial enlargement confers normal contractility. As the LV unloads a portion of its stroke volume into the LA, wall stress is lowered, thus sustaining normal or supernormal LV ejection fraction in mild to moderate MR. However, when the LV dilates and its end-diastolic volume (EDV) rises, symptoms evolve and functional status worsens.

■ Etiology

The relative frequency of different diseases causing MR is shown in Figure 34.1. In myxomatous degenera-

tion with mitral valve prolapse, the most common cause of **primary MR,** an abnormality of collagen tissue leads to loss of fiber orientation, thinning, and fragmentation of the normal fibrosa of the valve and its appendages. The affected valvular leaflet is stretched, redundant chordae elongate, and the mitral valve leaflet(s) prolapses into the left atrium. The ensuing MR is mild and mostly benign, but it may cause severe valvular leak and therefore congestive heart failure in some elderly patients.

A new systolic murmur and sudden development of congestive heart failure immediately following a myocardial infarction (MI) (especially after an inferior-wall MI) may signify acute MR due to papillary muscle dysfunction and/or chordal rupture. Ischemic papillary muscle dysfunction may also cause chronic MR.

"Secondary" MR results from LV dilatation and malalignment of the chordae tendineae-papillary muscle apparatus. Here, the normal mitral valve leaflets are unable to coapt normally owing to the dilated ring. The degree of MR varies with the severity of LV dysfunction.

■ Clinical Features

An accurate history is a key element in distinguishing whether MR is the cause or effect of LV dysfunction. A previous history of rheumatic fever, MI, angina, endocarditis, or murmur are helpful. With acute MR, dyspnea is acute, and pulmonary edema is usually present. In chronic primary MR, the murmur usually precedes congestive heart failure by a long interval. Palpitations related to the onset of atrial fibrillation and fatigue due to low cardiac output are frequent symptoms. Some patients never develop dyspnea, despite severely impaired LV function.

In acute MR with heart failure, rapid respirations, end-inspiratory rales, and bilateral or unilateral right-

TABLE 34.1.	Longitudinal Changes in LV Mechanics in Mitral Regurgitation							
Type of MR	**Preload**	**Afterload**	**Contractility**	**EDV**	**ESV**	**EF**	**SV**	**LAP**
Acute	↑↑↑	↓	Normal	↑	↓	↑↑	↓↓	↑↑↑
Chronic compensated	↑↑↑	N	Normal	↑↑	N	↑	N	↑
Chronic decompensated	↑↑↑	↑	↓↓	↑↑↑	↑	N	↓	↑↑

EDV = end-diastolic volume; EF = ejection fraction; ESV = end-systolic volume; LAP = left atrial pressure; MR = mitral regurgitation; SV = forward stroke volume; ↑, ↑↑, ↑↑↑ = degrees of increase from normal; ↓, ↓↓ = degrees of decrease from normal; N = normal.
(From: Carabello BA. Curr Probl Cardiol 1993;18:423–478. Reprinted with permission.)

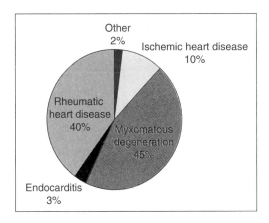

FIGURE 34.1. Causes of mitral regurgitation.
(Redrawn from: Fenster MS et al. Curr Probl Cardiol 1995;
20:211, Figure 13. Used with permission.)

sided pleural effusions may be noted. Tachycardia and a loud, usually blowing apical systolic murmur are typical; the rhythm is generally regular, and an atrial (S_4) gallop is present. In chronic MR, features of ventricular and atrial dilatation predominate, with a hyperdynamic precordium, an LV lift and a laterally displaced apical impulse, a diffuse parasternal lift from systolic "ballooning" of the left atrium, and, with atrial fibrillation, an irregular rhythm. The S_1 is soft and S_2 widely split due to early aortic valve closure. An S_3 gallop is common but does not inevitably mean LV systolic dysfunction. Brief middiastolic murmurs may denote excess diastolic flow across the mitral valve.

The typical MR murmur is apical and holosystolic (see Figure 24.7), and it radiates to the left axilla, its intensity not always indicating the degree of MR. A midsystolic click and a late systolic murmur may occur in mitral valve prolapse, duly augmented by standing or a Valsalva maneuver, measures that lower ventricular volume. With heart failure, the click may vanish; with severe MR or ruptured chordae, the murmur turns holosystolic. Systolic murmurs may radiate to the spine in MR due to a flail anterior leaflet or to the base of the heart with a ruptured or perforated posterior leaflet.

■ Ancillary Studies

In MI-related acute MR, the ECG may show signs of myocardial infarction or ischemia. Chronic MR lacks unique ECG findings other than atrial fibrillation, left atrial enlargement (P mitrale), LV hypertrophy, and nonspecific ST-T changes. In chronic MR, chest radiographs may show cardiomegaly, pulmonary vascular congestion, and a double density at the right heart border

due to left atrial enlargement. Mitral valvular or annular calcification may also be seen, but fluoroscopy may better illustrate these findings.

Besides defining the etiology (flail leaflet, endocarditis, prolapse) and estimating the severity of MR, transthoracic Doppler echocardiography (Figure 34.2) may also provide important prognostic data regarding LV function. A hyperdynamic LV with normal end-systolic volume and supernormal ejection fraction characterize early MR, but as disease progresses, end-systolic diameter increases greatly. An LV end-systolic diameter >55 mm denotes significant LV deterioration, and valve repair or replacement should be considered. Potential surgical candidates should undergo right and left heart catheterization to confirm the cause and severity of MR, identify other valvular disorders, assess LV function, and detect coexistent coronary artery disease.

■ Management

Both the altered pathophysiology and the primary disorder need to be addressed. In acute MR, treatment goals are to reduce pulmonary venous pressures, decrease the regurgitant fraction, and increase forward cardiac output, which can usually be attained with a vasodilator-diuretic combination. Sodium nitroprusside, given its ability to lower afterload and to dilate venous capacitance vessels, is especially useful. Surgery should be considered in symptomatic patients with acute MR and normal LV function before the LV dilates greatly or its systolic function declines. In severe cases of acute MR, especially the post-MI type, temporary stabilization may be needed with an intra-aortic balloon pump. Surgical repair should be performed at the earliest possible time after stabilization.

The usual cardiotonic regimen (diuretics and preload and afterload reduction) is given to patients with more long-standing MR and congestive heart failure. Digoxin is given to treat systolic dysfunction and to control ventricular response in patients with rapid atrial fibrillation. Endocarditis prophylaxis is warranted in all patients with documented MR. Long-term oral anticoagulation may be required in atrial fibrillation complicating MR.

Asymptomatic patients with significant MR should be followed regularly to detect heart failure or progressive ventricular deterioration early. Early LV dilatation can be detected by echocardiography. Mitral valve surgery is appropriate when end-systolic diameter exceeds 50 mm or the ejection fraction is below 50%. The decision regarding mitral valve surgery in chronic MR depends on both the symptoms and LV function. Optimally, surgery should precede severe, chronic irreversible heart failure.

In general, mitral valve repair or reconstruction

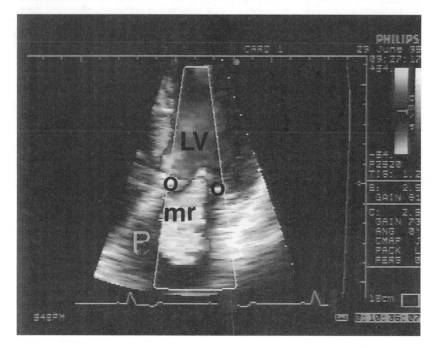

FIGURE 34.2. Mitral regurgitation. Doppler study showing turbulent, high-velocity flow across thickened mitral valve leaflets, indicating severe mitral regurgitation (mr). P = left atrium; o = mitral valve.

(Courtesy of Thomas Palmer, MD, and the Echocardiography Laboratory, St. Joseph's Hospital, Milwaukee, Wisconsin.)

should be attempted whenever possible. Potential candidates for valve repair include those with MR of nonrheumatic, noninfective, and nonischemic causes. Uncomplicated mitral valve repair is durable, has a low operative mortality, and because the chordae and supporting apparatus are preserved, it better preserves LV function. Since no prosthesis is used, infections, thrombosis and hemorrhage seem to be less.

Mitral Valve Prolapse

Mitral valve prolapse (MVP) is a common abnormality affecting about 2–3% of men and 4–6% of women. The exact prevalence depends on the population under study and the diagnostic test used to establish its presence; however, MVP affects both genders and all age groups.

■ Etiology

Although MVP is often inherited as an autosomal dominant trait, it may occur sporadically in normal persons or as part of a connective tissue anomaly (e.g., Marfan's or Ehlers-Danlos syndromes). MVP may also coexist with other clinical conditions, including atrial septal defect, autonomic dysfunction, Graves' disease, Wolff-Parkinson-White syndrome, and ischemic heart disease. Ascribing a cause and effect relationship to these associations is difficult.

■ Pathophysiology

MVP represents a myxomatous degeneration of the valve and its supporting structures histologically, leading to stretching of the affected leaflets, elongation of the chordae tendineae (which are often already redundant), and mid to late-systolic prolapse of one or both mitral valve leaflets into the left atrium. Myxomatous degeneration is the most common cause of acquired MR in the adult. Despite the mild MR and benign clinical course in most cases, MVP can predispose to cerebral thromboembolism, congestive heart failure, and infective endocarditis in some patients.

■ Clinical Features

Considerable controversy surrounds the actual prevalence of symptoms attributable to MVP. Almost

80% of patients report an assortment of nonspecific symptoms, including chest pain, dyspnea, fatigue, palpitations, dizziness, hyperventilation, and syncope. Anxiety, panic disorders, and other psychological disturbances are also common. The chest pain, being frequently nonexertional and prolonged, is usually unlike typical angina.

Physical examination may detect orthostatic hypotension or thoracic deformities (pectus excavatum, narrow anteroposterior diameter, loss of dorsal kyphosis and hypomastia) and classically, a mid to late-systolic click, murmur, or both. The click is loudest at the left sternal border and apex and is usually followed by a mid to late-systolic murmur (click-murmur syndrome). Valsalva maneuver or standing, by decreasing venous return, decreases the LV cavity size and hastens or worsens the prolapse of the mitral leaflets; thus, these move the click closer to S_1, prolonging the murmur and increasing its intensity. Squatting and handgrip have the opposite effect.

Ancillary Studies

Chest radiographs may show scoliosis, pectus excavatum or carinatum, or loss of normal thoracic kyphosis (straight-back syndrome) which, by distorting the cardiac silhouette, may feign cardiomegaly. The ECG may mimic myocardial ischemia in the inferior limb and lateral precordial leads, or it may exhibit paroxysms of supraventricular tachycardia and frequent premature atrial or ventricular beats at rest or exercise. The risk of sudden cardiac death is quite low, unless

the valves are markedly thickened or LV function is abnormal.

Transthoracic echocardiography typically shows superior displacement of one or both mitral valve leaflets (more commonly, the posterior leaflet) into the left atrium. Usually, the diagnosis is confirmed by this test (Figure 34.3). Doppler echocardiography can determine the extent and severity of MR and establish MVP as the cause of MR. Cardiac catheterization is usually not indicated.

Management

MVP mostly runs a benign course although complications may arise, especially in the elderly or those with marked thickening or redundancy of the valve leaflets with or without moderate to severe MR. Complications include endocarditis, chordal rupture, progressive MR, transient ischemic attacks, systemic emboli, and cardiac arrhythmias. Endocarditis prophylaxis is now recommended for all MVP patients with a MR murmur or those with great redundancy of mitral leaflets on echocardiography. β-blockers may relieve chest pain and/or palpitations. For those with transient ischemic attacks or other cerebral ischemic events, aspirin, 325 mg/day, is appropriate. Warfarin therapy (to produce an INR of 2–3) is reserved for those with recurrent emboli or associated atrial fibrillation. Patients with symptoms of congestive heart failure and severe MR due to MVP are candidates for mitral valve repair or replacement. Asymptomatic patients require reassurance.

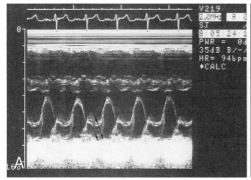 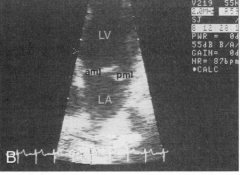

FIGURE **34.3. Mitral valve prolapse. A.** M-mode echocardiogram showing systolic separation of the anterior and posterior mitral leaflets (*arrows*). **B.** Transthoracic echocardiogram (apical view) showing prolapse of the posterior mitral valve leaflet (pml). LA = Left atrium; aml = anterior mitral leaflet.
(Courtesy of Thomas Palmer, MD, and the Echocardiography Laboratory, St. Joseph's Hospital, Milwaukee, Wisconsin.)

Mitral Stenosis

The normal cross-sectional area of the mitral valve orifice is 4–6 cm^2. Mitral stenosis is a narrowing or constriction of this orifice. Nearly all cases in the United States are presumably rheumatic, despite a past history of rheumatic fever being obtainable in only about half the cases. In rheumatic valvulitis, the valve leaflets scar and contract, the commissures fuse, and the chordae tendineae shorten. Mitral valve involvement is the hallmark of rheumatic heart disease. Mitral stenosis may less commonly follow severe mitral annular calcification and infective endocarditis. Left atrial myxoma or large left atrial thrombi may cause LV inflow obstruction that mimics mitral stenosis.

■ Pathophysiology

Mitral stenosis leads to obstructed LV inflow and left atrial hypertension and hypertrophy, which ultimately cause atrial fibrillation. A rising left atrial pressure also raises pulmonary venous and capillary wedge pressures; pulmonary congestion and dyspnea follow. In long-standing cases, the high pulmonary vascular resistance (PVR) finally leads to pulmonary arterial hypertension. When the PVR rises to about 5 times normal, signs of RV failure (venous and hepatic congestion) appear.

The impaired LV filling may so reduce preload as to compromise cardiac output. Because the early (passive) LV filling is relatively more impaired than late (active) filling, a forceful atrial contraction is crucial to push blood across the stenotic valve. Factors that prolong diastole (β-blockers, bradycardia) augment filling, while those that shorten it (fever, tachycardia) may compromise filling. Thus, "flash" pulmonary edema and low output states may follow tachycardias, especially atrial fibrillation.

■ Clinical Features

Mitral stenosis is 3–4 times more common in women than men. Nearly 50% of patients report slowly progressive symptoms, typically beginning in the fourth decade. Exertional dyspnea is the earliest and commonest symptom, with others including orthopnea, paroxysmal nocturnal dyspnea, fatigue (low output), palpitations, and edema. Bloody sputum occurs in about 50%, ranging from pink and frothy to frank hemoptysis. Chest pain occurs in about 10–15% of cases, often attributed to RV ischemia from pulmonary hypertension. Systemic emboli, sometimes the harbinger of mitral stenosis, occur in 15%, especially those with atrial fibrillation. In some, **tachyarrhythmias,** especially atrial fibrillation may cause an abrupt onset. Pulmonary edema may follow

exertion, excitement, fever, anemia, tachycardia, coitus, and pregnancy.

With atrial fibrillation, peripheral pulses may be weak and/or irregular. On auscultation (see Figure 24.9), an accentuated S$_1$ and an opening snap (OS) are heard, followed by a diastolic rumble of variable duration. S$_1$ may be soft if the mitral valve is heavily calcified or if there is coexistent mitral regurgitation, aortic insufficiency, heart failure, or atrial fibrillation. The closer the A$_2$—OS interval or longer the murmur, the worse is the stenosis. The murmur is confined to the apex, and if it is not heard with the stethoscope bell in the left lateral position, mild exercise may unmask it. When normal sinus rhythm prevails, the forceful left atrial contraction produces a presystolic accentuation. As pulmonary hypertension evolves, neck vein distension, an RV lift, loud P$_2$, murmurs of tricuspid leak and/or pulmonic insufficiency, and pedal edema appear.

■ Ancillary Studies

Chest radiograph shows a normal-sized LV. With significantly high left atrial pressures, signs of pulmonary vascular congestion emerge, and the distended interlobular septa cause Kerley's B lines (see Figure 26.2). The left atrial enlargement causes a "double density" (see

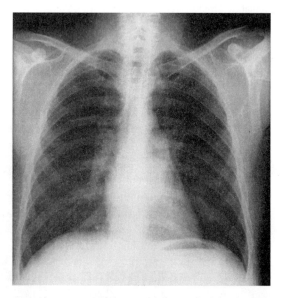

FIGURE 34.4. Mitral stenosis. "Mitralization" is evident on the left heart border—an enlarged left atrium is faintly seen as a double shadow.
(Courtesy of the Radiology Museum, St. Joseph's Hospital, Milwaukee, Wisconsin.)

Mitral Regurgitation), and the distended pulmonary arteries denote pulmonary hypertension. The small aortic knob, a bulging aortopulmonary window from a large central pulmonary artery, and a bulge below it from a large left auricle along with a small left ventricle together cause a straight left heart border (**mitralization, Figure 34.4**).

The ECG shows left atrial enlargement and with pulmonary hypertension, right axis deviation, and RV hypertrophy. Atrial fibrillation may be present. Transthoracic echocardiography is diagnostic.

Other associated valvular lesions may also be noted, as is common in rheumatic heart disease. Tricuspid regurgitation may be organic or functional due to dilated tricuspid annulus. The transvalvular gradient, the valve surface area, and pulmonary artery pressures can be estimated by Doppler echocardiography (Figure 34.5). When the valve orifice is 1 cm^2 or less, mitral stenosis is critical. Cardiac catheterization can confirm the severity of stenosis, diagnose other coexisting valve disease, and/or coronary artery disease, and quantitate the pulmonary hypertension.

TABLE 34.2.	Guidelines for the Diagnosis of an Initial Attack of Rheumatic Fever (Jones Criteria, 1992 Update)*
Major Criteria	**Minor Criteria**
Carditis	Clinical findings
Polyarthritis	Arthralgia
Chorea	Fever
Erythema marginatum	Laboratory findings
Subcutaneous nodules	↑ Acute phase reactants
	↑ Erythrocyte sedimentation rate
	↑ C-reactive protein
	Prolonged PR interval

Supporting evidence of preceding group A streptococcal infection

Positive throat culture or rapid streptococcal antigen test

Elevated or rising streptococcal antibody titer

*If a preceding group A streptococcal infection is proven, 2 major criteria or 1 major and 2 minor criteria denote a high probability of acute rheumatic fever.
(Adapted from: JAMA 1992; 268:2070. Used with permission.)

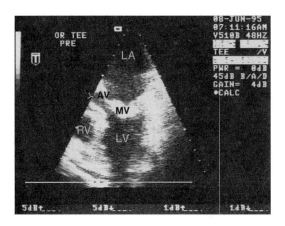

FIGURE 34.5. Mitral stenosis. Transesophageal echocardiogram showing an enlarged left atrium (LA), a small under-filled LV, and markedly thickened and fused mitral valve leaflets (MV). RV = right ventricle; AV = aortic valve.
(Courtesy of Thomas Palmer, MD, and the Echocardiography Laboratory and Cardiac Diagnostic Unit, St. Joseph's Hospital, Milwaukee, Wisconsin.)

■ Management

Correct diagnosis and therapy for streptococcal pharyngitis and acute rheumatic fever (Table 34.2), penicillin V (250 mg b.i.d) or erythromycin (250 mg b.i.d) to prevent rheumatic fever in known rheumatic heart disease until age 35, and lifelong endocarditis prophylaxis form the essentials of preventive care. Long-term oral anticoagulation with warfarin, maintaining an INR of 2–3, is indicated in atrial fibrillation to prevent systemic emboli. Although elective cardioversion may restore sinus rhythm, it prevails in less than one-half of cases after 1 year. In atrial fibrillation with a rapid ventricular rate, digoxin, β-blockers, verapamil, and diltiazem are quite useful.

Usually, only moderate to severe mitral stenosis and pulmonary venous hypertension with symptoms require intervention, either mitral commissurotomy, valvuloplasty, or mitral valve replacement. Atrial fibrillation or single systemic embolic event alone rarely suffice as indications.

Aortic Stenosis

Aortic stenosis (AS) is a narrowing of the aortic valve orifice from its normal 3–4 cm^2, causing obstruction to LV outflow. Most cases follow aortic valve disease due to a congenital bicuspid valve, calcific degeneration, or rheumatic valvulitis. Most congenital bicuspid aortic valves are not initially stenotic but narrow over several decades. Rheumatic AS almost always occurs with mitral valve disease, and so lone valvular AS is most likely nonrheumatic. Degenerative calcific AS, caused by wear and tear of normal valves, is common in the elderly, affecting men four times more often than women.

The etiology of AS varies with age (Figure 34.6). In persons under age 70, bicuspid valve disease is much more common; among those older than 70, calcific degenerative disease is more frequent. Dynamic LV outflow tract obstruction may occur in hypertrophic cardiomyopathy (chapter 37).

■ Pathophysiology

Progressive LV outflow tract obstruction results from a series of events, including accelerated fibrosis and degenerative changes in the valve due to mechanical stress and turbulent blood flow across the valve, rigidity of valve leaflets, and immobility of the cusps from calcification. This obstruction leads to increased LV wall stress and filling pressures, LV hypertrophy, and finally, chronic LV pressure overload. These, along with the impaired epicardial-to-endocardial blood flow, increased myocardial O_2 demands, and abnormal relaxation response of a stiff, hypertrophied ventricle (diastolic dysfunction) explain many of the manifestations of AS. LV dilatation, systolic or diastolic dysfunction, and clinical deterioration eventually supervene.

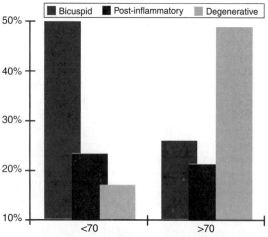

FIGURE 34.6. Influence of age on the etiology of aortic stenosis. Bicuspid aortic valves predominate in those younger than 70 years old when symptoms develop. Degenerative valve disease predominates in those whose age at onset of symptoms is 70. Postinflammatory conditions causing aortic stenosis are believed to be predominantly rheumatic. Congenital abnormalities become a major consideration if age at onset of symptoms is less than 30.

(Data from: Passik CS et al. Mayo Clin Proc 1987, 62:119. Used with permission.)

■ Clinical Features

AS is a slowly progressive disease. Angina, syncope, and dyspnea develop late in its course, as the valve area narrows to $1–1.5$ cm^2. Nearly one-third of patients present with dyspnea and angina, and 15% with syncope. Dyspnea is primarily from pulmonary venous hypertension caused by diastolic dysfunction. Angina may be due to LV hypertrophy or associated coronary artery disease. Syncope is usually exertional and follows global cerebral hypoperfusion, due to low cardiac output or arrhythmia. Atrial fibrillation, which afflicts nearly 10% of patients, is poorly tolerated and may evoke both pulmonary congestion and low cardiac output. In late, severe AS, congestive heart failure may be due to LV dilatation and systolic dysfunction.

The arterial pulse is typically low volume and slow rising *(pulsus parvus et tardus)*. Best appreciated in larger arteries, it may be absent in the elderly. A narrow pulse pressure is characteristic, with a blood pressure of 100/60 mm Hg being typical. However, given the very high LV intracavitary pressures, a systolic blood pressure of 160–170 mm Hg does not rule out critical AS.

The apical impulse may be sustained, forceful, and heaving, reflecting the LV pressure overload; a laterally displaced impulse signifies LV dilatation. A thrill is often felt in the aortic area. S_1 is generally normal and may be followed by an ejection click, which suggests mobile valve cusps; it is not specific for AS. The aortic valve closure (A_2) may be soft, absent, late, or reverse-split. The A_2 is key in helping to distinguish AS from aortic valve sclerosis (in which A_2 retains its normal intensity and timing). Because LV hypertrophy is common in AS, an S_4 is often heard with prevailing normal sinus rhythm. S_3 gallops are sporadic and usually indicate systolic dysfunction.

The usual murmur of AS (see Figure 24.6) is a harsh, diamond-shaped, systolic murmur that is often best heard at the aortic area and may radiate to the neck. The later it peaks, the more severe the stenosis. A faint early diastolic murmur, signifying mild aortic regurgitation, may also be heard. In the elderly with degenerative calcific AS, an apical holosystolic murmur may coexist, due to mitral annular calcification. Clinically diagnosing the cause of a systolic murmur is often difficult; helpful hemodynamic maneuvers are listed in Table 34.3.

■ Ancillary Studies

The ECG usually shows normal sinus rhythm, left atrial enlargement, and LV hypertrophy with associated ST-T wave changes. Conduction defects are common and left bundle branch block may be present. The chest radiograph often shows normal heart size, but cardiomegaly and poststenotic dilatation of aortic root may be present. Because the valve overlies the dorsal spine, aortic valve calcification may not be seen on posteroanterior projections, and lateral chest films and fluoroscopy may be more helpful in this regard.

Transthoracic echocardiography shows LV hypertrophy, thickened, calcific aortic valve cusps with decreased mobility, and the number of valve cusps (trileaflet or bicuspid). It also identifies any associated valvular disorders and assesses LV function (Figure 34.7). With Doppler echocardiography, the peak transvalvular (aortic valve [AV]-LV) gradient and valve surface area may be estimated. A peak AV-LV gradient of 50–75 mm Hg or a valve area of 0.5–0.8 cm²/m² indicates moderate stenosis. Cardiac catheterization confirms these findings and is indicated in symptomatic patients over age 40 to exclude coronary artery disease.

Management

The presence of any of the classic symptoms of AS dictates a thorough work-up so as to facilitate aortic

valve replacement if high-grade obstruction is found. Patients with symptoms of heart failure should avoid vigorous exercise. Vasodilators are risky in AS, since the systemic vasodilation in the face of fixed cardiac output lowers blood pressure so severely as to imperil cerebral perfusion. Endocarditis prophylaxis is required in all cases.

Aortic valve replacement is necessary in all symptomatic patients with an AV-LV gradient above 75 mm Hg and/or valve orifice below 0.5 cm², and it should be considered in symptomatic patients with AV-LV gradient above 50 mm Hg or valve orifice of 0.5–0.8 cm². The procedure carries a mortality of about 5%. The choice of a mechanical valve over bioprosthesis partly depends on the feasibility of long-term anticoagulation. Mechanical valves require warfarin in doses sufficient to keep the INR between 2.5–3.5. Aortic balloon valvuloplasty is palliative in nonoperable, high-risk patients with advanced symptoms, but restenosis and poor long-term survivals are valid concerns.

Angina, syncope, or heart failure each portends a

TABLE 34.3. Response of Systolic Murmur to Hemodynamic Maneuvers				
Maneuver	AS	HCM	MVP	MR
Standing upright	↓	↑	↑	±
Squatting	±	↓	↓	↑
Valsalva	↓	↑	↓↑	↓
Isometric hand grip	↓	↓	↓↑	↑
Post-premature beat	↑	↑	↓	±

↑ = Increased; ↓ = Decreased; ↓↑ = Variable; ± = No change; AS = Aortic stenosis; HCM = Hypertrophic obstructive cardiomyopathy; MVP = Mitral valve prolapse; MR = Mitral regurgitation.
(From: Duthie EH et al. J Am Geriatr Soc 1981; 29:500. Used with permission.)

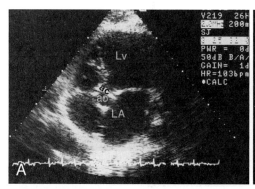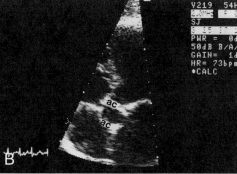

FIGURE 34.7. Aortic stenosis. A. Transthoracic echocardiogram showing thickened aortic valve cusps (ac) and stenosis of the valvular area (ao). B. Magnified view. LA = Left atrium.

(Courtesy of Thomas Palmer, MD, and the Echocardiography Laboratory and Cardiac Diagnostic Unit, St. Joseph's Hospital, Milwaukee, Wisconsin.)

very poor prognosis. With angina or syncope, the average survival declines to about 3–5 years, and heart failure reduces survival to 18 months. Independent preoperative predictors of mortality include patient age, emergency status, presence of significant LV dysfunction, and lack of sinus rhythm.

Aortic Regurgitation (Aortic Insufficiency)

Aortic regurgitation (AR) is the abnormal diastolic flow of blood from the aorta to the LV across an incompetent aortic valve. Most cases arise from two mechanisms: abnormalities of the aortic valve or the aortic root and its supporting structures. The former abnormalities, comprising cusp deformities (perforated or scarred cusps) and leaflet rupture or prolapse, include infective endocarditis, rheumatic valvulitis, myxomatous degeneration, and bicuspid aortic valve. Aortic root disorders include cystic medial necrosis, proximal aortic dissection, hypertension, aortoannular ectasia, and connective tissue diseases (ankylosing spondylitis, Reiter's syndrome, systemic lupus erythematosus, and rheumatoid arthritis). Ascending aortitis, another cause, was commonly caused by syphilis in the past.

■ Pathogenesis and Pathophysiology

Patients with AR are generally hypervolemic, but the presence or absence of compensatory mechanisms largely determines the pathophysiology in any given patient. In acute AR, the LV end-diastolic volume and thus the LV end-diastolic pressure increase acutely, followed by an abrupt and marked rise in left atrial, pulmonary venous, and pulmonary capillary wedge pressures. Thus, acute AR is poorly tolerated. In chronic cases, LV dilation and hypertrophy initially increase the stroke volume, but after a long asymptomatic period, contractility may worsen, ushering in symptoms of overt heart failure.

■ Clinical Features

AR has a clear predilection for men over women. Its clinical features largely depend on the underlying cause (e.g., endocarditis, dissection) and the presence of compensation for the hypervolemia. Symptoms of low cardiac output and pulmonary vascular congestion characterize acute AR, whereas a prolonged asymptomatic phase, often lasting decades, precedes the clinical presentation of most patients with chronic AR, even those with fairly severe AR. Symptoms, when they appear, often include palpitations, exertional dyspnea, and angina. Syncope is rare, but sudden death occurs in about 10%.

In acute AR, cardiac enlargement is minimal, and the apical impulse is only mildly displaced. Tachycardia is common, but the pulse pressure is normal. S_1 may be diminished in intensity or absent if the mitral valve closes prematurely. An early, high-pitched, diastolic murmur immediately follows S_2 and is heard best at the base and mid-left sternal border. When heard best to the right of the sternum, it may suggest aortic root disease. The murmur may be so faint as to be inaudible unless proper technique is used. A basilar systolic ejection murmur may also be present, due to excess forward flow across the aortic valve.

With long-standing AR, a wide pulse pressure, bounding peripheral pulses, and a bisferiens or "water hammer" pulse (see Figure 24.1) may be noted. Precordial palpation reveals a vigorously contracting and dilated LV. Heart sounds are generally normal. The typical murmur of AR is present. An S_3 gallop, a loud basilar systolic murmur, and occasionally, a mid-diastolic, low-pitched apical (Austin-Flint) murmur caused by vibrations from the regurgitant jet of blood on the anterior leaflets of the mitral valve may be noted.

■ Ancillary Studies

The ECG may show evidence of LV hypertrophy. The chest radiograph often shows cardiomegaly and a dilated aortic root. Marked aortic root dilatation should arouse suspicion of a primary aortic root abnormality (e.g., Marfan's syndrome or aortic dissection). Transthoracic echocardiography usually shows left atrial hypertrophy, LV enlargement, and fluttering of the mitral valve leaflets. Doppler echocardiography can detect and quantify the degree of AR as well as assess LV size and function. In suspected infective endocarditis, transesophageal echocardiography may be better to detect vegetations.

Cardiac catheterization is indicated if valve replacement is contemplated. It can assess LV function, identify other valvular abnormalities, and detect and assess the severity of any associated coronary artery disease.

■ Management

Long-term vasodilator therapy is recommended in AR, because it decreases the regurgitant volume and delays LV dilatation. Asymptomatic patients with severe AR and normal LV function may benefit from nifedipine, which may reduce or delay the need for aortic valve replacement.

Recently, enalapril was shown to decrease mean wall stress, LV mass, LV end-diastolic pressure, and the end-systolic volume. If heart failure develops, digitalis, diuretics, and vasodilators should be initiated. With onset of heart failure, rapid deterioration is the norm, with an average survival of about 2 years. Prompt evaluation for aortic valve replacement should follow. In asymptomatic patients, periodic transthoracic echocardiography is useful to evaluate the end-systolic diameter; when it exceeds 50 mm or signs of LV dysfunction appear, aortic valve replacement should be considered, even with only mild symptoms.

Tricuspid Regurgitation

Tricuspid regurgitation (TR) represents the abnormal systolic flow of blood from the RV into the right atrium across an incompetent tricuspid valve. Clinically significant primary TR is uncommon. It may exist with or without underlying pulmonary hypertension. When pulmonary hypertension is present, secondary TR develops as a result of RV failure and dilatation which stretch the tricuspid annulus. This type of "functional" TR commonly follows LV failure, mitral stenosis, and cor pulmonale due to chronic obstructive pulmonary disease. In the absence of pulmonary hypertension, acquired TR follows infective endocarditis (IV drug abuse), carcinoid syndrome, and RV dysfunction due to RV infarction. Tricuspid valve prolapse, Ebstein's anomaly, and atrial septal defect (ostium primum) are congenital lesions associated with TR.

The pathophysiologic consequences of TR include elevation of right atrial pressures, RV volume overload, and the development of signs and symptoms of systemic venous congestion. Symptoms of TR are primarily those of right heart failure and the underlying disease process responsible for TR. Physical examination shows jugular venous distension, prominent *v* wave with a rapid *y* descent and hyperdynamic parasternal impulse (RV lift), a holosystolic murmur along the lower left sternal border that waxes and wanes with respiration, an enlarged pulsatile liver, and peripheral edema.

The ECG may show right atrial enlargement and right ventricular hypertrophy. Atrial fibrillation and right bundle branch block are common. Transthoracic echocardiography may define the etiology of TR (prolapse, ruptured chordae, or vegetations). Doppler echocardiography, by measuring RV systolic and peak pulmonary artery pressures, can help assess its severity.

Except for endocarditis prophylaxis and the possible need for diuretics to manage peripheral edema, no specific treatment is indicated for mild to moderate TR. Tricuspid valve repair or annuloplasty may be performed in conjunction with mitral valve repair for severe TR due to mitral valve disease. In tricuspid valve endocarditis, excision of the tricuspid valve may be called for, especially for native valve infection due to *Staphylococcus aureus* or a fungal organism.

Tricuspid Stenosis

Tricuspid stenosis (TS) is a narrowing or constriction of the tricuspid valve orifice that leads to obstruction to RV inflow. Pathophysiologic sequelae of this obstruction include the development of right atrial hypertension and hypertrophy and decreased cardiac output due to decreased ventricular filling.

TS is rarely an isolated valvular lesion. In adults, it is almost always due to rheumatic valvulitis, for which the pathology is similar to mitral stenosis. Other causes of TS include carcinoid syndrome, congenital heart disease, and fibroelastosis. Right atrial myxoma occasionally mimics TS.

Because rheumatic heart disease causes most cases, most patients with TS are women. Patients may report easy fatigability, which may be due to the associated mitral stenosis. Physical findings are a large *a* wave in the jugular venous pulse with a slow *y* descent, a loud S_1, and a low-pitched diastolic rumble along the left sternal border. This murmur typically increases with inspiration and often has a presystolic accentuation. Hepatomegaly, jaundice, presystolic liver pulsation, ascites, and pedal edema may also occur.

ECG and chest radiographs show evidence of right atrial enlargement. Chest films may also show a distended superior vena cava. Transthoracic echocardiography confirms the diagnosis and may identify other associated valvular lesions. Valve repair or replacement is required for symptomatic patients with TS.

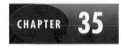

PERICARDIAL DISEASES

Pericarditis

Pericarditis refers to the acute or chronic inflammation of the visceral and parietal pericardium. Its causes are diverse (Table 35.1). Pericardial inflammation leads to fibrin deposition in the pericardium. The associated fluid exudation causes a pericardial effusion which, depending on the underlying disease process, may be serous, bloody, or purulent. Large or rapidly evolving effusions may evoke serious hemodynamic consequences that impair ventricular filling and compromise cardiac output. An epicardial extension of pericarditis may sometimes produce an associated myocarditis.

■ Clinical Features

The onset of pericarditis may be insidious or abrupt. Typical symptoms are fever and chest pain. The pain is variable in quality, location, and radiation, and it may be associated with dyspnea. Some report an intense, steady, crushing, substernal discomfort that radiates to the shoulder, or nape of the neck and may mimic an acute myocardial infarction. Typically worsened by a supine posture, coughing, or deep breathing, the pain is often relieved by sitting up and leaning forward—such posturing may reduce local pressure on inflamed pericardial surfaces.

Fever, tachycardia, and **pericardial friction rub** are classic findings. The rub is best heard with the diaphragm of the stethoscope pressed firmly on the chest wall and with the patient sitting up and leaning forward. Intermittent, fleeting, positional, and of variable intensity, it may have a coarse, scratchy ("leather on leather") quality. The classic 3-component rub conforming to

TABLE 35.1.	**Frequent Causes of Pericarditis**
Cause	**Comment**
Idiopathic	No unique features but resembles viral pericarditis.
Infectious/Infection-related	
Viral	Most cases are viral. Commonly due to Coxsackie B virus in young adults. Pneumonitis and pleuritis usually associated.
Bacterial	
Tuberculosis	Uncommon cause, but important in immunocompromised hosts. Pleural and/or systemic disease commonly associated. Eventually constrictive pericarditis may follow.
Purulent pericarditis	Follows pericardial "seeding" during bacteremia; extension of or contiguous infection; or penetrating chest wounds and esophageal perforation (Boerhaave's syndrome).
Rheumatic fever*	Pericarditis associated with valvulitis or myocarditis.
Non-infectious	
Uremia	Chronic end-stage renal disease generally present. Exuberant fibrinous pericardial reaction, often with hemorrhagic fluid. Reversible with dialysis.
Connective tissue diseases	Pericarditis part of panserositis in SLE, RA and PSS. Pericarditis and/or effusion develop sometime in the course of SLE and 30% of RA. May precede pancarditis in SLE.
Trauma	May follow significant closed chest trauma. Myocardial contusions and transient myopericarditis associated.
Post-MI	"Early" form commonly follows 10–15% of transmural MI in first few days, due to pericardial extension of epicardial inflammation directly from the injured myocardium. May be confused with recurrent ischemic pain and/or reinfarction. "Late" form (Dressler's syndrome) follows MI by 2 wks to 2 yrs; May be recurrent. Autoimmune basis. Associated hemorrhagic pleural effusion, high fever.
Postpericardiotomy syndrome	Follows open-heart surgery or procedures involving opening the pericardium. Features similar to Dressler's syndrome.

MI = myocardial infarction; PSS = progressive systemic sclerosis; RA = rheumatoid arthritis; SLE = systemic lupus erythematosus.
*Not actual infection of pericardium.

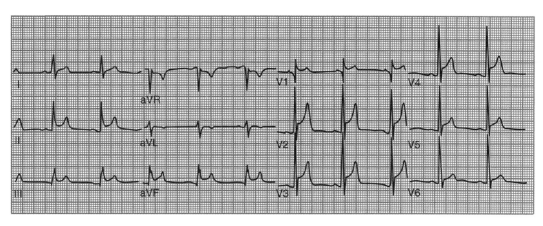

FIGURE **35.1.** ECG changes in acute pericarditis. Note the elevated ST segments with upward concavity in all the leads except aVR and aVL. There is no reciprocal ST depression.

TABLE **35.2.**	ECG Differentiation of Acute Pericarditis and Acute Myocardial Infarction (MI)	
	Pericarditis	**Acute MI**
ECG leads involved	Usually diffuse; spares aVR, V_1	Regional changes that correspond to distribution of coronary blood flow; may see reciprocal changes in other leads
PR segment	Usually depressed early	Normal
ST segments	Concave upwards	Convex upwards
Persistence of ST-segment changes	Days	Hours to days
Time course of T-wave changes	T waves invert after ST returns to baseline	T waves invert within hours while ST segment is still elevated
Q waves	Absent	Present unless non-Q wave infarct pattern
R-wave amplitude	Never lost	May be lost

ventricular systole, early diastole, and late diastole (atrial contraction) is less common. With only 1 or 2 components, the rub may easily simulate a murmur.

■ Ancillary Studies

Leukocytosis, elevated erythrocyte sedimentation rate, and high creatinine kinase (CK) levels are common. The CK-MB fraction rises when myocarditis is present. The chest radiograph shows cardiomegaly when a sizable pericardial effusion is present. Pleural effusions are common and are often left-sided.

ECG changes occur in about 90% of cases. Nearly one-half of these changes evolve through 3 phases. In phase I, the PR segment is depressed, the ST segment is diffusely elevated with an upward concavity, and the T waves are upright (Figure 35.1). The PR depression is an insensitive but specific ECG sign. Seen in two-thirds of

all cases, it may be the sole ECG change in some patients. In several days, phase II follows, with isoelectric ST segments and flattened T waves. In phase III, T waves are inverted widely, often with low-voltage QRS complexes. Although atrial extrasystoles and atrial fibrillation may occur, ventricular arrhythmias are uncommon. The ECG distinction from acute myocardial infarction is listed in Table 35.2.

Further diagnostic testing depends on the clinical picture (e.g., tuberculin skin test for suspected tuberculosis and antinuclear antibody and double-stranded DNA if systemic lupus erythematosus is suspected). Echocardiography has no role in uncomplicated cases, although it can detect even small amounts of pericardial fluid. Characterizing pericardial fluid as either transudative or exudative is not helpful diagnostically. Thus, pericardiocentesis for strictly diagnostic purposes should be avoided. Large-sized pericardial effusions in patients with incipient tamponade or shock may need to be drained to improve hemodynamics.

■ Management

The specific medical management of pericarditis has two goals: to provide symptom relief and to treat the etiologic process, if needed. Symptomatic patients are usually given bedrest and aspirin (or nonsteroidal anti-inflammatory agents). Although pericarditis has a self-limited course in most cases, nearly one-fourth, especially those with immunologically mediated processes, may have prolonged pain or recurrent symptoms. Colchicine and tapering doses of prednisone may benefit these patients.

Pericardial Effusion and Tamponade

The normal pericardium, an inelastic sac, contains less than 50 ml of fluid. Acutely, the pericardium can adjust to an accumulation of only about 100–200 ml of fluid without an abnormal rise in intrapericardial pressure (normally 0–3 mm Hg). With larger amounts, pericardial pressure rises sharply and intracardiac and pulmonary diastolic pressures rise. Chamber pressures equalize, and ventricular filling, and eventually cardiac output, decline. Ultimately, systemic blood pressure falls and shock supervenes. This condition is known as **cardiac tamponade.** With slower accumulations of fluid, the stretching pericardium blunts the rise in pericardial pressure. Thus, subacutely or chronically, relatively large amounts of pericardial fluid (>1 L) can accumulate before pericardial pressure rises sufficiently to impair cardiac filling.

■ Etiology

Although pericardial effusions and pericarditis share similar causes (Table 35.1), the relative frequency of diseases causing each is different. For example, malignancy, the commonest cause of pericardial tamponade, causes pericarditis only infrequently. Hemopericardium (blood in the pericardium) may follow blood dyscrasias, anticoagulation, chest trauma, cardiac perforation during procedures (e.g., catheterization, pacemaker insertion), cardiac rupture, or dissecting aortic aneurysm. Causes of cardiac tamponade are listed in Table 35.3.

■ Clinical Features

The clinical picture of pericardial effusion depends on the underlying disease as well as the compression and hemodynamic embarrassment due to the effusion. Hemodynamically trivial effusions are asymptomatic or evoke only vague, dull chest pain or dyspnea. Compression of adjacent organs, such as the major bronchi, recurrent laryngeal nerve, or esophagus, may evoke cough, hoarseness, or dysphagia, respectively. Only about one-third of patients with evidence of a pericardial effusion have a **pericardial friction rub.**

Patients with rapid accumulation of fluid may show classic signs of cardiac tamponade (Table 35.4). **Pulsus paradoxus** (a systolic BP on inspiration which is below that on expiration by ≥12mm Hg) is seen in almost 75% of these cases. Inspiration normally augments venous return to the RV and its end-diastolic volume. RV filling displaces the interventricular septum toward the LV, thereby decreasing LV end-diastolic volume. In pulsus paradoxus, the inspiratory RV expansion is exaggerated and RV filling occurs at the expense of LV filling. Although pulsus paradoxus is an important bedside clue, it is neither sensitive nor specific. Many of the findings may be absent or attenuated in patients with hypovolemia who experience "low-pressure tamponade."

■ Ancillary Studies

Evaluation of patients with pericardial effusion should include measurement of serum albumin, blood urea nitrogen, creatinine, thyroid-stimulating hormone

TABLE 35.3.	Common Causes of Pericardial Effusion: Mnemonic "VINDICATE"

Vascular (acute MI, hemopericardium) (6%)
Infectious (viral: Coxsackie B; bacterial: tuberculosis, *Staphylococcus aureus, Streptococcus pneumoniae,* Group A streptococcus, Enterobacteriaceae) (5%)
Neoplastic (metastatic, with most common primary sites being lung, breast, leukemia/lymphoma) (54%)
Drugs (procainamide, hydralazine) (2%)
Idiopathic (14%)
Connective tissue disease (systemic lupus erythematosus, rheumatoid arthritis) (2%)
Auto-immune (Dressler's and post-pericardiotomy) (2%)
Trauma (aortic dissection with tamponade, penetrating chest wound) (<1%)
Endocrine/metabolic (chronic renal failure, myxedema) (14%)

Figures in parentheses indicate approximate frequency of each category.

TABLE 35.4.	Classic Signs of Cardiac Tamponade

Dyspnea
Anxiety ("sense of impending doom")
Tachypnea
Signs of low cardiac output
  Fatigue, weakness, and confusion
  Tachycardia
  Hypotension (systolic BP often <100 mm Hg)
  Narrow pulse pressure
Marked neck vein distension (prominent *x* and absent *y* descents)
Pulsus paradoxus
Muffled heart sounds
Signs of compression of adjacent organs (see text)

(TSH), antinuclear antibody, urine protein, and tuberculin skin tests. Other diagnostic tests should be individualized to the clinical presentation.

At least 250 mL of fluid must accumulate in the pericardial sac before the chest x-ray shows cardiac enlargement. With more substantial accumulations, a symmetrically enlarged heart shadow may mimic a globular "water bottle". With large effusions, the ECG shows low-voltage QRS complexes and flattened T waves. Electrical alternans, a regular alteration of the amplitude of the QRS during sinus rhythm, seems to correlate specifically with hemodynamically important effusions.

Transthoracic echocardiography is the most sensitive and specific test in suspected, significant pericardial effusion. Small effusions (<300 mL) may appear on the subxiphoid view as an echo-free space between the posterior cardiac wall and parietal pericardium. Larger effusions may be seen both anteriorly and posteriorly. Right atrial compression and RV diastolic collapse are sensitive and specific echocardiographic signs of early tamponade (Figure 35.2). Because they appear before systemic hypotension and pulsus paradoxus and when the cardiac output is only modestly decreased, they foretell impending clinical cardiac tamponade with hemodynamic collapse.

Right-heart catheterization may detect coexistent conditions, such as LV failure or effusive-constrictive disease, and document hemodynamic improvement after pericardial drainage. Typically, the right atrial pressure is high with a preserved *x* descent and a decreased or absent *y* descent. Right-sided systolic pressures and the pulmonary capillary wedge pressure are moderately high. In tamponade, right atrial, RV, and LV end-diastolic pressures are all equal.

■ Management

Pericardiocentesis, usually performed at the bedside using local anesthesia and echocardiographic localization and following a subxiphoid approach, rapidly lowers right atrial pressures and pulsus paradoxus, increases cardiac output, and allows measurement of intrapericardial pressure. Its major risks are pneumothorax and cardiac laceration.

Patients presenting with hypotension and suspected tamponade should be given IV fluids to expand the intravascular volume. This may delay the echocardiographic appearance of RV diastolic collapse or the clinical onset of hemodynamic compromise. A single pericardiocentesis rapidly relieves tamponade in many patients. For recurrent, large effusions, additional options include the local instillation of nonresorbable steroids or creating a pleural-pericardial window. Persistently high right atrial pressure after effective pericardial drainage suggests combined effusive-constrictive disease, which may require a more complete surgical pericardiectomy. Urgent surgical drainage is warranted in hemopericardium to prevent cardiac tamponade.

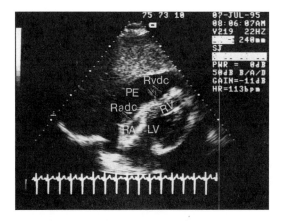

FIGURE 35.2. Cardiac tamponade. Two-dimensional echocardiogram (subcostal view) showing a large pericardial effusion (PE) and early-diastolic, concave indentation of right atrium (right atrial diastolic collapse, Radc) and right ventricle (right ventricular diastolic collapse, Rvdc), indicative of cardiac tamponade. LV = left ventricle. RA = right atrium. (Courtesy of Thomas Palmer, MD, and Echocardiography Laboratory of St. Joseph's Hospital, Milwaukee, Wisconsin.)

Constrictive Pericarditis

In constrictive pericarditis, the pericardial space is partially or completely obliterated by fibrous adhesions formed during a previous episode(s) of acute pericarditis. Its diagnosis requires evidence of systemic venous congestion without myocardial dysfunction or other causes of congestion. Pericardium is calcified in one-half of these patients, especially when the initial effusion is hemorrhagic or the etiology is tuberculosis.

Common causes of constrictive pericarditis are neoplasms, irradiation, post-cardiac surgery, idiopathic processes, infections, chronic renal failure, connective tissue diseases, and asbestos exposure. Radiation-induced changes may not appear for many years following thoracic irradiation. Constrictive pericarditis may follow open heart surgery, even though the pericardium is not closed primarily.

■ Pathophysiology

In constrictive pericarditis, because the heart is encased in a rigid shell, diastolic expansion is restricted and ventricular filling impaired. When the noncompliant pericardium is maximally stretched, systemic venous pressures rise and cardiac output eventually declines.

■ Clinical Features

The onset is usually insidious, and symptoms progress gradually over months to years. Typical early features include fatigue, weight gain, hepatomegaly, and peripheral edema. However, cardiac output and systemic blood pressure are usually maintained.

As pulmonary venous pressures rise, symptoms of pulmonary congestion evolve. Examination shows tachycardia and neck vein distension. The jugular venous waveform has a prominent and steep y descent along with a variable x descent (see Figure 24.3), which contrasts with pericardial tamponade (where the y descent is absent or blunted, and the x descent is prominent). **Kussmaul's sign,** a paradoxical inspiratory rise in jugular venous pressure, may occur with constriction but not with tamponade. It is difficult to appreciate when venous pressures are high. It is also nonspecific, being seen in restrictive cardiomyopathy and chronic RV failure. Pulsus paradoxus may occur but less commonly than in pericardial tamponade.

The apical impulse is not palpable. A pericardial knock is frequently heard at the apex. This sharp, high-frequency diastolic sound occurs earlier than an S_3 and corresponds to the sudden cessation of ventricular filling. Clear lung fields, ascites, and liver enzyme abnormalities are also common. Careful scrutiny of the neck veins is essential in differentiating constrictive pericarditis from chronic liver disease and nephrotic syndrome. Separating constriction from severe right heart failure is also a difficult feat.

■ Ancillary Studies

Chest radiographs may show extensive pericardial calcification in about one-half of cases, but alone, calcification is not pathognomonic of constriction. The ECG may show low-voltage QRS complexes and nonspecific ST-T changes. In severe cases, electrical alternans may occur. Atrial arrhythmias are common, and atrial fibrillation occurs in about 50% of patients.

Other than establishing normal LV function and ruling out cardiac tamponade and other causes of right heart failure, echocardiography has no diagnostic value. Cardiac catheterization may sometimes be necessary to assess hemodynamics. Computed tomography or magnetic resonance scans of the chest can document pericardial thickening and thus distinguish constrictive pericarditis from restrictive cardiomyopathy.

■ Management

Once symptoms develop, the patient's functional status declines slowly and inexorably. In symptomatic patients, surgical pericardiectomy provides relief. It carries an operative mortality of 10% and a 5-year survival of nearly 80%. Symptoms slowly improve after surgery; persistent symptoms may be due to comorbid cardiac conditions or an incomplete resection, a common sequel in those with heavy pericardial calcification.

CHAPTER 36

INFECTIVE ENDOCARDITIS

■ Definition and Epidemiology

Endocarditis, an inflammation of the endocardium, is referred to as either infective or nonbacterial. **Infective endocarditis** (IE) refers to bacterial or fungal infections of the endocardium, whereas infection is absent in **nonbacterial endocarditis** (syn. verrucous or nonbacterial thrombotic endocarditis [NBTE]). Irregular excrescences (vegetations) form on the surface of the cardiac valves in most cases of endocarditis. In the infective type, these consist of aggregates of platelets, fibrin, bacteria and rarely, neutrophils. Clots or shreds of fibrin form on an ulcerated valve surface in nonbacterial endocarditis.

■ Pathogenesis and Pathophysiology

The development of IE usually requires the interaction of two processes: an abnormal valve surface and transient bacteremia. Alterations of the endothelial surface, resulting from high-velocity flow across an abnormal valve, allow deposition of platelet and fibrin aggregates on the low-pressure side of the valve. During states of transient bacteremia, this sterile "vegetation" becomes a nidus onto which bacteria adhere. Bacterial colonization and further deposition of platelets and fibrin follow. These events lead to a bacterial "safe haven" where the microorganisms remain less accessible to the body's cellular and humoral defenses.

Valvular infection damages the architecture of the valve, and when progressive, these destructive changes cause or worsen valvular insufficiency. When infection extends locally into the annulus, ring abscesses and conduction disturbances result. Vegetations may detach and embolize systemically, involving the skin, brain, kidneys, and other organs. Emboli to the vasa vasorum of the brain may cause a mycotic aneurysm; these extracardiac aneurysms are prone to rupture. In patients with right-sided endocarditis, septic pulmonary emboli may bring about multiple cavitating pulmonary infiltrates.

The intense interaction between the host and microbe enhances production of circulating antibodies and immune complexes. A common example of this response is the formation of IgM antibody against IgG (rheumatoid factor), seen in about half the cases of endocarditis when the illness has lasted over 6 weeks.

■ Etiology

Despite traditional classification of IE as acute or subacute, the etiology of IE is probably better viewed in the context of the two major pathogenetic processes responsible for its development: characteristics of the infecting organism and host factors.

Characteristics of the microorganisms

The ability of bacteria to adhere to valve surfaces seems related to their ability to produce dextran, a complex extracellular polysaccharide. *Staphylococcus aureus, S. epidermidis,* viridans streptococci, and enterococci are common causes of IE, because of both the relatively high rate at which they cause transient bacteremia and their avid adherence to normal and abnormal valve surfaces.

Over half of the cases of culture-proven native-valve endocarditis are due to streptococci, typically the viridans streptococci, which are normal inhabitants of the gingival crevices. Minor trauma from dental manipulations can evoke fleeting bacteremia and endocarditis. Genitourinary disorders or manipulations are frequent precipitating events in enterococcal endocarditis. *Streptococcus bovis* bacteremia notably occurs with colonic polyps or colon cancer.

Staphylococcus aureus causes up to 25% of all cases of culture-proven endocarditis. Fungal endocarditis should be considered in IV drug abusers and those with recent cardiovascular surgery or prolonged IV antibiotic therapy. Finally, cultures are negative in less than 5% of cases of endocarditis. Recent antibiotic use and infections with slow-growing (HACEK group) or fastidious organisms (nutritionally deficient streptococci, fungi, Q fever, psittacosis, brucellosis, and chlamydiae) may be responsible.

Host factors

Several host factors, including underlying illnesses and immune competence, largely determine the clinical presentation of endocarditis and its microbiology. In this way, IE may be classified into native-valve or prosthetic-valve IE (bioprosthesis or mechanical) or that related to IV drug abuse (IVDA). The causative organisms differ significantly among these categories.

Native-valve endocarditis is most common in men over age 50, especially elderly diabetic men. Predisposing valvular lesions include mitral valve prolapse (30–50%), rheumatic heart disease (30%), and congenital heart disease (10–20%) with a bicuspid aortic valve, pulmonic stenosis, ventricular septal defect, aortic stenosis, IHSS or patent ductus arteriosus. In some elderly patients, degenerative disease of the aortic and mitral valves is responsible. No predisposing valve lesion is found in a few cases.

Prosthetic valve endocarditis is discussed separately. IE in IV drug abusers generally affects younger men and has a predilection for right-sided valves. Staphylococcus is the most common causative organism.

■ Clinical Features

IE affects persons of all age groups but mostly older men. Men predominate over women by a 2:1 ratio. The clinical features of IE may be constitutional, cardiac, embolic, and immunologic (Table 36.1).

Constitutional symptoms, being nonspecific, may actually delay diagnosis of IE. The most common cardiac symptom of IE is **dyspnea,** which is usually related to congestive heart failure. Major **emboli** occur in about one-third of patients, causing protean manifestations with involvement of different organs (skin, abdominal viscera, brain). Thus, sudden neurologic events in young patients should arouse suspicion of IE.

The virulence of the organism and its ability to adhere to the valve also influence the clinical picture. Thus, *Staphylococcus aureus* endocarditis presents as an acute, fulminant illness with high, hectic fever, predominant cardiovascular signs, and scant peripheral stigmata of endocarditis. Rapid valve destruction, hemodynamic instability, and extracardiac metastatic abscesses are its other features. Continuous, community-acquired *S. aureus* bacteremia should always be treated as endocarditis, especially if a primary nidus is not apparent. Enterococcal endocarditis has a subacute onset in men over 60 years of age. Endocarditis due to the viridans streptococci has an insidious onset with a low-grade fever and frequent extracardiac manifestations. A tendency for systemic emboli, ostensibly from large bulky vegetations, is typical of fungal endocarditis.

Fever and heart murmur are characteristic but not invariable. Fever may be absent in the elderly and in renal failure (urea has antipyretic properties), heart failure, and malnutrition. In many patients, particularly the elderly, the cardiac auscultatory findings of endocarditis are often inseparable from signs of prior valvular disease and high output (fever, anemia).

■ Ancillary Studies

A normochromic, normocytic anemia is very common. In subacute cases, the WBC count may be normal or modestly high. The erythrocyte sedimentation rate (ESR) is almost always high, but a normal ESR does not exclude IE. Rheumatoid factor may be present. Proteinuria, occasionally in the nephrotic range, and microscopic hematuria are generally noted; gross hematuria may follow renal emboli or infarcts. RBC and WBC casts, when present, reflect an immune-complex-mediated postinfectious glomerulonephritis.

Blood cultures are the key diagnostic test for IE, being positive in over 90% of cases. No more than 3 sets of cultures are routinely necessary in the first 24 hours unless antibiotics have been given in the preceding 2 weeks. The bacteremia is continuous, and therefore, in most patients, all sets of blood cultures will be positive. Persistent bacteremia without an identifiable source (e.g., an infected IV line) should arouse the suspicion of IE.

The chest x-ray may show heart failure. Septic pulmonary emboli (i.e, bilateral, multiple, small patchy infiltrates which may cavitate) are typical of right-sided endocarditis. In suspected prosthetic valve endocarditis, fluoroscopy typically shows abnormal valve motion or "rocking" by a loose prosthesis. With coronary artery

TABLE 36.1.	Clinical Features of Infective Endocarditis	
Type	**Common**	**Less Common**
Constitutional	Fever, chills, sweats, dyspnea, anorexia, weight loss, malaise, weakness	Nausea, vomiting, abdominal pain, myalgias/arthralgias, back pain, headache
Cardiac	Dyspnea, which may be acute or insidious; cardiac murmur (>85%)	Chest pain in 15%; myocardial infarctions due to emboli to coronary arteries from valvular vegetations; a new murmur/changing murmur very infrequent
Embolic	Major emboli to different organs (e.g., abdominal pain due to splenic or mesenteric infarction; focal neurologic symptoms)	Janeway lesions (non-tender, hemorrhagic, macules on the palmar and plantar surfaces) seen in about 10%
Immunologic	Splenomegaly, clubbing, and skin manifestations (each in up to 50% of cases)	Conjunctival, oral mucosal, and lower-extremity petechiae; splinter hemorrhages in about 15% (very nonspecific); Osler nodes (multiple, 2-5 mm, tender, nodular lesions on the fingers or toes, seen in 15% (nonspecific).

emboli and myocarditis, the ECG may show signs of myocardial infarction and ST-T changes, respectively. New conduction defects, the harbinger of a ring abscess, should be periodically sought in the ECG.

Transthoracic echocardiography, with a sensitivity of about 70% for large (>5 mm) vegetations and very few false-positives, can be used to assess the severity of valvular incompetence and detect vegetations and local complications (e.g., perforated leaflet, chordal rupture, myocardial ring abscesses). Nearly 80% of infected, native, left-sided valve vegetations may be detected. However, because small vegetations may be missed, a normal study does not rule out IE. **Transesophageal echocardiography,** with a sensitivity of nearly 90% for detecting vegetations, can detect smaller vegetations and identify periannular abscesses, mycotic aneurysms, and pulmonic valve vegetations.

■ Management

Newly proposed criteria for diagnosing IE incorporate pathologic (appearances of vegetations) and clinical aspects, which includes both major (typical organisms on blood culture, evidence of endocardial involvement on echocardiography) and minor (predisposing condition, fever, and vascular and immunologic manifestations) features. These criteria are summarized in the article by Bayer et al.

General principles of treating infective endocarditis include:

1. Using bactericidal and not bacteriostatic antibiotics (failure to sterilize the vegetations increases the risk of relapse)

2. Using IV therapy, which is almost always necessary

3. Ensuring high antibiotic concentrations for prolonged periods to eradicate slowly replicating organisms

Minimum inhibitory concentration (MIC) and minimum bactericidal concentration (MBC) should be measured in most cases to guide the choice and dose of antimicrobials. These provide critical data in patients who fail to respond to treatment or who harbor an unusual organism.

Antibiotic treatment

After appropriate cultures are obtained, empiric antibiotics may be given to patients with suspected IE, especially those who are acutely toxic or in heart failure. Ampicillin (3.0 g IV every 4 hrs) with nafcillin (2.0 g IV every 4 hrs) and gentamicin (1 mg/kg IM or IV every 8 hrs) is appropriate. Given the high rate of methicillin-resistant *Staphylococcus aureus* (MRSA), vancomycin (15 mg/kg IV every 12 hrs) may be used instead of ampicillin and nafcillin. Once blood culture results are

available, this regimen should be tailored to the specific organism and its in vitro sensitivities.

Because the MIC for viridans streptococci are low (usually <0.1 µg/ml) and the cure rate is high (95–99%), there are several successful treatment options (Table 36.2). Ceftriaxone is promising as a once-daily therapy.

TABLE 36.2.	Treatment of Infective Endocarditis Caused by Common Organisms

Viridans Streptococci and *S. bovis*
Penicillin-susceptible (MIC≤0.1µg/ml)
1. Penicillin G 12–18 MU/d in divided doses for 4 wks; OR
2. Penicillin G 12–18 MU/d in divided doses + Gentamicin 1 mg/kg IV q 8 h, both for 2 wks. OR
3. Vancomycin 15 mg/kg IV q 12h for 4 wks.
Relatively penicillin-resistant (MIC >0.1-≤0.5 µg/ml)
1. Penicillin G 12–18 MU/d in divided doses q 4 h + Gentamicin 1 mg/kg IV q 8 h, both for 2 wks. then continue penicillin G for 2 more wks; OR
2. Vancomycin 15 mg/kg IV q 12 h for 4 wks.

Enterococci and viridans Streptococci (MIC>0.5µg/ml)
1. Penicillin G 18–30 MU IV in divided doses q 4 h for 4 wks; OR
2. Ampicillin 12 g/d in divided doses 4 h + Gentamicin 1 mg/kg IV q 8 h both for 2 wks; OR
3. Vancomycin 15 mg/kg IV q 12 h + Gentamicin 1 mg/kg IV q 8 h for 4–6 wks

Staphylococci
Native valve
Methicillin-susceptible (S. epidermidis and S. aureus)
  Nafcillin 2 g IV q 4 h for 4–6 wks ± Gentamicin 1 mg/kg IV q 8 h for first 3–5 d.
Methicillin-resistant
  Vancomycin 15 mg/kg q 12 h for 4–6 wks.
Prosthetic Valve
Methicillin-susceptible
  Vancomycin 15 mg/kg q 12 h for 6–8 wks. + Gentamicin 1 mg/kg q 8 h for first 2 wks.
Methicillin-resistant
  Vancomycin 15 mg/kg q 12 h for 6–8 wks. + Gentamicin 1 mg/kg q 8 h for first 2 wks. If *S. epidermidis*, add Rifampin 300 mg q 8 h orally for 6–8 wks.

Culture-Negative
  Ampicillin 3 g IV q 4 h + Gentamicin 1 mg/ kg q 8 h.

d = days; h = hours; MIC = minimum inhibitory concentration; MU = million units; q = every; wks = weeks. In penicillin-allergic patients, one may give vancomycin or consider penicillin desensitization (Chapter 12). Gentamycin may be given IV or IM.
(Adapted from: Korzeniowski OM, Kaye D. Endocarditis. In: Gorbach SL, Bartlett JG, Blacklow NR (eds). Infectious Diseases 2nd ed. Philadelphia: WB Saunders, Co. 1998, p. 223.

Aminoglycoside resistance, seen in 5–30% of enterococci, creates serious treatment difficulties.

Patients with isolated *S. aureus* bacteremia, an identifiable focus or source of infection, and normal heart valves should be treated for 2 weeks with IV therapy. The vast majority of patients with disseminated *S. aureus* infections should be treated for 4–6 weeks with this regimen. Rifampin (600 mg/day orally) can be added if metastatic abscesses are suspected.

Endocarditis complicating intravenous drug abuse

Endocarditis may be responsible for 5–10% of hospital admissions for febrile intravenous drug abusers (IVDA). Despite the high rate of right-sided endocarditis among IVDA (primarily the tricuspid valve), predicting IE among these patients is difficult. Thus, patients with fever and IVDA should be observed closely (usually in the hospital) until blood cultures are reported sterile.

IE in IVDA often presents with pleuritic chest pain and cough. The responsible microorganisms are mostly *Staphylococcus aureus* (60–65%) and streptococci (15–25%). The geographical location (eastern vs western U.S.) may affect the microbial etiology. A murmur is common, but the classical triad of tricuspid regurgitation, a pulsatile liver, and the waxing-waning systolic murmur occurs in one-third of cases. Chest x-rays may show septic pulmonary emboli and/or pneumonia in about 50% of patients. Besides the tricuspid valve, mitral and aortic valve also may be involved.

Positive blood cultures are the cornerstone of diagnosis of IVDA-related IE. The cure rate in appropriately treated, right-sided *S. aureus* endocarditis exceeds 90%. The mortality in right-sided endocarditis averages 8–10%. Valve excision or debridement are usually reserved for those with persistent uncontrolled bacteremia. Persistent fever and septic emboli are not indications for surgical intervention.

Prosthetic valve endocarditis

Because of differences in pathogenesis and pathogens, prosthetic valve endocarditis (PVE) may be classified as early (within 60 days of valve surgery) or late (>60 days after surgery). *Staphylococcus epidermidis* is the most frequent organism in early PVE, suggesting an important role for intraoperative contamination. Causative organisms in late disease resemble those of native-valve endocarditis. Suggested

TABLE 36.3. Indications for Endocarditis Prophylaxis	
Prophylaxis Recommended	**Prophylaxis Not Recommended**
High-risk category	**Negligible risk category**
All prosthetic (including bioprosthetic and homograft) cardiac valves	Isolated secundum ASD
Previous bacterial endocarditis	Surgical repair of ASD, VSD or PDA without residua beyond 6 months
Complex cyanotic congenital heart disease	Previous coronary artery bypass graft surgery
Surgically constructed systemic pulmonary shunts or conduits	Mitral valve prolapse without valvular regurgitation**
Moderate risk category	Physiologic, functional, or innocent heart murmurs
Most other congenital cardiac malformations (other than above or below)	Previous Kawasaki disease without valvular dysfunction
Acquired valvular dysfunction	Previous rheumatic fever without valvular dysfunction
Hypertrophic cardiomyopathy	Cardiac pacemakers and implanted defibrillators
Mitral valve prolapse with valvular regurgitation and/or thickened leaflets	**Surgical procedures**
Surgical procedures	Endotracheal intubation; fiberoptic bronchoscopy[†]; tympanostomy tube insertion; transesophageal echocardiography; vaginal hysterectomy; vaginal delivery; Cesarian section; urethral catheterization, uterine dilatation and curettage, sterilization procedures, insertion or removal or IUDs and therapeutic abortion (all in uninfected tissue); cardiac catheterization; implanted pacemakers and defibrillators; circumcision; and incision or biopsy of surgically scrubbed skin
Tonsillectomy and adenoidectomy; procedures in the oral mucosa; rigid bronchoscopy; sclerotherapy for varices*; esophageal stricture dilation*; ERCP with biliary obstruction*; biliary tract surgery*; procedures involving intestinal mucosa*; prostate surgery, cystoscopy; urethral dilation	

ASD = atrial septal defect; ERCP = endoscopic retrograde cholangiopancreatography; PDA = patent ductus arteriosus; VSD = ventricular septal defect.
*Prophylaxis recommended in high-risk patients.
[†]Prophylaxis optional in high-risk patients.
**Individuals with prolapsing and/or myxomatous mitral valves that show regurgitation (audible on auscultation or shown on echocardiography) are at increased risk for bacterial endocarditis.
(Adapted from: Dajani AS et al. JAMA 1997; 277:1795-1801. Used with permission.)

TABLE 36.4. Endocarditis Prophylaxis for Dental, Oral, Respiratory Tract or Esophageal Procedures

Penicillin Allergy	Oral Intake	Agent	Dose, Route and Timing
None	Possible	Amoxicillin	2.0 g p.o. within 1 h before
None	Not Possible	Ampicillin	2.0 g IM or IV within 30 min before
Present	Possible	Clindamycin	600 mg p.o. within 1 h before, OR
		Cephalexin/Cefadroxil†	2.0 g p.o. within 1 h before, OR
		Azithromycin/Clarithromycin	500 mg p.o. within 1 h before
Present	Not Possible	Clindamycin	600 mg IV within 30 min before, OR
		Cefazolin	1.0 g IV within 1 h before

†Avoid if there is history of immediate hypersensitivity (urticaria, angioedema or anaphylaxis) to penicillin.
(Adapted from: Dajani AS et al. JAMA 1997; 277:1798. Used with permission.)

TABLE 36.5. Regimens for Endocarditis Prophylaxis for Procedures in Genitourinary/Gastrointestinal Tract (Excluding Esophagus)

Risk Category	Penicillin Allergy	Agents and Dosage	Comments
High	None	Ampicillin 2.0 g plus Gentamicin 1.5 mg/kg (not to exceed 120 mg)	First dose within 30 min; Ampicillin 1.0 g IV/IM or Amoxicillin 1.0 g p.o. 6 h later
High	Present	Vancomycin 1.0 g IV plus Gentamicin 1.5 mg/kg (not to exceed 120 mg)	Infuse vancomycin in 1–2 h; complete injection/infusion within 30 min before
Moderate	None	Amoxicillin 2.0 g p.o. OR Ampicillin, 2.0 g IM/IV	Amoxicillin 1 h before; Ampicillin within 30 min before
Moderate	Present	Vancomycin 1.0 g IV	Infuse vancomycin in 1–2 h; complete infusion within 30 min before

(Adapted from: Dajani AS et al. JAMA 1997; 277:1799. Used with permission.)

treatment of early PVE due to *S. epidermidis* (Table 36.2) takes into account the resistance patterns of this organism. Both early and late PVE often need reoperation for valve replacement.

Role of surgery

Valve surgery is required in about 25% of cases of IE. The most common indication is congestive heart failure (>70% of cases), with persistent infection or recurrent systemic emboli being less frequent indications. Ideally, patients are given antibiotics long enough to "sterilize" the vegetations before surgery, but hemodynamic issues often dictate the specific timing of surgery.

■ Prognosis and Course

The patient's age, comorbid conditions, the valve affected, virulence of the organism, and complications of treatment all influence the prognosis. With optimal treatment, most patients (>90%) with native-valve endocarditis attain a microbiologic cure. Recurrent fever may reflect local complications (e.g., myocardial or valve ring abscess, metastatic abscesses) or drug fever. Recurrences and relapses mostly occur within a few weeks to a month of cessation of treatment. Relapses should be distinguished from reinfection, which is more common with IVDA and those with periodontal disease.

■ Prevention

The use of **endocarditis prophylaxis** is rooted in medical practice, despite its empiric nature and documented failures. However, it is recommended for all high-risk patients undergoing procedures likely to cause transient bacteremia (Table 36.3). The selection of antibiotic depends on the nature of the procedure, the ability for oral intake, and the presence or absence of penicillin allergy (Tables 36.4 and 36.5).

CHAPTER 37   DISEASES OF THE MYOCARDIUM

Cardiomyopathies

The cardiomyopathies represent a group of primary myocardial diseases affecting the structure and function of heart muscle, but excluding ventricular dysfunction due to pericardial, valvular, hypertensive, or ischemic disease. Primary cardiomyopathies are generally divided into three clinical subgroups: dilated (congestive), hypertrophic, and restrictive (Figure 37.1). Dilated cardiomyopathies usually show features of ventricular systolic dysfunction, whereas hypertrophic and restrictive types feature mostly diastolic dysfunction.

Idiopathic Dilated (Congestive) Cardiomyopathy

Idiopathic dilated cardiomyopathy (IDC) is a primary myocardial disease of unknown etiology, with ventricular dilatation and impaired myocardial contractility.

■ Etiology, Pathology, and Pathogenesis

Dec and Fuster postulate four basic but not mutually exclusive mechanisms for IDC: (1) familial and genetic factors, (2) viral and other cytotoxic insults, (3) immune abnormalities, and (4) metabolic, energetic, and contractile abnormalities. IDC is believed to have a genetic predisposition, with the affected locus being involved with immunoregulation. Antibodies against coxsackie B virus, while common in IDC, do not prove this agent as the etiology; however, the virus may alter the MHC-antigen expression or activate T cells or specific HLA antigens. The metabolic, energetic, and contractile derangements mark the disease progression, rather than initiate the disease.

IDC lacks any anatomic or histologic characteristics that set it apart from other causes of dilated cardiomyopathy (Table 37.1). The coronary arteries are normal. The chief microscopic features are myocyte hypertrophy and degeneration, with varying degrees of interstitial fibrosis and inflammation. Inflammation is evident immunohistochemically in many cases, but this does not prove myocarditis.

Ventricular dilatation and impaired myocardial contractility eventually cause symptoms due to decreased ejection fraction, increased LV end-diastolic volumes, and pulmonary venous congestion. Excess circulating catecholamines chronically overstimulate cardiac β-receptors and damage an already-depressed myocardium.

■ Clinical Features

IDC has a distinct predilection for African Americans and men (by 2.5 times) compared to Caucasians and women. Signs and symptoms of advanced LV failure are the presenting features in most cases (Table 37.2). Despite normal coronary arteries, up to one-third of patients complain of angina-like chest pain. A minority experience atrial fibrillation or high-grade ventricular arrhythmias. Syncope strongly predicts sudden death. Pulmonary and/or systemic emboli may follow mural thrombi in the appropriate chambers.

Features of biventricular heart failure are typical, but signs of left heart failure are usually more prominent initially. Often, the blood pressure is low, and the pulse pressure is narrow. Tachycardia is common and pulsus alternans may occur. The apical impulse is diffuse and laterally displaced. Atrial (S_4) and ventricular (S_3) gallops as well as systolic murmurs are common, particularly during periods of symptomatic decompensation. The systolic murmurs often arise from secondary mitral or tricuspid regurgitation due to ventricular dilatation and chordal geometric distortion.

Bilateral end-inspiratory rales and pleural effusions signify left heart failure. Cool, pale extremities indicate poor peripheral perfusion. The neck veins are often distended; a prominent v wave follows tricuspid regurgitation. Ascites, tender hepatomegaly, and other signs of right heart failure occur in less than one-half of patients. Atrial fibrillation is tolerated poorly.

■ Ancillary Studies

The ECG typically shows tachycardia and nonspecific ST-T changes. Conduction delays occur in over three-fourth of all patients with IDC, their presence correlating with duration of symptoms and the extent of myocardial fibrosis. Sinus rhythm is mostly maintained, but in others, atrial fibrillation may prevail. The chest radiograph typically shows cardiomegaly and pulmonary vascular congestion. Pleural effusions, often bilateral, are common. Unilateral effusions are often right-sided.

Transthoracic echocardiogram shows ventricular di-

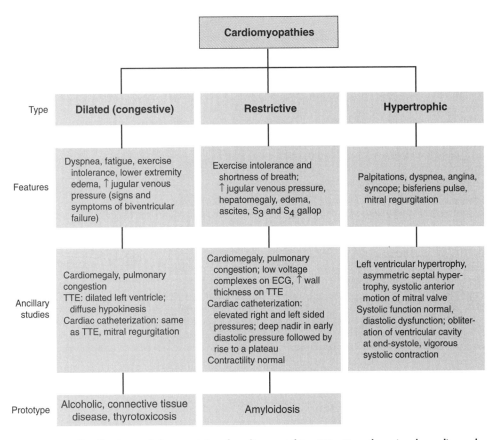

FIGURE **37.1.** Classification and characteristics of cardiomyopathies. TTE = Transthoracic echocardiography.

latation (often all 4 chambers may be enlarged), normal wall thickness, and a decreased ejection fraction. While global hypokinesis is common, segmental wall motion may be abnormal in over one-half of the cases, owing to altered regional wall stress.

Cardiac catheterization should be reserved for patients with strong risk profiles for, or symptoms of, ischemia (typical angina, suspected ischemic LV dysfunction). Endomyocardial biopsy is done only when a treatable underlying disorder, such as sarcoidosis or hypereosinophilic syndrome, is suspected.

■ Management

Nonpharmacologic therapy for IDC includes activity guidelines, salt restriction (2.0 g Na^+ diet), smoking cessation, and weight reduction. Vasodilators (either an ACE inhibitor or combined hydralazine-isosorbide dinitrate) improve symptoms and prolong survival in congestive heart failure. Digitalis not only controls resting heart rate in atrial fibrillation, but it also improves maximum exercise capacity and reduces

symptoms of heart failure, even in those with prevailing sinus rhythm.

Patients with atrial fibrillation, mural thrombus on echocardiography, or prior thromboembolism should receive adjusted-dose warfarin to keep the INR between 2–3. Antiarrhythmic agents are reserved for survivors of sudden death and symptomatic patients with proven, sustained ventricular arrhythmias, usually after electrophysiologic testing. These patients may also benefit from an automatic implantable cardioverter-defibrillator device.

■ Natural History

The overall prognosis in symptomatic IDC is poor, with 5-year mortality rates averaging 20–50%. Many deaths occur within the first year after symptoms appear. Although LV function may spontaneously improve in some patients, symptoms typically progress and LV failure worsens over time in most. Not surprisingly, IDC remains a common indication for heart transplantation.

TABLE 37.1.   **Known Causes of Dilated Cardiomyopathy**

Toxins	Infectious or inflammatory causes
Ethanol*	Infectious
Chemotherapeutic agents (doxorubicin, bleomycin)	Viral
Cobalt*	Coxsackie virus, cytomegalovirus*, human immuno-
Antiretroviral agents	deficiency virus
Zidovudine*, didanosine*, zalcitabine*	Rickettsial
Phenothiazines*	Bacterial (diphtheria*)
Carbon monoxide*	Mycobacterial
Lead*, Mercury*	Fungal
Cocaine*	Parasitic
Metabolic abnormalities	Toxoplasmosis*, trichinosis, Chagas' disease
Nutritional deficiencies	Noninfectious
Thiamine*, selenium*, carnitine*	Collagen vascular disorders
Endocrinologic disorders	Systemic lupus erythematosus, progressive systemic
Diabetes mellitus, hypothyroidism*, thyrotoxicosis*,	sclerosis, dermatomyositis
Cushing's disease, acromegaly*, pheochromocytoma*	Hypersensitivity myocarditis*
Electrolyte disturbances:	Sarcoidosis*
Hypocalcemia*, hypophosphatemia*	Peripartum dysfunction*
Familial cardiomyopathies	Neuromuscular causes
	Duchenne's muscular dystrophy, fascioscapulohumeral
	muscular dystrophy, Erb's limb girdle dystrophy,
	myotonic dystrophy, Fredreich's ataxia

*Potentially reversible either spontaneously or with treatment.
(Adapted from: Dec GW, Fuster V. N Engl J Med 1994; 331:1564. Used with permission.)

TABLE 37.2.   **Presenting Symptoms of Idiopathic Dilated Cardiomyopathy**

Dyspnea on exertion	86%
Heart failure	75–85%*
Peripheral edema	29%
Palpitations	30%
Exertional chest pain	8–20%†
Asymptomatic cardiomegaly	4–13%‡
Systemic/pulmonary emboli	1.5–4%
Syncope	Rare

*90% in NYHA Class III or IV.
†Chest pain eventually occurs in 35% of all patients.
‡Atrial fibrillation may be present in less than 25% of these.
(From: Dec GW, Fuster V. N Engl J Med 1994; 331:1564–1575.
Reprinted with permission.)

Hypertrophic Cardiomyopathy

■ Definition and Etiology

Hypertrophic cardiomyopathy (HCM), a heritable disorder, encompasses a wide spectrum of pathologic, clinical, and echocardiographic features, including a markedly hypertrophic, nondilated LV without systemic hypertension, aortic stenosis, or any other process capable of producing similar degrees of LV hypertrophy.

Although patients with HCM may exhibit variable degrees of LV outflow tract obstruction, nonobstructive forms are being increasingly recognized. Previously known as **idiopathic hypertrophic subaortic stenosis** (IHSS), this relatively uncommon disease is inherited as an autosomal dominant trait with a high degree of penetrance. Its specific etiology is unknown, but a familial-genetic abnormality of contractile proteins has been proposed.

■ Pathology and Pathogenesis

HCM is characterized pathologically by ventricular hypertrophy and, in almost 95% of cases, an endocardial biopsy showing myocardial cell disarray. This combination of myocyte degeneration and ventricular hypertrophy causes abnormal LV relaxation, excessive LV stiffness, and impaired LV filling. Consequently, the filling pressures rise, leading to pulmonary venous hypertension and dyspnea.

Decreased compliance and altered ventricular pressure/volume relationships also can jeopardize the cardiac output if the LV is "under-filled." For example, when effective atrial transport is lost (as in atrial fibrillation), the stiff and noncompliant LV does not fill adequately, thus compromising the preload.

Excessive myocardial O_2 demands or impaired perfusion of hypertrophied muscle may provoke myocardial ischemia. Small-vessel disease due to intimal thickening and medial fibrosis of the intramural coronary arteries may play a contributory role, with resultant subendocardial ischemia.

LV outflow tract obstruction is not universal in HCM. The obstruction, when present, is due to positioning of the anterior mitral valve leaflet against the adjacent hypertrophied ventricular septum during systole. Sudden death in HCM patients does not appear to be associated with the magnitude of LV outflow tract obstruction. Because HCM is the most common cause of sudden death in young athletes, its distinction from the ventricular hypertrophy that is common in well-trained athletes is crucial.

■ **Clinical Features**

Clinical features of HCM vary widely, ranging from no symptoms to progressive heart failure. Symptoms, when present, usually appear in the third or fourth decade. Predominant symptoms are exertional dyspnea, fatigue, and chest pain that may or may not resemble classic angina, palpitations, dizziness, and exertional syncope. Many of these symptoms are exacerbated by tachycardias and/or atrial arrhythmias.

Sudden death, which affects 2–3% of adults with HCM, may be the sole initial manifestation of HCM. Risk factors for sudden death are young age, history of syncope, family history of sudden death, marked LV wall thickening and perhaps, nonsustained ventricular tachycardia on ambulatory monitoring.

Typical findings in HCM include a fast-rising arterial pulse, left atrial and LV hypertrophy, and a systolic murmur accentuated by maneuvers that decrease LV cavity size (Valsalva, standing). Although a brisk carotid upstroke and bisferiens pulse are not specific for HCM, they are important bedside clues that help distinguish HCM from valvular aortic stenosis. Besides the harsh, diamond-shaped systolic murmur heard typically at the base, cardiac findings in HCM often include an S_4 gallop and an apical murmur of mitral regurgitation. In patients without any LV outflow tract obstruction, the murmur is usually absent, leaving an apical S_4 as the only auscultatory finding.

■ **Ancillary Studies**

The chest radiograph is normal in about one-half of cases, and in the others, it shows left atrial enlargement and cardiomegaly. The ECG is abnormal in over 90% of cases, with left atrial enlargement, LV hypertrophy, and

T wave inversion being frequent findings (however, these are not specific). Prominent, abnormal Q waves and diminished or absent R waves in lateral chest leads ("pseudoinfarct") often make the recognition of myocardial ischemia or infarction difficult. Giant T-wave inversion may be seen in some patients with asymmetric apical involvement. Atrial fibrillation is infrequent (<10%). Holter monitoring may show nonsustained ventricular tachycardia.

A nondilated, hypertrophied LV with a normal to supernormal ejection fraction and near-cavity obliteration at end systole are typical echocardiographic findings. Highly specific findings are asymmetrical septal hypertrophy, with a septal thickness exceeding 1.5 times the thickness of the posterior wall or an interventricular septal thickness exceeding 15 mm. The anterior mitral valve leaflet comes in contact with the ventricular septum during systole, producing dynamic outflow obstruction. This systolic anterior motion of the mitral valve, which is seen in about 50% of cases, is quite specific for LV outflow tract obstruction. Doppler echocardiography may show mitral regurgitation and signs of impaired ventricular filling.

Cardiac catheterization measures chamber pressures, quantitates the LV outflow tract gradient, and assesses the presence and severity of coexistent coronary artery disease. Left ventriculography in HCM often shows massive septal and free wall hypertrophy, large papillary muscles, and an almost obliterated LV cavity at end-systole.

■ **Management**

Patients with HCM should avoid strenuous exercise, dehydration, and hypovolemia. Medical management should aim to improve exercise capacity and decrease symptoms by slowing the heart rate and promoting ventricular relaxation. Although β-blockers or verapamil may relieve symptoms, their use prophylactically does not seem to prevent disease progression or sudden death. Vasodilators and inotropes are usually contraindicated, unless there is systolic dysfunction or digoxin is needed to control the ventricular response in atrial fibrillation. If not contraindicated, long-term anticoagulants should be instituted when atrial fibrillation develops. Mechanical alterations of the anterior mitral valve leaflet and the septal endocardial surface obligate endocarditis prophylaxis.

Surgery (septal myotomy-myectomy) is reserved only for severe, refractory symptoms or a LV outflow tract gradient exceeding 50 mm Hg. Because LV outflow tract obstruction is most often due to systolic anterior motion of the mitral valve, mitral valve replacement may also be beneficial. Hemodynamic improvement with dual-chamber pacing has also been noted.

Restrictive Cardiomyopathy

■ Definition, Etiology, and Pathophysiology

Restrictive cardiomyopathy (RCM) is a primary or secondary myocardial disease. In it, the stiff, but neither dilated nor hypertrophied, LV maintains a normal contractility. However, its increased stiffness creates diastolic dysfunction (i.e., impaired LV relaxation and filling and high pulmonary venous and right-sided pressures).

The major causes of RCM are summarized in Table 37.3. Among these unusual diseases, systemic **amyloidosis** (distinguished from senile cardiac amyloidosis) is one of the more common. Although **hemochromatosis** presents more often as a congestive cardiomyopathy, a subset of cases as well as **hypereosinophilic syndrome** (Loeffler's endocarditis) may present with a picture of RCM.

■ Clinical Features

Despite its rarity, the recognition of RCM is important since its causes are potentially reversible or

TABLE 37.3.   Common Causes of Restrictive Cardiomyopathy

Radiation
Amyloidosis
Idiopathic fibrosis
Scleroderma
Hemochromatosis
Infiltrative neoplasms
Sarcoidosis
Myocarditis
Endomyocardial fibrosis
Pseudoxanthoma elasticum

(From: Fowler NO. Heart Disease and Stroke 1992;1:94. Used with permission.

treatable (sarcoidosis, hemochromatosis). Features of biventricular failure are often the initial manifestation, and edema and ascites may sometimes become dominant. RCM may mimic constrictive pericarditis with neck vein distension and prominent x and y descents. Hepatomegaly, lung crackles, and a systolic murmur of tricuspid regurgitation are other common findings.

■ Ancillary Studies

Sinus tachycardia, low voltage in the limb leads, nonspecific ST-T changes, left bundle branch block, and arrhythmias are common ECG findings. Chest radiography often shows mild cardiomegaly and pulmonary venous congestion. On transthoracic echocardiography, the valves are normal, the LV has thickened walls and normal systolic function, and it is not dilated. Two-dimensional images, particularly in amyloidosis, may show biatrial enlargement, interatrial septal thickening, and a peculiar "speckled" pattern. Computed tomographic scans show no pericardial thickening, an important differentiating point from constrictive pericarditis.

Cardiac catheterization may be needed to distinguish RCM from constrictive pericarditis, but the findings may be inconclusive. Endomyocardial biopsy should be performed in patients with a high index of suspicion for potentially treatable causes of RCM (hemochromatosis, sarcoidosis).

■ Management

Diuretics and vasodilators should be used judiciously in RCM so that the LV preload is not compromised. Because systolic function is normal, digitalis is usually used only to treat atrial arrhythmias. Amyloidosis may predispose to digitalis toxicity. Calcium channel blockers and β-blockers may improve resting hemodynamics by promoting ventricular relaxation and prolonging filling time.

Myocarditis

Myocarditis is often clinically diagnosed when heart failure complicates a febrile illness and when LV dysfunction (LV ejection fraction <45%) occurs in the absence of coronary artery disease or another specific etiology. Histologic diagnosis of myocarditis requires demonstration of an "inflammatory infiltrate with necrosis and/or degeneration of adjacent myocytes not typical of the ischemic change seen in coronary artery disease" (Dallas criteria). However, only 10% patients with the clinical definition of myocarditis show confirmatory results on endomyocardial biopsy. This dichotomy between the clinical and histologic criteria makes an accurate definition of myocarditis difficult.

TABLE 37.4. Causes of Myocarditis

Infectious
    Bacterial: Diphtheria (toxin), infective endocarditis, Lyme disease (*Borrelia burgdorferi*)
    Fungal: Aspergillus
    Mycoplasma
    Parasitic: Toxoplasmosis, trypanosomiasis (Chagas' disease), trichinosis
    Rickettsial: Rocky mountain spotted fever
    Viral: Adenovirus, coxsackie virus groups A and B, cytomegalovirus, ECHO viruses, hepatitis B virus, HIV (may be
        opportunistic infections or drug effects also), influenza virus, poliomyelitis virus, rubella virus, rubeola virus
Inflammatory
    Idiopathic giant cell myocarditis, rheumatic fever, sarcoidosis
    Connective tissue diseases: Systemic lupus erythematosus, rheumatoid arthritis
    Vasculitis: Polyarteritis nodosa, Churg-Strauss vasculitis
    Hypereosinophilic syndrome
Toxic
    Drugs: Aerosol propellants, daunorubicin, emetine, phenothiazines, tricyclic antidepressants
    Physical agents: Radiation

■ Etiology, Pathology, and Pathophysiology

The causes of myocarditis are listed in Table 37.4. Coxsackie virus infections occur commonly in young adults, usually in association with pleurisy or pericarditis. Lyme carditis often presents with a predominance of cardiac conduction abnormalities.

Cytomegalovirus infection, usually a self-limited illness, may be a more serious process in immunocompromised patients. Up to 40% of AIDS patients exhibit focal myocarditis due to multiple factors, including HIV, opportunistic infections, or drug effects. While 20% show LV dilatation and dysfunction (decreased ejection fraction, global hypokinesis) clinically apparent heart failure develops in only a minority of AIDS patients.

■ Clinical Features

Myocarditis shows highly variable clinical features. Some patients are symptomatic during the early inflammatory phase and present acutely with fever, fatigue, palpitations, dyspnea, and chest pain. The chest pain may or may not simulate angina and, in some cases, results from associated pericarditis. Tachycardia is out of proportion to the fever. Signs of heart failure may be present.

The myocarditis may resolve uneventfully in some patients, but in others, it may evolve into a dilated cardiomyopathy. Thus, some patients may present initially with advanced heart failure and other complications of cardiomyopathy. An irregular rhythm, S_3 gallop, and signs of heart failure may be present.

■ Ancillary Studies

The WBC count and erythrocyte sedimentation rate may rise, but both are nonspecific findings. CK-MB rises in less than 15% of cases. Acute and convalescent viral antibody titers may help define a specific etiology.

The ECG often shows tachycardia, low voltage, nonspecific ST-T changes, and a long QT interval. Atrial and ventricular extrasystoles, intraventricular conduction delays, and fleeting, high-degree AV block are also common. The chest radiograph may be normal or show signs of heart failure. Cardiomegaly may be due to LV dilatation or pericardial effusion. Echocardiography shows depressed LV systolic function and possibly a pericardial effusion. The LV cavity size may be normal or increased with some segmental wall motion abnormalities. About 15% of cases may harbor LV mural thrombi. Coronary angiography shows normal findings. Biopsy evidence of definite myocardial damage and T-lymphocyte infiltration is seen in only a minority of cases.

■ Management

The usual treatment of myocarditis is supportive care. Because of concerns that exercise may enhance viral replication, physical activities should be limited in patients with suspected viral etiology. Congestive heart failure is treated with the usual measures.

Myocarditis does not appear to warrant immunosuppressive drug therapy. Therefore, routine gallium scanning and endomyocardial biopsy are not indicated.

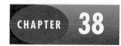

DISEASES OF THE AORTA

The normal aorta is a conduit vessel divided into 3 major segments: the ascending aorta, aortic arch, and descending aorta. The aortic arch, also called the transverse aorta, gives rise to brachiocephalic, left carotid, and left subclavian arteries. The thoracic and abdominal components of descending aorta are defined by their location above or below the diaphragm. The normal adult aorta is 3 cm wide at its origin and 1.8–2.0 cm wide at a level just below the renal arteries.

Aortic Aneurysms

An aneurysm is an abnormal widening of the vessel. Most aneurysms follow vessel wall degeneration, which is closely related to risk factors for atherosclerosis. Thus, hyperlipidemia, hypertension, smoking, and diabetes enhance the risk for forming an aneurysm, which is further aided by age-related changes (aortic elongation, tortuousity, inelasticity, and ectasia).

Cystic medial necrosis, the key pathologic finding, may occur prematurely in some cases (e.g., Marfan's syndrome) due to abnormalities of collagen and collagen cross-linking. Medial necrosis and/or atherosclerosis are pivotal in ascending aortic aneurysms, while the main factor in descending aortic aneurysms is atherosclerosis.

Abdominal Aortic Aneurysms

■ Clinical Features

Most (75–90%) aortic aneurysms are abdominal, the common site being the infrarenal segment between the renal arteries and aortic bifurcation. Abdominal aortic aneurysms (AAA) are often clinically silent and detected incidentally during the course of a routine physical examination or imaging. However, some patients may report a steady thoracic or lumbar spinal pain that is caused by local pressure or expansion of the aneurysm. A pulsatile abdominal mass may be present but not invariably so (Table 38.1).

Rupture of AAA, an ominous event, often leads to abrupt hypogastric or back pain. Lethal hypovolemic shock quickly sets in unless urgent surgical intervention follows. Hypotension, a pulsatile abdominal mass, and back pain, the classic triad of signs, are seen in only about one-half of patients with ruptured AAAs. In patients with a suspected aneurysm, a thorough examination of the peripheral vasculature is necessary. An associated femoral artery bruit may signify coexistent occlusive disease in that segment.

■ Ancillary Studies

Because physical examination inaccurately estimates aneurysm size, imaging is required to confirm the aneurysm and quantitate its size. A calcified aneurysmal wall is often noted incidentally on plain abdominal radiographs (Figure 38.1). Abdominal ultrasound is the imaging procedure of choice to detect an AAA and gauge its size. Computed tomography offers similar information, but at a higher cost and risk to the patient (radiation, contrast). Abdominal aortography is generally reserved for patients being considered for surgery. In addition to determining the extent of the aneurysm, it also can detect renal artery stenosis in hypertensive patients.

Aneurysm size has important prognostic and therapeutic implications. Aneurysms smaller than 4.0 cm in diameter rupture at a rate of 2% per year; the 5-year risk of rupture for aneurysms above 5.0 cm is 25–40%. Hypertension and smoking are other risk factors for rupture. Aneurysms expand by nearly 0.2–0.5 cm/yr, although the larger the aneurysm, the faster it dilates.

TABLE 38.1.	Clinical Features of Ruptured Abdominal Aortic Aneurysms

Common (>60%)
  Abdominal pain
  Abdominal tenderness
  Back or flank pain
  Leukocytosis (>11,000/mm^3)
Less Common (40-59%)
  Pulsatile mass
  Systolic BP <110 mm Hg or orthostatic drop
    >10 mm Hg
Infrequent (<40%)
  Vomiting
  Anemia (hemoglobin <11 g/dl)

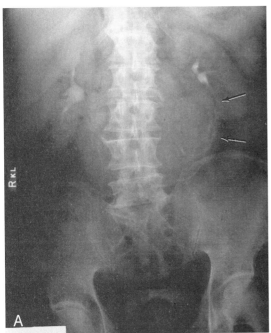

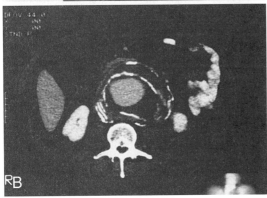

FIGURE **38.1. Abdominal aortic aneurysm. A,** A plain abdominal film shows the heavily calcified walls of a very large aneurysm (*arrows*). Aneurysms of this size, however, are quite uncommon. **B,** Computed tomographic scan confirms a large aneurysm with heavily calcified walls.
(Courtesy of the Radiology Museum, St. Joseph's Hospital, Milwaukee, Wisconsin.)

■ Management

All AAAs 6 cm or larger in diameter should be electively repaired unless surgery is strongly contraindicated. Aneurysms less than 4 cm can be followed with yearly ultrasound examination, and those between 4–6 cm with evidence of rapid expansion (>0.5 cm) should be electively repaired. The average surgical mortality for repair of nonruptured AAAs is near 4%, compared to 49% for repair of ruptured AAAs. Elective

AAA repair is contraindicated with recent myocardial infarction (past 6 months), unstable angina, refractory heart failure, severe lung disease (1 sec forced expiratory volume <50%), severe renal failure (serum creatinine >3 mg/dl), marked deficits from stroke, or life expectancy less than 2 years.

Successful aneurysm repair is followed by late complications (infection, aortoenteric fistula, false aneurysm, graft occlusion, and rupture) in about 10% of cases. Patients with graft infections may present with fever. Aortoenteric fistulae usually present with massive gastrointestinal (GI) hemorrhage. An aortoenteric fistula should generally be suspected in any patient with GI bleeding and a past history (even a remote past history) of AAA repair or aortoperipheral vascular bypass graft. False aneurysms are contained ruptures, presenting as expanding abdominal, back, or groin masses.

Thoracic Aortic Aneurysms

Nearly 25% of all aortic aneurysms involve the thoracic aorta, with the most common sites being the arch and descending aorta.

■ Clinical Features

Thoracic aortic aneurysms (TAAs) are easily diagnosed because the aneurysm is readily apparent on chest radiographs. Also, a TAA may compress adjacent structures and evoke symptoms before it expands to a critical size (e.g., hoarseness due to compression of the recurrent laryngeal nerve). Others may manifest deep, diffuse chest pain, dysphagia, hemoptysis, airflow obstruction, or cough. In ascending TAAs the aortic annulus may dilate, leading to aortic insufficiency; with severe valvular insufficiency, heart failure may evolve. Despite the common pathogenesis of abdominal and thoracic aortic aneurysms, spontaneous rupture of a TAA without warning is uncommon.

■ Ancillary Studies

Although one of several imaging studies (CT, MRI, or transesophageal echocardiography) can confirm a TAA, quantitate its dimensions, and clarify its relationship to adjacent structures, aortography and coronary angiography are generally necessary before elective TAA repair, given the high incidence of associated coronary artery disease.

■ Management

Patients with a dilated aortic root are liable to develop aortic valvular insufficiency, dissection, or rupture. β-blockers, by reducing heart rate and the rate of change of pressure in the aortic root, may decrease the rate of enlargement and prevent or delay the onset of complications.

Survival in TAA is also closely related to aneurysm diameter. Those exceeding 7 cm are more prone to rupture and should be electively repaired. Proximal TAA may require a composite graft with re-implantation of the coronary arteries.

TAA surgery involves a 10% mortality and other major complications, including hemorrhage and paraple-gia. Paraplegia occurs in about 5% of cases and is related to inadvertent interruption of the blood supply of the spinal cord. Early postoperative complications are related to advanced age, aneurysm size, coexisting diabetes mellitus, and technical factors (e.g., need for emergency surgery, prolonged aortic cross-clamp time). Early post-operative mortality is due to myocardial infarction, congestive heart failure, renal failure, respiratory failure, hemorrhage, and sepsis.

Aortic Dissection

■ Definition and Etiology

Aortic dissection develops from an aortic intimal tear that allows blood to dissect into the vessel wall. Although all dissections may be potentially lethal, classifying them into either proximal or distal sites has important thera-peutic and prognostic implications. **Proximal dissec-tions** (type A) involve the ascending aorta, with or without the descending aorta. **Distal dissections** (type B) involve only the descending aorta, usually beyond the left subclavian artery. Proximal dissections are twice as common as distal ones.

Distal dissections and proximal dissections of the ascending aorta just above the aortic valve together constitute over 95% of all aortic dissections. Because proximal dissections frequently involve the vicinity of the aortic valve, they often cause aortic insufficiency, hemopericardium, cardiac tamponade, and disrupted arch vessels. Hypertension and cystic medial necrosis cause proximal dissections more often; atherosclerosis and hypertension more often cause distal dissections.

■ Pathogenesis

Damage to the aortic media is a necessary prerequi-site for aortic dissection. This damage, caused by cystic medial necrosis a degenerative process that affects the collagen and elastin substrate of the vessel wall, is determined by chronic aortic wall stress and accelerated by long-standing hypertension. With a sudden intimal tear, blood under systemic pressure further disrupts the media and "dissects" the intima from adventitium.

■ Clinical Features

Dissection affects men twice as frequently as it does women, except for women in the last trimester of pregnancy, who are prone to dissection. Other predis-posing factors for aortic dissection are listed in Table 38.2. The typical patient is a 50 to 60-year-old man with long-standing hypertension who develops severe chest or back pain. The pain is described as tearing, ripping, stabbing, or sharp and is unaffected by respiration or change in position. It is severe and of maximal intensity from the very beginning, which contrasts with the pain of angina or myocardial infarction, which typically follows a more crescendo pattern. Proximal dissections tend to cause anterior chest pain, and almost all distal dissections involve back or interscapular pain. The migration of pain may signify extension of dissection.

Systemic blood pressure is often high despite apparent shock. Rapid, weak, and asymmetric peripheral pulses are typical. In one-half to two-thirds of patients with proximal dissection, aortic insufficiency may be present, manifest by syncope, cardiac tamponade (hemo-pericardium), or congestive heart failure. Focal neuro-logic deficits or hemiplegia are also common in proximal dissections, owing to involvement of the brachiocephalic vessels. In distal dissections, the left brachial and femoral pulses may be diminished or absent.

■ Ancillary Studies

The ECG frequently shows LV hypertrophy due to the long-standing underlying hypertension. Chest films show:

TABLE 38.2.	Predisposing Factors for Aortic Dissection

Risk factors for atherosclerosis
Long-standing hypertension (50% of cases)
Hereditary connective tissue defects with premature cystic
  medial necrosis (Marfan's syndrome, Ehlers-Danlos
  syndrome)
Coarctation of the aorta, with or without associated bi-
  cuspid aortic valve
Aortic stenosis (abnormally high aortic wall stress)
Trauma
  Blunt chest wall
  Iatrogenic (arteriography, cannulation, or intra-aortic
    balloon pump insertion)
Inflammatory conditions (e.g., syphilis, giant cell arteritis)

- Left-sided pleural effusions (due to either rupture of the dissection into the pleural space or by an inflammatory reaction).

In patients with chest trauma, these findings or a blurred aortic knob, left apical capping, mediastinal emphysema, or fracture of the first or second ribs should suggest traumatic aortic dissection.

Imaging studies (CT, MRI, transesophageal echocardiography, or aortography) can all visualize the intimal flap, delineate areas involved in the dissection, and identify the connections between true and false lumen (Figure 38.2, Table 38.3). Even in unstable patients with presumed traumatic dissections, transesophageal echocardiography can accurately, rapidly, and less invasively diagnose dissection (Figure 38.3). However, a later aortogram may be necessary to define the full extent of the dissection and to assess involvement of branch vessels, coronary arteries, and the aortic valve.

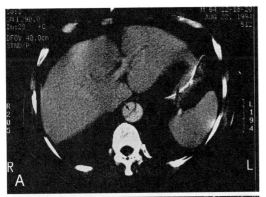
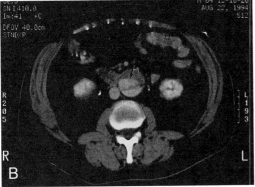

FIGURE 38.2. Aortic dissection. Computed tomographic scans showing a raised intimal flap (panel A) and false lumen (panel B).
(Courtesy of the Radiology Museum, St. Joseph's Hospital, Milwaukee, Wisconsin.)

- A widened mediastinum, aortic shadow, or dilated aortic root;
- Separation of intimal calcification from the adventitial border by 1-cm or greater in older persons with prior calcifications in the vessel wall (calcium sign); and

■ Management

All patients with dissection need emergent medical therapy (Table 38.4). The patients should be admitted to the intensive care unit with the goal of reducing the systolic blood pressure to 100–120 mm Hg and keeping the heart rate below 90 beats/min. Lowering the blood pressure and heart rate, attained by IV infusions of small incremental IV doses of β-blockers and sodium nitroprusside respectively, decreases the shear force on the aortic wall by lowering the velocity of LV ejection. Direct-acting vasodilators (hydralazine) should be avoided because they reflexly stimulate cardiac output, increase heart rate, and thus worsen the dissection.

Proximal dissections require immediate surgery, and those with aortic insufficiency may need placement of a composite graft with prosthetic valve and reimplantation of the coronary arteries. Stable, uncomplicated distal

TABLE 38.3.	Usefulness of Various Diagnostic Tests in Evaluating Suspected Aortic Dissection				
Variable	Aortography	CT	MRI	TEE
Sensitivity	++	++	+++	+++
Specificity	+++	+++	+++	++/+++
Site of intimal tear	++	+	+++	++
Presence of thrombus	+++	++	+++	+
Presence of AR	+++	−	+	+++
Pericardial effusion	−	++	+++	+++
Branch vessel involvement	+++	+	++	+
Coronary artery involvement	++	−	−	++

AR = aortic regurgitation (aortic valvular insufficiency); CT = computed tomography; MRI = magnetic resonance imaging; TEE = transesophageal echocardiography; +++ = excellent results; ++ = good results; + = fair results; − = not detected.
(From: Cigarroa JE et al. N Engl J Med 1993;328:42. Used with permission.)

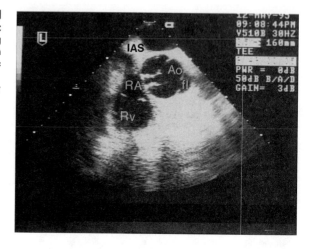

FIGURE 38.3. Aortic dissection. Transesophageal echocardiogram (TEE) obtained at the level of the aortic (Ao) root, showing a false lumen (FL) of the ascending aorta (Ao) posterior to the true lumen, indicative of an ascending aortic dissection. (RV = right ventricle; IAS = Interatrial septum.)

(Courtesy of Thomas Palmer, MD, and the Echocardiography Laboratory, St. Joseph's Hospital, Milwaukee, Wisconsin.)

TABLE 38.4.	Parenteral Drugs for Treatment of Acute Aortic Dissection*			
Drug	**Dose**	**Onset of Action**	**Duration of Action**	**Adverse Effects**
Vasodilators				
Nitroprusside	0.25–10 µg/kg/min	inst	1–2 min	Nausea, vomiting sweating, muscle twitching, thiocyanate and cyanide intoxication
Adrenergic inhibitors				
Trimethaphan	0.5–5 mg/min	1–5 min	10 min	Orthostatic hypotension, paresis of bowel and bladder, blurred vision, dry mouth
Esmolol	200–500 µg/kg/min for first 4 min; then 50–300 µg/kg/min	1–2 min	10–20 min	Hypotension, nausea
Labetalol	20–80 mg IV bolus over 10 min; then 2 mg/min	5–10 min	3–6 hrs	Nausea, vomiting, postural hypotension, dizziness, burning in throat, scalp tingling

*All are given as IV infusion.
Abbreviations: inst. = instantaneous.
(From: Kaplan NM (ed.). Clinical Hypertension. 6th ed. Baltimore: Williams & Wilkins, 1994, p. 290. Used with permission.)

dissections can be medically treated initially and repaired electively later. A subset of patients with chronic dissections (i.e., stable dissections of >2 weeks) or those with only distal descending aortic dissections may be given chronic medical therapy alone.

■ Prognosis

Untreated, aortic dissection has a 1-year mortality of 90%. Half of these deaths occur in the first week after presentation. With prompt, appropriate therapy, survival rises to 80%.

CHAPTER 39

PERIPHERAL VASCULAR DISEASE

Occlusive arterial disease of the lower extremities is an extremely common disorder that increases in prevalence with advancing age. In persons over age 50, 2–3% of men and 1% of women report symptoms of vascular occlusion. Each year in the United States, over 400,000 hospitalizations are for peripheral vascular disease (PVD), with an estimated 110,000 bypass operations, 50,000 angioplasties, and 69,000 foot or lower-limb amputations.

Although many patients with PVD have a chronic, stable course, almost one-third develop progressive symptoms. Over 5–10 years of follow-up, intermittent claudication may worsen in 15–30% of patients. Incidence rates of vascular surgery for necrosis or rest pain average 2.5–5% per year.

■ Etiology

Despite a component of impaired vascular reactivity, most patients with PVD have fixed atherosclerotic obstruction. Major risk factors for development of PVD are smoking, diabetes, hyperlipidemia, and hypertension.

Thromboangiitis obliterans (Buerger's disease) is a condition characterized by an inflammatory reaction that affects the small arteries and veins, typically in young male smokers, who display extensive, premature vascular disease. This inflammatory reaction leads to superficial thrombosis and arterial obstruction in the small, medium, and large-sized arteries of both the upper and lower extremities.

■ Clinical Features

Patients with PVD present a wide spectrum, from asymptomatic to limb-threatening ischemia. Most patients with PVD report **claudication,** defined as muscle fatigue, pain, or cramping, provoked by exercise and relieved by rest. Quantitating the walking distance of patients with claudication is helpful to track the progression of their symptoms. With progressive vascular occlusion and inadequate collateral circulation, symptoms occur on minimal exertion or even rest. **Rest pain,** a burning discomfort in the affected extremity, is disabling and entails a high risk of gangrene and limb loss. Claudication should be distinguished from nocturnal leg cramps, which are not of vascular origin.

The site of claudication pain may help localize the site of obstruction. For example, stenosis of the proximal iliac vessels (Leriche syndrome) evokes exertional discomfort in the buttocks and thighs. Loss of morning erections and impotence in men are early clues to pelvic vascular disease. Patients with femoral-popliteal system disease often report exertional calf pain.

Given the systemic nature of atherosclerosis, one should search for its signs elsewhere when PVD is suspected. PVD is associated with high-grade (>75%) carotid artery stenosis and severe coronary artery disease in up to one-half of patients.

Although PVD may be discovered in asymptomatic patients during a routine physical examination, normal pulses do not exclude PVD. Other clues to PVD include a decreased capillary refill time (normally <1 sec), decreased hair distribution, dependent rubor, and chronic atrophic skin changes. With advanced PVD, extremities become cool and mottled, nonhealing ulcers develop, and acrocyanosis and digital gangrene may evolve.

Vasospastic conditions can also compromise blood flow. **Raynaud's phenomenon** (or Raynaud's disease) is a triphasic response to cold exposure: blanching followed by cyanosis, and then redness. Raynaud's phenomenon is usually benign, but underlying disease should be excluded in older patients and those who present with unilateral signs and symptoms.

■ Ancillary Studies

Ankle-brachial index (ABI) is a simple, noninvasive, office-based procedure that can be used as a screening tool in suspected PVD. In it, the systolic blood pressure is measured with a Doppler probe from both brachial arteries and the dorsalis pedis or posterior tibial arteries. The ABI is then calculated by dividing the lower-extremity systolic blood pressure by the upper-extremity reading. Because normal ankle blood pressure exceeds the brachial by 10–15 mm Hg, the normal ABI exceeds 1. The ABI may be defined as mildly (0.8–0.9), moderately (0.5–0.8), or severely diminished (<0.5).

Besides confirming the clinical diagnosis, ABI can also help to localize the site of obstruction (proximal versus distal) and track progression in patients with established disease. The ABI also provides prognostic information and helps to predict limb survival. Values below 0.5 indicate limb-threatening ischemia; ischemic rest pain is common, and ulceration and gangrene are likely with values below 0.4. Stiff, calcified, and noncompressible arteries render the ABI inaccurate, and in these cases, other diagnostic tests, such as measurement of toe blood pressures, might be useful.

Limb radiographs may show osteomyelitis with nonhealing ulcers. Arterial calcification is common, particularly in diabetics. In selected patients, Doppler ultrasound before and after exercise, duplex scanning, and transcutaneous oximetry may add important diagnostic information. Contrast angiography is generally reserved for patients in whom surgical reconstruction or balloon angioplasty is being considered. Neurologic and/or musculoskeletal conditions (radiculopathies, neuropathies, and "pseudoclaudication" due to spinal stenosis) can occasionally cause sufficient diagnostic confusion to warrant additional testing.

■ Management

Patients with PVD should be advised to "stop smoking and keep walking." Profound deconditioning is common with severe PVD, and so exercise should be encouraged to the point of claudication. With a steady exercise training program, pain-free walking time is increased substantially.

Besides exercise, a vigorous risk-factor-modification program should be adopted. Smoking cessation is especially important. Good foot care is important in everyone, but especially in diabetic patients with sensory neuropathy. Patients should wear well-fitting, protective shoes, avoid injury, and inspect their feet daily for signs of skin breakdown or early ulceration.

Significant coronary artery disease is present in 75% of patients with PVD; thus, aspirin (325 mg/day) should be given to lower the risk of stroke, myocardial infarction, and vascular death. Presently, **pentoxifylline** (400 mg three times daily for at least 3 months) is the only approved drug for alleviating claudication. Pentoxifylline may act by decreasing blood viscosity and reducing the rigidity of red blood cells.

Chronic vasodilators and long-term anticoagulation appear to confer only minimal benefits. Concerns of potential harm from β-blockers in claudication have not been validated. Although Raynaud's phenomenon may improve with calcium channel blockers, avoiding cold exposure is very important.

Tissue necrosis (nonhealing foot ulcers, digital gangrene), rest pain, or disabling claudication with an ABI below 0.35 or toe pressure below 30 mm Hg warrants interventional therapy. **Angioplasty** may be the preferred initial step when limb claudication is due to a femoropopliteal stenosis. With proximal (below-the-knee) angioplasty, the long-term results are good, but the restenosis rate is generally high. Long-term patency with **surgical revascularization** depends on several factors, including the indication (intermittent claudication, limb-threatening ischemia), type of graft, site (axillary-femoral, femoral-femoral, femoral-popliteal, or more distal), and vessel characteristics (inflow, runoff distal to graft).

Acute Arterial Occlusion

Acute arterial occlusion, due to either thrombosis or embolism, is a surgical emergency. Such patients often present with the sudden onset of features of acute ischemic limb (i.e., the "5 Ps": pain, pallor, paresthesia, paralysis, and pulselessness). The pulseless, involved extremity is cold, pale, mottled, and occasionally "cadaveric" in appearance. Ischemic neuropathy is commonly present, with paralysis, decreased or absent reflexes, and loss of sensations. Untreated, myonecrosis quickly follows.

Acute **embolectomy** using a Fogarty catheter or infusion of **urokinase** results in 80–90 % limb salvage rates. Re-embolization occurs in about 25%. All patients should receive full heparinization sufficient to prolong the activated partial thromboplastin time to 1.5–2.0 times control. However, the role of long-term anticoagulation in such patients is less certain. Surgical revascularization should be considered when the anatomy is suitable and the stenosis is high-grade.

Atheroembolism

In patients with PVD, both large-vessel thrombosis and smaller atheromatous emboli may cause arteriolar occlusions and distal vessel infarctions. The resultant **"blue-toe syndrome"** is commonly due to atheroembolism, cardiac emboli, hyperviscosity states, systemic vasculitis, and hypercoagulable states. The atheroemboli are often composed of fibrin-platelet aggregates or cholesterol crystals. Disrupted atherosclerotic plaques in

the more proximal vessels, especially the abdominal aorta, are frequently the source. Atheroemboli may follow catheterization or vascular surgery, and anticoagulation may sometimes be a cause by promoting hemorrhage into atherosclerotic plaques which leads to their disruption.

Patients with lower-extremity atheroemboli may report bilateral limb pain and display a clinical picture resembling systemic vasculitis. Microinfarctions of the pancreas, kidneys, or bowel may result in pancreatitis, renal failure, or gastrointestinal bleeding. Physical findings include **livedo reticularis,** muscle tenderness, purpuric and ecchymotic skin lesions, acrocyanosis (blue toes), and occasionally digital gangrene. Laboratory findings are anemia, elevated sedimentation rate, leukocytosis, eosinophilia, and hyperamylasemia (all nonspecific findings). Wright's stain of the urine may reveal excess eosinophils.

A strong independent association exists between atherosclerosis of the ascending aorta or aortic arch and the risk of ischemic stroke. Ultrasonically detected atherosclerotic plaques exceeding 4 mm in thickness are risk factors for ischemic brain infarct and a possible source of cerebral embolism.

The management of atheroembolic disease and the response to therapy depend on the nature and severity of the underlying disease. Patients with operable and hemodynamically significant disease should undergo surgery. Antiplatelet agents or anticoagulants may be given on a long-term basis to patients with less severe or nonoperable disease (although anticoagulants may sometimes precipitate cholesterol embolism).

| CHAPTER | 40 | CARDIOGENIC SHOCK |

■ Definition and Etiology

Cardiogenic shock is a major abnormality of cardiac function that leads to systemic hypotension and severe, peripheral hypoperfusion. Its hemodynamic correlates are:

- Systemic hypotension (defined as a sustained [>30 min] and spontaneous drop in systolic blood pressure to below 90 mm Hg),
- Elevated intracardiac filling pressures (pulmonary capillary wedge pressure >18 mm Hg),
- Low cardiac output (cardiac index <2.2 L/min/m^2), and
- Low urinary output (<20 ml/hr).

With a patient in circulatory shock, it is critical to distinguish **hypovolemic shock** (preload failure) and **vasogenic shock** (afterload failure) from **cardiogenic shock** (pump failure) (Table 40.1). Frequent causes of hypovolemic shock are hemorrhage and excessive fluid losses from diarrhea, vomiting, and polyuria. Vasogenic shock may be due to a systemic inflammatory response syndrome (SIRS, previously called septic shock), neurogenic injury (spinal cord injury), anaphylactoid reactions, and vasodilator excess.

Although hypotension and hypoperfusion usually develop in patients with irreversible damage to over 40% of their myocardial mass, other conditions that decrease preload, increase afterload, or cause abnormal heart rate and rhythm can also cause cardiogenic shock. The etiology of cardiogenic shock is commonly subdivided into 3 categories: impaired contractility, decreased preload, and increased afterload (Table 40.2).

■ Pathophysiology

Unless the hemodynamic status is rapidly restored to normal, the low cardiac output in cardiogenic shock quickly leads to multiple organ system dysfunction. In patients with acute myocardial infarction, decreased myocardial compliance causes both LV end-diastolic volume and pressure to rise. Accordingly, the pulmonary capillary wedge pressure increases, leading to pulmonary edema when the pressure exceeds 18 mm Hg.

Compensatory mechanisms, such as increased sympathetic tone and decreased parasympathetic tone, enhance myocardial contractility, heart rate, and central blood volume and produce peripheral arteriolar and venous constriction. Although some of these effects are clearly advantageous, others are not, if they lead to an

TABLE 40.1.	Hemodynamic Profile in Circulatory Shock		
	Hypovolemic (preload failure)	**Cardiogenic (pump failure)**	**Vasogenic (afterload failure)**
Central venous pressure	↓	↑	N or ↓
Pulmonary capillary wedge pressure	↓	↑	N or ↓
Cardiac index	↓	↓	N or ↑
LV stroke work index	↓	↓	↓
Systemic vascular resistance	↑	↑	↓
Total O$_2$ consumption index	↓	↓	↓

(Adapted from: Teba L et al. Postgrad Med 1992;91:123. Used with permission.)

TABLE 40.2.   Causes of Cardiogenic Shock

Impaired contractility/excessive preload
  Acute myocardial infarction with markedly reduced
    LV function*
  Mechanical complications of acute myocardial
    infarction
    Acute mitral regurgitation due to papillary muscle
      dysfunction/rupture, Ventricular septal rupture
  Dilated cardiomyopathy (end–stage)
  Mitral insufficiency (subacute, chronic)
  Aortic insufficiency (subacute, chronic)
  Tachyarrhythmias
  Bradyarrhythmia including heart block
  Myocardial contusion
  Myocarditis, severe
  Myocardial dysfunction in septic shock
  Sequelae of cardiopulmonary bypass
Decreased preload
  RV infarction with RV pump failure
  Pericardial tamponade
    Ventricular free wall rupture
    Proximal aortic dissection (type 1)
  Pulmonary embolism, massive
  Pulmonary hypertension, severe
  Tension pneumothorax
  LV inflow tract obstruction
    Mitral stenosis
    Atrial myxoma
Excessive afterload
  LV outflow tract obstruction
    Aortic stenosis
    Hypertrophic cardiomyopathy (preload may also be
      reduced)
  Malignant hypertension
  Coarctation of the aorta

*Due to a massive infarction, preexisting LV dysfunction, associated dysrhythmias, and/or associated ischemic dysfunction.
(Data from: Grella RD, Becker RC. Current Probl Cardiol 1994; 19:693–742. Califf RM, Bengtson JR. N Engl J Med 1994; 330: 175.)

imbalance between myocardial O_2 supply and demand. Counter-regulatory mechanisms—including acidemia, circulating myocardial depressant factors, and decreased coronary artery perfusion—also lead to decreased myocardial performance in the setting of cardiogenic shock.

■ Clinical Features

The clinical evolution of circulatory shock is summarized in Table 40.3. Sustained systemic hypotension and peripheral hypoperfusion characterize cardiogenic shock. Systemic hypotension is also present when **systolic blood pressure** is maintained at or above 90 mm Hg by vasopressors or inotropes. Some patients can present with a picture of clinical shock with a "normal" blood pressure, especially if prior hypertension has been present. Conversely, a systolic blood pressure below 90 mm Hg is not necessarily shock, as end-organ hypoperfusion also should be present, manifested by general fatigue and weakness and features of hypoperfusion of the kidneys, central nervous system, and skin.

Coronary hypoperfusion further worsens cardiac ischemia, predisposing to infarct extension and perpetuation of shock. Urine output below 20 ml/hr or less than 500 ml/24 hrs represents **oliguria,** which indicates renal hypoperfusion. Dyspnea, another common finding in cardiogenic shock, arises from the high pulmonary capillary wedge pressure, reflecting the severe LV dysfunction.

Physical examination discloses tachypnea and tachycardia, often with weak and thready peripheral pulses. Asymmetric peripheral pulses (aortic dissection) and pulsus paradoxus (cardiac tamponade) may provide important clues for specific causes. In hypovolemic shock, the neck veins are flat, but in cardiogenic shock, they may be distended. In inferoposterior wall myocardial infarction, distended neck veins, systemic hypotension, and clear lung fields together strongly suggest RV infarction. Atrial (S_4) and ventricular (S_3) gallops, as well as crackles, are heard. A new, holosystolic murmur in a

TABLE 40.3.   Clinical Stages of Circulatory Shock

	Stage I (preshock)	Stage II (organ hypoperfusion)	Stage III (end-organ failure)
Mental State	Clear but distress present	Confusion, restlessness	Apathy, agitation or coma
Skin	Pale and cool	Cool and clammy	Cool, cyanotic, and mottled
Peripheral vasoconstriction	Mild	Marked	Intense
BP	Normal or slightly low	Hypotension	Undetectable by cuff
Urine output	Oliguria	Oliguria	Anuria
Heart Rate	Tachycardia	Tachycardia	Tachycardia
Other	Tachypnea, respiratory alkalosis	Respiratory failure; lactic acidosis; possible angina	Severe metabolic acidosis; multiple organ failure

(From: Teba L et al. Postgrad Med 1992;91:124. Used with permission.)

post-infarct patient suggests a ventricular septal rupture or mitral regurgitation (due to papillary muscle rupture). An early diastolic murmur of aortic insufficiency is a key finding in suspected proximal aortic dissection.

■ Ancillary Studies

Arterial blood gas analysis typically shows hypoxemia, hypocapnia, and metabolic acidemia from lactic acidosis. Leukocytosis, attributable to a stress response, is frequent. The ECG may show low-voltage complexes (tamponade), acute infarction, right heart strain (pulmonary embolism), conduction disturbances, or arrhythmias. Right-sided precordial leads may help confirm RV infarction.

The chest radiograph may show pulmonary vascular congestion or pulmonary edema. Pneumothorax with tracheal shift (tension pneumothorax), or widening of the mediastinal and aortic silhouette with a positive calcium sign (aortic dissection) are examples of important radiographic clues to the etiology of shock. Bedside echocardiography may detect pericardial tamponade, acute valvular insufficiency, or RV hypokinesis.

■ Management

The general approach to diagnosing an etiology for circulatory shock is outlined in Figure 40.1, and the therapeutic approach to cardiogenic shock is shown in Table 40.4. The first priority in managing cardiogenic

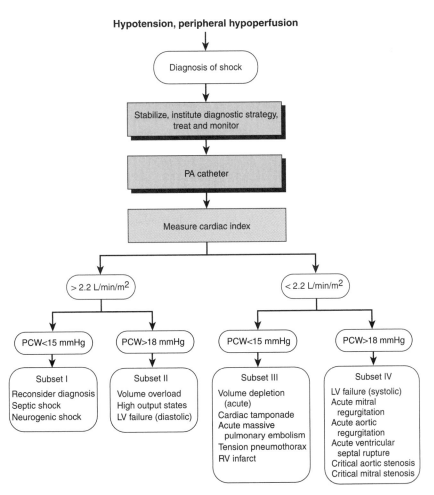

FIGURE 40.1. Determination of hemodynamic subgroups in cardiogenic shock. Patients with a clinical diagnosis of shock can be characterized using the pulmonary artery catheter to provide hemodynamic information. (PA Catheter = pulmonary artery catheter; PCW = pulmonary capillary wedge pressure.)

(Adapted from: Grella RD, Becker RC. Curr Probl Cardiol 1994; 19:693–742. Used with permission.)

TABLE 40.4. Therapeutic Approach to Cardiogenic Shock

1. **General resuscitation.**
   Monitor rhythm and blood pressure.
   Correct hypoxia, electrolytes abnormalities, and acid-base imbalance.
   Manage intravascular volume.
2. **Improve systolic function.**
   Administer catecholamines.
   Intra-aortic balloon pumping.
   Restore coronary blood flow.
   Angioplasty (PTCA)
   Thrombolysis
   Surgery
3. **Maximize preload and afterload.**
   Administer saline or produce diuresis.
   Vasodilation.
4. **Diagnose and manage mechanical dysfunction of an intracardiac structure.**
   Mitral valve
   Ventricular septum (rupture)
   Free wall (rupture, RV infarct)

PTCA = percutaneous transluminal angioplasty.
(Adapted from: Califf RM, Bengtson JR. N Engl J Med 1994; 330:1725. Used with permission.)

shock is to stabilize the hemodynamic status and restore perfusion. With a recent myocardial infarction and acute heart failure, aggressive restoration of coronary blood flow and limiting of infarct size are attained by thrombolysis, angioplasty, and bypass surgery (chapter 32). Successful opening of the infarct-related coronary vessel can reduce the mortality from cardiogenic shock significantly.

Systemic hypotension should be aggressively treated with IV fluids and, if necessary, inotropes. Hypoxemia, electrolyte abnormalities, and acid-base imbalances must be quickly recognized and corrected. Through cardiac monitoring, one may detect arrhythmias that require medications, temporary pacemaker support, or electrical cardioversion. Placement of a pulmonary artery (Swan-Ganz) catheter can stratify patients into one of the hemodynamic subsets (Table 40.5) and initiate the diagnostic algorithm of shock (Figure 40.1). Patients with RV infarcts may require large volumes of fluid to raise their central venous pressure, so as to provide adequate preload to the LV.

Afterload reduction is usually accomplished by continuously infusing **sodium nitroprusside** (0.25–10 µg/kg/min). Adverse effects include nausea, vomiting, sweating, muscle twitching, and, with long-term administration, thiocyanate and cyanide toxicity. Nitroprusside has balanced arteriolar and venous effects. IV

nitroglycerin, primarily a venodilator, may be substituted for nitroprusside in some patients who have signs or symptoms of ongoing cardiac ischemia. Inotropic therapy in this setting specifically aims to improve myocardial contractility, increase cardiac output, and provide adequate systemic perfusion without increasing myocardial O_2 demands (Table 40.6).

Dopamine affects all adrenoreceptor sites in a markedly dose-dependent fashion. At low doses of 2–5 µg/kg/min (renal dose), it stimulates the DA1 receptors and increases the glomerular filtration rate and renal tubular sodium excretion. Slightly higher doses (5–10 µg/kg/min) stimulate β-1 and DA2 receptors, producing cardiac inotropic and chronotropic effects. At 10–20 µg/kg/min, peripheral vasoconstriction follows stimulation of α-1 receptors.

Dobutamine, a synthetic inotrope, lacks α-1-adrenergic-mediated vasoconstriction. Because it has no activity at the dopaminergic receptor sites, it also lacks any DA1 or DA2 effects. By stimulating cardiac β-1 and peripheral β-2 receptors, it increases myocardial contractility and evokes peripheral vasodilation. The latter, along with the lack of significant vasoconstriction leads to net vasodilatation. Initial dose is 2–5 µg/kg/min.

Norepinephrine is a powerful vasopressor that has a limited role in the treatment of most patients with cardiogenic shock. Its main clinical indication is severe hypotension (<70 mm Hg) with normal or reduced systemic vascular resistance. Usually started at 1–4 µg/kg/min, its dose is further titrated according to the initial clinical and hemodynamic response.

In cardiogenic shock, dobutamine is often the "inotrope of choice" since it increases cardiac output with a smaller increase in heart rate and myocardial O_2 demands, and lowers systemic vascular resistance and pulmonary capillary wedge pressures. Because it is not a vasopressor, dobutamine should not be used as the sole inotrope in a severely hypotensive patient. Such patients require higher-dose dopamine or norepinephrine. Because it raises systemic blood pressure without incurring arrhythmias (unlike higher-dose dopamine), norepinephrine may be preferable.

All inotropic agents should be started at low doses and titrated upward to achieve the desired clinical response. Adverse effects include tachycardia, arrhythmias, provocation of myocardial ischemia, and local tissue necrosis (especially with extravasation into subcutaneous tissues). Dopamine and norepinephrine also have the potential to induce excessive vasoconstriction. Vomiting tends to be a more common side effect with dopamine because of stimulation of central dopaminergic receptors.

Cardiogenic shock not responding to appropriate pharmacologic therapy with IV vasodilators and inotro-

TABLE 40.5. Clinical and Hemodynamic Subsets of Patients With Acute Myocardial Infarction and Their Respective Mortality Rates

Hemodynamic Subset	Clinical subset		Mortality (%)	
	Pulmonary congestion	Peripheral hypoperfusion	Clinical	Hemodynamic
I.	–	–	1	3
II.	+	–	11	9
III.	–	+	18	23
IV.	+	+	60	51

Subsets: I = no pulmonary congestion or peripheral hypoperfusion; II = pulmonary congestion without hypoperfusion; III = peripheral hypoperfusion without pulmonary congestion; IV = both peripheral hypoperfusion and pulmonary congestion.
(Adapted from Forrester JS, et al. N Engl J Med 1976;295:1356–1362.)

TABLE 40.6. Adrenoreceptor Sites and Actions of Commonly used Inotropic Agents

Agent	Adrenoceptor sites				
	α-1	β-1	β-2	DA1	DA2
Norepinephrine	++++	++++	0	0	0
Dopamine	++++	++++	++	++++	++++
Dobutamine	+	++++	++	0	0

Actions of various adrenoceptor sites: α-1 = vasoconstriction causing increased systemic arterial resistance; β-1 = increased cardiac index, contractility, and rate; β-2 = vasodilation of the systemic arterial resistance vessels; = DA1 = increase renal blood flow, decrease renal tubular resorption of sodium and water; DA2 = presynaptically regulate norepinephrine release from sympathetic nerve terminals.
(From: DiBona GF. Semin Nephrol 1994;14:34. Used with permission.)

pic agents requires placement of an **intra-aortic balloon pump** to temporarily stabilize the clinical status. Patients with mechanical complications of myocardial infarction (rupture of papillary muscle or ventricular septum) often need prompt referral for urgent surgery.

Despite aggressive and appropriate therapy, the in-hospital mortality of cardiogenic shock remains high, averaging about 70% in most large series. Successful PTCA has reduced the mortality of cardiogenic shock to about 40% in patients with acute myocardial infarction.

CHAPTER 41 ASSESSMENT OF CARDIAC RISK FOR NONCARDIAC SURGERY

Cardiac complications, especially those related to coronary artery disease (CAD), are the leading cause of death following anesthesia and surgery. Patients with known or suspected cardiac disease commonly undergo risk assessment by internists or cardiologists before undergoing noncardiac surgical procedures. Through a detailed history and physical examination, combined with the use of selective testing procedures, the physician can identify individuals at low- and high-risk (risk stratification) for perioperative cardiac morbidity (PCM) (Table 41.1).

■ Risk Stratification

Risk stratification serves important goals:

1. Avoids the risk and expense of specialized cardiac testing procedures in patients who are found to be at low-risk for PCM after a simple history, physical examination, and routine laboratory tests.

2. Defines a subset of patients at high risk for PCM. These patients have acute but correctable medical problems and may benefit from further medical or

TABLE 41.1. Preoperative Cardiovascular Evaluation
• Begin with complete history, physical examination, ECG and chest radiograph.
• Specific questions to address:
1. Is angina pectoris or an anginal equivalent present?
2. What is the functional capacity?
3. Is there historical/ECG evidence of MI? If so, when did MI occur?
4. Is there prior or current CHF? Is it systolic or diastolic? Define functional capacity.
5. Is valvular disease or prosthetic valve present?
6. Is antibiotic prophylaxis required?
7. Is a temporary/permanent pacemaker present?
8. Is there chronic obstructive pulmonary disease? If so, is the $FEV_{1.0}$ less than 1 liter?
9. What is the general medical condition of the patient?
10. What operation is planned? Assess risk:benefit.
11. Is the current medical regimen appropriate/optimal?
12. If surgery is risky, what are the alternatives?
13. Is surgery necessary?

CHF = congestive heart failure; $FEV_{1.0}$ = 1-second forced expiratory volume.

surgical treatment prior to the planned noncardiac surgical procedure.

3. In some patients at high-risk for PCM, modification of the proposed noncardiac surgical procedure to one that entails a lower risk or cancellation of the procedure may be appropriate.

■ **Noncardiac Predictors of Risk**

Age

Older patients are more likely to have associated CAD, comorbid medical problems, and depressed cardiac responses to catecholamine stress. Many studies have demonstrated a greater surgical mortality among the elderly when age is the only variable studied. However, functional status (i.e., physiological status or physiological age) is probably a significant factor to be considered besides chronological age.

Type of anesthesia

Regional anesthesia offers no consistent advantage over general anesthesia in terms of improved surgical outcome. The one possible exception occurs in patients with a history of congestive heart failure, in whom regional anesthesia may be associated with a lesser incidence of postoperative pulmonary congestion.

Site and type of surgery

Emergency surgery is associated with a 2- to 5-fold increased risk of perioperative cardiac complications, including postoperative myocardial infarction (MI) or cardiac death. In addition, intrathoracic, intraperitoneal, orthopedic, aortic, and peripheral vascular procedures (particularly involving aortic cross-clamping) all also entail a higher risk of postoperative cardiac complications.

■ **Cardiac Predictors of Risk**

Ischemic heart disease

In general, the presence of CAD increases the mortality of noncardiac surgery by 3- to 5-fold. In patients with CAD, important considerations include the presence of symptoms of myocardial ischemia and the workload that provokes them, the overall anginal pattern and its stability over time, the patient's overall functional capacity, a past history of MI (and if so, when it occurred), and the presence of any symptoms or signs of heart failure. However, the absence of angina and the presence of a normal resting ECG do not exclude significant CAD.

Noninvasive testing for CAD in the preoperative patient

Younger patients (<70 years of age) with no angina, prior MI, or heart failure and whose functional status is class I or II by the Canadian Cardiovascular Society angina scale are at **low-risk** for most surgical procedures and need no further specialized testing for myocardial ischemia (Figure 41.1).

Similarly, a **high-risk** subset of patients can also be defined by history, physical findings, and ECG characteristics who do not need further specialized noninvasive testing. This high-risk subset includes patients who have had refractory or poorly controlled congestive heart failure, unstable angina, or a recent non–Q-wave MI with evidence for a large amount of jeopardized myocardium, or a recent MI complicated by heart failure or followed by angina. The majority of these patients can proceed directly to coronary angiography, assuming that they are candidates for potential revascularization.

The remaining large group of patients, who cannot be classified initially as low- or high-risk, form an **intermediate-risk** subset in which exercise stress testing or vasodilator perfusion imaging is helpful for risk stratification. This group consists of patients with known or suspected CAD but whose symptoms are currently stable, patients with a remote MI, patients with currently well-compensated congestive heart failure, or patients with diabetes mellitus. If these patients can exercise adequately, then **exercise stress testing** is generally performed. Exercise stress tests are most helpful when they provide clear evidence of myocardial ischemia at a low workload (<5 mets), indicating the patient is at high risk for PCM, or alternatively, when they are negative for ischemia at a high workload (>7 mets), indicating the patient is at low risk for PCM.

Unfortunately, many exercise test results do not fall into either category, and such patients carry an indeterminate risk of PCM. In these patients, as well as those whose history clearly precludes adequate exercise, **vasodilator perfusion imaging** may be used to test for the presence of significant CAD. Vasodilator perfusion imaging is most commonly performed with dipyridamole infusion, followed by either thallium-201 or technetium-99m sestamibi.

Numerous studies have demonstrated that the absence of reversible defects on vasodilator perfusion imaging is associated with a >95% negative predictive value for the occurrence of PCM (i.e., <5% of patients with no reversible defects will experience perioperative cardiac complications). The positive predictive value of reversible defects for PCM is only 20–30% (i.e., 70–80% of patients with reversible perfusion defects will not experience perioperative cardiac complications, but 20–30% will). It is up to the physician to decide which patients with reversible defects merit further investigation with, for instance, coronary angiography.

History of previous myocardial infarction

A history of previous MI is a risk factor for recurrent, perioperative MI, but the risk is decreasing. Recent data suggest that the risk of perioperative MI ranges from 1.5% in patients whose MI occurred over 6 months before the current planned surgery to 5.7% in patients whose MI

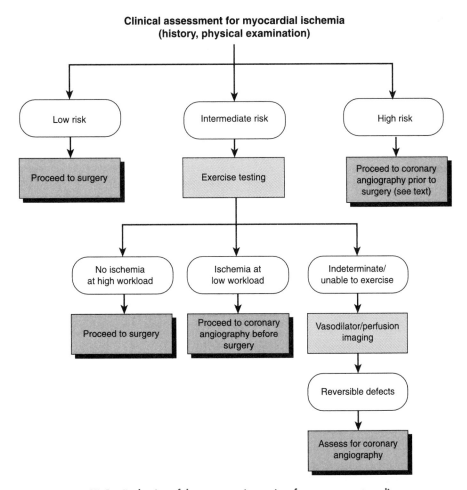

FIGURE 41.1. Evaluation of the preoperative patient for coronary artery disease.

occurred less than 3 months previously. The incidence of perioperative MIs tends to peak on the third postoperative day and entails a 40–70% mortality rate. Elective noncardiac surgery should be postponed for a minimum of 3 months following an MI.

Congestive heart failure

Congestive heart failure (CHF) is a major risk factor for PCM. The risk of postoperative pulmonary edema is negligible (<2%) when a prior history of CHF is absent, modest (6%) when clinical findings suggest well-compensated CHF, and moderate (16%) when active heart failure is present preoperatively. Thus, it is important to resolve heart failure fully prior to surgery, as well as avoid hypokalemia and volume depletion from over-diuresis. Additionally, one must determine whether CHF is due to diastolic or systolic dysfunction, since management of these conditions differs greatly.

Valvular disease

The risk of perioperative complications depends on the specific valve lesion, its degree of dysfunction, the state of LV systolic and diastolic function, and the patient's functional class. In general, significant aortic stenosis carries the highest mortality risk (10–15%) in patients undergoing noncardiac surgery.

Alterations in perioperative hemodynamics affect specific valvular/subvalvular lesions. For example, in patients with hypertrophic obstructive cardiomyopathy, careful fluid management (avoiding volume depletion) and avoidance of β-adrenergic agonists are both important, since these would increase the outflow obstruction. A relative tachycardia, by reducing regurgitant fraction, might benefit significant aortic regurgitation but could precipitate pulmonary edema in mitral stenosis. Perioperative hemodynamic monitoring with a pulmonary artery catheter is often helpful in patients with valvular disease.

Hypertension

In patients with mild to moderate, well-controlled hypertension and no evidence of serious end-organ damage, general anesthesia is well tolerated. Medications should not be discontinued at the time of surgery, but rather, they should be continued up until surgery. There is no benefit in postponing surgery to gain better blood pressure control as long as the diastolic blood pressure is at or below 100 mm Hg.

Arrhythmias

Ventricular and supraventricular arrhythmias commonly complicate the perioperative period. In general, the risk that arrhythmias pose to the patient is more closely related to the underlying heart disease. Ventricu-

lar arrhythmias discovered preoperatively should prompt a search for electrolyte abnormalities, ventricular or valvular dysfunction, pulmonary congestion, or myocardial ischemia. Medications such as digitalis, β-agonists, or theophylline may cause ventricular (or supraventricular) arrhythmias, and occasionally, an indwelling pulmonary artery catheter may cause mechanical irritation and hence ectopy.

If no reversible factor is evident, there are no data to support the prophylactic suppression of asymptomatic ventricular ectopy in the perioperative period. However, increased or new-onset ventricular ectopy in the postoperative patient with known or suspected CAD may reflect myocardial infarction or ischemia.

Other issues

Coronary revascularization

The choice between coronary artery bypass graft (CABG) surgery or percutaneous transluminal coronary angioplasty (PTCA) prior to a proposed noncardiac surgical procedure must be made carefully. Besides exposing the patient to a higher risk of morbidity and mortality, **CABG** entails the additional risk of delaying the noncardiac surgical procedure. Additionally, some groups of patients, notably prospective vascular surgical patients, have a higher-than-usual mortality risk from CABG. Patients who survive CABG, however, tolerate the subsequent noncardiac surgery well. Often, however, the mortality risk of the prophylactic CABG offsets the survival advantage it confers on the patient during the subsequent noncardiac surgery. Thus, although CABG in the preoperative patient may not confer a short-term survival advantage, it likely does confer a long-term survival benefit.

In general, the decision for CABG should rest on standard guidelines for CABG, rather than on a perceived need for it to meet the needs of the proposed noncardiac surgery. The severity of ischemic symptoms, amount of jeopardized tissue, degree of functional limitation, state of LV function, patient age, and comorbid conditions all affect subsequent management decisions, including the need for myocardial revascularization.

PTCA is an additional option, although there is no definitive proof that performing PTCA prior to noncardiac surgery improves surgical outcome.

■ Questions

Instructions: For each question below, select only **one** lettered answer that is the **best** for that question.

1. A 50-year old man complains of epigastric discomfort along with dyspnea during exercise and relief

after several minutes of rest. Which ONE of the following diagnoses best represents his condition?

A. Hiatus hernia
B. Angina pectoris
C. Aneurysm of the descending thoracic aorta
D. Gastric ulcer
E. Intestinal ischemia due to mesenteric arterial stenosis

2. A 45-year-old woman has episodic anterior chest pain, palpitations, and dyspnea occurring almost daily at 4–5 AM for the past 3 months. Physical findings, the ECG, and chest radiograph are normal. Which of the following laboratory tests is appropriate now?

A. Repeat ECG
B. Echocardiogram
C. Exercise ECG
D. Upper gastrointestinal series
E. ECG during chest pain
F. Coronary angiography

3. All of the following factors enhance the myocardial O_2 demand, with the exception of which of the following?

A. Enlarged LV chamber
B. Slow heart rate
C. Increased contractility
D. Hypertension

4. A. 60-year-old man enters the coronary care unit (CCU) with an acute inferior-wall myocardial infarction. Physical findings include a shallow pulse at 107 beats/min, blood pressure (BP) of 78/60 mm Hg, grossly distended neck veins, no apical S_3, and no lung crackles. Chest radiograph is normal. Which of the following statements is correct?

A. Patient has right heart failure and digitalis and diuretics are indicated.
B. Patient has cardiogenic shock and IV infusion of dopamine is indicated.
C. IV digitalis is indicated to slow down heart rate.
D. Pulmonary artery (Swan-Ganz) catheter should be inserted; the pulmonary artery wedge pressure is likely to be low or normal, and fluid therapy should then follow.
E. Patient is in cardiogenic shock, and insertion of an intra-aortic balloon for counterpulsation is indicated.

5. A known hypertensive is admitted to the CCU with an acute anterior-wall myocardial infarction. He is diaphoretic and tachypneic. Pulse is 156 beats/min and BP is 98/50 mm Hg. The ECG reveals atrial flutter with 2:1 AV block. Which of the following is indicated now?

A. Patient is in cardiogenic shock; start IV dopamine.
B. Rapid heart rate is probably a major contributor for cardiogenic shock; immediate electrical cardioversion should follow.
C. Ventricular rate is rapid; give IV propranolol.
D. Start oral digoxin to improve contractility and slow the ventricular rate.

6. A 45-year-old man is hospitalized for acute inferior-wall myocardial infarction. His BP is 80/50 mm Hg, and the ECG rhythm strip shows sinus bradycardia (40 beats/min.). Which of the following is indicated now?

A. Fluid challenge
B. IV isoproterenol
C. IV dopamine
D. IV atropine
E. Temporary pacemaker

7. His clinical status improves markedly after appropriate treatment. On the next day, the BP is 110/70 mm Hg and the ECG rhythm strip shows 5:4 Wenckebach type of second degree AV block. Which of the following is indicated now?

A. Temporary pacemaker
B. IV isoproterenol
C. IV atropine
D. Oral ephedrine
E. Observation

8. Sinus rhythm resumes on the fourth hospital day. On the same afternoon, sudden diaphoresis develops with dyspnea and rales at lung bases. His BP is 70/40 mm Hg. A faint, grade 2/6 systolic murmur is heard over the left lower sternal border. Which of the following conditions should be considered in the differential diagnosis?

A. Rupture of chordae tendineae
B. Rupture of ventricular septum or papillary muscle
C. Rupture of LV free wall
D. All of the above
E. None of the above

9. Which of the following will you do to diagnose and manage the above condition?

A. Pulmonary artery catheter; multiple blood samples for oximetry
B. LV and coronary angiograms
C. Administer IV dopamine
D. Intra-aortic balloon counterpulsation
E. Surgical repair
F. All of the above

10. A 50-year-old man has a history of exertional anterior chest discomfort for the last 2 years. During the last

2 months, he reports increasing exercise-related chest discomfort and some chest pain at night and at rest. Some of these episodes lasted over 20 minutes and only partly responded to sublingual nitroglycerin. Which of the following steps should be taken now?

A. Exercise stress test
B. Exercise
   Tl scintigraphy
C. Emergency coronary angiography and coronary artery bypass surgery
D. Continue with sublingual nitroglycerin and start oral propranolol and isosorbide dinitrate as an outpatient.
E. Hospitalize and start aspirin, β-blockers, and nitrates in progressively increasing doses. Plan an early coronary angiography, and if there are critical narrowings, consider myocardial revascularization.

11. A 72-year-old man presents to the emergency department after 2 hours of anterior chest pain, profuse sweating, and confusion. The systolic BP is 80 mm Hg, and the chest reveals bilateral rales. The 12-lead ECG shows sinus tachycardia at 118 beats/min and 2 mm ST-segment elevation in leads V_1 through V_4. Which of the following steps are appropriate for this patient's management?

A. Give IV esmolol to reduce the rapid heart rate.
B. Give soluble aspirin, 325 mg PO, and consult the cardiologist for emergent coronary angioplasty.
C. IV tissue plasminogen activator for a total dose of 100 mg in the next 3 hours.
D. Admit to the CCU and give IV fluids to treat hypotension.

12. A 55-year-old man is recovering from an inferior-wall MI in the CCU. On the third hospital day, he reports pleuritic-type chest pain, unrelieved by nitroglycerin. Examination shows a pericardial friction rub. Which of the following medications may be contraindicated?

A. Aspirin
B. β-blockers
C. Anticoagulants
D. Nonsteroidal anti-inflammatory agents

13. A 45-year-old man is admitted to the CCU with anterior crushing chest pain for 2 hours. Serial ECGs show ST-segment depression in leads V_2–V_4 and fourfold rise in CK-MB. The patient is asymptomatic; however, the repeat ECG continues to show ST-segment depression. Which one of the following statements is true?

A. The patient has no evidence of arrhythmia or heart failure and therefore has an excellent long-term prognosis.
B. The short-term prognosis is excellent; therefore, coronary arteriography is not indicated.
C. The patient is in an intermediate- or high-risk category; therefore, coronary arteriography is indicated to delineate the coronary anatomy.
D. β-blockers are expected to provide cardioprotection.
E. Diltiazem and aspirin are of no use for secondary prophylaxis

14. All of the following physical signs indicate the presence of a large intracardiac left-to-right shunt, except:

A. Loud S_3
B. Loud S_4
C. Mid-diastolic rumble across atrioventricular valves
D. Hyperkinetic precordium

15. Which of the following physical signs and laboratory tests indicate the development of pulmonary vascular disease and pulmonary hypertension in a patient previously known to have left-to-right shunt?

A. Prominent a waves in the jugular venous pulse
B. Loud pulmonary component of S_2
C. High-frequency early diastolic murmur along left upper sternal border
D. Progressively diminishing intensity and duration of previously loud systolic murmur
E. All of the above

16. *All* of the following statements concerning an atrial septal defect of the secundum variety are correct, EXCEPT:

A. Second heart sound is widely split and varies little with phases of respiration.
B. Precordial systolic murmur is usually produced by left-to-right shunt occurring at the atrial level.
C. Precordial systolic murmur is usually produced by augmented pulmonary blood flow across the pulmonary valve.
D. In young adults, large left-to-right shunt causes high pulmonary arterial pressure but the pulmonary vascular resistance is usually normal.
E. Mid-diastolic rumble at left lower sternal border showing an inspiratory increase in intensity usually indicates >2:1 left-to-right shunt.

17. A 19-year old man has a heart murmur. His BP is 110/60 mm Hg, jugular venous pulse is normal, and pulse is regular. The apical impulse is displaced downward and leftward. There is a systolic thrill over

the left midsternal area. A grade 4/6 pansystolic murmur is audible over the left midsternal area. S_1 is covered by the murmur. S_2 is widely split with considerable respiratory variation. An S_3 followed by a mid-diastolic rumble is heard over the apex. ECG shows biventricular hypertrophy, and the chest radiograph shows increased pulmonary vascularity. Which of the following conditions are compatible with these findings?

A. Atrial septal defect
B. Ventricular septal defect
C. Patent ductus arteriosus
D. Aortopulmonary septal defect (window)
E. Transposition of great vessels

18. Which of the following conditions can develop in the natural history of a ventricular septal defect?

A. Aortic regurgitation
B. Congestive heart failure
C. Infective endocarditis
D. Progressive decrease in the size of the defect
E. Eisenmenger's syndrome
F. Infundibular stenosis
G. All of the above

19. A 14-year-old girl is found to have a moderate left-to-right shunt through a patent ductus arteriosus (PDA). She is quite active in several sports and is entirely asymptomatic. What would you recommend?

A. Antibiotic prophylaxis against infective endocarditis until surgical division of PDA
B. Long-term antirheumatic prophylaxis
C. Curtailment of physical activity
D. Regular observation until the development of cardiac symptoms, and then recommend surgical treatment

20. A 32-year-old man is brought to the emergency department with complaints of substernal chest pain. Physical findings are essentially normal, except for some midabdominal obesity. The ECG is shown in Figure IV.1. Which one of the following is the best treatment?

A. Admit to the hospital and start nitroglycerin, heparin, and β-blockers.
B. Admit to the hospital and start nitroglycerin and heparin; schedule for exercise stress test.
C. Obtain a computed tomographic scan of the chest and start short-acting β-blockers to keep systolic BP around 110–120 mm Hg; obtain immediate thoracic surgical consultation.
D. Start indomethacin, 25–50 mg three times daily; give narcotics if pain is severe.

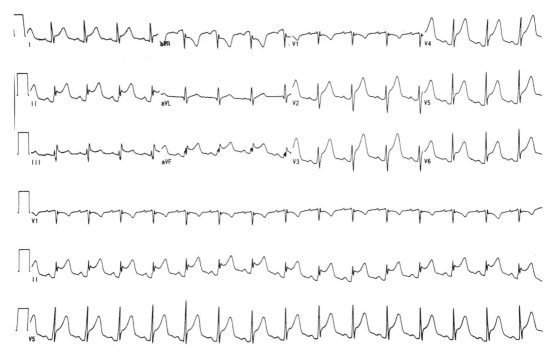

FIGURE IV.1

Answers

1. B	2. E	3. B	4. D	5. B
6. D	7. E	8. D	9. F	10. E
11. B	12. C	13. C	14. B	15. E
16. B	17. B	18. G	19. A	20. D

SUGGESTED READING

Textbooks and Monographs

Agency for Health Care Policy and Research. Unstable Angina: Diagnosis and Management. Clinical Practice Guidelines. Rockville, MD: U.S.Department of Health and Human Services; 1994.

Alpert JS, Becker RC. Pathophysiology, diagnosis and management of cardiogenic shock. In: Schlant RC, Alexander RW, O'Rourke RA, Roberts R, Sonnenblick EH (eds.). The Heart, Arteries and Veins. 8th ed. New York: McGraw-Hill, 1994:907–925.

Braunwald E. Heart Disease: A Textbook of Cardiovascular Medicine. 5th ed. Philadelphia: W.B Saunders, 1997.

Chou TC. Electrocardiography in Clinical Practice. 3rd ed. Philadelphia: W.B. Saunders, 1991.

Constant J. Bedside Cardiology. 4th ed. Boston: Little, Brown & Company, 1993.

The Criteria Committee of the New York Heart Association. Nomenclature and Criteria for Diagnosis of Diseases of the Heart and Great Vessels. 9th ed. Boston: Little Brown & Company; 1994.

Nugent EW, Plantar WH, Edwards JE, et al. The pathology, abnormal physiology, clinical recognition, and medical and surgical treatment of congenital heart disease. In: Hurst JW, Schlant RC, Rackley CE, et al (eds.). The Heart. 7th ed. New York: McGraw-Hill, 1990.

Perloff JK. Physical Examination of the Heart and Circulation. 2nd ed. Philadelphia: W. B. Saunders Company; 1990.

Scheld WM, Sande MA. Endocarditis and intravascular infections. In: Mandell GL, Bennett JE, Dolin R (eds.). Principles and Practice of Infectious Disease. 4th ed. New York: Churchill Livingstone, 1995:740–783.

Tresch DD, Aronow WS. Cardiovascular Disease in the Elderly Patient. New York: Marcel Dekker, Inc., 1994.

Wagner GS. Marriott's Practical Electrocardiography. 9th ed. Baltimore: Williams & Wilkins, 1994.

Willms JL, Schneiderman H, Algranati PS. Physical Diagnosis: Bedside Evaluation of Diagnosis and Function. Baltimore: Williams & Wilkins, 1994.

Articles
Common presentations of heart disease in adults

Manning HL, Schwartzstein RM. Mechanisms of disease: pathophysiology of dyspnea. N Engl J Med 1995;333: 1547–1553.

Cardiovascular examination

Duthie EH, Gambert SR, Tresch D. Evaluation of the systolic murmur in the elderly. J Am Geriatr Soc 1981;29:498–502.

Lembro NJ, Dell'Italia L, Crawford MH, et al. Bedside diagnosis of systolic murmurs. N Engl J Med 1988;318:1572.

Reddy PS, Salerni R, Shaver JA. Normal and abnormal heart sounds in cardiac diagnosis. Part II. Diastolic sounds. Curr Probl Cardiol 1985;10(4):1–55.

Shaver JA, Salerni R, Reddy PS. Normal and abnormal heart sounds in cardiac diagnosis. Part I. Systolic sounds. Curr Probl Cardiol 1985;10(3):1–68.

Swartz MH. Jugular venous pressure pulse: Its value in cardiac diagnosis. Prim Cardiol 1982;8:197.

Willms JL, Schneiderman H, Algranati PS. Physical Diagnosis: Bedside Evaluation of Diagnosis and Function. Baltimore: Williams & Wilkins, 1994.

Other noninvasive techniques of cardiac diagnosis

Conversano A, Walsh JF, Geltmann EM, et al. Delineation of myocardial stunning and hibernation by positron emission tomography in advanced coronary artery disease. Am Heart J 1996; 131:440–450.

Popp RL. Echocardiography (pts 1 and 2). N Engl J Med 1990;323:101,165.

Sansoy V, Glover DK, Watson DD et al. Comparison of thallium-^{201} resting redistribution with technetium ^{99m}sestamibi uptake and functional response to dobutamine for assessment of myocardial viability. Circulation 1995; 92:994–1004.

Schiller NB. Doppler echocardiography. Cardiol Clin 1990;8: 173–389.

Schiller NB. Transesophageal echocardiography. Cardiol Clin 1993;11:355–537.

Verani MS. Pharmacologic stress myocardial perfusion imaging. Curr Probl Cardiol 1993;18:481–528.

Disorders of cardiac rhythm and conduction

Akhtar M, Shenasa M, Jazayeri M, et al. Wide QRS tachycardia: reappraisal of a common clinical problem. Ann Intern Med 1988;109:905–912.

Binah O, Rosen MR. Mechanisms of ventricular arrhythmias. Circulation 1992;85:25–35.

Dreifus LS, ACC/AHA Task Force. Guidelines for implantation of cardiac pacemakers and antiarrhythmia devices. J Am Coll Cardiol 1991;18:1.

Josephson ME, Wellens HJJ. Differential diagnosis of supraventricular tachycardia. Cardiol Clin 1990;8:411–441.

Kudenchuk PJ. Atrial fibrillation: pearls and perils of management. West J Med 1996;164:425–434.

Prystowsky EN, Benson DW Jr., Fuster V, et al. Management of patients with atrial fibrillation. Circulation 1996;93:1262–1277.

Reiffel JA, Estes NAM, Waldo AL, et al. A consensus report on antiarrhythmic drug use. Clin Cardiol 1994;17: 103–116.

Schweitzer P, Teichholz LE. Carotid sinus massage: its diagnostic and therapeutic value in arrhythmias. Am J Med 1985;78:645–654.

Zipes DP, Akhtar M, Denes P, et al. Guidelines for clinical intracardiac electrophysiologic studies. J Am Coll Cardiol 1989;14:1827–1842.

Syncope

Abi-Samra F, Maloney JD, et al. The usefulness of headup tilt testing and hemodynamic investigations in the workup of syncope of unknown origin. PACE 1988;11:1201–1214.

Kapoor WN. Diagnostic evaluation of syncope. Am J Med 1991;90:91–106.

Linzer M. Syncope. Am J Med 1991;90:1–5.

Meissner MD, Akhtar M, Lehmann MD. Nonischemic sudden tachyarrhythmic death in atherosclerotic disease. Circulation 1991;84:905–912.

Congestive heart failure

Cohn JN. Structural basis for heart failure: ventricular remodeling and its pharmacological inhibition. Circulation 1995; 91:2504–2507.

Georghiade M, Bonow RO. Chronic heart failure in the United

States: a manifestation of coronary artery disease. Circulation 1998;97:282–289.

Groden DL. Vasodilator therapy for congestive heart failure. Arch Intern Med 1993;153:445.

Krum H, Sackner-Bernstein JD, Goldsmith RL, et al. Double-blind, placebo-controlled study of the long-term efficacy of carvedilol in patients with severe chronic heart failure. Circulation 1995;92:1499–1506.

Lenihan DJ, Gerson MC, Hoit BD, et al. Mechanisms, diagnosis, and treatment of diastolic heart failure. Am Heart J 1995; 130:153–166.

Stevenson LW, Miller LW. Cardiac transplantation or therapy for heart failure. Curr Probl Cardiol 1991;16:223–305.

Williams JF Jr., Bristow MR, Fowler MB, et al. Guidelines for the evaluation and management of heart failure. J Am Coll Cardiol 1995;26:1376.

Coronary artery disease

DeServi S, Arbustini E, Marsico F, et al. Correlation between clinical and morphologic findings in unstable angina. Am J Cardiol 1996;77:128–132.

Glasser SP, Selwyn AF, Ganz P. Atherosclerosis: Risk factors and the vascular endothelium. Am Heart J 1996;131: 379–384.

Gotto AM Jr.: Cholesterol management in theory and practice. Circulation 1997;96:4424–4430.

Opie LH. Calcium channel antagonists in the treatment of coronary artery disease: fundamental pharmacological properties relevant to clinical use. Prog Cardiovasc Dis 1996;38: 273–290.

Pattillo RW, Fuchs S, Johnson J, et al. Predictors of prognosis by quantitative assessment of coronary angiography, single photon emission computed tomography, thallium imaging and treadmill exercise testing. Am Heart J 1996;131: 582–590.

Summary of the second report of the National Cholesterol Education Program (NCEP) expert panel on detection, evaluation, and treatment of high blood cholesterol in adults (adult treatment panel II). JAMA 1993;269:3015.

Topol EJ: Toward a new frontier in myocardial reperfusion therapy. Circulation 1998;97:211–218.

Acute myocardial infarction

Cairns JA, Hirsh J, Lewis HD, et al. Antithrombotic agents in coronary artery disease. Chest (suppl) 1995;108:380S–400S.

Fletcher GF. Curent status of cardiac rehabilitation. Curr Probl Cardiol 1992;17:143–198.

Hamm CW, Katus HA. New biochemical markers for myocardial injury. Curr Opin Cardiol 1995;10:355.

Parker AB III, Waller BF, Gering LE. Usefulness of the 12-lead electrocardiogram in detection of myocardial infarction: electrocardiographic-anatomic correlations. Part I. Clin Cardiol 1996;19:55–61.

Pitt B. Evaluation of the postinfarct patient. Circulation 1995;91:1855.

Reeder GS. Identification and treatment of complications of myocardial infarction. Curr Prob Cardiol 1996;21:585–667.

Smith SM. Current management of acute myocardial infarction. Dis Mon 1995;41:363–433.

Congenital heart disease and valvular heart disease

Duncan AK, Vittone J, Fleming KC, et al. Cardiovascular disease in elderly patients. Mayo Clin Proc 1996;71:184–96.

Feldman T. Rheumatic heart disease. Curr Opin Cardiol 1996;11(2):126–30.

Fenster MS, Feldman MD. Mitral regurgitation: an overview. Curr Probl Cardiol 1995;20:193–280.

Katz NM. Current surgical treatment of valvular heart disease. Am Fam Phys 1995;52(2):559–68.

Passik CS, Ackermann DM, Pluth JR, et al. Temporal changes in the causes of aortic stenosis: a surgical pathologic study of 646 cases. Mayo Clin Proc 1987;62:119–123.

Scognamiglio R, Rahimotoola SH, Fasolii G, et al. Nifedipine in asymptomatic patients with severe aortic regurgitation and normal left ventricular function. N Eng J Med 1994;331:689–694.

Skorton DJ, Garson A Jr. Congenital heart disease in adolescents and adults. Cardiology Clinics 1993;11:543.

Infective endocarditis

Bayer AS, Ward JI, Ginzton LE, et al. Evaluation of new clinical criteria for the diagnosis of infective endocarditis. Am J Med 1994;96:211–219.

Durack DT. Prevention of infective endocarditis. N Eng J Med 1995;332:38–44.

Diseases of the pericardium and myocardium

Dec GW, Fuster V. Idiopathic dilated cardiomyopathy. N Engl J Med 1994;331:1564–1575.

Fowler NO. Pulsus paradoxus. Heart Disease and Stroke 1994;3:68–69.

Maisch B. Pericardial diseases, with a focus on etiology, pathogenesis, pathophysiology, new diagnostic imaging methods, and treatment. Curr Opin Cardiol 1994;9:379–388.

Diseases of the aorta

Amarenco P, Cohen A, Tzourio C. Atherosclerotic disease of the aortic arch and the risk of ischemic stroke. N Engl J Med 1994;331:1474–1479.

Cigarroa JE, Isselbacher EM, DeSanctis RW, et al. Diagnostic imaging in the evaluation of suspected aortic dissection: Old standards and new directions. N Engl J Med 1993;328:35–43.

Ernst CB: Abdominal aortic aneurysms. N Engl J Med 1993; 328:1167–1172.

Hollier LH, Taylor LM, Ochsner J. Recommended indications for operative treatment of abdominal aortic aneurysms. J Vasc Surg 1992;15:1046–1056.

Lederle FA, Parenti CM, Chute EP. Ruptured abdominal aortic aneurysm: the internist as diagnostician. Am J Med 1994;96:163–167.

Peripheral vascular disease

Hertzer NR. The natural history of peripheral vascular disease: Implications for its management. Circulation. 1991;83:I12–I19.

Newman AB, Sutton-Tyrel K, Vogt MT, et al. Morbidity and mortality in hypertensive adults with a low ankle/arm blood pressure index. JAMA 1993;270:487–489.

O'Keeffe ST, Woods BOB, Breslin DJ, et al. Blue-toe syndrome: causes and management. Arch Intern Med 1992; 152:2197–2202.

Cardiogenic shock

Califf RM, Bengtson JR. Cardiogenic shock. N Engl J Med 1994;330:1724–1730.

Teba L, Banks DE, Balaan MR. Understanding circulatory shock. Is it hypovolemic, cardiogenic, or vasogenic? Postgrad Med 1992;91:121–129.

Assessment of Cardiac Risk for Noncardiac Surgery

Guidelines for perioperative cardiovascular evaluation for non-cardiac surgery: report of the American College of Cardiology/American Heart Association Task Force on Practice Guidelines. J Am Coll Cardiol 1996;27:910–948.

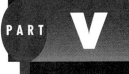

PART **V**

Melinda McCord
Janet A. Fairley

DERMATOLOGIC DISORDERS

While 4–5% of outpatient visits are specifically for skin disorders, up to 20% of patients have some symptom related to the skin.

History

The history should focus on specific aspects of the current skin problem and the relevant general characteristics of the patient (Table 42.1). Also important is the history of the lesions, their chronicity, and previous therapy. The latter may alter the appearance of some skin disorders or affect the findings of clinical tests. For example, use of over-the-counter antifungals not only alters the morphology of tinea infections, but also renders a potassium hydroxide (KOH) preparation negative. General information about age, gender, and race can also be helpful because some disorders show predilections related to those factors.

Physical Examination

Examination of the skin can be divided into the following three phases: 1) an overview of the patient, 2) a general inspection of the skin, and 3) a careful study of the morphology of the individual lesion(s). The purpose of the general overview is to look for signs of systemic illness, which may suggest that the skin lesion is a manifestation of a systemic disorder. A general inspection of the skin involves examining it for overall color, texture, and hydration (dry versus well-hydrated). A melanoma could be detected incidentally during such general inspection. Morphologic diagnosis of skin disorders depends on identifying 1) the primary lesion; 2) secondary changes; 3) the configuration, extent, and distribution of the lesion; 4) the color of the lesion; and 5) changes in the rest of the skin and/or skin appendages including the nails, scalp, and oral mucosa.

A primary lesion arises from the disease process, without alteration by the environment or by patient intervention (e.g., scratching), and its characteristics are the most important in determining a correct diagnosis; see Table 42.2 for common morphological terms. The *morphology* of the primary lesion forms the basis for classifying skin disorders into broad groups, a process that helps determine a correct diagnosis. These broad groups are 1) papulosquamous, 2) vesicobullous, 3) tumor-nodule, 4) vascular reaction, and 5) dermatitis-eczema. Not all disorders are amenable to this classification, such groups help narrow the differential diagnosis. Secondary changes (Table 42.3) evolve from

environmental or patient factors, and often reflect the "history" of the lesion (e.g., lichenification, erosions from scratching, or crusting from secondary infection).

Configuration describes the shape of the lesions, which may sometimes be characteristic (e.g., "target" lesions of erythema multiforme). **Discoid** usually refers to discoid lupus erythematosus, whereas **nummular** usually implies a type of eczema. Likewise, **guttate** refers to the guttate form of psoriasis. The *distribution* of a lesion is generally less helpful for diagnosis than its morphology; however, in some instances, the distribution is so striking that it may suggest the cause—for example, the characteristic dermatomal distribution of herpes zoster. The *color* within skin lesions is generally due to melanin, oxyhemoglobin, reduced hemoglobin, carotene, and cellular infiltration. Other causes may be foreign substances such as deposition of a drug or tattoo. Palpation of the skin can help the clinician notice the subtle depression of an atrophic skin lesion, identify an infiltrated lesion, or better evaluate the texture and hydration of the skin.

Diagnostic Procedures and Techniques

Once a differential diagnosis has been generated, specific diagnostic methods can follow. In general, nondermatologists tend to overdiagnose infectious disorders and underdiagnose inflammatory diseases. A few basic diagnostic techniques can help the physician avoid this pitfall.

Potassium hydroxide preparation

A potassium hydroxide (KOH) preparation identifies fungal elements present on the skin. Scrapings are obtained from the skin, nails, or scalp and placed on a glass slide. A drop of 10–20% KOH is added, a coverslip is placed over the KOH, and the slide is gently warmed by passing it through the flame of an alcohol lamp. The KOH should not boil. If allowed to stand for 5–10 minutes, KOH dissolves much of the keratin from the skin scrapings, thus enabling the clinician to see fungal hyphae and/or spores more clearly. Care should be taken to avoid getting KOH on the microscope because it will etch the lens. In **dermatophyte infections,** branched, segmented hyphae are present (see Color Plate 1, located in the color plate section at the end of the book); in **tinea versicolor** (a superficial fungal infection caused by Pityrosporum), shorter hyphae and spores cause a "spaghetti and meatballs" appearance.

Tinea capitis is more difficult to confirm with the

TABLE 42.1.	Pertinent Aspects of Dermatologic History

Questions specific to the skin problem
Acute or chronic?
  What was the initial site of involvement and the
    pattern of spread?
  Has there been any change of individual lesions from
    their initial appearance?
  Does anything seem to cause or irritate the lesions in
    the patient's view?
  Are the lesions symptomatic — itching or pain?
  Has the patient had any prior therapy (physician or
    over-the-counter preparations)
General information needed about the patient
  Age
  Gender
  Ethnic/racial background
  Geographic origin and travel
  Occupation and hobbies
  Family history — do any other family members have
    skin problems?
General medical history
  Allergies, asthma, diabetes, or other metabolic or
    chronic diseases
Medications, including over-the-counter ones

KOH preparation. Even in experienced hands, a KOH test has an accuracy of only 60%; therefore, a culture of the scalp should supplement a KOH test to diagnose tinea capitis. Both scales and hairs plucked from an involved site should be examined. The spores in endothrix infections are found inside the distorted hair shaft whereas in ectothrix infections, the spores and hyphae are outside of the hair shaft.

Wood's lamp examination

A Wood's lamp emits light at a wavelength of 365 nm; it enhances the presence of hypopigmented and hyperpigmented epidermal lesions and causes fluorescence of certain superficial bacteria, fungi, and chemicals. A Wood's lamp is used to determine the depth of pigmentary disorders because it enhances epidermal pigmentary changes and diminishes dermal pigmentary changes. **Vitiligo** is enhanced, and the ash leaf macules of tuberous sclerosis are rendered visible. Another classic use of the Wood's lamp is for determining tinea capitis. Ectothrix infections due to *Microsporum audouinii* or *Microsporum canis* elicit green fluorescence. However, over 90% of tinea scalp infections in the United States are caused by *Trichophyton tonsurans*, an endothrix infection that fails to fluoresce—which greatly diminishes the role of Wood's lamp in determining tinea capitis.

Other infections that can be detected with a Wood's

lamp include erythrasma and tinea versicolor. **Erythrasma,** a superficial, cutaneous bacterial infection caused by the corynebacterium species, mimics tinea cruris. Upon examination using a Wood's lamp, erythrasma fluoresces a coral red due to the presence of porphyrins in the corynebacterium; **tinea versicolor** fluoresces yellow-green. In **porphyria cutanea tarda,** the urine, feces, and blister fluid may fluoresce a pinkish-orange. Since spot-testing of the urine does not always elicit fluorescence, it does not supplant quantitative measurement of the porphyrins.

Cytologic (Tzanck) smear

The **Tzanck smear** can rapidly confirm herpes infections. Despite being positive in herpes simplex type I and II and in varicella/zoster infections, the smear

TABLE 42.2.	Morphologic Terms in Dermatology

Primary Lesions
  Macule — flat, circumscribed area of color change
  Papule — an elevated, palpable lesion <5 mm in
    diameter
  Nodule — an elevated lesion >5 mm in diameter
  Tumor — large nodule, usually >2 cm in diameter; may
    be either benign or malignant
  Plaque — a broad-based, elevated lesion in which the
    diameter of the lesion is greater than its height
  Wheal — transient swelling caused by edema of skin
  Vesicle — palpable, fluid-filled lesion <1 cm in diameter
  Bulla — a fluid-filled lesion >1 cm in diameter
  Cyst — circumscribed tumor containing semi-solid or
    liquid material
  Pustule — an elevated lesion containing a focal accumu-
    lation of inflammatory cells and serum (pus)
  Purpura — leakage of blood into the skin
  Burrow — linear lesion caused by parasites in the skin
Secondary Changes
  Scale — accumulation of squamous debris from the
    epidermis
  Crust — collection of dried serum, cellular, or bacterial
    debris overlying damaged epidermis
  Fissure — cleft in epidermis extending into the dermis
  Excoriation — loss of epidermis induced by scratching
  Lichenification — exaggeration of skin markings associ-
    ated with epidermal thickening and usually caused
    by scratching
  Erosion — loss of epidermis; heals without scarring
  Ulcer — loss of epidermis and at least part of the
    dermis; heals with scarring
  Atrophy — loss of substance of skin; can be either
    superficial (epidermal) or deeper (dermal or sub-
    cutaneous)
  Scar — new formation of connective tissue that replaces
    loss of the dermis or subcutaneous tissue

TABLE 42.3.	Descriptive Terms for the Configuration and Distribution of Skin Lesions

Configuration
Circinate — circular lesions
Discoid — disk-shaped
Nummular — coin-shaped
Annular — ring-shaped with clearing in the center
Polycyclic — annular but not forming complete rings
Guttate — multiple, small teardrop-shaped lesions
Serpiginous — snake-like
Iris or target — shaped like a bull's-eye with concentric rings
Herpetiform — grouped vesicles, papules, or erosions; similar to herpes
Zosteriform — a dermatomal distribution
Reticulated — interlacing, net-like
Distribution
Symmetry
Extensor vs. flexural surfaces
Contact areas — confined to areas of contact with an exogenous agent
Seborrheic distribution — face, upper chest, and back
Photo distribution — in areas exposed to sunlight; spares the area under the chin and in the deep creases of the eyelid; also often shows some sparing in the shaded area below the nose
Koebnerization — formation of lesions in an area that has been traumatized (see Figure 44.1)

cannot differentiate between these organisms. The test is done by removing the top of an intact blister and scraping its base with a scalpel blade. The scraping is smeared onto a glass slide, air-dried, and stained, usually with methylene blue, Giemsa, or Wright stains. A coverglass is applied, and the smear is examined under the microscope. A positive test requires finding the presence of multinucleated giant cells (see Color Plate 2), a task that is observer-dependent.

The Tzanck test requires an intact vesicle for accurate diagnosis. With intact vesicles, it is positive in over 70% of the cases, but the yield is much lower with crusted lesions. The Tzanck preparation correlates well with viral cultures in experienced hands; its other advantages are rapid results and almost universal availability. As an alternative to the Tzanck smear, many laboratories now offer rapid screening tests that rely on immunologic techniques and are usually available within 4–5 hours. Viral isolation, perhaps the most definitive test, is not 100% sensitive and the results take several days.

Scabies preparations

Scabies, caused by the mite *Sarcoptes scabiei*, is a common infestation, and skin scrapings are extremely helpful in its diagnosis. Mites are most successfully detected from a site that has not been excessively scratched. For help with identifying a burrow, the clinician can apply washable ink to the affected areas, wash off the excess, and then look for burrows that retain the ink. Using a #15 scalpel blade on which a drop of mineral oil has been placed, the clinician scrapes open an intact burrow and smears the contents on a slide. A common error is not scraping deeply enough because the scraping must be deeper than is required for fungal preparations. A coverslip is placed over the smear, and the preparation is examined with a microscope under low power. Identification of a mite, egg case, or feces is diagnostic (see Color Plate 3). Some prefer the use of KOH in identifying scabies as it helps dissolve the keratotic debris and thus improves the visibility of the mite; however, KOH will destroy any feces present.

Diascopy

Diascopy is a simple procedure that can provide information regarding the cause of a color change within a lesion. A clear glass or plastic slide is used to apply firm pressure to the surface of a skin lesion. Blanching of lesions implies that any erythema is due to vasodilation. Conversely, hemorrhage into the skin will not blanch. Exclusion of blood from the lesion may also reveal unusual color changes, such as a brownish-yellow hue in granulomatous disorders.

Skin biopsy

Taking a skin biopsy is one of the most definitive ways to establish the diagnosis of skin disorders. The selection of the site, the technique used, and the interpretation of the report in light of the clinical examination are crucial to the success of such a biopsy. In most disorders, a sample from a well-developed, representative lesion is most helpful. In bullous disorders, a biopsy from the margin of a lesion is usually more helpful in determining the level of separation; secondarily infected or excoriated lesions should not be selected. Discoid lupus erythematosus and vasculitis are often identified by routine histology in slightly older lesions, but biopsies for immunofluorescence testing for vasculitis should be obtained from recent lesions.

An **incisional biopsy** samples only a portion of the lesion, and an **excisional biopsy** removes it entirely. The most commonly used technique is the **punch biopsy,** which involves using a 3 to 4-mm punch (trephine). Following local asepsis and local anesthesia, the punch is rotated while pressure is applied to "drill" it through the skin. The specimen is gently lifted and snipped from the underlying subcutaneous fat. The specimen should be handled gently because damage from forceps can cause artifacts that can make histologic interpretation difficult. The site is closed with a suture and treated with a hemostatic agent such as 30% aluminum chloride or packed with Gelfoam to stop the bleeding.

Sometimes, the need for microbiologic studies may dictate that a larger piece of tissue, such as a **wedge biopsy,** be obtained. A narrow, elliptical sample of skin and the subcutaneous fat are removed, and the wound is closed with a suture, which causes a linear scar. Biopsy specimens for routine histologic examination should be fixed immediately in 10% neutral buffered formalin. However, immunofluorescence testing, electron microscopy, and many immunohistochemical techniques require special fixatives. Therefore, the reference laboratory should be consulted regarding the appropriate handling of the tissue prior to the biopsy.

<table>
<tr><td>**CHAPTER 43**</td><td># PRINCIPLES OF TOPICAL TREATMENT</td></tr>
</table>

Dermatologic therapy emphasizes topical treatment, the advantage of which is that the affected site receives direct treatment, generally without systemic side effects. However, to the nondermatologist, the many topical agents and vehicles may make the choice of an appropriate medication a daunting task.

Although the skin is a barrier, the epidermis does permit selective transport of some molecules through it. Drugs are absorbed into the skin via passive diffusion, and the major barrier to absorption is the **stratum corneum.** Percutaneous absorption of medications is affected by many factors. Absorption of a medication is proportional to the *concentration* of the molecule applied up to a point, beyond which it plateaus. However, the percutaneous absorption of many compounds cannot be predicted on the basis of simple diffusion. Lipids and **polar solvents**—for example, acetone, alcohol, and dimethyl sulfoxide (DMSO)—enhance percutaneous absorption via alteration of the stratum corneum. Increased skin temperature results in increased absorption. Occlusion of medications will raise the *surface temperature* and enhance percutaneous absorption. Finally, maximum *hydration* increases percutaneous absorption fivefold. Ironically, by damaging the barrier, excessive dryness may also enhance percutaneous absorption.

Percutaneous absorption also varies with the body site and age. For example, palmar and plantar skin absorbs much less than the skin of the trunk. The stratum corneum of a premature infant is only two to three cell layers thick whereas that of a full-term infant is four to six cell layers thick. Within 2–3 weeks after delivery, the premature infant's stratum corneum matures to that of a full-term infant. However, infants and children may exhibit increased toxicity to some topically applied compounds due to their increased surface-to-volume ratio compared with adults. On the other hand, old age does not seem to impose any demonstrable changes on percutaneous absorption.

Effective topical therapy depends on four major factors: the active ingredient, the vehicle, the condition being treated, and the patient (other medical problems, medications, compliance). The choice of the active ingredient and its vehicle—the two variables in the topical preparation—are most amenable to physician control. The choice of the correct active ingredient is dictated by the disorder being treated. A guide for the appropriate amount of topical preparations to prescribe is provided in Table 43.1.

The adage "If it is wet, dry it; if it is dry, wet it" has some general truth in that the selection of the vehicle has a significant impact on the response to therapy (Table 43.2). An eruption may be either *wet* (weeping, crusted, maceration, vesiculation) or *dry* (scale, lichenification, fissuring, and cracking). Vehicles can be divided into three groups: those that promote drying (wet dressings, powders, lotions, and sprays), those that moisturize (ointments and oils), and those with an intermediate effect (creams and gels). Table 43.3 lists the relative potency of topical steroids.

TABLE 43.1.	**Amounts of Creams for a Two-Week Course of Therapy**		
Area of Application		**Lotions**	**Creams, Ointments**
Localized application		1 oz	15–30 gm
Hands or feet		2 oz	60 gm
Trunk		4–8 oz	120 gm
Whole body		6 oz	480 gm

Note: Estimates based on twice-daily application.

TABLE 43.2. Summary of Vehicles in Dermatologic Therapy

Treatment	Principle	Ingredients	Advantages	Disadvantages
Open wet dressings	Moisturize areas by loosely wrapping many layers of moistened soft gauze or sheeting around them, leave in place for ½ h to 2 h, remove and remoisten	Normal saline, aluminum acetate (Burrow's solution), aluminum diacetate (Domeboro), KMnO$_4$, or 5% acetic acid in *Pseudomonas* infections	Dries and cools by evaporation, decreases local blood flow in inflammation by vasoconstriction, cleanses the area, and removes crust and debris; increases skin hydration to foster cutaneous drug absorption	Simultaneously compressing large amounts of the body may lead to excessive evaporative heat loss; can apply compresses to only about one-third of the body at a time
Closed wet dressings	Dressings covered by an impermeable wrap; otherwise same as above	Same as above	Same as above	May cause maceration and bacterial overgrowth; lacks the cooling effect of open dressings
Soaks	Useful for immersing extremities	Aluminum acetate, aluminum diacetate, and colloidal oatmeal (Aveeno)	Useful in treating widespread skin lesions; oatmeal soothes and is antipruritic; its oilated forms provide extra moisture	Useful in extremities only
Baths	Useful in immersing almost the entire body	Same as soaks Cornstarch (½ box in 6 in of tub water) is inexpensive, soothing, and antipruritic	Same as soaks; oil may be added to the bath, which coats, lubricates, and moisturizes dry skin conditions	Oil could coat the bath tub and make it slippery
Lotions	A suspension or solution; liquid base cools by evaporation	Inert or active agents; liquid base of water, alcohol, or propylene glycol	Ideal in hair-bearing or intertriginous areas because it is easy to apply and does not cause occlusion folliculitis	Not helpful as lubricants for dry skin conditions owing to high water and/or alcohol content
Ointments	Moisturize using a *small amount*, which is rubbed in	Emulsion of water droplets in oil; many agents	Gray or clear; have a greasy feel; very dry skin conditions can benefit from these	Patient acceptance is lower
Creams	Same as above	Emulsion of oil droplets in water; many agents	Patient acceptance is better; usually, a lighter and oilier base than ointment	Not as good at moisturizing as ointments because of volatile solvent or a high water content
Gels	Evaporate on contact and cause drying	Semisolid emulsions of agents in water, alcohol, or glycols	Useful in hair-bearing areas because they are not greasy or occlusive	Newer gels may lack the drying component seen in older types

Pastes	Often used to protect a localized area — e.g., ZnO$_2$ paste in diaper area	A powder in an ointment base; many agents	Useful in localized lesions only
Powders	Promote drying and minimize friction between opposing folds of skin	May be inert — e.g., talc, cornstarch, and ZnO$_2$ powder; or active — e.g., nystatin	High powder content provides more drying than ointment	Foreign body reactions from insoluble powders near open wounds; a sticky mess may result if residual powder is not removed before reapplying
			Best used in intertriginous areas that are normally moist and may potentially macerate	
Topical steroids	Anti-inflammatory, antiproliferative and immunosuppressive; suppress the mitotic activity of both keratinocytes and fibroblasts	Many agents (see Table 43.3); potency relates to the vehicle and concentration of active ingredient; ointments more potent than cream or lotions	Class VII steroids are generally preferred for use in areas such as the face and groin (least likely to cause atrophy)	May cause steroid acne, purpura, and easy bruising (see Figure 43.1), acneiform eruptions, perioral dermatitis or skin atrophy; may delay wound healing; fluorinated steroids are highly atrophogenic; use near eye can cause glaucoma, ocular hypertension, or cataracts if agents get in the eye

TABLE 43.3. Relative Potency of Selected Topical Steroids*	
Class I	**Class IV**
Betamethasone dipropionate	Desoximetasone
Clobetasol propionate††	Fluocinolone acetonide — ointment
Diflorasone diacetate	Flurandrenolide
Halobetasol propionate	Mometasone furoate
Class II	Triamcinolone acetonide 0.1%
Amcinonide — ointment	**Class V**
Betamethasone dipropionate — ointment	Betamethasone valerate — cream
Desoximetasone	Desonide
Diflorasone diacetate	Flurandrenolide
Fluocinonide — cream	Fluocinolone acetonide — ointment
Halcinonide	Hydrocortisone butyrate
Mometasone furoate	Hydrocortisone valerate
Class III	Triamcinolone acetonide 0.05%
Amcinonide — cream	**Class VI**
Betamethasone dipropionate — cream	Alclometasone dipropionate
Betamethasone valerate	Desonide
Diflorasone diacetate	Flumethasone pivolate
Triamcinolone acetonide	Fluocinolone acetonide cream — .01%
	Hydrocortisone butyrate
	Triamcinolone acetonide 0.025%
	Class VII
	Hydrocortisone Acetate 1 — 2.5%

†Suppression of hypothalamic-pituitary axis (HPA) is most common with use of higher potency (class I, II or III) steroids under occlusion or in small children. Class I agents can cause HPA suppression, even without occlusion.

††Maximum dose: 60 grams per week for a total of 2 weeks for clobetasol dipropionate to avoid HPA suppression. Occlusion should be avoided with these agents for the same reason.

*(Adapted from: Stoughton RB. Vasoconstrictor assay-specific applications. In: Maibach HI, Surber C (eds.). Topical Corticosteroids. Basel, Switzerland: Karger AG, 1992, pp. 42–53.

CHAPTER 44 PAPULOSQUAMOUS DISORDERS

Papulosquamous disorders are characterized by primary lesions consisting of papules or plaques, which are generally multiple and usually sharply marginated with secondary scaling. Among the papulosquamous disorders shown in Table 44.1, the more common ones are psoriasis, pityriasis rosea (PR), and lichen planus; others are secondary syphilis, dermatophytosis, pityriasis rubra pilaris, and parapsoriasis.

Psoriasis

■ Definition

Psoriasis is a common, chronic inflammatory skin disorder, which causes red papules and plaques covered by thick, silvery white scales. The integral features of psoriasis are increased keratinocyte proliferation, altered keratinocyte maturation, and inflammation.

■ Epidemiology, Etiology, and Pathogenesis

Psoriasis affects 1–2% of the U.S. population, without any gender predilection. The age of onset, although it is younger in women, has a bimodal distribution, with a larger peak between 15 and 25 years, and the other in the fifth decade and beyond. The primary defect is unknown but multiple factors seem to play a role, including local T-cell activation, induction of keratinocyte receptors, and altered cytokine production in a genetically susceptible host.

Although psoriasis appears to be a heritable disorder, its exact mode of transmission remains elusive. It shows an association with the genes of the HLA loci HLA-Cw6 and HLA-DR7. An autosomal dominant pattern, with reduced penetrance, is recognized in several large kindreds. In some of these families, a psoriasis susceptibility gene has been located on chromosome 17q; its identity is unknown and this linkage is apparent in only a subset of patients.

Psoriasis can be triggered or exacerbated by stress, excess solar irradiation, irritating topical therapy, infections (most commonly streptococcal), pregnancy, HIV infection, or drugs—the common medications in this context being ß-blockers, antimalarials, lithium, and perhaps nonsteroidal anti-inflammatory drugs (NSAIDs). Because systemic steroids can precipitate pustular psoriasis when their use is withdrawn, they should be used with extreme caution.

■ Clinical Features

The hallmarks of psoriasis are the red, sharply demarcated papules and plaques covered by thick, silvery white scales. Individual lesions can number anywhere from one to hundreds, and they vary in size and shape from small guttate papules to large circinate plaques (see Color Plate 5). Symmetrically distributed, the lesions show a predilection for the scalp, genitals, nails, and extensor aspects of the arms and legs. Secondary excoriations or lichenification may develop with pruritic eruptions. The nails may develop pitting (see Color Plate 6), onycholysis (lifting of the nail plate from the nail bed), brown "oil spots," subungual hyperkeratosis, grooving, and crumbling. The **Koebner phenomenon,** in which typical lesions form at the site of minor trauma, is characteristic (see Color Plate 5).

Psoriasis has numerous clinical variants including eruptive or guttate, inverse, pustular, and erythrodermic types. Guttate psoriasis is characterized by 0.5 to 1.5-cm red papules and plaques that may be provoked by infections, particularly streptococcal ones. Inverse psoriasis is localized to the axilla, groin, and skin folds rather than the classic sites. Pustular psoriasis may be localized or generalized. The generalized form has an acute onset with crops of pustules and associated fever and leukocytosis. **Erythroderma** of any cause, including psoriasis, disrupts thermoregulation and fluid balance, and thus signals a potential emergency. **Erythrodermic psoriasis** has many of the constitutional features of generalized pustular psoriasis. An inflammatory arthropathy, which is described in chapter 257, occurs in 5–7% of patients with psoriasis.

■ Differential Diagnosis

Chronic plaque-type psoriasis may resemble nummular eczema, mycosis fungoides, or tinea corporis. Guttate psoriasis should be distinguished from pityriasis rosea, secondary syphilis, and superficial tinea infections. Erythroderma may follow contact or atopic dermatitis, Sézary syndrome, drug eruptions, pityriasis rubra pilaris, or seborrheic dermatitis. *Inverse psoriasis* may resemble contact dermatitis, candidiasis, or Darier's disease.

■ Management

Psoriasis is a chronic disease with remissions and exacerbations. For limited disease, topical therapy may suffice. Commonly used preparations are topical steroids, tar preparations, anthralin, and the vitamin D analog, calcipotriene. Natural sunlight may sometimes be helpful, and ultraviolet light (UV), either UVB or UVA, combined with psoralen (PUVA) may be used in patients who do not respond to topical compounds. UV should be administered in a supervised setting by personnel experienced with the treatment of psoriasis.

Systemic therapy is reserved for extensive disease, disease in sites that may affect one's ability to work (palms and soles), or psoriasis with severe associated arthritis. Low-dose methotrexate (2.5–35 mg) is given orally once a week. Given the risk for bone marrow or liver toxicity, patients who receive methotrexate must be carefully monitored. Etretinate is especially useful in pustular psoriasis, usually stopping pustule formation within a few days. Because etretinate is highly teratogenic, its metabolites may remain in the bloodstream for several years after cessation of therapy. It should not be given to women of childbearing age. Other systemic agents such as cyclosporin, hydroxyurea, and sulfasalazine may also improve psoriasis.

TABLE 44.1.	Papulosquamous Disorders
Psoriasis	
Pityriasis rosea	
Lichen planus	
Secondary syphilis	
Dermatophytosis	
Pityriasis rubra pilaris	
Parapsoriasis	

Pityriasis Rosea

■ Definition, Epidemiology, and Etiology

Pityriasis rosea, which affects nearly 0.14% of the population, is a common, self-limited eruption occurring most frequently in children and young adults. Most frequently seen during the spring in the United States, pityriasis rosea has neither a gender nor a racial predilection. Its etiology is unknown, but its seasonal occurrence, its tendency to cluster in close social groups, and the rare reports of particles resembling picornavirus on electron microscopy all suggest an infectious etiology.

■ Clinical Features

The initial lesion, a "herald patch," is a 2 to 5-cm oval, pink plaque or patch with fine peripheral scales. This precedes the remainder of the eruption and commonly occurs on the trunk but may involve the extremities also. Within hours or days, crops of oval, pink macules and papules with fine white peripheral scales arise symmetrically on the trunk, neck, and proximal extremities. The lesions form along the lines of cleavage on the trunk and usually spare the sun-exposed sites, eliciting a "Christmas tree" pattern (see Color Plate 7). The herald patch is not always evident. Other than mild pruritus, symptoms or prodrome are usually absent.

Lichen Planus

■ Definition and Epidemiology

Lichen planus is a common papulosquamous disease involving the skin, mucous membranes, and the nails and affecting fewer than 1% of adults worldwide, most frequently those between 30 and 60 years of age.

■ Etiology

The etiology of lichen planus is unknown. It has been suggested that an unknown antigen, presumably an epidermal protein, altered by a virus or drug and processed by the Langerhans cells, stimulates the migration and activation of lymphocytes. Lichen planus is more frequently associated with certain HLA types, especially HLA-DR1 type. A certain complement of genes may predispose a given individual to a lichenoid reaction to a given antigen. Recently, an association with hepatitis C in 10% of patients has been reported. Although hepatitis B surface antigen may be associated, lichen planus is not considered a direct result of hepatitis B infection.

■ Clinical Features

The skin eruption consists of flat-topped, polygonal, purple papules arranged in a symmetric distribution on the extremities, commonly on the flexor surface of the wrists (see Color Plate 8). Fine, lacy lines on the surface of the papules are called **Wickham's stria.** Despite the associated severe pruritus, excoriations are rare. Mucous membrane lesions occur in 50% of patients and may occur without cutaneous disease. These consist of whitish, reticulated plaques that are most common on the buccal mucosa (see Color Plate 9) but may involve other

■ Differential Diagnosis and Management

While the herald patch may be confused with tinea corporis, nummular eczema, psoriasis, or contact dermatitis, the most important disease in the differential diagnosis of the generalized eruption is secondary syphilis. Syphilis should be excluded by appropriate tests whenever pityriasis rosea is suspected. Other conditions include viral exanthem, nummular eczema, guttate psoriasis, seborrheic dermatitis, and dermatophyte infections. Many drugs—including bismuth, barbiturates, captopril, ketotifen, metronidazole, d-penicillamine, gold, mercury, isotretinoin, and arsenicals—may cause a similar eruption.

For most patients, the eruption requires only reassurance that it will eventually clear up. Some antihistamines or topical steroids may relieve mild pruritus, but the severe pruritus of generalized PR improves with UVB treatment.

sites such as the mouth, vagina, and penis. In almost 25% of men with lichen planus, the genitals are affected. Nail dystrophy occurs in 1–10% of patients, consisting of thinning, grooving, splitting, longitudinal ridging, or pitting of the nail plate. Onycholysis and **distal subungual hyperkeratosis** may also occur. **Pterygium formation** (adhesion of the nail fold to the nail bed) may cause permanent scarring of the nail bed and nail dystrophy. These changes are not diagnostic; definitive diagnosis requires a nail biopsy.

Lichen planus has several morphologic variants: hypertrophic or verrucous (wartlike) plaques, follicular papules, vesicular or bullous lesions seen in conjunction with typical papules, actinic lichen planus involving sun-exposed sites, atrophy, and erosive mucosal lesions. In lichen planus of the scalp (lichen planopilaris), hyperkeratotic follicular papules progress to atrophy, scarring, and alopecia.

Most patients with lichen planus, although otherwise healthy, have a higher incidence of impaired glucose tolerance and liver disease or liver function abnormalities, including cirrhosis, elevated transaminases, presence of hepatitis B antigens and antibodies, chronic active hepatitis, and primary biliary cirrhosis. These may imply autoimmunity or a viral etiology for lichen planus and/or suggest a genetic susceptibility to infection with hepatotoxic viruses.

■ Differential Diagnosis

The distribution and morphology of the eruption often suggest the diagnosis. Many drugs (gold, penicillamine, antimalarials, arsenicals, hypoglycemic agents, tetracycline, thiazide diuretics, and angiotensin-converting enzyme inhibitors) and other agents (e.g., color film developers) may produce a lichenoid eruption. The other papulosquamous diseases should be considered in the differential diagnosis of the skin eruption. When lesions involve the palms and soles, syphilis should be excluded. The nail dystrophy may resemble psoriasis, onychomycosis, or alopecia areata. The mucous membrane lesions mimic lupus, leukoplakia, candidiasis, and syphilis.

■ **Management**

In about half the cases, the disease remits on its own in 6–18 months; in the remainder, it remains active for a prolonged period. Mild pruritus may be treated with antihistamines and topical steroids. With severe symptoms and extensive involvement, oral corticosteroids may be effective in a tapering dose over 2–6 weeks. However, activity often recurs when steroids are discontinued. They are best avoided in patients with chronic disease. PUVA therapy and retinoids can also be quite effective. For oral lesions, a potent topical steroid may be given in gel form or mixed in an adherent vehicle—for example, Orabase or topical retinoid (Retin-A).

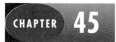

VESICOBULLOUS DISORDERS

Pemphigus

■ **Definition and Epidemiology**

Pemphigus refers to a group of autoimmune blistering diseases of the skin. In all forms of pemphigus, blisters arise due to the loss of cell-to-cell adhesion (**acantholysis**) within the epidermis. The onset of **pemphigus vulgaris** (PV) is typically in the fourth to sixth decades of life. While no ethnic group is exempt, it is more common among Ashkenazi Jews, and is associated with the HLA-DR4 or DRW6 haplotypes. The Brazilian endemic form of PV, **Fogo Selvagem** (FS), occurs in the forested regions of Brazil and is associated with the HLA -DR1-Dw20 haplotype. An environmental factor is strongly suspected in its pathogenesis. **Pemphigus foliaceus** (PF) is sporadic in the United States and shows no predilection for any specific group.

■ **Etiology and Pathogenesis**

Both forms of pemphigus (PV and PF) are characterized by the presence of IgG directed against the cell surface of keratinocytes. The stimulus for the development of these autoantibodies is unknown. They may be detected bound to the skin or in the circulation by various immunofluorescence techniques. These autoantibodies are pathogenic by passive transfer into neonatal mice. Some cases of pemphigus appear to be drug-induced; the more common offenders are penicillamine, captopril, rifampin, phenobarbital, and piroxicam.

The histological and clinical features of different forms of pemphigus are related to the level at which the keratinocytes detach (Table 45.1). For example, in PV, acantholysis occurs at the suprabasilar level of the epidermis, but in PF and FS, acantholytic lesions are more superficial at the subcorneal level. Using molecular biologic methods, researchers have found the targets of the autoantibodies in PV and PF to be the cadherin type of cell adhesion molecules that are localized to the desmosomes of the epidermis. PF autoantibodies are directed against the desmosomal cadherin, desmoglein 1, and PV autoantibodies are directed against a closely related protein, desmoglein 3. Desmoglein 3 is strongly expressed in the basal layer of the epidermis, and desmoglein 1, in the upper layers of the epidermis, which may explain these differences in the level of acantholysis and blister formation in PV and PF.

■ **Clinical Features**

Pemphigus vulgaris is characterized by the formation of flaccid bullae that arise on noninflamed skin. Pressure applied to the edge of the blister or the adjacent normal skin will cause these bullae to spread, termed **Nikolsky's sign**. The blisters rupture, leaving erosions and large areas of denuded skin. The mouth is usually the first affected site. The scalp is another common site of early involvement. Although PV may remain localized for

TABLE 45.1.   Characteristics of the Major Vesicobullous Disorders

Disease	Epidemiology	Clinical Features	Immunopathology and Histopathology	Therapy
Pemphigus vulgaris	Onset in fourth to sixth decade	Flaccid bullae arising on noninflamed skin; oral involvement common	IgG, C3 deposited on the cell surface of keratinocytes; suprabasilar acantholysis	Prednisone, 60–100 mg/day to suppress the blistering; add azathioprine (50–150 mg/d) or cyclophosphamide (50–200 mg/d) if necessary
Pemphigus foliaceus	Onset in fourth to sixth decade	Flaccid bullae, crusting, and erosions mainly on the head, neck, and upper trunk; oral mucosa spared	IgG, C3 deposited on the cell surface of keratinocytes; acantholysis at the upper layers of the epidermis	Same as above
Bullous pemphigoid	Onset >60 years	Tense bullae (Figure 45.1) on an erythematous base; often worse in the intertriginous areas	IgG, C3 deposited at the basement membrane zone; subepidermal blisters	Compresses of Burrow's solution, plus a high-potency topical steroid for localized disease; prednisone (0.6–1.2 mg/kg/d, initially; taper and use q.o.d dosing when disease is under control), with or without immunosuppressives (same as pemphigus vulgaris); tetracycline (500 mg qid) nicotinamide (500 mg tid) combination may be useful in selected cases
Dermatitis herpetiformis	Onset in second to fourth decade	Grouped vesicles on extensor surfaces; extreme pruritus	IgA in the dermal papillae; separation between tips of dermal papillae and the epidermis	Dapsone

prolonged periods, it becomes widespread if untreated. Prior to the development of immunosuppressants, PV was frequently fatal due to extensive loss of the epidermal barrier.

In contrast, in PF the blisters are more superficial and easily rupture, leaving erosions. Erythema and crusting are often prominent. Unlike PV, the PF lesions are most frequent on the head and neck, and spare the oral mucosa; despite its chronic course, PF has a better prognosis.

■ Diagnosis and Differential Diagnosis

PV and PF may be differentiated from each other clinically and histologically. They may at times resemble pemphigoid, dermatitis herpetiformis, and erythema multiforme (EM). The oral lesions of PV may be mistaken for EM, erosive lichen planus, herpes, and cicatricial pemphigoid. In both PV and PF, circulating antibodies directed against the keratinocyte cell surface can be detected by indirect immunofluorescence (IF). In addition, lesional epidermis exhibits autoantibodies bound to the keratinocyte surface by direct IF. The titers of serum autoantibodies roughly correlate with disease activity. However, differentiating PV from PF by this method is difficult because the IF staining patterns are similar for both diseases.

■ Management

The goal of therapy for all forms of pemphigus is to lower the autoantibody production, primarily through using high-dose corticosteroids, which are often combined with a steroid-sparing agent. Treatment is generally initiated with prednisone (Table 45.1). If steroids alone do not produce an adequate response, or if their dose cannot be adequately tapered, azathioprine, cyclophosphamide, or methotrexate is added. Plasmapheresis may reduce the levels of circulating autoantibodies; however, unless antibody formation is suppressed, their titers may rebound when plasmapheresis is completed.

While untreated PV is highly lethal (50% within the first year), therapy lowers the mortality significantly to almost 10% over 5 years. Morbidity and mortality in the treated patient are usually due to complications of therapy. Disease control and monitoring for these side effects are best done through close follow-up.

Bullous Pemphigoid

■ Definition and Epidemiology

Bullous pemphigoid, the most common of the autoimmune bullous disorders, is generally a disease of the elderly, with no racial or gender predilections. **Herpes gestationis,** a related disorder that shares the histologic and immunologic features of bullous pemphigoid, occurs during the second and third trimesters of pregnancy and generally resolves soon postpartum. A proposed link between bullous pemphigoid and cancer has not been proven. Other autoimmune diseases (pernicious anemia, diabetes, and rheumatoid arthritis) are often associated with bullous pemphigoid.

■ Etiology, Pathogenesis, and Pathology

The autoantibodies in BP patients are directed against two epidermal antigens of 230 kD and 180 kD (BP230 and BP180), both components of the hemidesmosome, an organelle of epithelial cells that functions in cell-substrate adhesion. Recent studies using a mouse model suggest that BP180 may be the more important target of autoantibodies in human BP. The initial trigger for autoantibody formation is unknown. Histologically, these blisters show separation of the epidermis from the dermis through the basement membrane zone of the dermo-epidermal junction. Binding of IgG and C3 is also demonstrable at the basement membrane zone by direct immunofluorescence.

■ Clinical Features

An urticarial phase may precede the vesico-bullous eruption of bullous pemphigoid, in which patients develop plaques of erythema that mimic true urticaria but persist longer than 24 hours. Generalized pruritus may also precede the eruption. Although the lesions may be widespread, they most commonly affect the intertriginous areas, the flexor surface of the arms and legs, and the lower abdomen (see Color Plate 10). Mucous membranes may be affected in up to 40% of patients, but are rarely severe or a major feature. Bullous pemphigoid often has a chronic course, usually 2–6 years.

■ Diagnosis and Management

Although the clinical features of bullous pemphigoid are distinctive, biopsies for routine histology and direct immunofluorescence are used to confirm the diagnosis. Nearly 80% of patients will have detectable circulating autoantibodies against the basement membrane zone of the epidermis. Bullous pemphigoid may be confused with pemphigus, epidermolysis bullosa acquisita, erythema multiforme, or dermatitis herpetiformis. In the urticarial phase, it may resemble true urticaria. Untreated, bullous pemphigoid may become widespread, causing the patient considerable discomfort and increasing the risk of infection. The majority of bullous pemphigoid patients will require systemic steroids (Table 45.1) and perhaps other immunosuppressives.

Dermatitis Herpetiformis

■ Definition and Epidemiology

Dermatitis herpetiformis (DH) is a chronic, autoimmune blistering disease, preferentially affecting men in their second to fourth decades. It is more frequent among Caucasians of Scandinavia, Ireland, and Great Britain than among African Americans or Asians. Initial studies revealed that 58% of patients with DH expressed HLA-B8 compared with 20–30% of normal controls. In patients with histologically confirmed DH, however, the frequency of HLA-B8 expression was 80–90%. Recent studies reveal an even stronger association with HLA class II antigens: 90–95% of patients with DH express HLA-DR3 and DQw2 antigens and 42% express the HLA-DPw1 antigen.

■ Etiology and Pathogenesis

In skin biopsy sections of patients with DH, the dermal papillae contain granular deposits of IgA; it is polyclonal and predominantly IgA1. However, the origin of the immunoglobulin or the antigenic site to which it is bound remains elusive. The association of the cutaneous eruption of DH with gluten-sensitive enteropathy suggests a role for the mucosal immune response in immunoglobulin production. Circulating immune complexes and an increased frequency of antireticulin, antiendomysial, antinuclear, and thyroid microsomal antibodies exist in the sera of patients with DH, but circulating antibodies against basement membrane (antibasement membrane antibodies) are absent.

■ Clinical Features

The most notable feature of DH is the severe pruritus, which burns or stings and often precedes the primary lesion—a tense subepidermal blister—by 8–10 hours. However, examination rarely discloses blisters because the trauma of scratching causes excoriations, erosions, and crusting. Pruritus may be relieved as the blisters rupture. The lesions are symmetric with herpetiform clustering, and most often affect the extensor surfaces, including the knees, elbows, buttocks, sacrum, back, shoulders, and nuchal region. Mucosal surfaces are rarely affected. The course is one of remissions and exacerbations. Although spontaneous resolution does occur, remissions may be long-lasting.

Small bowel biopsy may demonstrate histologic changes of gluten-sensitive enteropathy. However, this enteropathy is often clinically silent, and laboratory evidence of malabsorption occurs in only 20–30% of patients. Intestinal lymphoma, and less commonly an extraintestinal lymphoma, may complicate DH.

■ Differential Diagnosis

A definitive diagnosis of DH depends on the correlation of the clinical features with histologic and immunologic data. Clinically, DH may mimic scabies, neurotic excoriations, erythema multiforme, linear IgA disease, transient acantholytic dermatosis, bullous pemphigoid, and herpes gestationis. Characteristically, direct immunofluorescent examination of biopsy sections reveals granular IgA deposition in the dermal papillae.

■ Management

Medical management and adherence to a gluten-free diet are two approaches to therapy of DH. Often, the skin manifestations alone respond to dapsone (100–200 mg/day). Symptoms improve within hours of therapy, which confirms the diagnosis. Patients who do not tolerate dapsone may be given sulfapyridine (1–1.5 g/day). A gluten-free diet allows most patients to discontinue or reduce dapsone and clearly improves both the skin and bowel pathology, but patients are generally intolerant to such a diet.

CHAPTER 46

HYPERSENSITIVITY DISORDERS

This group of disorders consists of urticaria, angioedema, erythema multiforme (EM), vasculitis, and erythema nodosum. Urticaria is characterized by raised, usually pruritic lesions of variable size.

Angioedema, occurring as indurated areas of swelling, most commonly affects areas of loose tissue (e.g., lips and eyelids). Urticaria and angioedema are discussed in chapter 13.

Erythema Multiforme

■ Definition, Epidemiology, and Etiology

Erythema multiforme (EM), an acute hypersensitivity reaction with variable severity and manifestations, involves the skin and mucous membranes. Most common in persons in their second to fourth decades, EM increases during the spring and fall, paralleling the flux of infectious organisms. No age or race is exempt, and women are affected slightly more often than men.

Subclassified as EM major or minor, EM is triggered by infections, drugs, collagen vascular diseases, neoplasms, endocrinopathies, and environmental factors. EM minor is most commonly caused by the herpes simplex virus, with even subclinical herpes infections suspected in some cases. Other causes are contact sensitization and pregnancy. EM major most frequently follows *Mycoplasma pneumoniae* infections and the use of some drugs, which commonly include sulfa compounds, anticonvulsants (e.g., phenytoin), and NSAIDs (e.g., butazones and salicylates). **Toxic epidermal necrolysis** (TEN), a rare form of EM, is triggered by allopurinol, ethambutol, phenolphthalein, and pentazocine, in addition to the drugs previously listed. The interval between the exposure to the imputed drug and the onset of EM is variable and may be as long as 6 weeks.

■ Clinical Features

Clinical features of EM minor and major and TEN are compared in Table 46.1. EM major (**Stevens-Johnson syndrome**) is the severe variant of EM minor. During its initial prodrome, many patients are given antibiotics or other drugs that obscure the diagnosis. The loss of the cutaneous barrier produces abnormalities of fluid regulation and creates a risk of infection. TEN, a severe, progressive hypersensitivity reaction, is considered by some to be a variant of EM. The initial management problems involve fluid and protein losses, electrolyte imbalance, thermoregulatory failure, and infection.

■ Diagnosis and Differential Diagnosis

EM major and minor are usually identified by the typical, symmetric target lesions on acral sites (see Color Plate 11). EM major (Stevens-Johnson syndrome) is separated from EM minor by the involvement of two or more mucous membranes. Bullous lesions are also more likely to be present in EM major. An early eruption or an unusual presentation may make EM major difficult to distinguish from urticaria, urticarial vasculitis, bullous pemphigoid, viral exanthems, staphylococcal scalded-skin syndrome, or toxic erythemas due to drugs or infections. The distinction between EM major and TEN may also pose a diagnostic problem. TEN is more extensive and rapidly progressive, the skin is characteristically tender, and the initial eruption is morbilliform with early evidence of necrosis. TEN may be confused with burns, exposure to caustic substances, staphylococcus scalded-skin syndrome, and toxic shock syndrome. Cultures and histologic examination of a biopsy specimen or frozen section of denuded skin will establish the diagnosis.

■ Management

The important management issues in EM are to identify and eradicate the causative agent. All drugs used prior to the onset of the eruption should be discontinued, and inciting herpetic, bacterial, and fungal infections should be treated. EM minor frequently responds to antihistamines and local care. Because oral lesions may make eating and drinking difficult, nutritional status should be monitored. With herpetic infections, recurrences of EM minor are not unusual.

The primary treatment for EM and TEN is supportive. Severe disease is best treated in a burn unit. Frequent assessment of the hematocrit, fluid, and electrolyte balance and pulmonary, renal, and hepatic function will allow early treatment of systemic complications. Cultures will indicate the need for antibiotic therapy. An

TABLE 46.1.	Features of Erythema Multiforme and Toxic Epidermal Necrolysis		
	EM Minor	**EM Major**	**Toxic Epidermal Necrolysis**
Prodrome	Absent/mild; fever, malaise, cough	Acute prodrome in 50%, fever, malaise, rhinorrhea, cough, diarrhea, vomiting, myalgia and arthralgia, lasts 1–14 days	Similar to EM major
Lesions	Asymptomatic; symmetric, dull red macules and urticarial plaques that rapidly enlarge and develop central vesicles or papules; target/iris lesions; interior of each ring becomes violaceous or purpuric (Figure 46.1); there may be prominent hemorrhagic bullae	Initial lesions resemble EM minor but rapidly enlarge and become extensive; blistering and necrosis of skin and mucous membranes	Occur within 2 days of onset of initial symptoms; discrete, violaceous papules and macules; target lesions; lesions rapidly coalesce; minimal friction or pressure causes epidermis to slough (Nikolsky's sign); tender erythema evolves into bullae
Location of lesions	Extensor surfaces of extremities and the dorsa of hands and feet, sites of trauma or sun exposure; trunk, face and neck less involved; one or multiple crops of lesions	Similar to EM minor; conjunctiva and perianal areas; conjunctivitis, keratitis, corneal ulcers, uveitis, 2 mucosal sites must be involved to diagnose EM major	Extensive, but predominantly face and trunk; rapid epidermal necrosis and exfoliation
Mucosal lesions	Oral lesions in 25%; only in the buccal mucosa, tongue and lips; dehydration may develop	Most common mucosal site is oral cavity; thick crusts cover bleeding oral lesions	Large portions of mucosa may be affected
Other organ involvement	None; lymphadenopathy may occur	Pneumonitis, myositis, pericarditis, hepatitis, changes in mentation	Pneumonia, GI bleed, hepatitis, shock, renal failure, sepsis
Course	2–3 weeks; multiple crops of lesions develop; individual lesions last 1–2 weeks	2–4 weeks	4–6 weeks
Mortality	None	5–20%	15–20%

ophthalmologic consultation should be obtained. Biologic dressings (e.g., Vigilon) will enhance healing, which occurs in 2–6 weeks with pigmentary changes but without scarring. Neutropenia, old age, renal failure, extensive skin involvement, and multiple medications are poor prognostic signs. The use of systemic corticosteroids is controversial. Whether early, high-dose corticosteroid therapy in EM will halt the progression of blistering is uncertain—given the paucity of controlled studies—and it may increase the risk of infection.

Vasculitis

■ Definition and Epidemiology

Hypersensitivity vasculitis includes a number of distinct clinical entities characterized histologically by inflammation and necrosis of small arterioles and postcapillary venules. This vascular destruction is neutrophil-mediated and the neutrophils' nuclear remnants are observed in a perivascular location. (The term "leukocytoclasis" describes the neutrophilic nuclear fragmentation.) Except for Henoch-Schönlein purpura, which is more frequent in children, neither an ethnic nor an age-group predilection has been noted.

■ Etiology and Pathogenesis

Hypersensitivity vasculitis may result from many antigens, the sources of which include drugs (penicillin, sulfonamides, thiazide diuretics, and NSAIDs), bacteria (streptococci, staphylococci, mycobacteria), viruses (HIV and hepatitis B), and endogenous proteins (cryoglobulins). It is immune complex-mediated and may be idiopathic or associated with collagen-vascular diseases and neoplasms. In states of antigen excess, soluble antigen-antibody complexes are deposited in postcapillary venules, causing complement activation, release of chemotactic factors, mast cell degranulation, and neutrophil influx. Release of proteolytic enzymes and oxygen-free radicals cause tissue destruction. Edema follows excess vascular permeability caused by vasoactive mast cell mediators.

■ Clinical Features

Cutaneous symptoms are often mild and consist of burning or pruritus. Fever, malaise, arthralgias, and myalgias may occur. Palpable purpura (see Color Plate 12), the hallmark of leukocytoclastic vasculitis, is due to extravasation of RBC and plasma from pathologically permeable venules. Angioedema, urticaria, nodules, pustules, hemorrhagic vesicles or bullae, ulcers, gangrene, livedo reticularis, and subcutaneous edema are less common. The lesions usually arise in crops on the lower extremities or dependent sites, and heal in 1–4 weeks; residual hyperpigmentation or scarring may follow. With systemic disease, the gastrointestinal tract, kidneys, joints, muscles, heart, and nerves may be involved. Usually self-limited, the vasculitis may be recurrent or chronic.

■ Diagnosis and Differential Diagnosis

In early cases, disorders causing nonpalpable purpura must be distinguished from those with palpable hemorrhage. Nonpalpable purpura may occur in thrombocytopenia, coagulopathies, thrombocythemia, systemic diseases (amyloidosis, diabetes, and uremia), trauma, stasis, and vascular fragility. The progressive pigmented purpuras (forms of capillaritis), distributed on the lower extremity, may cause confusion. A skin biopsy is diagnostic for hypersensitivity vasculitis; it reveals vascular wall disruption, fibrin deposition, neutrophils, and nuclear dust. Biopsy is most reliable when the specimen is acquired within 48 hours of onset of the eruption. Perivascular complement and immunoglobulin deposition shown by direct immunofluorescence studies can confirm an otherwise questionable diagnosis. Initial screening tests may include a complete blood count, sedimentation rate, urinalysis, and liver and renal function tests. Other studies (total complement [CH 50], antinuclear antibody, rheumatoid factor, hepatitis B antibody and antigen, and serum protein electrophoresis) may be used selectively.

■ Management

The essentials of therapy are the removal of the suspected drug and the treatment of associated diseases. Vasculitis often resolves spontaneously in 1–4 months with supportive measures such as NSAIDs, rest, leg elevation, and antibiotics for infections. Some patients with renal involvement or extensive necrosis respond to systemic corticosteroids, dapsone, or colchicine.

Erythema Nodosum

■ Definition and Epidemiology

Erythema nodosum, a **panniculitis,** presents with tender, red subcutaneous nodules on the extensor surfaces of the lower extremities. The peak age of onset is between 20 and 30 years, and women are affected more often than men.

■ Etiology and Pathogenesis

Erythema nodosum represents a reaction to a wide range of conditions (Table 46.2). An immune mechanism has been suspected, but not proven. ß-hemolytic streptococcal upper respiratory tract infections represent the most common and well-documented trigger, with erythema nodosum developing within 3 weeks after the infection. The most frequently implicated medications are oral contraceptives, sulfonamides, and bromides.

■ Clinical Features

Prior to the onset of the cutaneous eruption, some patients experience a mild prodrome consisting of fever, chills, malaise, arthralgias, and myalgias, often reflecting the underlying disorder. Tender, red, single or grouped, 1–5-cm subcutaneous nodules are symmetrically distributed on the extensor surfaces of the lower extremities. They resolve after a few days or weeks, leaving brown-red to purple macules. Crops of nodules continue to occur for 3–6 weeks until they spontaneously resolve. In 20% of cases, the lesions are recurrent and, in a few, may be chronic.

TABLE **46.2.**	Common Causes of Erythema Nodosum (partial listing)	

Infections	*Sarcoidosis*
Bacterial	*Inflammatory bowel disease*
β-hemolytic (upper respiratory)	Ulcerative colitis
streptococcal infections	Regional enteritis
Primary tuberculosis	*Medications*
Fungal	Penicillin
Histoplasmosis	Sulfonamides
Coccidioidomycosis	Some oral contraceptives
	Bromides

■ Differential Diagnosis and Management

Other entities that may pose a diagnostic problem are nodular vasculitis, subcutaneous fat necrosis, erythema induratum, and other forms of panniculitis. Biopsy is frequently required to confirm the diagnosis. Erythema nodosum often responds rapidly to treatment of the primary disease. Bed rest and salicylates or NSAIDs can adequately mitigate symptoms and enhance resolution of this self-limited disease. Indomethacin and naproxen are especially effective. Corticosteroids, colchicine, potassium iodide, and support stockings may be useful in chronic or recalcitrant cases.

CHAPTER **47** # DERMATITIS-ECZEMA

Broadly defined, dermatitis is inflammation of the skin. The dermatitis group consists of many disorders (Table 47.1). Eczematous processes primarily consist of vesicles and, rarely, bullae, erythematous papules, and plaques. In acute eczema, exemplified by rhus dermatitis (poison ivy, oak, or sumac), weeping vesicles and erythematous papules with secondary excoriations and crusting predominate whereas chronic eczema typically has poorly marginated plaques and papules with scaling and lichenification.

Atopic Dermatitis

■ Definition and Epidemiology

Atopic dermatitis is a relatively common, chronic cutaneous disorder with a worldwide distribution affecting almost 7 in 1000 adults and 24 in 1000 children. Men are affected slightly more frequently than are women. The onset is rarely before 2 months of age.

■ Etiology and Pathogenesis

The cause of atopic dermatitis is unknown. In genetically predisposed persons, environmental, immunologic, and physiologic factors contribute to the onset and perpetuation of the disease. Both cell-mediated and humoral factors are involved in its pathogenesis. Cell-mediated immunity is defective in almost three-fourths of patients, with increased susceptibility to cutaneous viral and dermatophyte infections and decreased delayed hypersensitivity. T helper cells are increased relative to T suppressor cells. The predominant subset of T helper cells

TABLE **47.1.**	Component Disorders in the Dermatitis — Eczema Group

Contact dermatitis
Dyshidrotic eczema
Atopic dermatitis
Neurodermatitis
Photoallergic dermatitis
Nummular eczema
Stasis dermatitis
Lichen simplex chronicus
Drug reaction

in atopic dermatitis secretes interleukin (IL)-4, IL-5, IL-6, and IL-10, and not γ-interferon. Serum IgE levels are high in 40–80% of patients, but its exact role in the pathogenesis of this disease is unknown.

The skin of atopic persons is heavily colonized with *Staphylococcus aureus*. In some studies, *Staphylococcus* has been isolated from lesional skin in more than 90% of patients compared with less than 10% of normal controls.

■ **Clinical Features**

Clinical features vary with the age of onset; thus, three patterns exist. **Infantile eczema** is characterized by acute dermatitis with an age of onset between 2 months and 2 years. Weeping, oozing, erythematous papules and plaques, which may become generalized, occur on the scalp, face, neck, and buttocks. Pruritus is severe with secondary excoriation, crusting, and infection. Exacerbations may follow immunizations, exposure to wool, and changes in the ambient humidity. In some cases, the severity of skin disease correlates with the consumption of certain foods. In most cases, the process is self-limited and resolves in 1–5 years.

Atopic childhood eczema is characterized by papular lesions in the antecubital and popliteal fossae, face, neck, and wrists. This dry eruption is very pruritic, and scratching leads to lichenification and secondary infection. Increased sensitivity to wool, animal hair, feathers, pollen, nickel, and neomycin may be noted. **Adult (and adolescent) eczema** is characterized by symmetric, erythematous, poorly demarcated plaques and patches preferentially localized to flexural sites. The plaques may consist of coalescent papules or vesicles and have scaling and lichenification. Hand dermatitis is more frequent among atopic individuals; rarely, the eruption may become generalized. Pruritus is intermittent and leads to excoriated, thickened, fissured skin. This symptom may improve with age if the cycle of itching and scratching is broken.

Patients with atopic dermatitis have frequent personal and family histories of allergic rhinitis and asthma. Anaphylactic reaction to penicillin is also more frequent. Other features include infraorbital folds, called **Dennie-Morgan folds,** allergic "shiners," facial pallor, follicular prominence or keratosis pilaris, hyperlinear palms and soles, ichthyosis vulgaris, and xerosis (dry skin). Cataracts occur in almost 20% of patients with severe disease. The excoriated, lichenified skin is more prone to disseminated viral (herpes simplex or vaccinia) infections. Other common, secondary infections are verruca vulgaris, molluscum contagiosum, and dermatophytosis.

■ **Management**

Daily bathing for 10–15 minutes, followed immediately by application of moisturizers, help rehydrate the skin and prevent cutaneous evaporation. Petroleum jelly and viscous creams such as Eucerin and Nivea are more effective than lotions and should be applied frequently. A nonsoap cleanser or a gentle moisturizing soap is preferable to ordinary soaps. During the acute phase, compresses soaked in Domeboro solution are used to cool and dry oozing eczematous skin. Topical steroids are the most commonly used agents for atopic dermatitis; other topical agents are tar preparations. Antihistamines may help with pruritus. Secondary colonization may often develop with staphylococci; therefore, those with erosions and crusting should be considered for culture and antibiotics. Severe disease has been treated with PUVA and immunosuppressives (e.g., cyclosporin).

Stasis Dermatitis

■ **Definition, Epidemiology, and Etiology**

Stasis dermatitis, an eczematous eruption occurring on the lower extremities of middle-aged and elderly adults with venous insufficiency, has a multifactorial etiology that is somewhat elusive. Patients with a history of deep venous thrombosis and venous varicosities are at risk.

■ **Clinical Features**

Erythematous patches develop above the medial and lateral malleoli, which become scaly and pruritic. Frequently, excoriations cause erosions. Rarely, autoeczematization produces a generalized eczematous or vesicular eruption due to cutaneous hyperirritability. Subacute and chronic inflammation evolves from xerotic, scaly, pruritic skin that is scratched. Hydrostatic pressure causes extravasation of red blood cells from the vessels and the gradual deposition of hemosiderin, a brown pigment.

Seborrheic Dermatitis

▪ Definition and Epidemiology

Seborrheic dermatitis is a common inflammatory skin disorder characterized by red macules and irregular patches surmounted by yellow-white, fine, greasy scales.

▪ Etiology and Pathogenesis

The cause of seborrheic dermatitis remains elusive. Because of the abundant isolation of **Pityrosporum ovale**—a lipophilic, pleomorphic fungus from the scalp lesions—and because of the observed improvement with ketoconazole treatment, this fungus may have a role in the pathogenesis of this disease. Patients with HIV infection demonstrate severe seborrheic dermatitis, which supports a role for immune dysregulation and Pityrosporum overgrowth in these patients.

▪ Clinical Features

The most common presentation is fine, greasy scaling of the scalp. Other sites include nasolabial folds, eyelids, eyebrows, ears, chest, inframammary creases, axilla, and groin. Scaly red patches on the edges of the eyelids (marginal blepharitis) may be accompanied by conjunctivitis. In severe cases, an acute eczematous eruption develops on the trunk, which may evolve into erythroderma. The course is chronic with exacerbations and remissions. The lesions often improve after exposure to sunlight during the summer, and the disease is aggravated by cold winter weather and stress.

▪ Differential Diagnosis and Management

The differential diagnosis includes atopic dermatitis, psoriasis, tinea capitis, nutritional deficiencies, and inborn errors of metabolism. A KOH examination will distinguish an atypical dermatophyte infection; with eyelid involvement, contact dermatitis should be considered.

While usually well controlled with intermittent treatment, seborrheic dermatitis frequently recurs. Scalp lesions respond to shampoos containing selenium sulfide, salicylic acid, zinc pyrithione, chloroxine, tar, or ketoconazole. Topical corticosteroid solutions are applied once or twice daily in resistant cases. Facial and intertriginous lesions respond to low-potency topical corticosteroids (e.g., 1% hydrocortisone cream). The risk of atrophy of thin skin restricts the use of more potent steroids. Ketoconazole 2% cream is used as a single agent or combined with topical corticosteroid creams.

Lichen Simplex Chronicus

▪ Definition and Epidemiology

Lichen simplex chronicus, or **neurodermatitis circumscripta,** is a chronic, pruritic disorder featuring localized, red, lichenified, scaly patches or plaques. Women aged between 30 and 50 years are more susceptible than others.

▪ Etiology

A cycle of itching and scratching is central to this disorder. The reason for the original pruritic sensation is rarely manifest. In some, the pruritus may be related to an atopic diathesis (asthma, hay fever, allergic rhinitis, and seasonal allergies) with inherent dry pruritic skin. Chronic mechanical trauma to the skin defines and perpetuates the cutaneous eruption. Chronic rubbing and scratching can induce the formation of additional nerve fibers, and this enhanced sensitivity sustains the cycle of itching and scratching.

▪ Clinical Features

Some lesions are papular or nodular and many are excoriated with overlying crusts. Common sites of involvement are the neck, extensor surfaces of the arms and legs, inner thighs, wrists, ankles, and anogenital region. Pruritus may be constant or paroxysmal. Patients report a pleasurable, comforting sensation when rubbing their skin; the cause of this reaction is unknown. In a variant of lichen simplex chronicus, known as **prurigo nodularis,** the lesions are pruritic, pink, or brown nodules localized to the extremities. The severe pruritus is relieved only by vigorous scratching that may produce bleeding and scarring.

▪ Differential Diagnosis

One helpful feature is the localization of lesions to sites within the patient's reach. Psoriasis, superficial dermatophytoses, and atopic eczema may cause diagnostic confusion. Psoriasis has characteristic white, coarse, silvery scale and pinpoint bleeding with its removal. Dermatophyte infections are evaluated with a KOH examination. Atopic dermatitis is seen in patients with an atopic diathesis and is localized to the flexor aspects of the extremities.

■ **Management**

Management of the pruritus, which perpetuates the cycle of itching and scratching, is critical. Antihistamines with topical corticosteroids or intralesional corticosteroids are the most effective; mid-potency or high-potency topical steroids are used initially. In recalcitrant cases, they may be applied topically with occlusion. Compresses with tepid water provide symptomatic relief and hasten healing. Doxepin, a tricyclic antidepressant and potent antihistamine, may also be useful in small doses. Oral or topical antibiotics are used for secondary infection.

Contact Dermatitis

■ **Definition and Epidemiology**

Contact dermatitis is an eczematous dermatitis caused by exogenous agents. The dermatitis may be immunologically mediated (allergic contact) or may be a primary irritant response (irritant contact). The former requires a sensitization phase and is limited to persons who are genetically capable of being sensitized to that particular agent. Irritants, however, may elicit a reaction in any person who is exposed. Many more agents elicit irritant contact than allergic, and many others may cause either type. Approximately 80% are irritant reactions and the remainder are allergic. Contact dermatitis is common, affecting nearly 1% of the population and accounting for almost one-fourth of all occupational disorders.

■ **Etiology and Pathogenesis**

The pathogenesis of allergic contact dermatitis has been the focus of the majority of studies. It is a delayed (cell-mediated) type of hypersensitivity reaction. Sensitization to a compound involves three steps: formation of a protein-hapten conjugate, recognition of the conjugated antigen, and proliferation of sensitized lymphocytes upon further exposure to the antigen. Memory and effector T lymphocytes then evoke an inflammatory cutaneous response. Since sensitization is involved, a period of 7–14 days may elapse between initial contact and a rash, thus often creating confusion regarding the cause. On re-exposure, the rash may manifest within 24–48 hours. Irritant dermatitis, in contrast, follows contact within 24 hours.

A myriad of environmental agents can cause contact dermatitis. Irritant dermatitis is most frequently due to acid or alkali compounds, detergents, and soaps. Poison ivy (rhus) dermatitis is the prototype of allergic contact dermatitis (see Color Plate 13).

■ **Clinical Features**

The acute phase of contact dermatitis consists of a pruritic, erythematous, weeping eruption, with occasional frank vesicles or bullae. The dermatitis is usually limited to areas of contact with the offending agent. With subacute or chronic dermatitis, the vesicles and weeping subside, and a scaly, lichenified appearance develops. Fissuring may be seen in chronic cases. While irritants may elicit more burning and pain, and allergic reactions more pruritus, physical examination alone can rarely distinguish the two.

■ **Diagnosis and Management**

A good history and the pattern of localization give the most valuable clue to the correct diagnosis of contact dermatitis. Allergic contact dermatitis may be confirmed by patch testing. Dyshidrotic hand dermatitis, tinea pedis or manum, palmar-plantar psoriasis, or atopic dermatitis may cause diagnostic confusion.

In acute contact dermatitis, use of soaks or compresses combined with a potent topical steroid cream or lotion is the first step. An ointment-based steroid may be more appropriate as the vesiculation or weeping subsides and where scaling and lichenification are prominent features, as in more chronic cases. In some cases of widespread acute contact dermatitis, especially those involving the face, a short course of systemic steroids may be indicated. Oral antihistamines or topical anesthetic lotions (Sarna™, pramoxine) will help with pruritus. Secondary staphylococcal infection is not uncommon, and should be appropriately treated. Identification and elimination of the offending agent is key to successfully treating contact dermatitis.

CHAPTER 48 BENIGN TUMORS OF THE SKIN

Seborrheic Keratosis

■ Definition, Etiology, and Pathogenesis

Seborrheic keratoses are benign cutaneous tumors usually involving the trunk and commonly affecting individuals in the fourth decade and beyond. Reports of patients with numerous lesions in familial clusters suggest but do not establish a genetic predisposition. Altered cytokeratin expression in seborrheic keratoses has been documented, but the significance is unknown.

■ Clinical Features

Single or multiple lesions are most often observed on the trunk but also on the face, scalp, neck, and extremities. The palms, soles, and oral mucosa are spared. Initially, the lesions are well-demarcated, brown macules. They evolve into papillated plaques with prominent follicular plugs. The "stuck-on" appearance and the greasy irregular surface are classic findings. When removed, the base is moist and pink. Usually, they are 2 mm to 3 cm and brown but may appear black or flesh-colored. Some patients experience intermittent pruritus with these lesions and remove them by scratching.

The abrupt appearance of numerous pruritic seborrheic keratoses (the sign of Leser-Trélat) in adults may signal an internal malignancy. Slightly over half the reported cancers are adenocarcinomas, the leading site being the stomach, followed by malignancies of the breast and lung, and leukemias. However, studies using controls have not proven such a relationship.

■ Differential Diagnosis and Management

While the clinical findings often suggest the diagnosis, some deeply pigmented lesions simulate malignant melanoma or a compound nevus. The sharp demarcation and the verrucous surface suggest seborrheic keratosis. Differentiation is also needed from verruca and solar keratoses. Seborrheic keratoses are effectively removed with liquid nitrogen or curettage. Atypical lesions and those resembling melanoma should be excised surgically.

Actinic (Solar) Keratosis

■ Definition and Epidemiology

Actinic keratoses are common premalignant lesions that develop on chronically sun-exposed areas. Related to cumulative sun exposure, they are the first clinical stage in the evolution of a squamous cell carcinoma. Risk factors for their development include fair skin type, failure to protect the skin with sun screens, and exposure to high-intensity solar irradiation. Older adults with blue eyes, freckling, and a fair complexion who live in sunny, warm regions are at greatest risk for developing actinic keratoses and skin cancer. In high-risk persons, these keratoses may occur even at the age of 20 or 30 years.

■ Clinical Features

Unless irritated or traumatized, the lesions usually cause no symptoms. The face, ears, dorsal hands, and forearms are the most commonly involved sites. The 1–10-mm flesh-colored, pink, or red macules or scaly papules are more easily felt by palpation than identified visually. The surface is verrucous or hyperkeratotic with variable amounts of fine white scale. Hypertrophic actinic keratoses may form cutaneous horns; squamous cell cancer may develop later in the base. Other signs of excessive sun exposure may also be seen—for example, telangiectases, lentigines, and excessive wrinkling.

The rate of neoplastic transformation of actinic keratoses ranges from 5% to 15%. These squamous cell cancers are generally not aggressive, and their metastatic potential is limited. However, lesions in specific sites (e.g., the hands, ears, and lips) may be more aggressive, thus having a higher metastatic potential.

■ Differential Diagnosis

The clinical findings usually suggest the diagnosis. Seborrheic keratoses, disseminated superficial actinic porokeratoses, Bowen's disease, and squamous cell cancer may cause diagnostic confusion. Seborrheic keratosis has distinctive plugs on its surface and a "stuck on" appearance. In porokeratosis, the lesion has an elevated rim at the periphery. Bowen's disease is more finely demarcated, and squamous cell cancers are more indurated. Erosion, ulceration, and progressive enlargement are more typical of squamous cell cancer.

Management

Daily use of broad-spectrum sunscreens should be recommended to all patients with actinic keratoses. Lesions in limited numbers are often treatable with cryo-ablation with liquid nitrogen. Surgical excision, although rarely indicated as primary therapy, may sometimes be needed to establish the diagnosis. Topical 5-fluorouracil (T5-FU), 1% or 5% cream, applied twice daily, is the most effective therapy for multiple lesions or large areas of involvement. T5-FU elicits an inflammatory reaction at the site of precancerous and cancerous lesions. Generally, the T5-FU creams are used for 2 to 3 weeks, or for 3 days after the most intense inflammation; topical steroids may be applied in conjunction with the T5-FU to reduce the severity of the reaction. As an alternative, masoprocol cream, applied for 4 weeks, may significantly reduce the number of lesions. Masoprocol, which is an irritant, may cause contact sensitization.

Melanocytic Nevi

Definition and Epidemiology

Melanocytic nevi are congenital or acquired benign neoplasms of melanocytes or nevus cells. Melanocytes are single, fusiform, or dendritic, and nevus cells are round or oval and grouped into nests; both are derived from the neural crest and may be distinguished by size and distribution.

Pigmented nevi are the most common tumors in adults and children. Benign melanocytic nevi are acquired from 6–12 months of age until almost 25 years. The number of nevi is highest, averaging 40, at around age 25, after which they decline to almost zero by age 90. Caucasians and women acquire more nevi than persons of African descent and men, respectively. Nevi may be rapidly acquired during pregnancy, after intense sun exposure, or following therapy with corticosteroids, ACTH, or estrogen.

Etiology and Pathology

The exact origin of the nevus cell is uncertain. Based on their anatomic location, three primary variant nevi exist: junctional, compound, and intradermal types. Microscopically, **junctional nevi** show nests of nevus cells in the lower epidermis above the basement membrane zone. **Compound nevi** have both epidermal and dermal nests of nevus cells. In **intradermal nevi,** the cells are confined entirely to the dermis. Eventually, nevi regress with fibrous, fatty, or mucinous degeneration.

Clinical Features

Benign, pigmented lesions are characterized by a smooth border, even color, and sharp circumscription. Any cutaneous or mucosal site may be affected, but lesions in the oral cavity are unusual. A nevus enlarges proportionate to body growth, with eventual regression. The junctional nevus, the most common type of nevus found on palms, soles, and scrotum, is a smooth, brown or tan, 1-10-mm macule without terminal hairs. Round or oval, it has a uniform pigment and sharp borders, and retains skin markings on its surface. A compound nevus is a brown, black, or flesh-colored papule with a smooth or gently papillated surface. It tends to be only slightly raised from the surrounding skin. Occasionally, its central portion is more darkly pigmented. Coarse, dark hair may be present. An intradermal nevus is either a dome-shaped or a soft pedunculated papule, which may have hair. Although often flesh-colored, it may be brown or black. Usually smaller than 5 mm in diameter, intradermal nevi occur in adults.

Differential Diagnosis and Management

Junctional melanocytic nevi may be difficult to distinguish from freckles, lentigines, or *café au lait* macules. Other entities in this differential diagnosis include a blue nevus, seborrheic keratosis, epidermal nevus, angiofibroma, Becker's nevus, dermatofibroma, molluscum contagiosum, and early melanoma.

Most cases of benign melanocytic nevi require no treatment; the primary reason for removal is cosmetic. Symptomatic nevi from frequent trauma and features indicating possible malignancy may also warrant treatment. If a personal or family history of malignant melanoma is present, selected nevi may be excised if they are in a location that is difficult to follow. Giant congenital nevi carry a significant risk for melanoma and require staged excision, if possible.

Acrochordon

Acrochordons (skin tags) are flesh-colored to brown papules located on the neck, eyelids, and axilla. Less frequently, these pedunculated or sessile lesions occur on the trunk and groin. They are soft and usually measure

1–3 mm. Giant acrochordons may be several centimeters long. Their appearance or their tendency to become traumatized by clothing or jewelry may cause patients to request their removal, which may be done by electrodesiccation or excision.

Keloids

■ Definition and Etiology

A keloid is an excessive overgrowth of fibrous tissue at the site of a previous wound; it presents as a firm, smooth, red to pink tumor. Persons of African and Hispanic descent tend to develop keloids, but the reasons are unclear.

■ Clinical Features

Keloids have well-demarcated and angular borders with irregular extensions beyond the site of the original wound. The outline depends on the type of injury, the more common ones being burns and lacerations. Less often, they occur as sequelae of inflammatory acne. The sites of predilection are the sternum, neck, ear lobes, trunk, and extremities. **Telangiectases** may be evident through the thinned epidermis, and ulceration may occur. Patients often complain of tenderness or pruritus in early lesions.

■ Differential Diagnosis and Management

The diagnosis of keloid is usually evident from the distinctive clinical features. The only entity that is likely to cause confusion is a hypertrophic scar, which spontaneously improves within the first 6 months of formation and lacks fibrous projections beyond the original site.

No treatment is uniformly effective. In many cases, intralesional injection of triamcinolone suspension produces flattening of the lesions and may be used every 6 to 8 weeks. Some keloids are amenable to surgical excision, but at a significant chance of recurrence—which may be lessened by instilling triamcinolone into the suture site at the time of surgery. Other, less frequently used treatment options are x-ray therapy and methotrexate, which may be combined with surgery and silastic gel sheeting.

Epidermal Cyst

■ Definition, Epidemiology, and Etiology

Epidermal cysts are known by various terms, including sebaceous cysts, keratin cysts, and epidermoid cysts. "Sebaceous cyst" is a misnomer because it involves differentiation toward keratin and not sebaceous gland lobules. These cysts are discrete, firm, elevated tumors located in the dermis or subcutis, and usually observed after puberty. Their etiology is uncertain. Although some lesions may be attributed to the traumatic inoculation of epidermal fragments into the dermis or embryonic entrapment of epidermal cells, most arise spontaneously from occlusion of pilosebaceous follicles. The cyst has an epidermal lining and is filled with keratin and lipid debris, which are white, malodorous, and rarely drain from its punctum. Enlargement occurs due to keratin production in a space that cannot drain to the surface.

■ Clinical Features

The most common sites of involvement are the face, scalp, neck, back, and scrotum. With gradual enlargement, these cysts reach a final size of 0.5–5.0 cm. The epidermis above the lesion is normal or thinned from increasing pressure. The punctum in the skin represents the remnants of a ductal structure. Although adherent to the epidermis, the cyst is freely movable in the dermis. It is asymptomatic unless traumatized, infected, or ruptured, in which case intense inflammation and tenderness ensue.

■ Differential Diagnosis and Management

The diagnosis, which is usually based on clinical information, may be made definitively with a biopsy. Lipomas, metastatic cancer, and occasionally neurofibromas may cause some confusion.

Both medical and surgical treatments are applicable. Inflamed cysts often diminish in size with the intralesional injection of corticosteroids. Ruptured and inflamed cysts may be incised and drained. At times, the cyst wall may be removed after the inflammation subsides. Surgical excision, the definitive treatment, is difficult if the lesion has been inflamed because fibrosis causes the cyst wall to adhere to the surrounding tissue. Unless the cyst wall is fully excised, the cyst will recur and inflammation will follow.

Lipomas

■ Definition and Clinical Features

Lipomas are benign subcutaneous tumors composed of fatty tissue, commonly seen on the trunk, forearms, posterior neck, buttocks, and thighs. These soft, rubbery, poorly demarcated, and freely movable nodules are generally less than 2 cm but can become large (10 cm). Single or multiple, the lesions are asymptomatic unless traumatized due to the location or size. The onset is usually between the ages of 30 and 40 years. Malignant change is rare but may occur in large lesions. Midline lipomas may indicate spinal dysraphism and should be evaluated by magnetic resonance imaging of the spine prior to excision.

■ Differential Diagnosis and Management

A lipoma may need to be distinguished from its variant forms (angiolipoma, hibernoma) or from an epidermoid cyst. An **angiolipoma** contains vascular elements and is tender to palpation. A **hibernoma** contains embryonic brown fat. Firm, well-demarcated borders are suggestive of a cyst. Lipoma is reliably diagnosed by examination of a tissue specimen. Unless cosmetic concerns or symptoms exist, treatment is not needed. Surgical excision with a primary closure is the treatment of choice.

CHAPTER **49**   # MALIGNANT TUMORS OF THE SKIN

Malignant Melanoma

■ Definition and Epidemiology

Malignant melanoma, a cutaneous neoplasm with a rising incidence in the United States and and a rising mortality rate, may develop in any tissue in which **melanocytes** are found, including the skin, mucous membranes, retina, and the site of a benign nevus. The common phenotype is a fair-skinned, sun-sensitive person with red or blond hair, blue eyes, abundant moles, and a tendency to freckle. Blistering sunburns in childhood indicate increased risk for melanoma. Intense sun exposure enhances the risk of melanoma for anyone.

Race is also strongly associated with melanoma, with Caucasians more frequently affected than African Americans or Hispanics. In Europe, melanoma afflicts Celtic or Nordic populations more often than Mediterraneans, again because of skin type and patterns of sun exposure. African Americans tend to develop melanoma in the palms, soles, nail beds, and mucosal surfaces.

The incidence of melanoma rises with decreasing latitude, as shown in the United States and Australia. Socioeconomic status indirectly influences the development of melanoma as the more affluent are more likely to develop a melanoma. It has been hypothesized that the affluent are more likely to receive intermittent, intense sun exposure through recreational activities, and this type of exposure may be more influential in the development of melanoma than chronic exposure.

■ Etiology

Malignant melanoma is caused by multiple factors. Most investigators believe that tumor formation requires at least two separate genetic events. **Oncogenes** and **anti-oncogenes** are implicated in the cause of melanoma, with the anti-oncogenes that suppress neoplasia being the most important. Other genes that determine the susceptible phenotypes (e.g., those controlling pigmentation, DNA repair, and response to solar irradiation) probably also play a role. Although specific genes have been isolated, the involvement has been inconsistent. Genetic alterations may follow an environmental stimulus such as sun exposure and lead to **lentigo maligna melanoma,** but superficial spreading melanomas can arise in sun-protected sites. Thus, genetic factors are pivotal in the causation of melanoma as determinants of a phenotype with particular susceptibility, and as steps in tumor formation.

■ Clinical Features

Features of a melanocytic lesion suggesting malignant melanoma are asymmetry; irregular notched borders; multiple shades of tan, brown, and black; and a diameter exceeding 6 mm. Among the four primary clinical subtypes with divergent histologic findings and

TABLE 49.1.	Clinical Subtypes of Malignant Melanoma and Their Characteristics			
Subtype	**Characteristics**	**Appearance of Lesions**	**Frequency**	**Comments**
Superficial spreading melanoma (Color Plate 14)	Radial growth phase 1–5 yrs; predilection for the trunk in men and the lower extremities in women; median age at diagnosis is the fifth decade.	Flat papule or plaque, <3 cm in diameter, irregular borders, and patches of pink, brown, black, or white and areas of regression.	70% of all cases	Dysplastic or congenital nevi are precursor lesions. Regression may also reflect depth inaccurately and underestimate the tumor growth.
Nodular melanoma	Brief or absent radial growth and rapid vertical extension; most develop in 6–18 months. Men more affected than women; the trunk, head, and neck are the favored sites; the mean age of onset is in the sixth decade.	Symmetric blue, gray, or black dome-shaped nodules or pedunculated papules, with average size, 1–2 cm. Pedunculated ones are particularly aggressive. A small fraction are amelanotic.	15–30%	Aggressive lesions
Lentigo maligna melanoma	Slowly evolving. Present for 3–15 years at diagnosis. Most common in older women on the sun-exposed skin of the head and neck. Patients usually in the seventh decade of life.	Initially a tan macule, gradually enlarges to >3 cm. Exhibits asymmetry and varied color, and flecks of pigment may be noted within the brown or tan areas. After years of progression, the surface becomes irregularly elevated.	5% of all cases	Low risk of metastasis. Some clinicians designate the flat lesion as lentigo maligna and the elevated lesion as lentigo maligna melanoma.
Acral lentiginous variant	Involves the palms, soles, mucosa, nail bed, and periungual regions. The sole is the most frequently described location. Affects older individuals of both genders.	Nail bed melanomas produce a visible, pigmented band. Pigmentation of the proximal nail fold (Hutchinson's sign) is useful diagnostically. Diameter often >3 cm. May initially resemble lentigo maligna type. Ulceration and hyperkeratosis observed in the nodular sections of the neoplasm.	1–10% among Caucasians. Most common type in Asians, Hispanics, and American Indians.	Aggressive lesions. Often develop in 6 months.

clinical courses (Table 49.1), the outcome best correlates with the depth of tumor invasion (using the Breslow scale or Clark's correlation measurement; see the following) at diagnosis. Superficial spreading melanoma (see Color Plate 14) may show signs of regression; because both favorable and adverse outcomes are related to regression, its relevance is controversial. Nodular melanoma often has a worse prognosis, probably because of the melanoma's greater depth at diagnosis. The acral lentiginous variant also has a poor outcome because its recognition is often delayed. Metastases in melanoma follow local extension and occur by lymphatic or hematogenous invasion.

■ Differential Diagnosis and Management

All the previously described characteristics of malignancy may not be present in an individual lesion. Entities that may cause confusion include seborrheic keratosis, solar lentigo, pyogenic granuloma, metastatic renal cell carcinoma, pigmented basal cell carcinoma, blue nevus, hemangioma, and pigmented Spitz nevus.

The rapid diagnosis of malignant melanoma is crucial to the survival of the patient because early detection and treatment lead to frequent cures. However, the rate of cure declines with the degree of vertical growth. Two classification systems were developed to provide estimates of survival. The **Breslow scale** relies on tumor thickness, and **Clark's correlation** links survival with the anatomic level of invasion. Favorable prognostic features include a thickness less than 0.76 mm, low mitotic rate, brisk infiltration of the tumor by lymphocytes, feminine gender, location on the extremities, and absence of regression or ulceration.

Any suspicious pigmented lesion should be excised with adequate borders of normal skin (1–2 mm). Photographs provide excellent documentation for subsequent examination. Some advocate excising uninvolved regional lymph nodes when the primary lesion is treated as a means of inhibiting subsequent dissemination. Although applicable for melanomas exceeding 0.76 mm, this approach is not suitable for lesions with a high probability of metastasis at diagnosis. Regional lymph node or skin metastases are treated by surgical excision. The therapy for widely metastatic disease may relieve symptoms but only slightly extends survival. Irradiation, dacarbazine or combination chemotherapy, regional limb perfusion, or high-dose chemotherapy followed by bone marrow transplantation are other options. IL-2 has been approved for treating advanced melanomas.

After treatment, patients with confirmed malignant melanoma should be monitored regularly, using the depth of the lesion as the guide for the interval between visits. At each visit, the skin and lymph nodes should be thoroughly examined and the liver span assessed as an indicator of metastatic disease. Chest roentgenograms should be obtained yearly.

Dysplastic Nevus Syndrome

■ Definition and Epidemiology

A dysplastic nevus is a large, irregular, melanocytic nevus with cytologic atypia and specific architectural features. The term "dysplastic nevus syndrome" continues to generate controversy because of incomplete agreement about the histologic definition of this lesion and its natural history. Most dermatopathologists use strict criteria to identify this entity but emphasize either architectural or cytologic features. A sporadic form and a familial variety are now recognized; the latter is inherited in an autosomal dominant mode. The risk of a melanoma developing is far greater in persons with an inherited predisposition for dysplastic nevi than for those who have the sporadic form.

An NIH Consensus Conference in 1984 recommended categorizing those individuals with dysplastic nevi into four groups that correlated with risk of melanoma. The criteria considered in this classification were the following: personal history of melanoma and family history of multiple nevi and melanoma. Patients with the highest risk for the development of melanoma are those with a personal history of melanoma and two or more family members with a history of melanoma and multiple nevi. Those with the lowest risk have none of the pertinent criteria.

■ Clinical Features

Dysplastic nevi measure 6–15 mm in diameter and are variegated with shades of pink, tan, and brown. The pink color is usually peripheral to the central tan and brown (creating a "fried egg" configuration). Often, the lesions are flat, but central papules or a cobblestone surface is not unusual. The border is irregular and poorly defined but lacks the scalloping of a malignant melanoma. While commonly located on the back, they are also typically seen on the chest, abdomen, and extremities. Greater numbers of dysplastic nevi develop on sun-protected skin such as the buttocks, scalp, and breasts. They arise during puberty and continue to develop during adulthood. Many patients acquire more than 100 lesions.

■ Differential Diagnosis and Management

The diagnosis of a dysplastic nevus and the dysplastic nevus syndrome is based on the characteristic clinical features, histologic criteria, and medical history. The differential diagnosis is mainly between a compound nevus and melanoma. The initial management for a patient with suspected dysplastic nevi includes a thorough family history and a full skin examination with attention to the scalp, feet, buttocks, and breasts. Compared with common nevi, these are not only the sites where dysplastic nevi most abound but also those that are unlikely to be routinely examined. The measurements of all atypical nevi should be recorded. Most authorities advocate removing two representative lesions for histology. Biopsies should be taken from those nevi that have reportedly changed or are difficult to examine due to their location in hair-bearing areas. The patient should be told about the importance of sun protection and regular examination of the skin as well as the role of dysplastic nevi as potential markers for high risk of malignant melanoma. High-risk patients are examined every 3–6 months; low-risk patients are examined yearly.

Basal Cell Carcinoma

■ Definition, Epidemiology, and Etiology

Basal cell carcinoma derives from the basal layer of the epidermis and outer root sheath of the hair follicle. Strongly associated with excessive, chronic sun exposure, this carcinoma usually affects older persons with fair skin. Its higher frequency among men may be explained by the fact that men have traditionally done outdoor work. This carcinoma is not usual in African Americans. The histologic features determine the natural history of an individual lesion. For poorly defined reasons, basal cell carcinomas are associated with scars and exposure to ultraviolet light, X-rays, and arsenic. Some recent studies implicate oncogenes and anti-oncogenes in the pathogenesis of this cancer.

■ Clinical Features

Basal cell carcinoma has many clinical and histologic variants. The **nodular basal cell carcinoma** arises on the face or other sun-exposed (usually sun-damaged) site as a dome-shaped papule or nodule with a raised, pearly border and often with telangiectases (see Color Plate 15). The surface is generally smooth and shiny but may be ulcerated, scaly, and crusted. The **pigmented basal cell carcinoma,** with a color ranging from shades of tan or brown to black, may mimic malignant melanoma. The sclerosing or morpheaform type is a pink, flesh-colored, or white flat-topped papule or plaque that often extends beyond the visible borders. Superficial basal cell carcinomas are clinically subtle; these red, scaly plaques are often mistaken for solar keratoses, eczema, or psoriasis; untreated, they may cause extensive local destruction—despite the rarity of metastases. Periorbitally located invasive lesions may imperil vision by infiltrating the nerves and muscles. Nerve involvement and invasion of dermis by small discrete strands of cells signal a poor prognosis. Tumor size, location, and histologic features influence rates of recurrence and the odds of metastases, which occur by lymphatic spread.

■ Diagnosis and Management

Although the nodular basal cell carcinoma is easily identified, the recognition of the pigmented or scaly nodules and plaques is more difficult. Solar keratosis, psoriasis, melanoma, morphea, sebaceous hyperplasia, Bowen's disease, and seborrheic keratosis frequently must be distinguished from a basal cell carcinoma. Definitive diagnosis requires a biopsy.

Treatment of a basal cell carcinoma varies with its size, site, and histology as well as its status as a primary tumor, local recurrence, or metastasis. The goal of any treatment is histologic cure with optimal cosmetic results. For the primary tumor, available methods are surgery, electrodesiccation and curettage, radiation, or cryotherapy. In **Mohs micrographic surgery,** the tumor mass is removed by serial tangential sections that are examined histologically for residual neoplastic cells at the time of surgery. This surgery is used for large, recurrent cancers that exhibit aggressive histologic patterns or present on sites with high recurrence rates. Selected patients may also benefit from retinoids, immunotherapy with α-interferon, photodynamic therapy, and topical or systemic chemotherapy. The latter (with cisplatin and doxorubicin) is used for metastatic lesions. The role of education about protection from sun exposure cannot be overemphasized.

Squamous Cell Carcinoma

■ Definition and Epidemiology

Squamous cell carcinoma, an epithelial neoplasm, evolves from a clone of atypical keratinocytes. Some tumors are confined to the thickness of the epidermis and are called squamous cell carcinoma-in-situ or **Bowen's disease;** others penetrate the basement membrane, extend into the dermis and subcuticular tissue, and metastasize. Squamous cell carcinomas represent nearly 20% of all nonmelanoma skin cancers. They most commonly afflict older persons, persons with a fair complexion, and men. Many factors, particularly ultraviolet radiation, influence the incidence of squamous cell carcinoma. Increased recreational tanning is believed to cause many new cases.

■ Etiology and Pathogenesis

Squamous cell carcinoma of the skin evolves when a vulnerable host is exposed to carcinogens. Intrinsic risk factors are age, skin type, immune status, xeroderma pigmentosum, and lymphoproliferative disorders. Burn scars, chronic ulcers, or sinuses and premalignant lesions such as solar keratoses have a high rate of malignant degeneration. External risk factors are arsenic, UVA exposure with PUVA therapy, immunosuppressive agents, x-rays, hydrocarbons, human *papillomavirus* infection, and solar irradiation. Some of these factors cause direct damage to cellular DNA. The damaged, atypical cells divide for months or years until a clinical lesion is visible. For many of the other factors, the mechanism of carcinogenesis remains elusive.

■ Clinical Features

Squamous cell carcinomas frequently arise on sun-exposed sites as well-demarcated red plaques or nodules with a scaly, verrucous, or papillated surface. Compared with basal cell carcinomas, a predilection exists for the dorsal hands, scalp, and pinna. As the cancer cells invade the dermis and subcutis, the plaques become firm, indurated, and fixed to underlying structures. Ulceration and bleeding are common (see Color Plate 16). These lesions often run an indolent course with many years of radial growth. Solar lentigines, actinic keratoses, and other signs of sun damage are usually seen on the surrounding skin.

The other common settings that harbor these cancers are scarred or chronically inflamed tissues. Lesions originating within burn scars, radiation ports, chronic ulcers, or sinuses behave aggressively, despite their frequent presence for many months or years prior to diagnosis. The rate of metastasis is much greater in these patients. Invasive squamous cell carcinoma occurs in 5–15% of solar keratoses.

Many of the same factors that are predictive of recurrence and metastasis for basal cell carcinomas apply also to squamous cell carcinomas. Large, deep, and poorly differentiated lesions are more likely to be aggressive. The ear, lip, and inner canthus of the eye are sites with particularly high rates of recurrence and increased metastatic potential. Other poor prognostic factors are perineural spread, previous recurrence with adequate treatment, and formation within a scar. Patients treated with immunosuppressive drugs, especially for renal transplants, acquire greater numbers of tumors with an aggressive course. Widespread disease begins with lymph node involvement.

■ Diagnosis and Differential Diagnosis

The diagnosis frequently requires a biopsy. Clinical suspicion is aroused by the appropriate setting and presentation but squamous cell carcinomas may resemble superficial basal cell carcinomas, keratoacanthoma, verrucous lesions (warts and seborrheic keratoses), metastatic neoplasms, pyogenic granulomas, plaques of psoriasis or eczema, amelanotic or verrucous melanomas, and other papulosquamous disorders.

■ Management

The treatment of squamous cell carcinoma is similar to that of basal cell carcinoma. Superficial lesions may be removed by excision, electrodesiccation and curettage, or cryosurgery using probes to assess the depth of tissue necrosis with freezing. Tumors that are large, deep, or localized to sites with a high risk of invasion are treated with Mohs micrographic surgery, which is also preferred for lesions with neurotropism or basosquamous histology.

CHAPTER **50** ACNE

Acne Vulgaris

■ Definition and Epidemiology

Acne vulgaris, a very common skin disorder, is a self-limited inflammatory disorder of the pilosebaceous unit. Usually beginning at puberty and affecting mostly adolescents (85% of persons between 12 and 25 years of age), acne predominantly appears in areas where the pilosebaceous follicles are the most dense—namely, the face, neck, and upper trunk. In girls, it may precede menarche. The peak prevalence is age 14–17 years in girls and 16–19 years in boys, with a higher frequency and severity in boys. Most patients note significant improvement by age 20–23 years, but in 8–10% some activity continues into the fifth decade.

The inheritance pattern of acne vulgaris has not been established, but most experts invoke an autosomal dominant trait with variable penetrance or a polygenic trait involving many genes. Since Caucasian Americans are affected more often than Japanese or African Americans, genetics may play a role.

■ Etiology and Pathogenesis

Acne develops from the interaction of multiple factors. Lipid is released into the follicular canal as part of a complex mixture called sebum that lubricates the skin. In acne, sebum is produced in excess, perhaps due to changes in androgen levels. The sebum composition is altered compared to those without acne, with a significantly lower level of linoleic acid. This abnormality may encourage the cohesion of cornified cells; their accumulation in sebaceous follicles results in comedones. These noninflammatory lesions are transformed into inflammatory lesions by *Propionibacterium acnes* in the follicular canal. *P. acnes* incites inflammation by generating free fatty acids and by recruiting lymphocytes and neutrophils, which release inflammatory mediators. The inflammatory products and sebum exert pressure on the epithelial wall, causing the follicle to rupture; inflammatory papules, pustules, and nodules follow.

■ Clinical Features

Acne vulgaris has a number of clinical variants, with combinations of comedones, papules, pustules, nodules, and cysts. An open comedone is black due to the oxidation of accumulated material and the presence of melanin. A closed comedone is a flesh-colored papule with a minute ostium that inhibits the discharge of keratin debris. This is the primary lesion in the formation of inflammatory papules and pustules. In severe cases, nodules, cysts, and granulomatous lesions develop progressively. This intense inflammation finally leads to fibrosis, scars, and keloids. Individual papules and pustules resolve with transient erythema and postinflammatory hyperpigmentation, which can be particularly prominent in African Americans and takes months to improve.

■ Diagnosis and Differential Diagnosis

A complete history should be obtained to establish the cause, duration, localization, and severity. In susceptible individuals, the onset or exacerbation of acne is influenced by a family history of acne; menses; occupational exposure to oils, tars, greases, chlorinated hydrocarbons, and waxes; medications such as oral contra-ceptives, corticosteroids, iodides, isoniazid, lithium, phenytoin, and trimethadione; and cosmetics or hair preparations and androgen excess denoted by hirsutism or menstrual irregularities. While typically distributed eruptions are diagnostic, acneiform lesions may occur in rosacea, perioral dermatitis, miliaria rubra, impetigo contagiosa, and folliculitis.

■ Management

The treatment regimen is determined by the severity of the disease and the predominant type of lesion. Topical (Table 50.1) and systemic agents can reduce bacterial load, inhibit inflammation, decrease sebaceous gland activity, and impede corneocyte adhesion. Dietary restrictions have no role.

Inflammatory papules, pustules, and nodules are controlled with systemic antibiotics. They eliminate *P. acne* from the skin, thus decreasing the free fatty acids in the sebaceous glands. Tetracycline, 1.0 g daily, tapered as clinical improvement occurs, is a safe, effective, and inexpensive initial choice. Significant response may take 4–6 weeks. Alternative agents are erythromycin, doxycycline, and sulfonamides. Persons receiving tetracycline should avoid sun exposure.

The only medication likely to produce a remission in patients with recalcitrant severe acne is isotretinoin or Accutane, a vitamin-A derivative. All forms of acne respond to it but the side-effect profile restricts its use to only the most severe cases. Isotretinoin is given in a dose of 0.5–2 mg/kg/day; doses less than 1 mg/kg/day enhance the likelihood of recurrence. Its teratogenicity precludes its use in pregnancy. Other common complications are dry skin and mucous membranes, hyperlipidemia, mucositis, cheilitis, conjunctivitis, skin fragility, impaired night vision, desquamation of palms and soles, headache, and myalgia. An increased risk of pseudotumor cerebri exists, especially when tetracyclines are given simultaneously.

Comedonal acne is best treated by the topical vitamin A derivative, tretinoin (Retin A™), which normalizes keratinization in the follicles and suppresses bacterial proliferation. The formation of new follicular plugs is inhibited and existing plugs are eliminated. Tretinoin is applied in a thin layer every night to dry skin. Early complications include burning, erythema, and peeling. The concentration of the preparation is increased according to response and tolerance. It is indicated for all types of acne because comedones are a common component.

The use of Benzoyl peroxide as a topical bactericidal agent either alone or combined with tretinoin or antibiotics significantly reduces the density of *P. acne* on the skin. Many different preparations contain benzoyl peroxide, with concentrations varying between 2.5% and

TABLE 50.1.	Commonly Used Topical Products for Acne			
Agent	**Formulation**	**Use**	**Action**	**Side Effects**
Benzoyl peroxide	5, 10% gel; 2.5, 4% wash	1–2 times daily	Keratolytic; some antibacterial action	Irritation; allergic contact dermatitis
Tretinoin (Retin A®)	0.025, 0.05, 0.1% cream 0.01, 0.025% gel; 0.05% liquid	Once daily at bedtime	Comedolytic	Irritation; allergic contact dermatitis (rare); increased susceptibility to sunburn
Topical antibiotics	1% clindamycin; 2% erythromycin	1–2 time(s) daily	Antibacterial	Irritation; allergic contact dermatitis (rare); GI disturbances, including colitis (clindamycin, extremely rare)
Salicylic acid	2% wash	2–3 times daily	Keratolytic as a cleanser	Irritation

10%. Irritation is the most important side effect, related to the concentration of benzoyl peroxide and the vehicle. Another treatment option in mild to moderate acne vulgaris is topical antibiotics to decrease the population of *P. acne*, the most effective ones being 1% clindamycin and 2% erythromycin. Bacterial resistance may follow topical and systemic antibiotic use. Selected patients may use oral corticosteroids, oral contraceptives, and dapsone. Other ingredients included in topical preparations are salicylic acid, resorcinol, sulfur, and metronidazole.

Acne surgery is the physical removal of the contents of comedones, pustules, and cysts to promote rapid improvement while the patient awaits the gradual effects of topical or systemic therapy. The intralesional injection of triamcinolone acetonide into large inflammatory cysts, pustules, and nodules leads to resolution of lesions with less scarring.

Acne Rosacea

■ Definition, Epidemiology, and Etiology

Rosacea, a chronic vascular and inflammatory disorder, occurs primarily on the central region of the face and has two primary components: (1) the vascular component consists of erythema and telangiectases; (2) the acneiform component consists of papules, pustules, and sebaceous gland hyperplasia. The inflammatory lesions exacerbate and remit and, when deep, often heal with scarring. Although associated with menopause and observed most commonly in women aged 30 to 50 years, rosacea is more severe in men. It is rare in African American patients.

The cause of rosacea is unknown. Vascular instability, with a consistent tendency to blush and flush easily, is an important element. Celtic origin and a fair complexion are also risk factors. Vasodilators (e.g., hot liquids, alcohol, spicy foods, and sun exposure) exacerbate it. Although patients with increased numbers of Demodex folliculorum mites improve as the organism is eliminated by treatment, the association with Demodex is inconsistent. Sebaceous gland activity is stimulated, but not as the primary event. Unlike acne vulgaris, abnormal keratinization is absent.

■ Clinical Features

The cheeks, chin, nose, forehead, eyes, and, less often, the seborrheic areas of the chest, scalp, and posterior ears are involved. The disease evolves from intermittent episodes of flushing and blushing to persistent erythema and telangiectasia on the nose and cheeks. This may occur as early as the second decade. Crops of papules and pustules develop and the orifices of sebaceous glands become prominent. In severe cases, the nose becomes thickened and disfigured with the formation of rhinophyma. Rarely, inflammatory nodules are seen, which may be granulomatous or connected by sinus tracts, furuncles, and abscesses. The eyes are commonly involved, and blepharitis, conjunctivitis, iritis, keratitis, iridocyclitis, and hypopyon are common. Early eye involvement may be unnoticed by the treating physician.

■ Differential Diagnosis

Acne vulgaris, seborrheic dermatitis, lupus erythematosus, and carcinoid syndrome simulate rosacea. Lack of comedones and distribution in the medial face help distinguish it from acne vulgaris. The lesions of seborrheic dermatitis are red or pink macules covered with greasy yellow scales and localized to the eyebrows, nasolabial folds, scalp, chest, and ears. Lupus erythematosus and carcinoid syndrome can be established by estimating antinuclear antibodies and 5-hydroxyindoleacetic acid, respectively, especially in atypical cases.

■ Management

Rosacea has a spectrum of severity and its course is punctuated by exacerbations and remissions. However, even aggressive therapy rarely resolves all lesions completely. The use of a broad-spectrum sun screen should always be encouraged. Mild disease needs no treatment except avoiding sun exposure and other vasodilatory agents. Moderate disease often responds well to oral tetracycline with or without topical metronidazole. Usually, tetracycline (1.0 g/d) for 4–6 weeks will suffice until the flare remits; it is then tapered to the smallest maintenance dose. Alternative agents are erythromycin, minocycline, or oral metronidazole. Traditional acne therapy with benzoyl peroxide and topical erythromycin or clindamycin solutions may benefit some, but the benzoyl peroxide and the alcohol vehicle of these solutions may irritate sensitive, fair skin. Although topical steroids will initially help in cases of erythema, they should be used cautiously because their long-term use may worsen the telangiectases.

Rhinophyma and granulomatous lesions respond to isotretinoin, but relapses are frequent when the drug is discontinued. Additional options are pulsed dye laser or electrosurgery for telangiectases, laser or surgical therapy for rhinophyma, and antiparasitic drugs for exacerbations of rosacea due to Demodex infestation. Ketoconazole cream sometimes elicits good results owing to its anti-inflammatory and antibiotic properties.

CHAPTER **51** FUNGAL INFECTIONS OF THE SKIN

Dermatophyte Infections

■ Definition and Epidemiology

Dermatophytosis (tinea or ringworm) is a superficial fungal infection of the skin, hair, or nails. The primary types of dermatophytoses are tinea capitis, tinea faciei, tinea barbae, tinea pedis, tinea manus, tinea corporis, tinea cruris, and onychomycosis. Some infections are inflammatory with fluctuant plaques and pustules, and others cause minimal scaling and erythema.

■ Etiology and Pathogenesis

Dermatophytes live in the superficial, cornified epidermal cells. They are ubiquitous in the environment and the source of an individual infection may be difficult to determine if there has not been family or animal contact. The host response to the infection in humans is influenced by the origin of the organism; species acquired from the soil or from animals induce a vigorous response, but those acquired from humans induce little inflammation.

Three genera of dermatophytes exist: Microsporum, Trichophyton, and Epidermophyton. The organisms causing a given type of infection vary with time and geographic location. Most cases of tinea capitis are caused by *Trichophyton tonsurans, Microsporum canis,* and *Trichophyton violaceum,* and most cases of tinea corporis arise from *Trichophyton rubrum, Microsporum canis,* and *T. tonsurans.* Tinea pedis, tinea manum, and tinea cruris are caused by *T. rubrum, T. mentagrophytes,* and *Epidermophyton floccosum.* Tinea barbae is most commonly caused by *T. mentagrophytes* and *T. verrucosum. T. rubrum* and *T. mentagrophytes* are also present in onychomycosis.

■ Clinical Features

Tinea pedis is the most prevalent adult dermatophytosis and has several distinct clinical presentations: the interdigital form; a sharply circumscribed "moccasin" distribution; and an acute inflammatory, vesiculobullous eruption on the soles of the feet. Tinea manum often coexists with bilateral tinea pedis or fingernail involvement and resembles the dry, scaly noninflammatory form of tinea pedis. (See Table 51.1 and Color Plates 17 and 18.)

Dermatophytoses elicit two reaction patterns. The **id reaction,** representing hypersensitivity to fungal proteins, is the most common, with pruritic vesicles or papules on the trunk or extremities. **Erythema annulare centrifugum,** a chronic and recurrent disorder, consists of polycyclic, red plaques with central trailing scales localized to the trunk. Both eruptions respond to topical corticosteroid creams and ointments.

■ Diagnosis and Differential Diagnosis

Dermatophyte infections are diagnosed with a potassium hydroxide preparation using scales from the surface of the lesion. When tinea capitis is suspected, hairs from the periphery of the patches are inspected for spores. However, the KOH examination is rarely helpful without **alopecia** (hair loss) or with intense inflammation. A fungal culture will confirm the diagnosis. When *M. audouinii* and *M. canis* commonly caused tinea in the past, the Wood's lamp examination rapidly diagnosed tinea by observing a blue fluorescence. Because these are less common etiologic agents in tinea currently, the Wood's lamp is now rarely used to diagnose tinea.

In addition to folliculitis, impetigo, seborrheic dermatitis, trichotillomania, psoriasis, and lupus erythematosus, other entities to be differentiated from tinea corporis are seborrheic and contact dermatitis, nummular eczema, psoriasis, secondary syphilis, and pityriasis rosea. Tinea faciei is frequently mistaken for contact dermatitis, seborrheic dermatitis, or lupus erythematosus. Tinea barbae may be mistaken for bacterial and herpetic infections and contact dermatitis. Candidal intertrigo, erythrasma, seborrheic dermatitis, psoriasis, and irritant dermatitis resemble tinea cruris. Tinea pedis and tinea manum may mimic psoriasis, contact dermatitis, irritant dermatitis, dyshidrotic eczema, xerosis, or candidiasis. The differential diagnosis of tinea unguium includes trauma, lichen planus, psoriasis, damage from nail polish, and other primary nail dystrophies.

■ Management

Tinea capitis, unguium, and barbae, and severe or recalcitrant infections of the palms, soles, groin, or glabrous skin, require systemic antifungal therapy. Topical therapy usually suffices for tinea pedis, tinea manum, tinea corporis, and tinea cruris. Overall therapy of dermatophytoses and the role of local therapy such as soaks, solutions, and topical steroids are shown in Table 51.2.

Tinea Versicolor

■ Definition, Epidemiology, and Etiology

One of the most common dermatophytes causing superficial infections is *Malassezia furfur* (syn., *Pityrosporum orbiculare)*, the agent causing tinea versicolor. Nearly 5% of persons in the United States have had an episode of tinea versicolor. Although no age is exempt, this infection is most common in adolescents and young adults (15–30 years of age). *M. furfur* is found on normal skin in the yeast phase in small numbers. Clinical disease occurs when conditions enhance the growth of hyphal forms in large numbers. What stimulates this growth is uncertain, but such growth may be related to nutrition, immune competence, or genetic factors.

■ Clinical Features

Tinea versicolor presents as multiple, oval, hypopigmented or hyperpigmented patches with fine scale distributed on the trunk, proximal arms, and face. Although mild pruritus may occur, tinea versicolor is asymptomatic in most cases. Many patients present during the summer months when they note the contrast between tanned and lesional skin. The race and complexion of the individual influence the color of the lesions. The inhibition of melanin production and transfer by azelaic acid produced by the fungus causes hypopigmentation, and the stimulation of melanogenesis by the inflammatory response causes hyperpigmentation.

■ Differential Diagnosis

The diagnosis of tinea versicolor is usually evident by the characteristic cutaneous eruption. When the findings are subtle, the skin may be viewed in a darkened room with a Wood's lamp, which will enhance the differences in the lesional and uninvolved skin. The best confirmatory test is the KOH examination. Attempts to culture *M. furfur* are usually futile. Tinea versicolor should be distinguished from other papulosquamous diseases, seborrheic dermatitis, leprosy, pityriasis alba, and vitiligo. Pityriasis rosea and secondary syphilis are the most likely papulosquamous diseases to cause confusion.

■ Management

Tinea versicolor may be effectively treated with selenium sulfide 2.5% lotion or antifungal creams

TABLE 51.1. Characteristic Clinical Features of Dermatophytoses

Subtype	Characteristics	Comments	Causative Organism
Tinea pedis Interdigital form	The most prevalent dermatophyte infection in adults Maceration, scaling, and fissuring between the fourth and fifth toes; painful infection	May be complicated by lymphangitis and cellulitis Most common subtype; often extends to involve additional web spaces	*Trichophyton rubrum* *Trichophyton rubrum*
Vesiculobullous type	Sharply circumscribed, red, scaly plaques with a hyperkeratotic surface on the soles and lateral aspects of the feet in a "moccasin" distribution Vesicles/bullae and eczematous changes in the soles of the feet		*Trichophyton mentagrophyte*
Tinea manum	Lesions most frequent on the palms and thumb web space in a unilateral distribution	Acute inflammatory eruption; likely to be symptomatic with pruritus, burning, and tenderness Resembles the dry, scaly noninflammatory form of tinea pedis; often seen in conjunction with bilateral tinea pedis or fingernail involvement	*Trichophyton mentagrophytes* *Trichophyton mentagrophyte*
Tinea cruris (jock itch)	Arcuate, red, sharply marginated, generally symmetric, scaling patches, involving the inner thighs, inguinal folds, and rarely the perineum, buttocks, and scrotum; the enlarging rings are macerated, crusted, vesicular, or scaly	Heat and humidity perpetuate the infection; men affected more frequently than women; risk factors are obesity, tightly fitted clothing, and frequent, strenuous activity	*Epidermophyton floccosum*
Tinea capitis (Color Plate 17)	Initial lesions are erythematous, scaling patches of alopecia; variable inflammation; small patches of alopecia; hairs broken at the level of the skin, creating "black dots" (black-dot tinea); sharply circumscribed, boggy, highly inflammatory, tender mass (kerion); onset acute; papules and pustules often cover the surface	Superficial fungal infection of the scalp; occurs primarily in children Less common in infants, adolescents, or adults; incidence greater in boys and African-American children; lymphadenopathy often present even with subtle cutaneous findings (important diagnostic clue for tinea capitis)	Most cases due to *Trichophyton tonsurans*, *Microsporum canis*, and *Trichophyton violaceum*
Tinea corporis	Single or multiple annular, erythematous plaques with fine white scale; vesicles or pustules may be present on the surface of some acute inflammatory plaques; sharply demarcated, raised borders; they enlarge progressively	Lesions are localized to glabrous (non-hairbearing) skin (palms, soles, groin, and beard area excluded)	Most cases due to *Trichophyton rubrum*, *Microsporum canis*, and *Trichophyton tonsurans*
Tinea faciei	Erythematous lesions often have ill-defined borders; the scaling may be minimal	Unusual fungal infection to the cheeks and forehead	*Trichophyton rubrum*
Tinea barbae	Papules, pustules, nodules, and erythematous plaques in the beard area; with established infection, loosened and broken hairs form irregular patches of alopecia and crusting; fluctuant draining abscesses occur in some cases	Uncommon disorder, seen almost exclusively among male farm workers; spread by contaminated razors	*Trichophyton mentagrophyte*, *Trichophyton verrucosum*
Tinea unguium (Color Plate 18)	Gradual onset with a small patch of yellow, white or brown discoloration forming at the edge of the nail; onycholysis develops as the nail plate lifts from the nail bed with the creation of crumbly subungual debris; with further infection, the nail becomes thickened and broken	Chronic dermatophyte infection of the fingernails or the toenails	*Trichophyton rubrum*, *Trichophyton mentagrophyte*

TABLE 51.2.	Therapy of Dermatophytoses (partial listing)	
Type	**Comments**	**Therapy**
Tinea capitis, Tenia unguium, Tinea barbae	Require systemic antifungal therapy; severe or recalcitrant infections of the palms, soles, groin, or glabrous skin are also treated with oral agents	Drug of choice: Griseofulvin Duration: 6–8 week course for tinea capitis and barbae; 12–18 months for onychomycosis Response: more rapid in fingernails; duration of therapy may be a year or less. Alternative drugs: ketoconazole, itraconazole, and fluconazole
Tinea pedis, Tinea manum, Tinea corporis, Tinea cruris	Usually resolves with topical preparations of ketoconazole, miconazole, ciclopirox, clotrimazole, econazole, oxiconazole, and terbinafine	Improvement occurs in 2 weeks with topical agents but most cases require a full 4-week treatment; those with tinea corporis or tinea cruris who fail to improve in 4 weeks should be given griseofulvin; patients with tinea pedis and tinea cruris should keep these sites cool and dry with powder containing miconazole or tolnaftate and nonocclusive clothing and shoes; compresses with Burrow's solution and use of a low-potency topical corticosteroid cream are useful in acute vesicular eruptions of tinea pedis.

including miconazole, clotrimazole, ketoconazole, or econazole. Selenium sulfide lotion is applied to all involved areas and the bordering normal skin at night and scrubbed off in the morning. This may be repeated once a week for 4 weeks and then as needed to maintain complete clearing. Many different treatment schedules have been used with equal efficacy. Selenium sulfide should not be used in pregnancy. Patients with recalcitrant disease or poor compliance with a topical regimen are given oral ketoconazole. Ketoconazole, in a single 400 mg dose, is often curative, but some

advocate a second dose after 1 week and further doses as needed. An alternative method is 200 mg per day for 2 weeks. An acidic environment is required for ketoconazole absorption; thus, it should be taken with orange juice or cola. Because this drug is excreted in the sweat, efficacy is enhanced by consuming it before exercising.

The response to therapy may be evaluated by reexamination of lesional scales dissolved in KOH. Relapses follow hot humid weather, immunosuppression, selective immunodeficiency, and pregnancy.

Candidiasis

■ Definition and Epidemiology

Candidiasis, or **moniliasis,** encompasses a variety of infections of the skin, mucous membranes, viscera, and nails. *Candida albicans* is the most common cause of these disorders but other species may be identified, especially in immunocompromised patients. *Candida,* a normal inhabitant of the mouth, gastrointestinal tract, and vagina, will proliferate on other moist, warm, and macerated cutaneous sites such as the perianal region, intertriginous areas, digital web spaces, and nail folds. It acts as a pathogen when the cutaneous barrier is locally disrupted or the systemic immunologic defenses are altered.

■ Clinical Features

Susceptibility to candidiasis is enhanced by obesity, endocrinopathies (diabetes mellitus and hypoparathyroidism), malignancies (leukemia and lymphoma), drugs (oral contraceptives, corticosteroids, antibiotics, and immunosuppressive agents), and inherited disorders (Down's syndrome and chronic granulomatous disease of childhood). In addition, neonates are inherently predisposed to candidal infections and readily develop thrush, perlèche, or diaper dermatitis.

The most common cutaneous presentations of candidiasis are thrush, perlèche, diaper dermatitis, candidal vulvovaginitis, chronic paronychia, candidal intertrigo, and perianal candidiasis. Thrush, or oral candidiasis, is characterized by white, adherent plaques on the tongue, gingiva, palate, buccal mucosa, and oropharynx. The base of the plaque is red and tender and the organism is identified by examination of scrapings from the surface, using a KOH solution. The most commonly affected are neonates (who acquire the fungus from the vagina at birth), the elderly, the malnourished, diabetics, persons receiving inhaled corticosteroid (asthmatics) or antibiotic therapy, and the HIV-infected.

Perlèche, or **angular cheilitis,** consists of superficial fissures, maceration, erythema, and pustules at the corners of the mouth. An inflammatory response in which moist, abraded skin is secondarily invaded by *Candida albicans,* angular albicans is observed in children who drool because of braces, who lick their lips, or who suck their thumbs. Older adults are at risk for perlèche due to poorly fitting dentures and drooling from malocclusion. Perlèche is also present in patients with diabetes mellitus or HIV infection.

Several forms of cutaneous candidiasis are localized to intertriginous areas. In infants, moisture, maceration, and irritation from urine and stool in the diaper create an ideal habitat for candidal proliferation. The distinctive features of candidal diaper dermatitis are the formation of bright red patches with sharp borders, the involvement of the inguinal folds, and the presence of satellite macules or pustules peripheral to the initial lesion. The groin is tender and pruritic. A similar process leads to the development of smooth, red, pruritic patches with peripheral scale in skin folds of the axilla, groin, buttocks, umbilicus, and beneath the breasts. The pruritic patches are moist or dry with satellite pustules and fissuring. This form is called **candidal intertrigo.**

Although *Candida albicans* is a component of the normal flora of the vagina and bowel, it often proliferates with pregnancy, diabetes mellitus, and therapy with oral contraceptives and systemic corticosteroids. Candidal vulvovaginitis is associated with edematous, red, pruritic labia; painful urination; and a gelatinous white discharge.

Candida albicans is the most common pathogen in chronic paronychia. The proximal and lateral nail folds are red, swollen, painful, and raised from the nail plate. A purulent discharge may exude from the nail folds, and the nails become ridged and discolored in untreated infections. Workers at risk for this condition are food handlers, health care workers, launderers, and bartenders, whose hands are in water for many hours a day. Trauma sustained during nail care or other periungual disease creates a portal of entry for bacteria and fungi.

■ Diagnosis and Differential Diagnosis

Candidal infections are diagnosed by microscopic examination of KOH preparations of scrapings from white plaques, scaly patches, pustules, or discharge. Pseudohyphae and spores are diagnostic of Candida. Fungal cultures are obtained to confirm the diagnosis if the clinician is uncertain.

Many of these disorders (chronic mucocutaneous candidiasis and candidal vulvovaginitis) have distinctive clinical presentations, but others require confirmation. Oral candidiasis should be distinguished from leukoplakia and lichen planus. Perlèche and riboflavin deficiency have similar clinical features. Diaper dermatitis must be distinguished from tinea cruris, irritant dermatitis, acrodermatitis enteropathica, seborrheic dermatitis, and histiocytosis. Candidal intertrigo may resemble an irritant dermatitis, superficial bacterial, or dermatophyte infection. Chronic paronychia may be confused with acute bacterial paronychia, onychomycosis, or psoriasis.

The diagnosis of systemic candidiasis requires the isolation of Candida from the blood or other body fluid. Multiple fungal cultures should be obtained in all immunocompromised or debilitated patients having intermittent fevers that are unresponsive to broad-spectrum antibiotics. The differential diagnosis includes systemic infections with bacteria or viruses.

■ Management

To successfully treat candidal infections, the underlying risk factors should be adequately addressed. Although these infections will clear up when treated with antifungal agents, they will recur if chronic damage to the cutaneous barrier function exists. Thrush is treated with nystatin suspension or clotrimazole troches. Children and adults either swish nystatin liquid against their oral mucosa prior to swallowing or they slowly dissolve a clotrimazole troche in their mouths.

The treatment of perlèche depends on the cause. Macerated skin should be protected with petrolatum or zinc oxide. Fungi or bacteria should be treated with the appropriate topical antifungal or antibacterial agents. For intertrigo and diaper dermatitis, the principles of therapy are similar. The sites are kept cool and dry using powder, loose-fitting clothing, and compresses on the acutely inflamed areas. Use topical antifungals along with 1% or 2.5% hydrocortisone cream to relieve pruritus and inflammation, and use an antibiotic for suspected concomitant bacterial infection.

Topical antifungal agents, protective gloves, and avoidance of chronic moisture are pivotal to the successful treatment of paronychia. Occasionally, patients are treated with ketoconazole and oral antibiotics when evidence of superinfection is seen in recalcitrant cases. Vulvovaginitis is treated with intravaginal antifungal creams and suppositories of nystatin, clotrimazole, or miconazole. Most infections will resolve after 1 week of nightly therapy but some require 2 weeks. In resistant cases, the candidal source is eliminated from the gastrointestinal tract with nystatin oral suspension, or the patient is given IV/IM therapy for 2–4 weeks.

For chronic mucocutaneous candidiasis and candidemia, employing systemic treatment is also necessary. The drug of choice for systemic candidiasis is amphotericin B, which is often given along with 5-fluorocytosine for synergy. Although fluconazole is an effective, safer alternative, it may cause hepatotoxicity, which requires close monitoring with liver function testing. The nephrotoxicity caused by extended courses of amphotericin B limits its use in chronic mucocutaneous candidiasis, making oral ketoconazole the mainstay of therapy; oral itraconazole, clotrimazole, and IV miconazole are other options.

CHAPTER 52 — BACTERIAL INFECTIONS OF THE SKIN

Impetigo

■ Definition, Epidemiology, and Etiology

Impetigo, also called **impetigo contagiosa,** is a common superficial cutaneous infection with two basic subtypes: bullous and nonbullous. Both subtypes, exacerbated by hot, humid weather, are more frequent in children than in adults. Bullous impetigo, in which the blistered and denuded areas are a cutaneous response to the bacterial toxin, is caused by *Staphylococcus aureus* of phage group II and commonly with type 71. Nonbullous impetigo is due to group A ß-hemolytic streptococci *(Streptococcus pyogenes),* often along with *S. aureus.*

■ Clinical Features

Nonbullous impetigo is the most frequent skin infection in children, with lesions developing at sites of injury—for example, insect bites, abrasions, or other trauma. Poor hygiene, overcrowding, humidity, and warm environments favor its development. The highest incidence is during the summer, when a higher likelihood of injuries and factors that favor the development of lesions exists. Preferred sites of involvement are the face, extremities, and neck. The primary lesion, a red macule, evolves into a papule or vesicle and rapidly becomes crusted. Typical findings are multiple, thick, honey-colored crusts, ulcers, and erosions. Fever and lymphadenopathy are common. An uncommon but important late sequela is glomerulonephritis, which is caused by certain nephritogenic strains of streptococci. Superficial impetigo rarely causes scarlet fever.

Bullous impetigo is less common. Lesions develop on normal skin, most commonly in the axillae, groin, and hands. They consist of superficial, fragile, subcorneal bullae containing yellow-white opaque fluid. The bullae rupture rapidly, exposing erosions that are covered by thin, yellow-brown crusts.

■ Diagnosis and Differential Diagnosis

Although the thick, honey-colored crusts of nonbullous impetigo are pathognomonic, the lesions of bullous impetigo, with their thinner amber crusts, are less distinctive. The Nikolsky's sign (see chapter 45) is negative, which distinguishes bullous impetigo from primary blistering diseases with secondary infection. Ecthyma may mimic impetigo but on removal of the thick crust it reveals a deep ulcer with a halo of erythema. A culture of the blister fluid or base confirms the diagnosis.

■ Management

Impetigo is effectively treated by suitable antibiotics and topical skin care. A semisynthetic penicillin (dicloxacillin for 14 days) is recommended, given the need to treat staphylococci and streptococci. Erythromycin is an alternative, but resistance to it is emerging. For superficial impetigo, topical mupirocin ointment is as effective as oral antibiotics. Extensive or deep lesions mandate oral agents. Gentle cleansing and warm compresses can remove crusts. To minimize autoinoculation and contagion, patients should practice good hygiene.

Erysipelas

■ Definition and Epidemiology

Erysipelas is a form of superficial cellulitis caused by group A ß-hemolytic streptococci. Lymphatic involvement is a prominent feature. Erysipelas, in its most common form, occurs on the bridge of the nose and the cheeks. Chronic edema caused by venous or lymphatic insufficiency predisposes persons to recurrent episodes of erysipelas. Other predisposing conditions are immuno-deficiency syndromes, cachexia, malnutrition, diabetes mellitus, and poor general hygiene.

■ Etiology and Pathogenesis

The most common pathogen is group A ß-hemolytic streptococci. Other rarely isolated organisms are groups B, C, or G streptococci. The pathogen enters through an abrasion, surgical incision, puncture wound, ulcer, injury, or fissure in the nose, ears, or perineum. Any draining site may serve as a source of infection, but sometimes no portal of entry is apparent.

■ Clinical Features

Fever, chills, headache, and malaise precede and accompany the onset of the skin eruption, and the patient appears toxic. Some report gastrointestinal symptoms, arthralgias, and changes in mental status. Typically, the lesions are sharply circumscribed, red, and tender in-filtrated plaques localized to the face and scalp (see Color Plate 19); infrequently, they occur on the hands and genitalia. However, the infection is not limited to these areas. Leukocytosis is common, and often exceeds 20,000/mm³. The lesions progress rapidly by peripheral

extension of the raised indurated borders. In severe cases, the warm edematous plaques become blisters.

■ Diagnosis and Differential Diagnosis

When erysipelas presents in its classic form (bright red, indurated facial plaque with distinct borders), little diagnostic difficulty results. Sometimes, the lesions may resemble allergic contact dermatitis, urticaria, scarlet fever, systemic lupus erythematosus, tuberculoid leprosy, or relapsing polychondritis. Culture of this closed infection is difficult to obtain and rarely of use in initial management.

■ Management

Penicillin is the drug of choice for erysipelas. Improvement is rapid and dramatic. Penicillin-allergic patients are given erythromycin or clindamycin. A semi-synthetic penicillin or cephalosporin is used when *S. aureus* is a potential second pathogen. Cool compresses provide symptom relief for tender, warm, blistered plaques, and swelling is controlled with immobilization and elevation. With chronic or recurrent infection, a bacterial reservoir and a possible portal of entry (e.g., macerated skin of tinea pedis) should be determined.

Folliculitis

■ Definition and Etiology

Bacterial folliculitis is an infection of the hair follicles, commonly due to coagulase-positive staphylococci. While *S. aureus* is the most frequent cause of superficial and deep folliculitis, superficial folliculitis is caused by streptococcus, proteus, pseudomonas, or other Gram-negative organisms.

■ Clinical Features

The clinical features depend on the age of the patient, the depth of infection and the site of involvement. Superficial folliculitis (Bockhart's impetigo) is a follicular pyoderma occurring most frequently on the scalps of children and extremities and buttocks in adults. Small, dome-shaped pustules and red papules form in crops at the follicular ostia and resolve in 1–2 weeks. Hair growth continues and lesions heal without scarring. Untreated infections may evolve into a deeper process with perifollicular extension of inflammation. Common variants of superficial folliculitis are *Pseudomonas aeruginosa* folliculitis, *Pityrosporum* folliculitis and Gram-negative folliculitis. *P. aeruginosa* is usually acquired in a hot tub or whirlpool and causes an eruption within days of exposure. Papules and pustules occur on the trunk,

buttocks, arms, and legs. *Pityrosporum* folliculitis is a chronic pruritic infection of *Malassezia furfur* on the back, proximal arms, legs, face, and scalp. Gram-negative folliculitis occurs in patients with acne vulgaris after extensive courses of systemic antibiotics.

The prototype of deep folliculitis is sycosis barbae (folliculitis barbae). Follicular pustules and papules with central hairs form in the beard area. Men with dense facial hair are most predisposed. Without prompt therapy, the infection becomes chronic and recurrent. Crops of pustules recur at the same sites and rupture with shaving or cause excoriation. The trauma sustains and spreads the infection. Follicular papules coalesce into tender, red, crusted plaques.

■ Diagnosis and Differential Diagnosis

The appearance of pustules in the appropriate distribution is usually characteristic. Lesions in recalcitrant disease should be cultured before initiating another course of antibiotics. Tinea barbae and pseudofolliculitis barbae may mimic sycosis barbae. Tinea barbae consists of erythematous nodules and plaques with distorted, damaged hairs, and rarely involves the upper lip. In pseudofolliculitis barbae, the curly facial hairs of black men curve back and pierce the skin.

Furuncles and Carbuncles

■ Definition and Etiology

Furuncles (boils) and carbuncles are inflammatory lesions of the hair follicles. A furuncle is a tender red nodule that often develops from a previous superficial folliculitis. A carbuncle forms when several furuncles coalesce into a larger, deeper abscess; *S. aureus* is the most common pathogen. Autoinoculation is an important mechanism in perpetuating the infection. Reservoirs of staphylococci for further infections derive from material draining from follicular openings, infected towels and linens, or nasal carriage of bacteria.

■ Clinical Features

As the furuncle enlarges during the first 2–4 days, it is firm and red. Then it becomes fluctuant, and yellow-white material is visible through the thinned epidermis. As the nodule ruptures, pus and necrotic material are released onto the surrounding skin. The pressure and pain are reduced and healing follows, causing **fibrosis.** Furunculosis develops in areas with abundant hair follicles that are prone to friction and sweating—that is, the neck, face, axilla, and buttocks. Infestations and other pruritic disorders may be accompanied by impetiginization (the development of a contagious, superficial **pyoderma**) and furuncle formation. Malnutrition, diabetes mellitus, obesity, defective neutrophil function, alcoholism, immunosuppression, and hematologic disorders enhance susceptibility to the formation of furuncles and carbuncles, but these lesions usually occur in healthy patients.

Carbuncles are larger, deeper, and a source of greater morbidity than furuncles. Red, indurated plaques surmounted by multiple pustules evolve into very painful draining abscesses on the neck, back, and thighs. Fever, malaise, and leukocytosis may be present. After drainage, healing is slow and is accompanied by scarring. Complications, although rare, include bacteremia and cellulitis with either furuncles or carbuncles. Lesions on the lips or tip of the nose may cause bacteria to enter the cavernous sinus via the facial and angular veins, leading to its thrombosis.

■ Diagnosis and Management

Both furuncles and carbuncles have deep, red, suppurative nodules. The lesions in folliculitis are more superficial; perifollicular induration and systemic symptoms are absent.

Aside from warm compresses, initial therapy consists of systemic antibiotics to cover *S. aureus*; its frequent penicillin resistance dictates use of a semisynthetic penicillin (e.g., dicloxacillin). Rifampin is added to potentiate the antimicrobial effect. Furuncles and carbuncles should not be incised and drained until lesions are fluctuant and the thinned epidermis reveals pus below. Mupirocin ointment and a sterile dressing are placed locally after drainage to prevent autoinoculation.

In recurrent or recalcitrant cases, a culture should be obtained to ensure that the organism is not methicillin-resistant Staphylococcus or some other form of bacteria that is not susceptible to the previous antibiotic regimen. The predisposing factors should be explored. Potential staphylococcal sources (e.g., the nasal carriage) are treated with mupirocin ointment and chlorhexidine or another antimicrobial soap for daily bathing. The patient's linen and clothing are laundered in hot water to eliminate the transmission of bacteria to other family members.

Syphilis

■ Definition and Epidemiology

Caused by *Treponema pallidum*, syphilis is an infectious disease with both cutaneous and visceral manifestations. It most commonly affects sexually active young adults and teenagers, but no age, race, or gender is exempt. Although sexual activity is the most common mode of transmission, any direct contact with its highly contagious lesions may cause infection. Congenital syphilis is transplacentally acquired. Other sexually transmitted diseases (STDs)—HIV, chlamydia, and gonorrhea—may coexist with syphilis; the diagnosis of any one of these should prompt a search for the others.

■ Etiology

Treponema pallidum, the etiologic agent of syphilis, is a spirochete less than 20 μm in length. Identifiable with dark-field microscopy, it has a cell envelope, an axial filament, and a protoplast. These **treponemes** will not grow on culture media. Antibacterial drugs that impair cell wall synthesis are effective against *T. pallidum*. Spirochetes migrate through minute fissures in mucous membranes or skin in adults and can cross the placenta to infect a fetus.

■ Clinical Features

The course is divided into early and late stages. Early syphilis is defined as the first 2 years of disease and encompasses primary syphilis, secondary syphilis, and early latent syphilis. Late syphilis includes late latent and tertiary syphilis.

The **chancre** is the hallmark of primary syphilis. Usually developing at the site of contact with the treponemes 3–4 weeks after exposure, a chancre is accompanied by bilateral, nontender regional adenopathy and resolves in 6 weeks, evolving from a red papule into an indurated, oval plaque with a superficial erosion and serous exudate.

Although usually solitary and localized to the genitals, chancres may be multiple and involve oral mucosa, rectum, face, axilla, breasts, or distal extremities. In women, a chancre may be overlooked because it may occur on the cervix. It can occur as a mixed infection with chancroid or become superinfected.

Syphilids, the skin signs of secondary syphilis, occur an average of 6 weeks after the onset of the chancre, which may not have resolved by then. The initial eruption may be transient, rapidly progressive red-brown macules, and the fully developed **exanthem** (skin eruption) is diffuse, symmetric, and polymorphous, consisting of macules, papules, and, less often, nodules and pustules. Scaling is common and lesions may follow the lines of cleavage in the skin. While this suggests pityriasis rosea, involvement of the palms and soles suggests syphilis (see Color Plate 20). The distribution of the lesions may be annular, follicular, or lichenoid. Other lesions observed at this stage are mucous patches, condyloma lata, syphilitic pharyngitis, and patchy "moth-eaten" alopecia. Characteristically, none of these lesions is pruritic. Mucous patches are white, eroded papules that arise on the tongue, tonsils, gingival, buccal, and labial mucosa, cervix, vagina, labia minora, glans, and corona of the penis. Condyloma lata are pink, exophytic papules that are most infectious, affect moist intertriginous sites, and should be distinguished from condyloma acuminata. Fatigue, malaise, headache, nasal congestion, arthralgia, sore throat, and lymphadenopathy are usual symptoms. The gastrointestinal tract, kidneys, liver, central nervous system, prostate, lungs, and bones may be infected. Anemia, elevated sedimentation rate, leukocytosis, and increased alkaline phosphatase are notable. Resolution follows within 10 weeks and lesions heal with pigmentary changes.

During the latent period, the disease manifestations are absent and the diagnosis is by reactive serologic tests. Tertiary syphilis, which usually follows after 3 or more years of latency, has three basic forms: benign, neurosyphilis, and cardiovascular syphilis. In benign disease, patients develop red, coalescent nodules (gummas) that may ulcerate. These indolent, asymptomatic lesions are distributed on the extensor arms, face, and back. Healing occurs with scarring and destruction of soft tissue.

■ Diagnosis and Differential Diagnosis

Syphilis is diagnosed by correlation of the clinical findings and the results of serologic tests for syphilis (STS). Observing treponemes by dark-field examination provides an immediate diagnosis of primary, secondary, and congenital syphilis. STS are divided into nontreponemal or treponemal tests. The former detects reagins or phospholipids released from infected cells, the most common ones being the rapid plasma reagin (RPR) and the venereal diseases reference laboratory (VDRL) tests. These nonspecific flocculation tests are used to screen patients with risk factors for syphilis. Quantitative antibody titers are used to follow response to therapy. False negative results may occur in patients with very high antibody titers **(prozone phenomena).** Treponemal tests use *T. pallidum* components as the antigen. The fluorescent treponemal antibody (FTA-ABS) test and the microhemagglutination test (MHA-TP) are the most useful. In the FTA-ABS, a visible reaction results from the mixture of human serum with a fluorescein-labeled antihuman globulin on a slide to which *T. pallidum* has been adsorbed. The MHA-TP is less expensive and easier to perform.

T. pallidum induces a wide variety of different lesions and thus the vast differential diagnosis. The syphilitic chancre resembles the ulcers of chancroid or lymphogranuloma venereum, the eroded nodules of granuloma inguinale, and the blister base of herpes simplex virus infection. Chancroid produces soft, painful ulcers with inflamed, undermined borders, a superficial membrane, and unilateral adenopathy. The friable granulation tissue of granuloma inguinale is characteristic. The lesions of lymphogranuloma venereum are painless, fleeting, and followed by lymphadenopathy. Pain or a burning sensation often precedes the grouped vesicles of herpes simplex infection. Secondary syphilis may be confused with other papulosquamous disorders such as pityriasis rosea, lichen planus, dermatophytosis, guttate psoriasis, and mycosis fungoides. Syphilids may be mimicked by drug eruptions, sarcoidosis, leprosy, urticaria pigmentosa, tinea versicolor, and streptococcal infections. Syphilitic cutaneous lesions are asymptomatic. Mucous patches may be confused with erythema multiforme, candidiasis, leukoplakia, herpetic gingivostomatitis, erosive lichen planus, and aphthous stomatitis. Ulcerated oral gumma may mimic a squamous cell cancer.

■ Management

Parenteral penicillin G is the most effective treatment for all forms of syphilis. The treatment for syphilis is shown in Table 150.4 (chapter 150). Penicillin-allergic patients are given tetracycline hydrochloride 500 mg q.i.d for 2 weeks or erythromycin (the same dose), but these alternate agents are less effective. Ceftriaxone may be useful in persons with neurosyphilis owing to its penetration of the central nervous system. The management of pregnant patients depends on the same criteria for antibiotic selection. Patients with concurrent HIV infection and syphilis may not be cured with the standard regimens. Many physicians treat these patients with higher doses or treatment of longer duration to prevent the potential neurologic involvement that results from inadequate therapy. Reevaluation of patients with early-stage syphilis is scheduled at 3, 6, and 9 months following treatment. HIV-positive individuals are reassessed more frequently.

For more information on syphilis, see chapter 150, Sexually Transmitted Diseases.

CHAPTER 53 VIRAL INFECTIONS OF THE SKIN

Verrucae

■ Definition and Epidemiology

Warts, or verrucae, are common epidermal growths induced by a local infection with the human papilloma virus. Their characteristic appearance depends on the site of involvement and the viral type. Warts usually occur in children and adolescents, although no age is exempt. Patients with impaired cell-mediated immunity (e.g., immunosuppressive therapy) are particularly vulnerable and usually experience a protracted course. Patients with atopic dermatitis, AIDS, and lymphoma are also vulnerable. *Condyloma acuminata* (see the following) occurs most frequently in sexually active adolescents and young adults, and its incidence has significantly risen since the 1970s.

■ Etiology

The human papilloma virus (HPV), a member of the Papova virus family, contains double-stranded DNA. These viral particles lack a lipoprotein envelope that confers greater resistance to freezing, chemicals, higher temperatures, and desiccation. They remain viable even without a human host and, therefore, are transmissible by fomites. HPV is not pathogenic in other species.

Classified on the basis of the outer protein capsid antigens, more than 65 different types of HPV have been identified. Some these have been associated with malignant transformation in the involved lesion. DNA hybridization techniques, which are rarely clinically used unless concern exists regarding carcinogenic potential, allow identification of the viral type from a biopsy specimen. Current evidence suggests that HPV may inhibit the function of anti-oncogenes.

■ Clinical Features

Verruca vulgaris (common warts) are flesh-colored papules with a rough, scaly gray or white surface; these warts are associated with HPV types 1, 2, 4, and 7. Single or multiple and of variable size (a few millimeters to several centimeters), they most frequently are found on the dorsa of the hands, but no epithelial site is exempt. Easily spread from the hands to the face or extremities, these warts may be inoculated into sites of trauma. Periungual and subungual warts are not uncommon and usually are difficult to eradicate. They can become irritated, fissured, and tender. Filiform or digitate warts occur on the head and neck. They have rough projections from the surface and are attached to the skin by a broad stalk.

Verruca plantaris (plantar warts) grow into the thick skin of the sole and appear as flat or slightly elevated papules or plaques. HPV types 1, 2, and 4 are usually isolated from these. Because these firm, coarse keratotic lesions localize to sites of pressure, walking is painful. Mosaic warts form when multiple single papules coalesce into a plaque. These may enlarge to several centimeters. Upon removal, superficial keratoses exhibit a soft core with multiple bleeding points.

Verruca plana (flat warts) are 1–3-mm, pink or tan, flat-topped papules. The most common HPV types are 3, 10, 28, and 41. Variable numbers are distributed on the face, dorsal hands, wrists, and legs. Occurring in groups, they often coalesce into plaques, and they spread through autoinoculation. Shaving or other trauma induces new lesions in a linear distribution.

Condyloma acuminata arise in men on the penile shaft and in women on the vulva, perineum, or cervix; they also arise on the anal canal or the perianal skin. The soft, fleshy, clustered papules are tan, pink, or gray. Early lesions are minute, and diagnosed by applying dilute acetic acid compresses that whiten the altered epidermal surface. They may enlarge to form cauliflower-like masses. These larger lesions are frequently tender from recurrent trauma. HPV infection may be accompanied by a vaginal discharge, which may be malodorous because of secondary bacterial colonization. Pregnancy or immunodeficiency cause genital warts to become numerous. Transmission is via sexual contact or inoculation from a cutaneous site. Condylomata in children should prompt suspicion of sexual abuse and a workup for other STDs.

Genital warts have the following HPV types: 6, 11, 13, 16, 18, 30–33, 42–44, and 51–55. The isolation of HPV from penile, vulvar, and anal cancers, and the finding of HPV 6, 11, 16, 18, and other types in most cases of cervical cancer attest to its malignant potential. In women who have condyloma of the vulva or sexual partners with condyloma, gynecological examination and Papanicolaou smears should be performed to detect internal condyloma or neoplasia.

■ Diagnosis and Differential Diagnosis

Generally, the clinical appearance is diagnostic. Two important clues for the identification of skin warts are the presence of dilated, thrombosed capillaries that appear as brown or black dots and the disruption of the superficial skin lines. Lichen planus, lichen planus-like keratoses, molluscum contagiosum, and an epidermal nevus may be confused with verruca plana. Warts on the sole resemble corns or clavi. Paring the lesion will reveal a hard core of a clavus but a softer center with thrombosed vessels in a wart. Common warts occasionally need to be differentiated from seborrheic keratoses, nevi, acrochordons, and squamous cell cancer. Condyloma lata require differentiation from anogenital warts; syphilis serology is diagnostic. Condyloma acuminata may coexist with other STDs, which should be appropriately excluded.

■ Management

Not all HPV infections require therapy because many types of warts will resolve on their own. Treatment depends on the age and the immune status of the patient; the extent, site, and duration of the lesions; presence of symptoms; and the patient's wishes. Because all modes of therapy are not equally effective in all persons, individualization is important. Most measures destroy the epidermal cells that harbor the virus. All methods carry high rates of recurrence because viral particles may be present even in skin that appears normal.

Cryotherapy is frequently used in treating all forms of HPV infection. Liquid nitrogen, which is effective without scarring, is sprayed on the lesion or applied with a swab for 2–15 seconds. Flat warts or condyloma require a shorter application, and verruca vulgaris requires a longer application; multiple applications may also be needed. Rarely, superficial digital nerves or vessels are damaged. Electrodesiccation and curettage rapidly reduces the size of the lesions but has a high rate of recurrence and scarring with healing. In contrast, the CO_2 laser can vaporize the infected keratinocytes without scarring. Both the operator and patient should be appropriately protected from the aerosolized viral particles in the laser plume. Cantharidin solution (Cantharone), a blistering agent, separates the infected cells of the epidermis from the dermis. The application is painless, and the site is simply washed to remove the infected cells.

Condylomata and warts without a highly keratinized surface are often treated with podophyllum resin (available in a 25% solution with tincture of benzoin or as a less concentrated solution for home treatment). This irritating compound, which halts epidermal proliferation of virally infected cells, is carefully applied to individual lesions and removed in 4–6 hours. Other useful agents for verruca vulgaris or verruca plantaris include salicylic and lactic acid solutions and plasters, formalin, and 5-fluorouracil ointment. Resistant cases are treated with intralesional interferon or bleomycin, laser ablation, and—rarely—retinoids.

Molluscum Contagiosum

■ Definition, Epidemiology, and Etiology

Molluscum contagiosum is a common childhood viral disease, featuring single or multiple dome-shaped papules with central umbilication and a white core. The disorder is distributed worldwide and has a widely variable incidence. It is most commonly seen in children between the ages of 3 and 16 years and in sexually active adults. Persons with immunodeficiencies are especially susceptible and men are more often affected. Patients with AIDS can develop generalized lesions that are very difficult to treat. The causative agent is *Molluscum contagiosum*, a unique member of the poxvirus group. These are large, brick-shaped DNA viruses that measure 200–300 nm. There are two distinct pathogenic strains.

■ Clinical Features

Initially, the papules are firm and flesh-colored or pink and, with time, become waxy and white or pearly gray. The lesions range from 2–5 mm in diameter but may exceed a centimeter. The most frequently involved sites are the face, trunk, and extremities in children and the anogenital region in adults. Mucous membrane involvement is not uncommon. In adults, transmission is associated with sexual activity. Generally, the eruption lacks symptoms except, perhaps, mild pruritus. With rubbing, eczematous patches develop around some lesions. Eyelid lesions may incite conjunctivitis or keratitis.

■ Diagnosis and Management

The shiny, dome-shape papules with central umbilication are characteristic. Sometimes, they resemble milia, warts, varicella, papillomas, acne, epithelioma, and herpes virus infection. The diagnosis is confirmed by finding the viral inclusions (molluscum bodies or Henderson-Paterson bodies), which is accomplished by expressing the contents of a lesion onto a slide, flattening the material, and staining with Wright's stain.

In immunocompetent persons, the disease is generally self-limited and resolves in 6–9 months. Not all cases require therapy; however, hundreds of lesions may form before spontaneous remission. Once the central keratin core is removed or destroyed, the lesions will heal. The disease is most reliably treated by curettage following topical anesthesia. Children tolerate this procedure poorly and are best treated with a brief application of liquid nitrogen or cantharidin. Light electrodesiccation, application of 50% trichloroacetic acid until whitening, or daily treatment with Duofilm are other options. Because new lesions may continually evolve from self-inoculation, all these treatment regimens require multiple visits.

Molluscum contagiosum affecting immunocompromised persons is very difficult to treat. Trichloroacetic acid peels are useful in treating numerous facial, neck, and chest lesions in AIDS patients.

Herpes Simplex

■ Definition and Etiology

The herpesvirus group includes the herpes simplex viruses, human herpesvirus-6, cytomegaloviruses, Epstein-Barr virus, and varicella-zoster virus. Herpes simplex is a cutaneous viral infection that causes superficial, clustered vesicles on an erythematous base (see Color Plate 21). Herpesvirus hominis, the causative agent, is a large virus containing double-stranded DNA enclosed in a protein coat and lipid envelope. Its two distinct antigenic forms, herpes simplex type 1 and type 2 (HSV-1 and HSV-2), may be distinguished by their different surface glycoproteins, which induce distinct neutralizing antibodies. HSV-1 has a proclivity for the face and oral mucosa, and HSV-2, for the genital skin and mucosa. The lesion distribution shows significant overlap owing to orogenital sexual practices. The other main viral proteins are viral thymidine kinase and DNA polymerase, which play a key role in the antiviral drug therapy.

■ Clinical Features

Transmission follows direct contact with lesional skin or secretions. The incubation period is 1–26 days, often 1 week. HSV infections may be primary or recurrent. Primary infections occur in persons without antibodies to HSV. In some, a prodrome of burning, tingling pruritus or neuralgia is followed by symptomatic localized or generalized eruptions or systemic involvement. The eruptions are superficial, clustered vesicles on an erythematous base. Most lesions resolve without scarring unless bacterial superinfection has prevailed. In others, the infection is subclinical, with a humoral response and without any cold sores. Serologic evidence of exposure to the virus is present in over 85% of some populations. After primary infection, the virus remains dormant in the sensory nerve ganglia until reactivation. Symptomatic primary infections are more severe than recurrent infections. Although herpes infection stimulates both humoral and cell-mediated immunity, the severity of the disease in the immunodeficient underscores the importance of cell-mediated immunity.

Gingivostomatitis is the most common clinical expression of primary HSV-1 infection in children, most of whom are 1–6 years old. Often, associated malaise, fever, salivation, irritability, fetid breath, and tender cervical lymph nodes exist. The gingival mucosa is red, edematous, and friable. Vesicles appear on the tongue, palate, buccal mucosa, and pharynx within 1 week of exposure to the virus. These evolve into gray ulcers with surrounding erythema. Oral pain inhibits eating and drinking, but the lesions resolve in 2–3 weeks. **Primary ocular herpes simplex infections** lead to a purulent conjunctivitis and superficial keratitis. Vesicles arise on edematous and erythematous eyelid margins. Pain, photophobia, lacrimation, discharge, and preauricular lymphadenopathy may be present. Generally, herpetic keratoconjunctivitis heals uneventfully in 2 weeks; scarring and blindness are rare.

In contrast, HSV-2 infection occurs most frequently in adolescents and young adults through sexual contact. **Genital herpes** evokes symptoms much more often than its oral counterpart. HSV-1 is isolated from 20–40% of genital lesions. Genital herpes in children is suggestive of sexual abuse.

Genital herpes infections are subdivided into herpes progenitalis and herpetic vulvovaginitis. Herpes simplex is the most common cause of genital ulceration in sexually active individuals. The most frequently involved site in men is the penis (glans, foreskin, and the shaft) and, rarely, the scrotum or urethra. In women, the external genitalia and the mucosal surfaces of the vulva, cervix, and vagina are commonly involved. The vesicular eruption rapidly gives place to painful, superficial ulcers covered with gray exudate. Single or multiple 3-mm lesions develop on swollen, erythematous tissue and often coalesce into large, ulcerated plaques. Constitutional symptoms are severe in some patients, but resolution occurs in 3 weeks or less.

Several other forms of primary herpes virus infection exist. Inoculation of HSV directly into a skin fissure or abrasion induces vesicles, indurated papules, or bullae with regional adenopathy. Dentists may develop such herpetic whitlows on their fingers. In herpes gladiatorum, wrestlers and participants of contact sports may develop similar lesions on their face, scalp, and upper trunk through contact with the skin and mucous membranes of other players. Severe systemic symptoms often accompany the scattered, grouped vesicles and lymphadenopathy. Kaposi's varicelliform eruption arises from the introduction of HSV into skin affected by atopic dermatitis or **Darier's disease.** Neonates may develop a herpetic infection at the time of delivery from contact with lesions in the maternal genital tract (neonatal herpes).

Recurrent episodes of herpes virus infection have a shorter course and less severe symptoms than the primary infection. The vesicles are smaller and the distribution is more limited. A burning or tingling sensation often precedes the eruption, which resolves in 7–10 days without residual scarring. Common triggers include trauma, stress, menstruation, and ultraviolet radiation. In women, significant tenderness accompanies recurrent genital infections. Herpes may recur on the buttocks;

regional lymphadenopathy and neurologic complaints may be associated. Eczema herpeticum, keratoconjunctivitis, and inoculation herpes are other primary infections that recur less often. Herpes infections may be complicated by erythema multiforme with herpes labialis, cranial nerve or Bell's palsy, neuralgia, disseminated disease, arthritis, and lymphedema with involvement of the extremities.

■ Diagnosis and Differential Diagnosis

In most cases, the distinctive appearance of grouped vesicles on an erythematous base makes the diagnosis of herpes infection obvious. The most rapid method to confirm HSV is the Tzanck smear, which shows multinucleated giant cells among the keratinocytes scraped from the base of a vesicle. A viral culture is necessary to distinguish the viral type with certainty. Primary infections may be identified by the rise in antibody titer using the complement fixation test. Herpetic gingivostomatitis should be differentiated from hand-foot-and-mouth disease, aphthous stomatitis, erythema multiforme, herpangina, diphtheria, and Behcet's syndrome. Impetigo may be confused with herpes labialis, and the two may occur together. Herpes progenitalis resembles a syphilitic chancre or chancroid; however, the lesions of syphilis are painless.

■ Management

Uncomplicated, localized herpetic infections do not require treatment. Acyclovir or famciclovir, orally or intravenously, shortens the duration of each episode and reduces recurrences. Both are effective in primary infections and recurrences, regardless of immune status. They have few significant adverse effects, but the dose should be reduced for patients with renal failure. Although acyclovir ointment may reduce viral shedding, it does not affect recurrence rate. Primary infections respond to oral acyclovir, 200 mg five times a day for 7–10 days. Acyclovir is given intravenously for neonatal herpes and severe infections. Recurrent disease is not suppressed unless the episodes are frequent or unless the cellular immunity is impaired. The most common regimen is acyclovir, 400 mg twice a day. Among the immunocompromised with HSV, acyclovir resistance is well known and is attributed to thymidine kinase-deficient viral clones. Foscarnet or vidarabine are useful in these cases.

Adjunctive treatment consists of compresses with Burrow's solution to dry weeping lesions and therapy for superimposed bacterial infections. Factors that trigger recurrent episodes should be identified.

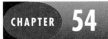

INFESTATIONS OF THE SKIN

Parasitic infestations are a common cause of pruritic eruptions. Primary lesions are often effaced by secondary changes, thereby obscuring diagnosis. The distribution of the lesions and a history of multiple affected persons within the same living group should arouse suspicion of these entities.

Scabies

■ Definition and Epidemiology

Scabies, an infestation of the skin with *Sarcoptes scabiei*, is contracted by close personal contact. Reported worldwide, scabies occurs in epidemics, with overcrowding and institutionalization perpetuating the disease. Scabies is rarely transmitted by fomites such as towels or linen because the organism cannot live for more than 5 days away from a warm human host. Thus, close human contact is essential for transmission. The two most common variants are nodular and crusted (Norwegian) scabies. Crusted scabies occurs most frequently among people with immune deficiencies and mental and physical disabilities (Down's syndrome, neurologic disorders, and malnutrition).

■ Etiology

Sarcoptes scabiei (var. hominis) is an arachnid that prefers a human host. Having an oval, gray, or translucent body, this arachnid measures 0.3–0.5 mm. After fertilization, the male mite dies; the female then enters the human stratum corneum where she forms a tunnel and lays two to three eggs daily for 4–8 weeks. She dies after the egg-laying is complete. The eggs hatch within 3–4 days of deposition, producing larvae, which develop into nymphs and then adults. An infested person who bathes frequently will have from 2–50 mites in the skin. Thousands of mites may exist on a person with Norwegian scabies.

■ Clinical Features

The eruption consists of pruritic papules, vesicles, and burrows with pronounced secondary changes of crusting, infection, excoriation, and eczematization. Asymptomatic for the first 4–6 weeks, the parasite causes pruritus after the host is sensitized to its foreign proteins. The intense pruritus is often worse at night, and it may persist for weeks after treatment. Burrows are 0.2–1-cm, raised, linear lesions. The axilla, groin, and the web spaces of the hands and feet are commonly infected. In children and the elderly, lesions may exist above the neck on the forehead, cheeks, and hairline. Buttocks, nipples, flexor arms, and the waist should also be examined.

The nodular type of scabies consists of 3–5-mm red nodules that remain for months or years after treatment and classically occur on the scrotum and penis, among other sites. In the crusted type, the large, scaly, crusted plaques resemble psoriatic plaques and may be accompanied by nail dystrophy, subungual and periungual hyperkeratosis, and fissuring. The genitals, buttocks, scalp, hands, feet, and areas of pressure are the sites of predilection.

■ Diagnosis and Differential Diagnosis

The differential diagnosis includes insect bite reaction, prurigo nodularis or neurodermatitis, atopic eczema, xerosis, or pruritus from systemic diseases with secondary excoriation. The history among multiple family members of a pruritic eruption that is present on the hands, wrists, axilla, and groin is suggestive of scabies. Although burrows are a reliable diagnostic clue, the frequency of secondary excoriations and crusting often makes them difficult to identify; applying black, washable ink to the skin and then wiping it off can outline these burrows and may help in their localization. Definitive diagnosis is through the recovery of a mite, eggs, or feces (see chapter 42, Color Plate 3). Mites are most likely to be recovered from new lesions or burrows on the web spaces of the hands, subungual region of the digits, and wrists. Rarely, a biopsy is required to ascertain the diagnosis.

■ Management

The two most frequently used therapeutic options are lindane (gamma benzene hexachloride) cream or lotion and Elimite™ cream (permethrin 5%). Lindane, the traditional treatment, is highly effective. However, due to its side-effect profile, its use has declined. Neurotoxicity may occur after its use in infants and children, owing to enhanced absorption. Inappropriate or frequent application may cause eczema, urticaria, and aplastic anemia. The cream or lotion is applied at night to all body surface areas below the neck in adults and older children, and washed off after 8 hours. Permethrin 5% cream is the treatment of choice in children and infants as young as 2 months of age; it is applied in the same manner but also on the face, neck, and hairline. All creases and folds should be carefully treated with all topical agents, and

crusts should be removed with tepid soaks. On the evening of the first treatment, all linens are laundered in hot water and other bedding or clothing is dry-cleaned or placed in plastic bags for 5 days. Sulfur (5–10%) in petrolatum and 10% crotamiton (Eurax™) are less effective alternatives. Other adjuncts include antihistamines and topical corticosteroid creams for relief of pruritus and antibiotics to treat bacterial superinfection. Family members and sexual contacts with or without pruritus should be treated to ensure eradication of the parasite.

Pediculosis

■ Definition and Epidemiology

Pediculosis is an infestation of the skin with lice that attack human hosts. Lice depend on their human hosts for blood. As they attach to the skin to obtain their meal, they inject noxious salivary secretions that are antigenic and may transmit some infectious diseases. Pediculosis affects both children and adults. Lice may be acquired by close human contact in a crowded environment and between individuals who share fomites such as combs, clothing, and upholstery. Poor hygiene contributes to the perpetuation of this disorder. Pediculosis capitis occurs most frequently in young girls and is rare in African Americans. Patients with pediculosis pubis tend to be adolescents and young adults who acquire the disease through sexual activity.

■ Etiology

The pediculi infecting humans are *Pthirus pubis* (the pubic or crab louse), *Pediculosis humanus corporis* (the body louse), and *Pediculosis humanus capitis* (the head louse). Each of these has a predilection for a defined site and rarely invades other areas. They have oval, gray, or translucent bodies with six legs and a proboscis for blood extraction. They range in size from 1–4 mm. The head louse is smaller than the body louse but both have a slender abdomen and legs of equal size. The pubic louse resembles a crab with a rounded body, a pair of smaller legs near the mouth, and two sets of large legs. The ova or nits are oval, gray, or white concretions that adhere to hair and clothing and measure 0.3–0.8 mm. The eggs are deposited within 48 hours of fertilization and require approximately 2 weeks to mature.

■ Clinical Features

Pediculosis capitis occurs in people of all ages but is most common in children. Severe pruritus leads to

scratching with frequent secondary infections and adenopathy. The hair is dull, and ova or nits adhere to the hair shafts. In pediculosis corporis ("Vagabond's disease" or "pediculosis vestimenti"), the lice live in the seams of clothing in areas that are warmed by the body, such as the neck, waist, and groin; acral sites, however, are spared. The lice puncture the skin for nourishment, and their bites produce pruritic macules, papules, and urticarial wheals with prominent central puncta. These lesions are usually obliterated by secondary excoriations, lichenification, eczematization, crusting, and infection. Healing occurs with hyperpigmentation. Severe pruritus with parallel scratches in the interscapular region is characteristic.

Pubic lice induce pruritic red papules on the thighs, abdomen, and chest. Pediculi may also adhere to the hair of the beard area, axilla, eyebrows, and eyelashes. Eyebrows and lashes are most often infested in older children and may be accompanied by **blepharitis** (inflamed eyelids). With abundant parasites, maculae ceruleae are seen; they are 3–15-mm, blue, nonblanching, asymptomatic macules on the thighs, proximal arms, and ventral trunk. Transmission occurs via sexual intercourse or less often through infested bedding or other fomites. Other sexually transmitted diseases may also exist.

■ Diagnosis and Differential Diagnosis

Pediculosis is usually diagnosed by the observation of nits and pediculi. Nits on scalp hair may resemble hair casts or scale, but nits adhere firmly to the hair shaft and fluoresce when a Wood's lamp is used. Examination of a hair with light microscopy should clarify the diagnosis of pediculosis capitis or pubis. At times, a superficial scalp infection is the only evidence of infestation. Pubic lice and their nits may be isolated near the skin surface in most cases. Body lice reside in the patient's clothes, not on the skin; an inspection of the clothing will reveal hundreds of eggs deposited in the seams.

■ Management

Several shampoos are effective in treating pediculosis capitis. Lindane shampoo (Kwell™, 1%) is the traditional treatment; it is applied to the scalp for 5 minutes and rinsed off, and this is repeated in 1 week. However, concerns about toxicity now limit its use. Both permethrin 1% cream rinse (NIX) and pyrethrin with piperonyl butoxide 1% (RID) are safe for children. After a 10-minute application, the agent is removed from the scalp and repeated in 1 week. A less convenient method is the use of crotamiton 10% cream or lotion for 24 hours. Nits are removed with a fine-toothed comb or tweezers after soaking the hair in a 5% solution of white vinegar. All items that come into contact with the scalp need to be cleaned or placed in plastic bags for 2 weeks.

Pediculosis pubis is treated with the same agents as above. Lindane is the treatment of choice and is applied to the affected area, adjacent normal skin, and perianal region. Sexual partners of infested individuals should be treated concurrently. Linen and clothing should be washed in hot water or dry-cleaned. If the eyelashes are infested, they should be treated with a thick coating of petrolatum 2 times a day for 1 week, followed by manual removal of the remaining lice. An alternative is physostigmine 0.25% ophthalmic ointment, 4 times a day for 3 days.

Body lice dwell in the clothing of the patient and remain on the skin only to feed. Frequent bathing and cleaning of clothing, bedding, carpets, upholstery, and mattresses should be sufficient to rid the host of this parasite.

CHAPTER **55** # PIGMENTARY DISORDERS OF THE SKIN

Pigmentary disorders are either (1) an acquired abnormality in melanin production and transfer or (2) a congenital absence of melanin or the constituents of its synthesis. The cosmetic consequences of these disorders can be psychologically devastating.

Vitiligo

■ Definition, Epidemiology, and Etiology

Vitiligo, which results from the loss of melanocytes, is a common disorder of patterned depigmentation affecting 1–2% of the population. It affects all races and both genders equally. The peak age of onset is between 10 and 30 years. Almost 30% of patients with vitiligo have another affected family member. In some families, the pattern of inheritance is autosomal dominant with incomplete penetrance. Further studies are likely to reveal a polygenic inheritance pattern.

Antibodies to melanocytes and melanoma cells have been observed in 80% of patients. It is proposed that an autoimmune process, by an antibody-mediated mechanism, causes melanocyte destruction. Melanocytes may be destroyed by a neurotransmitter released from nerve terminals or the accumulation of toxic intermediates in the synthesis of melanin. Another proposed factor in the pathogenesis of vitiligo is exposure to chemicals that produce depigmentation, such as thiols, phenol, derivatives of catechol, quinones, and mercaptoamines. Loss of pigment follows both inhibition of tyrosinase and direct injury to melanocytes.

■ Clinical Features

The lesions are symmetrically distributed, ivory-white, depigmented, round, oval, or irregularly shaped macules, with sharp and sometimes hyperpigmented borders. The initial hypopigmentation progresses to depigmentation, and enlargement occurs with peripheral extension. Exposed sites such as the hands, distal arms, and periorificial regions of the face are often the first to be involved. Other typical locations include the axilla, groin, gluteal cleft, areolae, elbows, knees, knuckles, umbilicus, and shins. Some patients have extensive loss of pigment on the oral mucosa and in areas of minor trauma. In many patients—especially those with diffuse disease—a severe sunburn, chemical exposure, emotional stress, or physical illness is the triggering event.

Vitiligo is most commonly associated with premature graying and **halo nevi**—normal melanocytic nevi with a peripheral depigmented rim. Pigment loss may be noted in the retina. Vitiligo may also occur in patients with malignant melanoma at the primary tumor site and as a widespread progressive process. Several autoimmune disorders are also associated with vitiligo, including alopecia areata, Hashimoto's thyroiditis, hyperthyroidism, hypothyroidism, parathyroid disease, myasthenia gravis, diabetes mellitus, pernicious anemia, and idiopathic adrenal insufficiency.

■ Diagnosis and Differential Diagnosis

The diagnosis is based on history and skin examination. Important clues are the distribution, history of potential precipitating events, associated endocrinopathies, and family history of vitiligo or early graying of the hair. A Wood's lamp examination is important to enhance early subtle lesions and establish an accurate baseline. The physician should inquire about changes in vision. If signs or symptoms suggest an endocrinopathy or collagen vascular disease, a TSH and antibody panel (antinuclear antibody, antiparietal cell, antithyroid antibodies) should be obtained. Other important entities in the differential diagnosis include tinea versicolor, lichen sclerosus et atrophicus, postinflammatory hypopigmentation, leprosy, lupus erythematosus, sarcoidosis, and mycosis fungoides.

■ Management

Treatment is neither required nor consistently effective. Spontaneous repigmentation occurs in less than 25% of cases—more commonly in children and in lesions younger than 2 years old. Usually, extended periods of stability occur and then exacerbations are triggered by stress or illness.

The two primary forms of treatment are topical steroids and phototherapy. Topical corticosteroids are most effective in early-stage vitiligo and in localized disease. Treatment should be initiated with high-potency topical steroids in a test area. PUVA consists of psoralens plus UVA phototherapy. The psoralens enhance the effect of the ultraviolet light, and therapy may be complicated by severe phototoxic reactions. A protracted treatment course is often required to induce repigmentation. Eye protection must be worn for 24 hours after ingestion of psoralens because of its deposition in the lens of the eye. Because compliance with these restrictions may be difficult with children, PUVA should be used with great caution in this age group. Patients treated with topical PUVA soak the involved area in a psoralen solution and then expose the skin to ultraviolet light.

■ Questions

Questions 1–3: For each of the patients described in questions 1–3, refer to items A through H below and select the procedure that is most appropriate. Each item in A–H may be selected once, more than once, or not at all.
  A. Potassium hydroxide (KOH) preparation
  B. Skin biopsy
  C. Darkfield examination
  D. Tzanck smear
  E. Wood's lamp examination
  F. Gram stain
  G. Scabies preparation
  H. Patch testing

1. A 16-year-old girl has had painful, tense vesicles on her groin for the past 2 days.

2. A 5-year-old black child has a 3-week history of a scaling, itchy scalp.

3. A 21-year-old man has an intensely itchy rash between his fingers and on the scrotum. The itching gets worse at night. Numerous excoriations and crusting are noted in the web spaces. The lesions on the scrotum are more nodular.

Questions 4–5: For questions 4 and 5, select the drug from A through H below that is MOST likely responsible for the condition described. Each item in A–H may be used once, more than once, or not at all.
  A. Clonidine
  B. Propranolol
  C. Trimethoprim-Sulfamethoxazole
  D. Phenytoin
  E. Methotrexate
  F. Penicillamine
  G. Dapsone
  H. Furosemide

4. A 56-year-old man with a long history of mild psoriasis of the elbows and knees has sudden, widespread exacerbation of psoriasis.

5. A 62-year-old woman has a 3-week-old eruption involving the head and neck. Erosions and blisters are seen in a seborrheic distribution. The oral mucosa is clear.

Questions 6–8: For each patient described in questions 6–8, identify the organism from the items listed in A through H below that is most likely to be responsible. Each item in A–H may be used once, more than once, or not at all.
  A. *Trichophyton tonsurans*
  B. Group A ß-hemolytic streptococci

C. *Pthirus pubis*
D. *Pediculosis hominis*
E. *Sarcoptes scabiei*
F. Herpes zoster
G. Herpes simplex
H. *Candida albicans*

6. A 43-year-old woman has a red face for 2 days. Well-demarcated, erythematous plaques are seen on the entire lower right side of the face and she has a fever of 102°F.

7. A 7-year-old girl has the sudden onset of guttate, papulosquamous lesions 2 weeks after an upper respiratory infection.

8. A 25-year-old man has intense pruritus localized to the groin. Excoriations in the groin and adherent, white lesions on the eyelashes are noted.

Questions 9–12: For each question below, select only **one** lettered answer that is the **best** for that question.

9. An 82-year-old woman has had a blistering eruption for 2 months. Tense blisters are seen on an erythematous base, localized to the intertriginous areas, with sparing of mucous membranes. These clinical findings are most compatible with which of the following:
A. Pemphigus vulgaris
B. Pemphigus foliaceus
C. Dermatitis herpetiformis
D. Bullous pemphigoid
E. Erythema multiforme

10. A 42-year-old man with lichen simplex chronicus is given a topical steroid for use. The major barrier to absorption of the medication into his skin will be which of the following:
A. Lamina lucida
B. Stratum basale
C. Dermis
D. Stratum corneum
E. Stratum granulosum

11. A 36-year-old man has an atrophic nail with pterygium formation. The papulosquamous disorder most likely to cause these findings is which of the following:
A. Psoriasis
B. Lichen planus
C. Pityriasis rosea
D. Mycosis fungoides
E. Discoid lupus

12. A 24-year-old man is placed on topical steroids for a rash in the periorbital region. You caution him not to

get the medication into his eye because this can lead to which of the following:
A. pseudotumor cerebri
B. hypopyon
C. keratitis
D. iritis
E. glaucoma

■ **Answers**

1. D   2. A   3. G   4. B   5. F
6. B   7. B   8. C   9. D   10. D
11. B   12. E

SUGGESTED READING

Textbooks and Monographs

Champion RH, Burton JL, Ebling FJG (eds.). Textbook of Dermatology. London: Blackwell Scientific Publications, 1992.
Fitzpatrick TB, Eisen AZ, Wolff IC, et al. Dermatology in General Medicine. New York: McGraw-Hill, 1993.
Sams WM, Lynch PJ (eds.). Principles and Practice of Dermatology. New York: Churchill Livingstone, 1990, pp. 235–238.

Articles
Therapy

Pierard GE, Pierard-Franchimont C, Ben Mosbah T, et al. Adverse effects of topical corticosteroids. *Acta Derm Venereol* 1989; 69:26–30.
Tanz RR, Hebert AA, Esterly NB. Treating tinea capitis: should ketoconazole replace griseofulvin? *J Pediatrics* 1988; 112:987–991.

Papulosquamous Disorders

Boyd AS, Nelder KH. Lichen planus. J Am Acad Dermatol 1991;25(4):593–619.
Fox BJ, Odom RB. Papulosquamous diseases: a review. J Am Acad Dermatol 1985;12(24):597–624.
Stern RS. Psoriasis. Lancet 1997;350(9074):349–353.
Simpson KR, Lowe NJ. Trends in topical psoriasis therapy. Int J Dermatol 1994; 33(5):333–336.

Vesiculobullous Disorders

Diaz LA, Provost TT. Pemphigus. In Lichenstein LA, Fauci AS (eds.). Current Therapy in Allergy and Immunology. St. Louis: C.V. Mosby, 1983, pp. 166–170.
Rye B, Webb JM. Autoimmune bullous diseases. Am Fam Physician 1997;55:2709–2718.
Wooldridge WE. Three blistering diseases. Why proper management is critical. Postgrad Med 1990;88:103–104.

Hypersensitivity Disorders

Calabrese LH. Cutaneous vasculitis, hypersensitivity vasculitis, erythema nodosum, and pyoderma gangrenosum. Curr Opin Rheum 1991;3(1):23–27.
Hurwitz S. Erythema multiforme: a review of its characteristics, diagnostic criteria, and management. Pediatr Rev 1990;11:217–222.
Parsons JM. Toxic epidermal necrolysis. Int J Dermatol 1992;31(11):749–768.

Dermatitis—Eczema

Fitzpatrick JE. Stasis ulcers: Update on a common geriatric problem. Geriatrics 1989;44:19–21, 25, 26, 31.

Rabinowitz LG, Esterly NB. Atopic dermatitis and ichthyosis vulgaris. Pediatr Rev 1994;15(6):220–226.

Rebora A, Rongioletti F. The red face: Seborrheic dermatitis. Clin Dermatol 1993;11(2):243–51

Rietschel RL, Ray MC. Nonatopic eczemas. J Am Acad Dermatol 1988;18(3):569–573.

Benign Tumors of the Skin

Banik R, Lubach D. Skin tags: localization and frequencies according to sex and age. Dermatologica 1987;174(4):180–183.

Gallagher RP, McLean DI, Yang CP, et al. Suntan, sunburn, and pigmentation factors and the frequency of acquired melanocytic nevi in children. Similarities to melanoma: the Vancouver mole study. Arch Dermatol 1990;126(6):770–776.

Lindelof B, Sigurgeirsson B, Melander S. Seborrheic keratoses and cancer. J Am Acad Dermatol 1992; 26: 947–950.

Murray JC. Keloids and hypertrophic scars. Clin Dermatol 1994;12(1):27–37.

Malignant Tumors of the Skin

Cohen LM. Lentigo maligna and lentigo maligna melanoma. J Am Acad Dermatol 1995;33:923–936.

Creagan ET. Malignant melanoma: an emerging and preventable medical catastrophe. Mayo Clin Proc 1997;72:570–574.

Preston DS, Stern RS. Nonmelanoma cancers of the skin. N Engl J Med 1992;327(23):1649–1662.

Sober AJ. Diagnosis and management of early melanoma: a consensus view. Semin Surg Oncol 1993;9(3):194–197.

Acne

Healy E, Simpson N. Acne vulgaris. BMJ 1994; 308:831–833.

Wilkin JK. Rosacea. Pathophysiology and treatment. Arch Dermatol 1994;130(3):359–362.

Fungal Infections of the Skin

Borelli D, Jacobs PH, Nall L. Tinea versicolor: epidemiologic, clinical, and therapeutic aspects. J Am Acad Dermatol 1991;25:300–305.

Brodell RT, Elewski B. Superficial fungal infections. Errors to avoid in diagnosis and treatment. Postgrad Med 1997;101:279–287.

Goldstein SM. Advances in the treatment of superficial candida infections. Semin Dermatol 1993;12(4):315–330.

Gupta AK, Sauder DN, Shear NH. Antifungal agents: an overview. J Am Acad Dermatol 1994;30(5):677–700; 30:911–933(2 parts).

Mehregan DA, Mehregan DR, Rinker A. Onychomycosis. Cutis 1997;59:247–248.

Bacterial Infections of the Skin

Dahl MV. Strategies for the management of recurrent furunculosis. South Med J 1987;80(3):352–356.

Elsner P. Treatment of bacterial sexually transmitted diseases. Semin Dermatol 1993;12(4):342–351.

Feingold DS. Staphylococcal and streptococcal pyodermas. Semin Dermatol 1993;12(4):296–300.

Grosshans EM. The red face: Erysipelas. Clin Dermatol 1993;11(2):307–313.

Johnson PC, Farnie MA. Testing for syphilis. Dermatol Clin 1994;12(1):9–12.

Kraus SJ. Diagnosis and management of acute genital ulcers in sexually active patients. *Semin Dermatol* 1990;9(2):160–166.

Schachner L, Gonzalez A. Diagnosis and treatment of impetigo. J Am Acad Dermatol 1989;20(1):132.

Viral Infections of the Skin

Cobb MW. Human papillomavirus infection. J Am Acad Dermatol 1990;22(4):547–566.

Corey L, Spear PG. Infections with herpes simplex viruses (I and II). N Engl J Med 1986;314:169–172, 686–691.

Green J. Therapy for genital warts. Dermatol Clin 1992;10(1):253–267.

Williams LR, Webster G. Warts and molluscum contagiosum. Clin Dermatol 1991;9(1):87–93.

Infestations of the Skin

Janniger CK. Kuflik AS. Pediculosis capitis. Cutis 1993; 51(6):407–408.

Rasmussen JE. Scabies. Pediatr Rev 1994; 15(3):110–114.

Pigmentary Disorders of the Skin

Grimes PE. Vitiligo. Dermatol Clin 1993; 11(3):325–338.

PART VI

Diana L. Maas
Albert L. Jochen
Irene M.
O'Shaughnessy
Russell Wilke

ENDOCRINE AND METABOLIC DISORDERS

CHAPTER 56

DISEASES OF THE ANTERIOR PITUITARY GLAND

The pituitary gland has three lobes: the anterior (adenohypophysis), the posterior (neurohypophysis), and the intermediate. It is surrounded by important structures that can be affected by its enlargement, including the optic chiasm, cranial nerves, and the internal carotid artery; the last two are contained within the cavernous sinuses. The infundibular stalk connects the pituitary gland with the hypothalamus and contains the portal plexus. The adenohypophyseal hormones are regulated by a neuroendocrine system of stimulatory and inhibitory peptides produced in the ventral hypothalamus and transported to the anterior lobe through the hypothalamic-hypophyseal portal system.

■ Production and Function of Adenohypophyseal Hormones

Six major hormones are synthesized and released by the anterior pituitary: corticotropin (ACTH), thyroid-stimulating hormone (TSH), prolactin (PRL), follicle-stimulating hormone (FSH), luteinizing hormone (LH),

and growth hormone (GH). Their major regulatory pathways and end organ products are shown in Figure 56.1. All of the anterior pituitary hormones, except possibly prolactin, are feedback-controlled by their end organ secretory products, at both the hypothalamic and pituitary levels. Prolactin is primarily regulated by an inhibitory factor, dopamine. GH secretion is pulsatile throughout the day, with the largest secretory peak in young, healthy adults occurring 60–120 minutes after the onset of stages 3 and 4 sleep. ACTH secretion and the levels of plasma cortisol that it evokes are widely pulsatile but strongly diurnal; both hormones peak at around 8 AM and ebb from 6 PM to midnight. The normally pulsatile gonadotropin-releasing hormone (GnRH) secretion stimulates release of LH and FSH; when infused continuously, however, it inhibits LH and FSH release.

The major site of action of the hormone prolactin is the mammary gland, where it stimulates postpartum lactation. Prolactin regulates dopamine and GnRH release in the hypothalamus. GH exerts its effects directly and indirectly through its synthesis of insulin-like growth

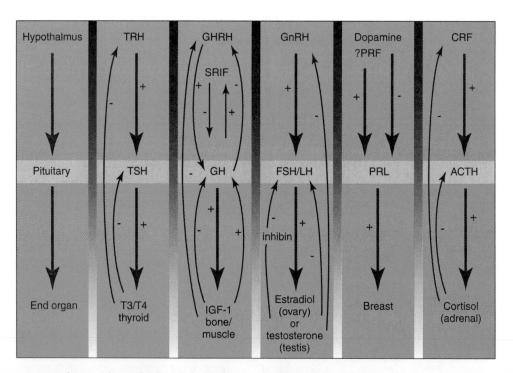

FIGURE 56.1. Regulatory pathways for the six major adenohypophyseal hormones. IGF-I = Insulin-like Growth Factor-I; SRIF = Somatostatin; PRF = Prolactin Releasing Factor; GHRH = Growth Hormone Releasing Hormone; CRH = Corticotropin Releasing Hormone; GnRH = Gonadotropin Releasing Hormone.

TABLE 56.1.   Evaluation of Pituitary Function

Pituitary Hormone	Laboratory Evaluation	Abnormal Results
ACTH	Insulin-induced hypoglycemia	Cortisol level <18 µg/dl in response to symptomatic hypoglycemia (plasma glucose <40 mg/dl)
	Overnight metyrapone: Drug that inhibits the enzyme 11 β-hydroxylase which catalyzes the conversion of 11-deoxycortisol (compound S) into cortisol (compound F)	Cortisol level <5 µg/dl and 11-deoxycortisol <7 µg/dl
FSH, LH	Simultaneous assessment of basal FSH/LH/17β-estradiol	Low 17 β-estradiol with low or inappropriately normal FSH and LH
	Simultaneous assessment of basal FSH/LH/Testosterone	Low total testosterone with low or inappropriately normal FSH and LH
TSH	Free T$_4$ measured, TSH	Low free T$_4$ with low or inappropriately normal TSH
GH	Insulin-induced hypoglycemia Levodopa Infusion Clonidine Exercise	GH level <7 ng/ml

TABLE 56.2.   Treatment of Panhypopituitarism

Pituitary Hormone	Hormone Replacement
ACTH	Cortisone acetate 25 mg AM, 12.5 mg PM; Hydrocortisone 20 mg AM, 10 mg PM
TSH	Thyroxine: Dosage adjusted to keep free T$_4$ in the normal range
FSH/LH	Men: Testosterone enanthate or cypionate, 200 mg IM q2 weeks: Testosterone patch
	Women: Estrogen therapy, oral or transdermal, adjusted to relieve symptoms
GH	In prepubertal children only: Synthetic GH subcutaneous injections 3×/week

factor I (IGF-I, somatomedin-C), mainly in the liver. GH stimulates skeletal and soft tissue growth, lipolysis in adipose tissue, protein synthesis (especially) in muscle, and lactotropic activity by breast tissue; by antagonizing insulin, it inhibits cellular glucose uptake and stimulates hepatic gluconeogenesis and glycogenolysis. The effects on skeletal growth may be partially mediated through IGF-I. In both genders, the major functional roles of the gonadotropins LH and FSH include pubertal sexual development, fertility, and sexual activity; most of these functions are mediated through estrogen and progesterone in women and through testosterone in men. ACTH has its major effect on the adrenal glands, where it stimulates synthesis and secretion of glucocorticoids and adrenal androgens. TSH stimulates all aspects of the synthesis and secretion of the thyroid hormones, thyroxine (T4) and triiodothyronine (T3).

Pituitary tumors, usually benign, comprise 10–15% of intracranial tumors. A pituitary adenoma is the most common cause of pituitary insufficiency and pituitary masses in adults. These tumors are considered microadenomas if the vertical height on magnetic resonance imaging (MRI) or computed tomography (CT) is 10 mm or less, or as macroadenomas if vertical height exceeds 10 mm. Typically, a pituitary tumor presents with signs and symptoms related to mass effect and/or endocrine dysfunction. The endocrine dysfunction may be due to hyposecretion or hypersecretion of a pituitary hormone by the tumor.

Common clinical features of a pituitary mass include headache, visual field deficits, and cranial nerve palsies. The headache is typically retro-orbital or bitemporal. Its pathogenesis is unknown, but may be due to stretching of dura mater. The classic visual field abnormality, which is formally tested by Goldman perimetry, is bitemporal hemianopsia; it results from suprasellar tumor extension and compression of the optic chiasm. A pituitary tumor laterally invading into the cavernous sinuses may lead to dysfunction of cranial nerves III, IV, and VI, causing ophthalmoplegia, and of cranial nerves V1 and V2, causing facial pain.

Hormonal insufficiency due to a pituitary tumor may involve any or all of the six major pituitary hormones; it usually results from compression of normal pituitary tissue by the tumor. The earliest and most common manifestation of pituitary hormonal deficiency is impotence in men and amenorrhea in women. The tumor may compress the pituitary gonadotrophs, thus directly decreasing gonadotropin secretion; the elevated blood levels of prolactin (**hyperprolactinemia**) produced by a prolactin-secreting pituitary tumor inhibit the hypothalamic-derived GnRH, thus indirectly decreasing gonadotropin secretion. Despite variations, pituitary hormones are lost in the following order: GH, FSH/LH,

TSH, ACTH; prolactin deficiency is rare. Rather, pituitary macroadenomas usually produce mild hyperprolactinemia (PRL 20–100 ng/ml), which results from decreased dopamine inhibition due to infundibular stalk interruption. In adults, GH deficiency evokes no major clinical consequences. In children with pituitary insufficiency, growth retardation and delayed puberty are common presenting signs. Anterior pituitary hormone insufficiency is diagnosed biochemically (Table 56.1) and clinically (e.g., gonadal failure, hypothyroidism, and adrenal insufficiency). Pituitary hormone replacement is discussed in Table 56.2. A functional morphological classification of pituitary adenomas, which has gained wide acceptance, is useful in predicting the biologic behavior of the various tumor types and in planning their appropriate treatment strategies. Types of pituitary adenomas and their prevalence are listed in Table 56.3. The initial laboratory workup of a newly diagnosed pituitary tumor is shown in Table 56.4.

TABLE 56.3.	Incidence of Pituitary Adenomas
Prolactin-secreting	27–29%
Nonsecretory or Null cell	25%
GH-secreting	13–16%
ACTH-secreting	10–14%
Plurihormonal	8–12%
LH/FSH/alpha subunit-secreting	2–9%
Silent adenomas (ACTH-staining)	5%
TSH-secreting	1%

TABLE 56.4.	Laboratory Evaluation of Pituitary Tumors
Pituitary Tumor	**Biochemical Features**
Prolactinoma	Serum prolactin level usually >200 ng/ml
Acromegaly	Somatomedin C elevated above normal level for age. Non-suppressible serum GH level >2 ng/ml 2 hours after 75 gram oral glucose load
Cushing's Disease	Elevated 24-hour urinary free cortisol (always obtain simultaneous urine creatinine to ensure specimen is sufficient)
	1 mg Dexamethasone (given at 11:00 PM the night before) suppression test: abnormal if 8:00 AM fasting serum cortisol >5 µg/dl
TSH-secreting	Serum TSH inappropriately normal or elevated with elevated free T_4 or total T_4 Serum alpha subunit elevated Alpha subunit/TSH >1
FSH/LH/alpha subunit-secreting	Elevated serum LH, FSH, and/or alpha-subunit

Lactotroph Adenomas and Hyperprolactinemia

■ Epidemiology

Hyperprolactinemia accounts for at least 20% of infertility in women and approximately 8% of sexual dysfunction in men, including infertility. The causes of pathological hyperprolactinemia are diverse (Table 56.5), but a prolactin-secreting pituitary tumor is, by far, the most common cause. The pathogenesis of these tumors is unknown.

■ Clinical Features and Diagnosis

The clinical presentation of prolactinomas varies with the patient's age and gender. Typically, young menstruating women report irregular menses (amenor-

rhea, oligomenorrhea, or delayed menarche), infertility, or galactorrhea. The galactorrhea occurs in 30–80% of these women. Hyperprolactinemia directly suppresses hypothalamic GnRH secretion, resulting in amenorrhea. Given this early disturbance in the menstrual cycle, prolactinomas are typically microadenomas at the time of diagnosis. In contrast, men and postmenopausal women usually present with macroprolactinomas that produce tumor mass-related effects. Approximately 80% of these men report decreased libido and the majority are fully or partially impotent; galactorrhea occurs in 20–30%.

A serum PRL level exceeding 200 ng/ml is diagnostic of a prolactinoma. While a slightly elevated PRL level (20–200 ng/ml) may be the result of a microprolacti-

TABLE 56.5. Causes of Hyperprolactinemia	
Category	**Examples/Disorders**
Physiologic	Pregnancy, nipple stimulation/suckling
	Stress, exercise, sleep
Pathologic	
Pituitary adenoma	Prolactin-secreting pituitary tumor
	Plurihormonal-secreting pituitary tumor (acromegaly)
Hypothalamic-pituitary disorders causing hyperprolactine-mia in the absence of a prolactinoma	Tumor (e.g. craniopharyngioma, germinoma)
	Histiocytosis X
	Sarcoidosis
	Pituitary stalk interruption/secretion
	Radiation involving neuraxis
	Surgery
Adrenal insufficiency	
Cirrhosis	
Primary hypothyroidism	
Renal failure	
Drug-induced	Estrogens/oral contraceptives
	Psychotropic drugs (e.g. phenothiazines, tricyclic antidepressants)
	Reserpine
	Methyldopa
	Metoclopramide
	Opiates
	Methadone
	Cimetidine
	Cocaine
Neurogenic	Chest wall lesions/surgery
	Spinal cord lesions
	Breast stimulation
"Functional"/idiopathic	

noma, mild PRL elevations can also result from one of several secondary causes (e.g., renal failure, primary hypothyroidism, or drugs).

■ Management and Prognosis

The dopamine agonists bromocriptine and cabergoline decrease serum prolactin levels consistently and rapidly and reduce tumor size in 80% of patients. Dopamine agonists are thus the treatment of choice for all clinically significant microprolactinomas and macroprolactinomas. Many clinicians advocate initial treatment with a dopamine agonist for all patients, even those with visual abnormalities. Surgical resection is reserved for prolactinomas that do not respond to medical therapy or for patients who cannot tolerate the side effects of the dopamine agonists. External radiation therapy is reserved for the occasional patient who is refractory to or intolerant of these conventional therapies. The ultimate goal of therapy, whether medical and/or surgical, is decompression of the optic chiasm, correction of cranial nerve abnormalities, and resumption of normal pituitary hormone function.

Somatotroph Adenoma or Acromegaly

■ Definition and Epidemiology

Acromegaly, abnormal enlargement of the extremities of the skeleton caused by hypersecretion of GH after maturity, has an estimated annual incidence of three to four cases per million, without any gender predilection. It can occur at any age, but is most frequently diagnosed in the fourth or fifth decade of life. Approximately 85% of cases result from a GH-secreting pituitary macroadenoma (Table 56.6). GH-producing pituitary tumors account for nearly 17% of all surgically resected pituitary tumors; about 30% of these tumors also secrete prolactin. Excessive GH secretion in a prepubertal child prior to the

TABLE 56.6.	Causes of Acromegaly

Pituitary adenoma
   Pure growth hormone secreting
   Mixed growth hormone/prolactin secreting
Ectopic pituitary tumor
   Sphenoid sinus
   Parapharyngeal sinus
Ectopic growth hormone-releasing hormone secreting
   Small cell carcinoma of the lung
   Carcinoid
   Pancreatic islet tumor
   Adrenal adenoma
   Pheochromocytoma
Ectopic growth hormone secreting (rare)
   Pancreas
   Lung
   Ovary
   Breast

TABLE 56.7.	Clinical Manifestations of Acromegaly

Coarsening facial features/soft tissue swelling
Frontal bossing
Dental malocclusion with increased spacing between teeth
Headaches
Excessive sweating
Soft tissue swelling in hands/feet
Increased ring/glove size
Increased shoe size/width with thick heel pad
Skin tags
Colon polyps/cancer
Carpal tunnel syndrome
Hypertension
Diabetes mellitus
Deep, resonant voice/laryngeal thickening
Obstructive sleep apnea
Galactorrhea
Osteoarthritis—especially knees and hips
Visceromegaly

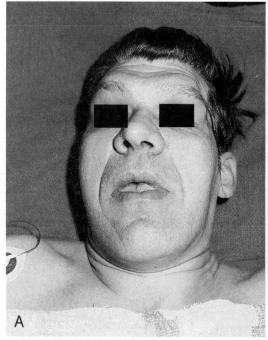
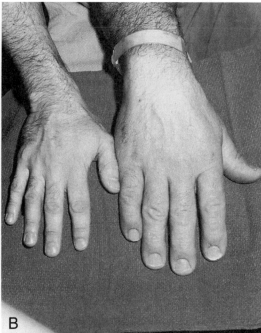

FIGURE **56.2.** **A.** Physical appearance of a 48-year-old acromegalic man. Note coarse facial features and prognathous. **B.** Acromegaly. The hand on the left is that of an adult normal man and the one on the right is that of the man with acromegaly shown in **A.**

closure of the epiphyseal growth plates leads to gigantism; this condition is very rare.

■ Clinical Features and Diagnosis

The manifestations of excessive GH secretion (Table 56.7 and Figure 56.2) usually develop gradually in older patients. Because they are insidious, these changes are often missed by the patient and are instead first noted by someone who has not seen the patient for a long time. In younger patients, these tumors are more aggressive; thus, the characteristic features evolve more rapidly. Besides the characteristic facial and acral soft tissue changes produced by excessive GH secretion, the sellar mass itself may also evoke symptoms from local effects. Nearly one-half of acromegalics harbor colonic polyps and about 5% develop colon cancer. Risk factors for neoplasia include age above 50, duration of acromegaly exceeding 10 years, and presence of three or more skin tags.

A serum somatomedin C level usually suffices as a screening test for acromegaly. Diagnostic biochemical criteria are elevated somatomedin C and nonsuppressible serum GH level above 2 ng/ml 2h after a 75 gram oral glucose load.

■ Management and Prognosis

Acromegaly is a difficult disease to cure. Treatment goals include lowering the serum GH level below 2 ng/ml two hours after a 75 gram oral glucose administration; normalizing the somatomedin C level; and reversing associated medical problems, including diabetes mellitus, hypertension, soft tissue hyperplasia, and hyperhidrosis. Management options include surgery, radiation therapy, and medications; most patients require all three. Surgical removal or debulkment of the tumor remains the first line of therapy. A surgical cure can be obtained in 80% of patients with microadenomas. Using the above biochemical criteria, surgery cures less than 30% of patients with macroadenomas. The somatostatin analogue, octreotide, and the dopamine agonists, bromocriptine and cabergoline, are used as medical therapy for acromegaly. Octreotide is useful as adjunctive therapy when cure is not achieved by surgery and/or radiation. It can also be used preoperatively to reduce the tumor size. Some patients respond to dopamine agonists; octreotide and a dopamine agonist can also be combined.

Corticotroph Adenoma or Cushing's Disease

■ Definition and Epidemiology

Cushing's syndrome is a condition caused by excess amounts of cortisol in the bloodstream **(hypercortisolemia)**, resulting from hypersecretion of the adrenal cortex or prolonged exposure to high therapeutic doses of glucocorticoids. It has widespread systemic effects, as summarized in Table 56.8. **Cushing's disease** refers to a subset of Cushing's syndrome, resulting from pituitary ACTH hypersecretion; it accounts for approximately 75–85% of adults with Cushing's syndrome. The underlying pathology of Cushing's disease in about 90% of cases is anterior pituitary microadenomas; pituitary hyperplasia underlies the remaining 10%. Cushing's disease is six times more common in women than in men; the mean age at diagnosis is in the fourth decade.

■ Etiology and Pathogenesis

Iatrogenic (exogenous) causes are the most frequent, owing to the widespread use of pharmacologic doses of glucocorticoids. Endogenous cases may be ACTH-dependent (e.g., ACTH-secreting pituitary adenoma or ectopic ACTH-secreting neoplasm) or ACTH-independent (e.g., adrenal adenoma, adrenal carcinoma). Benign adrenal tumors causing Cushing's syndrome predominantly produce glucocorticoids; adrenal cancers,

TABLE 56.8.	Clinical Manifestations of Hypercortisolemia

Truncal obesity
Hypertension
Facial plethora (round face)
Hirsutism/vellus type hair growth
Gonadal dysfunction
   Menstrual disorders
   Impotence/decreased libido
Osteopenia/back pain
Supraclavicular/dorsocervical fat pads
Neuropsychiatric disorders/depression
Violaceous abdominal striae >1 cm width
Proximal muscle weakness
Headache
Acne
Easy bruising
Superficial fungal infections
Poor wound healing
Hyperpigmentation
Glucose intolerance/diabetes mellitus
Nephrolithiasis

however, frequently secrete high levels of adrenal **androgens, mineralocorticoids,** and **glucocorticoids.** Ectopic ACTH secretion occurs in a few neoplasms,

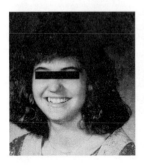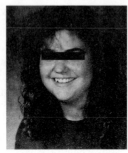

FIGURE 56.3. Photographs of a young woman with Cushing's syndrome showing subtle changes in the facial outlines over a three-year period.
(Photographs courtesy of James Findling, MD, St. Luke's Hospital, Milwaukee, Wisconsin.)

Cushing's syndrome must be further separated into a pituitary tumor or an ectopic ACTH-secreting neoplasm. A normal CT or MRI of the sella cannot make this distinction, since only 50–60% of patients with Cushing's disease have a sellar abnormality on MRI or CT.

■ Management and Prognosis

Transsphenoidal resection is the treatment of choice for the ACTH-secreting pituitary neoplasm; adrenalectomy is the preferred treatment in glucocorticoid-producing adrenal neoplasms. Remissions occur in approximately 80–90% of patients with Cushing's disease who undergo transsphenoidal adenoma resection. Conventional external radiotherapy is not effective as a primary treatment, but it may be combined with pituitary

(e.g., small cell carcinoma of the lung, carcinoid tumors, pancreatic islet cell tumors) usually afflicting men in the fifth decade and beyond.

■ Clinical Features

It is helpful to examine serial photographs of the patient (Figure 56.3), looking for evidence of progressive physical changes consistent with excessive cortisol exposure. The facial plethora (round face) may be subtle (Figure 56.3) or quite obvious (Figure 56.4). Cushing's syndrome can also be caused by ectopic production of ACTH by certain cancers, classically in small cell cancer of the lung. These patients more frequently present with severe proximal weakness, weight loss, and hypokalemia along with rapid development of the florid clinical manifestations of Cushing's syndrome.

■ Diagnosis

The evaluation of a patient with suspected Cushing's syndrome is outlined in Figure 56.5. Screening with the 24-hour urinary free cortisol has very few false positives; the 1 mg dexamethasone suppression test, however, may be false-positive from acute stress or illness, obesity, anticonvulsant agents, liver disease, high estrogen states, alcoholism, or affective disorders. Once hypercortisolemia is established, the distinction between ACTH-dependence and ACTH-independence should follow, based on measurement of plasma ACTH; levels exceeding 20 pg/ml indicate ACTH-dependent hypercortisolism. Patients with primary adrenal neoplasms have a suppressed or low plasma ACTH (<10 pg/ml) and adrenal mass on CT scan. ACTH-dependent

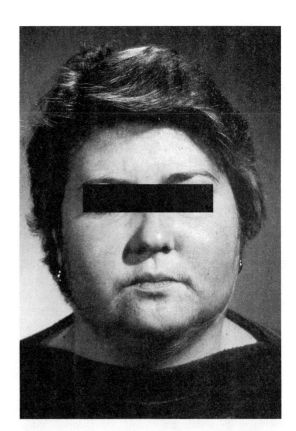

FIGURE 56.4. Photograph of a middle-aged woman with Cushing's syndrome demonstrating the characteristic plethoric facies.
(Photograph courtesy of James Findling, MD, St. Luke's Hospital, Milwaukee, Wisconsin.)

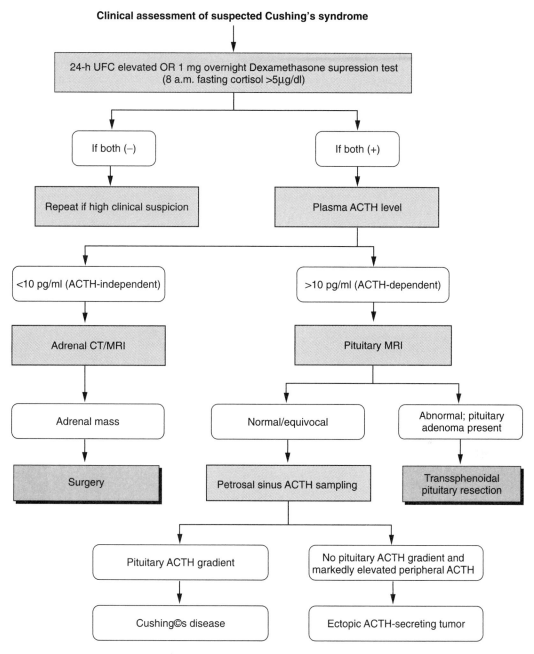

FIGURE 56.5. Work-up for the diagnosis and further differentiation of Cushing's syndrome. UFC = Urinary Free Cortisol.

surgery. Heavy charged-particle stereotactic radiosurgery is also used as initial therapy, but is not widely available and has a high complication rate (e.g., cranial nerve palsies, visual field defects, and hypopituitarism). Ec-topic ACTH production is managed by treating the primary tumor or by using adrenolytic agents such as mitotane, aminoglutethimide, or metyrapone. These agents are also useful in inoperable cases.

CHAPTER 57

DISORDERS OF THE POSTERIOR PITUITARY GLAND

The posterior lobe of the pituitary, which comprises only 20% of the total pituitary mass, is one of the three components of the neurohypophysis, the other two being the hypothalamic supraoptic and paraventricular neurons, and the supraopticohypophysial tract (Figure 57.1). The neurohypophyseal hormones are regulated by a direct neurosecretory pathway from the anterior hypothalamus.

The posterior pituitary secretes two major peptide hormones, **oxytocin** and **vasopressin** (known also as **antidiuretic hormone,** ADH). Both are synthesized in the hypothalamus, packaged into neurosecretory gran-ules, transported along axons to the posterior pituitary gland, and stored until released into the blood stream (Figure 57.1). Oxytocin stimulates uterine contraction, but its importance in normal parturition is unclear. Nipple stimulation by the suckling infant causes pituitary release of oxytocin, followed by milk ejection by the nipple. ADH is the major regulator of renal water excretion, and, therefore, of the total body water balance. Its deficiency causes diabetes insipidus (DI) with hypernatremia and polyuria; excess ADH leads to syndrome of inappropriate ADH (SIADH) with hy-ponatremia and oliguria.

FIGURE 57.1. A schematic illustration of the neurohypophysis, including the hypothalamic paraventricular and supraoptic nuclei, supraopti-cohypophysial tract, and posterior pituitary gland (neurohypophysis).

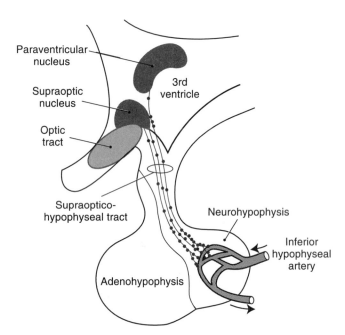

Diabetes Insipidus

■ Definition

Diabetes insipidus is characterized by **polyuria,** defined as the excretion of urine in excess of 2–3 L/24 hours. Large volumes of dilute urine are excreted, giving rise to severe **polydipsia** (excessive thirst) and a specific craving for ice water. Biochemical and clinical hallmarks of DI are shown in Table 57.1.

■ Etiology, Pathogenesis, and Clinical Features

The three major types of DI are **hypothalamic** (central), **nephrogenic** or renal-resistant, and **dipsogenic primary polydipsia** (Table 57.2). There are two primary differences between hypothalamic and nephrogenic DI: (1) the plasma ADH concentration and (2) the response

TABLE 57.1.	Biochemical and Clinical Hallmarks of Diabetes Insipidus (DI)
Clinical	
Polyuria	
Urine output	>200 ml/hr
Mild:	2–4L/day
Moderate:	4–6 L/day
Severe:	>6 L/day
Polydipsia:	
Especially crave very cold fluids/ice water	
Biochemical	
Urine	
Specific gravity	≤1.005
Osm_U	Inappropriately ↓ for ↑ Osm_{Pl}
Plasma	
*Hypernatremia	Serum Na^+ >145 mEq/L
*Osm_{Pl}	>290 mOsm/L
ADH level	
Central DI	↓ or inappropriately nl
Nephrogenic DI	↑
Water deprivation test	
Response to Vasopressin	
Central DI	(±) or full
Nephrogenic DI	(±) or none

Osm_U = Urine osmolality; Osm_{Pl} = Plasma osmolality; (±) = partial; ↑ = elevated; ↓ = decreased; *Present if inadequate hypotonic fluid replacement or uncompensated.

to vasopressin injection. Dipsogenic primary polydipsia results from overdrinking, with resultant polyuria and ADH suppression.

Hypothalamic DI is uncommon; it requires the destruction of at least 90% of ADH synthesizing hypothalamic neurons. DI caused by destruction of the posterior pituitary gland is not permanent, because the axons can regenerate new axon and capillary contacts to release ADH. While nearly two-thirds of traumatic and postsurgical DI are transient, idiopathic DI is almost always permanent. Postoperative DI has a rapid onset, usually developing within 24 hours following surgery. Some patients with postoperative or traumatic DI may exhibit a "triphasic" response. The first phase is DI due to axon shock or lack of release of vasopressin lasting 5–10 days. The second phase, lasting for about a week, is characterized by antidiuresis due to the release of excessive amounts of vasopressin from the degenerating axon terminals. During this phase, the patient may require fluid restriction and cessation of desmopressin therapy. The third or final phase, which may be permanent or transient, is the return of DI after the pool of stored vasopressin is exhausted.

The key abnormality in nephrogenic DI is a refractoriness to vasopressin on the part of the renal collecting ducts, resulting in the output of inappropriately hypotonic urine compared with a hypertonic plasma. Renal resistant DI is further characterized by normal renal filtration rate and solute excretion, normal (if partial nephrogenic DI is present) or elevated plasma ADH level, and a failure of exogenous vasopressin to raise urine osmolality by 50% or to reduce urine volume. Lithium-induced nephrogenic DI may not be reversible, unlike nephrogenic DI due to hypokalemia, hypercalcemia, and prolonged polyuria.

TABLE 57.2.	Causes of Diabetes Insipidus
Central/Hypothalamic	Idiopathic (30%)
	Post-cranial syndrome (20%)
	Tumors (20%)
	craniopharyngioma (most common)
	pituitary macroadenoma
	meningioma
	dysgerminoma
	metastatic carcinoma (lungs, breast)
	Head injury (16%)
	Vascular
	Sheehan's syndrome
	aneurysms
	cerebral hypoperfusion
	Granulomatous disease
	sarcoidosis
	histiocytosis
	Infections
	meningitis
	encephalitis
	Autoimmune
Nephrogenic/renal resistant	Idiopathic
	Chronic renal disease
	Hypokalemia
	Hypercalcemia
	Drug-induced
	lithium
	demeclocycline
	methoxyflurane
	Amyloidosis
	Post-obstructive uropathy
Dipsogenic primary polydipsia	Idiopathic
	Psychogenic
	Drug-induced
	tricyclic antidepressants
	anticholinergic

Primary or psychogenic polydipsia, usually seen in psychotic patients, is an uncommon condition, featuring excessive water intake and polyuria; genuine thirst is absent. It requires the intake of gallons of water. This excessive drinking leads to plasma dilution, physiologic ADH suppression, and resultant polyuria. This disorder is diagnosed by demonstrating a normal osmoregulated ADH secretion and renal function during a standard water deprivation test. The treatment is fluid restriction; no therapy other than that of the underlying psychosis is required.

■ Diagnosis

The diagnosis of DI and its etiology is established with a standard water deprivation test (Figure 57.2). The patient is deprived of all water intake until dehydration results, with a weight loss of at least 2% of body weight

and a rise in plasma osmolality above 300 mOsm/kg. If polyuria remits, it practically excludes DI; if it persists, osmolality of two plasma and consecutive voided urine samples is measured. Aqueous vasopressin (5U) is given subcutaneously and urine and plasma osmolality measurements are repeated. Typical results in patients with central and nephrogenic DI as well as normals are shown in Table 57.3.

■ Management and Prognosis

In acute postsurgical and traumatic hypothalamic DI, hypotonic oral or IV fluids are given to replace the losses and maintain hydration. Vasopressin, if needed, is given subcutaneously as a short-acting aqueous preparation. This procedure makes it possible to assess whether the DI is permanent while at the same time avoiding overtreatment, with resultant free water retention and hyponatre-

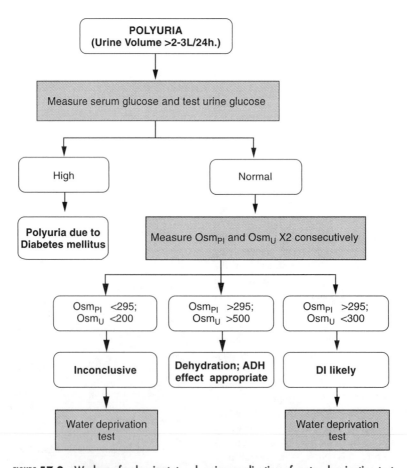

FIGURE **57.2.** Workup of polyuric states showing application of water deprivation test.

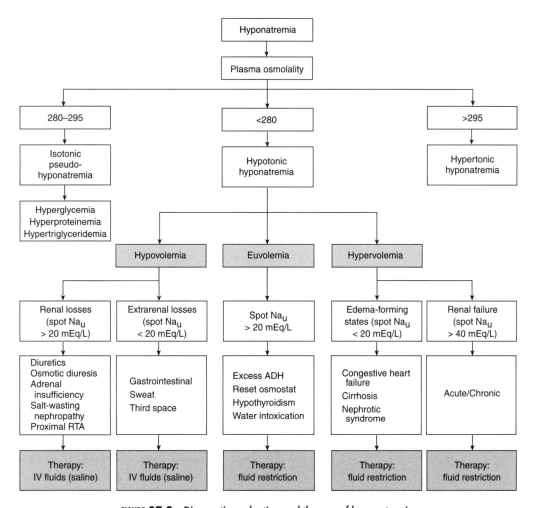

FIGURE 57.3. Diagnostic evaluation and therapy of hyponatremia.

TABLE 57.3.	Interpretation of the Standard Water Deprivation Test	
	Ability to Concentrate Urine with Dehydration	
State	**Before ADH**	**After ADH**
Normal	+++	$\uparrow$, <5%
Complete Central DI	+	$\uparrow$, >50%
Partial Central DI	+	$\uparrow$, >10%
Complete Nephrogenic DI	++	No response
Partial Nephrogenic DI	++	$\uparrow$, >10%
Primary Polydipsia	+++	$\uparrow$, <5%

+++ = marked; ++ = moderate; + = minimal; $\uparrow$ = increased; $\downarrow$ = decreased.

mia. Chronic central DI is usually treated with the long-acting synthetic analogue 1-desamino-8-D-arginine-vasopressin (DDAVP, 10-20 µg, 2-3 intranasal insufflations daily or 0.1–0.2 mg, 2–3 oral tablets daily). Other drugs (chlorpropamide, carbamazepine, and clofibrate) are most effective in patients with partial central DI. Chlorpropamide enhances the renal effects of vasopressin, while clofibrate and carbamazepine increase its release. Besides removal of the underlying cause and ensuring adequate hydration, no specific treatment exists for nephrogenic DI. Reducing the solute load by medications and restricting the patient's salt intake help reduce polyuria and minimize nocturia; thiazides are the most effective agents in this context.

Syndrome of Inappropriate Antidiuretic Hormone Secretion

■ Definition and Epidemiology

SIADH is characterized by continual vasopressin release in the face of subnormal plasma osmolality or in the absence of either osmotic or nonosmotic stimuli. It accounts for over 95% of hyponatremia in the hospital population.

■ Etiology

Small cell lung cancer is the most common malignancy causing SIADH. Other underlying conditions are listed in Table 57.4.

■ Clinical Features and Diagnosis

Clinical features are usually those of hyponatremia (lethargy, confusion, muscle cramps, coma, seizures), those of the underlying etiology, and generally, diminished urine output. Significant thirst, edema, hypo-

TABLE 57.4. Conditions Associated with SIADH	
Physiologic	Nausea, pain
Pathologic	
Tumors	Carcinoma (lung, pancreas, duodenum, urinary tract)
	Thymoma
	Lymphoma/leukemia
	Mesothelioma
Pulmonary	Tuberculosis
	Pneumonia/empyema/abscess
	Chronic obstructive pulmonary disease
Intracranial conditions	Meningitis/encephalitis/abscess
	Head injury
	Brain tumor
	Cerebral hemorrhage/subdural hematoma
	Guillain-Barré syndrome
	Seizures
Drug-Induced	Vasopressin preparations, carbamazepine, chlorpropamide, clofibrate, thiazides, vincristine, vinblastine, cisplatin, narcotics, phenothiazines

volemia, and orthostatic hypotension, diuretic use and excessive water intake are absent. Biochemical criteria for the diagnosis of SIADH are Serum Na^+ below 136 mmol/L; normal renal, adrenal, and thyroid function; normal triglycerides and glucose; urine osmolality exceeding that of serum; and excessive urinary Na^+ excretion (>20 mEq/L). Plasma ADH levels may be clearly elevated or inappropriately normal in relation to the plasma osmolality.

■ Management

The diagnostic evaluation and treatment of hyponatremia are discussed in chapter 170. Determination of osmolality is critical: beyond osmolality, the diagnostic strategy to assess the cause of hypotonic hyponatremia is based on an initial evaluation of volume status.

Treatment of hyponatremia depends on the severity, the rate of evolution and the underlying etiology of the hyponatremia as well as the presence or absence of symptoms. **Severe symptomatic hyponatremia** (serum Na^+ <120 mmol/L, with significant neurologic manifestations, i.e., confusion, seizures, coma) requires immediate therapy (see chapter 170). Rapid or overcorrection of serum sodium can be very detrimental, resulting in **central pontine myelinolysis.** This condition is most liable to develop in patients undergoing rapid correction of **chronic asymptomatic hyponatremia** (duration of hyponatremia exceeds 48 hours). Central pontine myelinolysis, a demyelinating lesion of the pons with destruction of the myelin sheaths, features flaccid quadriplegia or paraplegia, facial weakness, dysphagia, dysarthria, and coma.

Mild to moderate, asymptomatic SIADH is treated by restricting fluid intake to less than the urine output, approximately 1000–1500 mL daily. If fluid restriction is unsuccessful, the antibiotic demeclocycline can be given. This agent inhibits the action of ADH at the level of the collecting duct. Persons with a light complexion should avoid direct sun exposure while receiving demeclocycline due to the photosensitivity caused by the medication.

THYROID DISEASES

Thyroid Physiology and Thyroid Function

The thyroid gland, located anteriorly in the neck, weighs 15–20 gm. It consists of a right and left lobe connected by an isthmus. A palpable pyramidal lobe extending upward from the isthmus occurs as a normal variant in many people. Accessory thyroid tissue is occasionally found along the course of the thyroglossal duct. Histologically, the structural unit of the thyroid is the follicle; the follicle consists of a single layer of cuboidal follicular cells enclosing a cavity filled with colloid, a gel-like material that serves as a reservoir of thyroid hormone. The thyroid gland also contains a small number of parafollicular cells (**C cells**) that secrete

calcitonin and are unrelated to thyroid hormone metabolism. The gland receives its blood supply from superior and inferior thyroidal arteries.

Thyroid gland produces two thyroid hormones, **thyroxine** (T_4) and **triiodothyronine** (T_3), which are iodinated metabolites of tyrosine. The first step of their synthesis involves active transport and trapping of circulating iodides into the follicular cell (Figure 58.1). The iodine is oxidized and incorporated (by a process called organification) into the tyrosine residues of thyroglobulin (TG) by thyroid peroxidase, to form monoiodotyrosine (MIT) and diiodotyrosine (DIT). Most of the TG-bound MIT and DIT are later condensed to

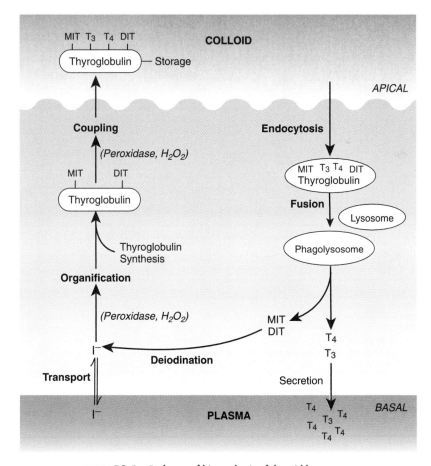

FIGURE 58.1. Pathway of biosynthesis of thyroid hormones.
(From: Best and Taylor's Physiological Basis of Medical Practice. 12th ed. West JB (ed.). Baltimore: Williams & Wilkins, 1991, Fig 8.26, p. 813.)

form T_3 and T_4 (coupling). The T_4 and T_3 are stored in the colloid of the thyroid gland, combined with TG. The final step involves resorption of colloid by the follicular cell and proteolysis of TG, releasing T_4 and T_3 into the circulation. The amount of T_4 released exceeds that of T_3 by nearly ten-fold. Each of these steps is physiologically regulated by TSH and is liable to inhibition by pharmacologic agents. Propylthiouracil and methimazole, drugs used to treat hyperthyroidism, block organification, and iodide in large doses inhibits thyroid peroxidase activity.

■ Peripheral Circulation and Metabolism of Thyroid Hormones

T_4 and T_3 circulate in the bloodstream tightly bound to three serum proteins: thyroxine-binding globulin (TBG), albumin, and transthyretin (also called thyroxine-binding prealbumin). TBG is quantitatively the most important of the binding proteins, accounting for 70% of the total thyroid binding capacity of the serum. Greater than 99% of both T_4 and T_3 are protein-bound. Although T_4 is more abundant than T_3 in the circulation, T_3 interacts with intranuclear receptors at a higher affinity and is more important in producing the biologic effects of thyroid hormone. T_4 is converted to T_3 intracellularly in its target cells by the action of 5'-deiodinase. T_4 may also be metabolized to metabolically inactive reverse T_3 by 5-deiodinase (Figure 58.2).

■ Laboratory Testing of Thyroid Function

Serum free T_4 and TSH levels are the best tests of thyroid function. These tests, along with the traditional thyroid tests used in diagnosing hyperthyroidism, hypothyroidism, and thyroid hormone binding abnormalities, are summarized in Table 58.1. Assays to test for the autoimmune etiology of thyroid disease are also available. Commonly used laboratory tests of thyroid function are described below.

The **free T_4** is in reversible equilibrium with the bound hormone and represents the fraction of hormone that is biologically active. The changes in serum T_4-binding proteins (as in pregnancy, oral contraceptive therapy, nephrotic syndrome, etc.) that affect total T_4 concentration do not affect the concentration of free T_4. Therefore, the free T_4 concentration remains normal even in the presence of binding protein abnormalities. Free T_4 is measured by immunoextraction/enzyme immunoassay or by equilibrium dialysis. **Serum TSH** is the best individual test of thyroid function. Except in secondary hypothyroidism due to pituitary insufficiency and the rare TSH-secreting pituitary adenomas, TSH is more sensitive than either total T_4 or free T_4 in diagnosing mild hypothyroidism or hyperthyroidism. **Total T_3 by radioimmunoassay (T_3RIA)** is used in the diagnosis of mild hyperthyroidism when the TSH is suppressed but the free T_4 is normal ("T_3 thyrotoxicosis"). Because many

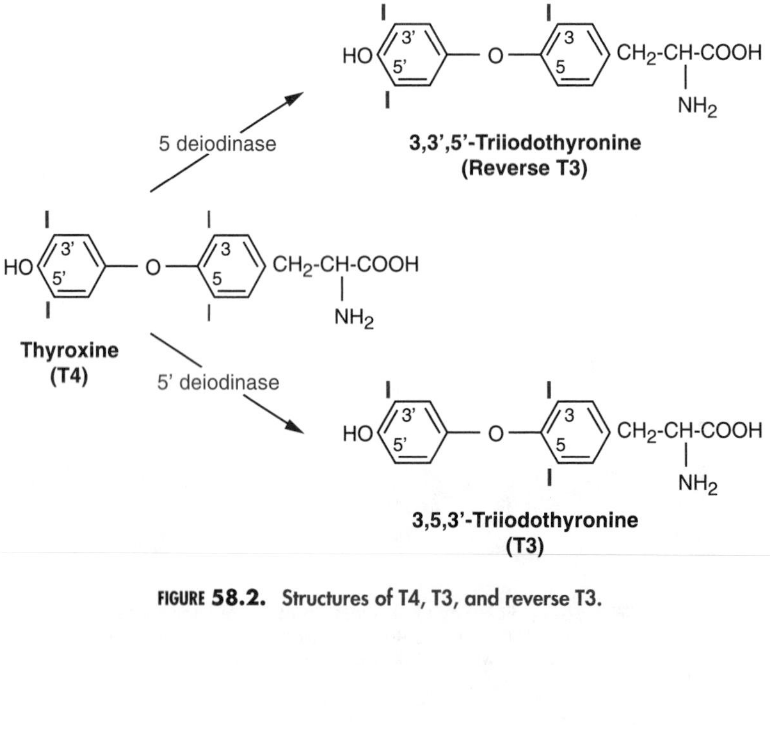

FIGURE 58.2. Structures of T4, T3, and reverse T3.

TABLE 58.1. Laboratory Evaluation of Hyperthyroidism and Primary Hypothyroidism	Euthyroid, Normal TBG	Hyperthyroid, Normal TBG	Hypothyroid, Normal TBG	Euthyroid, ↓ TBG	Euthyroid, ↑TBG
Total T_4 (normal 5–12 µg/dl)	↔	↑	↓	↓	↑
T_3RU (normal 30–40%)	↔	↑	↓	↑	↓
FTI (free thyroxine index)	↔	↑	↓	↔	↔
Free T_4	↔	↑	↓	↔	↔
TSH	↔	↓	↑	↔	↔

Abbreviations: See text.

TABLE 58.2. Thyroid Imaging Studies	Ability to Differentiate …				Detecting Substernal Extension		
Test	Cold vs. Hot	Solid vs. Cystic	Benign vs. Malignant	Resolution	Detecting Substernal Extension	Cost	Comments
Radionuclide Scan	+++	–	+	++	+	$300	Most nodules are cold
Ultrasound	–	++++	–	++++	+	$200	Supplements physical examination
CT	–	++++	–	++++	++++	$600	Excellent for evaluating mass lesions
MRI	–	++++	–	++++	++++	$800	Same as CT

factors can affect the T_4 to T_3 conversion, measurement of T_3RIA is not useful in diagnosing hypothyroidism.

The 24-hour **radioactive iodide uptake** (RAIU) helps differentiate among the common causes of hyperthyroidism. The RAIU is an *in vivo* test involving the oral administration of a small dose of radioactive iodide, such as ^{123}I or ^{131}I, with subsequent gamma counting over the thyroid bed to determine the percentage of administered counts concentrated in the thyroid after a specified period of time, generally 24 hours.

Many thyroid diseases are autoimmune. Thyroglobulin and thyroid microsomal proteins are common antigens involved in this process. Serum titers of **anti-thyroglobulin and antimicrosomal antibodies** can be quantitated and used to document the autoimmune etiology of primary hypothyroidism and goiters. Given that thyroid peroxidase is the microsomal antigen targeted by antimicrosomal enzymes, antimicrosomal antibodies are also called antithyroid peroxidase antibodies.

Available thyroid imaging techniques include high-resolution ultrasound, radionuclide scan, computed tomography, and magnetic resonance imaging. Their relative merits, limitations, and indications are compared in Table 58.2. Imaging studies are rarely indicated in the hyperthyroid or hypothyroid patient. They are used more in evaluating thyroid nodules and masses in euthyroid patients.

Hyperthyroidism

In **hyperthyroidism,** excessive activity of the thyroid hormones causes a hypermetabolic state. It arises from excess circulating quantities of free T_4 or free T_3. The causes of hyperthyroidism (Table 58.3) belong to three categories: conditions where the thyroid gland is actively synthesizing and releasing excess thyroid hormone; conditions due to thyroid inflammation; and exogenous sources of thyroid hormone. (In the latter two categories, the thyroid itself is not synthesizing new T_4 or T_3 and takes up low amounts of iodide.) The first category is distinguished diagnostically by demonstrating an elevated 24-hour RAIU. Conditions with a "high uptake" include Graves' disease, toxic multinodular goiter, toxic adenoma, TSH-secreting pituitary tumor, and human chorionic gonadotropin (HCG) secreting tumor. Hyperthyroidism with a "low uptake" includes thyroid hormone use, struma ovarii, and various forms of thyroiditis or following exposure to exogenous iodine, e.g., radiocontrast agents.

The three most common causes of hyperthyroidism—Graves' disease, toxic multinodular goiter

(Plummer's disease), and thyroiditis—have distinctive clinical features (Table 58.3).

Graves' Disease

■ Pathogenesis

Graves' disease is the most common cause of hyperthyroidism. It is an autoimmune disease arising from the production of thyroid-stimulating immunoglobulins capable of interacting with the TSH receptors on thyroid follicular cells and mimicking the actions of TSH. Pathways of thyroid hormone synthesis and release are markedly increased despite the absence of TSH itself. Graves' disease is more common in women than in men, with an estimated incidence of 37 women and 8 men per 100,000 population. Histologically, the thyroid shows

TABLE 58.3. Characteristics of Common Causes of Hyperthyroidism

	Demographics	Thyroid gland	Ophthalmopathy	24 h RAIU	Need for Definitive Therapy
Graves' Disease	Predominantly young to middle-aged women	Firm, diffusely enlarged with a bruit	Frequent	↑	Yes
Toxic Multi-nodular Goiter	Middle-aged and elderly	Small to massive goiters with multiple nodules	Absent	↑	Yes
Subacute Thyroiditis	Young and middle-aged patients	Tender, modestly enlarged	Absent	↓	No

RAIU = Radioactive Iodine uptake; ↑ = elevated; ↓ = diminished.

TABLE 58.4. Clinical Manifestations of Graves' Disease

Symptoms	Frequency (%)	Signs	Frequency (%)
Nervousness	99	Tachycardia	100
Increased sweating	91	Goiter	100
Heat intolerance	89	Skin changes	97
Palpitations	89	Bruit over thyroid	77
Fatigue	88	Eye signs	71
Weight loss	85	Atrial fibrillation	10
Tachycardia	82	Splenomegaly	10
Dyspnea	75	Gynecomastia	10
Weakness	70	Liver palms	8
Increased appetite	65		
Eye complaints	54		
Swelling of legs	35		
Hyperdefecation (without diarrhea)	33		
Diarrhea	23		
Anorexia	9		
Constipation	4		
Weight gain	3		

(Adapted from: Williams RH. J Clin Endocrinol 1946;6:1.)

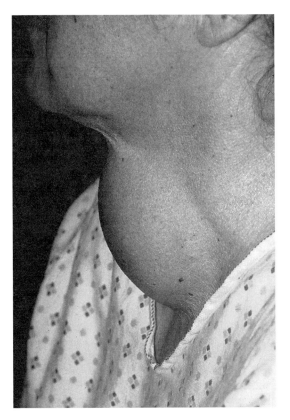

FIGURE 58.3. A large, diffuse goiter as seen in Graves' disease.
(Photograph courtesy of James M. Cerletty, MD, Department of Medicine, The Medical College of Wisconsin.)

evidence of lymphocytic infiltration and a plethora of active, intact follicles.

Clinical Features

The presentation of Graves' disease is influenced by the age of the patient, the severity of hyperthyroidism, and the presence of coexisting medical conditions (Table 58.4). Younger patients are apt to manifest heat intolerance, hyperhidrosis, anxiety, emotional lability, and tremors early in the course of their disease. In contrast, elderly patients often fail to manifest these symptoms, but rather, tend to present only with atrial fibrillation, weight loss, or depression—a subtle and limited presentation, called **apathetic hyperthyroidism.** The thyroid is diffusely enlarged, firm and nontender (Figure 58.3). In contrast to goiters from other causes, a bruit is often audible over the gland.

Patients with Graves' disease often have specific autoimmune diseases of selected nonthyroid tissues.

Ophthalmopathy is especially common and results from inflammation of the tissues of the eye and the orbit. It includes conjunctival inflammation (chemosis), infiltration and swelling of the eye muscles, producing ophthalmoplegia, corneal ulcerations, and proptosis (Figure 58.4). Retrobulbar swelling and edema cause the proptosis. Dermopathy and acropachy are much rarer. **Dermopathy** results from mucopolysaccharide infiltration of the dermis and manifests localized myxedema, characterized by elevated, firm, thickened, erythematous patches usually involving pretibial areas. Itching and pain may be present. **Acropachy** is clubbing and osteoarthropathy of the distal phalanges of the fingers, due to periosteal bone formation and associated soft tissue reaction.

Diagnosis and Management

When thyrotoxicosis is suspected clinically, the diagnosis is confirmed by demonstrating a suppressed TSH level along with either increased "classical" thyroid function tests or an increased free T_4. The 24-h RAIU is measured to confirm the presence of "high uptake" hyperthyroidism.

Spontaneous remission is unusual for the hyperthyroidism of Graves' disease. Thus, definitive treatment is indicated. Among the three available modes of therapy, thyroid ablation with radioactive iodine (^{131}I) is most commonly employed; prolonged therapy with antithyroid drugs and surgery are alternatives in selected patient subsets. The patient should be apprised of the benefits and limitations of all three modes. Regardless of the mode elected, and unless contraindicated, all patients are given β-blockers (e.g., propranolol 20–40 mg q.i.d.) to reduce the adrenergic symptoms.

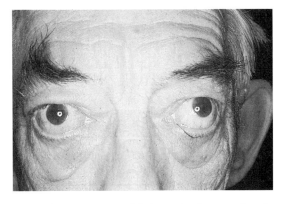

FIGURE 58.4. Graves' ophthalmopathy (see text for description).
(Photograph courtesy of James M. Cerletty, MD, Department of Medicine, The Medical College of Wisconsin.)

The treatment of choice for hyperthyroidism in adult men is radioablation with ^{131}I. The treatment sometimes produces euthyroidism, but more often results in permanent hypothyroidism, requiring life-long thyroxine replacement. Cumulative experience with ^{131}I use suggests no increase in the incidence of leukemias or other cancers. Its use is contraindicated in pregnancy; fears over its gonadal effects make its use in children and women of child-bearing age rather controversial. Destruction of the overactive thyroid gland with ^{131}I causes rapid release of the stored thyroid hormone, and the hyperthyroidism worsens transiently but significantly (radiation thyroiditis). Therefore, depending upon the age and the general health of the patient and the severity of the thyrotoxicosis, treatment with antithyroid drugs for one or two months can be given before treatment with ^{131}I, so as to deplete the gland of its stored thyroid hormone. In less severe hyperthyroidism, such pretreatment is not needed, but β-blockers are given.

Subtotal thyroidectomy in children and in women of child-bearing age is often advocated. Prior to surgery, the patient must be rendered clinically and biochemically euthyroid, using β-blockers, antithyroid drugs, and large amounts of nonradioactive iodine.

In mild hyperthyroidism with relatively small goiters, prolonged therapy with **antithyroid drugs** (propylthiouracil or methimazole) for 6–18 months will sometimes induce a spontaneous remission in the hyperthyroidism. About one-third of this select group maintain euthyroidism after the antithyroid drugs are discontinued. Hyperthyroidism relapses in the remaining two-thirds.

■ Course and Prognosis

Most subjects become permanently hypothyroid as a result of therapy with ^{131}I, generally over 3–5 months. Subtotal thyroidectomy will also usually produce the same result, either immediately postoperatively or more gradually as the thyroid remnant is finally destroyed by the autoimmune process. Thus, the majority of patients with treated Graves' disease will require life-long thyroid hormone replacement. A small minority will develop euthyroid state without need for thyroid hormone replacement. Extrathyroidal autoimmune features of Graves' disease (e.g., ophthalmopathy) run a largely independent course; thus, ophthalmopathy may remain stable or even worsen upon treating the hyperthyroidism.

Plummer's Disease

Plummer's disease is a toxic multinodular goiter, where hyperthyroidism develops secondarily in a multinodular goiter of long-standing.

■ Pathogenesis and Pathology

Evidence of inflammation in Plummer's disease is scant or absent. The nodular hyperplasia is of uncertain cause, but local growth-stimulating factors, growth-stimulating immunoglobulins, or neoplastic characteristics intrinsic to the cells themselves may be responsible. Iodine deficiency contributes in some geographical areas. Hyperthyroidism develops when the follicles become autonomous (when TSH is no longer required to stimulate thyroid hormone production). The overactivity of these nodules results in increased iodine trapping as well as the characteristic appearance of the Plummer's gland on radionuclide scanning, showing "hot" nodules and areas of increased activity interspersed with "cold" zones; the latter arises from the low TSH levels, which suppress the iodine uptake in the remaining normal tissue.

■ Clinical Features

Hyperthyroidism typically develops slowly in patients with toxic multinodular goiters. In these patients, hyperthyroidism can be precipitated by iodine in iodide-containing IV radiologic contrast dyes or medications (e.g., amiodarone and saturated solutions of potassium iodide). While most features are similar to those in hyperthyroidism of Graves' disease, the presentation of Plummer's disease is more subtle, owing to the more elderly population that it afflicts and the gradual onset of thyrotoxicosis. Unexplained weight loss, atrial fibrillation, and depression may thus dominate the clinical picture. The extrathyroidal autoimmune manifestations of Graves' disease are absent.

■ Management and Prognosis

Plummer's disease is most commonly treated with ^{131}I ablation of the gland. The 24-h RAIU, while generally elevated, is usually not as high as that in Graves' disease. Thus, the usual ^{131}I dose for Plummer's disease generally exceeds that for Graves' disease. The hyperfunctioning follicles take up ^{131}I much more avidly than the normal, suppressed follicles. The latter may regain normal function after ^{131}I therapy. Thus, euthyroid state is more often restored in Plummer's disease relative to Graves' disease. It is also prudent to administer β-blockers until hyperthyroidism is resolved and to give antithyroid drugs before ^{131}I therapy. Subtotal thyroidectomy is also an option in selected cases.

Thyroiditis

■ Definition and Etiology

Thyroid inflammation, by disrupting normal follicular architecture and releasing the stored hormone, can cause **thyrotoxicosis** of limited severity and duration. Based upon clinical features and thyroid histopathology, three types of thyroiditis can be recognized: subacute, postpartum, and silent. Subacute (syn. painful, de Quervain's, or granulomatous thyroiditis) thyroiditis is probably viral, whereas postpartum thyroiditis is autoimmune. A subset of patients with silent thyroiditis manifest antithyroid antibodies, also implying an autoimmune etiology.

■ **Clinical Features**

Subacute thyroiditis is a painful inflammation of the thyroid; acute onset of pain in the region of the thyroid is sometimes preceded by an upper respiratory infection. The pain may be severe and radiate to the jaw or ear. General malaise, muscle aches, fatigue, and fever may be associated. Nearly one-half of patients with subacute thyroiditis develop symptoms of mild or moderate thyrotoxicosis. The thyroid may be moderately enlarged and tender to palpation. Cervical adenopathy is usually absent. The **erythrocyte sedimentation rate** (ESR) is typically high. The painful thyroid and the elevated ESR clinically differentiate subacute thyroiditis from silent thyroiditis. **Silent** (or painless) **thyroiditis,** less common than subacute thyroiditis, evokes mild, self-limited hyperthyroidism without neck pain. A normal ESR and the lack of neck pain and systemic symptoms differentiate it from subacute thyroiditis. Hyperthyroidism, which occurs with increased frequency postpartum, is at times due to a relapse of Graves' disease, but often it is due to postpartum thyroiditis, a form of painless thyroiditis. Often, thyroiditis has followed earlier pregnancies.

■ **Diagnosis and Management**

Thyroiditis may be suspected when thyrotoxicosis is mild and occurs in a compatible clinical setting, as described above. The diagnosis is confirmed by obtaining a 24-h RAIU showing low uptake or by measuring serum thyroglobulin.

Thyrotoxicosis in thyroiditis is treated symptomatically. Adrenergic symptoms (tachycardia, etc.) can be treated with propranolol. All other therapies previously cited for thyrotoxicosis are ineffective and contraindicated. The pain of subacute thyroiditis is treated with analgesics (aspirin and nonsteroidal anti-inflammatory drugs); high doses of glucocorticoids are required for severe pain.

■ **Course and Prognosis**

The hyperthyroid stage of thyroiditis is self-limited (weeks). Hyperthyroid symptoms and TSH levels should be assessed monthly so that β-blockers can be discontinued when appropriate. The hyperthyroidism often leads to a hypothyroid phase, which is occasionally permanent and requires levothyroxine replacement. Therefore, patients should be closely monitored.

Hypothyroidism

Hypothyroidism results from the functional inactivity of the thyroid gland. **Primary hypothyroidism** resulting from diseases intrinsic to the thyroid gland is much more frequent than hypothyroidism secondary to TSH deficiency. The causes of hypothyroidism are shown in Table 58.5.

■ **Pathogenesis**

Primary hypothyroidism usually follows destruction of normal thyroid follicles by **chronic autoimmune thyroiditis;** this form of thyroiditis has two forms: with atrophy of the gland, known as **idiopathic** (atrophic) variant, or with a goiter, called **Hashimoto's disease.** Both disorders have a high incidence of antibodies against thyroid antigens, specifically thyroglobulin and thyroid peroxidase; therapy for the two disorders is thyroid hormone replacement. Thus, it is not usually clinically useful to distinguish between these two variants.

TABLE 58.5.	Differential Diagnosis of Primary Hypothyroidism

1. Common causes
   Autoimmune hypothyroidism
      Hashimoto's disease and atrophic variants
   Iatrogenic
      Radioactive iodine
      Thyroidectomy
      External radiation therapy
2. Less common causes
   Iodine deficiency
   Inherited enzyme defects
   Medications
      e.g., lithium, amiodarone, anti-thyroid drugs
   Infiltrative diseases
      e.g., cystinosis, hemochromatosis, scleroderma, amyloidosis

■ Clinical Features

Symptoms of primary hypothyroidism include fatigue, lethargy, increased sleeping, cold intolerance, coarsening of the hair, and dry skin. Weight gain, also typical, may be accompanied by nonpitting edema of the lower extremities and generalized puffiness of the face, particularly periorbitally. Also common are generalized cramps and aches in the lower back muscles. The thyroid may be enlarged, or may not be palpable. In Hashimoto's disease, the goiter is typically firm to rock-hard; its texture is multinodular or bosselated.

■ Diagnosis and Management

Primary hypothyroidism is definitively diagnosed by a high TSH level in conjunction with a decreased free T_4. Thyroid antibodies, while positive in 70–90% of cases, need not be checked routinely. Treatment consists of oral administration of synthetic levothyroxine (T_4). The goal of T_4 therapy is to provide sufficient levels of thyroid hormone (starting dose of 75–100 μg/d in a young person and 50 μg/d in the middle-aged; usual maintenance dose, 75–150 μg/d) to maintain a normal TSH level. Treatment markedly improves the symptoms, although it may take several weeks to months. T_4 replacement raises cardiac oxygen consumption; in a patient with significant coronary artery disease (CAD), it can precipitate crescendo angina or even a myocardial infarction. Thus, in older patients and in those with known CAD, T_4 is started in lower doses (25 μg/d); the biochemical and clinical euthyroid state is attained over a longer period of time and with close monitoring.

■ Iatrogenic Primary Hypothyroidism and Secondary Hypothyroidism

The second most common cause of primary hypothyroidism is iatrogenic. It arises from a variety of causes: destruction of the thyroid gland by ^{131}I in treating Graves' disease, thyroidectomy for thyroid cancer or other reasons, and neck irradiation for lymphoma and other head and neck cancers. Therapy with T_4 replacement is identical to that of chronic autoimmune thyroiditis.

Destruction of the pituitary gland or the hypothalamus can cause TSH deficiency. Hypothyroidism follows, along with thyroid gland atrophy. Clinically, these patients differ from those with primary hypothyroidism because other pituitary hormones are also deficient, most notably ACTH. Because treating hypothyroidism with T_4 in the setting of unrecognized **panhypopituitarism** (a state of inadequacy or absence of all anterior pituitary hormones) can precipitate an adrenal crisis, secondary hypothyroidism should be excluded.

Thyroid Nodules and Thyroid Cancer

Thyroid Nodules

Both benign and malignant conditions can produce thyroid nodules and goiters. Hyperthyroidism and hypothyroidism are routinely associated with benign goiters as a natural consequence of their pathogenesis; they are rarely associated with malignancies. Benign nodules are more common than malignant, even in euthyroid patients (Table 58.6). Consequently, it is impractical and unnecessary to surgically resect all thyroid nodules. Benign and malignant lesions can be differentiated by taking the patient's risk factors in conjunction with the cytology of thyroid cells obtained by fine needle aspiration. Imaging is not used routinely; when selectively applied, it can provide additional useful information.

TABLE 58.6.	Differential Diagnosis of Thyroid Nodules/Masses

1. Colloid goiter (multinodular goiter)
2. Chronic autoimmune thyroiditis
   Hashimoto's disease
   Euthyroid Graves' disease
3. Benign follicular adenoma
4. Simple cyst
5. Thyroid cancers
   Papillary
   Follicular
   Medullary
   Anaplastic
   Lymphoma

■ Evaluation of Thyroid Nodules

Periodic palpation of the thyroid is all that is needed for evaluating a patient with a stable multinodular goiter and no worrisome risk factors such as history of neck irradiation. High-resolution ultrasound, by accurately quantitating the size and number of nodules, can supplement palpation. CT, by defining the relation of the goiter to the trachea and esophagus, is useful in assessing mass symptoms (e.g., dysphagia or hoarseness). An approach to thyroid nodules is shown in Figure 58.5.

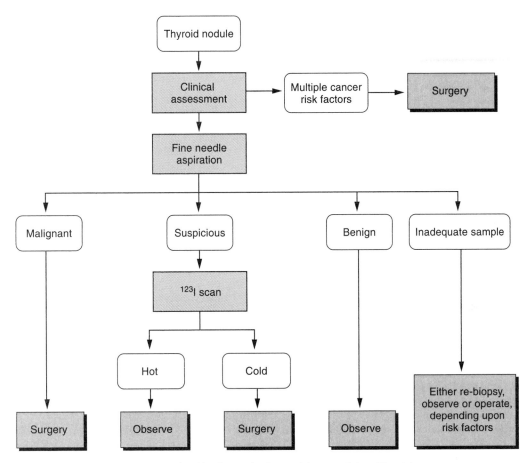

FIGURE 58.5. Algorithm for evaluation and therapy of thyroid nodules.

Thyroid Cancer

■ Epidemiology, Etiology, and Risk Factors

The incidence of thyroid cancer is 5 per 100,000. Because the most frequent thyroid cancers are the low-grade papillary (60%) and follicular (25%) types with an excellent prognosis, overall mortality is low. Medullary cancer accounts for 10%; anaplastic and lymphoma account for less than 5% each. Risk factors for thyroid cancer are listed in Table 58.7. Less than 15% of all solitary nodules are malignant.

■ Specific Types of Thyroid Cancer and Their Management

Cancers that are histologically predominantly follicular but contain papillary elements behave biologically like papillary carcinomas—the least aggressive thyroid cancers. They tend either to remain localized in the thyroid gland or to metastasize to local lymph nodes. The prognosis of papillary cancers is not materially affected by localized lymph node metastasis at diagnosis. The follicular type, while still indolent, is more aggressive than papillary cancer and tends to metastasize more readily to distant locations, including the bone and lung. Overall, about 3% of patients with these two types of cancer (usually those with larger tumors or extrathyroidal extension at initial presentation, or those in whom the thyroid cancer develops after age 70) will eventually succumb to the malignancy.

Papillary and follicular carcinomas are treated by an individualized combination of surgery, ^{131}I therapy, and suppressive doses of T_4. The most appropriate regimen for a given patient remains controversial. Thus, lobectomy alone may suffice for small (<1.5 cm) papillary and

TABLE 58.7.	Features of Solitary Thyroid Nodules Associated With Increased Risk of Malignancy

History:
   Age <20 or >60 (~30% malignant)
   Gender: Men > Women
   Compression symptoms (dysphagia, hoarseness)
   History of neck irradiation (~30% malignant)
   Family history of medullary cancer
Physical Examination:
   Rapid growth
   Presence of fixation
   Presence of lymphadenopathy
Course:
   Growth while on thyroid hormone suppression
Laboratory:
   Euthyroid clinical status
Imaging:
   Cold on radionuclide scanning (10–15% malignant)

follicular carcinomas, while total or near-total thyroidectomy is typically required for large tumors. Residual benign and malignant thyroid tissue can be ablated with large doses of ^{131}I. Because papillary and follicular cancer cells possess TSH receptors, growth of residual tissue can also be slowed by T_4 given in sufficient doses to suppress the TSH to nonmeasurable levels.

Medullary carcinoma of the thyroid (MCT) arises from the parafollicular cells of the thyroid gland. While a sporadic form is well known, it is frequently familial and inherited as part of the **multiple endocrine neoplasia-II syndrome.** The characteristic feature of MCT is the production of calcitonin. Because MCT is not derived from thyroid epithelial follicular cells, it does not take up iodine, nor does it depend on TSH as a growth factor; thus, therapy with ^{131}I or with suppressive doses of T_4 is ineffective. Surgical resection is the treatment; if it is not curative, other modalities of therapy include medical therapy with octreotide, chemotherapy, and external irradiation, none of which are successful in completely stopping the usually slow growth of residual tumor tissue.

Anaplastic carcinoma accounts for less than 5% of all thyroid carcinomas. This highly aggressive lesion grows rapidly, invading surrounding structures, thereby causing compression symptoms in the neck, such as stridor, dysphagia, and hoarseness. Although surgery is usually attempted for diagnostic purposes and for initial tumor debulking, it rarely cures this aggressive cancer. As with MCT, ^{131}I and T_4 suppression are ineffective. External radiation therapy and chemotherapy have been used as palliative therapies for the compression symptoms. The overall prognosis is very poor. Survival exceeding six months after the diagnosis of anaplastic carcinoma is rare.

Primary (non-Hodgkin's) lymphomas of the thyroid are being recognized with increasing frequency. The incidence of thyroid lymphoma is increased greater than fifty-fold in patients with Hashimoto's disease, suggesting that the lymphoma arises from the intrathyroidal lymphocytes present as a result of the chronic autoimmune process. Thyroid lymphoma should be suspected when a patient with known Hashimoto's disease develops a rapidly growing thyroid mass accompanied by symptoms of local compression. In this setting, needle aspiration can be helpful in identifying the lymphoma. In patients with localized disease or in those experiencing significant localized compression, surgical resection may be used. Subsequent therapy is similar to that used for other lymphomas and includes external radiation therapy and chemotherapy. Surgery is not the primary therapy in cases where subsequent staging with CT and bone marrow biopsy demonstrate extrathyroidal lymphoma.

Miscellaneous Thyroid Disorders

Thyroid crisis (thyroid storm) is life-threatening hyperthyroidism. In most instances, it is ushered in by a precipitating event in previously untreated, severe hyperthyroidism. Precipitating events include infections, surgery, and trauma. The majority of patients have Graves' disease. The features include fever, which may be high, restlessness, confusion, and, possibly, frank psychosis. Cardiac arrhythmias are common and cardiovascular collapse may supervene. Treatment includes propylthiouracil (800–1200 mg) or methimazole (80–120 mg/day) given orally or by nasogastric tube. Iodide (10 drops of Lugol's iodine every 8 hours orally or as IV radiological contrast, sodium ipodate 1 g/d) is given to block thyroid hormone synthesis and peripheral T_4 to T_3 conversion.

Antithyroid drugs must precede the iodide, since iodide is also a substrate for thyroid hormone synthesis. β-blockers (propranolol 1–5 mg IV or 20–80 mg orally every 4 hours) are a critical component of the therapy. Glucocorticoids (hydrocortisone, 200–300 mg/day or dexamethasone in equivalent doses) are administered to offset a relative adrenal insufficiency. Both propranolol and corticosteroids also lower the peripheral conversion of T_4 to T_3. A precipitating event should be carefully searched for and, if found, appropriately treated.

Myxedema coma, a medical emergency, is the end-stage of advanced, untreated hypothyroidism. Its hallmarks are hypothermia, mental status changes, hypoventilation, and bradycardia. Paralytic ileus (generalized hypomotility of intestinal smooth muscle) and hyponatremia may occur. Precipitating events are exposure to cold weather, surgery, congestive heart failure, infection, and drugs, including anesthetics, tranquilizers, and narcotics. Diagnosis is based on classic signs and symptoms of severe hypothyroidism, hypothermia, and the above features. In myxedema coma, a relative adrenal insufficiency may prevail, due to the suppression of the pituitary-adrenal axis by advanced hypothyroidism. Therapy consists of aggressive T_4 replacement (200–500 µg initial IV bolus, followed by 50–100 µg daily, IV), glucocorticoids, (hydrocortisone IV, 100 mg every 8 hours for the first several days), and general measures. Precipitating factors should be sought and treated if present. IV preparations of triiodothyronine are available now and may be used instead of T_4. Supportive measures are IV hydration, passive rewarming, and ventilatory support for hypoxemia and CO_2 retention. Rapid rewarming by external electric warming blankets ushers in vasodilatation and exacerbates hypotension.

In **euthyroid hyperthyroxinemia,** the serum total or free T_4 level is high, but without hyperthyroidism. It most commonly occurs with excess thyroid hormone binding proteins, in which case, measurement of free T_4 and serum TSH readily excludes hyperthyroidism. Iodine-containing medications (e.g., amiodarone) block peripheral T_4 to T_3 conversion, thus leading to high T_4. In acute psychiatric illness and hyperemesis gravidarum, free T_4 is also high.

Many medical and surgical illnesses affect thyroid function tests. In some, the serum T_3 level is low and is attributed to impaired conversion of T_4 to T_3, resulting in high reverse T_3. T_4 is also slightly reduced in most patients. This state is called **euthyroid sick syndrome.** Very low T_4 levels correlate with a high mortality. Serum TSH is typically normal, ruling out primary hypothyroidism.

CHAPTER 59 — DISEASES OF THE PARATHYROID GLANDS, VITAMIN D METABOLISM, AND CALCIUM HOMEOSTASIS

Calcium has two major physiologic functions: 1) calcium salts provide the rigidity and strength of the skeleton and 2) ionized calcium plays critical roles in blood clotting, neuromuscular and membrane physiology, and signal transduction. Calcium kinetics are shown in Figure 59.1. Despite the high variability in dietary calcium intake, overall calcium balance is maintained principally by efficient regulation of intestinal calcium absorption. Circulating serum calcium takes three forms: free (ionized), albumin-bound, or complexed to citrate or phosphate. Only the ionized calcium is hormonally regulated and biologically active. Changes in serum albumin level affect the serum calcium level, but not the biological activity of calcium. When the albumin level is abnormal, it is possible to measure ionized calcium directly or to correct the total serum calcium by subtracting 0.8 mg/dl for each gram/dl the serum albumin level is below 4 g/dl.

The parathyroid gland secretes **parathyroid hormone** (PTH), an 84-amino acid polypeptide, in close and inverse relation to serum calcium level. Binding of extracellular calcium to the calcium-sensing receptor regulates PTH secretion. PTH maintains serum calcium levels in five ways: by stimulating (Figure 59.1) osteoclast activity, causing bone resorption, effecting release of calcium into the circulation, increasing the distal tubular reabsorption of calcium in the kidney, and stimulating renal 1α-hydroxylase. PTH also increases urinary phosphate secretion.

The active form of vitamin D, 1,25-dihydroxyvitamin D, increases small intestinal absorption of dietary calcium and maintains calcification of the bone matrix. Its two precursors are ergocalciferol (synthetically derived from vegetable sterols) and the naturally occurring 7-dehydrocholesterol, both of which are activated sequentially in the skin, liver, and kidneys (Figure 59.1). 25-hydroxyvitamin D is the major storage form of vitamin D; its production is not homeostatically regulated. The conversion of 25-hydroxyvitamin D to 1,25-dihydroxyvitamin D is by a specific 1α-hydroxylase in the kidney, which is regulated primarily by PTH. 1,25-dihydroxyvitamin D acts by binding to high-affinity receptors in its target cells.

Hypercalcemia

■ Definition and Clinical Features

Hypercalcemia exists when the serum calcium level exceeds 10.4 mg/dl or when the ionized calcium exceeds 5.2 mg/dl. Hypercalcemia that is acute and severe (>14 mg/dl) can cause fatigue, anorexia, nausea, vomiting, and dehydration. When these symptoms are advanced or accompanied by confusion or coma, the diagnosis is **hypercalcemic crisis.** Hypercalcemia that is more chronic and mild evokes a variety of systemic signs (Table 59.1). The features of the underlying disease that cause the hypercalcemia also often influence the presentation.

■ Diagnosis and Differential Diagnosis

Recognition of hypercalcemia has increased markedly in recent years with the advent of routine, automated laboratory testing. The differential diagnosis of hypercalcemia is shown in Table 59.2. The underlying disorders are often **primary hyperparathyroidism** or

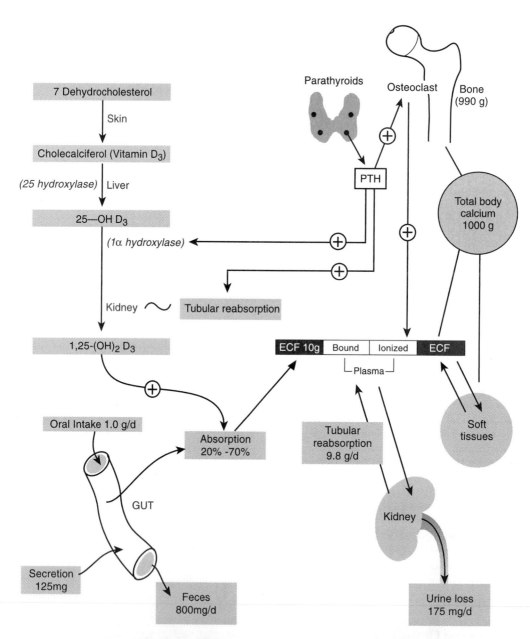

FIGURE 59.1. Calcium balance on an average diet. Stimulatory pathways are indicated by ⊕. PTH = parathyroid hormone.

TABLE 59.1.	Clinical Manifestations of Hypercalcemia

Renal	Neuromuscular
Nephrolithiasis	Muscle weakness
Impaired concentrating ability	Lethargy
(polyuria, polydipsia, and	Somnolence
dehydration)	Coma
Renal tubular defects (natriuresis)	Hyporeflexia
Interstitial nephritis	Psychiatric
Nephrocalcinosis	Apathy
Renal failure	Depression
Gastrointestinal	Psychosis
Constipation	Ectopic calcification
Anorexia	Pruritus (calcium deposition within the skin)
Nausea	Band keratopathy (calcium deposition within
Peptic ulcer	the cornea)
Pancreatitis	Cardiovascular
	Shortened QT interval on ECG (characteristic)
	Increased sensitivity to digoxin

TABLE 59.2.	Differential Diagnosis of Hypercalcemia

Common	Less Common	Factitious
Primary hyperparathyroidism	Medications (lithium, thiazides)	Acute hemoconcentration
Malignancy	Vitamin D intoxication	Increased calcium-binding proteins (e.g.,
	Familial hypocalciuric hypercalcemia	hypergammaglobulinemia)
	Sarcoidosis (and other granulomatous	
	diseases)	
	Acute immobilization	
	Renal failure	
	Hyperthyroidism	
	Milk-alkali syndrome	

malignancy, which together account for 90–95% of hypercalcemia cases. The two can usually be differentiated by the clinical presentations. Most patients with primary hyperparathyroidism have mild hypercalcemia (<13 mg/dl) and are either asymptomatic or manifest a complication of **chronic hypercalcemia,** such as **nephrolithiasis.** Patients with malignancy, however, usually present with advanced cancer and manifest more acute, severe hypercalcemia.

■ Laboratory Evaluation of Hypercalcemia

The etiology of hypercalcemia is usually found through the core tests listed in Table 59.3. Patients with primary hyperparathyroidism usually have significantly elevated intact PTH level; it is low-normal or nondetectable in patients with hypercalcemia of malignancy.

TABLE 59.3.	Laboratory Evaluation of Hypercalcemia

1. Core Studies
   Serum calcium, albumin, phosphate, and creatinine
   Parathyroid hormone level (PTH)
   Urine calcium excretion (24-hour urine collection)
2. Additional Tests Sometimes Useful
   Ionized calcium
   SPEP, UPEP
   Chest X-ray
   CT/MRI of chest/abdomen
   Parathyroid hormone-related protein
   (PTH-rp)

CT = Computed tomography; MRI = magnetic resonance imaging; SPEP = Serum protein electrophoresis; UPEP = Urine protein electrophoresis.

Measurement of urinary calcium excretion is useful 1) to definitively exclude **familial hypocalciuric hypercalcemia** when clinical and laboratory features suggest mild

primary hyperparathyroidism, and 2) to determine the long-term risk for nephrolithiasis and **nephrocalcinosis** in patients with mild hyperparathyroidism.

Primary Hyperparathyroidism

■ Epidemiology and Pathogenesis

Primary hyperparathyroidism is the most common cause of hypercalcemia. It is seen more frequently in women than in men and its peak incidence is around the sixth decade. Primary hyperparathyroidism results from one of three pathologic conditions: a **single benign parathyroid adenoma** (85%) that produces excessive PTH; **diffuse hyperplasia** of all four glands, accounting for most of the remaining 15% and often occurring in the setting of the MEN (multiple endocrine neoplasia) syndromes; and **parathyroid carcinoma,** accounting for less than 1% of cases.

■ Clinical Features

Patients with primary hyperparathyroidism can be completely asymptomatic or manifest symptoms of either the hypercalcemia itself, or those of end organ damage. Serum calcium level typically ranges from 10.5–13 mg/dl; occasionally it is severely elevated. The bones and kidneys are typical targets for long-term complications. Nephrolithiasis is common and is the harbinger in many patients. **Hypercalciuria** can be severe and chronic so as to lead to nephrocalcinosis and renal failure. Increased bone resorption causes demineralization and osteopenia. Advanced, primary hyperparathyroidism classically leads to **osteitis fibrosa cystica** (Figure 59.2), with bone cysts, pathological fractures, and brown tumors.

■ Management

Preoperative localization is usually not indicated. Single adenomas are definitely treated by surgical removal. In cases of four gland hyperplasia, three of the glands are usually removed. A portion of the remaining gland is either left in place or transplanted to the forearm to foster access, if hypercalcemia persists and reoperation is needed. Serum calcium falls postoperatively within several hours of successful surgery. Owing to the suppressed function of the remaining normal glands by the adenoma, transient postoperative hypocalcemia may ensue. Because permanent hypoparathyroidism can follow if all four glands are inadvertently removed surgically, observation for postoperative hypocalcemia is critical.

The treatment of asymptomatic hyperparathyroidism is not clearly defined. Some advocate deferring surgery in asymptomatic patients with mild hypercalcemia

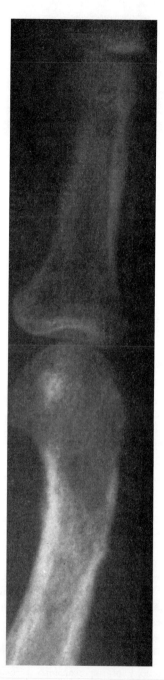

FIGURE 59.2. Radiographs showing subperiosteal bone resorption in primary hyperparathyroidism. Excessive resorption of bone leads to an imperceptible blending of the cortex into the cancellous bone.

(Courtesy, Radiology Museum, St. Joseph's Hospital, Milwaukee, Wisconsin.)

(<11 mg/dl), especially those who are elderly or frail and poorly suited for general anesthesia. If medical manage-

Hypercalcemia of Malignancy

▪ Pathogenesis

Malignancies are commonly associated with disorders of calcium metabolism, including hypercalciuria and hypercalcemia. Neoplasms may secrete PTHrP (**PTH-related protein**) which, while distinct from PTH, has amino-terminal homology with PTH and can mimic its effects on PTH receptors. PTHrP is produced most commonly by squamous cell cancers (head, neck, lung, and esophagus), renal cell carcinoma, and breast cancer. Metastases with extensive localized bone destruction constitute the second most common mechanism of tumor-related hypercalcemia. Hematologic neoplasms (e.g., multiple myeloma and lymphoma) cause hypercalcemia by releasing osteoclast-activating cytokines, and occasionally (in lymphomas), 1,25-dihydroxyvitamin D.

▪ Clinical Features and Management

Most cancer-related hypercalcemia complicate an advanced malignancy, already diagnosed and associated with a poor prognosis. Uncommonly, the tumor is occult and requires an extensive workup to unmask it (Table 59.3). The features of advanced cancer dominate the presentation, with weight loss, anorexia, fatigue, and pain from bone metastases. The hypercalcemia is more acute

ment without surgical intervention is selected, bone mass and renal function should be closely monitored.

and severe (**hypercalcemic crisis**) than is typical for primary hyperparathyroidism and is more likely to cause nausea, vomiting, dehydration, and changes in mentation.

When possible, treatment is directed toward the primary tumor. Hypercalcemic crisis is treated medically (Table 59.4 and chapter 207). One may elect not to treat the hypercalcemia in many patients with terminal cancer, but to provide only palliative and supportive care.

TABLE 59.4.	Medical Therapy of Hypercalcemic Crisis
Step I:	Intravenous normal saline to reverse dehydration and establish brisk urine output
Step II:	Cautious use of furosemide (e.g., 20 mg B.I.D.) to promote further urine calcium excretion *Note: Furosemide should be started only after adequate hydration has been established*
Step III:	Individualized use of calcitonin or pamidronate Less commonly indicated are plicamycin, glucocorticoids, oral phosphate, indomethacin, dialysis, or gallium

Hypocalcemia

▪ Definition and Etiology

Hypocalcemia is defined as a corrected serum calcium less than 8.2 mg/dl or ionized calcium less than 4.0 mg/dl. It can be due to a decrease in the albumin-bound and/or ionized (free) fraction of the serum calcium. Alterations in blood pH affect the ionized serum calcium without altering the total serum calcium. For example, acute acidosis increases ionized calcium by decreasing its binding to albumin, while acute alkalosis has the opposite effect. In true hypocalcemia, however, both the total and the ionized serum fractions are reduced.

Hypocalcemia is usually due to a deficiency in the production, secretion, or action of PTH or of 1,25-dihydroxy vitamin D. The serum phosphorus level is a key to its etiology. Since PTH decreases renal tubular phosphate reabsorption, PTH-related hypocalcemia is associated with hyperphosphatemia. In contrast, 1,25-dihydroxy vitamin D normally increases renal tubular

phosphate reabsorption. Thus, vitamin D-related hypocalcemia is associated with hypophosphatemia.

▪ Clinical Features

Hypocalcemia often elicits no symptoms. Its clinical manifestations depend on the degree, rate of development, and duration of hypocalcemia. Among the many features in Table 59.5, two important ones are Chvostek's and Trousseau's signs. **Chvostek's sign** is elicited by tapping the facial nerve approximately 2 cm in front of the ear lobe and just below the zygomatic arch (Figure 59.4A). A positive response is a twitching of the lip at the angle of the mouth. **Trousseau's sign** is tested by inflating a blood pressure cuff 10–20 mm Hg above the patient's systolic BP for 3–5 minutes, thus reducing the blood supply to the ulnar nerve. In hypocalcemia, this maneuver causes the classical **obstetrician's hand** (main d'accoucheur, Figure 59.4B). While Chvostek's sign is

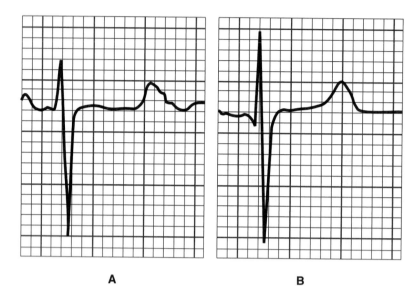

A   B

FIGURE 59.3. Prolonged QT interval in hypocalcemia. **A.** Baseline QT interval and the same corrected for rate (QTc) are 492 msec and 599 msec respectively. **B.** After treatment, the QT and QTc are 432 and 442 msec respectively.

TABLE 59.5.	Clinical Manifestations of Hypocalcemia

Cardiac
  Decreased myocardial contractility
  Congestive heart failure
  Prolonged QT interval (Figure 59.3A and Figure 59.3B)
Dental
  Hypoplasia of teeth/enamel
  Dental caries
  Delayed eruption of teeth
Neurologic
  Paresthesias (toes, fingers and perioral regions)
  Muscle cramps/fasciculations
  Chvostek's sign (Figure 59.4 A)
  Trousseau's sign (Figure 59.4B)
  Tetany
  Seizures
  Basal ganglia calcifications
  Mental changes
Ophthalmologic
  Cataracts
  Optic neuritis
  Papilledema

positive in 10–20% of normal persons, Trousseau's sign is rarely present normally. The hallmark of severe hypocalcemia is tetany, caused by spontaneous sensory and motor discharges in peripheral nerves and featuring muscular twitching, spasms, or seizure. Acute respiratory distress may occur from laryngospasm and bronchospasm.

■ Differential Diagnosis

The differential diagnosis of hypocalcemia based on the serum phosphate level is addressed in Table 59.6. Renal failure is the most common cause of endogenously produced **hyperphosphatemia** and subsequent hypocalcemia. As the glomerular filtration rate falls below 30 ml/min, PTH can no longer produce phosphaturia. Chronic **hypomagnesemia** can precipitate hypocalcemia by decreasing PTH secretion and by causing renal and skeletal resistance to the actions of PTH. In general, hypocalcemia does not develop until the serum magnesium is below 1.0 mg/dl.

PTH resistance most commonly results from **pseudohypoparathyroidism** (PHP), a hereditary condition. In PHP, PTH administration does not raise serum calcium or evoke **phosphaturia.** Inheritance of PHP can be autosomal dominant or recessive and X-linked dominant. The classic biochemical and clinical features of PHP are hypocalcemia, hyperphosphatemia, elevated PTH, peripheral PTH resistance, parathyroid hyperplasia, and **Albright's hereditary osteodystrophy** (AHO, Table 59.7, Figure 59.5A, B). The newer subtypes of PHP, however, present with different phenotypic appearances and different urinary biochemical responses to PTH infusion. In pseudopseudohypoparathyroidism, patients are normocalcemic but do harbor the physical features of AHO.

Hypocalcemia with hypophosphatemia usually implies a deficiency in or resistance to vitamin D. Vitamin D absorption depends on intact gastrointestinal function. Therefore, malabsorptive gastrointestinal disorders and

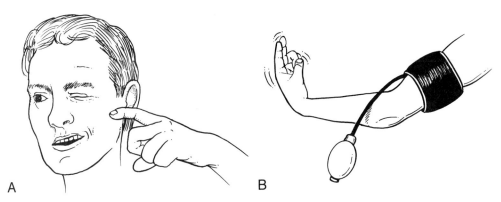

FIGURE 59.4. **A.** Illustration of a positive Chvostek's sign. **B.** Illustration of a positive Trousseau's sign.

TABLE 59.6.	Causes of Hypocalcemia as Integrated With Serum Phosphate Level	
Hyperphosphatemia	**Hypophosphatemia**	**Variable Phosphate Levels**
Parathyroid hormone–related	Vitamin D–related	Osteoblastic metastasis
PTH Deficiency	Deficient Vitamin D	Acute pancreatitis
Congenital	Poor diet/no sun exposure	Hungry bone syndrome
Acquired	Malabsorption	Drugs
Post surgical	Impaired 25-hydroxylation of Vitamin D	Critical illness/Gram-negative
Autoimmune	Impaired 1-hydroxylation of 25 (OH)	sepsis
Infiltrative	Vitamin D	Toxic shock syndrome
Chronic hypomagnesemia	Resistance to Vitamin D	
Idiopathic	Vitamin D-dependent rickets, type 1	
(may cause PTH	and type 2	
resistance also)		
PTH Resistance		
Pseudohypoparathyroidism		
Parathyroid hormone-unrelated		
Endogenous Phosphate Load		
Renal failure		
Hemolysis		
Rhabdomyolysis		
Tumor lysis syndrome		
Exogenous phosphate load		
Laxatives and enemas		

TABLE 59.7.	Clinical Features of Albright's Hereditary Osteodystrophy

Short stature
Rounded facies
Obesity
Mental retardation
Subcutaneous ossification
Skeletal abnormalities
Thickened calvarium
Shortening and widening of the metacarpals, metatarsals, and phalanges of the hands and feet
Short neck

some medications, including cholestyramine, can impair vitamin D absorption. Because the liver is the site of 25-hydroxylation, liver disease impairs this stage of vitamin D metabolism; similarly, formation of the biologically active metabolite 1,25-dihydroxy vitamin D is impaired in advanced renal disease. **Vitamin D dependent rickets** (VDDR) types 1 and 2 are autosomal recessive syndromes of vitamin D resistance. Patients with type 1 VDDR have a selective resistance to vitamin D due to an isolated defect in 1-α hydroxylase activity, causing a deficiency in 1,25-dihydroxy vitamin D; patients with type 2 VDDR have a generalized vitamin D resistance owing to a mutation in the vitamin D receptor.

Thus, in type 1 VDDR, circulating 1,25-dihydroxy vitamin D level is low, whereas in type 2, the level is high due to end organ resistance. High-dose calcium supplementation and 1,25-dihydroxy vitamin D are the primary therapy for type 2 and type 1 VDDR, respectively.

Pancreatic lipase, which is released in acute pancreatitis, liberates free fatty acids from the surrounding retroperitoneal and omental fat. These free fatty acids chelate calcium ions, resulting in hypocalcemia—a poor prognostic sign. The **hungry bone syndrome** occurs when calcium and phosphorus are acutely deposited into bones causing hypocalcemia; it is typically seen within hours after a **parathyroidectomy** (excision of a parathyroid gland) for primary hyperparathyroidism. This condition may last for at least a month or until the remaining suppressed parathyroid glands resume functioning. Patients typically have a low serum phosphorus level in contrast to patients with true PTH deficiency, who exhibit hyperphosphatemia. Several therapeutic agents can also cause hypocalcemia. Diphenylhydantoin, phenobarbital, and glutethimide impair 25-α hydroxylation of vitamin D; foscarnet may chelate circulating calcium; and cholestyramine may interfere with vitamin D absorption. Finally, cisplatinum and pentamidine may produce urinary magnesium wasting.

■ Diagnosis

Once hypocalcemia is detected, measuring the serum phosphorus guides the subsequent evaluation. A high level indicates either PTH deficiency or PTH resistance. A low level indicates a vitamin D-related disorder. Generally, when vitamin D deficiency is suspected, it is only necessary to measure the metabolite 25-hydroxyvitamin D, because it is consistently low in states of vitamin D deficiency. Circulating 1,25-

TABLE 59.8.	Therapy for Hypocalcemia

Acute Symptomatic Hypocalcemia (Tetany)
1. 10% Calcium gluconate (90 mg of elemental Ca^{++}/10 ml ampule)
   - Dilute 2 × 10 ml amps of calcium gluconate (2 mg/kg body weight) in 50–100 ml of D_5 solution and infuse over 5–10 min.
   - Continue IV calcium until overt tetany is controlled
   This rapid infusion may ameliorate symptoms for 15 min. to several hours
   - Follow rapid loading infusion by a slower infusion of 15 mg/kg of calcium gluconate mixed with D_5 infused over 6–12 hours
2. Calcium chloride (272 mg of elemental calcium/ 10 ml ampule of 10% calcium chloride)
   - Dilute 1 × 10 ml ampule in 50–100 ml of D_5 solution. Rapidly infuse 2 mg/kg over 5–10 minutes

Chronic Hypocalcemia
1. Mild vitamin D deficiency
   Multivitamin containing 400 IU of vitamin D daily
   Oral calcium, 800–1200 mg daily
2. Hypoparathyroidism
   Oral elemental calcium 1–2 g in 3 divided doses
   Vitamin D replacement (approximate doses only)
   1,25 $(OH)_2$ vit. D: 0.25 to 2.0 μg/day
   Vitamin D_2: 25,000 to 100,000 IU/day

D_5 = Dextrose in water.

dihydroxyvitamin D levels are less consistently depressed.

■ Management

Acute hypocalcemia is treated by IV calcium gluconate or calcium chloride (Table 59.8). Vitamin D

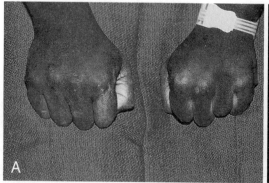
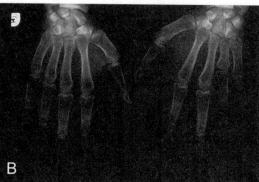

FIGURE 59.5A, B. Albright's hereditary osteodystrophy: Photograph and radiograph of hands.
(Courtesy of James M. Cerletty, MD, Department of Medicine, Medical College of Wisconsin.)

and calcium supplements are therapeutic mainstays of all forms of parathyroid hormone and vitamin D deficiencies. If possible, the pharmacotherapy of vitamin D should allow for regulated production of 1,25-dihydroxyvitamin D. For example, if a hypocalcemic patient has normal renal function, a simple vegetable-derived vitamin D preparation should be used. Alternatively, 25-hydroxyvitamin D is used to treat patients with normal kidney function and liver disease, while 1,25-dihydroxyvitamin D is used for hypocalcemic subjects with advanced renal disease.

CHAPTER **60** ## METABOLIC BONE DISEASE

Bone provides mechanical support for the body and is integrally involved in calcium homeostasis. There are two major forms of bone. The majority of skeletal mass is **cortical** or compact bone, found principally in the shafts of long bones. **Trabecular** or cancellous bone, found in vertebral bodies and at the ends of long bones, is less dense. Bone is composed of matrix, mineral, and cells. The **matrix** is the intercellular substance of bone tissue, consisting of collagen fibers, ground substance, and inorganic bone salts. The primary component of the matrix is type I collagen. Other glycoproteins, proteoglycans, and enzymes are present in the matrix, contributing to its mechanical strength and mediating its calcification. The rigidity of bone is derived from the calcium salts; hydroxyapatite $[Ca_{10}(PO_4)_6[OH]_2]$ is the most common calcium salt. Three specialized cells form and regulate the bone matrix and its calcification: the osteoblast, osteoclast, and osteocyte. The **osteoblast** synthesizes the enzymes involved in bone formation as well as most of the proteins of the bone matrix. **Osteocytes,** a matured form of osteoblasts, become embedded within the bone structure. **Osteoclasts,** giant multinucleated cells, are primarily responsible for bone resorption. The bone matrix and calcium salts are constantly remodeled and turned over by these cellular elements.

The three most prevalent metabolic bone diseases are osteoporosis, osteomalacia, and Paget's disease.

Osteoporosis and Osteopenia

■ Definition and Epidemiology

Osteoporosis is a common, age-related disorder, characterized by reduced bone mass. Bone mineral and bone matrix are proportionally decreased. Decreased bone mass and decreased bone strength are correlated with fracture risk. **Osteopenia** is a more general term for radiographically decreased bone mass; besides osteoporosis, it also encompasses primary hyperparathyroidism, **osteomalacia** (vitamin D deficiency), and other metabolic bone diseases.

Osteoporosis may be a primary disorder or it may follow a chronic disease. **Primary osteoporosis** is sometimes divided into **postmenopausal osteoporosis,** in which trabecular bone loss and vertebral fractures predominate, and **senile osteoporosis,** in which cortical and trabecular bone are lost equally and both vertebral and hip fractures occur. Multiple factors can cause primary osteoporosis (Table 60.1). Estrogen deficiency is an important factor in most women. For several years following menopause, the decline of bone mass accelerates. Therefore, early menopause is one of the strongest predictors for the development of osteoporosis. Because bone mass is higher in men than in women and in blacks than in whites, women and whites and Asians are at greater risk of developing osteoporosis.

TABLE 60.1. Risk Factors for Post-Menopausal Osteoporosis
Early menopause
Race (White and Asian)
Thin body habitus
Low calcium intake
Heavy alcohol use
Cigarette smoking
Physical inactivity

■ Clinical Features

Uncomplicated osteoporosis is asymptomatic. Symptoms, when they occur, are related to fractures and their complications. Fractures most commonly involve the thoracic or lumbar vertebral bodies, the ribs, the proximal femur, and the distal radius; they result from minimal trauma and falls that ordinarily would not cause fractures. Fractures may cause local pain and loss of

TABLE 60.2.	Common Causes of Secondary Osteopenia/Osteoporosis

Endocrine
   Hyperthyroidism
   Cushing's syndrome
   Primary hyperparathyroidism
   Hypogonadism
   Diabetes mellitus
Gastrointestinal Disease/Malabsorption
Drugs
   Anticonvulsants
   Glucocorticoids
   Levothyroxine (overreplacement)
   Heparin
Neoplastic Disease
   Multiple myeloma
   Diffuse metastatic disease

height, and they can lead to functional disabilities. Chronic pain from vertebral body collapse is especially common; it may be unremitting and disabling. Morbidity and mortality are high following hip fractures, particularly from venous thromboembolism.

■ Differential Diagnosis

Several diseases can accelerate primary osteoporosis or can cause osteoporosis in patients otherwise at minimal risk (Table 60.2). In many of these conditions, an element of vitamin D deficiency is present, and patients may have a combination of osteoporosis and early osteomalacia (described in the following).

■ Ancillary Studies

Because approximately one-third of skeletal mass must be lost before it is appreciable on standard radiographs, they are insensitive indicators of bone loss. Bone mass can be more accurately quantitated by specific bone densitometry techniques. **Single** and **dual photon absorptiometry** measure bone density in the radius, a largely cortical bone. **Dual energy x-ray absorptiometry** is a newer technique that images the spine and hip with minimal radiation exposure. Bone densitometry is indicated in women with a history of early menopause, in patients with evidence of osteopenia on routine radiographs, and in most patients with diseases listed as secondary causes of osteoporosis (Table 60.2). In general, patients with bone density exceeding 1.0 gm/cm have a low risk for fractures, whereas those with less than 0.6 gm/cm are at very high risk.

Secondary forms of bone loss should be excluded before primary osteoporosis is diagnosed. As part of the evaluation, vitamin D deficiency (**osteomalacia**) should be excluded. A careful review of systems can suggest the need for work-up for other conditions. Bone turnover markers (e.g., urine hydroxyproline and serum osteocalcin) are not useful in managing osteoporosis.

■ Management

In established, advanced osteoporosis, therapy is more effective in preventing future bone loss than in restoring bone density to normal premenopausal levels. Thus, preventing bone loss in healthy women with normal bone density is a primary goal of therapy; the first step is to identify patients at risk (Table 60.1 and Table 60.2), including menopausal women. Treatment strategies include increasing physical activity, eliminating alcohol and smoking, and ensuring adequate dietary calcium. Unless there is history of nephrolithiasis, calcium supplement of 1000 mg/day is reasonable in most patients at risk. Supplementation with a daily multivitamin containing 200–400 units of vitamin D is also reasonable. Estrogen replacement can lower the rates of bone loss and fracture, particularly if it is begun within three years of menopause. The minimum effective dose for this purpose is 0.625 mg of conjugated equine estrogens.

Treatment of **established osteoporosis** (low bone mass complicated by a history of nontraumatic fractures) also includes estrogen replacement, calcium supplementation, and addressing risk factors related to lifestyle (Table 60.3). In frail, elderly patients, it is of critical importance to assess for risk of falls and to undertake appropriate intervention(s). While the efficacy of estrogen replacement is proven, and newer bisphosphonates, such as alendronate, are proving to be effective, efficacy of other pharmacologic interventions is more modest or negligible. Calcitonin inhibits osteoclast activity and either improves bone mass or slows rates of bone loss in established osteoporosis.

TABLE 60.3.	Treatment of Primary Osteoporosis

Core Therapy
   Estrogen replacement
   Reverse risk factors where possible
   Oral calcium supplement (1000 mg/d)
   Calcitonin
   Alendronate
   Low-dose vitamin D
Occupational/Physical Therapy
Unproven Therapies
   Sodium fluoride

■ Osteoporosis in Men

While less common in men than women, osteoporosis with vertebral and hip fractures is highly prevalent in elderly men, particularly in those with low bone densities. Osteoporotic men are more likely than women to have a definable condition (e.g., hypogonadism) listed in Table 60.2.

Osteomalacia and Rickets

Osteomalacia, a disease characterized by a softening and bending of the bones, results when inadequate calcium is available for bone matrix calcification, owing to vitamin D deficiency. Therefore, in contrast to osteoporosis, where the decreases in bone mineral and matrix are proportional, osteomalacia is characterized histologically by decreased mineralization with increased bone matrix. It is caused by either vitamin D deficiency (inadequate diet, malabsorptive gastrointestinal disorders) or diseases or other factors that impair conversion of vitamin D to 1,25-dihydroxyvitamin D (liver or renal disease, or anticonvulsant therapy). The decreased intestinal absorption of calcium reduces its availability to mineralize bone matrix. A compensatory increase in parathyroid hormone levels leads to increased bone mineral resorption by osteoclasts.

Clinical features vary depending upon the age at onset, the precipitating causes, and the presence or absence of concomitant hypocalcemia. **Rickets** is osteomalacia occurring in children prior to epiphyseal closure. Children with rickets develop bowing of long bones, growth retardation, bone pain, and delayed dentition. Adults with osteomalacia present with bone pain and pathological fractures. Associated hypocalcemia leads to hypotonia, muscle weakness, and tetany.

Imaging studies show diffuse demineralization (osteopenia), increased trabecular markings, and pseudofractures (Figure 60.1). Serum calcium and phosphate are often low, and alkaline phosphatase is high. The two latter findings reflect secondary hyperparathyroidism. Therapy of osteomalacia includes administration of vitamin D or its active metabolite, 1,25-dihydroxy vitamin D, and,

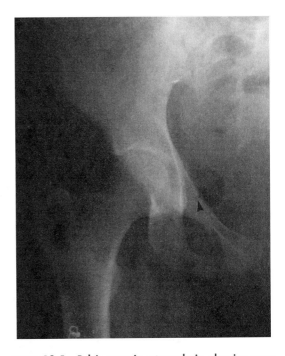

FIGURE 60.1. Pelvic x-ray in osteomalacia, showing pseudofracture (Looser's zones). These are generally best seen on the concave side of the affected bones.
(Courtesy of the Radiology Museum, St. Joseph's Hospital, Milwaukee, Wisconsin.)

where possible, identification and treatment of the underlying disease(s).

Paget's Disease of Bone

■ Definition and Etiology

The hallmark of **Paget's disease** (osteitis deformans) is disordered bone remodeling with an increase in the rate of bone turnover. While usually focal, Paget's disease may be widespread. The pelvic bones are most commonly involved, followed by skull, femur, lumbosacral spine, clavicles, ribs, and tibia. Excessive bone resorption results in areas of radiolucency on x-rays (**osteoporosis circumscripta**). The normal marrow is replaced by fibrovascular connective tissue. Excessive osteoblastic activity replaces resorbed bone, but new bone is organized haphazardly, with multiple, irregular cement lines; histologically, it has a characteristic mosaic pattern. While the coarse, dense Pagetic bone appears abnormally dense on x-rays, its strength is not enhanced; the irregular structure makes it weaker than normal bone, thus causing fractures and/or deformities. The etiology of Paget's disease is unknown, but it may be caused by a slow virus infection.

■ Clinical Features

Paget's disease is rare before middle age, but estimates suggest that it may be present in 3% of persons over age 40. Because most patients are asymptomatic, the disease is usually first found incidentally on x-rays or by an isolated, otherwise unexplained rise in alkaline phosphatase. It can also present with swelling, deformity, or pain in a long bone. Skull enlargement may increase hat size over the years. Temporal bone involvement may cause hearing loss, and Pagetic bone growth and basal skull compression may evoke other neurologic symptoms. Vertebral and long-bone fractures may result from structural bone abnormalities; these fractures and deformities together may cause loss of height. With widespread disease, the high skeletal blood flow raises cardiac output, thus leading to heart failure. Osteogenic sarcoma occurs in less than 1% of cases.

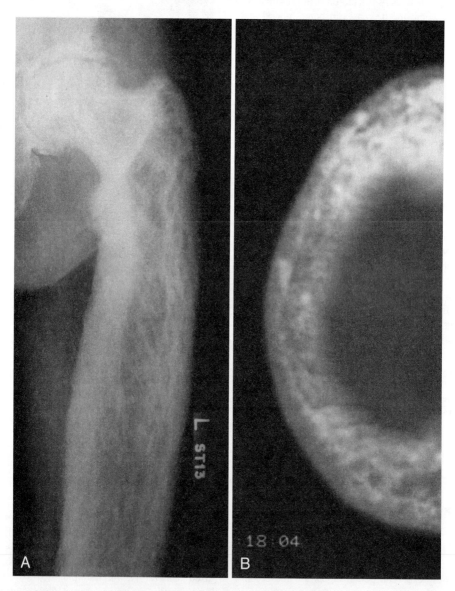

FIGURE 60.2. **A.** X-ray of the femur in a patient with advanced Paget's disease. **B.** CT scan of the skull of the same patient, showing coarse, dense, Pagetic bone.
(Radiograph courtesy of the Radiology Museum, St. Joseph's Hospital, Milwaukee, Wisconsin.)

Laboratory and Radiologic Evaluation

Bone turnover in Paget's disease is focally increased. Therefore, markers of osteoblast activity (serum alkaline phosphatase) and of osteoclast activity (urine hydroxyproline) are usually high in active disease; observing changes in them can be helpful in monitoring response to therapy. Serum calcium and phosphate are usually normal. However, hypercalcemia can follow immobilization in patients with Paget's disease. Skeletal x-rays, especially of the pelvis, skull, femur and lower spine, are useful in diagnosis (Figure 60.2). Bone scans, which are more sensitive than x-rays, can define the extent of Paget's disease, but the findings are nonspecific and overlap with degenerative arthritis and metastatic cancer.

Management

The major goals of drug therapy are to reduce pain, limit the development of further deformities, and prevent neurologic complications. Aspirin or nonsteroidal antiinflammatory agents can help relieve pain. If symptoms are clearly attributable to Paget's disease, more specific therapy can be given, but it can be difficult to judge whether back pain in a patient with Paget's disease is due to Paget's disease or to coexisting degenerative disc disease. The use of calcitonin or diphosphonate may suppress disease activity. Human or salmon calcitonin, 100 units daily, may be started subcutaneously, daily. Following symptomatic improvement, the dose can be tapered to about 50 units 3 times per week; therapy can eventually be totally discontinued. The bisphosphonate etidronate is given orally cyclically (200–400 mg qD, 6 months on and 6 months off); pamidronate is given in a series of IV infusions to produce a prolonged remission in symptoms. Mithramycin is less useful because of its hepatic, renal, and hematologic toxicity. Disease activity should be monitored during therapy.

CHAPTER 61 · DISEASES OF THE ADRENAL CORTEX

The adrenal glands, located at the superior pole of each kidney, consist of two concentric layers: the cortex and the medulla. The cortex is subdivided into three histological zones: the subcapsular **zona glomerulosa,** which secretes mineralocorticoids, and the **zona fasciculata** and **zona reticularis,** both of which secrete glucocorticoids and androgens.

The synthetic pathways for the steroid hormones produced in the adrenal cortex are shown in Figure 61.1. The major regulatory system for cortisol is through **hypothalamic corticotropin-releasing factor** (CRF) and **pituitary adrenocorticotropic hormone** (ACTH). Secretion of ACTH is pulsatile, creating a daily diurnal variation in cortisol secretion with maximal release in the morning. Cortisol circulates in plasma, bound to **corticosteroid-binding globulin** (CBG), a protein synthesized in the liver; only a small fraction occurs in the biologically active free form.

The renin-angiotensin system, hyperkalemia, and hyponatremia strongly stimulate aldosterone synthesis and release. Renin is produced by the juxtaglomerular cells of the kidney. It catalyzes the conversion of renin substrate to **angiotensin I** (A-I). The regulation of renin depends on intravascular volume. Upright posture, hemorrhage, diuretics, salt/sodium restriction, and edematous states increase renin secretion by decreasing effective plasma volume. **Angiotensin-converting enzyme** (ACE) converts A-I to A-II, which upregulates the enzyme that converts cholesterol to pregnenolone, the first step in adrenal steroid synthesis, and the conversion of corticosterone to aldosterone. Aldosterone promotes renal tubular Na^+ reabsorption as well as excretion of K^+ and H^+ ions.

Dehydroepiandrosterone (DHEA), **DHEA-sulfate** (DHEAS), and **androstenedione** are the major androgens synthesized in the adrenals. They exert their androgenic activity after peripheral conversion to the more potent androgens, **testosterone** and **dihydrotestosterone.** ACTH is the major stimulator of adrenal androgen secretion, but additional adrenocortical or other circulating regulators may also play a role in controlling their synthesis and release.

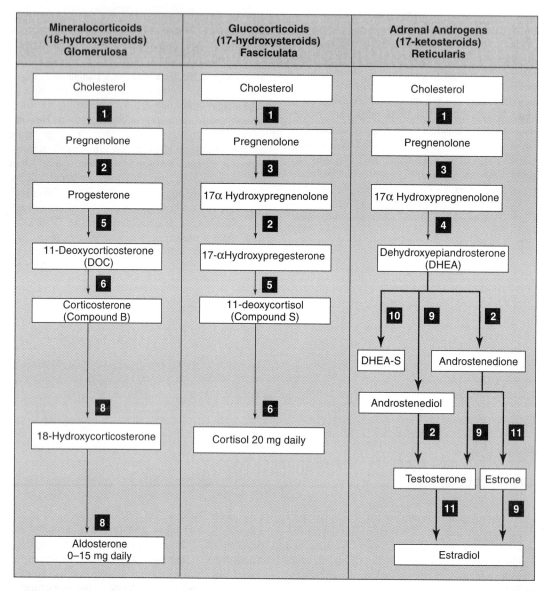

FIGURE 61.1. Synthetic pathways of adrenocortical steroids. Boxed numbers represent enzymes. Key: 1 = 20,22 hydroxylase, desmolase; 2 = 3β-hydroxysteroid dehydrogenase; 3 = 17-hydroxylase; 4 = 17,20-desmolase; 5 = 21-hydroxylase; 6 = 11ß-hydroxylase; 7 = 18-hydroxylase; 8 = 18-aldehyde synthetase; 9 = 17-ketosteroid reductase; 10 = 3ß-hydroxysteroid sulfotransferase; 11 = P-450 aromatase.

Adrenal Insufficiency

■ Definition

Adrenocortical insufficiency (Addison's disease), first described by Thomas Addison in 1885, has an estimated incidence of approximately 50 cases per million adults in Western countries. The development of the clinical manifestations of adrenocortical insufficiency requires loss or destruction of 90% or more of both adrenal cortices. Its treatment is simple, but if left undiagnosed and untreated, its consequences are devastating and often lethal.

Etiology and Pathogenesis

Adrenocortical hormone insufficiency can result from primary destruction of adrenal cortices (**primary adrenal insufficiency**), insufficient pituitary ACTH (**secondary adrenal insufficiency**), or decreased hypothalamic CRF secretion (**tertiary adrenal insufficiency**). **Acute adrenal insufficiency** most commonly occurs in a patient who is exposed to stress, such as sepsis, trauma or surgery, and who requires increased glucocorticoids that the underactive glands cannot provide. It can also follow acute bilateral destruction of the adrenal glands. The most common cause of adrenal insufficiency is **iatrogenic tertiary adrenal insufficiency;** this condition follows suppression of endogenous CRF/ACTH/cortisol owing to use of exogenous glucocorticoids in pharmacologic doses to treat unrelated diseases.

The **idiopathic** type is the most common primary adrenal insufficiency in the United States; it results from autoimmune destruction of all three layers of the cortex. Idiopathic primary adrenal insufficiency is more common in women; it may be familial, and it is usually diagnosed in the third to fifth decades of life. Nearly 60% of patients have circulating adrenal antibodies, and lymphocytic infiltration of the gland is noted early on. Addison's disease shows a high association with autoimmune disorders of other endocrine glands (Table 61.1), known as the **polyglandular autoimmune syndrome** (e.g., Addison's disease and Hashimoto's hypothyroidism). The causes of primary adrenal insufficiency are listed in Table 61.2. Tuberculosis (TB) is the second most frequent cause in the United States and is also a common cause in developing countries. TB manifests with adrenal calcification on abdominal x-rays. The remaining listed entities are rare.

Clinical Features

Clinical features of adrenal insufficiency are shown in Table 61.3; its evolution may be gradual or catastrophically sudden. The major physiologic derangements of adrenal insufficiency are fluid and sodium depletion. Mineralocorticoid and glucocorticoid loss reduce the ability to retain Na^+ and excrete K^+ and H^+ ions; cardiac output and renal perfusion are decreased. In acute adrenal insufficiency, intravascular volume, vascular tone, and cardiac output are all decreased; hypotension and, potentially, vascular collapse and shock follow. Characteristically, the skin pigmentation is absent when the adrenal failure is acute, secondary, or tertiary. Among the laboratory features summarized in Table 61.4, hyponatremia is primarily due to an impaired ability to excrete free water; thus it is common to any type of adrenal insufficiency. However, hyperkalemia and metabolic

TABLE 61.1.	Disorders Associated With Autoimmune Addison's Disease
Thyroid disease	
Hashimoto's hypothyroidism	
Graves' hyperthyroidism	
Diabetes mellitus (Type I)	
Primary gonadal failure	
Pernicious anemia	
Myasthenia gravis	
Hypoparathyroidism	
Chronic mucocutaneous candidiasis	
Alopecia	
Vitiligo	
Chronic active hepatitis	
Malabsorption syndrome	

TABLE 61.2. Etiology of Adrenal Insufficiency	
Primary Adrenal Gland Failure	**Secondary and Tertiary Adrenal Insufficiency**
Idiopathic/Autoimmune	Long-term glucocorticosteroid use
Tuberculosis	Congenital hormonal or releasing factor deficiencies
Adrenal hemorrhage	Neoplasms
Bilateral infarction	Inflammatory lesions
Fungal infection	Granulomatous disease
HIV/AIDS	Degenerative disease
Invasive disorders	Trauma (in fundibular stalk section)
Bilateral adrenalectomy	Radiation
Cytotoxic agents (mitotane)	Vascular lesions
Congenital adrenal hypoplasia	Necrosis (Sheehan's syndrome)
Congenital adrenocortical hyporesponsiveness	
Congenital adrenal hyperplasia	
Adrenoleukodystrophy	
Drugs	

TABLE 61.3.	Clinical Features of Adrenal Insufficiency

Gastrointestinal
  Anorexia
  Nausea, vomiting
  Diarrhea
  Abdominal cramping
Cardiovascular
  Hypotension
  Tachycardia
Signs of dehydration
Fever
Muscle weakness
Restlessness
Hyperpigmentation of skin

TABLE 61.4.	Typical Laboratory Abnormalities in Adrenal Insufficiency

Hyponatremia
Hyperkalemia
Hypoglycemia
Metabolic acidosis
Azotemia
Na/K ratio usually <20
Eosinophilia/lymphocytosis/anemia
Hypercalcemia

acidosis are absent in secondary or tertiary adrenal failure, because aldosterone secretion is preserved.

■ Diagnosis

In the case of **shock** with dehydration and intact adrenal function, a random plasma cortisol level should be at least 20 µg/dl; in most cases, the level will exceed 30 µg/dl. Adrenal insufficiency is best diagnosed by a rapid **cosyntropin stimulation test**. **Cosyntropin,** a synthetic fragment of ACTH, contains the first 24 amino acids of ACTH from the amino terminal end. Neither a fasting state nor the time of day is critical for the test. Plasma samples are drawn for cortisol before and 60 minutes after administering 250 µg of cosyntropin IV. Normally, the plasma cortisol rises 7 µg/dl above the baseline and should exceed 20 µg/dl at 60 minutes. The plasma ACTH level separates primary from secondary adrenal failure; ACTH typically exceeds 250 pg/ml in the primary type, but it is low or inappropriately normal in other types.

■ Management

The management of acute adrenal insufficiency is shown in Table 61.5. The most important point to

remember in treating acute adrenal crisis is that if the diagnosis is considered, the patient should be treated immediately without waiting for confirmation. Once basal blood specimens have been obtained for diagnosis, fluid restoration and hormone substitution should follow promptly. IV glucocorticoids should be given in large quantities. If a cosyntropin stimulation test is performed, the patient initially receives an injection of dexamethasone, which does not affect plasma cortisol measurement. Hydrocortisone is the preferred glucocorticoid in the treatment of Addisonian crisis because it inherently exhibits the greatest mineralocorticoid activity. Mineralocorticoid replacement is unnecessary if the total daily hydrocortisone dose exceeds 100 mg. With proper treatment, patients with adrenal insufficiency, even in Addisonian crisis, have a very good prognosis. Left untreated, acute adrenal crisis is lethal.

In managing chronic adrenal insufficiency (Table 61.6), it is important to educate the patient on three points: the need to take the glucocorticoid replacement regularly, to increase its dose twofold to threefold for the few days of intercurrent illness or stress, and to revert to regular maintenance doses once the illness has resolved. It is not necessary to alter the mineralocorticoid dose. Cues for the patient to contact the physician include signs of dehydration, worsening of the illness, or its persistence beyond three days.

TABLE 61.5.	Managing Acute Adrenal Crisis

1. IV fluid replacement
   Use normal saline (NS) or D5 NS if hypoglycemia is present.
   Infuse rapidly initially to stabilize blood pressure.
   Never infuse hypotonic saline or dextrose in water alone; life-threatening hyponatremia can be induced in this manner.
   Monitor for signs and symptoms of fluid overload.
   Monitor serum K^+ carefully, because K^+ will drop precipitously. Replace as needed.
2. Glucocorticoid replacement
   Dexamethasone 4 mg IV for initial dose.
   Hydrocortisone 100 mg IV immediately after cosyntropin stimulation test is completed and every 8 hours thereafter.
   Taper glucocorticoids rapidly to a maintenance dose, usually decreasing the dose by one half each day, if precipitating illness permits.
3. Treat the precipitating stress
   Search for and treat the precipitating illness that caused the adrenal crisis.

TABLE 61.6.	Management of Chronic Primary Adrenal Insufficiency

1. Maintenance glucocorticoid replacement (any 1 of these regimens)
   Cortisone acetate 25 mg in AM and 12.5 mg in PM
   Hydrocortisone 20 mg in AM and 10 mg in PM
   Prednisone 5–10 mg daily
   Monitor weight, clinical signs and symptoms of fluid retention and appearance of Cushingoid features; adjust
      dosage accordingly.
2. Maintenance mineralocorticoid replacement
   Fludrocortisone 0.05–0.2 mg daily
   Monitor standing and recumbent BP and serum electrolytes.
3. Educate the patient about the disease, and how to manage minor illnesses and major stresses.
4. Obtain a Medical Alert™ bracelet or necklace and an emergency medical information card.

Cushing's Syndrome

Cushing's syndrome (see detailed discussion in Chapter 56) is a clinical disorder resulting from excessive cortisol production. The focus here will be on Cushing's syndrome due to an adrenal neoplasm (**ACTH-independent hypercortisolemia**). **Functioning benign adrenal adenomas** and **adrenocortical cancers** each give rise to less than 10% of cases of Cushing's syndrome. Generally, benign adenomas are small (<100 gm at diagnosis) and synthesize cortisol very efficiently. In contrast, functioning adrenocortical cancers are very large at diagnosis and frequently produce adrenal steroids inefficiently. Because adrenal cancer is virulent, patients almost always present with a palpable abdominal mass and metastatic spread, but lacking Cushingoid features.

Clinical features of hypercortisolemia are described in Table 56.8. In benign adrenocortical adenoma, the signs of cortisol excess usually begin gradually. Hyperpigmentation of the skin, hirsutism, and other virilizing signs are often absent. However, in functioning adrenocortical carcinomas, the course tends to be more acute and rapidly progressive, with hyperandrogenic effects predominating. Patients also report abdominal, back, and flank pain caused by the large tumor size. Hypercortisolemia with concomitant ACTH suppression (ACTH less than 10 pg/ml) and an adrenal mass seen on CT or MRI are diagnostic.

Surgical removal of the benign adrenocortical adenoma through a **unilateral adrenalectomy** of the affected gland is curative. Glucocorticoid replacement is required to avoid acute adrenal crisis due to suppression and atrophy of the hypothalamus, pituitary, and contralateral adrenal. It may take as long as 1–2 years for these suppressed glands to resume functioning, so such replacement therapy must be tapered slowly. The prognosis for most adrenal carcinomas is dismal. These malignant tumors are usually treated with debulking surgery followed by chemotherapy with mitotane. Median survival

after diagnosis in adults is 14–36 months; untreated, survival averages 3 months. While mitotane lowers steroid production in 75% of patients and measurably reduces tumor size in 30%, there is no clear evidence that it actually prolongs life.

Primary Hyperaldosteronism

▪ Definition and Epidemiology

Mineralocorticoid excess causes hypertension by three patterns: aldosterone excess (primary hyperaldosteronism), real or apparent mineralocorticoid excess independent of aldosterone, and secondary hyperaldosteronism (Table 61.7). In 1955, Conn described primary hyperaldosteronism—a syndrome of hypertension and spontaneous hypokalemia due to aldosterone excess. Occurring in less than 1% of hypertensives, primary hyperaldosteronism is rare. It is most often seen in the third through fifth decades. In hypertensives with spontaneous hypokalemia (K^+ <3.5 mEq/L), 40% have a variant of primary hyperaldosteronism.

▪ Etiology and Pathogenesis

Primary hyperaldosteronism most often results from **aldosterone-producing adenomas** (APA) and idiopathic hyperaldosteronism (IHA). Rarely, it may be due to **glucocorticoid-suppressible hyperaldosteronism** or an **aldosterone-secreting adrenal carcinoma.** APAs are typically solitary, unilateral, small (<2 cm in diameter), and benign. In IHA, there is bilateral hyperplasia of the zona glomerulosa, possibly from hyperstimulation by an unidentified aldosterone-releasing factor. In primary hyperaldosteronism, the intravascular volume is typically high. Secondary hyperaldosteronism is hyperreninemic (elevated renin); patients may be normotensive or hypertensive. In normotensives with secondary hyperaldosteronism, the elevated circulating renin and aldosterone levels are due to decreased effective intravascular volume, whereas the hypertension in secondary hyperaldosteronism is more likely related to increased angiotensin II than to aldosterone.

■ Clinical Features and Diagnosis

Key manifestations of primary hyperaldosteronism include hypertension, spontaneous hypokalemia, alkalosis, low plasma renin activity, and an elevated plasma aldosterone level. The hypertension is usually moderate and is due to the sodium-retaining effects of the mineralocorticoid. Rarely, the hypokalemia may evoke polyuria, easy fatigability, anorexia, muscle weakness, and cramps.

Generally, a screening for primary hyperaldosteronism is required for a hypertensive with spontaneous hypokalemia, a serum K^+ below 3.5 mEq/L, or a serum K^+ below 3.0 mEq/L while taking a diuretic. The first step is to confirm primary hyperaldosteronism, then to determine its etiology. Testing is optimal when the individual is salt loaded and when the hypokalemia is corrected. Before biochemical testing, the following medications should be discontinued: all antihypertensive

agents except peripheral α-1 antagonists and central α-2 agonists, for at least 1 week; diuretics, for 4 weeks, and estrogen and spironolactone, for 6 weeks. The first phase of the workup includes screening tests followed by multiple tests to confirm the diagnosis (Table 61.8). Approximately 80% of the cases of primary hyperaldosteronism are due to either APA or IHA, so the second phase involves differentiating between these two causes. Imaging and bilateral adrenal vein catheterization are used to make the distinction. High-resolution CT is performed initially, because it localizes the APA in 70–80% of cases. If further testing is necessary, cortisol and aldosterone levels are determined; an aldosterone ratio exceeding 10 with a symmetrical ACTH-induced cortisol response is consistent with APA. Bilateral adrenal vein catheterization is the most effective means to distinguish between APA and IHA, but it is reserved for patients with equivocal CT scans and posture studies.

■ Management and Prognosis

Patients with an APA who are at low surgical risk should undergo adrenalectomy. One year following a successful surgery, 80–90% of patients remain normotensive and normokalemic; after five years, however, 50% develop recurrence of the hypertension while remaining normokalemic. Because bilateral adrenalectomy is usually ineffective in controlling hypertension, medical management is chosen in all patients with IHA and for patients with APA whose surgical risk precludes an operation. Patients should follow a low sodium diet (<80 mEq/d), exercise regularly and maintain an ideal body weight. Spironolactone, amiloride, and triamterene are the usual pharmaceutical agents for treating the hypokalemia of primary hyperaldosteronism. Spironolactone, the drug of choice, is often combined with Nifedipine or an ACE inhibitor to adequately control blood pressure. If this therapy does not control the

TABLE 61.7. Causes of Secondary Hyperaldosteronism	
Hypertensive	**Normotensive**
Renal artery stenosis	Cardiac failure
Renin-secreting tumors	Gastrointestinal disorders
Malignant hypertension	Renal tubular acidosis
Chronic renal disease	Renal tubulopathies (Bartter's syndrome)
	Hepatic cirrhosis
	Diuretic abuse
	Nephrotic syndrome

TABLE 61.8 Diagnostic Tests for Primary Hyperaldosteronism Due to Aldosterone-Producing Adenoma and Idiopathic Hyperaldosteronism		
Screening	**Confirmatory**	**Localizing**
24-h (U) K^+ >30 mEq PRA (ng/mL/h) <2	4-h upright PAC/PRA >20 Captopril suppression test PAC/PRA >50 PAC (ng/dL) >15	CT of the adrenals Adrenal vein catheterization
PAC (ng/dL) >15	4-h saline infusion test PAC (ng/L) >10	

PAC = plasma aldosterone concentration; PRA = plasma renin activity; (U) = Urinary.

TABLE 61.9. Clinical and Biochemical Characteristics, Diagnosis and Management of the CAH Syndromes				
Enzymatic Defect	Phenotypic Presentation	Adrenal Hormone	Clinical/Biochemical Features	Diagnosis
21-hydroxylase	NM VF to AG	GD, MD, AE	±SW, ↑K+A	↑ Plasma 17-OH progesterone
11-hydroxylase	NM VF to AG	GD ME (↑DOC) AE	HBP ↓K+Alk	↑ Plasma 11-deoxycortisol
3β-hydroxysteroid dehydrogenase	UM to AG, VF to AG	GD MD AE	±SW ↑K+A	↑ Plasma pregnenolone ↑ Plasma 17-OH pregnenolone ↓ Plasma progesterone ↓ Plasma 17-OH progesterone ↑ DHEA ↓ Androstenedione
17-hydroxylase	UM to AGF: lack of SSC	GD ME (↑ DOC) AD	HBP ↓K+Alk	↑ Plasma progesterone ↑ Plasma pregnenolone ↓ Plasma 17-OH progesterone ↓ Plasma 17-OH pregnenolone
20,22 desmolase	UM to AG NF	GD MD AD	±SW ↑K+ A Massive adrenal enlargement	Deficiency of all adrenocortical steroids

↑ = High; ↓ = low; ↑K+A = hyperkalemic acidosis; ↓K+Alk = hypokalemic alkalosis; AD = Androgen deficiency; AE = Androgen excess; AG = Ambiguous genitalia; AGF = Ambiguous genitalia female; DOC = 11-deoxycorticosterone; DHEA = dehydroepiandrosterone; GD = glucocorticoid deficiency; HBP = hypertension; MD = mineralocorticoid deficiency; ME = Mineralocorticoid excess; NF = Normal female; NM = Normal male; SSC = Secondary sexual characteristics; SW = Salt-wasting; UM = Undervirilized male; VF = Virilized female.
Measurement of the plasma steroid precursor after exogenous ACTH stimulation may be necessary to diagnose mild or late-onset forms.

hypertension, the next step is to try empirically other antihypertensive drugs, which are generally equally effective.

Congenital Adrenal Hyperplasia

■ Definition and Epidemiology

Congenital adrenal hyperplasia (CAH) is a family of autosomal recessive disorders resulting from defects in cortisol production; they involve five enzymes: 21-hydroxylase, 11-hydroxylase, 3ß-hydroxysteroid dehydrogenase, 17-hydroxylase, and 20,22-desmolase. Figure 61.1 shows the biosynthetic steps in the adrenal cortex that are catalyzed by these five enzymes. Deficient cortisol biosynthesis causes a compensatory rise in pituitary ACTH; therefore, adrenocortical hyperplasia and overproduction of the steroids precede the enzymatic defect. CAH can take two forms: a classic, congenital form with nearly total enzymatic deficiency; or, more often, a late onset form with a partial enzymatic deficiency and onset after puberty.

■ Clinical Features and Management

Clinical manifestations of each of the five enzymatic deficiencies depend on which steroids are deficient or in excess, as well as the absolute degree of deficiency or excess. The clinical and biochemical characteristics and diagnosis of the five forms of CAH are reviewed in Table 61.9. Classic 21-hydroxylase deficiency, the only HLA-linked type, accounts for more than 90% of cases of CAH. The next most common, 11-hydroxylase deficiency, accounts for nearly 5% of all CAH cases.

The enzymatic defects that impair cortisol and mineralocorticoid synthesis are treated respectively with glucocorticoids and mineralocorticoids. The consequent reduction in release of pituitary ACTH results in suppression of the overproduced adrenocortical steroids.

The Incidental Adrenal Mass

■ Definition and Epidemiology

Since the advent of abdominal CT scanning, the unsuspected (incidental) adrenal mass (**adrenal incidentaloma**) has become a common diagnostic dilemma. The incidence of adrenal masses thus detected ranges from 0.5–10%. Since most of these masses have been found to be nonfunctional, and because primary adrenocortical cancer is exceedingly rare in adrenal masses below 5 cm, a small, adrenal incidentaloma is usually benign and nonfunctional.

■ Etiology and Pathogenesis

Frequent causes of an adrenal mass can be found in Table 61.10. Thirty to fifty percent of primary adrenocortical carcinomas are nonfunctional; the remaining are functional. Excessive cortisol is the most common secretory product for both benign and malignant adenomas. Primary malignancies that most commonly metastasize to the adrenals include breast, lung, lymphoma, melanoma, and colon.

■ Clinical Manifestations

The clinical characteristics of adrenal incidentalomas depend on their functional nature. A primary adrenal cortical carcinoma most commonly presents with abdominal pain and an easily palpable mass. The mean

TABLE 61.11.	Screening Laboratory Assessment

1. Overnight 1 mg Dexamethasone suppression test and 24-hour urinary free cortisol
2. Serum total testosterone and serum dehydroepiandrosterone sulfate
3. Serum 17-β estradiol
4. Serum potassium
   Aldosterone: Plasma renin activity (if serum potassium <3.5 mEq/L)
5. 24-hour urine metanephrines, VMA and catecholamines

duration of symptoms prior to diagnosis is 6–9.5 months; most patients present in an advanced stage with a five-year survival ranging between 15–25%, independent of the stage at diagnosis. Typical sites of metastases include lung, lymph nodes, liver, bone, and gastrointestinal tract.

■ Diagnosis and Management

The appropriate diagnostic approach to patients with an incidentally discovered adrenal mass is unresolved. Initially, the CT or MRI appearance taken in context with a thorough history and physical examination may provide clues to the nature of the mass. **Myelolipomas** contain fat and are easily recognized on CT and MRI. Clinically, evidence is sought for Cushing's syndrome, **pheochromocytoma,** nonadrenal malignancies, virilization in a girl or woman, and feminization in a man or boy. Additional studies obtained to rule out the more common metastatic primaries include mammogram, chest x-ray, stool occult blood series, and flexible sigmoidoscopy/colonoscopy. Cortical and medullary dysfunction should be determined using the screening tests shown in Table 61.11. Large masses should be removed. Needle aspiration is useful in cystic lesions and to help stage an extra-adrenal neoplasm (e.g., lung).

TABLE 61.10.	Differential Diagnosis of Adrenal Mass

Benign nonfunctional adrenal cortical adenoma
Benign functional adrenal cortical adenoma
  Cushing's syndrome
  Virilizing
  Feminizing
  Hyperaldosteronism
Primary adrenal cortical carcinoma
  Nonfunctional
  Functional
Tumors of the adrenal medulla
  Pheochromocytoma
  Ganglioneuromas/neuroblastoma
Benign adrenal cyst
Myelolipoma
Intraadrenal hemorrhage
Metastases from other primary malignancies
Congenital adrenal hyperplasia

CHAPTER **62**

DISEASES OF THE ADRENAL MEDULLA

The main secretion of the adrenal medulla is **epinephrine** (EPI) rather than **norepinephrine** (NE), owing to the presence of **phenylethanolamine-N-methyl transferase** (PNMT), which converts NE to EPI. **Epinephrine, norepinephrine,** and **dopamine,** collectively called **catecholamines,** are derived from tyrosine, the dietary amino acid; these structurally similar compounds are contained within the same biosynthetic pathway. All neurons and cells of the catecholaminergic lineage contain the enzyme **tyrosine hydroxylase.** Once tyrosine is hydroxylated to DOPA, the nature of the final hormonal product released by these cells is determined by their respective set of biosynthetic enzymes. Since most adrenomedullary chromaffin cells contain a full complement of all the enzymes outlined above, EPI is the main secretion of these cells. Approximately 10% of the adrenal catecholamines are excreted directly into the urine as free EPI. All the remaining catecholamine derivatives are renally excreted (Figure 62.1).

The systemic effects of adrenomedullary catecholamine release are mediated through the activation of peripheral α- and β-adrenergic and dopaminergic receptors. The catecholamines are important mediators of central nervous system and autonomic nerve functions, and they are important regulators of the cardiovascular system. Since EPI has a slightly higher affinity for β-adrenergic receptors, the main hemodynamic effect of chromaffin cell secretion is cardiac, increasing both heart rate and contractility. Venous return, and, thus, preload to the heart, increase from α_1-mediated vasoconstriction of capacitance vessels. Combined with an α_1-mediated vasoconstriction of resistance vessels, these collective effects significantly raise the blood pressure. Catecholamines directly or indirectly affect all other endocrine systems. Circulating EPI levels alter fluid and electrolyte balance, because a β-mediated sympathetic mechanism controls the renin-angiotensin-aldosterone axis. Increased circulating EPI levels also enhance basal metabolism and facilitate the breakdown of stored fuels by directly stimulating lipolysis and enhancing glucagon-mediated glycogenolysis and gluconeogenesis.

Neoplasms are the most significant of all the adrenal medullary disorders. Their histology and functionality reflect the cell type of derivation. Tumors arise more often from the catecholamine-secreting cells of neural crest origin, presenting as pheochromocytomas in adults and as neuroblastomas in children (one of the common solid tumors of childhood).

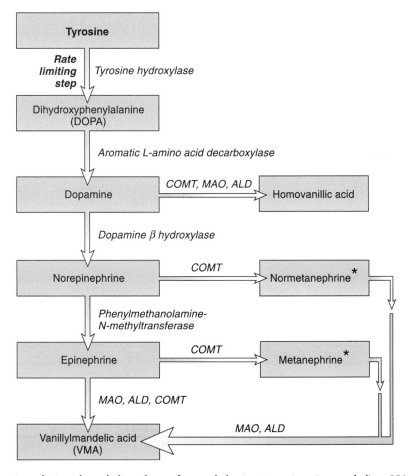

FIGURE 62.1. Biosynthetic and metabolic pathways for catecholamines * = major urine metabolites; COMT = Catechol O-methyl transferase; MAO = Monoamine oxidase; ALD = Aldehyde dehydrogenase.

Pheochromocytoma

■ Definition and Etiology

Pheochromocytomas are autonomously functioning, catecholamine-secreting, chromaffin-cell neoplasms. About 90% are benign solitary nodules found within the adrenal medulla itself. However, they can arise anywhere that neural crest tissue has migrated during the course of embryonic development; nearly 10% are located intra-abdominally in close proximity to the celiac or mesenteric sympathetic ganglia. Adrenal medullary pheochromocytomas are almost always (90%) unilateral. Bilateral lesions usually occur only as familial neoplasms, as in type IIa (**Sipple's syndrome**) or type IIb (**multiple endocrine neoplasia**) (MEN, Table 62.1).

■ Clinical Features

The hallmark of a pheochromocytoma is hypertension. The clinical triad of severe headache, palpitations, and excessive diaphoresis occurring with hypertension provides the best clinical clue for this tumor (Table 62.2). If this triad and hypertension are absent, the diagnosis of a pheochromocytoma can be confidently set aside. While 80% or more of these patients are hypertensive on examination, nearly one-half exhibit normotensive, symptom-free periods, interspersed with episodic and transient symptoms. Spectacular fluctuations in blood pressure are quite common. Excessive catecholamine secretion causing the constellation of these symptoms appears to be paroxysmal. During an attack, if BP and pulse rate both rise, the tumor is primarily releasing EPI. In contrast, if pulse rate declines as BP rises, the tumor is secreting mainly NE.

■ Diagnosis

Pheochromocytomas are diagnosed biochemically. The most useful screening test is a 24-hour urine measurement of the levels of catecholamines (NE and EPI) and of their metabolites, metanephrine and vanillylmandelic acid (see Table 62.3 for normal values). The quantitation of total urinary metanephrines and catecholamines, especially NE, provides the most sensitive and specific proof of pheochromocytoma. Recently, the determination of free NE in a 24-hour urine sample was shown to be 100% sensitive and 98% specific for diagnosis. In most cases of pheochromocytoma, the **total urinary metanephrines and catecholamines** (NE + EPI) exceed 1000 µg/24 h and 150 µg/24 h, respectively. Because many medications influence the test results, they should be withheld, if possible, before collecting the urine sample. **Plasma NE,** another useful screening test in pheochromocytomas, typically exceeds 2000 pg/ml. However, since the catecholamine secretion may be intermittent, single plasma catecholamine measurements

TABLE 62.1.	Classification of the Multiple Endocrine Neoplasia (MEN) Syndromes
MEN Syndrome	**Associated Disorders**
MEN Type I (Wermer's syndrome)	Hyperparathyroidism
	Pituitary adenomas
	Pancreatic islet cell tumor
	Gastrinoma
	VIPoma
	Insulinoma
	Glucagonoma
MEN Type IIa (Sipple's syndrome)	Medullary carcinoma of thyroid
	Pheochromocytoma
	Hyperparathyroidism
MEN Type IIb	Marfanoid habitus
	Pheochromocytoma
	Medullary carcinoma of thyroid
	Mucosal and intestinal neuromas

TABLE 62.2.	Clinical Manifestations Associated With Pheochromocytomas		
Symptoms	**Incidence**	**Signs**	**Incidence**
Headache	75–100%	Hypertension	75–100%
Palpitations	50–75%	Tachycardia	50–75%
Diaphoresis	50–75%	Postural hypotension	50–75%
Anxiety	25–50%	Paroxysmal hypertension	25–50%
Tremulousness	25–50%	Weight loss	25–50%
Chest pain	25–50%	Tremor	25–50%
Abdominal pain	25–50%	Pallor	25–50%
Nausea/emesis	25–50%		
Weakness/fatigue	25–50%		

TABLE 62.3. **Normal Urine Levels of Catecholamines and Their Metabolites**

Substance in Urine	Upper Limit of Normal
Total catecholamines	100 µg/d
Norepinephrine	75 µg/d
Epinephrine	25 µg/d
Dopamine	525 µg/d
Metanephrines	1.1 mg/d
Vanillylmandelic acid	7 mg/d

may be less sensitive than urinary levels. Specific pharmacologic stimulation/suppression tests are often used when the clinical features are equivocal and when urinary/plasma catecholamines are only slightly elevated. Provocative testing with IV glucagon bolus in these patients will often elicit an exaggerated pressor response; agents that normally attenuate adrenomedullary catecholamine release (clonidine, α_2-agonist) have no effect.

Once a pheochromocytoma is confirmed biochemically, its localization should follow with CT or MRI. CT is often not the best initial imaging study when extra-adrenal or metastatic pheochromocytomas are suspected. Radionuclide tests with ^{131}**I-meta-iodobenzylguanidine** (MIBG), a radioactive amine taken up and concentrated by adrenergic cromattin cells, are quite useful in this setting.

■ Management and Prognosis

Pheochromocytoma is almost always cured by surgical excision of the tumor. The five-year postoperative survival rate exceeds 95%. An α-adrenergic blocking agent (phenoxybenzamine, 10 mg b.i.d.) is administered 7–10 days prior to surgery, in order to avoid an intraoperative hypertensive crisis. Unless **tachyarrhythmias** develop from complete α-blockade, preoperative β-blocking agents are not routinely given. **Phentolamine** (a reversible α-blocker) and **nitroprusside** (a direct-acting arterial vasodilator) are usually used to manage any hypertensive crises that arise during the induction of anesthesia or during surgery. Severe hypotension after tumor excision is usually avoided by perioperative plasma volume expansion with normal saline. Inoperable or malignant pheochromocytomas are medically managed, using both α- and β-adrenergic blockade. **Metyrosine**, a tyrosine hydroxylase inhibitor, may be added if these agents fail to produce adequate symptom relief. In these rare patients, the five-year survival rate is less than 50%.

Unrecognized pheochromocytomas are potentially lethal. Hypertensive crisis or lethal shock may be precipitated by drugs, anesthetic agents, surgery for unrelated conditions, or parturition. However, with early diagnosis, these patients enjoy an extremely high cure rate.

CHAPTER 63

DISORDERS OF OVARIAN FUNCTION

■ Ovarian Physiology

The ovary has two distinct regions: the **outer cortex** with the **germinal epithelium** and **follicles,** and the **central medulla,** consisting of supportive stroma, blood vessels, nerves, and lymphatics. The **graafian follicle** contains both theca and granulosa cells. The interstitial and stromal ovarian cells arise from degenerating atretic follicles.

The ovaries have two major functions: cyclic **steroidogenesis** (the biosynthesis of steroids) and **ovulation** (oocyte maturation and release). **Estrogens, progestins,** and **androgens** are the major sex steroids synthesized by the three main functional components of the ovary: the **follicles,** corpus luteum, and **ovarian stroma** (Figure 63.1). Ovarian hormone production is controlled by the anterior pituitary gonadotropins, FSH and LH, which are necessary for follicle stimulation. Follicle stimulation results in estrogen production by the **theca interna** and **granulosa** cells found in the follicular wall. The main and most important estrogen produced by the germinal epithelium is **17β-estradiol.** The mid-cycle LH surge causes **ovulation** (discharge of the ovum from the graafian follicle), after which the corpus luteum secretes primarily progesterone. Androgens are produced mainly by the interstitial thecal cells and to a lesser degree by the ovarian stroma. The androgens include **dehydroepiandrosterone** (DHEA), **androstenedione,** and **testosterone.** While the role of the ovarian androgens is not clear, the functions of the other ovarian hormones are shown in Table 63.1.

■ Normal Menstrual Physiology

Menses is the monthly flow of blood from the female genital tract. **Menarche** (the onset of menses) occurs between 10–15 years. Menses cease **(menopause)** between 45–53 years. Normal menses occur every 28 days

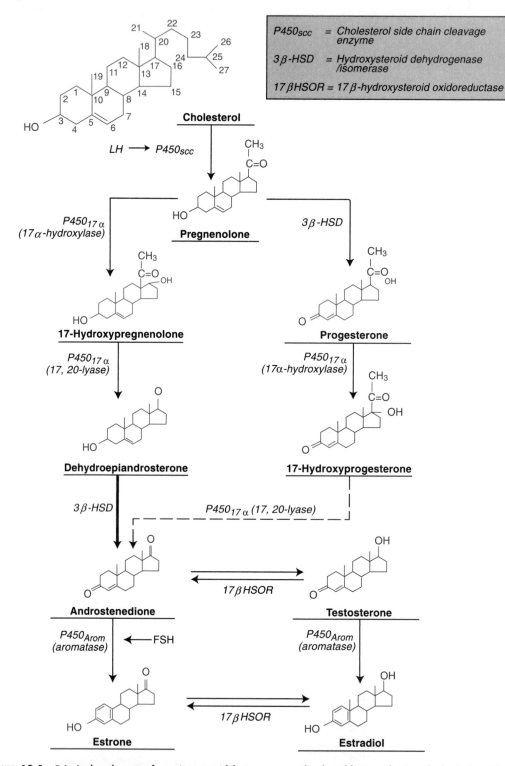

$P450_{scc}$ = Cholesterol side chain cleavage enzyme

3β-HSD = Hydroxysterol dehydrogenase /isomerase

$17\beta HSOR$ = 17β-hydroxysteroid oxidoreductase

Cholesterol

$LH \longrightarrow P450_{scc}$

$P450_{17\alpha}$
(17α-hydroxylase)

Pregnenolone

3β-HSD

17-Hydroxypregnenolone

$P450_{17\alpha}$
(17, 20-lyase)

Progesterone

$P450_{17\alpha}$
(17α-hydroxylase)

Dehydroepiandrosterone

17-Hydroxyprogesterone

3β-HSD

$P450_{17\alpha}$ (17, 20-lyase)

Androstenedione

$17\beta HSOR$

Testosterone

$P450_{Arom}$
(aromatase)

$\longleftarrow$ FSH

$P450_{Arom}$
(aromatase)

Estrone

$17\beta HSOR$

Estradiol

FIGURE 63.1. Principal pathways of ovarian steroid hormone biosynthesis. The major enzyme complements for the corpus luteum, theca, and granulosa cells are shown; these cells produce predominantly progesterone and 17-hydroxyprogesterone (corpus luteum); androgen (theca); and estrogen (granulosa). The horizontal arrows indicate the major sites of action of LH and FSH in mediating this pathway. The dotted line emphasizes the limited metabolism of 17-hydroxyprogesterone in the human ovary.

(Redrawn with permission from: Carr BR. In: Wilson JD, Foster DW (eds.). Williams Textbook of Endocrinology. 8th ed. Philadelphia: WB Saunders Company, 1992, p. 745.)

TABLE 63.1.	Actions of the Sex Steroids
Sex Steroid	**Major Actions**
Estrogen	Promotes development of secondary sexual characteristics in women
	Promotes uterine, vaginal, and fallopian tube development and thickening of vaginal mucosa
	Promotes thinning of cervical mucus
	Promotes development of breast ductal system
Progesterone	Induces secretory activity in the endometrium of the estrogen-primed uterus
	Required for implantation of the fertilized ovum
	Required for maintenance of pregnancy
	Induces decidualization of the endometrium
	Inhibits uterine contraction
	Increases viscosity of cervical mucus
	Promotes glandular development of breasts
	Increases basal body temperature

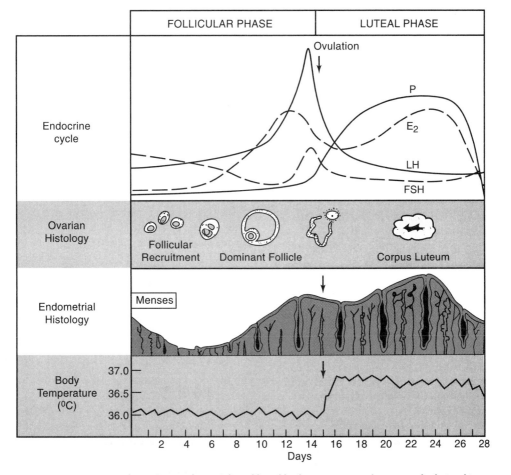

FIGURE 63.2. Hormonal, ovarian, endometrial, and basal body temperature changes and relationship throughout the normal menstrual cycle.

(Redrawn from: Carr BR, Wilson JD. In: Isselbacher KJ, Braunwald E, Wilson JD, et al (eds.). Harrison's Principles of Internal Medicine. 13th ed. New York: McGraw-Hill, 1994, p. 2022, fig. 340.5. Reproduced with permission.)

TABLE 63.2.	**Major Androgens in Women**			
	Sites of Formation			
Androgen	Ovary (%)[b]	Adrenal (%)	Conversion (%)	Relative Androgen Activity[a]
Testosterone	5–25	5–25	50–90	100
Androstenedione	45–50	30–45	5–25	10–20
Dehydroepiandrosterone (DHEA)	20	80	—	5
DHEA-Sulfate	<5	>95	—	minimal
Dihydrotestosterone	—	—	100	250

[a]Relative to testosterone (100 = 100 × relative to testosterone).
[b]Percent of a particular androgen produced at each site.

(with a range of 21–40 days) and last 2–7 days, with a blood loss of 30–100 ml during each cycle. The **menstrual cycle** is the interval between two consecutive menstrual periods. It is the response of the uterus to the cyclic changes and interactions of hypothalamic GnRH, pituitary gonadotropins, and the secretion of ovarian estradiol and progesterone (Figure 63.2). The menstrual cycle is divided into the **follicular** (proliferative) and the **luteal** (secretory) phases. The follicular phase marks the first half of the cycle; ovulation occurs at midcycle, and the luteal phase follows ovulation.

Amenorrhea

■ Definition and Etiology

Amenorrhea is defined as the absence of menses by age 16 (**primary**) in a nonpregnant woman or as no menses for over 3 months in a woman with previously regular cycles (**secondary**). The differential diagnosis of amenorrhea is based on the anatomic structure primarily responsible for the problem (Table 63.3). **Oligomenorrhea** is infrequent menstruation. A defect at any level of the hypothalamic-pituitary-ovarian-genital tract axis may be responsible. Hypothalamic **hypogonadism** may follow tumors and infections; pituitary adenomas, craniopharyngiomas, germinomas, hamartomas, and teratomas are the most common underlying tumors. Infections that can have this effect include tuberculosis, syphilis, encephalitis, and meningitis. Almost 15% of cases of amenorrhea result from hyperprolactinemia, which inhibits hypothalamic GnRH release. Hyperprolactinemia is discussed in Chapter 56.

Hypergonadotropic hypogonadism is seen in patients with **gonadal dysgenesis** or Turner's syndrome who have a defect or absence of one of the two X chromosomes. **Turner's syndrome,** the most common cause of primary amenorrhea, occurs in about 1 in 2000 female births. These girls typically have characteristic

■ Physiology of Androgen Secretion

The major circulating androgens in women are shown in Table 63.2. **Dihydrotestosterone,** formed from the conversion of testosterone by the enzyme 5α-reductase, appears to be the androgen responsible for androgen-dependent hair growth. Androstenedione, DHEA, and DHEA-Sulfate possess little intrinsic direct androgenic activity until after conversion to testosterone and dihydrotestosterone (Table 63.2).

somatic abnormalities, including sexual infantilism, short stature, webbing of the neck, shieldlike chest, low-set ears with low posterior hairline, high arched palate, and **cubitus valgus** (increased carrying angle of the elbows). They also commonly manifest transient lymphedema of the hands and feet at birth (30%), cardiovascular anomalies (50%), renal defects (35%) and gonadal failure (95–100%). Other causes of hypergonadotropic hypogonadism include ovarian enzymatic deficiencies and premature ovarian failure. Besides the conditions listed in Table 63.3, patients with polycystic ovarian syndrome (Stein-Leventhal syndrome), adult-onset congenital adrenal hyperplasia, Cushing's syndrome, and hypothyroidism or hyperthyroidism often will have amenorrhea with estrogen present.

■ Evaluation

In assessing both primary or secondary amenorrhea, it is first necessary to exclude pregnancy. A thorough history and physical examination, as shown in Table 63.4, will reveal the cause in most patients with amenorrhea. After assessing for the signs of Cushing's syndrome, hyperprolactinemia, and acromegaly, supportive laboratory tests should be scheduled. Besides the quintessential pregnancy test, basal serum measurements of TSH, prolactin, 17-β estradiol FSH, and LH are also generally required in all amenorrheic women, especially with a normal physical examination. The workup of amenorrhea is outlined in Figure 63.3. The progesterone withdrawal test or progestin challenge is a bioassay for estrogen production; it is performed by giving 5–10 mg of oral medroxyprogesterone acetate for 5–10 days or 100–200 mg of progesterone in oil IM. Any vaginal bleeding within 7–10 days indicates **adequate estradiol** (estradiol level of at least 40 pg/ml) and confirms integrity of the uterine/vaginal tract. If withdrawal bleeding does not occur, cyclic estrogen followed by progesterone is given. Patients with normal or low FSH and LH who initially fail to bleed with progesterone alone, but who respond to sequential estrogen and progesterone, most likely have a hypothalamic or pituitary abnormality. Women who also

TABLE 63.3.	Causes of Amenorrhea
Pregnancy and/or Breast-Feeding	
Hypogonadotrophic Hypogonadism	
Hypothalamus	Tumors/infection
	Hand-Schuller-Christian disease
	Kallmann syndrome
	Sarcoidosis
	Idiopathic hypogonadotropic hypogonadism
	Chronic debilitating disease
	Anorexia, malnutrition, weight loss
	Exercise-associated
	Emotional trauma/stress
Pituitary	Tumor compression
	Hyperprolactinemia
	Empty sella
	Sheehan syndrome
	Sarcoidosis
	Hemochromatosis
	Post-surgical, irradiation, trauma
Hypergonadotropic Hypogonadism	
Ovarian	Gonadal agenesis/dysgenesis
	Ovarian enzymatic deficiency
	Premature ovarian failure
Normal Gonadotropins and Estrogen	
Uterus/Vagina	Mullerian agenesis
	Endometrial hypoplasia/ aplasia
	Labial fusion/imperforate hymen
	Cervical stenosis/agenesis
	Vaginal agenesis
	Uterine scarring
	Testicular feminization

TABLE 63.4.	Clinical Evaluation of Amenorrhea
HISTORY	
General	
Significant medical illness	
Emotional stress	
Weight loss	
Exercise	
Exposure to toxic chemicals/drugs/radiation	
Past surgeries	
Symptoms of estrogen deficiency (hot flashes)	
Headaches	
Visual field changes	
Galactorrhea	
Symptoms of hypothyroidism	
Developmental	
Age and sequence of secondary sexual characteristics	
Menarche	
Menstrual history	
Sexual history	
Family History	
Reproductive problems	
Time of mother's menarche and menopause	
PHYSICAL EXAMINATION	
Body habitus	Muscle mass and fat distribution
Skin	Pigment, acne, hair distribution and type, striae
Eye	Visual fields
Thyroid	Size and consistency
Breasts	Tanner stage, galactorrhea, atrophy
Pubic hair	Tanner stage
Pelvic	Presence/absence/normalcy of internal and external genitalia, vaginal estrogenization, cervical mucus

fail to respond to the sequential estrogen and progesterone regimen usually have an outflow tract obstruction. High serum FSH levels (>40 mIU/ml) indicate ovarian failure. A karyotype should be analyzed in young women (<30 years old) with elevated FSH levels looking for Turner's syndrome.

Management

The treatment of amenorrhea depends on the diagnosis and on patient goals. Influential factors include reversibility of the abnormality, adequacy of feminization, desire for fertility, need for contraception, problems due to estrogen deprivation, risk of endometrial hyperplasia and cancer with unopposed estrogen, and associated hirsutism and virilization. If **functional hypothalamic amenorrhea** is induced by stress, weight loss or excessive exercise, important treatment strategies include counseling, and lifestyle changes. Women with a positive progesterone withdrawal test should be given

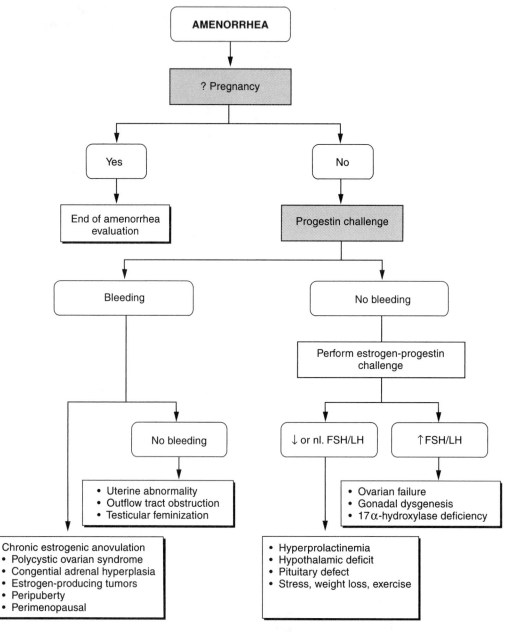

FIGURE 63.3. Assessment of amenorrhea.

oral progesterone (medroxyprogesterone acetate 5–10 mg daily) for 5–10 days every 1–3 months or an oral contraceptive pill to induce periodic bleeding, avoiding endometrial hyperplasia. Combined estrogen/progester-one therapy should be given when response to progesterone is remiss, as in patients with ovarian failure and women with irreversible hypothalamic or pituitary disorders.

Hirsutism and Virilization

■ Definition

Hirsutism is defined as the presence in women of excessive body hair in areas associated with a masculine pattern of hair growth. There are two types of hair, vellus and terminal. **Vellus hair** is fine, soft, generally unpigmented hair that is not androgen-stimulated and is found diffusely over the body. **Terminal hair** is coarse, pigmented, androgen-dependent, and normally localized (in a masculine pattern) to the back, face, chest, abdomen, axilla, and pubic area. Hirsutism is generally more of a cosmetic problem capable of causing severe psychosocial difficulties than a pathological disorder. It is common, with 15–35% of normal women developing terminal hairs on the lower abdomen, upper lip and chest. Terminal hair on the face, periareolar, and lower abdomen is normal, but that on the upper back, shoulders, sternum, and upper abdomen suggests a more marked androgen effect. **Virilization** is both decreased feminine secondary sexual characteristics (breast and vaginal mucosal atrophy) and increased masculine secondary sexual characteristics (hirsutism, temporal balding, voice deepening, clitoromegaly, and increased muscle mass). Virilization usually implies more significant hyperandrogenism.

■ Etiology and Pathogenesis

Hirsutism in women results from increased androgen production and/or action, and its etiology may be androgen-dependent or androgen-independent. **Androgen-dependent hirsutism** has a male pattern of hair growth and is typically due to excessive adrenal or ovarian androgen production (Table 63.5) or increased follicle sensitivity to androgen. **Androgen-independent hirsutism** is characterized by increased growth of vellus-type hair.

Virilizing adrenal and ovarian tumors may be benign or malignant. Adrenal tumors produce primarily DHEA and DHEA-S; ovarian tumors primarily produce testosterone. Benign tumors generally produce androgens efficiently; therefore, they are small when diagnosed. In contrast, malignant tumors are usually inefficient in steroid hormone biosynthesis; they are large (>6 cm in diameter) and easily palpable at diagnosis.

Polycystic ovarian syndrome (PCOS) is a heterogeneous disorder characterized by some or all of the following: oligomenorrhea, obesity, hirsutism, and infertility. More than 90% of adult women presenting with clinical androgen excess have PCOS. Virtually all circulating androgens (adrenal and ovarian) are mildly to moderately elevated in these women. Despite the name, enlarged, cystic ovaries are not essential for diagnosis. Additionally, obesity with associated hyperinsulinemia and insulin resistance is a clear predisposing factor for the development of PCOS. While the cause of PCOS is elusive, many biochemical and physiological abnormalities of the ovaries, pituitary gonadotropins, and adrenal androgens have been described.

■ Clinical and Laboratory Evaluation

The primary goal in the diagnostic evaluation of a hirsute/virilized woman is to exclude a serious underlying cause. A thorough history and physical examination is the first step, with biochemical testing to pursue the clues thus obtained (Table 63.6). Abrupt, nonperipubertal onset, rapid advance of hirsutism, and additional signs and symptoms of virilization suggest serious disease. It is important to inquire about anabolic steroid use, especially in athletic women. Constitutional symptoms (malaise, weight loss, and anorexia) suggest a malignancy. A thorough skin examination is essential, looking specifically for acne, **acanthosis nigricans** (diffuse, velvety, dark brown/black skin pigmentation chiefly on

TABLE 63.5.	Causes of Hirsutism and Virilization

Androgen-Dependent
  Adrenal Causes
    Virilizing adrenal neoplasms
    Congenital adrenal hyperplasia
    Cushing's syndrome
  Ovarian Causes
    Virilizing ovarian tumors
    Severe insulin resistance
  Combined Adrenal and Ovarian
    Polycystic ovarian syndrome
    Idiopathic or functional hirsutism
    Exogenous androgens
Androgen-Independent
  Drugs
    Phenytoin
    Diazoxide
    Minoxidil
    Glucocorticoids
    Cyclosporine
  Starvation/Anorexia Nervosa
  Inherited/Ethnic Background
Miscellaneous Causes
  Acromegaly
  Hyperprolactinemia
  Hyper- and hypothyroidism

TABLE 63.6. Clinical and Laboratory Evaluation of Hirsutism and Virilization

History
Time of onset
Rate of progression
Ethnic background
Menstrual history
Careful drug history
Past medical history (hypertension and diabetes mellitus)
Presence of constitutional symptoms
History of weight gain

Physical Examination
Deepening of the voice
Amount and distribution of hair
Temporal balding
Skin changes
Obesity (truncal)
Galactorrhea
Dorsocervical and supraclavicular fat pads
Proximal muscle weakness
Pectoral muscle development
Abdominal mass
Pelvic mass
Clitoromegaly

Laboratory Evaluation

Ovulatory menses; mild to moderate hirsutism
Routine hormonal evaluation not needed

Oligo/amenorrhea; mild to severe hirsutism
Total testosterone
Dehydroepiandrosterone sulfate
Prolactin
LH, FSH
Thyroid function tests
24-hour urinary free cortisol
or
1 mg dexamethasone suppression test
ACTH-stimulated 17-hydroxyprogesterone

the back of the neck, axillae, and other body folds, thought to reflect the hyperinsulinemia accompanying PCOS), signs of Cushing's syndrome (wide violaceous abdominal striae, thin skin, facial plethora, and ecchymoses), and the quality and distribution of hair growth and virilization. Abdominal and pelvic masses should be noted.

Generally, a serum testosterone level above 200 ng/ml suggests a virilizing ovarian tumor; an ultrasound should be obtained. If the DHEA-S level is above twice normal, an abdominal CT should follow, to search for a virilizing adrenal tumor. A 17-hydroxyprogesterone level should be done 60 minutes after IV Cosyntropin to exclude partial 21-hydroxylase deficiency; a poststimulation level above 1500 ng/dl diagnoses a homozygous deficiency. A mildly elevated prolactin frequently goes with PCOS, but if its level is above 50 ng/ml, it is necessary to rule out a pituitary tumor. LH and FSH are used to evaluate for primary ovarian failure and PCOS. An LH:FSH above 2 or 3 is consistent with PCOS.

■ **Management and Prognosis**

Therapy for hirsutism and virilization is directed toward correcting the underlying specific cause and at suppressing abnormal androgen secretion. Hirsutism

TABLE 63.7. Therapeutic Approaches to Hirsutism

Mechanical	Drug Therapy
Shaving	Oral contraceptive agents
Bleaching	Spironolactone
Electrolysis	GnRH analogues
Laser hair removal	Cyproterone acetate
Weight loss	Flutamide

due to idiopathic hirsutism, PCOS, and attenuated congenital adrenal hyperplasia is usually treated with a combination of mechanical and drug therapy (Table 63.7). Oral contraceptive agents alone are usually ineffective for treating hirsutism; they are used in combination with spironolactone, which blocks the androgen receptor and is the drug of choice in the United States for treating hirsutism. However, drug therapy is not a cure, and it generally takes at least six months to evaluate the efficacy of any given agent. Lifelong therapy is usually required to prevent recurrence. Hirsutism does not resolve completely with combination therapy in most cases, but the majority will report a satisfactory improvement.

Menopause

■ Definition and Etiology

Menopause is defined as the final episode of menstrual bleeding in a woman. Its median age of onset is 50 years. Menopause occurs when the ovaries are depleted of primordial follicles, resulting in decreasing estrogen secretion. Pituitary gonadotropins rise in response (FSH >40 mIU/ml). Not all women experience an abrupt cessation of menses; many will experience variable cycles with skipped periods and increasing intervals between cycles. Therefore, menopause usually cannot be diagnosed clinically unless menses have been absent for 6–12 months in women over 45 years of age.

■ Clinical Features

Loss of estrogen leads to a number of signs and symptoms (Table 63.8). Although the prevalence decreases with time, nearly 50% of untreated women continue to experience flushing five years after menopause. The flushing may occur frequently throughout the day and night, leading to insomnia, irritability, and fatigue. The effects of estrogen deprivation on the cardiovascular and skeletal systems are of far greater medical significance. Estrogen replacement therapy leads to a 50% reduction in cardiovascular risk in women, possibly due to improved lipid levels. Bone mass begins to decrease after age 40 in both sexes, but this process rapidly accelerates at menopause. While the beneficial effect of long-term estrogens in preventing bone demineralization and in reducing hip, wrist, and vertebral fracture rates is now well-documented, the potential risks of estrogen replacement therapy include uterine cancer, breast, cholelithiasis, hypertension, and venous thrombosis.

■ Management

Estrogen replacement therapy (ERT) should be given to women with symptoms of estrogen deficiency and to those at high risk for osteoporosis and coronary artery disease. ERT is usually contraindicated in women with estrogen-dependent tumors, undiagnosed genital bleeding, active liver disease, active thromboembolic disorders, porphyria, and pregnancy. For women with a uterus, an estrogen-progestin combination is used to prevent endometrial hyperplasia and cancer. Most clinicians use a cyclic or intermittent regimen: the estrogen is given for the first 25 days of the month and the progestin for the last 10 days of the ERT (Table 63.9). In patients who receive combined continuous estrogen and progesterone therapy, endometrial atrophy with absence of bleeding will eventually occur. This state is usually reached in about six months. These women experience unpredictable intermittent bleeding, which may require endometrial biopsies. ERT and progestins may commonly produce breast tenderness, bloating, weight gain, and depression.

TABLE 63.8.	Clinical Features of Post-Menopausal Estrogen Deficiency

Vasomotor Instability
  Hot flashes
  Sweating
Decreased libido
Vaginal dryness
Urinary difficulties (e.g., incontinence)
Osteoporosis
Increased cardiovascular disease
Atrophy of urogenital epithelium and skin
Decreased size of reproductive organs and breasts

TABLE 63.9.	Hormonal Replacement Regimens for Post-Menopausal Women				
Estrogen	**Dose (mg)**	**Progestin**		**Intermittent (mg)**	**Continuous (mg)**
Conjugated estrogens	0.625	Medroxyprogesterone acetate		5–10	2.5
Micronized estradiol	1.0				
Transdermal estradiol	0.05–0.1tw				

Note: Any of the estrogens could be paired with any of the progestins shown in the table.
Intermittent = cyclic therapy; continuous = daily, without cycling; tw = twice weekly.

CHAPTER **64** DISORDERS OF TESTICULAR FUNCTION

The **testicles** (the male gonads) are paired organs located in the scrotum, which acts as a temperature regulator and protects the gonads from physical injuries. The **testicular parenchyma** consists of the seminiferous tubules, which are embedded in a connective tissue matrix containing scattered Leydig cells, blood vessels, and lymphatics. The seminiferous tubules and the Leydig cells make up the two functional units of the testis. The **tubules** are a highly complex, convoluted network, duly responsible for spermatogenesis and transport of sperm to the excretory-ejaculatory ducts. The **Leydig cell,** the primary endocrine organ of the testes, produces testosterone. **Sertoli or nurse cells,** also located in the seminiferous epithelium, function as a supporting matrix for the germ cells; they also synthesize and secrete inhibin and clear damaged germ cells from the epithelium.

Spermatogenesis is the progressive maturation of the germ cell from **spermatogonia** (an undifferentiated male germ cell) to mature spermatozoa through the processes of mitosis, meiosis, and spermiogenesis; it takes approximately 70 days to complete and requires an intact hypothalamic-pituitary axis (Figure 64.1). Transport of sperm through the epididymis to the ejaculatory duct takes about 12–21 days. The spermatozoa are initially released with fluid secreted by the Sertoli cells into the lumen of the seminiferous tubules.

From here, they pass through the straight tubules to the Rete testis, then to the efferent ducts and into the ductus epididymis. During their transit through the epididymis, the spermatozoa undergo further maturation to become motile and attain fertilizing capacity. After passing through the epididymis, the sperm enter the **vas deferens,** which empties into the ejaculatory duct. There the semen is prepared for ejaculation through the urethra. The seminal vesicles and prostate add additional secretory factors to the semen before it is emptied into the ejaculatory duct.

Most testosterone is transported in the circulation protein-bound, with only 2% free (active). Almost 44% is bound to testosterone-binding globulin; another 54% binds to albumin and other proteins. Estradiol and dihydrotestosterone are the two major biologically active metabolites (Figure 64.2) of testosterone. **Estradiol** is yielded by the aromatization of testosterone at extraglandular sites in peripheral tissues, catalyzed by aromatase. The conversion of testosterone to **dihydrotestosterone** is catalyzed by 5-α reductase. Dihydrotestosterone is localized to distinct tissues such as liver, skin, and accessory organs of reproduction (seminal vesicles and prostate); it leads to male sexual differentiation, including, external virilization, and sexual maturation at puberty. The physiologic role of estradiol in men is unknown.

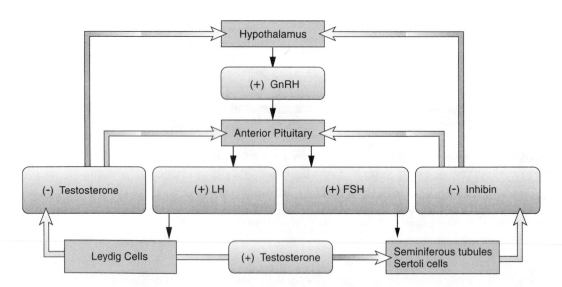

FIGURE 64.1. The hypothalamic-pituitary-gonadal axis. (−) = negative influence; (+) = positive influence.

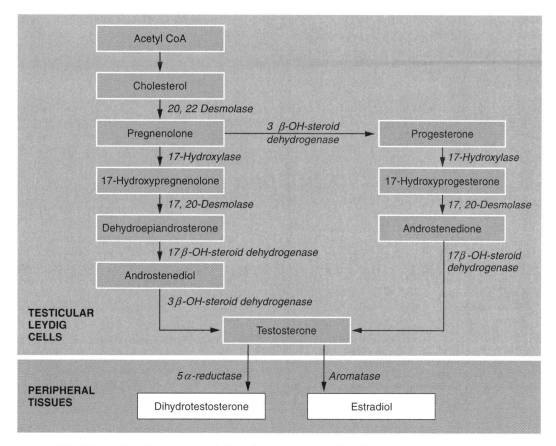

FIGURE 64.2. Biosynthesis and metabolism of testosterone. The first side-chain cleavage of cholesterol to pregnenolone is the rate-limiting reaction and is probably regulated by LH.

Hypogonadism/Testicular Failure

■ Definition

Hypogonadism, or testicular dysfunction, can be classified as **primary hypogonadism** (due to a defect of the testes), **secondary hypogonadism** (due to a hypothalamic-pituitary defect), or androgen resistance. Abnormal testicular function has different clinical presentations depending on the phase of sexual life in which they appear. The focus of this chapter will be on adult abnormalities.

■ Etiology and Pathogenesis

The causes of hypogonadism based on hypogonadotropic or hypergonadotropic etiology are listed in Table 64.1. **Hypogonadotropic hypogonadism** can be due to a deficiency in hypothalamic GnRH and/or pituitary gonadotropins, FSH and LH. Permanent GnRH deficiency is seen with congenital disorders such as Kall-

mann and Prader-Willi syndromes, external hypothalamic irradiation, and idiopathic acquired GnRH deficiency. **Primary or hypergonadotropic hypogonadism** can be congenital or acquired. **Klinefelter's syndrome,** affecting 1 in 500 male infants, is the most common cause of congenital testicular disease; it is caused by an early meiotic nondisjunction that leads to a 47 XXY karyotype. The syndrome is characterized by small testes, tall stature, increased arm span, long legs, gynecomastia, and azoospermia. Primary testicular failure may be associated with renal failure, liver disease, sickle cell anemia, febrile illness, paraplegia, and myotonic dystrophy. Spironolactone, ketoconazole, alcohol, and cyclophosphamide decrease androgen production.

Androgen resistance, an uncommon cause of hypogonadism, can arise from one of two different mechanisms. The first involves an abnormality of the enzyme 5α-reductase, which converts testosterone to

TABLE 64.1.	Causes of Hypogonadism

Primary Hypogonadism
Autoimmune
Chemotherapy
Chromosomal abnormalities
Cryptorchidism
Drugs/Alcohol
Radiation therapy
Systemic diseases
Trauma/Castration
Viral orchitis (mumps)
Secondary Hypogonadism
Hyperprolactinemia
Pituitary tumors
Benign sellar tumors
Metastatic sellar tumors
Kallmann syndrome
Infiltrative disorders
Idiopathic hypogonadotropic hypogonadism
Panhypopituitarism
Granulomatous disease
Autoimmune hypophysitis
Primary hyperthyroidism
Androgen Resistance
5α-reductase deficiency
Androgen receptor defect

dihydrotestosterone; the second involves an intrinsic abnormality of the androgen receptor. This latter defect has variable severity; the mildest forms cause only infertility, whereas severe forms lead to ambiguous genitalia. Recent studies of patients with androgen receptor abnormalities or testicular feminization syndrome (a condition in which a genetic male, with 46 chromosomes and an XY karyotype, develops as a female) reveal that most patients have a single base substitution within the androgen receptor gene.

■ Clinical Features and Diagnosis

Symptoms and signs of hypogonadism vary depending on whether the age of onset is before or after puberty. Adult men with androgen deficiency report decreased libido, infertility, impotence or erectile dysfunction, impaired masculinization, gynecomastia, and facial flushing. Physical examination should assess testicular size and consistency and look for signs of undervirilization, a palpable testicular mass and gynecomastia. Laboratory tests should include serum testosterone, LH, FSH, TSH, and prolactin, semen analysis if fertility is an issue, and a karyotype if Klinefelter's syndrome is suspected.

■ Management

Treatment of male androgen deficiency depends on whether the hypogonadism is primary or secondary and on whether the goal is only to normalize serum testosterone levels or also to stimulate spermatogenesis. Whether the problem is due to hypo-or hypergonadotropic hypogonadism, the serum testosterone can be increased by using transdermal or IM testosterone. However, spermatogenesis can be induced only in individuals with secondary hypogonadism. It requires IM injections of human chorionic gonadotropin and/or human menotropin or pulsatile GnRH injections.

Gynecomastia

■ Definition and Epidemiology

In normal adult men, no breast tissue is palpable. Remnants of a duct system can be detected histologically, but the lining cells are atrophic. **Gynecomastia** is defined as the unilateral or bilateral enlargement of the male breast. It may be asymmetric, with one side larger than the other; the tissue may be a discrete subareolar plate or a diffuse mass of fibroadipose tissue. Gynecomastia is common, reportedly affecting 30–50% of normal men between the ages of 17–80 years and 70% of hospitalized men.

■ Etiology and Pathogenesis

Generally, any palpable breast tissue in men is abnormal except during three stages of life: the transient gynecomastia of neonates, the breast enlargement at puberty, and the gynecomastia of senescence. In neonates, it is due to maternal estrogens and usually lasts a few weeks. Pubertal gynecomastia, which is likely due to testicular production of estradiol (which peaks initially before testosterone), affects 70% of pubertal boys and resolves within 2–3 years. In the 7th–8th decade of life, the increased adipose tissue increases peripheral conversion of testosterone to estradiol (andropause); testosterone decreases slightly, and gynecomastia results.

Besides these three physiologic circumstances, any gynecomastia in an adult is more likely to represent an underlying disease (Table 64.2). The growth, division, and elongation of the tubular duct system of the female breast is normally caused by estrogen and inhibited by androgens. Gynecomastia can, therefore, follow an alteration in the balance between these two opposing

TABLE 64.2.	Causes of Gynecomastia
Mechanism	**Causes**
Exposure to exogenous estrogens	Vaginal creams
	Occupational exposure
	Anti-balding creams
Deficient production or action of testosterone	Anorchism (46,XY)
	Klinefelter's syndrome (47, XXY)
	Androgen resistance syndrome
	Defects in testosterone synthesis
	Gonadal Toxins (drugs, radiation)
	Viral orchitis (mumps)
	Trauma
	Castration
	Renal failure
Increased endogenous estrogen production	True hermaphroditism
	Testicular tumors
	Germinal cell tumors (HCG-producing stimulate estrogen)
	Stromal cell tumors (estradiol and testosterone-secreting)
	Bronchogenic carcinoma and other HCG-producing tumors
Increased peripheral conversion of androgens to estrogen	Hyperthyroidism
	Cirrhosis
	Obesity
	Senescence
	Adrenal carcinoma
	Refeeding/starvation

TABLE 64.3.	Medications Commonly Associated With Gynecomastia
Method of Action	**Drug**
Inhibits testosterone production	Chemotherapeutic agents (alkylating agents, vincristine, methotrexate)
	Ketoconazole
	Metronidazole
Androgen receptor antagonist	Spironolactone
	Cimetidine
	Marijuana
	Digoxin
Increase peripheral conversion of testosterone to estrogen	Testosterone
Increase testicular estrogen production	HCG
Has estrogen-like actions	Estrogen
	Diethylstilbestrol
Uncertain	Amiodarone
	Calcium-channel blockers
	Heroin
	Phenothiazines
	Methyldopa
	Tricyclic antidepressants
	Isoniazid
	Theophylline
	Diazepam

influences. Prolactin directly causes galactorrhea, but it does not directly stimulate breast enlargement; however, it may do so indirectly by inhibiting GnRH secretion. History of recent sudden breast enlargement with pain and tenderness usually implies an underlying disorder. Medications causing gynecomastia are listed separately in Table 64.3. Breast cancer is rare in men. However, gynecomastia in a patient with Klinefelter's syndrome is

TABLE 64.4.	Biochemical Work-Up of Gynecomastia

Laboratory Studies
Liver function tests
TSH
Testosterone
Estradiol
LH, FSH
HCG
Androstenedione
Prolactin
Karyotype

Laboratory Interpretation

↑ LH with ↓ /normal testosterone	Suggests primary testicular insufficiency
↓ LH with ↓ testosterone	Suggests estrogen-producing tumor or hypothalamic/pituitary deficiency
↑ LH with ↑ testosterone	Suggests androgen resistance or pituitary gonadotropin-secreting tumor

associated with a 10–20 fold increase in the incidence of breast cancer.

■ **Diagnosis**

Mild asymptomatic breast enlargement is common in normal men. Generally, symptomatic and progressive

cases warrant evaluation, the major goal being to exclude breast cancer. For this purpose, it is usually sufficient to conduct a careful physical examination, observing for characteristics typically seen in women with breast malignancy, such as irregularity, hardness, fixation, eccentric location, ulceration, and axillary adenopathy. Mammography or ultrasonography can be helpful. Any suspicious finding on physical or radiologic examination should be biopsied.

Once breast cancer is ruled out, most causes of gynecomastia can be identified by careful clinical assessment and workup. It is important to review medications carefully, and note the age of onset and duration of gynecomastia, and check for the presence of impotence and subnormal virilization, galactorrhea and headaches, and symptoms of thyroid disease. Physical examination should stress breasts and testes (size, consistency, atrophy and masses) and search for signs of liver disease and thyroid disease. Helpful laboratory studies (if dictated by clinical assessment) and their interpretations are shown in Table 64.4.

■ **Management and Prognosis**

The initial emphasis is on correcting the underlying disorder (e.g., withdrawal of an offending medication). Unfortunately, long-standing gynecomastia may evoke significant fibrosis, which does not regress even after removing the cause. Regression may take many years; therefore, surgery is the mainstay of therapy and is frequently indicated for psychological and cosmetic reasons.

CHAPTER **65** HYPOGLYCEMIA AND DIABETES MELLITUS

The plasma glucose concentration normally fluctuates between 80–120 mg/dl (4.4–6.7 mM). This normal blood level of glucose (**Euglycemia**) is maintained by the interplay of three separate processes: dietary carbohydrate intake, endogenous glucose production, and peripheral glucose utilization. In the **postabsorptive "fasting" state** (5–6 hours after a meal), with dietary intake no longer a factor, the model is simply an equilibrium between glucose production and utilization. Under these conditions, most glucose utilization is by obligatory oxidative processes within tissues that function primarily on glycolysis; these include brain tissue and formed elements of the blood.

In the early post-absorptive state, **hepatic glycogenolysis** accounts for most of the endogenous glucose

production. **Gluconeogenesis** is responsible for the balance; its importance increases as the fast continues. The quantity of hepatic glycogen available for mobilization as a potential source of circulating glucose is only about 70 g (an amount that is exhausted within 8 hours at the usual glucose utilization rate); consequently, gluconeogenesis becomes the only source of glucose with prolonged fasting. Because amino acids are the substrates for gluconeogenesis, muscle wasting eventually occurs. Fat tissue provides the largest source of stored calories as **triglycerides.** After about 48 hours, as the rates of lipolysis and ketogenesis increase, the brain adapts to ketone bodies as an alternative metabolic fuel. Because the brain utilizes most of the glucose at the cellular level, this adaptation allows lowering the rate of gluconeogenesis. After refeeding, glucose is absorbed across the intestinal mucosa at more than twice the rate of fasting endogenous glucose production. Glycogenolysis, gluconeogenesis, and lipolysis are then inhibited, and the many intracellular storage forms of metabolic fuel are repleted within the liver, muscle, and fat tissues.

Five hormones are key to maintaining euglycemia: insulin, glucagon, epinephrine, cortisol, and growth hormone. **Insulin** lowers blood glucose level by stimulating its cellular uptake and utilization, and by curbing its endogenous production. Glucagon, epinephrine, cortisol and growth hormone all oppose insulin metabolically, and are thus referred to as **counter-regulatory hormones.**

Insulin is synthesized, stored and released by the β cells of the pancreatic islets. It is initially synthesized as a pre-prohormone, then converted to **proinsulin** as it is stored within the intracellular secretory granules. Before its release systemically, proinsulin is further modified proteolytically, producing the final form of insulin and a cleavage fragment called **C-peptide.** The insulin molecule has two disulfide linked subunits: a 21-amino acid A chain and a 30-amino acid B chain. (Figure 65.1).

Pancreatic β cells secrete equimolar concentrations of C-peptide and insulin, at a basal rate of 0.5 units/h. Despite the islet innervation by both sympathetic and parasympathetic postganglionic fibers, β cells function largely independently, releasing insulin primarily in response to the local delivery of substrate; the most potent stimulus is the glucose level. Other substrates (arginine, free fatty acids, and ketone bodies) also stimulate insulin secretion. Following direct release into the portal circulation, insulin stimulates hepatic glycogen synthesis and inhibits hepatic glycogenolysis and gluconeogenesis. It also stimulates glucose uptake and utilization by other tissues (such as muscle and fat). Insulin possesses overall anticatabolic and anabolic effects. Collectively, these effects of insulin lower circulating blood glucose levels (Table 65.1).

All body tissues are capable of utilizing glucose. Glucose is transported across cell membranes by a facilitative diffusion mechanism, through several molecular subtypes of the **glucose transporter** (GLUT 1 through 5). Hepatocytes, pancreatic β-cells, and the absorptive epithelial cells of the intestinal mucosa all express GLUT 2, which facilitates free bidirectional movement of glucose across their plasma membranes; consequently, their intracellular glucose levels can be in continual equilibrium with ambient glucose levels. Tissues with a constant high level of metabolic activity (brain, kidney, smooth muscle, and RBC) express GLUTs independently, regardless of insulin availability. Tissues whose activity levels fluctuate dramatically, most notably skeletal muscle and adipose tissue, require the presence of insulin to express their major GLUT on the cell surface.

Glucagon, a 29-amino acid polypeptide synthesized and secreted by the alpha cells of the pancreatic islets, is released into the portal circulation, with primarily hepatic effects. By increasing cAMP through G-protein activation of adenylate cyclase, glucagon strongly stimulates hepatic glycogenolysis and gluconeogenesis, effects directly opposed by insulin. Glucagon is the primary counter-regulatory hormone. It is released from the α-cells in response to decreases in circulating glucose level; the resultant increase in hepatic glucose output

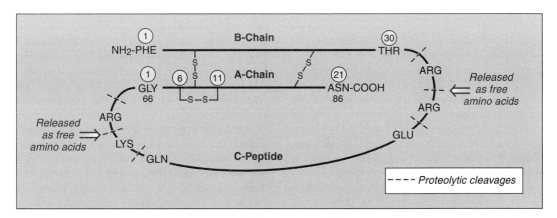

FIGURE 65.1. Structure of proinsulin and insulin. Proinsulin is an 86 amino acid protein that is cleaved at two sites to yield insulin, which is composed of A and B chains. An equal quantity of biologically inert C-peptide is produced as a byproduct.
(From West JB (ed.). Best and Taylor's Physiological Basis of Medical Practice. 12th ed. Baltimore: Williams & Wilkins, 1991, p. 820. Used with permission.)

TABLE 65.1.	Metabolic Effects of Insulin		
	Liver	Adipose Tissue	Muscle
Anticatabolic	↓ glycogenolysis ↓ gluconeogenesis ↓ ketogenesis	↓ lipolysis	↓ protein catabolism ↓ amino acid output
Anabolic	↑ glycogen synthesis ↑ fatty acid synthesis	↑ glucose uptake ↑ glycerol synthesis ↑ fatty acid synthesis	↑ glucose and amino acid uptake ↑ protein synthesis ↑ glycogen synthesis

↑ = increased; ↓ = decreased.

occurs within minutes. The main stimulant for glucagon release appears to be alterations in the local delivery of substrate to the islets, as is the case with insulin secretion.

Epinephrine, like glucagon, is an acute-acting counter-regulatory hormone. Its secretion is neurally controlled in response to circulating glucose levels. By inducing β_2-adrenergic receptor-mediated increase in hepatocyte cAMP levels, epinephrine increases hepatic glycogenolysis and gluconeogenesis. Epinephrine also indirectly affects the hepatic manipulation of glucose storage by inhibiting insulin secretion (α_2-receptors on pancreatic β cells). Besides, the activation of β_1-receptors on adipocytes stimulates lipolysis and generates free fatty acids, which can be used by the liver for ketogenesis. Glycogenolysis within skeletal muscle is also stimulated.

Cortisol and **growth hormone** are also counter-regulatory hormones, but neither appears to have a primary role in correcting hypoglycemia. Mobilization of glucose does not occur until several hours following a rise in their circulating levels. Growth hormone initially has a paradoxical insulin-like effect, causing a transient lowering of blood glucose. Despite their tardy hyperglycemic effect, both these hormones appear to serve an integral role in glucose homeostasis.

Hypoglycemia

Hypoglycemia, a deficiency of glucose concentration in the blood, manifests clinically by symptoms of catecholamine release and/or neuroglycopenia (Table 65.2). Catecholamine release-related symptoms predominate when the blood glucose falls precipitously. With a more gradual decrease, the initial symptoms may be a reflection of inadequate substrate delivery to the central nervous system **(neuroglycopenia).** Although hypoglycemic symptoms often develop when blood glucose drops below 45 mg/dl (2.5 mM), many healthy adults are asymptomatic at this level, thus making it difficult to define precisely and numerically, clinically significant hypoglycemia. Rather, definitive diagnosis depends on the presence of **Whipple's triad:** adrenergic and/or neuroglycopenic symptoms consistent with hypoglycemia, low blood glucose level, and relief of the symptoms when blood glucose is restored to within normal limits.

Hypoglycemia has diverse and numerous causes. It can be divided into one of two types, based upon the temporal relationship between ingestion of a meal and the onset of clinically relevant symptoms (Table 65.3). **Postprandial** *(reactive)* hypoglycemia often occurs within the first few hours after food intake. On the other hand, **postabsorptive** *(fasting)* hypoglycemia is not seen until several hours later, after the meal has been fully digested and absorbed.

The best documented form of postprandial hypoglycemia in adults is ***alimentary hypoglycemia,*** caused by surgical procedures leading to the rapid movement of ingested food into the small intestine (e.g., pyloroplasty, gastric bypass, gastrectomy). An ***idiopathic*** *(functional)* form of reactive hypoglycemia remains debatable; it is often erroneously diagnosed by both physicians and patients. These persons tend to be thin, anxious, and emotionally labile, with somatic features of autonomic hyperactivity, such as gastric hypermotility and irritable bowel syndrome. In most cases, insulin responds appropriately to a glucose load and the onset of symptoms correlates poorly with the nadir in blood glucose. Early type II diabetes is occasionally seen with postprandial hypoglycemia.

Fasting hypoglycemia is far more prevalent than the postprandial type, and most cases are **drug-induced.** Insulin and the sulfonylureas cause most episodes. **Iatrogenic hypoglycemia** is seen frequently in Type I diabetics attempting to maintain tight control with insulin. It is also seen, albeit less frequently, in Type II diabetics taking oral hypoglycemic agents. Ethanol potentiates the hypoglycemic effects of both of these agents, and can also induce hypoglycemia by itself, by directly inhibiting gluconeogenesis. Salicylates and β-blockers inhibit the mobilization of endogenous glu-

TABLE 65.2.	Symptoms of Hypoglycemia
Adrenergic	Neuroglycopenic
Sweating	Headache
Tremors	Irritability
Palpitations	Confusion
Pallor	Seizure
Hunger	Coma

cose stores. Quinine, pentamidine, sulfamethoxazole, and disopyramide promote release of excessive amounts of endogenous insulin.

Insulinomas (pancreatic β-cell tumors), are a rare but important cause of fasting hypoglycemia. Most of these tumors are benign and extremely small; they usually cause neuroglycopenic symptoms following a missed meal or exercise. The diagnosis of the insulinomas is often delayed because patients learn to avoid symptoms by eating frequently. As a result, many patients with insulinomas are obese. The evidence for insulinoma is an inappropriately high, fasting level of insulin. During symptomatic episodes, blood glucose level tends to be below 45 mg/dl (2.5 mM) and the plasma insulin level is above 10 μU/ml (72 pmol/L). Some *nonpancreatic neoplasms,* which tend to be large, retroperitoneal, and mesenchymal, can also cause fasting hypoglycemia. Most of these tumors probably cause hypoglycemia due to the production of aberrant IGF-II, which has poor affinity for IGF-II binding protein 3 and therefore, circulates disproportionately in the free form, with resultant hypoglycemia. The poor nutrition and inanition, which are often associated, are additional factors.

Factitious hypoglycemia has also been observed in nondiabetic psychiatric patients who have access to syringes and insulin. The presence of insulin antibodies, an inappropriately low C-peptide level, and high levels of circulating insulin is often diagnostic. Prescription errors can lead to inadvertent use of oral sulfonylureas, a possibility easily excluded by a negative urine screen for sulfonylurea metabolites.

The treatment of hypoglycemia depends on the cause. In adults, reactive hypoglycemia can be managed with small, frequent meals and reassurance. Anticholinergic drugs, by slowing GI transit, are sometimes useful in managing alimentary hypoglycemia. If an insulinoma is diagnosed biochemically, CT, preoperative and intra-operative ultrasound, and selective arteriography may help in anatomic localization. In most cases, surgical excision is curative. Diazoxide can help control hypoglycemia in multiple or metastatic insulinomas; it blocks insulin release from pancreatic β-cells by opening the same K⁺ATP channels known to be blocked by sulfonylureas. In drug-induced hypoglycemia, therapy is directed toward the offending agent. Hypoglycemia from sulfonylureas, notably chlorpropamide, can be insidious and protracted. Because the brain is vulnerable to prolonged hypoglycemia, patients who develop severe hypoglycemia due to these drugs should be hospitalized and given IV glucose until stable.

TABLE 65.3.	Differential Diagnosis of Hypoglycemia	
Fasting		**Post-prandial**
Insulin		Alimentary
		Idiopathic
Oral Sulfonylurea agents		Early Non-insulin
Ethanol		dependent diabetes
Medications:		mellitus (NIDDM)
Pentamidine		
Salicylates		
Propranolol		
Sulfamethoxazole		
Disopyramide		
Tumor hypoglycemia		
Insulinomas		
Adrenal Insufficiency		
Prolonged starvation		
Liver failure		
Uremia		

Diabetes Mellitus

Diabetes mellitus is a syndrome of altered carbohydrate, fat, and protein metabolism resulting from an absolute or relative deficiency of insulin. The most common biochemical abnormality is hyperglycemia. Long-standing diabetes is commonly associated with chronic complications of retinopathy, nephropathy, neuropathy, and accelerated atherosclerosis.

■ Epidemiology and Classification

Diabetes mellitus affects approximately 3–4% of the U.S. population. It is a heterogeneous disorder with two subtypes. Type I or **insulin-dependent diabetes mellitus (IDDM)**, caused by autoimmune destruction of the islet cells, accounts for approximately 10% of cases. It is characterized by a sudden onset of symptoms, insulin insufficiency, ketoacidosis, and dependence on insulin for maintenance of life. Because it typically occurs in young subjects, IDDM was previously called juvenile diabetes. Type II or **noninsulin-dependent diabetes mellitus** (NIDDM) is the most common type; it is characterized by a more gradual and insidious onset of hyperglycemia and lack of susceptibility to ketoacidosis. While insulin may be needed for optimal control of hyperglycemia, patients are not dependent on it to maintain life. Endogenous insulin levels may be high, low, or normal in these patients. Peripheral tissues, such as muscle, fat, and liver, are abnormally resistant to the effects of insulin; the result is decreased glucose uptake and inappropriate hepatic gluconeogenesis, despite insulin levels that may be normal. Because NIDDM often debuts after the age of 40, it was formerly called maturity (adult) onset diabetes. In other types of diabetes, entities such as pancreatic insufficiency (e.g., chronic pancreatitis, hemochromatosis, and pancreatectomy), Cushing's syndrome, and acromegaly are the underlying cause. Drugs, including glucocorticoids and nicotinic acid, can produce hyperglycemia in patients predisposed to NIDDM.

■ Clinical Features and Diagnosis

The classic triad of polyuria, polydipsia, and polyphagia (excessive eating) arise from hyperglycemia, which leads to glycosuria upon exceeding the renal threshold. Glucose acts as an osmotic diuretic, leading to polyuria and, hence, polydipsia. Loss of calories evokes a sensation of excess hunger and polyphagia. Weight loss occurs frequently, despite excess food intake. These symptoms arise classically in patients with IDDM. Diabetic ketoacidosis may also be the initial manifestation of IDDM. Skin infections, vulvovaginitis (inflammation of the vulva and the vagina), and balanitis (inflammation of the glans penis) may cause the patient to seek medical care. NIDDM is frequently detected by screening examinations or because of fatigue accompanied by polyuria and polydipsia, albeit less severe than in IDDM. Peripheral neuropathy (pathological changes to the peripheral nervous system), often present when NIDDM is diagnosed, may be the presenting feature in some cases. Less commonly,

NIDDM presents with vascular complications, such as myocardial infarction, peripheral vascular disease, or chronic renal failure.

Table 65.4 shows the accepted criteria for the diagnosis of diabetes in the nonpregnant adult as developed by the National Diabetes Data Group. Commonly, IDDM patients are diagnosed by the first criterion; NIDDM patients are diagnosed by the second. Oral GTT is reserved for individuals with potential symptoms of diabetes or its complications as well as FBS below 125 mg/dl.

■ Management

Goals of therapy

The aims of treatment are twofold: first, to relieve the symptoms of hyperglycemia, and second, to prevent or delay the onset of chronic complications. These goals should be accomplished while avoiding severe, recurrent hypoglycemia. Symptoms of hyperglycemia (thirst, polyuria, fatigue, blurred vision, etc.) are alleviated when the glucose level is generally maintained below the renal threshold for glucose of 180–200 mg%. Because glucose values in this range are associated with a high rate of long-term microvascular complications, the second goal of therapy is to further lower the glucose to achieve near-euglycemia. For optimal control, guidelines of the American Diabetes Association include fasting and premeal glucose levels of 70–120 mg% with postprandial excursions to less than 180 mg%. Glycated hemoglobin levels should be maintained below 8%.

Diet

Dietary therapy is a key part of the treatment, irrespective of the type of diabetes and whether or not oral hypoglycemic agents or insulin is administered. The principle of dietary therapy is to provide an adequate number of calories to meet energy needs. Depending on physical activity, nonobese adults require 25–40 calories/kg for weight maintenance. Patients with NIDDM are usually obese and should be encouraged to lose weight by prescribing lower-calorie diets. Once the total caloric requirement has been determined, the distribution of calories should be decided, taking into account food preferences, work schedule, and other personal factors. Carbohydrates should provide 50–60% of total calories, protein, 15–20%, and fat, the remainder. Generally, the

TABLE 65.4. Diagnosis of Diabetes Mellitus in Non-Pregnant Adults
1. Random glucose exceeding 200 mg/dl with symptoms of hyperglycemia
2. Fasting venous, plasma glucose (FBS) ≥126 mg/dl on two or more occasions
3. Oral glucose (75 gm) tolerance test (GTT) showing a 2-hr glucose level of >200 mg/dl

daily caloric intake is prescribed as 3 major meals with 2–3 snacks during a 24-hour period.

Insulin therapy

Before 1982, insulin preparations were mixtures of beef and pork insulin. In 1982, human insulin, produced by recombinant molecular technology, became available and has largely replaced animal source insulins. Human, pork, and beef insulin have similar biopotencies and pharmacokinetics. The regular unmodified insulin acts rapidly. A newer insulin, lispro, contains amino acid substitutions that accelerate insulin absorption and action relative to regular insulin. The other insulin preparations have been modified to prolong the insulin action (Table 65.5). NPH and Lente may be mixed with regular insulin, if required, but the activity of regular insulin is better preserved when mixed with NPH insulin alone.

TABLE 65.5.	Insulin preparations		
	Action profile (hr)		
Type	**Onset**	**Peak**	**Duration**
Rapid			
Lispro	0.25	0.5–1	2–3
Regular	0.5	2–5	6–8
Semilente	1–2	3–6	10–12
Intermediate			
Lente	1–2	4–12	18–26
NPH	4–6	8–30	24–36
Long-acting			
Ultralente	1–3	6–15	18–26

NPH = Neutral Protamine Hagedorn.

Insulin is given in a manner to roughly approximate the idealized profile of insulin secretion in a nondiabetic (Figure 65.2). This profile arises from **basal insulin secretion** (occurring in the absence of eating) and nutrient-stimulated insulin secretion with meals. Short-acting regular insulin is given before two or more meals to mimic nutrient-stimulated insulin secretion and to promote metabolism of the ingested calories. Intermediate- or long-acting insulin is given once or twice daily to mimic basal insulin secretion. Most diabetics require intermediate- or long-acting insulin in the evening in order to suppress the nocturnal hepatic gluconeogenesis that will otherwise occur in both types of diabetics; when unrestrained, it leads to prebreakfast hyperglycemia (Table 65.6). The standard **split-mixed regimen** is a mixture of NPH (or lente) and regular insulin before breakfast and before supper (dinner). In many patients, the presupper NPH peaks at 2–4 AM causing overnight reactions. These reactions can be avoided by giving the NPH (or lente) at bedtime. By also adding a dose of regular insulin prelunch, the morning NPH (lente) can often be eliminated in many patients.

The most appropriate insulin dose for a given patient cannot be predicted. Rather, insulin adjustments are made prospectively based on the patient's glucose levels. Therefore, most diabetics should be encouraged to self-monitor capillary blood glucose *(fingersticks);* the frequency of testing is individualized, based on the stability of the glucose level and the goals of insulin therapy. In nonuremic patients, the prebreakfast and presupper levels predominantly reflect the adequacy of the PM (or bedtime [h.s.]) and AM intermediate-acting insulin doses, respectively. The prelunch level can help adjust the AM regular insulin dose, just as the h.s. level can

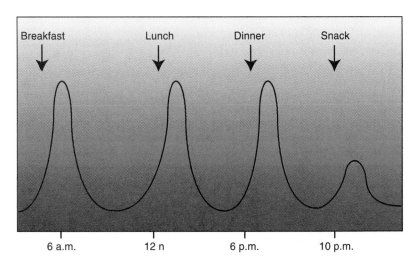

FIGURE 65.2. Idealized profile of a 24-hour insulin secretion pattern in a non-diabetic individual.

TABLE 65.6.	Common Insulin Regimens		
Pre-Breakfast	**Pre-Lunch**	**Pre-Supper (PM)**	**Bedtime (h.s.)**
NPH/Reg		NPH/Reg	
NPH/Reg		Reg	NPH
Reg	Reg	Reg	NPH

NPH = Neutral Protamine Hagedorn; Reg = regular insulin.

TABLE 65.7.	Insulin Side-Effects

Hypoglycemia
Insulin atrophy
Lipoatrophy
Lipohypertrophy
Insulin edema
Weight gain

help adjust the P.M. regular insulin dose. **Glycosylated hemoglobin** (Hb a1c) is covalent modification of hemoglobin by glucose; its assay rests on the premise that its amount is proportional to the mean glucose level. Hb a1c is high in patients with sustained, prolonged hyperglycemia; thus, measurements help assess glycemic control during the two previous months. Measurements every 4–6 months can supplement self-monitoring and objectively document glycemic control.

Table 65.7 shows the complications of insulin therapy. The most common complication is hypoglycemia. Unfortunately, many insulin-dependent diabetics with long-standing diabetes cannot secrete adrenomedullary catecholamines following insulin-induced hypoglycemia. These catecholamines provide the adrenergic "warning" symptoms that prompt the diabetic to ingest carbohydrates immediately. Without this warning, the patient has *hypoglycemic unawareness*; as a result the first symptom of hypoglycemia may be cognitive impairment, seizures, or syncope. Catecholamine secretion depends on the extent and the rapidity with which hypoglycemia develops as well as the absolute level of hypoglycemia; thus, patients with good glycemic control can become hypoglycemic with smaller decreases in glucose than those with chronic hyperglycemia, and they are at heightened risk for hypoglycemic unawareness. Insulin allergy and lipoatrophy have decreased in frequency with improved, highly purified, insulin preparations.

Oral sulfonylurea agents

The sulfonylureas stimulate insulin secretion from the pancreatic β cells. They can be used only in NIDDM where blood sugar is not controlled by combined diet and exercise; they are contraindicated in IDDM and in pregnancy. (See Table 65.8 for dosages and duration of action.) Therapy with the sulfonylureas begins with the smallest dose, which is gradually increased until optimal control or maximum dose has been reached. If adequate glucose control does not follow the maximum dose, the drug should be discontinued and insulin therapy initiated. Side effects include anorexia, nausea, and diarrhea. Jaundice, skin rashes, and hematologic toxicity (**agranulocytosis**) have also been reported. The sulfonylureas may cause severe and prolonged hypoglycemia, especially when there is impaired kidney function or no oral intake. Therefore, sulfonylureas should not be given under these conditions. Because they have far fewer side effects, the second-generation sulfonylureas now dominate the oral sulfonylurea market.

Metformin is the only member of a class of drugs called biguanides that is approved for use in the United States. Biguanides decrease glucose levels by multiple potential mechanisms, including anorexia, decreased intestinal glucose absorption, and potentiation of insulin action in its target tissues. Metformin is used in combination with either insulin or sulfonylureas in type II diabetes. It is contraindicated in type I diabetes and pregnancy. Metformin's side effects are primarily gastrointestinal. Lactic acidosis, sometimes fatal, has been reported. Metformin-associated lactic acidosis occurs primarily, if not solely, in patients with renal failure, hepatic dysfunction, or advanced cardiac disease. For this reason, use of metformin in these patients is contraindicated. Metformin should be withheld for two days before patients undergo radiographic contrast studies.

Troglitazone is the first approved compound of the thiazolidinedione class of insulin-sensitizing agents.

TABLE 65.8.	Oral Anti-Diabetic Agents		
Agent	**Starting Dose (mg/day)**	**Maximum Dose (mg/day)**	**Duration of Action (hr.)**
Sulfonylurea agents			
Tolbutamide	500	3000	6–8
Chlorpropamide	100–250	750	36
Acetohexamide	100–250	1500	12–18
Tolazamide	250	1000	24
Glyburide	1.25–5	20	24
Glipizide	2.5–5	40	12
Glimepiride	1–2	8	12
Other anti-diabetic agents			
Metformin	1000	2500	8
Troglitazone	200	600	16
Acarbose	75	300	6

Acarbose delays the absorption of carbohydrates from the gastrointestinal tract, significantly reducing postprandial hyperglycemia. Metformin, troglitazone, and acarbose can each lower mean blood glucose levels by approximately 50%.

■ Acute Complications of Diabetes: Diabetic Ketoacidosis and Hyperosmolar Coma

The term **diabetic coma** is loosely applied to diabetic ketoacidosis and hyperosmolar coma, but most patients are conscious and many have no alteration in mental status. The distinction between ketoacidosis and nonketotic diabetic coma is not absolute; mild ketonemia may be present in patients with a hyperosmolar state. Diabetic ketoacidosis generally occurs in type I diabetics, whereas nonketotic hyperosmolar coma occurs in type II diabetics.

The pathophysiology of diabetic ketoacidosis is summarized in Figures 65.3 and 65.4. The most important pathogenetic aspect is insufficient insulin action, further complicated by the unopposed action of anti-insulin hormones, namely, catecholamines, growth hormone, glucocorticoids, and glucagon. As a consequence of insulin deficiency and counter-regulatory hormone excess, hyperglycemia and ketoacidosis evolve. Hyperglycemia leads to osmotic diuresis; dehydration and shock follow.

Insulin inhibits lipolysis by its effect on hormone sensitive lipase. This action of insulin is very sensitive, requiring less insulin than is needed to maintain euglycemia through increased cellular glucose uptake. Without insulin, increased lipolysis makes increased amounts of free fatty acids available to the liver; they are oxidized, and ketone bodies (acetoacetate and β-hydroxybutyrate)

are formed as by-products. Ketone bodies can be utilized as a source of energy, but they accumulate in the blood if they are produced at a rate beyond which they can be excreted or oxidized. Ketone bodies are organic acids that readily dissociate and release hydrogen ions into the body fluids, causing the pH to fall, a metabolic state known as **ketoacidosis.**

Diabetic ketoacidosis

The onset of diabetic ketoacidosis is characterized by an increase in symptoms of hyperglycemia, such as polyuria and polydipsia. Patients with previously undiagnosed diabetes may give a history of weight loss. Nausea, vomiting, and abdominal pain are common. Lethargy and some alteration of consciousness is generally present. Although most patients are not comatose at the time of admission, deep coma may result. On physical examination, signs of dehydration are evident (dry skin, a dry tongue, and hypotension). Increasing H^+ ion concentration leads to an increased rate and depth of respiration (**Kussmaul's respiration**). Hypovolemia and shock or electrolyte abnormalities may be lethal. Precipitating events, such as infection, myocardial infarction, injury, or, often, noncompliance with insulin, may be present. Many patients either do not know of or ignore the need to continue insulin during a flu-like illness when they are eating poorly. In this setting, patients often discontinue insulin. Combined insulin deficiency and stress rapidly ushers in diabetic ketoacidosis.

Diagnosis

Ketoacidosis is diagnosed biochemically; its features are marked hyperglycemia, ketonemia, and acidosis. Blood glucose generally ranges between 400–800 mg%. The concentration of ketone bodies can be obtained

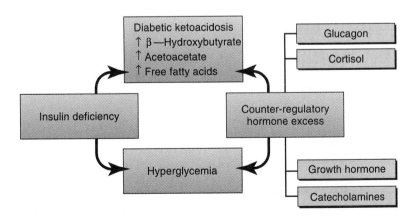

FIGURE 65.3. The pathophysiology of diabetic ketoacidosis.
(Adapted from: Shade DS, Eaton RP. Diabetes 1977;26:597. Used with permission of American Diabetes Association, Alexandria, VA.)

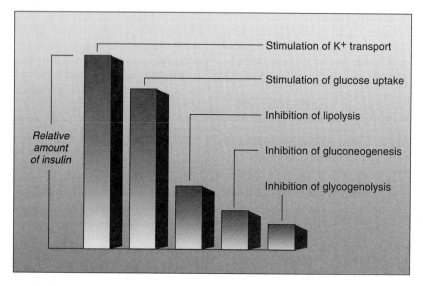

FIGURE 65.4. Metabolic processes as dependent on relative levels of insulin. Gluconeogenesis is inhibited by minimal levels of insulin, whereas pharmacological levels of insulin are needed to mobilize K⁺ into the cells.
(Adapted from: Alberti KGMM, Nattras M. Med Clin North Am 1978;62:804.
Used with permission of WB Saunders Co., Philadelphia, PA.)

semiquantitatively by using the Acetest™ tablet (**nitro-prusside reaction**) with progressive dilutions of plasma. This reaction is sensitive to acetoacetate, but not to β-hydroxybutyrate. Measurement of electrolytes and pH reveals an **anion gap acidosis.** Normal anion gap ($[Na^+] - [Cl^- + HCO_3-]$) is below 12 mEq/L; in general, the higher it is above 16 mEq/L, the greater the severity of ketoacidosis. (Some laboratories derive the anion gap by subtracting the total anions $[Cl^- + HCO_3]$ from the sum of cations $[Na^+$ and $K^+]$; the normal value then is below 16 mEq/L.)

Management

It should be emphasized that diabetic ketoacidosis is a life-threatening situation. Its management requires close observation and careful attention to details to achieve an optimal outcome. The essentials of treatment are insulin administration, replacement of fluid and electrolytes, and management of precipitating events. Only regular insulin is used in the treatment of patients with ketoacidosis. Low-dose insulin regimens, compared to high-dose regimens, evoke less frequent and less severe late hypoglycemia. Following an initial IV bolus of 10–20 units, insulin is administered preferentially as a continuous IV infusion, with an initial rate of 0.1 unit/kg/h. If no response to treatment is evident in two hours, the insulin infusion rate is doubled. In the presence of insulin resistance, larger insulin doses should be given. Plasma glucose should be monitored hourly; when it reaches approximately 250 mg/dl, the IV fluid is changed from normal or half-normal saline

to 5% glucose. It is imperative to avoid hypoglycemia, as it may predispose to cerebral edema and brain damage.

The fluid losses in diabetic ketoacidosis range between 4–10 L. Although the fluid loss is hypotonic in ketoacidosis, fluid therapy is started with normal saline, so as to achieve a prompt re-expansion of the circulating blood volume. In the first hour, 1 liter of normal saline is administered rapidly, followed by a liter of normal or half-normal saline in the next hour. The remainder of the fluids can be given more slowly until the patient's volume status is restored. Total body potassium is depleted, despite the deceptively normal or even high serum levels that appear initially. Hyperkalemia occurs when acidosis shifts potassium from the intracellular to the extracellular compartment. Insulin administration and correction of acidosis will reverse this shift, therefore, hypokalemia should be anticipated. Consequently, it is necessary to begin potassium administration at the rate of 20–30 mEq/l of fluid after adequate urinary output has been established. Potassium administration should be started at initiation of therapy if the initial serum K^+ is low or in the lower end of the normal range. Hypophosphatemia is common during therapy for ketoacidosis; because it reverses with refeeding, however, phosphate administration is not generally required. Most cases do not require administration of sodium bicarbonate, but it should be administered if the pH is below 7.0; some consider a pH below 7.1 as the indication.

A diligent search for precipitating causes should follow. If a bacterial infection is detected, appropriate antibiotics are required. It is necessary to rule out silent myocardial infarction by serial ECG and appropriate blood tests. Gastric dilatation in the semiconscious patient requires nasogastric suction of the stomach contents.

Nonketotic hyperosmolar coma

Hyperosmolar coma is much less common than diabetic ketoacidosis and usually occurs in older, type II patients. Conceptually, these patients have enough insulin to prevent ketosis and acidosis, but not enough to prevent hyperglycemia. (See Figures 65.4 and 65.5 for pathophysiology.) The evolution of the hyperglycemia, glycosuria, dehydration, and shock is similar to that in diabetic ketoacidosis. The patients usually present with a history of polyuria, polydipsia, and progressive fatigue of several days' or weeks' duration. The condition is typically precipitated by an associated illness, such as acute infection, myocardial infarction, cerebrovascular accident, heat stroke, hip fracture, or exacerbation of an underlying chronic illness. Precipitating events occur at a higher frequency in nonketotic hyperosmolar coma than in diabetic ketoacidosis.

Physical examination reveals evidence of dehydration and impaired mentation. Focal neurologic signs, while frequent, usually resolve with treatment. Severe hyperglycemia is present; the blood glucose usually ranges from 800–1300 mg/dl. Plasma ketones are usually absent or, if present, occur in small amounts. The serum osmolarity is greatly increased, as measured directly or estimated by the following formula: serum osmolarity = 2(Na + K) + glucose/18 + BUN/2.8 (with serum osmolarity expressed in mOsm/L, sodium and potassium in mEq/L, glucose in mg/dL, and BUN in mg/dL). The principles of treatment are similar to those of diabetic ketoacidosis. The dehydration is usually more profound than in diabetic ketoacidosis. It must be emphasized that the initial priority is to ensure adequate hydration.

■ Chronic Complications of Diabetes

The availability of insulin has dramatically reduced the mortality from diabetic coma. The major morbidity and mortality due to diabetes now result from chronic complications, which consist of macrovascular disease (accelerated atherosclerosis) and microvascular disease (retinopathy, neuropathy, and nephropathy).

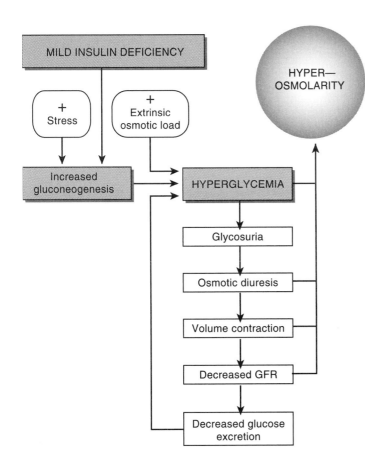

FIGURE 65.5. Pathogenesis of hyperosmolar hyperglycemic non-ketotic state. GFR = Glomerular filtration rate.
(Adapted from: Greene DA. Top Emerg Med 1984; 5:49. Used with permission of Aspen Publishers, Inc., Gaithersburg, MD.)

A major emphasis in the treatment of diabetes is to prevent or delay the onset of complications by modifying risk factors that increase the rate of complications. Tobacco use is forbidden and hypertension is aggressively treated. Because hyperlipidemia is very prevalent in diabetes, cholesterol, HDL-cholesterol, and triglycerides should be measured annually; hyperlipidemia, if present, should be treated. Obesity and inactivity portend risk of macrovascular disease. Suboptimal glucose control has a proven relationship with long-term complications, particularly of the microvasculature. Finally, most serious eye and foot problems can be avoided by proper preventive care by ophthalmologists and podiatrists, respectively.

Macrovascular disease

Coronary artery disease

Atherosclerosis occurs more frequently, at an earlier age, and with greater severity in diabetic patients than in nondiabetics. Even patients with impaired glucose tolerance are at a greater risk for the development of atherosclerosis. Similar to the general population, coronary artery disease is the leading cause of mortality in diabetes. Because of autonomic neuropathy, **myocardial infarction** in diabetes may be painless; it may present as diabetic ketoacidosis, and it is often diagnosed incidentally at a later date by a routine ECG.

Peripheral vascular disease

Involvement of large-sized or medium-sized blood vessels in the lower limbs is a common complication of diabetes. Its prevalence is particularly high in older, type II diabetics. A diagnosis of arterial insufficiency is suggested by a history of **claudication**. Physical examination reveals absent or weak peripheral pulses. Noninvasive vascular testing involving measurement of arterial blood pressure and flow is used to confirm the diagnosis. Patients with peripheral vascular disease often cannot supply the increased blood flow needed to heal foot infections. The inability to heal these infections leads to **osteomyelitis**, **gangrene**, and **amputations**. Most foot infections are preceded by calluses. Therefore, routine foot care including podiatric evaluation and proper foot wear is critical in preventing foot infections.

Microvascular disease

Retinopathy

Diabetic retinopathy is a leading cause of blindness in the United States. However, it is important to emphasize that with yearly ophthalmological examinations and preventive eye care, significant vision loss is prevented in all but a small fraction of patients. Some degree of diabetic retinopathy is detectable in more than 90% of patients who have had diabetes for 20–25 years. Diabetic retinopathy has two stages: **background retinopathy** and **proliferative retinopathy**. The earliest visible lesions of background retinopathy are exudates and microaneurysms. Capillary degeneration with fluid leakage and edema lead to exudates. Macular edema or a plaque of hard exudate may cause **visual loss**. In some patients, background retinopathy may progress to the proliferative stage; new vessels arise from the disc or from the retinal periphery. Traction on these new vessels may induce **vitreous hemorrhage** and visual impairment. Organization of these hemorrhages with fibrosis ultimately leads to **retinal detachment**. Careful follow-up is required in mild background retinopathy; if proliferative changes develop, appropriate treatment should follow readily.

Proliferative diabetic retinopathy is treated by either xenon arc or laser beam photocoagulation to prevent vitreous hemorrhages and retinal detachments. The high-intensity light beam produces small spots of scarring. The rationale of this treatment is based on the theory that new vessel growth is a response to areas of poor perfusion, releasing angiogenic growth factors. Controlled, scattered destruction of a portion of the retina prevents new blood vessels by eliminating their growth factor. In addition to retinopathy, **cataracts** and **glaucoma** are present at increased prevalence in the diabetic population.

Diabetic nephropathy

Diabetic nephropathy is frequently present along with retinopathy, and occurs in approximately one-third of patients. Nephropathy does not usually occur until 15–30 years after the initial diagnosis of diabetes. The specific lesion of diabetic nephropathy is nodular sclerosis (Kimmelstiel-Wilson lesion), visible on light microscopy as a rounded hyaline mass at the center of the glomerular lobules. More frequent, but less specific, is the diffuse glomerulosclerosis with thickening of the glomerular basement membrane and an increased mesangial matrix. Nephropathy is first clinically evident by **proteinuria** (24-h urine protein >500 mg). It is at first intermittent, but later becomes constant. **Microalbuminuria** (20–200 μg/min of albumin) heralds future development of gross proteinuria. Progressive nephropathy results in heavy proteinuria and the development of nephrotic syndrome, which typically progresses to renal failure within five years.

Besides good glycemic control, the treatment of diabetic nephropathy should be aimed at strict control of hypertension. Uncontrolled hypertension exacerbates worsening of renal function. A decrease in protein intake may slow the progression of nephropathy. Progression of proteinuria to overt renal failure may also be slowed by angiotensin converting enzyme inhibitors. Insulin requirements fall as renal failure becomes manifest, and hypoglycemia may be frequent. Hemodialysis, peritoneal dialysis, and renal transplantation are used to manage end-stage renal disease.

Diabetic neuropathy

Diabetic neuropathy affects both the somatic and the autonomic nervous systems. Somatic neuropathy most commonly presents as symmetric peripheral neuropathy, with initial symptoms of numbness and tingling, usually in the feet and legs. Painful, burning, and aching variants occur and are especially bothersome at night. Tendon reflexes and response to sensory stimuli, particularly vibration, are decreased. Distal weakness may be noted. Peripheral neuropathy markedly worsens the risk of infection and amputation in patients with peripheral vascular disease and underscores the need for preventive foot care. Therapy of uncomfortable peripheral neuropathy involves the use of drugs with combined analgesic and sedative properties (e.g., tricyclic antidepressants, carbamazepine, phenytoin, and, in severe cases, narcotic analgesics). Topical agents (e.g., capsaicin) are effective at times. Neuropathy may less often involve a single peripheral nerve, causing motor or sensory deficit in the distribution of the affected nerve (mononeuropathy). Peripheral nerves may be affected either singly or in combination, producing a mononeuritis multiplex. Cranial nerves may be similarly affected, especially the third nerve.

Autonomic neuropathies can affect nearly all organs. The more notable examples include skin (anhidrosis), cardiovascular system (orthostatic hypotension and absence of reflex tachycardia), and genitourinary system (neurogenic bladder dysfunction, impotence, and retrograde ejaculation). Impotence has a prevalence of 75% among diabetic men 60–65 years old. Gastrointestinal autonomic neuropathy has varied features, including delayed emptying of the stomach (gastroparesis), symptoms of which are early satiety, nausea, and vomiting. Irregular gastric emptying complicates efforts at glycemic control. Therapy of gastroparesis with metoclopramide is partially effective in some patients. Constipation or frequent, profuse, nocturnal watery urgent bowel movements (nocturnal diabetic diarrhea) may also occur. In some instances, diabetic diarrhea may respond to a broad-spectrum antibiotic, but the treatment is mostly symptomatic. Evaluation for other causes of diarrhea is important.

CHAPTER 66

NUTRITIONAL DISORDERS

■ Estimating Energy Requirements

An understanding of the body's basal energy requirements is a prerequisite to an effective nutritional assessment. Factors that contribute to the body's total energy requirements include the **basal metabolic rate** (BMR), the energy required for activity, and the thermic effect of food. The BMR, the energy expended by the body at rest and without food, is estimated by the **Harris-Benedict equation** (Table 66.1). The energy expended during various types of physical activity is **energy of activity;** it accounts for nearly one-third of total energy expenditure, but varies with the type of activity. Sedentary activities (sleeping, reading) utilize 72 kcal/h, whereas running or construction work expends 60kcal/h.

Thermic energy is the amount of energy required to carry out the digestion, absorption, and metabolism of food. The metabolism of all foods produces heat **(thermic effect of food);** the extent varies with different

TABLE 66.1.	Estimation of BMR and Ideal Body Weight	
	BMR[a]	**Ideal Body Weight[b]**
Women	$655 + (9.5 \times W) + (1.8 \times H) - (4.7 \times A)$	100 lb (45kg) for the first 5 ft (152cm) + 5 lb (2.2kg) for every inch (2.54cm) of H >5 ft (152cm)
Men	$66 + (13.7 \times W) + (5 \times H) - (6.8 \times A)$	110 lb (2.2kg) for the first 5 ft (152cm) + 5 lb (2.2kg) for every 1 inch (2.54cm) of H >5 ft (152cm).

W = Weight in kg; H = Height in meters; A = Age in years.
[a] Harris-Benedict equation; Source: Harris JA and Benedict FG: A Biometric Study of Basal Metabolism in Man, Carnegie Institute of Washington, Publ. No. 279, 1919. Used with permission.
[b] (Adapted from Krause and Mahan. Food, Nutrition and Diet Therapy. 7th ed. Philadelphia: W.B. Saunders Company, 1984. Used with permission of publisher.)

foods. These differences are expressed quantitatively as the **specific dynamic action** (SDA) or **calorigenic effect** of foods. Carbohydrate or fat increases heat production by approximately 5% of the meal's caloric content; protein has the highest thermogenic effect, approximately 30%. Inflammatory, febrile diseases increase BMR according to severity—mild illness by 10%, moderate, by 25%, and severe, by 50%.

Thus, the total daily energy requirement can be estimated by adding together the BMR, a compensation for the severity of illness, an allowance for physical activity and the SDA. A less precise, but easier, method, multiplies the estimated ideal body weight (Table 66.1) by a factor that takes into account physical activity and SDA (sedentary = 30 kcal/kg; moderately active = 35–40 kcal/kg, and very active = 45 kcal/kg). Thus, a moder-

ately active, healthy 70-kg man requires 2450–2800 kcal/d.

■ **Clinical Nutritional Assessment**

An individual's nutritional status reflects the degree to which the physiologic need for nutrients is being met. Nutritional assessment consists of gathering data: 1) to identify persons who will require specialized nutritional care, 2) to ascertain the cause and degree of malnutrition, if present, and 3) to judge the potential risk for the development of malnutrition. A careful history, a physical examination, and appropriate laboratory data are essential. The different methods of assessing nutritional status have the same aims: to identify persons at nutritional risk and to intervene quickly with appropriate nutritional therapy.

TABLE 66.2.	1983 Metropolitan Height and Weight Tables			
Height		**Weight (lb)**		
Feet	**Inches**	**Small Frame**	**Medium Frame**	**Large Frame**
Men				
5	2	128–131	131–141	138–150
5	3	130–136	133–143	138–153
5	4	132–138	135–145	142–156
5	5	134–140	137–146	144–160
5	6	136–142	139–151	146–164
5	7	138–145	142–154	149–168
5	8	140–148	145–157	152–172
5	9	142–151	148–160	155–176
5	10	144–154	151–163	158–180
5	11	146–157	154–166	161–184
6	0	149–160	157–170	164–188
6	1	152–164	160–174	168–192
6	2	155–168	164–178	172–197
6	3	158–172	167–182	176–202
6	4	162–176	171–187	181–207
Women				
4	10	102–111	109–121	118–131
4	11	103–113	111–123	120–134
5	0	104–115	113–126	122–137
5	1	106–118	115–129	125–140
5	2	108–121	118–132	128–143
5	3	111–124	121–135	131–147
5	4	114–127	124–138	134–151
5	5	117–130	127–141	137–155
5	6	120–133	130–144	140–159
5	7	123–136	133–147	143–163
5	8	126–139	136–150	146–167
5	9	129–142	139–153	149–170
5	10	132–145	142–156	152–173
5	11	135–148	145–159	156–176
6	0	138–151	148–162	158–179

Source of basic data: 1979 Build Study, Society of Actuaries and Association of Life Insurance Medical Directors of America. 1980. Courtesy of Statistical Bulletin, Metropolitan Life Insurance Company. Used with permission.

TABLE 66.3.	Pathophysiologic Response to Protein-Calorie Malnutrition

Decrease in energy expenditure
Muscle wasting
Mobilization of body fat
Endocrine changes
   Euthyroid sick syndrome
   Decreased insulin and somatomedin
   Increased growth hormone, catecholamines, glucocorticoids, and aldosterone
Reduced red cell mass and oxygen transport
Decreased cardiac work and GFR
Reduced T-lymphocytes
Electrolyte abnormalities
Malabsorption of lipids
Decreased absorption of glucose
Diarrhea (due to bacterial overgrowth and abnormal intestinal motility)
Impaired central and peripheral nervous system(s)

History and Physical Examination

Historical data should include appetite, recent weight change, physical activity, dental and oral health, and food and drug allergies. Additional inquiries relate to gastrointestinal illness, chronic diseases, medications, eating disorders and nutritional problems, and a history of substance abuse. The patient's general appearance should be carefully noted. **Protein-energy status** is generally assessed by anthropometric and biochemical means. Height and weight are compared with standardized population tables (such as life insurance tables) (Table 66.2). The **body mass index** (BMI) is calculated by dividing weight (in kg) by height (in meters) squared and expressed as kg/M^2. BMI correlates well with body fatness. A BMI of 24–27 for women or 24–25 for men indicates excess weight; a BMI above 30 indicates obesity.

Ancillary Studies

Nutritional assessment also includes several biochemical measurements that primarily assess visceral (nonstructural) protein. Serum albumin is often included in these tests, but these levels may fluctuate for reasons other than nutritional depletion. Also the relatively long half-life (about 14 days) limits its usefulness in evaluating malnutrition of short duration. Therefore, prealbumin (2-day half-life), is a better screening test for malnutrition. A total lymphocyte count below 1200 cells/mm^3 may indicate poor nutrition.

Malnutrition

Malnutrition represents inadequate total calorie or protein intake to meet nutrient needs. Protein-energy malnutrition is common in as many as 50% of hospitalized patients; world-wide, it most commonly affects infants and preschool children. However, no age group is exempt. Pathophysiologic changes that follow protein-energy malnutrition are listed in Table 66.3.

The treatment of protein-calorie malnutrition requires identification of patients at risk, often by hospital-based staff dietitians. Various grading systems categorize a patient's nutritional risk as mild, moderate, or severe, based on history, anthropometric indices, and laboratory testing, the patient's primary disease, anticipated duration of illness, and accessibility to nutrition (illnesses may limit patients' access to oral nutrition for protracted periods).

After careful nutritional assessment, a diet prescription must be created for each patient. Planning a diet begins with a review of the patient's usual food intake and a determination of its adequacy. Decisions regarding the route of feeding and the consistency of food are made based upon the patient's ability to chew, swallow and digest. No standard diet will meet every individual's needs, and modifications must often be made based on underlying conditions such as dysphagia, hypertension, diabetes, and hyperlipidemia (Table 66.4). For example, the diabetic should receive approximately 55–60% calories from complex carbohydrates, 20% from protein, and less than 30% from fat. The exchange list describing serving sizes of various foods in groups of similar nutrient value is a useful teaching tool for diabetics.

The American Heart Association and National Cholesterol Education Program have provided nutritional guidelines for patients with hyperlipidemia and coronary artery disease; they are used for both the primary prevention and the secondary treatment of established cardiovascular disease. The Phase 1 diet, a moderately low-fat, low-cholesterol diet for persons with normal lipids who wish to follow a preventive eating plan, is also useful in persons at moderate to high risk for the development of coronary heart disease. In general, the Phase 1 diet is continued for 2–4 months, at the end of which the serum cholesterol is reevaluated; if there is insufficient response to the Phase 1, the Phase 2 diet is initiated. It further reduces saturated fatty acid intake (to less than 7% of calories) and cholesterol (to less than 200 mg/day). If serum cholesterol levels still do not sufficiently respond, drug therapy is added.

In the malnourished patient or one at risk for malnutrition, the necessary nutrition can be effectively provided by two routes: enteral (by tube feeding through the **gastrointestinal** [GI] tract) and **parenteral** (by IV infusion, bypassing the GI tract). The decision-making regarding specialized nutrition support is shown in Figure 66.1.

Enteral feeding is preferred if the GI tract is functional. It is easier, less expensive, and safer, and it

TABLE 66.4.	Summary of Usual Hospital Diets		
Diet	Purpose	Nutritional Value	Comments
General[a]	For adult patients who do not require diet modifications.	Can be adequate in meeting all needs based on menu selection.	Can be modified by personal taste in food.
Soft	Provides food which requires little or no chewing.	Can be adequate in meeting all needs based on menu selection.	Texture can be determined on individual needs from pureed to chopped.
Full liquid	Supplies fluid and nutrients for patients who are between clear liquid and solid foods.	May be deficient in niacin, folic acid, and iron. Snacks may be needed to increase caloric intake.	For postoperative or acutely ill patients; or those with gastrointestinal diseases and in those unable to chew. Can serve as transitional diet.
Clear liquid	Short-term administration of fluid and 600–900 kcal/day.	Falls short of providing adequate nutrition.	Generally should not be continued more than 3–5 days.

[a] Contains 1600–2200 kcal, with 60–80 g protein, 80–100 g fat, and 180–300 g carbohydrate.

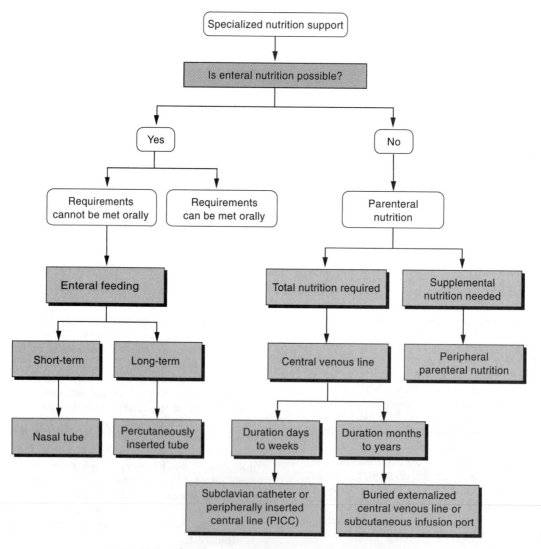

FIGURE 66.1. Algorithm for evaluation of specialized nutrition support.

prevents intestinal atrophy and stress-induced gastritis. Many types of enteral feeding tubes are available (Table 66.5). Nasogastric and nasoduodenal or nasojejunal tubes may be placed nonsurgically. Introduced nasally, they can be left in place for several weeks. Ensuring accurate tube placement is essential before initiating feeding. This can be done by aspirating gastric contents and by X-ray evaluation for tubes with metallic weights at their tips. For long-term enteral feeding, surgically placed tubes are preferable. Gastrostomy and jejunostomy tubes can be placed via surgical, fluoroscopic, and endoscopic means.

A wide range of formulations are available for enteral feeding; with variable osmolality, caloric density, and composition. Disease-specific formulas are also available. When more specific nutritional support is required, a custom-made diet can be prescribed using commercially available components of carbohydrate, protein, and fat. Tube feeding is usually given full strength, but may need to be initiated in a diluted form, and increased incrementally to full strength. Feeding is administered continuously by pump or intermittently by gravity or pump over 30–60 minutes every 3–6 hours. Careful patient monitoring can help avoid the complications of enteral feeding (Table 66.6). Aspiration of gastric contents is often preventable (see Table 239.3).

Parenteral nutrition may supplement enteral feeding or be the sole source of nutrients. Parenteral nutrition is given by two routes. **Peripheral parenteral nutrition (PPN)** (injected into arm veins) is limited to patients who require partial or short-term parenteral nutrition, with only low osmolar solutions (<600 mOsm/L). Most patients receiving parenteral nutrition require **central parenteral nutrition (CPN)**, using external jugular, internal jugular, or subclavian veins. Subcutaneous tunneling of a central venous catheter is recommended when CPN is continued for over two weeks. Components and complications of total parenteral nutrition (TPN) are shown in Table 66.7 and Table 66.8 respectively. The presence of a terminal condition that precludes aggressive therapy and a functioning GI tract are relative contraindications to TPN.

TABLE 66.5. Enteral Feeding Tubes

Type of Tube	Comments	Complications
Nonsurgically Placed Tubes		
Nasogastric	For short-term use; easy to insert and reinsert	Tracheal intubation, aspiration, intestinal perforation, clogging
Nasoduodenal or nasojejunal	For short-term use; used when gastric emptying is impaired	Same as above
Surgically Placed Tubes		
Gastrostomy tube	Long-term use; used when swallowing is impaired	Irritation at tube site; diarrhea
Jejunostomy tube	Long-term use; used when gastric emptying is impaired; usually need continuous feeding	Same as above
Combined gastrojejunostomy tubes	Allows for simultaneous gastric suction and jejunal feeding	Same as above

TABLE 66.6. Complications of Enteral Feeding

Mechanical	Gastrointestinal	Metabolic
Erosions	Nausea	Overhydration
Abscesses	Vomiting	Dehydration
Esophageal ulcerations	Diarrhea	Nutrient imbalances
Tube obstruction	Constipation	Hyperglycemia
		Hypoglycemia
		Electrolyte imbalance

TABLE 66.7.	Components of Parenteral Nutrition	
Component	**Supplied As**	**Comments**
Carbohydrate	50% dextrose in water (D50W)	Monitor urine glucose; if positive, initiate plasma glucose monitoring
Protein	3–10% AA	Branched chain AA: in trauma and liver disease; essential AA: in renal failure
Fat	Weekly infusions of 0.5–1.0 liter of 10% and 20% emulsions of soybean or safflower oil	Required for supplying essential free fatty acids and if TPN is continued for over 7–10 days
Vitamins and minerals	Added to the infusate	Based on RDA and patient's specific needs
Fluid	Generally 30–50 ml/kg for maintenance	Replenish abnormal fluid losses; to avoid metabolic complications, check BUN and electrolytes daily for the first week; monitor intake, output, and daily weight

AA = amino acids; RDA = recommended daily allowance; TPN = total parenteral nutrition.

TABLE 66.8.	Potential Complications of Parenteral Nutrition	
Mechanical	**Infectious**	**Metabolic**
Pneumothorax (simple and tension)	Infection at catheter insertion site	Dehydration
Hemothorax	Seeding of catheter from distant infection	Hyperglycemia
Subclavian artery injury	Contamination of solution	Deficiencies of calcium, magnesium and/or phosphorus
Central venous thrombosis		Hyperphosphatemia
Air embolism		Hyperchloremic metabolic acidosis
Cardiac perforation/tamponade		Trace mineral deficiencies

Obesity

Obesity, an excess of **body fat** (adipose tissue), may be defined in terms of deviation from a presumed **ideal body weight** (IBW) for a given height (Table 66.9). Obesity is one of the most common health problems in the United States. An estimated 40 million Americans are obese, and the incidence is rising.

■ Etiology

Obesity has multiple causes and pathophysiologic mechanisms. Genetic, behavioral, environmental, and metabolic factors contribute to an energy imbalance. Specific genetic defects leading to obesity remain elusive in humans, but animal studies suggest that genetic factors influence energy balance and may increase susceptibility to obesity. Occasionally, obesity follows an underlying medical disorder.

Overeating (the ingestion of an amount of energy exceeding the body's needs) contributes to the development of obesity. Overeating is probably due to both biological and psychological factors. Obese individuals may harbor an aberration in one of many physiological signals that regulate feeding behavior, causing abnormal satiety; these signals may be metabolic (e.g., glucose, amino acids, and fatty acids), hormones (e.g., insulin), and GI events. A sedentary lifestyle may also cause obesity.

■ Clinical Features and Complications

Obesity significantly increases morbidity and decreases life expectancy. Hypertension occurs three to five times more often in the obese. Obesity, particularly abdominal obesity, frequently coexists with other risk factors for atherogenesis (hypertension and glucose intolerance); lipid abnormalities (including elevated total cholesterol, reduced **high density lipoprotein** (HDL) cholesterol, and increased triglyceride levels), coronary heart disease (for which it also increases the risk for thromboembolic events); non–insulin dependent diabetes mellitus; and respiratory abnormalities, including hypoventilation and sleep apnea. In obesity, the risk of certain cancers (breast and endometrial) is enhanced; excess estrogens may be partly responsible. For unknown reasons, overweight men suffer a higher risk of fatal prostatic cancer; dietary factors (e.g., excess saturated fat in the diet) are suspected.

Liver abnormalities include abnormal liver tests and fatty liver. Cholelithiasis is strongly associated with obesity, with a prevalence of 30% among obese women. Many endocrine abnormalities complicate obesity, including adrenocortical hyperactivity. Cortisol production and cortisol turnover are high; however, 24-hour urine free cortisol levels are normal. In obese women, menstrual disorders (oligomenorrhea, amenorrhea, and dysfunctional uterine bleeding) and hirsutism are common. Obese men may have decreased libido and impotence; total testosterone levels are often low. The severity of these abnormalities parallels the degree of obesity and often, they can be reversed with weight loss. The obese commonly report joint pain, especially in the lumbosacral spine, hips, knees, and ankles. Excess weight contributes to the evolution of degenerative joint disease.

■ Management

Because obesity has multiple causes, prevention and treatment are difficult. Obesity due to a medical cause (e.g., hypothyroidism, hypercortisolism, male hypogonadism, hypopituitarism, or hypothalamic abnormalities) should receive specific therapy.

If no underlying disorder is identified, treatment is then directed at weight reduction measures. Although short-term weight loss is often achieved, long-term weight reduction frequently fails: only 20% of obese persons maintain their weight loss 5–15 years after initial treatment. Thus, obesity should be considered a medical condition requiring lifelong therapy, the cornerstone of which is dietary therapy. In general, weight loss occurs when energy expenditure exceeds energy intake. While many calorie-restricted diets exist, moderate calorie restriction using normal foods can be an effective and safe way to lose weight; the patient's age, medical condition, level of physical activity and degree of obesity determine the degree of calorie restriction. While a weekly weight loss of two pounds (1 kg) is normally a reasonable goal, underlying medical complications of severe obesity (heart failure, hypoventilation, or severe

hyperglycemia), may require faster weight loss. Exercise (daily walking or swimming), initiated gradually, is also part of an effective weight reduction program. In severely obese persons, some weight loss may be necessary before exercise can be initiated. Long-term success in therapy also requires behavioral modifications, often involving attitudes toward eating, physical activity, socializing, and entertaining.

At present, drug therapy plays a limited role in the treatment of obesity. Thyroid hormone and diuretics should be used only when medically indicated. Amphetamines should never be prescribed to treat obesity. With the development of newer appetite suppressing agents, however, drug therapy may play a more significant role in the future treatment of obesity. A number of different brain receptors (including noradrenergic and serotoninergic receptors) can modulate appetite. Phenylpropanolamine (Dexatrim) and phentermine suppress appetite by stimulating $\alpha 1$ and $\beta 2$ adrenergic receptors, respectively. Fenfluramine and fluoxetine stimulate serotonin release and block its reuptake although fenfluramine is no longer available due to safety concerns.

Occasionally, morbid obesity requires surgical treatment, most commonly gastroplasty and gastric bypass. Both procedures cause patients to limit food intake by delaying gastric emptying and causing the sensation of fullness after a small meal. Surgery should also be combined with behavior modification.

Anorexia nervosa and bulimia, are discussed in Chapter 20.

■ Vitamins and Trace Elements

Vitamins are a group of unrelated organic compounds that share at least two common features: the body cannot synthesize them at all, or only to a very limited extent, and minute quantities are needed in the diet. Many vitamins act as coenzymes or as catalytic cofactors for biologic reactions. Single vitamin deficiencies now occur rarely; they appear more commonly with general malnutrition. Vitamin deficiencies occur in states of malabsorption, in individuals who follow radical diets or suffer from alcoholism, as a complication of total parenteral nutrition, and in inborn errors of metabolism. Vitamin excess states are now more common than vitamin deficiency because of increased public use of vitamin supplements.

Vitamins are generally divided in two groups: fat soluble and water soluble. The fat soluble vitamins—A, D, E, and K—are found in foods in association with lipids. Conditions that interfere with fat absorption also interfere with the absorption of these vitamins. They can be stored in the body to some extent. The water soluble vitamins include vitamin C and vitamins of the B complex. Water soluble vitamins are not normally stored

TABLE 66.9.	Classification of Obesity Based on Ideal Body Weight
Overweight	0–20% above IBW BMI 25–30 kg/m²
Obesity	20% or more above IBW BMI greater than 30 kg/m²
Morbid Obesity	100% or more above IBW BMI greater than 40 kg/m²

BMI = Body mass index; IBW = Ideal body weight.

TABLE 66.10.   Vitamin Deficiency and Excess

	Function	Signs of Deficiency	Signs of Excess
I Fat Soluble Vitamins			
Vitamin A	Vision Growth Reproduction, anti-cancer	Night blindness Corneal ulcerations Dryness and hyperkeratosis of skin	Fatigue, malaise Lethargy, bone pain and fragility. Hepatomegaly, headaches, vomiting
Vitamin D	Calcium homeostasis Bone mineralization	Rickets Osteomalacia Costochondral beading	Hypercalcemia Vomiting, anorexia Irritability, diarrhea, sei- zures
Vitamin E	Antioxidant Absorption of Vitamin A	Hemolytic anemia in pre- mature and newborns, red blood cell fragility	None known
Vitamin K	Production of prothrombin and clotting factors VIII, IX, and X	Hemorrhage Cirrhosis	Hemolytic anemia, Nerve palsy
II Water Soluble Vitamins			
Vitamin C	Collagen cross-links Wound healing Antioxidant Utilization of iron	Joint tenderness, Scurvy (capillary hemorrhage), Impaired wound healing, Acute periodontal gingivitis, Petechiae	Risk of renal oxalate stones
Thiamin (B1)	Metabolism of carbohy- drates, fats and protein, nervous system function, coenzyme for carboxyla- tion of 2-keto acids	Beriberi, neuritis, edema, cardiac failure, anorexia, muscle weakness, con- fusion	None known
Riboflavin (B2)	Reactive portion of fla- voproteins included in oxidation	Photophobia, cheilosis, glossitis, scrotal skin changes	None known
Niacin	Coenzyme in fat synthesis, tissue respiration and car- bohydrate utilization, Digestion	Pellagra (dementia, derma- titis, diarrhea), muscle weakness, Tremors, glossitis	Flushing, tingling of skin, head throbbing
Pyridoxine (B6)	Coenzyme in synthesis and breakdown of amino acids. Synthesis of unsaturated fatty acids	Depression, nausea, vomit- ing, ataxia, convulsions, peripheral neuritis, hypo- chromic and macrocytic anemia	None known
Folic Acid	Synthesis of nucleic acids. Normal maturation of red blood cells. Coenzyme	Megaloblastic anemia, Subacute combined degen- eration of the cord	None known
Cyanocobalamin (B12)	Biosynthesis of nucleic acids and nucleoproteins; recy- cling of tetrahydrofolate	Megaloblastic anemia Subacute combined degen- eration of the cord	None known
Biotin	Synthesis and breakdown of fatty acids and amino acids	Anorexia, nausea, vomit- ing, glossitis, depression, skin and hair changes	None known
Pantothenic Acid	Part of coenzyme A inter- mediate metabolism of carbohydrate, fat and protein	Infertility, abortion, depres- sion, slowed growth	None known

in the body in appreciable amounts, so a daily supply is desirable. Information regarding the various vitamins, their biologic functions, and symptoms of their deficiency and excess are shown in Table 66.10.

Trace elements are metals present in minute amounts in biologic fluids that are considered essential for optimal growth and development. They are constituents of, or interact with, larger molecules, such as enzymes or hormones. Many enzymes require a small amount of a trace metal for full activity. Metals can cause disease through deficiency, excess, or imbalance. Deficiency states can result from inadequate dietary intake, malabsorption states, and excessive loss through the urine, pancreatic juice or other exocrine losses. Deficiencies may also follow imbalances between metals. Trace element deficiencies can also occur in patients receiving total parenteral nutrition.

Metal toxicity, involving a number of metals including aluminum, copper, nickel, and zinc, can occur in several settings, including chronic renal dialysis. Its early recognition can avoid significant neurologic, hematologic, and skeletal complications.

CHAPTER 67 DISORDERS OF LIPID METABOLISM

The two major circulating lipids are triglycerides and cholesterol. Triglycerides, composed of three fatty acids esterified to glycerol, are stored in adipose tissue in the fed state and are mobilized during fasting; they provide the body's primary fuel reserves. Cholesterol serves several functions. It is a major structural component of the cell membrane and the synthetic precursor of steroid hormones and bile salts. Cholesterol and triglycerides must be efficiently transferred between their organs of origin (principally the liver and intestine) and their peripheral destinations. Because both lipids are highly hydrophobic and essentially insoluble in water, they are transported in spherical particles called lipoproteins; nonpolar triglycerides and cholesterol esters are concentrated in the central core of these lipoproteins. Phospholipids and apolipoproteins (apoproteins) make up a polar shell that allows the lipoprotein particle to remain suspended in the plasma. Apoproteins are specialized proteins that confer specific properties to the lipoprotein particles of which they are a part, permitting them to interact appropriately with their target tissues and with other lipoprotein particles. Six major lipoproteins are recognized, based upon their functional roles, lipid composition, constituent apoproteins, electrophoretic mobilities, and particle density (Table 67.1).

Lipoprotein metabolism can be simplified into three interdependent pathways: the exogenous pathway, endogenous pathway, and reverse cholesterol transport. These pathways interface with one another either at the hepatic level or via direct exchange of lipids and apoproteins between lipoproteins in the plasma. The exogenous pathway starts with the absorption of dietary fats from the small bowel; they are assembled into chylomicrons, stable droplets containing triglyceride fat, cholesterol, phospholipids, and protein (Figure 67.1). After entering the systemic circulation, the chylomicrons interact with lipoprotein lipase, an enzyme which lines the capillaries of adipose and muscle tissues. Lipoprotein lipase hydrolyzes chylomicron triglycerides into fatty acids and glycerol, which are then used by peripheral tissues. The triglyceride-depleted chylomicron remnants are removed from the circulation by the liver and catabolized.

In the endogenous pathway, hepatically derived triglycerides and cholesterol are secreted into the circulation in the form of very low density lipoproteins (VLDL, Figure 67.2). The lipid of VLDL is approximately 80% triglycerides and 20% cholesterol. VLDL also interacts with endothelial lipoprotein lipase, producing a triglyceride-depleted particle, the intermediate density lipoprotein (IDL). Further catabolism and modification of IDL in the plasma largely yields low density

TABLE 67.1. Properties of Lipoprotein Classes				
Class	Density (g/ml)	Diameter (nm)	Triglyceride: Cholesterol Ester	Characteristic Apoproteins
Chylomicrons	0.93	75–1200	30:1	B-48, C-II, E
VLDL	0.93–1.006	30–80	4:1	B-100, C-II, E
IDL	1.006–1.019	25–35	1:1	B-100, E
LDL	1.019–1.063	18–25	1:7	B-100, E
HDL	1.063–1.210	5–12	1:4	A, C, D, E
Lp(a)	1.040–1.090	25–30	1:7	B-100, apo[a]

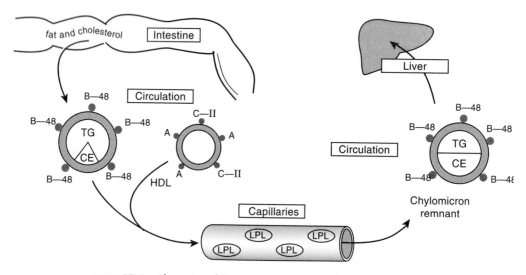

FIGURE 67.1. Absorption of dietary fat and its assembly into chylomicrons.

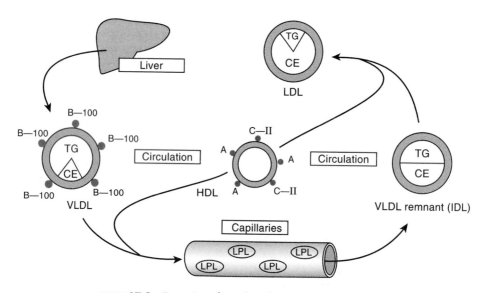

FIGURE 67.2. Formation of very low density lipoproteins (VLDL).

lipoprotein (LDL); LDL is taken up by the LDL receptor, a specific plasma membrane receptor in the liver. Extrahepatic tissues also possess LDL receptors. LDL thus provides cholesterol to the gonads and adrenal cortex for steroidogenesis. LDL can also be taken up by a less specific scavenger pathway by other cells, such as macrophages. In reverse cholesterol transport, the third basic lipoprotein pathway, the HDL takes up free cholesterol from peripheral tissues; it esterifies the free cholesterol with the enzyme lecithin-acyl cholesterol transferase (LCAT), then transfers the cholesterol ester to LDL in the plasma. Because HDL removes free choles-

terol from tissue and plasma, high HDL levels tend to protect against atherosclerosis. The major morbidity of dyslipidemias results from the atherogenic nature of lipoproteins enriched with cholesterol-esters; elevated LDL is most strongly associated with atherosclerosis and coronary heart disease.

Hyperlipidemias were originally classified according to the profile of lipoprotein particles analyzed by electrophoresis or density ultracentrifugation. Thus, syndrome categories were based on which combination of chylomicrons, VLDL, LDL, and remnant particles (IDL) was present (Table 67.2). It is now recognized that each syndrome category is made of multiple genetic syndromes and that a patient with a single defined genetic syndrome can be moved between them by diet and other secondary factors. Therefore, it is more useful to consider hyperlipidemias according to their primary genetic disorder, as discussed below.

■ Chylomicronemia Syndrome

The clearance of chylomicrons is defective in chylomicronemia syndrome, leading to a marked rise in fasting plasma triglycerides above 1000 mg/dl and sometimes as high as 10,000–20,000 mg/dl. Mild elevations usually cause no symptoms, but higher levels increase the chances of evoking one or more symptoms of the chylomicronemia syndrome (i.e., recurrent pancreatitis, eruptive xanthomas, lipemia retinalis, dyspnea, and changes in mentation). The xanthomas, which are nontender, yellowish papules, typically occur on the buttocks, elbows, and knees. They can slowly resolve as the triglyceride level is lowered. Accelerated atherosclerosis is absent.

Chylomicronemia is found either as a primary, full-blown, familial disorder or resulting from secondary factors superimposed on a milder, genetic predisposition to hypertriglyceridemia. The secondary disorders are more common (Table 67.3). Treatment of the disorder successfully lowers triglyceride levels in most patients, but some hypertriglyceridemia generally persists.

■ Familial Hypercholesterolemia

Familial hypercholesterolemia results from defects in the gene coding for the plasma membrane receptor for LDL. Patients with one defective gene have heterozygous familial hypercholesterolemia and possess half the number of normal, functional LDL receptors. LDL is approximately twice normal, and total serum cholesterol varies from 300–600 mg/dl. Heterozygous familial hypercholesterolemia, which afflicts 1 in 500

TABLE 67.3.	Causes of Secondary Hypertriglyceridemia

Diabetes mellitus
Obesity
Alcohol
Nephrotic syndrome
Uremia
Dysglobulinemia
Estrogens
Glucocorticoid excess
Systemic lupus erythematosus

persons, is associated with markedly accelerated atherosclerosis; most patients manifest clinically apparent coronary artery disease by age 40—many, by age 20. Tendon xanthomas, usually noted on the Achilles tendon and the extensor tendon of the hands and forearms, are virtually diagnostic. Tuberous xanthomas occur over extensor surfaces of elbows, knees, and hands. Premature arcus senilis (an opaque ring) is noted in the eyes at the corneal periphery. In homozygous familial hypercholesterolemia, LDL receptors are absent because both alleles encoding for the LDL receptor are defective; serum cholesterol is typically 600–1200 mg/dl. Aggressive atherosclerosis is apparent by early childhood. Response is poor to medical therapy, but extracorporeal LDL apheresis or plasma exchange may be partially effective. Portocaval anastomosis and liver transplantation are potential surgical approaches.

■ Polygenic Hypercholesterolemia

Patients with polygenic hypercholesterolemia have a mixture of genetic and environmental factors, leading to hypercholesterolemia of 200–350 mg/dl. Triglyceride levels are generally normal or modestly increased. Inheritance is not clearly autosomal dominant as in familial heterozygous hypercholesterolemia. Nonetheless, premature atherosclerosis is often present in first-degree relatives; significant hypercholesterolemia is noted in some first-degree relatives on screening.

■ Familial Dysbetalipoproteinemia

Clearance of both chylomicron and VLDL remnants is defective in familial dysbetalipoproteinemia, causing remnant particles to accumulate. Cholesterol and triglycerides are symmetrically elevated to 300–450 mg/dl. Premature coronary artery disease occurs, and the clinical phenotype is characterized by planar xanthomas.

■ Familial Combined Hyperlipidemia

Familial combined hyperlipidemia is the most common disorder in patients with premature coronary artery

TABLE 67.2.	Classification of Lipoprotein Profiles in Hyperlipidemia		
Type	Lipoprotein Elevated	Cholesterol Level	Triglyceride Level
Type 1	Chylomicrons	↑	↑↑↑
Type 2a	LDL	↑↑↑	↔
Type 2b	LDL & VLDL	↑↑	↔ or ↑
Type 3	Chylomicron and VLDL remnants	↑↑	↑↑
Type 4	VLDL	↔ or ↑	↑↑
Type 5	VLDL and chylomicrons	↑	↑↑↑

TABLE 67.4.	Target LDL-Cholesterol Levels
Risk Factors	**Target Level**
CHD Absent	
0 or 1 CHD risk factor	<130 mg/dl
CHD Present or	
≥2 CHD risk factors	<100 mg/dl

disease. It is characterized by variable increases in both LDL and VLDL levels. Depending on diet, exercise, and the presence of secondary aggravating factors, patients may have elevated triglyceride levels, elevated cholesterol levels, or both. Decreased HDL levels are common. In this polygenic disorder, many genetic causes are likely.

■ **Primary Hypertriglyceridemia**

Primary hypertriglyceridemia is characterized by elevated triglycerides in the range of 200–500 mg/dl. Plasma VLDL is elevated. The underlying genetic defects are heterogeneous and related to either overproduction or defective clearance of VLDL. The presence of secondary factors (such as diabetes, obesity and alcohol) can markedly increase triglycerides in this disorder. In primary hypertriglyceridemia, plasma HDL levels are often low. In some families, premature atherosclerosis is present.

■ **Treatment of Hypercholesterolemia**

Goals

Goals for treating hypercholesterolemia are based upon recommendations by the National Cholesterol Education Program Adult Treatment Panel (NCEPII). The LDL cholesterol targets differ, depending on the presence of pre-existing coronary atherosclerosis and the number of other risk factors for it (Table 67.4 and Table 67.5). The positive benefits of lowering cholesterol on reducing myocardial infarctions is well established. Secondary causes of hypercholesterolemia (hypothyroidism, nephrotic syndrome, acute intermittent porphyria, glucocorticoid excess, and dysglobulinemia) should be excluded in all patients with hypercholesterolemia. LDL cholesterol is generally not measured directly, but is calculated after quantitating triglycerides, total cholesterol, and HDL-cholesterol. The following formula is used to calculate LDL-cholesterol, provided fasting triglyceride levels are less than 400 mg/dl:

$$LDL\text{-}Cholesterol = Total\ Cholesterol - (HDL\text{-}Cholesterol + Triglycerides/5)$$

Diet

Many patients with mildly elevated LDL cholesterol are treated with diet therapy alone. The initial Step 1 NCEP diet contains less than 300 mg/day of cholesterol and 30% or less of total fat calories. Saturated fats are restricted to 10% of total daily calories, and most dietary triglycerides are polyunsaturated. The Step 2 NCEP diet is more restrictive; it contains less than 200 mg per day of cholesterol and 7% or less saturated fats. Because diet alone will usually reduce LDL cholesterol by no more than 25%, significant hypercholesterolemia requires drug therapy along with a continued Step 2 NCEP diet.

Drug therapy

Table 67.6 shows the drugs used to treat cholesterol problems. The major drugs for lowering LDL cholesterol are bile acid resins, HMG CoA-reductase inhibitors, and nicotinic acid. Bile acid resins (cholestyramine and colestipol) bind bile acids in the intestine, preventing their reabsorption. Plasma LDL cholesterol is lowered as hepatic cholesterol is diverted to increased bile acid synthesis. Given in high doses (20 g/d), bile acid resins will reduce LDL cholesterol by approximately 20%. Long-term compliance is limited by gastrointestinal side effects. The HMG CoA-reductase inhibitors (lovastatin, pravastatin, simvastatin, atorvastatin, and fluvastatin) inhibit the rate-limiting enzyme for cholesterol synthesis in the liver. These agents are usually well tolerated and are the most potent LDL cholesterol lowering agents, typically reducing LDL cholesterol by approximately one-third. Nicotinic acid successfully lowers LDL cholesterol by approximately 25% in most patients. As with the bile acid resins, significant side effects impair long-term compliance. The most bothersome side effects—flushing and pruritus—can be partially blunted with aspirin and by starting with low doses (100 mg T.I.D.). Given in the short-acting crystalline form, in 2–3 divided doses, the total dose is gradually increased to 2–3 g/day.

Secondary drugs used to treat hypercholesterolemia are fibric acids and probucol. Fibric acid derivatives more effectively treat hypertriglyceridemia, but they will lower LDL cholesterol in a subset of patients. Probucol typically reduces LDL cholesterol by 10–20%, but it also lowers HDL levels.

TABLE 67.5.	Risk Factors For Coronary Atherosclerosis (CHD)

Current cigarette smoking
Hypertension
High LDL cholesterol
Low HDL cholesterol (<35 mg/dL)
Diabetes mellitus
Age
  Men ≥45 years
  Women ≥55 or premature menopause without
    estrogen replacement therapy
Positive familial history of premature CHD (men ≤55 years, women ≤65 years) in first-degree relatives

TABLE 67.6.	Summary of Lipid-Lowering Drugs			
	LDL-C	**VLDL-TG**	**HDL-C**	**Side Effects**
Bile acid resins	↓	↑	↔	Dyspepsia, constipation, proctitis
Fibric acids	↑ or ↓	↓↓	↑	Gallstones
HMG CoA-reductase inhibitor	↓↓	↓ or ↑	↑	Myositis, abnormal LFTs
Nicotinic Acid	↓	↓	↑	Glucose intolerance, Abnormal LFTS, flushing, pruritus
Probucol	↓	↔	↓	Decreased HDL

HMG CoA = 3-hydroxy-3-methylglutaryl coenzyme A; LFT = Liver function tests. For others, see text.

■ Treatment of Hypertriglyceridemia

Goals

Treatment goals in hypertriglyceridemia are twofold, depending on the triglyceride level. In patients with the chylomicronemic syndrome and triglyceride levels above 1000 mg/dl, the goal is to reduce the levels below 1000 mg/dl in order to prevent immediate complications (such as recurrent pancreatitis and eruptive xanthomas). In patients with a more modest hypertriglyceridemia, there is an increased association with coronary heart disease (due largely to the relationship of hypertriglyceridemia with low HDL levels). In these patients, the goal is to lower triglyceride levels to as close to normal as possible, thus reciprocally raising HDL reducing long-term risk for coronary heart disease.

Diet

Because the triglycerides within chylomicrons originate from dietary fat, diet is the only effective therapy for patients with the chylomicronemic syndrome. Dietary fat is restricted to 20% or less of total daily calories and, if need be, to 10%. It is essential to identify and correct causes of secondary hypertriglyceridemia (Table 67.3). There are no drugs that effectively promote chylomicron metabolism. Milder hypertriglyceridemia resulting from VLDL is often associated with hypercholesterolemia as well. Dietary management follows the NCEP 1 and 2 diets described above, duly modified as needed to lower the fat below 30%.

Drug therapy

The major drugs for reducing triglyceride levels are the fibric acids and nicotinic acid. Fibric acids, gemfibrozil and clofibrate, decrease the production of VLDL triglyceride and also enhance VLDL clearance by increasing lipoprotein lipase activity. Gemfibrozil is given at a dosage of 600 mg once or twice daily. Fibric acids are generally well tolerated, despite an increased incidence of gallstones. Nicotinic acid also reduces triglyceride levels. Its use in hypertriglyceridemia is somewhat limited due to its side effects and the high incidence of glucose intolerance and overt diabetes present in the hypertriglyceridemic population.

■ Questions

INSTRUCTIONS: For each question below, select only **one** lettered answer that is the **best** for that question.

Questions 1–4: A 50-year-old woman gained 20 lb and noted increased fatigue and cold intolerance. Her symptoms started approximately one year ago and have gradually worsened. She also reports constipation, dry skin, coarsening hair, deepening of her voice, and amenorrhea. Physical examination shows bradycardia (pulse 52), pale, dry skin, dry, brittle hair, infraorbital edema, diffuse thyromegaly with a firm consistency to the gland, white milky nipple discharge (galactorrhea), normal pelvic exam, and delayed relaxation phase of the Achilles tendon reflex.

Laboratory studies included:

		Normal range
Total T4	3.0 μg/dl	5–11 μg/dl)
T3 resin uptake	19%	(25–35%)
TSH	52μU/ml	(0.4–4.8 μU/ml)
Prolactin	56 ng/ml	(<20 mg/ml)

1. What is the most likely diagnosis in this patient?
   A. Secondary hypothyroidism
   B. Primary hypothyroidism
   C. TSH-secreting pituitary tumor
   D. None of the above

2. The best explanation for the hyperprolactinemia is:
   A. Presence of a prolactin-secreting pituitary tumor.

B. TRH that is elevated in primary hypothyroidism and stimulates pituitary prolactin release.

C. Infundibular stalk compression from a nonsecretory pituitary tumor.

D. Decreased levels of dopamine.

3. Her amenorrhea is most likely due to which of the following?
A. Pregnancy
B. Hypothyroidism
C. Polycystic ovarian syndrome
D. Hyperprolactinemia

4. How would you treat this patient?
A. Bromocriptine
B. Combined estrogen/progestin therapy
C. Levothyroxine
D. All of the above

Questions 5–7: A 64-year-old man reports constipation, mild abdominal pain, thirst, polyuria, weakness, and fatigue. He has hypertension (10 years), peptic ulcer disease (10 years), depression (5 years), and two renal stones (5 and 3 years ago). There is no family history of hypercalcemia. His only medication was a thiazide diuretic. Complete physical examination was significant only for BP of 154/95.

Laboratory studies included:

		Normal
Total calcium	12.5 mg/dl	(8.2–10.4 mg/dl)
Phosphorus	2.5 mg/dl	(3.0–4.5 mg/dl)
Creatinine	0.8 mg/dl	(0.7–1.2 mg/dl)
Intact PTH	75.0 pg/ml	(10–60 pg/ml)
24 hr urine		
Calcium	350 mg/d	
Creatinine	1.2 g/d	

5. What is the most likely cause of this patient's hypercalcemia?
A. Primary hyperparathyroidism
B. Malignancy-associated hypercalcemia
C. Sarcoidosis
D. Familial hypocalciuric hypercalcemia

6. What laboratory study best distinguishes between (5 a) and (5 d) above?
A. Intact PTH
B. Fractional excretion of calcium
C. Serum phosphorus
D. Serum creatinine

7. Production of PTH-related protein is most commonly associated with which of the following?
A. Lymphoma
B. Melanoma
C. Colon cancer
D. Squamous cell carcinoma of lung

8. A 22-year-old woman has decreased peripheral vision, frontal headaches, and milky breast discharge. She has never had any menses. She takes no medications. The serum prolactin is 650 ng/ml (normal <20 ng/ml). The most likely diagnosis is which of the following?
A. Pituitary tumor
B. Turner's syndrome
C. Craniopharyngioma
D. Congenital adrenal hyperplasia

9. A 42-year-old diabetic woman has secondary amenorrhea. She takes insulin and metoclopramide. Her serum prolactin is 85 ng/ml (normal <20 ng/ml). If pregnancy is excluded, what is the most likely cause of her hyperprolactinemia?
A. Prolactin-secreting pituitary tumor
B. Metoclopramide
C. Chronic renal failure
D. Insulin

10. During the past 6 months, a 47-year-old man has noted fatigue, 20-lb weight gain, proximal muscle weakness, and ankle swelling. His BP is mildly elevated. You note plethoric facies, truncal obesity, abdominal striae, and supraclavicular fullness. Which of the following tests would you now order?
A. High-dose (8 mg) dexamethasone suppression test
B. MRI of the pituitary gland
C. Overnight 1 mg dexamethasone suppression test
D. Random serum cortisol and ACTH levels.

11. A 27-year-old woman with progressive visual loss undergoes transsphenoidal resection of a nonsecretory pituitary macroadenoma. On the first postoperative day her urine output rises dramatically to 500–1000 ml per hour, and she reports polydipsia. Her polyuria is best explained by:
A. Central diabetes insipidus.
B. Syndrome of inappropriate ADH secretion.
C. Intravenous fluids.
D. Nephrogenic diabetes insipidus.

Questions 12–15: A 37-year-old woman reports increased anxiety, tremulousness, diarrhea, palpitations, and heat intolerance over the last six months. Her appetite is reportedly "too good". She is on no medications. Her pulse is 120/min and BP, 122/76 mm Hg. She is thin and anxious, with warm and extremely moist skin; Proptosis is noted; extraocular muscle movements are normal. The thyroid gland is firm and diffusely enlarged with a bruit; fine tremor of distal upper extremities and a shortened relaxation phase of her deep tendon reflexes are noted.

12. What is the most likely cause of this woman's signs and symptoms?

A. Graves' hyperthyroidism
B. Toxic solitary nodule
C. Iodine-induced hyperthyroidism
D. TSH-secreting pituitary adenoma

13. If you were to order a 24-hour radioactive iodine uptake (RAIU) in this patient, which of the following results would you expect?
A. Normal
B. Decreased
C. Increased
D. Nondetectable

14. The patient is placed on propranolol and propylthiouracil. One month later she develops a sore throat and fever of 103°F. What test should be obtained?
A. Throat culture
B. Chest x-ray
C. TSH
D. WBC count

15. Possible therapeutic agents used to treat thyroid storm include which of the following?
A. Propranolol
B. Propylthiouracil
C. Dexamethasone
D. All of the above

16. In a patient with hypertension and paroxysms of diaphoresis, palpitations and headache, which of the following is the best initial test to perform?
A. CT scan of the adrenal glands
B. Measurement of urinary catecholamines and metanephrine levels
C. Measurement of plasma renin activity and plasma aldosterone concentration
D. Measurement of plasma catecholamines

17. A 29-year-old woman notes progressive acne, weight gain, and increasing hair growth on the face, chest and shoulders for one year. A physical examination confirms these. The plasma testosterone level is 396 ng/dl. Which of the following is the most likely diagnosis?
A. Ovarian tumor
B. Adrenal tumor
C. 21-hydroxylase deficiency
D. Polycystic ovarian disease

18. Conditions that predispose patients to develop vitamin D deficiency include:
A. Renal failure.
B. Malabsorption (steatorrhea).
C. Being house-bound.
D. All of the above.

19. Conditions associated with osteoporosis include which of the following?
A. Cushing's syndrome

B. Thyrotoxicosis
C. Postmenopausal
D. All of the above

20. A 24-year-old woman with anorexia nervosa has not had any menses for the last several months. What is the most likely cause?
A. Diminished GnRH secretion
B. Primary ovarian failure
C. Pregnancy
D. Polycystic ovarian disease

21. What is the best drug therapy for a 45-year-old man with hypertriglyceridemia who is unresponsive to diet?
A. Bile-acid binding resin
B. Nicotinic acid
C. Gemfibrozil
D. Probucol

22. A 58-year-old woman, previously healthy, has persistent low back pain following a fall. A CT scan reveals an incidental 3-cm solid adrenal mass. What is the next step in the evaluation of this mass?
A. Needle biopsy of the mass
B. Hormonal assessment of adrenal function
C. Repeat CT scan in 6 months
D. Right adrenalectomy

23. A 64-year-old man has widely metastatic small cell lung carcinoma. His serum sodium is 119 mEq/L, spot urine sodium is 40 mEq/L and plasma osmolality is 260 mOsm and urine osmolality is 320 mOsm. He has no neurologic symptoms. What is the most likely diagnosis?
A. Primary polydipsia
B. Syndrome of inappropriate ADH secretion
C. Central diabetes insipidus
D. Nephrogenic diabetes insipidus

24. What is the most appropriate therapy for the patient described in question 23?
A. Fluid restriction
B. Infusion of hypertonic saline
C. Demeclocycline
D. Intranasal DDAVP

■ Answers

1. b	2. b	3. d	4. c	5. a
6. b	7. d	8. a	9. b	10. c
11. a	12. a	13. c	14. d	15. d
16. b	17. a	18. d	19. d	20. a
21. c	22. b	23. b	24. a	

SUGGESTED READING

Textbooks and Monographs

Maas DL, Kochar MS. Primary aldosteronism. In: Rakel RE (ed.). Conn's Current Therapy. Philadelphia: W.B. Saunders Company, 1995.

West JB (ed.). Best and Taylor's Physiologic Basis of Medical Practice. 11th ed. Baltimore: Williams & Wilkins, 1985.

Wilson JD, Foster DW (eds.). Williams Textbook of Endocrinology. 8th ed. Philadelphia: W.B. Saunders Company, 1992.

Articles

Disorders of the Anterior Pituitary

Klibanski A, Zervas NT. Diagnosis and management of hormone-secreting pituitary adenomas. N Engl J Med 1991; 324:822–831.

Melmed S. Acromegaly. N Engl J Med 1990;322:966–977.

Molitch ME. Gonadotroph-cell pituitary adenomas. N Engl J Med. 1991;324:626-627.

Sarapura V, Schlaff WD. Recent advances in the understanding of the pathophysiology and treatment of hyperprolactinemia. Curr Sci 1993;5:360–367.

Snyder PJ. Clinically nonfunctioning pituitary adenomas. Endocrinol Metab Clin North Am 1993;22:163–175.

Vance ML. Hypopituitarism. N Engl J Med 1994;330: 1651–1662.

Disorders of the Posterior Pituitary

Fraser CL, Arieff AI. Epidemiology, pathophysiology, and management of hyponatremic encephalopathy. Am J Med 1997;102:67–77.

Robertson GL. Physiology of ADH secretion. Kidney Int 1987;32:S20–S26.

Verbalis JG. Hyponatremia: Endocrinologic causes and consequences of therapy. Topics in Endocrinol & Metab 1992;3: 1–7.

zRA, Thier SO. Pathophysiologic approach to hyponatremia. Arch Intern Med 1980;140:897–902.

Thyroid Diseases

Hamburger JI. The autonomously functioning thyroid nodule: Goetsch's disease. Endocrinol Rev 8:439, 1987.

Magner JA. TSH-mediated hyperthyroidism. The Endocrinologist. 1993;3:289–296.

McDougal IR. Graves' disease: Current concepts. Med Clin North Am 1991;75:79.

Ridgway EC. Clinician's evaluation of a solitary thyroid nodule. J Clin Endocrinol Metab 1992;74:231.

Disorders of Parathyroid Glands, Vitamin D Metabolism, and Calcium Homeostasis

Bilezikian JP. Management of acute hypercalcemia. N Engl J Med 1992;326:1196–1203.

Potts JT Jr. Management of asymptomatic hyperparathyroidism. J Clin Endocrinol Metab 1990;70:1489–1493.

Riggs BL, Melton LJ, III. The prevention and treatment of osteoporosis. N Engl J Med 1992;327:620–627.

Diseases of the Adrenal Cortex

Aron DC, Findling JW, Tyrrell JB. Cushing's disease. Endocrinol Metab Clin 1987;16:705–730.

Chodosh LA, Daniels GH. Addison's disease. The Endocrinologist 1993;3:166–181.

Gill JR Jr. Primary hyperaldosteronism: Strategies for diagnosis and treatment. The Endocrinologist 1991;1:365–369.

Ross NS, Aron DC. Hormonal evaluation of the patient with an incidentally discovered adrenal mass. N Engl J Med 1990;323:1401–1405.

Diseases of the Adrenal Medulla

Werbel SS, Ober KP. Pheochromocytoma. Update on diagnosis, localization, and management. Med Clin North Am 1995; 79:131–153.

Disorders of Ovarian Function

Barnes R, Rosenfield RL. The polycystic ovary syndrome: Pathogenesis and treatment. Ann Intern Med 1989;110:386–399.

Barret-Connor E, Bush TL. Estrogen and coronary heart disease in women. JAMA 1991;265:1861–1867.

McDonough PG. Amenorrhea—an etiology approach to diagnosis. Fertil Steril 1978;30:1.

Rittmaster RS, Loriaux DL. Hirsutism. Ann Intern Med 1987;106:95–107.

Disorders of Testicular Function

Braunstein GD. Gynecomastia. N Engl J Med 1993;328:490–495.

Krane RJ, Goldstein I, Saenz De Tejada. Impotence. N Engl J Med 1989;321:1648–1656.

Hypoglycemia and Diabetes Mellitus

Davidson MB. Clinical implications of insulin resistance syndromes. Am J Med 1995;99:420–426.

Gerich JE, Mokan M, Veneman T, et al. Hypoglycemia unawareness. Endocr Rev 1991;12:356–371.

Gearhart JG, Forbes RC. Initial management of the patient with newly diagnosed diabetes. Am Fam Phys 1995;51:1953–1962, 1966–1968.

Jaspan JB. Taking control of diabetes. Hosp Pract (Office Edition) 1995;30:55–62.

Konen JC, Shihabi ZK. Microalbuminuria and diabetes mellitus. Am Fam Phys 1993;48:1421–1428.

Laine C, Caro JF. Preventing complications in diabetes mellitus: the role of the primary care physician. Med Clin North Am 1996;80:457–474.

Raskin P, Arauz-Pacheco C. The treatment of diabetic retinopathy: a view for the internist. Ann Intern Med 1992;117:226–233.

Umpierrez GE, Khajavi M, Kitabchi AE. Review: diabetic ketoacidosis and hyperglycemic hyperosmolar nonketotic syndrome. Am J Med Sci 1996;311:225–233.

Valdovinos MA, Camilleri M, Zimmerman BR. Chronic diarrhea in diabetes mellitus: mechanisms and an approach to diagnosis and treatment. Mayo Clin Proc 1993;68:691–702.

Nutritional Disorders

Barrocas A, Belcher D, Champagne C, et al. Nutrition assessment: Practical approaches. Clin Ger Med 1995;11: 675–713.

Ham RJ. The signs and symptoms of poor nutritional status. Primary Care: Clin Off Pract 1994;21:33–54.

Lipkin EW, Bell S. Assessment of nutritional status. The clinician's perspective. Clin Lab Med 1993;13:329–52.

Manning EM, Shenkin A. Nutritional assessment in the critically ill. Crit Care Clin 1995;11:603–634.

McMahon MM, Rizza RA. Nutrition support in hospitalized patients with diabetes mellitus. Mayo Clin Proc 1996;71:587–594.

Reife CM. Involuntary weight loss. Med Clin North Am 1995;79:299–313.

Disorders of Lipid Metabolism

Jialal I. A practical approach to the laboratory diagnosis of dyslipidemia. Am J Clin Pathol 1996;106:128–138.

Larsen ML, Illingworth DR. Drug treatment of dyslipoproteinemia. Med Clin North Amer 1994;78: 225–245.

Rosenson RS, Frauenheim WA, Tangney CC. Dyslipidemias and the secondary prevention of coronary heart disease. DM 1994;40:369–464.

Summary of the Second Report of the National Cholesterol Education Program (NCEP) Expert Panel on detection, evaluation, and treatment of high blood cholesterol in adults (Adult Treatment Panel II). JAMA 1993;269:3015–3023.

PART VII

Konrad H. Soergel
Kulwinder S. Dua
Vincents J. Dindzans

GASTROENTEROLOGY AND DISEASES OF THE LIVER

CHAPTER 68

GENERAL APPROACH TO THE PATIENT WITH GASTROINTESTINAL DISEASES

The gastrointestinal (GI) tract extends from the mouth to the anal canal. Associated structures include the pancreas and the hepatobiliary system.

Some typical GI symptoms in relation to the organ involved are shown in Table 68.1. Since GI disorders can be associated with other diseases or may be inherited, the importance of a thorough history cannot be overemphasized. Complete physical examination should include all the principal methods of examination. The information thus gathered may need to be supplemented by general laboratory tests. In most instances, this may lead to a reasonable diagnosis, thus allowing initiation of treatment. In others, radiologic studies may be required. Patients with lesions requiring endoscopy, those with persistent symptoms despite therapy, and those defying diagnosis are best referred to a gastroenterologist. Some may require additional specialized evaluation—for example, those being considered for a liver transplant or those requiring endoscopic pancreatico-biliary intervention. These patients are best managed at specialized medical centers.

TABLE 68.1. Symptoms of Gastrointestinal Disease

General	*Colon/Rectum*
Anorexia	Diarrhea
Malaise	Constipation
Symptoms of anemia	Abdominal pain/colic
Weight loss	Abdominal distention
Pharyngeal	Tenesmus
Difficulty initiating swallowing	Blood per rectum
Choking attack	*Hepatobiliary*
Nasal regurgitation	Anorexia
Pharyngeal residues after swallowing	Epigastric/right upper quadrant pain
Esophageal	Yellow discoloration of sclera
Heartburn	Dark urine
Regurgitation	Pale stools
Dysphagia: solids, liquids	Itching
Odynophagia	*Pancreatic*
Chest pain	Abdominal pain
Gastroduodenal	Weight loss
Upper abdominal pain	Anorexia
Postprandial fullness	Diarrhea
Vomiting	Symptoms of biliary obstruction
Hematemesis	
Melena	
Small bowel	
Diarrhea	
Abdominal pain/colic	
Abdominal distention	
Melena	

Common Symptoms and Signs of Gastrointestinal Disease

Dysphagia

Dysphagia is difficulty swallowing solids or liquids, owing to conditions impeding orderly bolus transport from mouth to stomach (Table 68.2). In neuromuscular diseases, dysphagia results from dysfunction of the muscles of the mouth and pharynx involved in bolus formation and propulsion. This may lead to recurrent aspiration into the airway and nasal regurgitation of food. In cricopharyngeal muscle dysfunction, hypopharyngeal tumor, or Zenker's diverticulum, dysphagia resembles a neuromuscular disorder. Patients with dysphagia due to

TABLE 68.2.	Selected Causes of Dysphagia
Mechanism	**Diseases**
Neuromuscular	Brain stem neoplasms and vascular accidents
	Multiple sclerosis
	Poliomyelitis
	Muscular dystrophy
	Amyotrophic lateral sclerosis
	Myasthenia gravis
Abnormal peristalsis	Diffuse esophageal spasm
	Achalasia
	Cricopharyngeal dysfunction
Structural lesions of the esophagus	Stricture
	Web
	Ring
	Neoplasm
	Diverticulum
Extrinsic compression	Bronchogenic carcinoma
	Aberrant blood vessels
Psychogenic	

structural lesions or extrinsic compression of the esophagus feel as if the bolus is going "down the hatch" but then stops. The sensation produced by the arrested bolus may be felt substernally at the level of the obstruction, or may be referred, often up to the suprasternal notch. Patients with neuromuscular disorders usually report dysphagia for liquids and solids alike, while those with structural lesions have more difficulty with solids. A neoplasm is more likely when dysphagia is of recent onset. Dysphagia should be distinguished from *globus hystericus*, in which the patient feels a lump in the throat but has no actual difficulty swallowing.

Heartburn

The most common esophageal symptom is *heartburn* or *pyrosis*, a burning discomfort in the subxiphoid or epigastric region, radiating substernally to the neck, and diminishing at the upper reaches. Occasionally, gastric contents may regurgitate into the mouth. Often relieved by swallowing saliva, water, or an antacid, heartburn is a common symptom of **gastroesophageal (g-e) reflux.**

Odynophagia

Odynophagia refers to pain upon swallowing. The symptom may occur in the oropharynx (e.g., acute pharyngitis). Esophageal odynophagia is usually perceived substernally. Infective esophagitis and corrosive injury frequently cause odynophagia. Odynophagia may also be caused by motor disorders of the esophagus (e.g., diffuse esophageal spasm), but it is rarely due to g-e reflux disease.

Dyspepsia

Dyspepsia is a sensation of discomfort in the upper abdomen—often perceived as "indigestion" by the patient—which is thought to reflect a disorder of the upper gastrointestinal tract. Usually linked to eating, dyspepsia may involve epigastric pain, fullness or bloating after meals, belching, nausea, and heartburn. Detailed inquiry may reveal a pattern suggestive of g-e reflux, peptic ulcer disease, cholelithiasis, or chronic pancreatitis. Instances where diagnostic studies exclude an organic basis for chronic dyspepsia are termed **"functional dyspepsia."** Despite significant overlaps, symptoms of functional dyspepsia fall into three subgroups. In **ulcer-like dyspepsia,** symptoms mimic peptic ulcer disease including relief with food, antacids, or H_2-receptor antagonists. In **dysmotility or stasis-type dyspepsia,** patients report symptoms of gastroparesis—early satiety, nausea, belching and bloating after meals. In **flatulent or biliary-type dyspepsia,** the patients report postprandial fullness, epigastric discomfort, or flatulence. Despite the co-existence of dyspepsia and cholelithiasis, the two have no proven association.

Functional dyspepsia has no explainable pathophysiology at present. Basal and peak acid outputs are normal in the majority of these patients, although gastric acid suppression benefits some. Delayed gastric emptying and reduced postprandial antral motility have been noted in some; in others, a reduced threshold has been found for discomfort after gastric distention, suggesting visceral sensory abnormality. Functional dyspepsia is largely a diagnosis of exclusion of other organic causes for dyspepsia. Management should include diet and life-style counseling (e.g., avoiding alcohol, tobacco, caffeinated drinks, and spicy, greasy foods). Those with continuing symptoms can undergo empiric acid suppression with H_2-receptor antagonists (e.g., cimetidine, ranitidine) or gastroduodenal motility enhancing by prokinetic agents (e.g., metoclopramide, cisapride).

Abdominal Pain

Abdominal pain is one of the main symptoms of GI disorders for which patients seek medical help. Its expression and diagnostic evaluation are complex. The pain is best assessed using a sequence of dichotomous or similarly discrete descriptors. In this way, pain that is "terrible" and "all over" may be seen as acute or chronic, visceral or somatic, constant or intermittent, and centered in one area or another. Despite the frequent necessity for additional tests to make a diagnosis, in some instances, abdominal pain is the only dependable means of diagnosis—for example, the right lower quadrant pain of acute appendicitis.

Abdominal pain can be *visceral* or *parietal* (Table 68.3). Pain originating from GI organs is visceral, carried by sympathetic nerve fibers. Because visceral organs have multisegmental innervation from both sides of the spinal cord, visceral pain is generally felt in the midline, and has indistinct borders with poor localization. Visceral pain is believed to result from stretching of a hollow GI viscus or the capsule of a solid organ, or from mediators released during inflammation or ischemia of GI structures. Sympathetic pain fibers in splanchnic nerves enter the posterior horn of the spinal cord, which may cause the pain sensation to spread retrogradely in the somatic sensory nerve of the corresponding dermatome. Thus, referred pain may be felt in areas remote from the source (e.g., right scapular pain from biliary tract disease). Pain may be *referred* to the abdomen from diseases outside the abdomen—for example, myocardial ischemia may present as upper abdominal pain alone or abdominal pain with chest pain. Diseases that extend to involve peritoneum will exhibit *parietal pain*, which is sharper and more severe, usually more accurately localized, and aggravated by movement or coughing. Occasionally, systemic diseases like porphyria and diabetic ketoacidosis can present as abdominal pain.

The *location* of the pain, in terms of four quadrants, should be noted (Figure 68.1, Table 68.4); the nine-area section system may also be used. The *quality* of pain, as described by the patient, is also meaningful. Sharp and fairly localized parietal pain is secondary to peritoneal involvement by an inflamed GI viscus directly underlying the localized area. Generalized peritonitis due to perforation of a GI viscus could present as diffuse, severe abdominal pain. Visceral pain may be constant (e.g., right upper quadrant in acute hepatitis) or intermittent (e.g., colicky pain in small bowel obstruction).

The next consideration in the evaluation of abdominal pain is its *radiation*. Duodenal and pancreatic pain may radiate to the back, gallbladder pain to the right scapula, and pain from diaphragmatic irritation to the shoulder. The *timing* of abdominal pain and *factors aggravating or relieving* it also help in differential diagnosis. Nocturnal pain that interrupts sleep strongly indicates an organic cause for the pain. The effect of food, belching, passing flatus, defecation, and medications (e.g., antacids) on pain may help localize the pain to a specific viscus. *Change in pain* over time is particularly useful in the course of acute abdominal pain where sequential examinations will distinguish between acute illness requiring surgical or other intervention, and illness that is self-limited and often idiopathic. Finally, *other associated symptoms* should be noted. In the context of pain, vomiting may suggest bowel obstruction or gastric outlet obstruction; hematemesis or melena may suggest ulcer disease; and left lower-quadrant pain with rectal bleeding could be due to colitis.

Rebound tenderness and involuntary guarding on palpation implies localized or generalized peritonitis. Bowel sounds may be absent, owing to peritonitis-related ileus. The patient tends to avoid movement and generally keeps the abdominal muscles tense (rigidity). By contrast, patients with visceral pain, as in acute pancreatitis, may be in severe distress but may have minimal abdominal signs on palpation. However, visceral pain may evolve into parietal pain as the disease process extends to the peritoneum. Sequential physical examinations are useful in eliciting this change. Renal angles and hernial orifices should be systematically examined in patients with abdominal pain. Besides detecting lower rectal lesions and abnormalities in the pouch of Douglas, a digital rectal examination can help assess the tone of the anal sphincter and presence of frank or occult blood in the stool. The genitalia should also be examined. In women, a pelvic examination may be necessary.

TABLE 68.3.	**Some Distinctions Between Visceral and Parietal Pain**	
Characteristic	**Visceral**	**Parietal**
Localization	Generally midline	More accurate
Nature	Dull, burning, cramping, gnawing, indistinct borders	Sharp, severe
Associated autonomic activity (e.g., sweating, nausea, vomiting)	May be present	Uncommon
Increase with movements, coughing, deep inspiration	—	Present
Radiation to other areas	May be present	—

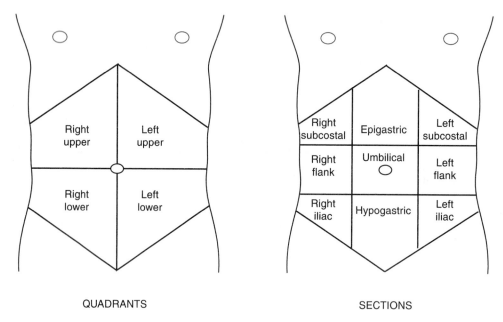

QUADRANTS

SECTIONS

FIGURE 68.1. Two methods of designating abdominal area for describing findings: A. Four quadrantic divisions. B. Nine sections.

TABLE 68.4.	Frequent Causes of Abdominal Pain			
Site	Acute		Chronic	Referred
Upper quadrants	Perforated gastric/duodenal ulcer Cholecystitis Biliary colic Acute pancreatitis Splenic rupture or infarction		Duodenal ulcer Gastric ulcer Non-ulcer dyspepsia Chronic pancreatitis Irritable bowel Liver diseases	Cardiac Pleuritic Spinal root
Periumbilical	Appendicitis Small bowel obstruction Small bowel infarction Dissecting aortic aneurysm		Inflammatory bowel disease Intestinal ischemia Irritable bowel	Spinal root
Lower Quadrants	Appendicitis Diverticulitis Colon obstruction Colon infarction		Inflammatory bowel disease Colon ischemia Irritable bowel	Spinal root Pelvic diseases

Despite a thorough clinical assessment, the etiology of the abdominal pain may remain elusive. General laboratory tests (a complete blood count with differential, liver tests and plain abdominal x-rays) may be required. Acute presentations may require urgent abdominal imaging with ultrasound or computed tomography (CT). While exploratory laparotomy may be urgently undertaken in some, a more deliberate and selective approach may be pursued in others, especially those with longstanding abdominal pain. Laparoscopy is being increas-

ingly used in the diagnosis of abdominal pain and cancer and in the evaluation of abdominal trauma.

Nausea and Vomiting

Nausea is the experience of revulsion to food and the anticipation of vomiting. Vomiting is a coordinated somatic and visceral motor activity, where prolonged contractions of the abdominal muscles and the diaphragm raise the intra-abdominal pressure sufficiently to overcome the opposing hydrostatic and muscular forces of the gastric cardia, g-e junction, and the esophagus. The proximal small bowel contents are thus moved into the stomach, and forcefully thereafter, into the mouth and beyond. With retching, spontaneous contractions occur without fluid propulsion above the g-e junction. Vomiting is controlled by the vomiting center in the medulla and triggered by afferent neural input to the medulla or stimulation of chemoreceptor trigger zone. Additional neural pathways are also involved. In contrast, g-e reflux leading to oral regurgitation of gastric contents lacks the autonomic or somatic features (sweating and emotional distress) of vomiting.

Nausea and vomiting may be provoked by a myriad of disorders, some of which are not primarily gastrointestinal. Fundamentally, obstructive vomiting must be distinguished from the more common vomiting caused by sensory stimulation of the GI tract. In small bowel obstruction, patients vomit large volumes of bilious material, consisting of gastric and pancreatic secretions besides bile. Colicky periumbilical pain and a tympanitic, distended abdomen are associated. In pyloroduodenal stenosis and gastric outlet obstruction from peptic ulcer, patients usually vomit bile-free material, often containing food eaten many hours before. A succussion splash may be elicited. In colonic obstruction, vomiting trails constipation, abdominal pain, and distension. Nonobstructive GI causes of nausea and vomiting cover a full range of GI disorders with mucosal irritation or dysmotility—e.g., esophagitis, gastritis, peptic ulcer disease, and diabetic gastroparesis. Vomiting may be due to non-GI causes—toxic, metabolic, neurologic, or cardiac conditions (e.g., uremia, medications, pregnancy, ketoacidosis, raised intracranial pressure, or myocardial infarction). In some patients, the cause is elusive; emotional or psychiatric problems may be implicated.

Sustained, large-volume vomiting may cause dehydration and electrolyte imbalance. Loss of gastric acid results in metabolic alkalosis, often with hypokalemia. Nausea is a very potent stimulator of antidiuretic hormone (ADH) secretion; therefore, nausea and vomiting may lead to hyponatremia. Thus, treatment must not only address the cause and symptomatic control of nausea and vomiting but also correct the fluid, electrolyte, and nutritional consequences. While antiemetics are not needed for controlling nausea and vomiting in patients with a treatable primary cause (e.g., gastric outlet obstruction), for those who do require them, various drugs are available that may act centrally (**antihistamines, anticholinergics, phenothiazines**), peripherally (**cisapride**), or in both domains (**dopaminergic antagonists**).

Diarrhea and Malabsorption

See chapters 69 and 70.

Radiographic Vs. Endoscopic Studies

Endoscopy is superior to radiography in several ways. It can directly demonstrate bleeding sites and detect flat or superficial mucosal lesions more readily. Endoscopically obtained biopsies can reliably separate malignant from benign ulcers. While a cancer or retained food material can both cause a filling defect in the esophagus on a barium swallow, one can directly inspect the area using esophagoscopy. G-e reflux seen on barium studies cannot exclude associated Barrett's esophagus. The ability for interventional therapy, the other facet of endoscopy, clearly makes it the procedure of choice in patients where such intervention is planned. Dilating strictures, placing endoprostheses and feeding tubes, controlling GI bleeding, removing polyps, and decompressing the colon are all possible during endoscopy.

Nonetheless, in some situations, radiologic studies are superior to endoscopy. Plain abdominal films, and not endoscopy, can reveal bowel gas patterns and intra-abdominal calcification. Whereas barium studies can assess GI motility, endoscopy cannot. Subtle strictures are better seen radiologically. In patients with suspected perforation, radiological studies are more informative and safer. Despite the availability of enteroscopy in some centers now, large areas of the small bowel are inaccessible to endoscopy. In instances where full endoscopic facilities are not readily available, radiological studies of the upper and the lower GI tracts are still excellent alternatives. Patients with dysphagia should have a barium swallow study first. Finally, x-ray studies are cheaper than endoscopy and carry a lower risk of complications.

In some situations, radiography and endoscopy are combined. For example, during endoscopic retrograde cholangiopancreatography (ERCP), biliary and pancreatic ducts are cannulated endoscopically and the cholangiopancreatogram is obtained radiologically. Prior transhepatic cholangiography may be required to gain bile duct access in difficult or failed ERCP attempts.

Newer imaging modalities play a major diagnostic and therapeutic role in GI diseases. Ultrasonography (US), computed tomography, and magnetic resonance imaging (MRI), can effectively image intra-abdominal structures not readily visualized otherwise (liver, gall bladder, pancreas, biliary system, kidneys, lymph nodes, masses, and fluid collections). The Doppler technique makes dynamic evaluation (blood flow pattern) possible. Endoscopes with an attached ultrasound probe (endoscopic ultrasound, EUS) can scan organs like the pancreas, liver, and bowel wall in close proximity, and through targeted fine needle, aspirate material for cytology. GI bleeding site(s) that cannot be located endoscopically can be identified by angiography, and occluded by intra-arterial emboliza-

tion or vasopressin injection. Available radionuclide imaging tests include 99^mTc-sulfur colloid (liver parenchyma), 99^mTc- HIDA (acute cholecystitis), 99^mTc-pertechnetate (ectopic gastric tissue—e.g., Meckel's diverticulum), and 99^mTc-labeled red cells (intermittent GI bleeding).

Diagnostic laparoscopy is sometimes indicated in the evaluation of patients with ascites where peritoneal disease is suspected. Occasionally it is used to biopsy hepatic surface lesions under direct visualization.

CHAPTER 69 DIARRHEA

▪ Definition

Diarrhea is defined as stool weight exceeding 200g/day in patients ingesting a typical Western diet (>300g/day on a high-fiber diet). The stool water content is approximately 80% and even higher in loose or watery stools. Therefore, diarrhea can be equated with increased fecal water loss. Symptoms may include increased stool frequency (>3/day), decreased stool consistency, abdominal pain, and fecal incontinence.

▪ Physiology and Pathophysiology

Of the 10–12 L of fluid that the intestines receive daily, oral intake is 2 L, the rest being salivary, gastric, biliary, pancreatic, and small bowel secretions. The duodenum, jejunum, and the ileum absorb about 9 L/day. The colon absorbs all but 0.1 L from the remaining 1.0–1.5 L. Water moves passively across the bowel mucosa to maintain isotonicity of its contents; the absorption and secretion of osmotically active solutes determine this flux. As shown in Figure 69.1, water transport is mainly *paracellular*, via the tight junction **(zonula occludens).** Solutes absorbed across the brush border exit into the lateral intercellular space (LIS), thus causing an osmotic gradient from LIS to the isotonic lumen contents. Water flows osmotically (hydraulic), so as to dispel this gradient; in the process, small solutes (MW <100) entrained in the water flow are absorbed by "solvent drag." This paracellular absorption of solutes depends on the permeability of the tight junction: jejunal tight junctions are "leaky", whereas those in the colon are much less permeable (Figure 69.1). When solutes are not absorbed, this obligates excess water in the lumen to maintain isotonicity; diarrhea results. The normal colon, with its ability to absorb up to 4 L/day, can partly compensate for increased fluid delivery to it from the small intestine. Diarrhea occurs when the

overall efficiency of intestinal water absorption falls below 99%. For flow rate and composition of bowel contents, see Table 69.1.

Inorganic ions and nutrients are absorbed through the mature cells on the villus tips in the small bowel and the surface epithelium in the colon. In both organs, the crypt cells secrete electrolytes and water. In the small bowel, Na^+ enters the enterocytes by two mechanisms: (a) by an Na^+/H^+ cation exchange and (b) in association with glucose, galactose, and most amino acids. The Na^+/H^+ exchanger is coupled to an anion transporter, which

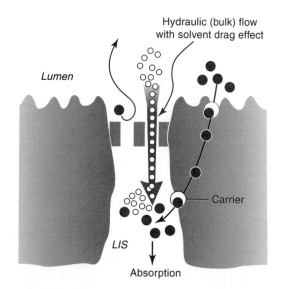

FIGURE 69.1 Paracellular water absorption in response to active, carrier-mediated transport of a solute (large filled circles) from lumen to the lateral intercellular space (LIS). The water flow is driven by the osmotic gradient between lumen and the LIS, across the junction. The water flow carries with it a second, smaller solute (open circles)—i.e., solvent drag. The solute transported by carriers is too large to pass the tight junction; it is reflected from it.

TABLE 69.1.	Intestinal Contents in the Postprandial State				
	Flow Rate (L/d)	Na (mEq/L)	K (mEq/L)	Cl (mEq/L)	HCO$_3$ (mEq/L)
Proximal jejunum^a	10	60	15	60	15
Mid-gut	5	140	5	100	30
Terminal ileum	1.5	140	8	60	50
Rectum/stool^b	0.1	15	85	15	30

^{a}Varies with meals.
^{b}Main anion: Short-chain fatty acids.

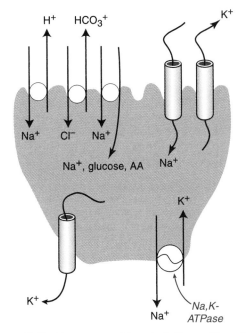

FIGURE 69.2. Transporters of intestinal villus and/or colon surface epithelial cells. Left side: present in small bowel and colon. Middle: Na$^+$ uptake coupled to glucose, galactose or to amino acids; present in small bowel only. Right side: apical K$^+$- and Na$^+$-channels: colon only. Only the basolateral Na, K-ATPase provides energy.

exchanges Cl$^-$ for HCO$_3^-$. This dual process (Figure 69.2), which occurs throughout the small bowel and colon, absorbs NaCl electroneutrally. Also, in the colonic brush border membrane, there are Na$^+$- selective channels that allow Na$^+$ to enter the cell by concentration gradients. Through the Na, K-ATPase ("sodium pump"), the Na$^+$ is ejected across the basolateral cell wall. This process leads to active Na$^+$ absorption and a low Na$^+$ in normal stool water. Potassium enters the colonic contents mainly by diffusion, and partly by active secretion. All active absorption in the entire bowel derives its energy from the sodium pump, which exchanges 3 Na$^+$ ions for 2 K$^+$ ions.

Multiple mechanisms regulate the intestinal absorption and secretion of electrolytes. These include mediators released from inflammatory and mast cells in the lamina propria (histamine, prostaglandins, leukotrienes, serotonin, interleukins, etc.), neurotransmitters which act through receptors on the basolateral wall of enterocytes, hormones in circulating blood, neuropeptides released by specialized cells within the mucosa and bacterial enterotoxins, such as cholera toxin and E. coli enterotoxin. The majority of these mechanisms decrease the absorption and/or increase the secretion of ions. Most mechanisms that produce gastrointestinal secretion inhibit the electroneutral absorption of NaCl by the villous cells, *and* open Cl$^-$ channels in the brush border membrane of crypt cells. Chloride ions enter the cell by basolaterally located Na$^+$ 2Cl$^-$ K$^+$ uptake; the excess intracellular K$^+$ exits via basolateral K$^+$ channels and the Na$^+$ by the sodium pump (Figure 69.3). By contrast, Na$^+$ absorption coupled to sugars and amino acids is unaffected in secretory diarrhea; this is the basis for oral rehydration therapy.

■ **Classification**

Diarrhea is traditionally classified according to the underlying pathophysiologic mechanism(s)—osmotic, secretory, and miscellaneous types. **Osmotic diarrhea** results when excessive, osmotically active solutes reach the rectum, accompanied by obligatory water to maintain isotonicity (Table 69.2). Carbohydrates are a common cause. Diarrhea results when intact sugars remain in the rectum and stool. Colonic bacteria anaerobically ferment carbohydrates to short-chain fatty acids (acetate, propionate, and n-butyrate) and H$_2$. The maximum fermentation capacity is 60g/meal of carbohydrates, of which 15g/meal is "physiologic" malabsorption. Carbohydrate-induced diarrhea occurs when the fermentation capacity of the colonic bacteria is surpassed—for example, during therapy with broad-spectrum antibiotics. The organic acids so produced are rapidly absorbed and play no role in the ensuing diarrhea.

Secretory diarrhea is due to reduced absorption and/or excess secretion of inorganic ions (Table 69.2). The 2-OH bile acids and some long-chain fatty acids

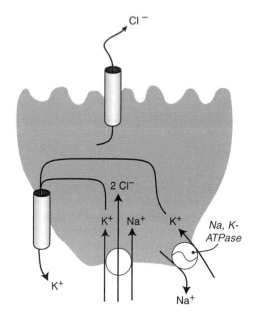

FIGURE 69.3. Chloride secretion by intestinal and colonic crypt cells. The rate of secretion depends on the activation (opening) of the apical Cl⁻ channel. The energy is provided by the Na, K-ATPase.

impede colonic ion absorption, thus causing secretion. Diarrhea follows resection or extensive disease of the terminal ileum where bile acids are normally actively absorbed. Oleic acid, and its bacterial hydroxylation product, 10-OH stearic acid, lead to excess stool water in steatorrhea. Stimulant laxatives (e.g., phenolphthalein, castor oil, bisacodyl, and cascara) induce colonic secretion and stimulate colonic motility. One-half of patients with gastrin-producing tumors have diarrhea, from excess gastric and pancreatic secretions that outstrip the absorptive ability of the entire gut. Serotonin, vasoactive intestinal polypeptide (VIP), and thyrocalcitonin bind to the enterocyte receptors, and incite secretory diarrhea.

Exudation from ulcerated ileal or colonic mucosa contributes to the diarrhea of **inflammatory bowel disease.** Increased luminal hydrostatic pressure proximal to a bowel obstruction lead to secretion, causing **"paradoxical diarrhea."** Rapid intestinal transit causes diarrhea after gastric surgery (dumping syndrome and postvagotomy diarrhea), and perhaps in hyperthyroidism also.

■ **Laboratory Tests**

In theory, two simple tests distinguish between secretory and osmotic diarrhea. First, osmotic diarrhea from poorly absorbed solutes stops during 48 hours of fasting. While secretory diarrhea from malabsorption of

bile or fatty acids does the same, continued diarrhea during fasting indicates a secretory cause. The second test is a stool water osmotic gap (stool water osmolality [290 mOsm/kg] − 2[measured stool Na⁺ + K⁺]). In secretory diarrhea, the gap is below 50 mOsm/kg. In osmotic diarrhea, the osmotic gap exceeds 50. However, these two tests have limited practical use since most diarrheas have more than one mechanism.

■ **Clinical Categories**

Clinically, diarrhea is divided into acute and chronic (>3 weeks' duration). **Acute diarrhea** is usually caused by a pathogen, toxin, or food component ingested hours to one week before the onset of symptoms. Onset with watery stools, nausea, vomiting, and little or no fever reflects predominant small bowel involvement by a pathogen, without epithelial invasion. "Dysenteric syndrome"—that is, abdominal cramping, fever, and frequent small-volume bloody stools, suggest infection by an invasive organism, usually afflicting the colon. **Chronic diarrhea** frequently has a gradual onset and persists for over 3 weeks.

■ **Diagnostic Evaluation**

Acute diarrhea is marked by signs of dehydration, such as acute weight loss, orthostatic hypotension, poor capillary perfusion, and oliguria. Next, to determine a cause, inquiries should be directed to

TABLE 69.2.	**Causes of Osmotic and Secretory Diarrhea**

I. Osmotic Diarrhea
A. Carbohydrates escaping absorption and colonic fermentation
   a) Disaccharidase deficiencies
   b) Poorly absorbed dietary sugars: sorbitol, fructose, mannitol, lactulose
   c) Broad-spectrum antibiotic therapy
B. Poorly absorbed inorganic ions
   a) Magnesium: antacids, laxatives, food supplements
   b) Anions: Na-sulfate, -phosphate, -citrate
C. Miscellaneous: Polyethylene glycol 3250 (GoLYTELY)
II. Secretory Diarrhea
Bacterial enterotoxins
Stimulant laxatives
Diffuse small intestinal disease
Bile acid and fatty acid malabsorption
Microscopic/collagenous colitis
Hormonally mediated:
   a) Increased digestive secretions: gastrinoma
   b) Intestinal secretion: carcinoid syndrome, VIP-oma, medullary carcinoma of the thyroid
Congenital ion transport defects

recent travel, similar illness among contacts, and food consumption. Stool tests for enteric pathogens, ova, and parasites are generally needed only in a dysenteric syndrome. Fecal leukocytes, when present, imply an invasive pathogen or inflammatory bowel disease. "False negatives" occur in enterohemorrhagic (O 157:H 7) E. coli, *C. difficile* and Yersinia infection, and amebic colitis. (See, also, chapter 79.)

A thorough medical history, the probability of specific causes (Figure 69.4), and the results of routine tests (complete blood count, serum electrolytes and albumin, sedimentation rate, stool testing for occult blood, ova, parasites, and enteric pathogens) are paramount in selecting tests for evaluating chronic diarrhea. **Functional diarrhea,** the most common cause, typically has a duration over 2 years, intermittent and daytime-only diarrhea, weight loss below 5 kg, normal routine tests, and a stool weight below 300g/day. A panoply of medications may cause diarrhea, including Mg citrate, phosphates, broad-spectrum antibiotics, antacids, colchicine, prostaglandins (Cytotec®), fluoxetine (Prozac®), olsalazine (Dipentum®), lactulose, and, occasionally, diuretics and nonsteroidal anti-inflammatory drugs (NSAIDs). **Surreptitious laxative and diuretic abuse** is frequently overlooked; the stool should be tested for phenolphthalein by adding 1N NaOH or KOH to observe the color change to a red-purple. When this is negative, urine can be analyzed for diuretics and for polyphenolic laxatives, including bisacodyl, and cascara. In some patients with acute, travel-related diarrhea, watery diarrhea continues, without a demonstrable pathogen. This post-infectious diarrhea abates within 6–24 months. Chronic watery diarrhea (Brainerd) syndrome is endemic in areas of the rural Midwest. The prognosis is good, although the pathogen remains elusive. Hormonally caused chronic diarrhea is rare—for example, carcinoid syndrome (elevated urine 5-HIAA), gastrinoma (Zollinger-Ellison and MEN-I syndrome), VIPoma, medullary thyroid carcinoma, adrenal insufficiency, and hyperthyroidism. These should not be sought routinely.

When initial evaluation does not yield a preliminary diagnosis, two studies are very helpful. The first is a 48- or 72-hour quantitative stool collection performed at home with the patient receiving a regular diet and no anti-diarrheal medications. Stool weight less than 200g/d rules out diarrhea; 200–300g/d suggests a functional cause, and a weight above 800g/d indicates small bowel involvement. Stool fat should be measured in order to detect steatorrhea (>7g fat/d) as a sign of generalized malabsorption. The second test is a proctosigmoidoscopy with no (or only saline) preparatory enemas. Brown-black mucosal discoloration (melanosis coli) is diagnostic of long-term use of anthraquinone-type laxatives (e.g., cascara sagrada, senna, aloe). Biopsies should be done to

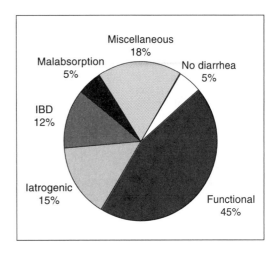

FIGURE 69.4. Diagnosis in patients referred for evaluation of chronic diarrhea. IBD: inflammatory bowel disease. Miscellaneous: systemic diseases (e.g., diabetes, amyloid, immunosuppression), 5%; self-induced (laxative abuse, long-distance running), 5%; food/travel related (e.g., lactose deficiency, sorbitol, fructose, postinfectious diarrhea), 5%; hormonal causes, congenital transport defects, 3%.

exclude lymphocytic, microscopic, and collagenous colitis. A schematic approach to the diagnosis of chronic diarrhea is shown in Figure 69.5.

■ Management

Rehydration and acid-base balance

Severe dehydration is defined as an estimated weight loss of over 4%—that is, an extracellular fluid deficit exceeding 2.5 L in a 60 kg patient. The deficit should be replaced in about 24 h with an IV solution of 0.45% NaCl (NaCl, 78 mEq/L) to which $NaHCO_3$, 50 mEq/L plus KCl, 10–20 mEq/L are added. For significant hypernatremia (>154 mEq/L), 1 L of 5% dextrose in water (D5W) is given for every 2 L of the above solution. Serum electrolytes, urine output, and BP should be monitored. Metabolic acidosis requires HCO_3 supplementation only with a serum HCO_3 below 15 mEq/L. Fluid should also be given for ongoing maintenance needs (about 2.5 L/d) as D5 0.45% NaCl, alternating with D5 0.25% NaCl; nearly 40 mEq of K^+ is added per 24 hours.

Oral rehydration solutions (ORS) are used to correct mild to moderate dehydration and for maintenance therapy of severe dehydration after initial rehydration (Table 69.3). In secretory diarrhea, glucose will stimulate Na^+ and water absorption; solvent drag will lead to absorption of K^+ and anions. ORS used for initial rehydration has a higher Na^+ level than that used for maintenance hydration. Saccharides (e.g., sucrose, glucose polymers, or boiled rice flour) may be used in lieu

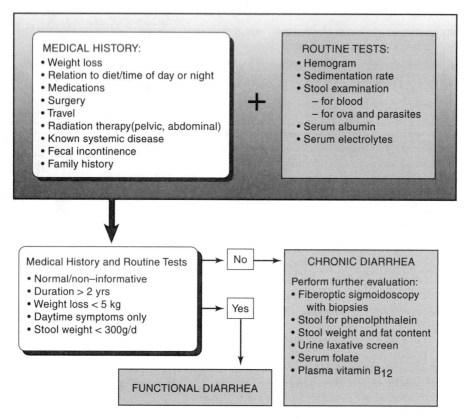

FIGURE 69.5. Evaluation of chronic diarrhea.

TABLE 69.3. Oral Rehydration Solutions							
	Source	Na	K	Cl	Base**	Glucose mmol/l
Rehydration							
WHO-UNICEF	—	90	20	80	30	111
Rehydralyte	Ross	75	20	65	30	140
Maintenance							
Pedialyte	Ross	45	20	35	30	140
Infalyte	Pennwalt	50	20	40	30	111

**Bicarbonate or citrate.

of glucose. The volume administered equals the sum of the fluid deficit and the ongoing losses. Additional fluid and food intake are encouraged. Acute diarrhea frequently features transient acquired lactose deficiency; thus, dietary lactose should be low. Fructose, sorbitol, and caffeine should also be avoided.

Anti-diarrheal medications

Anti-diarrheals are not indicated during acute, self-limited diarrhea, particularly when an invasive pathogen ("dysenteric syndrome") is suspected. Opiate-type

agents are the mainstay of symptomatic therapy of chronic diarrhea. Loperamide (Imodium®, 2 mg b.i.d.), diphenoxylate (Lomotil®, 5 mg q 6–8h), and codeine (30 mg q 6–8h) are equally effective. They delay small bowel transit, and by interaction with the δ-type opiate receptor on enterocytes, may facilitate absorption. They may cause nausea and abdominal cramps. A long duration of action and the lack of central nervous system (CNS) effects make Loperamide the preferred agent; doses up to 10 mg b.i.d. may have to be given. Bulk-forming agents (e.g., bran, methylcellulose, and calcium polycarbophil) do not reduce stool losses of water and salts. At best, they increase stool consistency. Anti-spasmodics are not recommended.

■ Special Situations

Immunosuppressed patients

Most patients with AIDS develop diarrhea eventually, manifested either by large-volume diarrhea and weight loss or as the dysenteric syndrome. The latter indicates colitis caused by *C. difficile*, cytomegalovirus, or common bacterial pathogens. The former type is associated with infection by *Giardia lamblia*, cryptosporidia, microsporidia, *Mycobacterium avium-intracellulare*, or viruses. A cause may be elusive in nearly 50% of this group. Stool studies for bacteria, parasites, and viral pathogens are indicated. Colonoscopy and duodenoscopy with biopsies may be dictated by the clinical presentation. Management should be directed at the cause.

Diabetic diarrhea

Rarely, chronic watery diarrhea complicates diabetes mellitus, usually with associated neuropathy and retinopathy. The autonomic neuropathy impairs intestinal motility and decreases Na^+ and Cl^- absorption. The absorptive defect is due to reduced catecholamine content in the ileal mucosa, thus reducing activation of α-2-adrenergic receptors on the enterocytes. Celiac sprue and intestinal bacterial overgrowth should be excluded, since both are more common in diabetics. Mild steatorrhea, found in nearly one-third of cases of diabetic diarrhea, is due to pancreatic atrophy. Treatment should be step-wise. "Sugar-free" diets with sorbitol or fructose are discontinued first. Opiate anti-diarrheal drugs are given next; abdominal cramps may limit their use. Third, α-adrenergic agonists (e.g., clonidine, 0.1 mg initially, with a maximum of 0.6 mg q 12h) may be tried, but their long-term efficacy is unknown. Pre-existing orthostatic hypotension may worsen. Oral antibiotics, pancreatic enzymes, and somatostatin should not be routinely used.

Post-vagotomy diarrhea

Diarrhea follows truncal or selective vagotomy in up to 25% of patients; it is severe in 1–8%. The precise cause is unclear, but rapid gastric emptying of liquids ("dumping syndrome," chapter 76), rapid intestinal transit, and bacterial overgrowth may all be involved. The onset may be delayed by several years and the course is commonly episodic. Treatment is with small meals of low sugar content and, frequently, high doses of anti-diarrheal opiates. Octeotide, a somatostatin analogue, may sometimes help.

Antibiotic-associated diarrhea

Diarrhea occurs in up to 30% of patients receiving antibiotics, particularly penicillins, cephalosporins, and clindamycin. Colitis due to toxin-producing strains of *C. difficile* accounts for only 15–20% of cases; osmotic diarrhea due to decreased bacterial carbohydrate fermentation occurs in the remaining. Those with *C. difficile* toxin in the stool are given appropriate antibiotics (chapter 91). In those without, antibiotics should be stopped, if possible; poorly absorbed carbohydrates should be omitted from the diet.

Tube-feeding diarrhea

Diarrhea may complicate liquid formula feedings through a nasogastric tube or a gastrostomy, with or without added fiber. Frequent causes include concurrent antibiotics or sorbitol-containing medications, a pre-existing intestinal disorder, or bolus feeding. Formula diets, including the elemental type, do not cause diarrhea when given by constant infusion into an otherwise normal intestinal tract.

CHAPTER **70**   # MALABSORPTION

S ince the colon does not absorb nutrients, malabsorption is the increased passage of single or multiple nutrients across the ileocecal valve, with or without diarrhea. Malabsorption of single nutrients includes vitamin B_{12}, glucose-galactose malabsorption, amino acid transport defects, and disaccharidase deficiencies. Generalized malabsorption consists of defects of digestion and of malabsorption due to resection or extensive disease of the small bowel (Table 70.1).

■ Physiology and Pathophysiology

Digestion and absorption are complex processes. The surface area available for absorption is limited to the top 10–20% of the intestinal villus surface. The pH of the fluid layer overlying the absorptive cells is 1–2 units below that of luminal contents; this fluid layer, about 40–100μ thick, does not mix with intestinal bulk contents. Solutes need to cross this "unstirred layer" by diffusion, a process that limits the absorption rate of substances with a slow

TABLE 70.1.	Causes of Malabsorption

Impaired intraluminal digestion
  Pancreatic enzyme deficiency
   — Deficient secretion in pancreatic disease; decreased CCK release
   — Enzyme inactivation: excess gastric acid secretion
   — Asynchrony: post-gastric surgery
  Defective fat solubilization: decreased bile salt concentration
   — Decreased synthesis: liver disease
   — Decreased bile flow: cholestasis
   — Excess bile salt inactivation: bacterial overgrowth, acid pH, binding (cholestyramine)
   — Bile salt loss: disease or resection of terminal ileum
Impaired mucosal function
  Brush border enzyme deficiency
   — Lactase, sucrase - isomaltase, trehalase deficiency: inherited or acquired
  Impaired mucosal transport
   — Global defect: diffuse intestinal disease, bypass or resection
   — Isolated defects: glucose-galactose malabsorption; Hartnup disease; cystinuria; congenital cobalamin deficiency
  Drug effects
   — Decreased crypt cell proliferation: colchicine, cytostatic drugs, neomycin
   — Decreased folate absorption: methotrexate, sulfasalazine, phenytoin
Miscellaneous
  Disorders of mesenteric lymphatics
   — Obstruction; primary ectasia
  Intestinal ischemia
  Serum protein loss
   — Menetrier's disease
   — Lymphatic obstruction
   — Diffuse inflammation
  Infiltrative disorders
   — Amyloid
   — Lymphoma
   — Mastocytosis
  Fibrosis
   — Diffuse systemic sclerosis
   — Chronic radiation injury

aqueous diffusion coefficient, such as the products of fat digestion. Digestion and absorption of carbohydrates is rapid and nearly complete in the jejunum; the ileum completes the fat and protein absorption. While the human digestive tract has considerable reserve capacity for digestion and absorption, it is limited in its capacity to absorb sorbitol and free fructose and to hydrolyze lactose to glucose and galactose.

Digestion and absorption of fat

In the stomach, gastric lipase hydrolyzes fat to glycerol and fatty acids. The remainder of the fat is emulsified with proteins and the products of gastric lipase activity. The amphipathic conjugated bile acids stabilize the fat emulsion droplets. After pancreatic lipase binds to these droplets in the presence of colipase, fatty acids are released from positions 1 and 3 of the triglyceride, leaving intact 2-monoglycerides (2MG). The lipolytic products are then solubilized in bile salt micelles, which form when duodenal bile salts exceed a "critical micellar concentration" of approximately 2mM. The products of lipolysis diffuse out of the micelles, through the unstirred layer and across the apical cell wall into the cytoplasm of enterocytes. Further steps in fat absorption are shown in Figure 70.1. Chylomicrons and very low-density lipoproteins (VLDL), the final products of the absorptive process enter the intestinal lymphatics. Fat-soluble vitamins, cholesterol, and phospholipids are absorbed in tandem with the products of lipolysis. Fat absorption is vulnerable at many steps, including duodenal acidification, which inactivates lipase and precipitates bile salts; duodenal bile salt concentrations below about 2mM, which precludes micelle formation; decreased lipase availability and a defective or reduced absorptive area. Further, lipase is the pancreatic enzyme most vulnerable to tryptic digestion within the intestinal lumen.

Digestion and absorption of proteins

The hydrolysis of proteins begins in the stomach, where pepsin digests collagen to OH-proline peptides. The action of pancreatic trypsin, chymotrypsin, and elastase produces oligopeptides, which are hydrolyzed at the brush border of the enterocytes to a mixture of tri- and dipeptides and amino acids. These small peptides are efficiently absorbed intact (Figure 70.1). Carboxypeptidases A and B liberate free amino acids, which are absorbed by several distinct Na-coupled transport systems.

Digestion and absorption of carbohydrates

Starch, the main dietary carbohydrate, consists of straight glucose chains connected by 1,6-glycosidic bonds. Salivary and pancreatic alpha-amylase splits starch, yielding maltose, maltotriose, and alpha-limit dextrins. Carbohydrate digestion, which involves several enzymes, is completed at the brush border membrane since only monosaccharides are absorbed. Glucose and galactose are actively absorbed by the Na-glucose co-transporter, termed SGLT 1. Fructose binds to a transporter termed glucose transporter (GLUT) 5, and is taken up by facilitated diffusion. The exit of fructose, glucose, and galactose across the basolateral cell well is mediated by GLUT 2, a high capacity, rapidly inducible transport protein (Figure 70.1).

Regional absorption

The brush border enzyme, pteroyl polyglutamate hydrolase, acts on dietary folates to produce pteroyl monoglutamate, which is then absorbed. Both activities take place in the duodenum and proximal jejunum. Folate absorption is inhibited by sulfasalazine, phenytoin, and methotrexate. Similarly, the absorption of inorganic ferrous ions and active, vitamin D-dependent Ca^{++} transport are limited to the proximal small intestine. By contrast, active reabsorption of bile salts and the uptake of the B_{12}-intrinsic factor complex (Figure 70.2) are located in the distal ileum.

■ Etiology

The most common cause of impaired intraluminal digestion is deficient pancreatic enzyme secretion due to chronic pancreatitis, cystic fibrosis, or obstruction to the flow of pancreatic juice (Table 70.1). The steatorrhea in high gastric acid secretory states (**Zollinger-Ellison syndrome**) results from acid inactivation of pancreatic enzymes. Rapid gastric emptying and the altered anatomy created by gastric operations may lead to poor mixing between pancreatic secretions and ingested food. The normal postprandial pancreatic enzyme output is 10 times what is required for food digestion; malabsorption

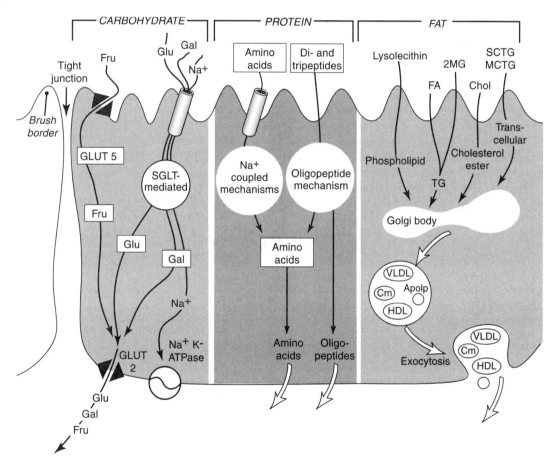

FIGURE 70.1. Schematic presentation of absorption of carbohydrate, protein and fat from the small bowel. Glucose transporters (GLUT), sodium-glucose transporters (SGLT) represent special transport mechanisms of absorption across the brush border. Components of absorbed lipid are reassembled in the Golgi body and transported across the cell using a process of exocytosis. 2MG = diglyceride; ApoLP = Apolipoprotein; Cm = chylomicron; FA = fatty acid; Fru = fructose; Gal = galactose; Glu = glucose; GLUT = glucose transporter; HDL = high-density lipoprotein; MCTG = medium-chain triglycerides; SCTG = short-chain triglycerides; SGLT = sodium-glucose co-transporter; TG = triglyceride; VLDL = very low-density lipoprotein.

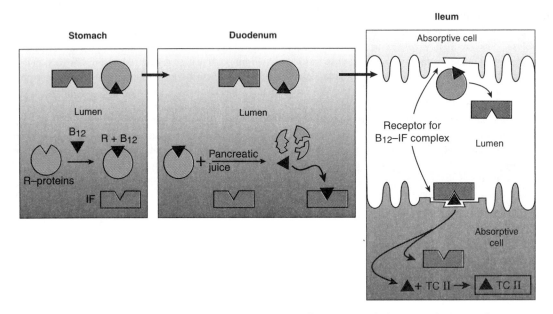

FIGURE 70.2. Schematic of vitamin B_{12} (cobalamin) absorption. Lower halves of the three panels show the normal process of B_{12} absorption. The top panels indicated by red lines represent B_{12} malabsorption in pancreatic exocrine insufficiency, in which tryptic digestion of R-proteins is absent. TC II = transcobalamin II; IF = intrinsic factor. Note that intrinsic factor binds vitamin B_{12} only in the absence of intact R-proteins.

occurs only when pancreatic enzyme output is below 10% of normal. Any process that reduces intraduodenal bile acid concentration may impair fat absorption.

Specific diseases causing malabsorption are discussed in chapter 80. **Disaccharidase deficiencies** are inherited, but may also be acquired with acute or chronic intestinal mucosal injury. Lactase is most vulnerable in this regard. **Diffuse small bowel disease** causes malabsorption of all nutrients, vitamins, and minerals. In contrast, **pancreatic enzyme deficiency** only affects the utilization of nutrients requiring digestion. **Bile salt deficiency**, in turn, impairs the absorption of fat as well as of fat-soluble vitamins (A, D, E, K).

■ Diagnostic Evaluation

Clues to malabsorption include **anemia** without apparent blood loss, but with low serum iron, folate, or B_{12}; **koilonychia** (spoon nails) seen in iron deficiency; glossitis and cheilitis with folate, B_{12}, and iron deficiency; paresthesias and **tetany** due to Ca^{++} or Mg^{++} deficiency; **bleeding diathesis** from vitamin K deficiency; **bulky, malodorous stools** (visible fat droplets suggest pancreatic insufficiency); **spontaneous fractures** due to Ca^{++} and vitamin D deficiency; and **edema** from **hypoproteinemia.** Weight loss is nonspecific, and more often due to poor food intake than to malabsorption.

Steatorrhea

Identifying excess fat excretion is central to evaluating malabsorption. Because long-chain triglycerides and fatty acids (FA) are not degraded in the colon, stool fat reliably and quantitatively indicates generalized malabsorption. Total FA is measured in a 2- or 3-day stool collection, while the patient receives a regular diet. A high-fat diet is generally neither needed nor feasible. Normal stool fat content is 6–7g/d, but may be as high as 15g/d during severe watery diarrhea. Thus, **steatorrhea** in patients with a stool weight over 600g/d is defined as a stool fat excretion exceeding 15g/d. Qualitative tests for fat malabsorption, while less onerous to perform, are also less accurate; they include Sudan III stain for fecal fat droplets, serum carotene, and breath tests for $^{14}CO_2$ after oral test doses of ^{14}C-labeled fat compounds.

Small intestinal biopsy

Mucosal biopsies can be obtained endoscopically or with special instruments from distal duodenum or proximal jejunum. When properly handled, biopsy is highly useful (Table 70.2).

Pancreatic exocrine function

In practice, pancreatic exocrine insufficiency is commonly inferred when pancreatic calcifications are noted on plain x-rays or atrophy on CT scans, or from abnormal pancreatic duct anatomy found during endoscopic retrograde pancreatography. The **secretin test,** the gold standard for assessing pancreatic exocrine function, involves aspiration and analysis of duodenal contents for volume and HCO_3 output following IV injection of secretin. It is expensive and requires specially trained personnel. In the **bentiromide (MBT-PABA) test,** pancreatic chymotrypsin hydrolyzes an orally administered peptide; the output of p-aminobenzoic acid thus liberated is measured in a 6-hour urine collection. In 80% of advanced pancreatic insufficiency and steatorrhea, less than 50% of the dose is excreted.

Vitamin B$_{12}$ (cobalamin) absorption

Schilling Test (Figure 128.4) is used to assess B_{12} absorption. Essentially, the 24-hour urinary excretion of orally administered, radio-labeled B_{12} is measured (Stage I). An abnormal Stage I establishes B_{12} malabsorption. In Stage II, intrinsic factor (IF) is added to the oral test dose. Its results will be normal if the defect is absence of gastric IF (pernicious anemia). Four additional possibilities may explain abnormal Stage I and Stage II test results: (1) ileal disease or resection; (2) congenital absence of the ileal receptor for the B_{12}-IF complex; (3) B_{12} uptake by bacterial overgrowth in the small intestine or by D. latum, the fish tapeworm; and (4) pancreatic insufficiency. Nonspecific salivary and gastric R-proteins successfully compete with IF for binding to B_{12} at the acidic gastric pH. Pancreatic proteases destroy the R-proteins in the duodenum; the liberated B_{12} then combines with IF, which resists digestion (Figure 70.2). In pancreatic exocrine insufficiency, where proteolytic activity in the duodenum is low, the B_{12}-R-protein complex remains intact, but no ileal receptor exists for the absorption of this complex. Therefore, stages I and II of the test may be abnormal in patients with pancreatic insufficiency; it normalizes when the test is repeated with the administration of adequate doses of pancreatic enzyme supplements.

Breath tests

Malabsorption of test compounds can be surmised if their breakdown by colonic bacteria produces highly diffusible, measurable, exhaled gases. Incremental rises in breath H_2 concentration during colonic carbohydrate fermentation is widely used to detect carbohydrate malabsorption—for example, lactose and sucrose breath tests for diagnosing lactase and sucrase-isomaltase deficiency, respectively, and a glucose breath test to detect anaerobic bacterial overgrowth in the small bowel. The time of the rise in breath H_2 after an oral dose of a poorly absorbed sugar, such as lactulose, gives an indication of the orocecal transit time.

Miscellaneous tests

While most serum proteins entering the GI tract are digested, reabsorbed, or degraded, serum α_1-antitrypsin largely appears intact in the stool. Its GI clearance can be measured using serum level and its daily output in the stool. Other tests can suggest the malabsorption of specific nutrients—for example, low serum folate, B_{12}, iron, albumin, calcium, and magnesium; serum vitamin D, urinary Ca^{++}, and elevated alkaline phosphatase (bone fraction), and prothrombin time.

■ Management

Treatment of malabsorption disorders is discussed in chapters 80 and 95. Dietary management is discussed here. Fat intake should be curtailed to 40–60 g daily because high stool fat causes diarrhea and abdominal discomfort. Carbohydrate restriction may be similarly needed in intestinal disease, but not in pancreatic insufficiency where little carbohydrate malabsorption occurs. Patients with infectious diarrhea and those with diffuse intestinal diseases frequently have transient lactase deficiency, and dairy products should be avoided. Medium chain triglycerides (MCT; fatty acids of C_8 and C_{10} chain length) can be absorbed intact, without the need for digestion and solubilization, and have theoretical advantages in pancreatic insufficiency and bile salt deficiency states. However, MCT substitution for dietary fat leads to weight gain only in patients with cystic fibrosis and may actually cause osmotic diarrhea. Vitamin, calcium, and iron deficits should first be corrected by the oral route, but parenteral supplementation may have to be employed when the underlying malabsorption prevents a therapeutic response.

TABLE 70.2.	Usefulness of Proximal Small Bowel Mucosal Biopsy

Diagnostic
 Whipple's disease
 Amyloidosis
 Giardiasis
 Eosinophilic enteritis
 Lymphangiectasia
 Mastocytosis
 Opportunistic pathogens (immunosuppressed patients)
 Immunoglobulin A (IgA) deficiency
 Lymphoma
Suggestive
 Tropical sprue
 Idiopathic intestinal pseudo-obstruction
 Celiac sprue
 Bacterial overgrowth (aspirated fluid)
 Antro-duodenal Crohn's disease

CHAPTER 71   GASTROINTESTINAL HEMORRHAGE

■ Definitions and Etiology

Blood loss from the gastrointestinal tract may be **gross** (obvious to the observer) or **occult** (not obvious). **Gross bleeding** is generally *acute* on presentation, with or without hemodynamic instability from volume depletion. **Chronic GI bleeding** is usually occult and generally without associated hypovolemia. GI bleeding may present as hematemesis, melena, hematochezia, or a combination of these. **Hematemesis** is vomiting blood that can be either red or acid-altered, appearing like "coffee grounds." It generally signifies bleeding proximal to the ligament of Treitz. **Melena** is black, tarry, foul-smelling stools, usually due to acute bleeding anywhere between the proximal GI tract and the right colon. **Hematochezia** is the passing of maroon or bright red stools originating from any site in the GI tract; when this site is proximal GI tract, the bleeding is brisk enough to advance rapidly to the rectum. Patients with chronic GI bleeding present with symptoms of anemia—for example, dyspnea, fatigue, syncope, and angina. Others are identified by a positive fecal occult blood test, or on screening tests showing iron deficiency anemia.

Among some of the causes of GI bleeding shown in Table 71.1, a few account for most of the bleeding episodes encountered clinically. More than 90% of upper-GI bleeds are secondary to peptic ulcer disease,

---

TABLE 71.1.   Some Causes of Gastrointestinal Bleeding

Esophagus
  Esophagitis, varices, ulcer, neoplasm
Stomach and Duodenum
  Gastric erosions, Mallory-Weiss tear, ulcer, varices, neoplasm, vascular anomalies
Small Bowel
  Meckel's diverticulum, Crohn's disease, infarction, vascular anomalies, aorto-enteric fistula
Colon
  Inflammatory bowel disease, infectious colitis, ischemia, neoplasm, vascular anomalies, diverticulosis
Rectum/Anus
  Proctitis, solitary ulcer, neoplasm, hemorrhoids
Systemic Conditions
  Thrombocytopenia, coagulopathies, chronic renal failure, swallowed blood

---

gastric erosions, Mallory-Weiss tears, and esophageal varices (Figure 71.1). Common lesions causing lower-GI bleeding are hemorrhoids, diverticula, neoplasms, and colitis (discussed below).

■ Management

Approach to a patient with acute GI bleeding begins with prompt **assessment of hemodynamic stability.** Patients with orthostatic hypotension or shock should first be stabilized with IV infusion of crystalloids; blood is sent for crossmatching, complete count including platelets, coagulation profile, liver tests, electrolytes, blood urea nitrogen, and creatinine before embarking on diagnostic investigations. Such patients are best managed in an intensive care unit with early surgical consultation. The amount of visible bleeding does not reliably indicate the degree of blood loss. For example, a little blood near the mouth or lower rectum might appear more impressive than bleeding that cannot be easily seen. In early, acute GI bleeding, hematocrit value is unreliable, because it does not decrease until the extracellular fluid shifts into the intravascular compartment, which takes several hours. The need for blood transfusion is dictated by the presence of ongoing bleeding, hemodynamic instability arising from volume loss, and pre-existing medical conditions that lower the patient's tolerance to blood loss. An initially low hematocrit with relatively stable vital signs suggests chronic GI blood loss, particularly if the mean corpuscular volume (MCV) is low. Such cases do not require urgent resuscitation unless the anemia has exacerbated an associated condition such as heart failure or angina pectoris. Since volume depletion is absent, packed RBC should be slowly transfused, with a close watch for volume overload.

The **timing of further diagnostic procedures** depends on the rate of ongoing bleeding and the need for urgent therapeutic intervention. After resuscitation, patients with acute, significant GI bleeding require immediate diagnostic procedures, which guide emergent endoscopic or surgical intervention. Patients with chronic GI blood loss can usually be investigated electively. A nasogastric tube may be passed first to examine the aspirate. A positive Gastroccult™ test on the gastric aspirate could be secondary to nasogastric tube-related trauma. However, an upper GI lesion is the likely source if the aspirate shows fresh or altered blood. Aspirate negative for visible blood, however, does not rule out an upper GI source, as seen, at times, with lesions distal to the pylorus. Endoscopy most accurately, rapidly, and

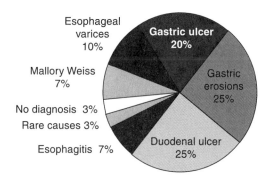

FIGURE 71.1. Etiology of upper GI bleeding.

safely identifies the bleeding site, with the additional advantage of allowing therapeutic interventions and obtaining tissue for histology. Upper GI endoscopy, anoscopy, proctosigmoidoscopy, and colonoscopy are some of the commonly performed endoscopic procedures. The small bowel can be evaluated by single- or double-contrast barium examination or by endoscopic enteroscopy.

In 5–10% of cases, endoscopy may not identify the site of bleeding, either because the lesion is beyond its reach or because brisk bleeding and large blood clots prevent adequate visualization. While angiography may be used in these patients, it will not detect slow or intermittent bleeding. A radioisotope labeled red cell scan, while more sensitive in this context, may not localize the bleeding site correctly.

Most patients with GI bleeding recover without active therapeutic intervention, especially those with esophagitis, gastritis, Mallory-Weiss tear, peptic ulcers, angiodysplasia, or diverticulosis. Those who continue to bleed or experience recurrent bleeding require urgent therapy. Active bleeding, a visible blood vessel, or a fresh blood clot in the ulcer base seen on endoscopy indicate high risk of continued or recurrent bleeding. Many highly effective, endoscopic therapies (e.g., thermocoagulation, electrocoagulation, laser photocoagulation, and submucosal injection of a sclerosant or epinephrine) can be applied in these patients. Bleeding esophageal and gastric varices may require either injection sclerotherapy or banding; other methods for controlling variceal bleeding include the insertion of an endoluminal compression device (Sengstaken-Blakemore- or Minnesota tube) and IV vasopressin or somatostatin analog and transjugular intrahepatic portosystemic shunting (TIPS). Neoplastic lesions, such as polyps, can be removed endoscopically. Selective arterial embolization or vasopressin injection are options when endoscopy fails. Early surgery is indicated for persistent and life-threatening bleeding and in patients over 60 years of age, in whom the mortality risk rises with every episode of re-bleeding.

CHAPTER 72

NONMALIGNANT DISEASES OF THE ESOPHAGUS

The esophagus is a hollow, muscular conduit that conveys swallowed material from the oropharynx to the stomach and prevents the reflux of gastric contents. Esophageal muscle, along with the cricopharyngeus, and the lower fibers of inferior pharyngeal constrictor function as the upper esophageal sphincter (UES), which marks the proximal end of the esophagus. The esophageal body, about 25 cm long, terminates in the lower esophageal sphincter (LES), which has important functional properties but no distinctive anatomic features.

Swallowing is initiated voluntarily by pressing the tip of the tongue against the hard palate, after which the tongue rises against the hard palate, propelling the bolus back into the pharynx. The rest of the swallowing action is a reflex. The muscles of the soft palate and nasopharynx contract, shutting off the posterior nasal opening. The larynx is pulled upward and forward, away from the path of the food bolus and toward the base of the tongue, closing the airway, as the epiglottis retroverts to occlude the laryngeal orifice. Pharyngeal contractions move the bolus toward the esophageal introitus. Muscle relaxation, pull by the anteriorly and superiorly moving larynx, and bolus pressure, open the UES. Peristaltic esophageal contraction wave continues downward while the LES relaxes to allow the bolus to pass into the stomach.

The normal swallow wave, or **primary peristalsis,** comprises sequential contractions of the body of the esophagus starting at the upper end and propagating downward. It is associated with complete relaxation of the LES (Figure 72.1). Propagating motility patterns induced by esophageal distention are termed **secondary peristalsis. Tertiary contractions** occur simultaneously and are nonpropagating; they may be spontaneous or swallow-induced.

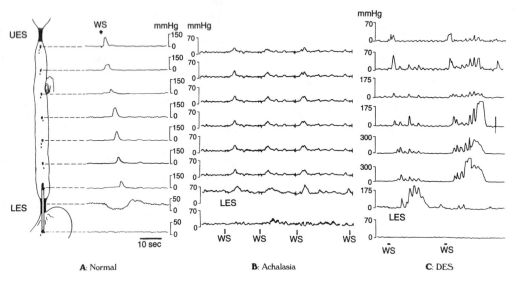

FIGURE 72.1. Esophageal manometry. A. Normal peristalsis showing propagating contractions in the body of the esophagus with complete LES relaxation. B. Patient with achalasia showing simultaneous low amplitude contractions in the body of the esophagus with incomplete LES relaxation.

C. Patient with diffuse esophageal spasm (DES) showing peristaltic contractions followed by simultaneous high amplitude contractions. UES = upper esophageal sphincter; LES = lower esophageal sphincter; WS = water swallow.

Gastroesophageal Reflux Disease

Gastroesophageal reflux disease (GERD), one of the most common GI disorders, includes conditions characterized by clinical symptoms and/or histopathological changes produced by episodes of gastroesophageal reflux (GER).

■ Etiology and Pathophysiology

Except when its tone is reduced, the LES closes by tonic contraction, producing a pressure of 15–30 mm Hg above intragastric pressure. Normally, the LES tone and the low frequency of spontaneous (inappropriate) LES relaxations mainly help prevent gastroesophageal reflux. During GER, gastric contents enter the esophagus through three major suggested mechanisms. During **transient lower esophageal sphincter relaxation** (tLESR), the LES relaxes without any antecedent swallow and the relaxation persists longer than with swallow-induced relaxation. This may predispose to GER, especially during the post-prandial period. **Hypotensive LES** (which is present in a few patients, including those with GERD due to scleroderma) allows free GER. Thirdly, sudden rises in **intra-abdominal pressure** may exceed the LES resting pressure and induce GER. When a hiatal hernia is present, the "pinchcock" effect of the crural diaphragm on the LES is absent, which facilitates GER with rises in intraluminal

pressure. Refluxed material may become trapped in the hernia sac and becomes available for return to the esophagus. Nearly all the refluxate is cleared by esophageal peristalsis. The minimal residual acidic material is eventually neutralized by swallowed saliva. The time that the esophagus remains acidified is called the **esophageal clearance time.**

Gastroesophageal reflux occurs regularly even in healthy people, mostly secondary to tLESRs. GERD develops when there is a disturbed balance between the potency of the refluxate and the ability of the esophagus to withstand (mucosal resistance) and clear the refluxate. GERD occurs in a variety of clinical settings. In scleroderma, the LES pressure is low and the amplitude of esophageal peristalsis decreased, predisposing to both GER *and* longer esophageal clearance time. Pregnancy-related reflux is secondary to raised intra-abdominal pressure and hormones lowering the LES pressure. Fatty meals, coffee, tea, alcohol, and smoking lower the LES pressure and delay gastric emptying. Certain drugs (calcium channel blockers and anticholinergics) also lower the LES pressure.

■ Clinical Features

Most patients with GERD report frequent heartburn. However, heartburn may be absent in some patients with esophagitis or with complications like esophageal stricture and Barrett's esophagus (where the native esophageal squamous epithelium is replaced by specialized columnar epithelium). Sour and bitter fluid, occasionally even food, may regurgitate into the pharynx or mouth. Often, these symptoms are induced or worsened by bending forward or lifting. While dysphagia is usually due to peptic stricture, it may also be secondary to esophagitis related dysmotility and decreased esophageal compliance. In some patients, esophageal acidification leads to hypersalivation (water brash), whereas others report chest pain. GER with aspiration also leads to chronic cough (chapter 208), pneumonia, pharyngitis, laryngitis, and worsening of asthma.

■ **Diagnosis**

In most cases, a careful history is sufficient to make a diagnosis. Differential diagnosis includes infections (e.g., candida, herpes, cytomegalovirus) or pill-induced esophagitis, dyspepsia secondary to peptic ulcer or biliary tract diseases, and chest pain due to coronary heart disease or esophageal motor disorders. Barium swallow may show GER, any associated motility disorder, and strictures. Endoscopy is indicated for symptoms refractory to medical therapy, evaluation and dilatation of peptic strictures, and to exclude Barrett's metaplasia. Patients with GERD may have normal-appearing esophageal mucosa although biopsy may show microscopic esophagitis. Two tests are useful in relating the symptoms of heartburn and chest pain to the reflux. One is the **Bernstein esophageal acid perfusion test.** Through a tube placed in the mid-esophagus, normal saline is infused and is switched to 0.1 N HCl without the patient's knowledge. If this reproduces the patient's usual symptoms, the HCl is replaced by normal saline, which should relieve the symptoms. The other test is **ambulatory esophageal pH monitoring** (usually 24 hours) using an intraluminal pH probe placed transnasally. Evaluation of the tracings includes the percent of time the esophageal pH was acidic (pH <4.0; normal: up to 5%) the number

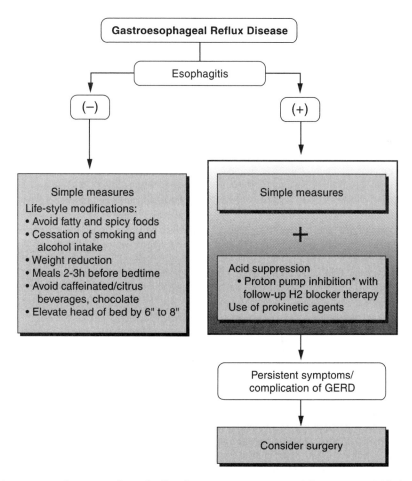

FIGURE **72.2.** Management of gastroesophageal reflux disease (GERD). * = In patients with erosive esophagitis whose symptoms recur while receiving H2 blockers, proton pump inhibitors can be used on a long-term basis.

of reflux episodes and the temporal relation between symptoms and the occurrence of reflux. Esophageal manometry is recommended prior to planned antireflux surgery.

■ Management

Treatment of GERD ranges from simple measures in uncomplicated cases to maximum acid suppression in patients with high-grade esophagitis (Figure 72.2). Acid suppression, using a proton pump inhibitor, initially for 6 weeks, is necessary in patients with persistent or severe symptoms and those with erosive esophagitis. Prokinetic drugs (metoclopramide, bethanechol, or cisapride) raise LES pressure, and increase gastric emptying; they can also be used either alone or with H2-receptor antagonists. Surgical management—that is, a fundoplication procedure—is reserved for those who have failed medical treatment, those who prefer not to be on long-term medications or are non-compliant (e.g., mentally retarded patients) or those with GERD-related complications (e.g., recurrent aspiration pneumonia, etc.).

Complications of GERD

Benign esophageal stricture most commonly results from peptic esophagitis. Most patients present with slowly progressive dysphagia, although some may present acutely with food impaction. Distinction is required from malignant strictures, motility disorders (achalasia), strictures from other causes (infection, pill-injury, lye ingestion), and esophageal webs, most commonly the Schatzki ring. Malignancy must be ruled out by biopsy and dysphagia relieved by mechanical dilatation. Vigorous antireflux measures are also needed. Patients with **esophageal ulcer** may report retrosternal chest pain, odynophagia, or epigastric pain. Some may have acute bleeding as the first and only symptom. Differential diagnosis includes ulcers caused by infection, pill injury, or malignancy. Endoscopic evaluation and biopsy are a must. Bleeding in GERD is usually chronic and due to esophagitis. **Acute bleeding** in GERD is usually due to esophageal ulcer. Rigorous medical therapy, as outlined, is called for. Occasionally, chronic bleeding arises from an ulcer within a sliding hiatal hernia at the level of the diaphragmatic hiatus.

In **Barrett's esophagus,** the native esophageal squamous epithelium is replaced by specialized columnar epithelium, most commonly with goblet cells and a villous pattern, representing incomplete intestinal metaplasia and, less commonly, with cardia- or fundic-type mucosa. This change starts at the g-e junction and progresses upward during the course of GERD. Barrett's mucosa by itself evokes no symptoms. While more resistant to the effects of acid reflux, the new mucosa is prone to dysplasia and adenocarcinoma. The risk of such neoplasia being 30–50 times that of the general population, it calls for regular surveillance endoscopic biopsies. Esophagectomy is recommended for high-grade dysplasia. The underlying GER calls for vigorous therapy; however, the presence and extent of Barrett's mucosa are not alleviated by medical or surgical anti-reflux therapy. Although photodynamic therapy (PDT) has been used with success for treating esophageal cancer, its role in ablating dysplasia associated with Barrett's esophagus requires further evaluation. In PDT, a photosensitizing agent (e.g., hematoporphyrin) is injected IV which then preferentially concentrates within the dysplastic tissue/tumor. Cytotoxic effect is achieved by activating the compound endoscopically, using a specific wavelength laser.

Motility Disorders of the Oropharynx and Esophagus

Oropharyngeal Disorders

Oropharyngeal motility disorders causing dysphagia can be due to any of the neuromuscular causes listed in Table 68.2. Symptoms may arise gradually or abruptly, depending on the etiology. Patients may report difficulty initiating a swallow, pharyngeal food residue after swallowing, nasal regurgitation, food getting held up in the throat, and coughing while swallowing. Some may have recurrent pneumonia. Video fluoroscopy during barium swallow, cine-esophagography, direct endoscopic visualization of the pharynx during swallowing, and pharyngeal manometry can be used to assess oropharyngeal dysphagia. Treatment is directed at the primary cause. Many patients with cerebrovascular accidents recover with time. Others may require training in swallowing exercises best supervised by a speech therapist.

Achalasia

Achalasia is a primary esophageal motility disorder featuring progressive dysphagia for liquids and solids, and delayed esophageal emptying, in the absence of an organic obstructing lesion. Postulated but unproven mechanisms include a viral etiology and defects in the esophageal neural pathways. Primarily, there is loss of ganglion cells in the esophageal myenteric plexus. Smooth muscle denervation leads to weak, nonprogressive, esophageal contractions, incomplete swallow-induced LES relaxation, and elevation of the basal LES pressure. An identical disorder occurs with chronic Chaga's disease, where *Trypanosoma cruzi* destroys the intramural ganglia. Although achalasia may present at any age, the onset of symptoms is usually in the fifth to sixth decade. The yearly incidence is about 1 per 100,000 population.

The slowly progressive dysphagia may be associated with weight loss. Regurgitation of food while bending or recumbent is common and may lead to pulmonary aspiration and pneumonia. Unlike gastroesophageal reflux, regurgitation in achalasia is usually not associated with heartburn. Some patients report chest pain (see "vigorous achalasia," below). Esophageal cancer may be associated, especially in those who have had no (or unsatisfactory) treatment. Plain x-rays may reveal a widened mediastinum with an air-fluid level and no gastric air bubble. Esophagogram shows no peristalsis in

the distal two-thirds of the esophagus, and the lower esophagus tapers to a beak-like ending (Figure 72.3A). The esophagus may be of normal caliber or dilated and tortuous, and may contain retained food. Endoscopy should be done to rule out a cancer (of the gastric cardia or fundus) that mimics achalasia-like symptoms, the so called **pseudo-achalasia.**

Characteristic findings on manometry (Figure 72.1) include absent peristalsis, weak or repetitive contractions in the esophageal body, incomplete LES relaxation, raised LES- and intraesophageal pressures. The LES pressure may rise paradoxically after cholecystokinin octapeptide injection. A subset of patients have chest pain and high-amplitude, nonpropagating esophageal contractions **(vigorous achalasia).** Calcium channel-blocking agents (e.g., nifedipine) or nitrates may bring mild or modest symptomatic improvement and may be tried initially. However, eventually patients will require pneumatic dilatation of the LES or surgery (Heller myotomy). Recently, success has been reported by endoscopically injecting a muscle-weakening toxin (botulinum toxin) into the LES.

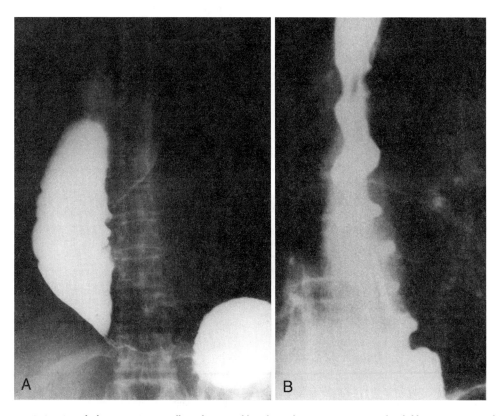

FIGURE **72.3.** A. Achalasia. Barium swallow showing dilated esophagus, tapering to a beak-like narrowing at the lower end. B. Diffuse esophageal spasm with tertiary contractions.

Diffuse Esophageal Spasm

Diffuse esophageal spasm (DES) is a rare, idiopathic primary esophageal motility disorder, where high-amplitude tertiary contractions occur with normal peristalsis. The lower two-thirds of the esophagus shows diffuse muscular thickening, but ganglion cells are preserved. Odynophagia, dysphagia, and substernal chest pain simulating angina, with radiation to the neck, jaw, shoulders, and back, and even relieved by nitroglycerin, are the main symptoms. The pain may be spontaneous or incited by emotional stress or drinking hot or cold liquids, but not related to exercise or relieved by rest. The dysphagia varies in severity and may not accompany chest pain. Esophagogram shows tertiary contractions (Figure 72.3B); manometry shows more than 10% simultaneous contractions during water swallows and intermittent normal peristalsis (Figure 72.1). Reducing stress, avoiding cold or hot foods, and therapy with long-acting nitrates and calcium channel-blockers may help. Nitroglycerin may relieve acute attacks of pain. Pneumatic dilatation may help some patients while a long esophagomyotomy may benefit those with severe, intractable symptoms.

Esophageal Webs, Rings

A **web** is a 2–3 mm thick structure comprised of mucosa and submucosa. A **ring** is a thicker structure containing mucosal and muscle tissue (except Schatzki's ring, which is really a web). An anterior web at the upper end of the esophagus is seen in **Plummer-Vinson syndrome (Patterson-Kelly syndrome).** If dysphagia and iron deficiency anemia are associated, it is termed **sideropenic dysphagia.** Most patients are middle-aged or elderly women. A predisposition to develop postcricoid carcinoma is present. Esophagogram shows these webs best in the lateral projection. Circumferential cervical webs may require forceful dilatation.

The lower esophageal web (**Schatzki's ring**) is a persistent, annular, thin narrowing of the esophagus at the squamocolumnar junction, with squamous epithelium above and columnar mucosa below. Patients present with intermittent dysphagia. Typically, a bolus of meat gets impacted, which is then regurgitated; the patient then continues eating without further dysphagia. Occasionally, sudden, total dysphagia may occur, requiring endoscopic disimpaction. Schatzki's rings are best demonstrated by barium swallow. Dysphagia due to subtle webs and rings can be evaluated by barium marshmallow swallow study. Thicker rings probably represent short strictures due to reflux disease. Endoscopy is required to differentiate between lower esophageal ring and an annular stricture, which can be secondary to cancer. Those causing symptoms require dilatation.

Other Conditions

Infectious Esophagitis

Candida albicans is part of normal gut flora. Conditions that alter the normal gut ecology lead to colonization. Invasion of tissue by candida, i.e., **Candida esophagitis,** usually occurs with defects in body immunity (AIDS, leukemia, lymphoma, congenital immunodeficiency states, and chemo- or immunosuppressive therapy). It can also follow medical conditions like diabetes mellitus, adrenal insufficiency, and malnutrition. Retention of food in the esophagus, as occurs in esophageal stricture, diverticula, and achalasia, can also predispose to Candida esophagitis. The condition may be asymptomatic or lead to retrosternal pain and odynophagia. Oral thrush occurs in most cases. If untreated, mucosal sloughing and perforation may occur. Stricture may follow ulcerative esophagitis. Double-contrast barium esophagogram shows mucosal lesions—plaques, inflammation, shaggy outline, ulcers, or strictures. Endoscopy may show white plaques, confluent pseudomembranes, mucosal friability, ulceration, bleeding, and sloughing. As the fungus is a normal commensal, brushing and cultures are not diagnostic.

Only biopsies can accurately diagnose tissue invasion. Based on the severity of the esophagitis, one may use luminally active drugs (nystatin, clotrimazole) systemically acting oral drugs (ketoconazole, fluconazole), or IV medications (amphotericin B, miconazole). Oral drugs are also used prophylactically in the immunosuppressed.

Herpes simplex virus (HSV) esophagitis can occur in normal or immunocompromised hosts. HSV invades the squamous epithelium, forming vesicles that slough. Discrete ulcers can coalesce, leading to widespread denudation of the esophageal mucosa. Patients usually report retrosternal pain, odynophagia, nausea, vomiting, and hematemesis. A presumptive diagnosis can be made if oral HSV infection is evident. Esophagogram shows multiple esophageal ulcers. As HSV primarily invades the squamous epithelium, endoscopic biopsies are taken from the edge of an ulcer. HSV is identified by histology, immunohistology, or culture. Patients with intact immunity heal spontaneously. Immunodeficient patients require prophylaxis or treatment with acyclovir. Acyclovir-resistant strains may require foscarnet.

Cytomegalovirus (CMV) esophagitis is seen in immunosuppressed patients. It may be acquired (blood product transfusion, organ transplant) or activated from a latent state. Unlike HSV that infects squamous epithelium, CMV invades submucosal fibroblasts and endothelial cells, thus making endoscopic biopsies from the center and not the edge of an ulcer more relevant for its diagnosis. CMV lesions start as serpiginous ulcers that coalesce to form giant ulcers, usually in the mid- and lower esophagus. Patients report nausea, vomiting, odynophagia, or hematemesis, but unlike candida or HSV, acute severe retrosternal pain is unusual. Barium study may show a large esophageal ulcer. Endoscopic biopsies should be examined by routine histology, immunohistology, and culture. Ganciclovir is effective for prevention and treatment of CMV infection. Those refractory to ganciclovir can be given foscarnet.

Esophageal Injuries

Accidental or suicidal ingestion of corrosive material (lye, drain cleaners, mineral acids such as HCl, H_2SO_4) can cause significant esophageal damage, leading to severe inflammation, bleeding, perforation, and long strictures. Presence or absence of oral burns correlates poorly with the degree of esophageal involvement. Urgent endoscopy is required to assess the extent of esophageal and upper GI tract injury. Treatment is generally supportive. Corticosteroids have been tried with variable success to reduce the degree of inflammation and subsequent fibrosis. Patients with lye injury are prone to develop esophageal cancer. **Pill injury** of the esophagus occurs when pills get held up in the esophagus, mostly at the level of the aortic arch, causing localized mucosal damage. Quinidine, iron salts, tetracycline, NSAIDs, and potassium are common offenders. The size, shape, and coating of the pill and the habit of swallowing them without or with only minimum water have all been implicated in the pathogenesis of pill injury. Most of these injuries occur in patients with a normal esophagus. Symptoms are chest pain, odynophagia, GI bleeding, perforation, or dysphagia secondary to a stricture. Most pill injuries resolve within 6 weeks. Esophageal injuries also follow radiation, chemotherapy, and sclerotherapy or banding of esophageal varices.

Mallory-Weiss Syndrome

Vomiting and retching generate high gastric pressures that can cause a longitudinal tear in the gastric mucosa just below the g-e junction that can extend into the lower esophagus. Patients frequently report vomiting gastric contents first, followed by bright red blood. Some patients lack a prior history of vomiting. Endoscopy is the best means of confirming the diagnosis although the lesion can easily be missed. If an active bleeding site is identified, it can be treated endoscopically. Some may require surgical exploration. In most cases, the bleeding stops spontaneously.

▪ Perforation

Esophageal perforation can either be spontaneous or traumatic. Spontaneous perforation could follow vomiting (Boerhaave syndrome), esophageal ulcers, caustic injuries, pill injuries, infections, or neoplasms. Traumatic perforation may follow blunt or penetrating injuries or could be iatrogenic (instrumentation or surgery). The most common sites are the cervical and lower thoracic esophagus. Patients report chest pain. Fever and signs of mediastinitis, subcutaneous emphysema, or pleural effusion may be noted. Pleural effusions characteristically have a low pH, high amylase (salivary), abundant bacteria, and sometimes, food particles. Lower esophageal perforation can mimic an acute upper abdominal crisis. Chest x-ray may reveal pleural effusion, pneumomediastinum, or subcutaneous air. Imaging with water-soluble contrast is invaluable in detecting intrathoracic perforation. Endoscopy is useless and unsafe, as it may extend an incomplete perforation during intubation or air insufflation.

Contamination by saliva and food is avoided by totally avoiding any food or fluids by mouth. Anticholinergics may be given to reduce salivary flow. Almost all patients require broad-spectrum antibiotics. Contaminated perforations and those communicating with the pleural space or abdominal cavity require immediate surgery. However, in practice, most spontaneous perforations do require surgery, given their late recognition and significant contamination. An instrumentation-related perforation can be conservatively treated, provided it is recognized early. Perforation complicating esophageal cancer can be treated by placing an esophageal endoprosthesis.

CHAPTER 73   CARCINOMA OF THE ESOPHAGUS

■ Epidemiology

Delayed diagnosis and resultant incurability make esophageal cancer one of the most dismal of all cancers. **Squamous cell carcinoma** and adenocarcinoma are the main types of esophageal cancers. While the squamous cell type is one of the most common cancers worldwide, it is relatively infrequent in North America. In the United States, it shows a distinct (3:1) preponderance among older (seventh decade) men. Black men are at higher risk. Predisposing factors are alcohol consumption, smoking, corrosive esophageal injury, Plummer-Vinson syndrome with anemia, and achalasia. **Adenocarcinoma,** which arises from Barrett's mucosa or esophageal mucous glands, accounts for one-third of esophageal cancers, and its incidence is rising among Caucasian men.

■ Clinical Features and Management

Most patients present with recent dysphagia for solids that rapidly progresses to dysphagia for liquids. Odynophagia and bleeding are also common. Over one-half of patients note significant weight loss. Some experience pulmonary symptoms related to esophageal obstruction and aspiration or to tracheoesophageal fistula, or hoarseness due to paralysis of the recurrent laryngeal nerve. Chest x-ray may show metastases or complications such as pneumonia. Esophagogram may show a stricturing, polypoid, or ulcerated lesion (Figure 73.1). Endoscopy is essential for tissue diagnosis. Endoscopic ultrasound, CT scan, bronchoscopy, lymph node biopsy, and mediastinoscopy may all be required for staging, which is TNM-based.

Because the esophagus lacks serosa, most esophageal tumors have spread by the time of diagnosis. Survival rate for adenocarcinoma of the esophagus is similar to that for squamous cell carcinoma. Only about 50% of patients with esophageal cancer are considered operable, and less than half of these are resectable, leaving palliation as the only viable option for the majority of these patients at initial presentation. The major goal of palliation is to relieve dysphagia, which is achieved by *surgical removal* of the primary lesion with esophagogastric anastomosis or colonic interposition, or, *nonsurgical options* of dilatation, endoprosthesis placement (also addresses esophagotracheal fistula), or tumor ablation with heat (bicap), laser, (including photodynamic therapy [PDT]) or alcohol injection and irradiation. These can be combined as, for example, surgery with irradiation. Chemotherapy confers limited benefit. Good nutritional support is essential, and in some cases, intensive therapy for pain.

With screening programs for conditions like Barrett's esophagus, an increasing number of esophageal cancers are now being diagnosed early. Esophagectomy in such patients has a 5-year survival rate above 90%. In patients with small esophageal cancer who pose a high surgical risk, PDT is being tried as an alternative therapy.

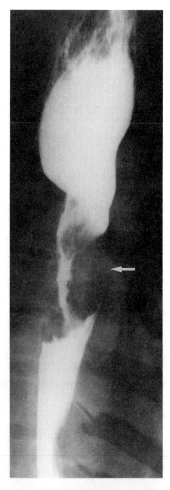

FIGURE 73.1. Esophageal cancer. Barium swallow showing an irregular, ulcerated stricture (arrow) in the esophagus.

CHAPTER 74 GASTRIC PHYSIOLOGY AND TESTS OF GASTRIC FUNCTION

The portion of the proximal stomach that is adjacent to the esophagogastric junction is the cardia, and the dome-shaped portion to the left of it and lying beneath the left hemidiaphragm is the fundus. Extending downward and to the right is the corpus, or body, the main portion of the stomach. The narrower distal stomach, or the antrum, ends in the pylorus, a narrow channel that connects with the first portion of the duodenum, known to radiologists as the "bulb."

Gastric motor functions include storage and volume adaptation, mixing of contents, trituration of solid food particles, and propulsion (emptying). The stomach has two distinct motor regions, each with a different functional role. The **proximal stomach** (the fundus and upper body) acts as a reservoir and is capable of receptive relaxation (increase in gastric volume without a corresponding increase in intragastric pressure). The proximal stomach exerts slow, sustained, or tonic contractions that, by steady pressure on its contents, gradually press them toward the distal stomach. This mechanism is largely responsible for emptying of liquids from stomach to duodenum. The **distal stomach,** which performs mixing and grinding, has a major regulatory role in the gastric emptying of solids; its motor activity is controlled by the gastric pacemaker, located in the smooth muscle cells in the midbody of the stomach.

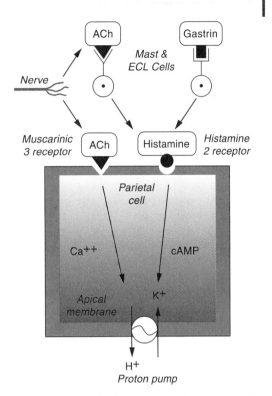

FIGURE **74.1.** Parietal cell and acid secretion. See text for details. ACh = Acetylcholine; cAMP: = cyclic adenosine monophosphate; ECL = enterochromaffin-like cells.

■ Gastric Acid Secretion

Gastric secretion is under neuroendocrine control, an integrated autoregulatory system with stimulatory and inhibitory influences acting to modulate and adjust gastric secretion to specific needs after food intake, as well as during the interdigestive period. The principal constituents of gastric juice are HCl, electrolytes (Na^+, K^+, Cl^-, HCO_3), mucus, digestive enzymes, and intrinsic factor. Gastrin, produced by G cells located mainly in the antrum, is the main hormone-stimulating gastric acid secretion under physiologic circumstances. The parietal cell secretes H^+-ions by an Mg-dependent H^+, K^+-ATPase (the proton pump), which is located exclusively in its luminal secretory membrane. The H^+ secretion is activated by histamine binding to H2- receptors and, to a lesser extent, by acetylcholine (ACh) binding to M_3-receptors, both located on the basolateral aspect of the parietal cell. Histamine is released from nearby enterochromaffin-like (ECL) and mast cells in response to the receptor binding of gastrin and ACh. The parietal cell secretion is down-regulated by paracrine release of somatostatin and prostaglandins. The histamine effect on the parietal cell is mediated by cyclic AMP-, and the ACh action by Ca^{++}- dependent mechanisms (Figure 74.1).

Neural stimulation is triggered at different stages of eating a meal. Anticipation, sight, and smell constitute the **cephalic phase.** The tasting, chewing, and swallowing of food, and food in the stomach (probably via distention), all cause acid secretion through neural reflexes; distention also leads to gastrin release that, in turn, stimulates parietal cells to produce HCl. Partially digested proteins on contact with antral mucosa, a neutral pH in the antral lumen, antral distention, and vagal impulses, also evoke gastrin release. Calcium, in the lumen or blood, stimulates acid production, through gastrin release and direct parietal cell stimulation. Caffeine, roast products in decaffeinated coffee, fermented alcoholic drinks, all stimulate acid production. Pure ethanol and distilled spirits have no effect on gastric secretion.

Inhibitory mechanisms for gastric secretion are located mainly beyond the pylorus. Secretin, cholecystokinin, and gastric inhibitory peptide (GIP) are released from duodenal or small bowel mucosa on stimulation variously by acid, fat, protein, and glucose in the lumen, and inhibit gastric acid secretion. Neural reflexes that originate in the duodenal bulb stimulated by acid inhibit acid secretion.

■ Pepsin and Intrinsic Factor

Pepsinogen, especially the pepsinogen I fraction, originates in chief cells and correlates well with acid secretory capacity. Stimuli that increase acid output also raise enzyme levels in the gastric juice. Pepsinogen, the proenzyme, is converted to pepsin by HCl and by pepsin. Intrinsic factor, a product of the parietal cell, depends only partially on stimuli for gastric acid secretion for its elaboration or secretion.

■ Procedures for Investigating Gastric/ Duodenal Disease

Measurement of gastric secretory capacity

Considerable inter- and intraindividual variation exists in measured acid secretory rates. Mean values are shown in Table 74.1. Secretory rates in patients with duodenal ulcer, as a group, exceed that of normals. Secretory rates for gastric ulcer patients, as a group, are about 60% of those for normals. Patients with gastrinomas (Zollinger-Ellison syndrome) show marked basal hypersecretion, with BAO over 15 mEq/h, and the BAO:MAO exceeding 0.66.

Gastric secretory assessment has little value in the routine diagnosis of peptic ulcer. It should be measured in patients suspected of having Zollinger-Ellison syndrome, and in patients with abdominal pain or GI bleeding following partial gastric resection and/or vago-

TABLE 74.1.	Mean Values of Gastric Acid Output (mEq/Hour)	
	Men	**Women**
Basal acid output (BAO)	4	2
Maximum acid output (MAO)	30	20
Peak acid output (PAO)	37	25
BAO/MAO Ratio	<.6	<.6

Modified sham feeding (MSF) test = 50% of PAO; lower limit = 10% of PAO.

tomy done for peptic ulcer disease. BAO or MAO values in the postoperative stomach exceeding 5 and 15 mEq/h, respectively, are highly predictive of recurrent ulcer. An intact response to modified sham feeding indicates persistent vagal innervation.

Serum Gastrin

The greatest value of determining serum gastrin is in identifying patients with ulcer disease due to hypergastrinemia, the hallmark of the Zollinger-Ellison syndrome. Hypergastrinemia also occurs in patients with achlorhydria (e.g., pernicious anemia, carcinoma of the stomach), renal insufficiency (mild to moderate hypergastrinemia), and may follow massive small bowel resection. The retention of antral mucosa in continuity with the duodenum following partial gastric resection and Billroth II anastomosis may lead to hypergastrinemia and stomal ulcer. Here, the antral gastrin cells are excluded from gastric acid or other inhibitory factors in the feedback regulation of antral gastrin release. Currently, the most common cause of hypergastrinemia is medication-induced hypo- or achlorhydria, particularly in patients treated with a "proton pump" inhibitor.

CHAPTER 75 GASTRITIS AND OTHER DISORDERS

Gastritis

The term "gastritis" has suffered from a looseness of definition and application, because it can be defined according to clinical presentation, endoscopic appearances, or histopathology. Moreover, gastritis does not always imply inflammatory changes. Gastropathy is a condition where epithelial and vascular changes predominate with minimum inflammatory cell reaction.

Erosive and Hemorrhagic Gastritis

An **erosion** is a break in the mucosa that does not penetrate the muscularis mucosae. Endoscopically, erosion appears as a whitish lesion with an erythematous halo. They are usually multiple. A black base implies recent bleeding. **Hemorrhagic gastritis** appears as petechiae, red streaks, or patches without any break in the mucosa. Patients with erosive or hemorrhagic gastritis may have no symptoms, or may report nausea, vomiting, GI bleeding, and upper abdominal pain. Endoscopy is the best means of diagnosis.

Aspirin and other NSAIDs cause gastritis, probably by topical mucosal effects and by suppressing endogenous prostaglandins. The fundic and corpus mucosa are more damaged than the antral mucosa. The onset is usually acute. Healing is rapid once the offending drug is withdrawn. Therapy with enteric coated NSAID preparations, or preventive therapy with synthetic prostaglandins (e.g., misoprostol) reduce NSAID-induced mucosal injuries. Gastritis may also follow alcohol intake, ingestion of corrosive agents, and drugs like potassium chloride. Severe stress, as in seriously ill patients, can compromise gastric mucosal defense and repair mechanisms, thus leading to lesions ranging from gastritis to complete ulcers. Gastritis may also follow radiation injury. Chronic erosive gastritis (diffuse varioliform gastritis), a disease of unclear etiology, has multiple erosions, seen endoscopically as small nodules with central umbilications. The condition may remit within months or persist for years.

Chronic Active Gastritis

With or without mucosal atrophy, chronic active gastritis (CAG) can involve the fundic mucosa (type A gastritis), antral mucosa (type B gastritis), the whole stomach (pangastritis), or be multifocal. Antral nodularity or thin folds with prominent vessels may be seen endoscopically. Histology is required for evaluating the type of mucosal involvement (superficial, full-thickness, atrophic), the existence of metaplasia (e.g., intestinal metaplasia), and the etiology (e.g., *Helicobacter pylori*). When atrophic gastritis spares the antrum, the low acid output evokes hypergastrinemia.

Helicobacter pylori (H. pylori) is a gram-negative, comma-shaped rod with potent urease activity. Its relationship with peptic ulcer disease is discussed later. Superficial chronic active gastritis is the most common type of gastritis associated with *H. pylori*. The exact mode of transmission is unknown. Intrafamilial clustering suggests person-to-person spread. Higher prevalence rates are seen with increasing age, lower socioeconomic status, and among Latinos/Latinas and African Americans. On histology, the organism is seen in the mucous layer near the surface and pit epithelial cells. Though the antral mucosa is predominantly affected, lesser degrees of inflammation are seen in the fundic and corpus mucosa. The organism can also be found in the duodenum in areas with gastric metaplasia. Diagnosis and treatment of *H. pylori* are addressed in chapter 76.

Chronic active gastritis can be seen in patients having alkaline (bile) reflux, usually following gastric resection and pyloroplasty. Atrophic gastritis is seen in elderly patients or in autoimmune conditions like pernicious anemia. Adenocarcinoma of the gastric antrum and body can be associated with multifocal atrophic gastritis and intestinal metaplasia.

Specific Gastritis

Cytomegalovirus, herpes virus, tuberculosis, and syphilis can cause gastritis. Gastritis can also occur in systemic conditions like sarcoidosis, Crohn's disease, chronic granulomatous disease, and graft-versus-host disease.

Menetrier's disease, a rare disease seen mostly in men over the age of 50, features giant folds in the proximal stomach, with a greatly thickened mucosa showing foveolar hyperplasia (abnormal pit epithelium with lengthening of pit) and glandular atrophy. Abnormal mucosa and superficial ulcers cause gastric protein loss leading to hypoproteinemia. A true link to cancer has not been shown. Clinical features include epigastric pain, diarrhea, microcytic anemia from chronic blood loss, and peripheral edema. Barium x-ray shows large and tortuous gastric folds. Diagnosis requires full-thickness mucosal biopsies by laparotomy or open biopsy. Mild symptoms may require no therapy; severe symptoms may dictate total gastrectomy. Acid suppression, corticosteroids, anticholinergics, and tranexamic have been tried with variable success.

Other Disorders of the Stomach

Diaphragmatic Hernias

The diaphragm separates the "low-pressure" thorax from the "high-pressure" abdomen. Therefore, defects in the diaphragm may predispose to herniation of stomach or other abdominal contents into the thorax. The most common type of diaphragmatic hernia is the **sliding hiatal hernia,** in which the gastroesophageal (g-e) junction and a portion of the stomach slide through the diaphragmatic hiatus into the posterior mediastinum. Occasionally, reflux esophagitis may cause longitudinal shortening of the esophagus. Although hiatal hernia is not synonymous with g-e reflux, it may predispose to reflux disease. Patients with sliding hiatal hernias may be asymptomatic. Those with large hiatal hernias may report vague chest pain or present with chronic anemia due to either associated g-e reflux disease, or "kissing" erosions/ulcers on the crest of the mucosal folds as they pass through the hiatus.

In **paraesophageal hernia,** the g-e junction retains its normal anatomic position, but the stomach herniates alongside the g-e junction through the diaphragmatic hiatus. The entire stomach, oriented in an upside-down position, can herniate into the thorax. Stasis of food and secretions in the herniated stomach lead to erosions and ulcerations. Patients may, therefore, present with GI blood loss. A rare but serious complication of paraesophageal hernia is gastric volvulus. Delay in diagnosis and futile attempts at gastric decompression by a nasogastric tube may cause incarceration or strangulation of the herniated stomach. Inability to swallow, retching, and progressive severe pain suggest incarceration. **Congenital diaphragmatic hernias** result when structures involved in the development of the diaphragm fuse defectively. The posterolaterally located **foramina of Bochdalek** is the most common such congenital defect. The **foramina of Morgagni** are located anteriorly and 90% of the time the hernia is on the right side. Symptoms, when present, include obstruction, incarceration, strangulation, and respiratory distress. Post-traumatic diaphragmatic hernias result from injuries like stab wound, gunshot wound, or blunt trauma. The left diaphragm is more susceptible to injury as the liver protects the right

diaphragm from blunt trauma, and as most assailants in stabbing incidents are right-handed. Rarely, the diaphragm may be injured during surgery or may rupture during coughing or severe straining.

Chest x-ray may show a mediastinal air fluid level. Barium x-rays, and not endoscopy, is the most useful means of diagnosis. Surgery is the treatment of choice for diaphragmatic hernias, except in the sliding type. When complications occur, surgery carries a higher risk; thus, it is advisable to consider it even in the asymptomatic patient. Management of GERD complicating sliding hiatal hernia is the same as that without hernia.

Foreign Body Ingestion

All kinds of foreign bodies may be ingested, particularly by children (80% of the total), edentulous (denture-wearing) adults, prisoners, and the mentally ill. Immediate or delayed impaction with obstruction, perforation, and bleeding are potential complications. While plain x-rays of neck, chest, and abdomen are useful, some ingested foreign bodies (chicken bones, glass, plastic) will not be detected because they are radiolucent. All retained esophageal foreign bodies should be removed by endoscopy. Small, smooth objects (e.g., coins) in the stomach usually pass on their own, but sharp, pointed or larger (>5 cm long or >2 cm thick) objects must be removed by endoscopy or surgery.

"Body packing" refers to smuggling drugs (cocaine, heroin) in rubber or latex bags that are either swallowed or inserted into the rectum or vagina. These patients are admitted to an ICU until all packets are passed by GI tract lavage. For fear of rupturing a packet while it is still within the body, instrumentation is strictly forbidden.

CHAPTER **76** PEPTIC ULCER DISEASE

Peptic ulcers are mucosal defects extending beyond the muscularis mucosae with implied pathogenic association with acid and pepsin ("no acid, no ulcer"). They can develop in the stomach, duodenum, lower esophagus, jejunum (after gastrojejunostomy), and in areas with ectopic gastric mucosa.

■ Etiology and Pathophysiology

The mucus/bicarbonate layer is the first line of mucosal defense, followed by the epithelial cells. Adequate blood flow clears the back-diffused H$^+$ and

supplies necessary nutrients to the cell. Prostaglandins enhance mucosal resistance to injury ("cytoprotection"). In simple terms, peptic ulcers follow when the balance between mucosal defense and acid-pepsin is disturbed. Duodenal ulcer is rare in persons with a maximal acid output less than 12–15 mEq/h. One-third of patients with duodenal ulcer also have increased basal acid output. However, gastric ulcer can occur even if acid secretion is low, although both gastric and duodenal ulcers heal with acid suppression. Acid with pepsin is more ulcerogenic than acid alone. A break in the mucosal defense by extraneous factors may be an additional, and possibly the primary, event in the pathogenesis of peptic ulcer. For example, NSAIDs cause peptic ulcers by their topical mucosal damaging effects or by their systemic effect of depleting mucosal prostaglandins.

An estimated 15% of persons with *H. pylori* will develop peptic ulcer. However, over 95% of patients with duodenal ulcer and around 75% of patients with gastric ulcer are infected with *H. pylori*. The exact mechanism by which *H. pylori* induces ulceration is unknown. The microbe itself or factors released by it may evoke inflammation that damages mucosal defense. *H. pylori* infection is also associated with elevated levels of gastrin and pepsinogen. As *H. pylori* is also found in a high percentage of people who never develop peptic ulcers, the exact pathogenesis of peptic ulcer is still unclear.

■ Risk Factors

Peptic ulcer disease is slightly more prevalent in men than in women; the lifetime prevalence is about 10%. Duodenal ulcers are more frequent than gastric ulcers. Peptic ulcer incidence rises with age, reflecting a cohort phenomenon, possibly due to higher use of NSAIDs or increased prevalence of *H. pylori* in the elderly. Epidemiologic studies show higher incidence of gastric and duodenal ulcers in first-degree relatives of patients with similar types of ulcers. Patients with blood group O and nonsecretors of ABO antigens in body fluids are also at a higher risk of developing duodenal ulcer. Smoking increases the risk for both gastric and duodenal ulcers, besides impairing ulcer healing and promoting recurrence. Although tea and coffee stimulate acid production and alcohol may damage the mucosa, evidence is lacking to implicate them as risk factors. The role of psychological stress in the pathogenesis of ulcer remains unclear. Other diseases like cirrhosis, renal failure, chronic obstructive pulmonary disease, polycythemia vera, and hyperparathyroidism, for elusive reasons, are associated with an increased incidence of duodenal ulcer.

■ Clinical Features

The most common symptom of duodenal ulcer is epigastric pain, which is usually burning, occurring 1–3 hours after meals, and relieved by food or antacids. Nocturnal pain may interrupt sleep. The pain may last for a few weeks followed by symptom-free intervals of weeks to months. Less typically, it may be a gnawing or crampy discomfort, or felt in the right or left upper quadrants, or may radiate to the back. While a sizable number of duodenal ulcer patients present initially with complications of ulcer, acute bleeding, or perforation, some report anorexia with nausea and vomiting, despite the lack of gastric outlet obstruction. Gastric ulcer patients are older and, more often than not, asymptom-

atic. They may present initially with GI bleeding or perforation. The typical pain-food-relief pattern may occur, but it is less distinct than with duodenal ulcer. In fact, food may worsen the pain. Vague or severe, diffuse upper abdominal pain may accompany nausea, anorexia, and weight loss. Nocturnal pain is less common. Except with complications or other associated diseases, physical examination is not generally very helpful for diagnosis. Epigastric tenderness may be noted.

Complications of peptic ulcer disease are shown in Table 76.1.

■ Diagnosis

Peptic ulcer disease should be distinguished from non-ulcer dyspepsia, esophagitis, biliary diseases, pancreatitis, carcinoma, and infectious, granulomatous, or infiltrative diseases of the stomach and duodenum. History and physical examination lack sensitivity and specificity as diagnostic tools. Expertly done upper-GI barium radiology has a diagnostic accuracy of 80–90% for duodenal and 80% for gastric ulcer. Endoscopy detects a further 5–10% of ulcers and many consider it the procedure of choice. In some, peptic ulcer is discovered on urgent laparotomy for complications (e.g., perforation). Benign gastric ulcer has a regular, rounded edge and a smooth base. However, despite appearances, multiple biopsies to rule out malignancy are essential.

Several tests are available for diagnosing H. pylori infection. Bacterial urease activity can be tested by either the ^{13}C-urea breath test (90–95% sensitivity) or rapid urease test (90–98% sensitivity). The latter is done by placing an endoscopically taken gastric biopsy specimen on a pellet containing urea and a pH color indicator. Urease produced by *H. pylori* converts urea to ammonia; the pH rises and color changes. The bacteria can also be found on histology or cultured (70–95% sensitivity).

TABLE 76.1. Complications of Peptic Ulcer Disease
Intractability
Bleeding
Perforation
Penetration
Gastric outlet obstruction
Complications of therapy (H2 blockers antacids or proton pump inhibitors)
Complications of surgery
Postgastrectomy syndrome
Dumping syndrome
Blind-loop syndrome
Anastomotic ulcer
Postvagotomy diarrhea

Serum antibodies, while highly sensitive (95%) cannot separate current from previous infection. Antral mucosal biopsy should be obtained on all endoscopically detected gastric or duodenal ulcers, to document H. pylori infection by rapid urease test. With eradication of H. pylori, antibody titers fall progressively. Serum gastrin and acid output studies have no role in the usual evaluation of peptic ulcer disease, unless hypersecretory states (e.g., Zollinger-Ellison syndrome) are suspected.

■ Medical Management

The objectives of ulcer therapy are to promote ulcer healing and to prevent recurrences and complications. The strategy includes general measures, acid suppression, and promoting mucosal protection. Smoking and NSAID intake should be forbidden, as both of these are strong risk factors for ulcer nonhealing, recurrence, and complications. A causal relationship between alcohol abuse and ulcer disease is not proven; nonetheless, alcohol should be discouraged as it hampers the patient's compliance with the treatment. Specific dietary advice is not necessary but regular food intake should be encouraged. Stressful life situations reportedly delay ulcer healing.

Gastric acid can be reduced by either neutralization or inhibition of secretion. While antacids, which neutralize gastric acid, have been replaced by other anti-ulcer drugs, patients may still use them; one should be familiar with their role and side effects. Patient compliance is a problem and so is diarrhea due to magnesium-containing antacids. Ionized calcium in calcium-containing antacids stimulates gastrin secretion. Prolonged use of absorbable calcium-containing antacids with large amounts of milk leads to milk-alkali syndrome: hypercalcemia, alkalosis, nephrocalcinosis, and azotemia.

H2-receptor antagonists (cimetidine, ranitidine, famotidine, and nizatidine), which selectively block histamine H2-receptors on the parietal cells have been the most popular class of drugs used in treating peptic ulcer disease. Ulcer healing rates following therapy with these agents are 70–80% after 4 weeks and 90% after 8 weeks. Maintenance therapy with a single bedtime dose is also effective in reducing recurrence. Some of the side effects of these drugs are antiandrogenic effects, CNS symptoms, T-lymphocyte suppression, and pancytopenia. Through its effect on hepatic cytochrome protein pump inhibitors P_{450}, cimetidine and lansoprazole can inhibit the metabolism of many drugs like warfarin, phenytoin, and theophylline, leading to toxicity from these agents.

Substituted benzimidazoles (protein pump inhibitors, e.g. omeprazole, lansoprazole) are the most potent inhibitors of acid secretion. Omeprazole (20 mg or 40 mg/d) will heal duodenal ulcers in 80–100% of cases at 4 weeks respectively, and unlike H2-receptor antagonists, has very few side effects. Hypergastrinemia caused by sustained hypochlorhydria leads to enterochromaffin-cell hyperplasia in the gastric corpus and fundic mucosa, with progression to gastric carcinoid tumors in rats. Despite no such reported complication in humans, it is advisable that omeprazole be discontinued in patients whose serum gastrin levels exceed 500 pg/ml after 1 year of therapy.

Sucralfate, a sulfated polysaccharide-aluminum complex, prevents mucosal injury and heals ulcers without altering gastric acid or pepsin secretion. Several mechanisms have been proposed for its anti-ulcer effect. It forms a viscous barrier over granulation tissue, thus preventing detrimental effects of acid and pepsin; it may also enhance healing by stimulating prostaglandin production, adsorbing pepsin, and reducing oxidant damage to epithelial cells. The usual dose is 1.0 g four times daily. **Prostaglandins** (E and I groups) inhibit acid secretion and are also cytoprotective. Their acid inhibitory effect is mediated by suppressing histamine-related c-AMP generation in the parietal cell. Misoprostol is one such agent and is used mainly to prevent NSAID-induced ulcers. Side effects include crampy abdominal pain and diarrhea. Because misoprostol also has uterotropic effect, it can induce abortion.

Approach to therapy

Nearly 30–40% of duodenal ulcers heal by 4–6 weeks spontaneously, and more than 75% heal with H2-receptor antagonists, and 80–100% with protein pump inhibitors. After initial healing, 70–80% of peptic ulcers recur within 6–12 months. Maintenance H2-blocker therapy greatly reduces recurrence, but the current emphasis is on eradicating H. pylori. As over 95% of duodenal ulcers are associated with H. pylori, and as eradication of H. pylori significantly lowers ulcer recurrence rate (to 0–21%), most of the newly diagnosed duodenal ulcers and H. pylori-positive gastric ulcer patients can also be treated against H. pylori initially. This approach, while more expensive than giving H2-receptor antagonist alone, is more cost-effective in the long run, given the significantly lowered recurrence rate. Several regimens are available. A bismuth drug (e.g., Pepto-Bismol) with two antibiotics (e.g., tetracycline and metronidazole; tetracycline and clarithromycin; or amoxicillin and clarithromycin) eradicates H. pylori by 90–96%; most instances call for an additional 4–6 weeks of follow-up treatment with ranitidine. Protein pump inhibitors with clarithromycin *and* amoxycillin or metronidazole given for 2 weeks also leads to excellent ulcer healing and eradication of *H. pylori.*

While it is unnecessary to document duodenal ulcer (they are rarely malignant) healing, endoscopy may be needed to obtain biopsies for *H. pylori* in patients with nonhealing ulcers. Ongoing *H. pylori* can also be determined using the breath test based on *H. pylori* urease activity. Other causes of nonhealing ulcers like NSAID use and hypersecretory states like Zollinger-Ellison syndrome should be excluded. One should also consider infection with *H. pylori* strains that are metronidazole-resistant and/or clarithromycin-resistant. All gastric ulcers should be followed up until healed. Cancer should always be excluded by biopsy in unhealed gastric ulcers. Slowly healing gastric ulcers may require additional courses of treatment.

With modern medical management of peptic ulcer disease, total refractoriness to medical treatment is quite uncommon. Some may prefer surgery, but surgery is indicated mainly for complications. However, medical treatment does not eliminate the risks of ulcer recurrence, and for those who need maintenance therapy, or those with poor drug compliance, surgery is an excellent, drug-free alternative. A few patients will develop recurrent ulcers or experience chronic morbidity postoperatively.

The main objective of surgery is to reduce gastric acid secretion. **Subtotal gastrectomy** removes the bulk of the parietal cell mass and has an ulcer recurrence rate of 4–5%. Subtotal gastric resection is coupled with a gastroduodenostomy (*Billroth I*) or gastrojejunostomy (*Billroth II*) to restore continuity. Interrupting the neural path of acid secretion (vagotomy) and removing the main source of gastrin (antrectomy) can also accomplish acid reduction. Since truncal vagotomy will delay gastric emptying, a drainage procedure (e.g., pyloroplasty, gastrojejunostomy) must be added to this approach. In *proximal gastric vagotomy* (highly selective or superselective vagotomy), the vagal innervation to the fundus is interrupted and that to the antrum is preserved. As antral motility is intact, a drainage procedure is obviated. This operation has an ulcer recurrence rate of around 10%. Subtotal gastrectomy or antrectomy may be required for gastric ulcers. Vagotomy is not necessary as most patients with gastric ulcer have normal or low acid output.

■ Complications

During their life-time, nearly one-third of patients with peptic ulcer will experience one or more complications. **Intractability** implies failure of the ulcer to heal despite 8–12 weeks of intensive therapy, ulcer recurrence, or development of complications despite maintenance therapy. Intractability may be due to hypersecre-

tory states, penetrating or obstructing ulcers, smoking, and NSAID use. Eradication of *H. pylori* has significantly reduced the ulcer recurrence rate. When no remediable cause can be found, surgery is indicated.

Bleeding can complicate 15–20% of peptic ulcer cases, being more frequent in duodenal ulcers than gastric ulcers. It may be the first sign of peptic ulcer in 20–30% of patients. NSAID use accounts for the increasingly high incidence of ulcer bleeding in the elderly. Mortality from peptic ulcer bleeding has remained at 6–10%, the risk being higher in those over 60 years of age, or with concomitant diseases or continued bleeding or rebleeding. Deep ulcers in the posterior duodenal bulb and high lesser curve tend to erode large arteries and thus bleed briskly. Bleeding stops on its own in most patients with ulcer disease. Those found to have active bleeding on endoscopy or those at high risk for rebleeding (nonbleeding visible vessel, adherent fresh clot in the base of an ulcer) can be treated by endoscopic interventions. (See chapter 71 for general management of acute GI bleeding.) Surgery may be necessary when bleeding continues or recurs. Those unable to undergo surgery should be considered for angiographic embolization. Medical management of peptic ulcer should follow in all cases. Maintenance therapy after ulcer healing and eradication of *H. pylori* may reduce the rebleeding risk.

Perforation of an ulcer is less common than bleeding, but can be the first manifestation of peptic ulcer disease. It occurs in 5–10% of cases with duodenal ulcer and 2–5% of gastric ulcer cases. Perforation is more common with lesser curve gastric ulcers and anterior duodenal bulb ulcers. The use of NSAIDs has also increased the incidence of perforation in the elderly. Typical presentation is with the abrupt transition of vague, visceral pain of ulcer disease to the sharp, acute pain of peritonitis. Signs of acute peritonitis (muscle rigidity, rebound tenderness) are present with hypotension and tachycardia. Upright abdominal x-ray will show free intra-abdominal air. Endoscopy must be avoided as air insufflation can extend the perforation and further contaminate the peritoneal cavity. Spillage of duodenal contents may lead to hyperamylasemia. While the perforation seals without any intervention in a small minority, prompt surgery is indicated once perforation is diagnosed. While simple closure of the perforation is often enough, many surgeons carry out a more definite ulcer operation to avert further complications. **Penetration** is full thickness erosion of the gastric or duodenal wall into the pancreas, liver, biliary tree, or colon, but without free perforation. Penetration is identified in 20% of cases requiring surgery for peptic ulcer. Patients may note an alteration in their typical pain pattern—for example, the classical duodenal ulcer pain will begin radiating to the back once the duodenal ulcer penetrates the pancreas. Penetrating ulcers can respond well to medical therapy. Complicated penetrating ulcers (e.g., gastrocolic fistula) will require surgery.

Nearly 2% of patients with ulcer disease develop **gastric outlet obstruction,** arising from either inflammatory edema or cicatricial narrowing of the pylorus due to chronically recurring ulcer. Since obstruction is insidious and the stomach dilates as a result, the syndrome takes many weeks to develop. Vomiting is the most frequent symptom, which may cause severe esophagitis. Typically profuse, the vomit contains retained food, consumed many hours earlier. Abdominal pain, vague fullness after meals, anorexia, and weight loss may be reported. A succussion splash is a common and valuable sign besides dehydration. Hemoconcentration, prerenal azotemia, anemia, hyponatremia, low serum albumin, and in severe cases, hypokalemic alkalosis are typical laboratory findings. Barium study is diagnostic, but endoscopy is required to define the cause, especially to exclude malignancy. Nasogastric tube drainage of the stomach, IV rehydration, and restoration of electrolytes are immediate priorities. Acid suppression (H2-blockers, omeprazole) may relieve obstruction due to inflammatory edema. Gastric retention persisting beyond 5–7 days requires either endoscopic balloon dilatation of the pylorus or surgery.

Zollinger-Ellison Syndrome

Zollinger-Ellison (ZE) syndrome is characterized by the autonomous production and release of gastrin by a tumor (gastrinoma) leading to severe ulcerative disease of the upper GI tract, diarrhea, hypergastrinemia, and hyperchlorhydria. Fewer than 1% of peptic ulcers are ZE syndrome-related. It mostly presents in patients between 30 and 50 years of age and is slightly more common in men.

Autonomous gastrin production by proliferating non-β islet cells leads to uncontrolled acid secretion by the parietal cells. Ninety percent of gastrinomas are found in the head of the pancreas and the wall of the duodenum. Slightly over one-half are multiple and a similar proportion are malignant. The tumor grows slowly and metastasizes mainly to regional lymph nodes and liver. About 30% of cases with gastrinomas have type I multiple endocrine neoplasia, and nearly all gastrinomas of this type are multiple.

The majority of patients have typical symptoms of peptic ulcer disease. Gastrinoma-related peptic ulcers tend to be persistent and poorly responsive to conventional therapy. Over one-third of patients report diarrhea, probably due to excess HCl in the small intestine that inactivates pancreatic digestive enzymes and thus reduces bile salt solubility. Some patients have diarrhea but no ulcer symptoms. In those with MEN-I syndrome, a family history—mainly of hyperparathyroidism with renal stones—is usually present. Most of the ulcers are located in the duodenal bulb or the stomach and may be multiple. However, ulcers may occur beyond the duodenal bulb (14%) and in the jejunum (11%). Recurrent ulcers may rapidly develop at or distal to the anastomotic site following conventional peptic ulcer surgery. Esophagitis and esophageal ulceration may also occur.

Severe, progressive, and recurrent peptic ulcer disease, peptic ulcers at unusual sites, and diarrhea should raise the suspicion of ZE syndrome. Besides demonstrating ulcers, barium study may show prominent gastric and duodenal folds, thickened and widened small intestinal folds, and excessive fluid in the small bowel lumen. Owing to the continuous stimulation of the parietal cells by gastrin, the ratio between basal and maximum pentagastrin-stimulated acid output is 0.66% or more. Both fasting serum gastrin levels and basal acid output are high. Gastrinomas thus confirmed are localized by CT, MR, ultrasound, or selective angiography with or without venous gastrin level sampling. Surgical resection is the ideal treatment for resectable tumors. If resection is not feasible, acid hypersecretion is suppressed by high doses of H2-blockers or omeprazole, or rarely, by total gastrectomy. Chemotherapy (e.g., streptozotocin) reduces tumor size and serum gastrin in metastatic gastrinomas.

Stress Ulcers

Severe physiological stress can result in gastroduodenal lesions ranging from mucosal erosions to life-threatening ulcers—for example, duodenal ulcers **(Curling's ulcers)** in severe burns, and gastroduodenal ulcers in CNS trauma or with other serious illnesses **(Cushing's ulcer).** The pathogenesis of stress ulcer is elusive. Physiological stress can compromise mucosal perfusion, and mucosal defense and repair. The usual presentation is acute GI bleeding in an ICU setting. Bleeding stress ulcers carry a high risk of rebleeding and mortality. Given the underlying serious illnesses, most of these patients respond inadequately to any form of therapy. Prevention is thus crucial. In clinical trials, keeping the gastric pH over 3.5–4 by antacid or sucralfate by nasogastric tube or by IV H2 blockers has lowered the rate of stress ulcer complications.

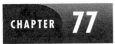

NEOPLASMS OF THE STOMACH

Gastric Cancer

■ Epidemiology and Etiology

This once-common cancer has declined in incidence since the 1940s. While most common in men older than 50 years, the gender difference is inapparent in cancers in younger persons. Gastric cancer has a striking geographic variation with a higher incidence in Costa Rica, Japan, and China. Dietary factors (e.g., high salt intake, pickled vegetables, smoked food, and salted fish) have been epidemiologically linked to its genesis. Patients with chronic atrophic gastritis with intestinal metaplasia, pernicious anemia, gastric polyps, hypertrophic gastropathy, and post-gastrectomy gastric remnant also share a higher risk. Nitrite-forming bacteria that colonize the stomach in patients with hypo- or achlorhydria help convert dietary nitrates to nitrites. Nitroso compounds formed in this process are carcinogenic in animals. Antioxidants (e.g., vitamin C) inhibit this conversion. An epidemiological link has been noted between *H. pylori* infection and later occurrence of gastric adenocarcinoma. Chronic atrophic gastritis due to *H. pylori* infection may be the precursor. Both first-degree relatives of gastric cancer patients and persons with blood group A have a higher risk of gastric cancer, suggesting a genetic basis. Gastric cancer may present as an ulcer, but chronic benign gastric ulcer does not seem to be precancerous.

■ Pathology

Over 90% of gastric cancers are adenocarcinomas. Cancers with intracellular mucus laterally displacing the nucleus (ring-like appearance) are termed **signet ring carcinomas. Colloid or mucinous carcinomas** are mucus-producing. Gastric carcinomas may also show glandular structures (papillary) or masses of cells (medullary). The cells can be highly, moderately, or poorly differentiated. Gastric carcinomas are also classified as *intestinal* or *diffuse* types. The former often arises from intestinal metaplasia. It is polypoidal or ulcerated, better circumscribed, and has a glandular structure resembling colon cancer. It is more common in older people. The diffuse type, more common in younger people, features rare glandular structures, indistinct margins, and frequent signet-ring cells. Early gastric cancer, which invades only the mucosa or submucosa, is diagnosed by combined endoscopy and histology.

■ Clinical Features and Diagnosis

Patients with *early gastric carcinoma* are generally asymptomatic or may report vague, nonspecific epigastric symptoms. Such cancers are usually found by screening techniques being used in countries endemic for gastric cancer (e.g., Japan). Symptoms of advanced gastric cancer are listed in Table 77.1.

With the double-contrast x-ray technique, 90–95% of cases of gastric cancers may be accurately diagnosed. Malignancy is suggested by an ulcer within a mass, polypoidal mass, interrupted or nodular folds approaching an ulcer, and rigidity with loss of peristalsis. However, appearances are deceptive; thus, all gastric ulcers, benign-looking or not, must be biopsied via endoscopy. Early gastric cancer may evoke only subtle changes; careful examination of the stomach is thus

TABLE 77.1. Manifestations of Gastric Cancer	
Category	**Symptoms**
Constitutional/systemic	Anorexia, weight loss, thrombophlebitis, neuropathy
Local	Abdominal pain, gastrocolic fistula
Obstruction	Dysphagia (cardiac), vomiting (antral)
Bleeding	Hematemesis, melena, anemia
Metastasis	Pleural effusion, Virchow's nodes, periumbilical infiltration (Sister Joseph's nodule), ascites, ovarian metastasis (Krukenberg tumor)

paramount. CT and endoscopic ultrasound can help define the depth of tumor invasion and presence or absence of metastases.

■ Management

For patients with localized disease (early gastric cancer), surgery is the only hope of a cure. Patients with nonmetastatic but locally advanced disease should also be offered surgery to seek curative resection. If surgery is not possible, and for those with disseminated disease, palliative surgery may be done to relieve symptoms (dysphagia, gastric outlet obstruction, bleeding); chemotherapy should also be considered. Using single agents like 5-fluorouracil or Mitomycin C, a 20–25% response rate (i.e., ≥50% reduction in size) has been observed, which increases to 25–50% when combination chemotherapy with the FAM regimen (5-fluorouracil, Adriamycin, and Mitomycin C) is used. Combining chemotherapy with radiotherapy confers no additional benefits. Because 10–50% of gastric cancers have estrogen receptors, giving tamoxifen with chemotherapy may have some advantage.

Gastric Lymphoma

Gastric lymphomas are rare (<5% of gastric neoplasms). Most are extranodal non-Hodgkin's lymphomas, arising from the submucosal lymphoid tissue, with a few arising from the mucosa-associated lymphoid tissue (MALT lymphoma). Epidemiological studies show a link between prior *H. pylori* infection and later development of MALT gastric lymphoma. Clinical features simulate those of peptic ulcer or gastric cancer. Systemic disease features lymphadenopathy and hepatosplenomegaly. Radiologic and endoscopic features can rarely differentiate lymphoma from adenocarcinoma. Thickened folds, duodenal extension, and multiple lesions with extensive ulcerations suggest lymphoma. Multiple biopsies are necessary for diagnosis. Ann Arbor system is used for staging. Early disease is treated by surgery; when surgery is not feasible, radiotherapy can be used instead as the primary therapy. For later stages, chemotherapy and radiotherapy can be combined. A few cases of gastric MALT lymphoma have been cured by eradication of *H. pylori* infection.

Ampullary Carcinoma

These cancers, which tend to occur in middle-aged persons, arise from either the ampulla of Vater itself or from adjacent structures like the distal common bile duct, pancreatic head, or the duodenum that involve the ampulla. A common presenting feature is jaundice due to biliary obstruction, which may remit as the tumor erodes into the duodenum. Ulceration can lead to overt or occult GI bleeding. Cholangitis or pancreatitis are other presentations. Biochemical studies may show features of cholestatic jaundice. The ampulla can be directly visualized and biopsied using a side-viewing endoscope. Endoscopic ultrasonography can define the depth of the lesion. Surgery is the treatment of choice with a cure rate of 30%. If surgery is not possible, biliary obstruction can be palliated endoscopically.

CHAPTER 78 ANATOMY AND PHYSIOLOGY OF THE SMALL INTESTINE

■ Anatomy

The small intestine, approximately 250 cm long, extends from the pylorus to the ileocecal valve, and consists of the duodenum (first 25–30 cm), the jejunum and the ileum. The small bowel is supplied by the celiac and the superior mesenteric arteries; anastomotic channels exist between the superior- and the inferior mesenteric arteries, thus providing a collateral circulation. The vagus nerves that terminate in the myenteric and submucosal plexuses of the bowel wall provide the parasympathetic innervation; postganglionic fibers from the celiac and superior mesenteric ganglia provide the sympathetic efferents.

The mucosal surface of the intestinal folds is studded with slender villi with their bases encircled by pit-like crypts. The crypts and villi are lined by a continuous layer of columnar absorptive and mucoglycoprotein-producing goblet cells. Cell renewal begins from the undifferentiated crypt cells. In about 3–5 days, these newly formed cells migrate up the walls of the crypts and onto the villi, and mature into absorptive cells. Upon reaching the villus tips, the cells slough off into the lumen. The crypt epithelium also contains Paneth and enterochromaffin (enteroendocrine) cells. Endocrine cells from the stomach to jejunum secrete gastrin, secretin, cholecystokinin, gastric inhibitory polypeptide, and motilin, while ileal and colonic cells produce peptide YY, enteroglucagon, and neurotensin. Somatostatin-producing cells are found throughout the GI tract.

The lamina propria, the loose cellular connective tissue beneath the epithelium, contains the capillaries, venules, and lymphatics serving the absorptive epithelium, besides lymphocytes and plasma cells. The lymphocytes are seen between the columnar epithelial absorptive cells, in the lamina propria, and in focal aggregates called lymphoid follicles and Peyer's patches. Covering these aggregates are specialized epithelial cells (M-cells), which can endocytose antigens, and present them to the underlying T and B lymphocytes. It is thought that the antigen-sensitized B lymphocytes migrate to the lamina propria, and evolve into immunoglobulin-synthesizing plasma cells. Eighty to 90% of these plasma cells synthesize and contain IgA; 12–16% contain IgM; and 2–4%, IgG. The IgA, locally synthesized and secreted into the gut lumen, contains antibodies developed after exposure to antigens entering from the lumen. The secretory IgA has two IgA molecules joined by a J-piece to which a glycoprotein secretory component is added. The secretory component, synthesized by the epithelial cells and attached to the IgA before it enters the lumen, probably protects IgA from intraluminal enzymatic digestion. Secretory IgA is felt to exert a critical role in regulating gut bacterial flora, preventing and controlling tissue invasion by enteroviruses, and in preventing the absorption of undesirable antigenic material.

■ Physiology

Motor Activity

An inherent, rhythmically fluctuating membrane potential occurs continuously and in synchrony in the adjacent cells of the longitudinal layer of small intestinal smooth muscle cells, known as the slow-wave activity (syn., basic electrical rhythm, or electrical control activity). These slow waves occur as a distally migrating signal at 12 cycles/min. in the duodenum to about 8 in the terminal ileum. On the peaks of slow waves are superimposed the spike potential; the smooth muscles contract only in relation to them. The frequency of spike potentials and muscle contractions varies in time and in relationship to food intake, as well as in response to neural and hormonal stimuli. Meanwhile, slow wave activity runs constantly, unaffected by fasting, feeding, or hormonal or nervous stimuli.

The most common form of small intestinal motor activity is the segmental contraction, a very brief, localized, ring-like contraction usually 1–2 cm in length. These recur and disappear rhythmically, leading to movement of intestinal contents back and forth for mixing and better exposure to the mucosal surface.

While fasting, the small bowel demonstrates a motor pattern, the interdigestive myoelectric complex (migrating motor complex), that starts concurrently in the stomach and upper small intestine (Figure 78.1). At first,

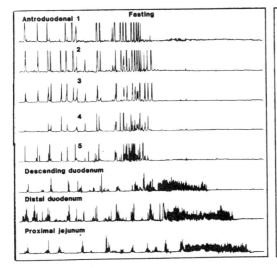
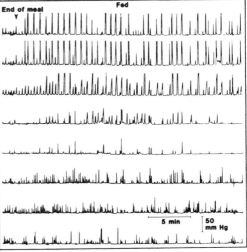

FIGURE 78.1. *Left:* Normal interdigestive migrating motor complex in the fasting state. *Right:* Normal fed motor activity.
(Source: Malagelada JR, Camilleri M, Stanghellini V. Manometric Diagnosis of Gastrointestinal Motility Disorders. New York: Thieme Medical Publishers, 1986. Used with permission.)

irregular segmental contractions occur (phase II), which slowly gather frequency and strength; then a slowly migrating contraction complex sweeps down to the ileum, with a velocity of 4–6 cm/min in the upper intestine, and 1 cm/min in the lower small intestine (phase III). A period of minimal, scattered contractions follows (phase I). As one complex reaches the ileum, another begins in the stomach or duodenum, thus repeating the cycle. After feeding, these complexes give place to frequent segmental contractions that are either stationary or migrate distally over short distances.

The act of vomiting also has a specific motor pattern. The medullary vomiting center receives signals from the chemoreceptor trigger zone. Receptors for serotonin (5-HT), dopamine, and histamine transmit the signals that trigger the vomiting act via vagal fibers. Following a brief period of motor inhibition, a retrograde migrating contraction from the midgut empties bowel contents into the stomach. The abdominal wall muscles then suddenly contract, propelling gastric contents to the mouth.

The epithelial cell and absorptive mechanisms

Digestion and absorption are discussed in chapters 69 and 70. Carbohydrates consisting of starch (60–70%), sucrose (30%), and lactose (0–10%) make up 40–50% of total daily calories. Fat, nearly all of which is long-chain triglycerides, comprises 30–40% of calories; the majority of fatty acids are palmitic, stearic, oleic, and linoleic. The remaining 5% of dietary fat consists of medium-chain triglycerides, phospholipids, fat-soluble vitamins, and cholesterol. Dietary protein averages 70 g/day. A nearly equal amount of endogenous protein, mostly secretions and desquamated mucosal cells and some plasma protein, enters the gut lumen.

Congenital Abnormalities

Most congenital anomalies are encountered during infancy and childhood, and only occasionally in adults.

Meckel's Diverticulum

Meckel's diverticulum, the most frequent congenital intestinal anomaly affects almost 1.5% of the population. It arises from incomplete obliteration of the vitelline duct at the intestinal end, leaving a sac or diverticulum that arises from the antimesenteric border of the ileum, about 80 cm proximal to the ileocecal valve. These diverticula contain ectopic gastric, duodenal, colonic, and pancreatic mucosa, but the gastric mucosa is the most common. While usually asymptomatic, problems related to the diverticulum tend to arise most commonly during the first 2 years of life. Among the complications of bleeding, diverticulitis, perforation, and bowel obstruction, bleed-ing from ileal mucosal ulceration adjacent to ectopic gastric mucosa is the most common. Meckel's diverticulitis may mimic acute appendicitis.

Nonsurgical detection of the diverticulum is difficult, because it seldom fills with barium. Radioactive pertechnetrate scanning may demonstrate those diverticula with gastric mucosa, but there are false negatives. Occasionally, mesenteric angiography or tagged RBC scan may be helpful when there is significant bleeding.

Miscellaneous

Incomplete duodenal atresia may appear as an intraluminal diaphragm causing bilious vomiting. Anomalies of embryologic rotation and fixation may present as intestinal obstruction and/or a dilated cecum in the left upper abdominal quadrant in the adult.

CHAPTER 79 INFECTIOUS ENTERITIS

■ Definition and Epidemiology

Infectious enteritis (syn., acute gastroenteritis) is an acute illness with diarrhea and, depending on the causative agent, nausea, vomiting, abdominal cramps, fever, bloody stools, and headache. In the United States, the incidence of diarrheal illness is 1.5–1.9 per person per year, causing 10,000–20,000 deaths annually. The majority of these enteritides occur in infants, particularly those living in areas with poor sanitation and a high incidence of malnutrition. Risk factors for acquiring infectious gastroenteritis are shown in Table 79.1. Additional information is given in chapter 151. Special problems in immu-

TABLE 79.1. Risk Factors for Infectious Enteritis

- Infants and preschoolers, especially in day care centers, kindergarten
- Travel to tropical and other areas with poor sanitation
- Contaminated food or drink
  - poorly refrigerated food
  - contaminated water supply
  - raw or undercooked meat, fish and shellfish
  - nonpasteurized milk
- Low or suppressed gastric acid secretion

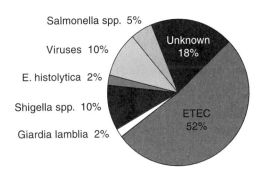

Salmonella spp. 5%
Viruses 10%
E. histolytica 2%
Shigella spp. 10%
Giardia lamblia 2%
Unknown 18%
ETEC 52%

FIGURE 79.1. Causes of traveler's diarrhea *(turista)* acquired in Central America. The incidence of Giardia varies from 0–50%, depending on the geographic location (see text). ETEC = enterotoxigenic *E. coli.*

nocompromised patients are discussed in chapters 157 and 158.

Etiology

In the United States, bacteria and unicellular parasites account for 20–30% of episodes of infectious diarrhea, viruses for 30–40%, and undetermined agents (probably food toxins and viruses) for the remainder. The epidemiologic setting dictates the relative role of these agents in enteric infections, particularly in sporadic outbreaks of large-scale epidemics. The major causes of traveler's diarrhea *(turista)* among travelers to Mexico and infectious enteritis are listed in Figure 79.1 and Table 79.2, respectively. The contribution of individual infectious agents differs with the country visited.

Pathogenesis

Gastric acidity provides an important initial defense by killing ingested organisms. Most pathogens need to attach to the epithelial brush border surface and to the specialized M-cells overlying Peyer's patches in order to proliferate, to produce toxins, and, for some pathogens, to invade the epithelium (Table 79.2). Specialized proteins in bacterial flagella and fimbriae interact with the epithelial cell membrane to effect attachment. Some pathogens invade the mucosa, causing inflammation, ulceration, bleeding, and, occasionally, bowel perforation. Others produce cytotoxins that destroy epithelial cells with or without ensuing tissue invasion (Table 79.2). *Vibrio cholerae,* enteropathogenic *E. coli,* and noninvasive Salmonella and Shigella release enterotoxins that bind to cell surface receptors, initiating active Cl⁻ ion secretion and reducing electroneutral NaCl absorption (see chapters 69 and 70).

Clinical Features

In broad terms, enteric infections cause either watery, secretory, **nonbloody diarrhea** with little abdominal pain and no fever, or the **dysenteric syndrome,** with cramps, bloody diarrhea, and fever. The incubation period may be hours (ingested toxins) to 2 weeks. Physical findings may include signs of dehydration (see chapter 69), diffuse abdominal tenderness without signs of peritoneal irritation (rigidity or rebound tenderness) and reduced, rather than absent bowel sounds. Sensory and motor neuropathy may accompany enteritis acquired via sea food ingestion. The stool should be tested for blood. In the dysenteric syndrome, proctosigmoidoscopy is needed in order to obtain biopsy and aspirated exudate for microscopy (e.g., amebic trophozoites). In suspected infectious enteritis, expensive stool studies should be efficiently used (Figure 79.2). In secretory diarrhea, stool tests for pathogens may help define the source of the outbreak, but not guide management.

TABLE 79.2. **Agents Commonly Causing Infectious Diarrhea**

	Comment
Bacteria	
E. coli	
enterotoxigenic	Common
enterohemorrhagic*	Serious. Undercooked beef, apple cider
enteroadherent	Rare
Shigella	Foodborne
dysenteriae[a,b]	Low infectious dose
other spp.	Common
Salmonella	High infectious dose
typhi (paratyphi)[a]	Rare
other spp.	Mild. Poultry, turtles
V. cholerae	
-0.1; El Tor	Life-threatening diarrhea
Other spp.	Less severe. Fish, shellfish
Campylobacter jejuni[a,b]	
Yersinia enterocolitica[a]	Milk, pork
C. difficile[b]	Antibiotic use; fecal-oral
Parasites	
Giardia lamblia	Camping; Russia. May cause prolonged illness and mild malabsorption
Cryptosporidium spp	Low infectious dose, contaminated water supply
Entameba histolytica[a]	Rare
Viruses	
Rotavirus[b]	Infants; in winter
Norwalk agent	Adults; water, food
Adenovirus spp.	All ages
Food toxins	Incubation period <12 hrs.
S. aureus	Food
C. perfringens[a]	Food
Fish toxins (ciguatera-, scromba)	Neurotoxins

[a] = Invasive.
[b] = Produces cytotoxin.

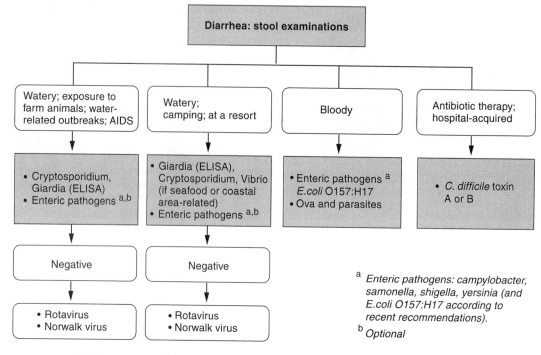

FIGURE 79.2. Recommended stool studies according to the clinical presentation of infectious diarrhea.

TABLE 79.3.	Guide to Antibiotic Therapy of Infectious Enteritis
Organism	**Treatment**
Shigella: dysenteric illness	TMP/SMX, 160/800* t.i.d. × 5 days
	Ciprofloxacin, 500 mg b.i.d. × 5 days
Salmonella: dysenteric illness	Chloramphenicol, 0.5-1.0 g q.i.d., ×10–14 days
	TMP/SMX, t.i.d. × 10–14 days
	Ciprofloxacin, 500 mg b.i.d. × 10-14 days
Campylobacter jejuni	Erythromycin, 250–500 mg b.i.d. × 7 days
	Ciprofloxacin, 500 mg b.i.d. × 7 days
Yersinia enterocolitica	Tetracycline, 500 mg q.i.d. (?)
Giardia lamblia	Quinacrine, 100 mg t.i.d. × 7 days
	Metronidazole, 250 mg t.i.d. × 7 days
Entameba histolytica	Metronidazole, 250 mg t.i.d. plus diiodohydroxyquin, 650 mg t.i.d. × 20 days
Cryptosporidium	Paromomycin, 500 mg q.i.d. × 14 days
	Clarithromycin, 250–500 mg b.i.d. × 14 days; efficacy not established
Acute infectious diarrhea with blood in stool; no pathogen identified or etiologic diagnosis	Ciprofloxacin, 500 mg b.i.d. × 3 days (?)

*TMP/SMX = trimethoprim-sulfamethoxazole.

■ Management and Prognosis

Hospitalization and infection (enteric) precautions are indicated in patients with moderate or severe dehydration and/or the dysenteric syndrome. A stool sample should be sent to the laboratory before antibiotics, radiologic contrast material, or enemas are given. The management of dehydration and the use of antidiarrheals are discussed in chapter 69. Antibiotic use in infectious diarrhea should be limited to specific situations (Table 79.3). Their empiric use is controversial and not generally endorsed. Two factors limit the efficacy of antibiotics: (1) by the time the pathogen is identified, not only is the illness subsiding, but the issue of specific therapy may be moot; (2) enteric bacterial pathogens frequently alter

their antibiotic susceptibility patterns. The prognosis is excellent in almost all patients. In the few where watery diarrhea lasts many months without a persistently identifiable pathogen, all that is needed besides antidiarrheals is reassurance that the diarrhea will eventually abate.

CHAPTER 80 SELECTED SMALL BOWEL DISEASES CAUSING MALABSORPTION

General aspects of absorption, malabsorption, and the use of various laboratory studies in diagnosing malabsorption are discussed in chapter 70. Among the many disorders that cause malab-

sorption, some specific small bowel diseases are considered here.

Disaccharidase Deficiency

Lactase deficiency

Lactose, a disaccharide present only in milk, is composed of glucose and galactose. **Lactase** is required in the luminal surface of enterocytes to digest lactose to these readily absorbable sugars. Lactase deficiency, which occurs in the majority of the world's population (Figure 80.1), is most commonly an autosomal recessive disorder where the enzyme disappears after the weaning period. Its symptoms are those of carbohydrate malabsorption—that is, abdominal dis-

tention, flatulence, and diarrhea. The relationship to ingestion of milk (cow's milk contains 5% lactose) and other dairy products—such as ice cream, pasteurized yogurt, and cheese—may be obvious. The diagnosis is established by a lactose-breath hydrogen test where breath H_2 rises above 20 ppm after a lactose test dose, or by a rise in plasma glucose not exceeding 20 mg/dl. Treatment is avoidance of nonfermented dairy products in the diet. Patients, particularly postmenopausal women, who need a constant source of

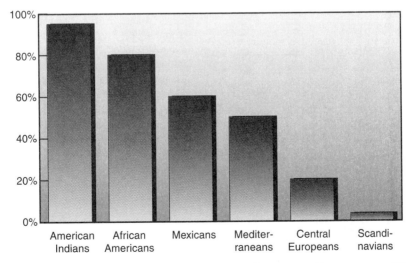

FIGURE 80.1. Prevalence of lactase deficiency in various populations of the world. Among Asians the prevalence ranges from 90 to 100%, among central Europeans from 15 to 25%, and among Scandinavians from 0 to 3%.

calcium, phosphorus, and vitamin D, may consume milk with an added microbial lactase preparation (Lactinase, Lactrase). Nonpasteurized yogurt is well tolerated. Secondary lactase deficiency may follow any intestinal disease causing widespread mucosal damage.

Celiac Sprue

Also known as **gluten-sensitive enteropathy,** this disease is a prime clinical example of a mucosal absorptive defect causing malabsorption. There is a poorly understood sensitivity to (or inability to metabolize) gluten, a glutamine-rich protein component of wheat, rye, and barley. The higher prevalence of HLA-B6 and HLA-DR3 antigens suggests a genetic basis. The current notion is that gluten, or some peptide fraction derived from it, may induce immunologically mediated intestinal mucosal injury. The disease is more prevalent (normally 1/1000–1/2000) among diabetics. In untreated celiac disease, the mucosa reveals flattened surface with total loss of villi, elongated crypts, and flattened epithelial cells with some loss of brush-border microvilli. The lamina propria and the surface epithelium are infiltrated by lymphocytes and plasma cells. In symptomatic cases, serum folate levels are low almost universally. Circulating antibodies to gliadin, reticulin, and endomysium occur in most patients; the anti-endomysial antibody has the highest diagnostic accuracy.

■ Clinical Features

Clinical manifestations vary widely depending on the extent of the disease beyond the pylorus. The onset may be in infancy, shortly after weaning, or in childhood. Not infrequently it remits in adolescence only to reappear later. Besides steatorrhea, diarrhea, weight loss, cramps, abdominal distention, and malaise, nutritional deficiency state(s) due to impaired absorption of iron, calcium, vitamin D, vitamin B_{12}, or vitamin K dominate the clinical picture. Physical examination may be normal or show signs of weight loss, decreased muscle mass, or signs of specific nutritional deficiencies, such as easy bruising, dependent edema, tetany, and glossitis. In severe cases, the abdomen is protuberant and has a doughy consistency.

■ Diagnosis and Management

Laboratory findings may reflect any of the above deficiencies. The small bowel series shows a coarse fold pattern, irregular dilatation of gut loops, and, occasionally, transient intussusceptions. The diagnosis depends on mucosal biopsy and then documenting clinical, biochemical, and morphologic remission after excluding dietary gluten. A sprue-like small bowel mucosa on biopsy, IgA deposits in the dermis, mild malabsorption, and even remission of intestinal and skin lesions after a gluten-free diet occur in most cases of *dermatitis herpetiformis.*

Treatment is life-long, with total gluten avoidance, best attained through careful patient education by an experienced dietitian, and by encouraging contact with the local chapter of a Celiac Disease or Sprue Society. Clinical and biochemical improvement follow within days or a few weeks of starting the diet, and bowel biopsies revert to normal within 3–12 months. Titers of circulating IgA antibodies to gliadin, endomysium, and reticulin also decline.

While the prognosis is generally excellent on a gluten-free diet, a favorable response is not universal in every patient with a compatible biopsy. This so-called **refractory sprue** usually responds to corticosteroids. **Ulcerative jejunitis,** a life-threatening complication, features worsening diarrhea and malabsorption, perforation, and occasional bleeding. In **collagenous sprue** that develops in a few, jejunal biopsy shows a collagenous deposit beneath the epithelial basement membrane, extending into the lamina propria. The associated clinical worsening (i.e., weight loss, increasing malabsorption and diarrhea, anemia, and hypoproteinemia) does not respond to steroids and gluten withdrawal. Life-long adherence to a gluten-free diet lessens the increased risk of malignancy in this disease (generalized and intestinal lymphoma, squamous cancer of oropharynx and esophagus, and adenocarcinoma of the small bowel).

Tropical Sprue

Tropical sprue occurs in discrete tropical areas (scattered islands in the Caribbean, the Indian subcontinent, and in Southern Africa). The disease can be acquired during lengthy visits to endemic areas. Chronic contamination of the bowel by pathogenic bacteria is believed to be the cause. Progressive malabsorption, weight loss, and anemia frequently follow a bout of nonspecific, acute diarrhea. The small bowel biopsy shows varying degrees of villus shortening, crypt hypertrophy, and chronic inflammation of the lamina propria. Pharmacologic doses of folate along with tetracycline are highly effective.

Intestinal Bacterial Overgrowth

Bacteria swallowed with saliva and food contaminate the normal small bowel only intermittently, an important bactericidal barrier being the gastric acid. Bacterial overgrowth, usually resulting from coliforms and enteric anaerobes, occurs in several conditions, as listed in Table 80.1. The gold standard of diagnosis, albeit expensive and not widely available for lack of laboratories with facilities, is quantitative aerobic and anaerobic culture of a fasting duodenal or proximal jejunal aspirate, showing in excess of 10^5 viable bacteria/ml. Several screening tests are available, although none carry an accuracy over 80%.

1. Glucose H_2 breath test: since a 50 g or 80 g glucose test dose should be totally absorbed, a rise in breath H_2 implies bacterial fermentation in the small bowel.

2. In the ^{14}C-D-xylose and ^{14}C-cholylglycine tests, bacterial D-xylose fermentation and bile acid deconjugation, respectively, cause ^{14}CO$_2$ to appear in the breath, signaling overgrowth.

In bacterial overgrowth, bacteria consume both the free vitamin B_{12} and the B_{12}-intrinsic factor complex, thus causing B_{12} malabsorption. Bacteria also deconjugate bile acids, which are then absorbed by passive diffusion; the reduced intestinal bile acid concentration may then lead to steatorrhea. H_2 and CO_2 produced by bacterial carbohydrate fermentation cause abdominal distention and pain, which leads patients to reduce their nutrient intake. Empiric antibiotics are used which may have to be altered over time as symptoms recur during therapy. Tetracycline or cephalexin (250 mg q.i.d.) elicit a response in 40%. Amoxicillin/potassium clavulanate, 250–500 mg t.i.d. or ciprofloxacin, 500 mg b.i.d., plus metronidazole, 250–500 mg t.i.d., lead to better results. Once clinical success is achieved, antibiotics are given monthly, for 10–14 days.

TABLE 80.1.	Conditions Associated with Bacterial Overgrowth in the Small Intestine
Reduced or absent gastric acid	Achlorhydria ± pernicious anemia
	Gastric operations, vagotomy, total gastrectomy
Intestinal stasis	Multiple duodenal and intestinal diverticula
	Afferent loop of Billroth II gastrectomy
	Proximal to intestinal strictures
	Pseudo-obstruction syndromes
Contamination by colonic contents	Resection of ileocecal valve
	Intestinal-colonic fistula

Whipple's Disease

This rare, progressive multisystem disease, seen mostly in middle-aged men, is an antibiotic-responsive bacterial infection. In untreated patients, even without diarrhea and malabsorption, jejunal biopsies show periodic acid-Schiff (PAS)-positive macrophages and intra- and extracellular rod-shaped organisms in the lamina propria of the jejunal villi. Many organs also contain PAS-positive macrophages. The organism appears to be a gram-positive actinomycete bacillus, *Tropheryma whippelii*, despite its lack of consistent isolation from cultures of affected tissues. A host defect is likely, as the phagocytized bacteria are not destroyed and since a strong inflammatory response is remiss, despite bacteria lying free in various organs.

Episodic arthralgias and nondeforming arthritis of large joints typically antedate GI symptoms by several years. Pneumonia, cough, and pleurisy occur, with occasional low-grade fever, anorexia, nausea, vomiting, diarrhea, edema, ascites, and lymphadenopathy. Hyperpigmentation occurs in the exposed skin in about 50% of patients. In 10–40% of cases, CNS symptoms are manifest, including headache, dementia, myoclonus, ataxia, supranuclear ophthalmoplegia, and blindness.

Laboratory manifestations of malabsorption commonly occur. Small bowel x-rays usually show dilated loops with coarse, irregular folds. Diagnosis is made by duodenal or jejunal biopsy showing swollen and distorted intestinal villi; abundant PAS-positive macrophages and, often, dilated lacteal vessels are seen in the lamina propria. Electron microscopy shows rod-shaped bacilli.

Penicillin, 1.2 million units/day, and streptomycin, 1 g/day for 14 days, are given initially, followed by oral trimethoprim-sulfamethoxazole (160/800 mg b.i.d.), or tetracycline, 1 gm/d for 1 year to ensure penetration of the antibiotic into the CNS. Complete remission regularly follows this regimen, but relapses occur in up to 35% of cases followed for at least 1 year. CNS involvement is very serious. Relapsed CNS disease is less amenable to retreatment.

Protein-Losing Enteropathy

This is a pathophysiologic process where excess plasma protein (>1.5 g/d) is lost by leakage into the gut. All plasma proteins participate in this process. Hypoproteinemia results when the proteins enter the distal GI tract, where they cannot be digested and absorbed, or when the liver's capacity for plasma protein synthesis from absorbed amino acids and oligopeptides is exceeded. Many clinical disorders exhibit this syndrome, including Ménétrier's disease, enteritis (allergic, viral, and bacterial), and diseases with increased pressure in the intestinal lymphatic system, such as inferior vena caval obstruction, constrictive pericarditis, and congestive heart failure. Some patients present with dependent edema or anasarca; others basically exhibit features of the primary disorder. The diagnosis is made by IV infusion of Cr-labeled albumin and collecting the stools for 96 hours to measure the radioactivity. Serum and stool α-1-antitrypsin is very useful for clearance tests, since it is not reabsorbed or digested after leakage from blood into bowel lumen.

Short Bowel Syndrome

This syndrome refers to losses of fluids and electrolytes as well as malabsorption following extensive intestinal resection. Several factors determine the clinical consequences: (1) *the length of the remnant*, the loss of up to 50% of intestinal length being generally well tolerated; (2) *adaptation by the remnant*, which increases absorptive capacity over the first 3–12 postoperative months; (3) *the site of resection*, which determines malabsorption of specific nutrients; (4) *the presence of colonic capacity* for water and salt absorption and for the bacterial production of short-chain fatty acids and their absorption, and (5) *the integrity of the remnant*.

Resection of under 100 cm of ileum from the ileocecal valve (e.g., for Crohn's disease), reduces bile salt absorption, which is offset by increased hepatic bile salt synthesis. Excess delivery of bile salts into the colon disturbs colonic water and salt absorption. However, resection of over 100 cm of terminal ileum leads to heavy losses of bile salts into the colon that outstrips the hepatic synthesis. The lowered bile salt levels in bile and small intestinal contents lead to steatorrhea and a predilection for cholesterol gallstones. Dietary fat restriction can minimize the diarrhea, since colonic water and salt absorption is compromised by long-chain fatty acids. However, vitamin B_{12} absorption is likely to suffer. Steatorrhea increases colonic absorption of dietary oxalate, resulting in urinary calcium oxalate stones.

Management of the short-bowel syndrome must address many issues. **Caloric losses** tend to decrease during the initial period of adaptation of the intestine remaining. Frequent, high-caloric feedings should be encouraged, but elemental diets are not indicated. Supplemental home parenteral nutrition may be needed in those with very little intestine remaining. **Water and electrolyte deficits** are more likely with small bowel stomas than with an intact colon. Minor deficits are correctable by daily use of an oral rehydration solution but electrolyte solutions may need to be infused overnight. It is necessary to monitor for and treat any **nutrient deficits** from excessive losses of minerals, especially calcium, magnesium, potassium, and zinc, and of fat-soluble vitamins. **Vitamin B_{12} malabsorption** is the rule after extensive ileal resections, thus necessitating B_{12} replacement by monthly injections. **Diarrhea** due to excess bile salt delivery can be abolished by a bile salt-binding resin (e.g., cholestyramine). Because calcium ions precipitate oxalate and prevent its intestinal absorption, dietary calcium should be increased and oxalate intake restricted. **D-lactic acidosis** with confusion and ataxia is a rare but serious complication, which resolves with antibiotics and cessation of carbohydrate intake.

CHAPTER 81   MESENTERIC VASCULAR DISEASE AND INSUFFICIENCY

Mesenteric arterial insufficiency is a formidable problem for the clinician, the surgeon, and the radiologist. The collateral interconnecting arteries between the celiac, superior mesenteric, and inferior mesenteric arteries endow the gut with a significant degree of protection from ischemia.

Chronic Intestinal Ischemia

Chronic mesenteric ischemia (abdominal angina) is due to atheromatous stenosis or occlusion of two of the three major gut arteries, often at or near their aortic origins. Patients report steady and often severe mid-abdominal or generalized pain, occurring 20–30 minutes after meals. However, the relation between food intake and pain is not always constant. Fear of pain on eating leads to decreased food intake and weight loss. Physical examination is usually unrevealing, save for abdominal bruits. However, the elderly often exhibit asymptomatic bruits. Angiography, the major diagnostic tool, also shows equivalent stenosis in asymptomatic persons. The more common causes of chronic abdominal pain must be excluded before diagnosing intestinal angina or embarking on surgical revascularization or balloon angioplasty.

Acute Mesenteric Ischemia

Acute bowel infarction, a life-threatening intra-abdominal calamity, is due to sudden compromise of the intestinal blood supply. Serious cardiovascular, renal, or other systemic disease is often associated. At least one-half of the cases represent nonocclusive intestinal ischemia and infarction, which particularly afflicts those above age 50, with chronic congestive heart failure, cardiac arrhythmias, recent myocardial infarction, hypotension, and hypovolemia. Splanchnic vasoconstriction is the central theme here. It may be brief but long enough to damage mucosa. Thromboembolic arterial occlusion leads to 35% of cases, with the clinical setting of emboli being arrhythmias (atrial fibrillation), recent myocardial infarction, or infective endocarditis. Aortic dissection, vasculitis, and venous thrombosis account for 15%.

Abdominal pain is the most common initial symptom, along with an urge to defecate. Early on, abdominal findings are sparse or absent. Bloody stools are common. With time, nausea, vomiting, and back pain appear, along with fever, peritoneal signs, leukocytosis, metabolic acidosis, hyperamylasemia, and blood-tinged peritoneal fluid that denotes progressive intestinal necrosis. The diagnosis of acute mesenteric ischemia must be considered in any older patient with persistent, acute abdominal pain without other abdominal findings or plain x-ray abnormalities, especially because this often indicates that the process is at an early stage. The diagnosis is difficult, but delays are fatal. In this setting, rapid assessment of the cardiovascular status and prompt resuscitation should be carried out to alleviate or correct congestive heart failure, pulmonary edema, or arrhythmias.

Abdominal x-rays are obtained to exclude other acute abdominal events and to detect signs of ischemic bowel. A duplex ultrasound can detect blood flow and its direction in the three major visceral arteries. With angiography, the diagnostic "gold standard," the state of the splanchnic vessels can be assessed; if the findings justify it, a vasodilator such as papaverine can be given. The decision for surgery is extremely difficult. At surgery, it is often not possible to confidently assess the limits of viable bowel, and a "second-look" laparotomy 12–36 hours later may help identify and resect any additional nonviable bowel. Atherosclerotic or thrombotic obstruction of the celiac and superior mesenteric artery, near their origin, may be treated by percutaneous balloon angioplasty but recurrent occlusion is common.

CHAPTER 82

NEOPLASMS OF THE SMALL INTESTINE

Neoplasms of the small bowel are infrequent. The majority are benign, and are quiescent or incidentally found. Polyposis syndromes involving the small bowel are discussed in chapter 93.

Adenocarcinoma

Occurring mainly in the duodenum and jejunum, adenocarcinoma is the most common small bowel cancer. It may rarely complicate the course of long-standing Crohn's ileitis. Symptoms occur due to obstruction, ulceration, bleeding and, occasionally, to intrussusception or perforation. Adenocarcinoma in the region of the papilla of Vater tends to develop from villous adenomas. It may produce ulcer-like symptoms but also frequently obstructs the common bile duct or ampulla, thus clinically simulating cancer of the head of the pancreas with jaundice. Most adenocarcinomas of the duodenum and small bowel are discovered too late for curative surgical resection. The prognosis is grim.

Lymphoma

Most GI lymphomas arise from monoclonal proliferation of intestinal B lymphocytes. Primary lymphoma of the small intestine occurs most commonly in the ileum and has several forms. The multifocal, nodular form can produce a picture resembling regional enteritis by producing localized polypoid, infiltrative, and ulcerative lesions affecting several segments. Diffuse involvement of the small bowel by lymphoma may mimic celiac disease, including x-ray and biopsy features, with evidence of malabsorption. Fever, abdominal pain, and anorexia are more suggestive of diffuse lymphoma. In a subset, an abnormal, IgA-type immunoglobulin is produced, composed of heavy chains of the α-1 subclass (**α-heavy chain disease**). It occurs among adolescents and young adults of Middle Eastern countries, Asia, and South America. New symptoms (e.g., pain, weight loss) occurring in established celiac disease or lack of response to a gluten-free diet could be an indication of lymphoma of the small intestine. Treatment and prognosis depend on the extent of bowel involvement and whether or not there is extraintestinal lymphoma. Localized or small-segment disease is best treated by surgery, with or without postoperative radiation and/or chemotherapy. Primary diffuse lymphoma of a long intestinal segment is less amenable to surgery; radiotherapy and chemotherapy are the mainstays.

Kaposi's sarcoma

Kaposi's sarcoma may involve any part of the GI tract. It presents as a submucosal infiltrative process and is usually clinically silent. The typical skin manifestations are present in nearly all, most of whom have AIDS. Metastases to the small intestine predominantly originate from malignant melanomas and lung cancer. Bleeding, obstruction, or perforation are the usual symptoms.

Carcinoid tumor

Carcinoid tumors are most common in the terminal ileum, appendix and the rectum. The great majority are small, asymptomatic, and found incidentally at surgery or autopsy. However, some are clinically malignant. Metastases, which seem to correlate best with size, occur in 20–30% of cases at diagnosis. These slow-growing neoplasms may cause partial bowel obstruction; liver metastases may produce the "carcinoid syndrome," with cramps and watery diarrhea, cutaneous flushing, bronchial constriction, telangiectasias, and right heart valvular lesions. Food and alcohol intake may precipitate flushing in foregut tumors. Carcinoid tumor cells hydroxylate and decarboxylate tryptophan to serotonin, which is later metabolized to 5-hydroxyindoleacetic acid (5-HIAA) and excreted abundantly in the urine.

Widespread metastases are rare. Although liver metastases may be present, tumor resection should be considered so as to prevent intestinal obstruction and bleeding. Combined 5-fluorouracil and streptozotocin chemotherapy has shown a 35–50% temporary response rate. Hepatic artery ligation or embolization followed by chemotherapy is another option. Diarrhea may respond to diphenoxylate and loperamide. Infusion of octreotide, a somatostatin analogue, can help prevent "carcinoid crises" during anesthesia and surgery. Carcinoid tumors and their metastases grow quite slowly, with many patients surviving 5–10 years or more; almost 25% survive 5 years, even with liver metastases. Death usually occurs from hepatic or cardiac failure.

INTESTINAL OBSTRUCTION AND PARALYTIC ILEUS

■ **Etiology and Clinical Features**

Mechanical obstruction or generalized hypomotility of intestinal smooth muscle (paralytic ileus) may cause intestinal and abdominal distension. Features of mechanical obstruction and paralytic ileus are compared in Table 83.1. In mechanical obstruction, rhythmic cramps reach a peak, causing the patient to writhe, and then recede. The cramps are accompanied by loud, often high-pitched or hollow bowel sounds (**borborygmi**). Abdominal distension is present unless obstruction is at a high level. Constipation depends on level of lesion; the lower the level and more complete the obstruction, the sooner the obstipation (severe constipation). Repeated vomiting and sequestered fluid in the bowel lumen cause dehydration. If strangulation, infarction, or peritonitis develops, signs of shock and sepsis will follow. Surgery is then urgently needed.

■ **Diagnosis**

Hernial orifices should be carefully checked for incarcerated or strangulated hernias. Metabolic acidosis or alkalosis, leukocytosis, hyperamylasemia, and hemoconcentration are seen, but these are nonspecific. Plain supine, upright, and lateral abdominal x-rays should be obtained, and if inconclusive, repeated in a few hours. Besides air-fluid levels (Figure 83.1), bowel gas patterns might suggest inguinal or other internal hernias, volvulus, or air in the biliary tree (a bilio-enteric fistula with gallstone passage) or in the portal vein (bowel infarction). A cautiously performed barium enema often shows the level and nature of mechanical colon obstruction. Treatment consists of correcting fluid and electrolyte imbalance, relieving emesis, and decompressing the small bowel of its fluid and swallowed air. In suspected mechanical obstruction, early surgery

TABLE **83.1.** Features of Mechanical Obstruction and Paralytic Ileus		
	Mechanical Obstruction	**Paralytic Ileus**
Etiology	Intraluminal blockage (tumors, foreign bodies, gallstones, or worms) or extrinsic compression and obstruction (adhesions, tumors, herniations, or volvulus)	Secondary to a primary derangement, e.g., trauma, peritonitis, uremia, sepsis, postoperative atony from manipulation of abdominal viscera; pelvic and spinal fractures, narcotics, anticholinergics, hypokalemia and hypocalcemia
Evolution	Rapid, with high obstruction and less rapid for lower levels	Slow. Clinical picture dominated by the underlying illness
Abdominal pain	Colicky, appears in bouts that reach a peak, borborygmi heard during contraction	Usually painless; discomfort and dyspnea depend on extent of distention
Other symptoms	Nausea, vomiting, distention, and obstipation	Nausea, vomiting, distention, and obstipation
Abdominal examination	Soft and tympanitic, visible outlines of dilated intestinal loops, borborygmi (early); bowel sounds are absent in late disease complicated by peritonitis	Abdomen may be distended but is characteristically silent
X-rays	Single or multiple loops of distended small bowel (figure 83.1) with air-fluid levels	Multiple, distended, gas-filled small and large intestinal loops with gas also in the lower colon and rectum.
Course and treatment	Progressive unless obstruction relieved; surgery needs to be considered early	Often self-limited. Responds to correction of the underlying illness through intestinal decompression and management of fluid/electrolyte problems

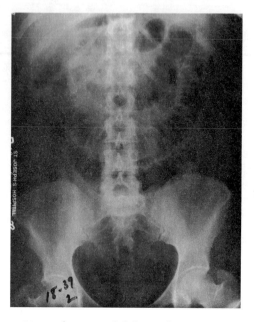

FIGURE 83.1. Plain x-ray of abdomen showing small bowel obstruction.

should be considered before strangulation (non-viable bowel segment) occurs.

Colonic obstruction is most often due to cancer (see chapter 93). Its course is gradual, but obstipation occurs early. Plain abdominal x-rays show a gas-filled colon, up to a point distal to which no gas is seen. In *cecal volvulus*, a large, left upper-quadrant gas-filled viscus is seen with a paucity of gas distal to it. In *sigmoid volvulus*, a large, dilated colonic loop arises from the pelvis. On a barium enema, a normal rectum and distal sigmoid taper to a "bird's beak" at the site of the volvulus. Barium enema or sigmoidoscopy can successfully reduce most cases of sigmoid volvulus.

CHAPTER 84   REGIONAL ENTERITIS

■ Definition and Epidemiology

Regional enteritis, or **Crohn's disease of the small intestine,** is a chronic inflammatory disorder of unknown cause, potentially involving the GI tract from mouth to anus with secondary involvement of regional lymph nodes, liver, skin, eyes, and joints. Crohn's colitis is discussed in chapter 88. The incidence of Crohn's disease has risen substantially during the past few decades; it is particularly common among Jews and people residing in areas with a cold or temperate climate. While no defined pattern of inheritance is apparent, first-degree relatives of index cases have a 5% life-time risk of acquiring this disease. The age at diagnosis is below 30 years in 75% and below 20 years in 30% of patients.

■ Pathology

The cellular reaction in the intestine is lymphoplasmacytoid; mononuclear cells aggregate to form non-caseating granulomas with giant cells in one-half of cases. This inflammation, along with edema and fibrosis, involves all layers of the gut wall. The initial lesion consists of micro-ulcers overlying mucosal lymph follicles (aphthae). Irregular ulcers and the formation of deep fissures typify evolving Crohn's disease. The inflamed and swollen intervening mucosa gives it a "cobblestone" appearance. Crohn's disease of the small bowel typically tends to form fistulae and single or multiple fibrotic strictures. The bowel wall is thick and stiff. Normal "skip areas" may be present between grossly diseased segments.

The small bowel, mainly the distal ileum, is solely involved in 30% of cases; in 50% ileitis contiguously extends into the colon; 20% involve only the colon. Duodenal and antral involvement occurs in 1–3% of cases. Perianal disease, with fistulae and abscesses, as well as deep anal and perineal ulcers, develops in 30% at some time and is the initial presentation in 1–3% of patients.

■ Clinical Features

The clinical picture is determined by the site of GI involvement. Given the distal ileal involvement in 80–90% of patients, nonbloody diarrhea is the rule; steatorrhea and vitamin B_{12} malabsorption is related to the length of the affected ileum. Abdominal pain (usually right lower quadrant) is very common. A steady ache

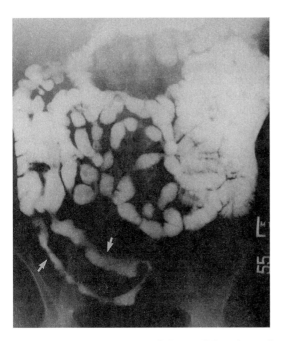

FIGURE 84.1. Crohn's disease of the small bowel. Small bowel barium x-ray shows the entire small bowel and the proximal and transverse colon; the transit time to the cecum was 55 min. Two separated loops (solid arrows) represent about 40 cm of terminal ileum with irregular narrowing and eccentric dilatation (pseudosacculations). The loops are separated by transmural inflammation and thickening of the mesentery. No abscess or intestinal fistula was found. The colon is spared.

(Courtesy of Edward Stewart, MD, Milwaukee, Wisconsin.)

indicates serosal extension and possible perforation; a palpable, tender inflammatory mass may form and evolve into an intra-abdominal abscess. Such perforations lead to sinus tracts, or fistulae into another viscus (bowel, urinary bladder, or vagina), or to the abdominal wall. Colicky pain with distention and its relief after bowel movements suggest partial ileal obstruction, due to inflammatory ileal swelling or fibrotic strictures. Weight loss may follow anorexia, fear of pain after eating, or malabsorption. Rectal bleeding is most often occult. Gross bleeding occasionally occurs, especially in young persons during their first attack with extensive Crohn's colitis.

Perineal disease may be severe, often with dusky, anal skin tags and perianal or ischiorectal abscess, draining perineal fistulas, and anorectal stricture. Antro-duodenal involvement may cause ulcer-like pain and pyloric or duodenal obstruction. Low-grade fever is usual; with spiking fever, an abscess is suspect. Extraintestinal complications are erythema nodosum, arthritis, uveitis, oral aphthous ulcers, and primary sclerosing

cholangitis. Malabsorption caused by ileal disease or resection leads to metabolic bone disease, anemia, bleeding diathesis, gallstones, renal oxalate stones, and weight loss (see chapter 80).

■ Diagnosis

Laboratory abnormalities reflect inflammation, malnutrition including hypoalbuminemia, blood loss, and malabsorption. Anemia has multiple causes including myelosuppression by chronic disease. Imaging of the ileum by a small bowel series or barium enema may show mucosal edema, aphthous ulceration, luminal narrowing ("string sign"), fistula formation, and inflammatory mass-effect (Figure 84.1). Crohn's disease of the small intestine must be distinguished from ileocecal tuberculosis, lymphoma, and ileal carcinoid. Colon x-rays or colonoscopy can identify colon and terminal ileal involvement. "Skip areas" in the colon and absence of rectal disease negate the diagnosis of ulcerative colitis. Work-up for intestinal obstruction is necessary if symptoms suggest it. Abdominal/pelvic CT can detect inflammatory masses, abscesses, fistulae, and extrinsic ureteral obstruction.

■ Management

The overriding treatment goal is to preserve the quality of life in patients with this chronic, recurrent disease, which has no specific treatment. Pain and diarrhea respond to codeine and antidiarrheal agents (loperamide). Nutritional support should correct vitamin and mineral deficiencies and ensure adequate caloric intake. Liquid formula diets are useful in some cases of severe and extensive disease. Patients with narrow strictures should avoid high-residue foods (e.g., corn, Chinese cabbage, pulp of citrus fruit, and enteric-coated tablets). Parenteral alimentation may be needed to prepare for surgery or as part of short-term therapy to induce a remission. The rare case of short bowel syndrome from extensive bowel resection will require home parenteral nutrition.

A few medications can help spur clinical remission but do not help in managing complications, such as abscesses and bowel strictures. Prednisone in daily doses of 20–40 mg is useful, but it does not prevent recurrences and its use should be limited to 2–4 months. Enteric-coated 5-ASA (mesalamine) products begin to release the active agent in the small bowel, while the release of 5-ASA from sulfasalazine and olsalazine (Dipentum®) occurs entirely within the colon. Concurrent use of steroids and 5-ASA-compounds may be additive. Immunosuppressive agents such as azathioprine and 6-mercaptopurine can be steroid-sparing and maintain remission for several years. Their use must be weighed against their serious side effects (bone marrow suppression, pancreatitis, predisposition to infections, allergies, and a higher risk of developing neoplasms). Long-term metronidazole may aid in closing fistulae. Maintenance therapy with therapeutic doses of mesalamine (5-ASA) products may lower the 1-year relapse rate from about 60% to nearly 35%. Surgery is indicated for complications that cannot be treated medically (e.g., abscesses, bowel obstruction, enterocutaneous fistulae and incapacitating pain unresponsive to medical measures, and the rare case of adenocarcinoma of the ileum). The life-time risk of requiring surgery is about 70%; 30–50% of these patients require further surgery. Disease recurrence following an ileocolonic resection regularly begins at the surgical anastomosis and extends proximally.

CHAPTER 85   PHYSIOLOGY OF THE COLON

■ Colonic Motility

Unlike the small bowel, the colon has no uniform pattern of fasting and postprandial motor activity. Its primary motor activity is the nonpropulsive, ring-like segmental contraction, which produces mixing and to-and-fro movement of contents. Coordinated but irregular contractions propel intraluminal contents aborally over varying distances. The cecum and ascending colon delay the transit of solids until liquefied. Segmental contractions, more frequent in the distal colon, retard the flow into the rectum, the distension of which with feces causes a sensation of fullness that evokes an urge to defecate. A normally distensible rectum can accommodate rather large volumes of material. Giant migrating contractions frequently accompany colonic inflammation; they rapidly fill the rectal ampulla, prompting urgent defecation.

Cholecystokinin (CCK), gastrin, and motilin stimulate colonic smooth muscle, whereas secretin, glucagon, and vasoactive intestinal polypeptide (VIP) inhibit it. The final step in the motor inhibition of the colon and its sphincters is believed to be the local release of nitric oxide (NO). Prostaglandins of the E type diminish segmental activity and increase propulsion.

■ Fluid and Electrolyte Transport in the Colon

Colonic epithelium differs functionally from that of the small bowel. The colonic mucosa is a tight membrane with lower effective pore size, lower osmotic permeability for water, higher electrical resistance and transmucosal potential difference and higher ability to absorb Na^+ against electrochemical gradients. Over 95% of the large amount of short-chain fatty acids (SCFA) produced by carbohydrate fermentation is absorbed, most of it in exchange for bicarbonate. Absorption of these organic acids (acetate, propionate, n-butyrate) also stimulates the colonic absorption of Na^+ and water. SCFA, especially n-butyrate, is the major and essential substrate of colonocyte metabolism. Most of the n-butyrate entering colonocytes are metabolized by the cells and do not enter the portal system. Decreased SCFA production causes colonic absorptive dysfunction and, possibly, inflammation.

Ileal flow into the colon in a healthy person approximates 1500 ml/24h, containing 200 mEq of Na^+. Stool output has 100–150 ml of water/24h and 1–5 mEq of Na^+. The maximal, estimated absorptive capacity of the colon is 4–5L of water and 800 mEq Na^+ daily, provided the inflow from the terminal ileum is constant. Thus, the colon can compensate for a two–threefold rise in the volume normally delivered to it.

■ Bacteriology of the Colon

Distal to the ileocecal valve there is an abundant, metabolically active bacterial population averaging 10^{10}–10^{12} bacteria/mL, composed mainly of strict anaerobes such as bacteroides and bifidobacteria. *E. coli* is the most common facultative aerobic organism; anaerobic gram-positive cocci are also common. One-third of fecal weight consists of bacteria. Their activities alter bowel contents in many ways, such as the fermentation of both simple and complex (e.g., fiber) carbohydrate, deamination and decarboxylation of proteins and amino acids, ammonia formation from urea, hydroxylation of fatty acids, degradation of bilirubin to urobilins, deconjugation and dehydroxylation of bile acids, and the synthesis of vitamin K and folate. Bacteria also deconjugate glucuronide conjugates or convert inert compounds to pharmacologically active metabolites (e.g., splitting sulfasalazine into 5-ASA and sulfapyridine).

PROCEDURES IN THE DIAGNOSIS OF COLONIC DISORDERS

■ Radiography

Plain films of the abdomen can detect "toxic" colonic dilatation (as in inflammatory bowel disease) and mechanical obstruction. Barium contrast enema is useful in detecting diverticulosis, inflammatory bowel disease, ischemic colitis, and motility disorders, such as Hirschsprung's disease.

■ Proctosigmoidoscopy

Proctosigmoidoscopy is indicated in patients with changes in bowel habit, rectal bleeding, anorectal pain, persistent constipation or diarrhea, weight loss, or anemia. Besides observing the mucosal appearance and the vascular pattern and looking for lesions such as polyps and tumors, it is possible to biopsy and to take specimens for parasitologic examination and bacterial culture. Biopsies should routinely be obtained in patients with chronic diarrhea. Rigid proctoscopy allows inspection of the distal 25 cm of rectosigmoid. However, prior pelvic surgery, irradiation, and diverticulosis may cause sufficient fixation and angulation to limit full passage of the rigid scope. Flexible sigmoidoscopes not only surmount these problems, but extend inspection to 60 cm; they are routinely used to screen for cancer and polyps.

■ Stool Examination

Stool obtained by routine digital examination should be inspected and tested for occult blood. A variety of products, using a color indicator method, can detect fecal occult blood. In the presence of hydrogen peroxide, the peroxidase activity of heme hastens the oxidation of guaiac to a quinone; a blue color develops, indicating the presence of blood. False-positive results may follow ingestion of raw or undercooked red meat, turnips, or horseradish. Finding RBCs and WBCs in the stool of patients with diarrhea may help recognize acute or chronic inflammatory colonic disease. Proper collection and handling of fresh stool samples are a must for successful bacteriologic and parasitologic examinations in evaluating diarrhea. Guidelines established by the clinical laboratory must be observed, and the stool collected before administering antibiotics and laxatives or barium x-rays.

■ Colonoscopy

Fiberoptic colonoscopy is invaluable for confirmation and biopsy of findings on barium enema, in detecting and removing colon polyps, and in evaluating known or suspected inflammatory bowel disease. It is widely used for screening individuals at high risk for bowel cancer. In some situations, it complements barium x-ray examination, but several reports indicate a higher yield of significant pathology than barium enemas, albeit at a higher cost.

■ Miscellaneous Tests

Defecography: Anorectal morphology and functional dynamics during defecation can be investigated by defecography. This radiology techniques involves using a stool-consistency barium paste and is a useful tool for evaluation of rectal prolapse, fecal continence, and to asses the rectoanal angle and perineal descent during rest and straining.

Colorectal Transit Time: In this technique, the subject ingests radiopaque markers (e.g. Sitzmarks) and progression of markers is monitored by abdominal X-rays until total expulsion of markers. Segmental transit times can be measured by counting markers in the right colon, left colon and rectosigmoid areas.

Anorectal manometry

Rectal distension evokes rectoanal inhibitory reflex—that is, brief relaxation of the internal anal sphincter and contraction of the striated muscle external sphincter. Recording pressures from the anal canal and rectum, before and during rectal balloon distention, can diagnose Hirschsprung's disease (absent rectoanal reflex), and detect the cause of fecal incontinence (by increased rectal sensation and reflex thresholds, decreased rectal compliance, or impaired internal or external sphincter function).

CHAPTER 87 MOTILITY DISORDERS OF THE COLON

Congenital Motility Disorder: Aganglionic Megacolon

This familial congenital disorder, known as **Hirschsprung's disease,** is thought to result from failure of the intramural ganglion cells to migrate into certain parts of the GI tract. Most commonly, a variable length of distal colon, involving the internal sphincter and adjacent rectum, is devoid of myenteric ganglion cells. Rarely, more extensive portions or the entire colon are involved. The aganglionic segment is narrowed and unable to transport fecal contents, causing constipation and progressive dilatation of the normal proximal bowel that eventually leads to abdominal distention. The clinical history is one of obstipation dating from birth.

On digital rectal examination, the ampulla is usually empty. X-rays show a narrowed distal colon and dilatation of the remainder of the bowel. Anorectal manometry reliably separates chronic idiopathic constipation from Hirschsprung's disease by demonstrating in the latter the absence of the **rectoanal inhibitory reflex** (see chapter 86). The confirmatory finding is the absence of myenteric ganglion cells on mucosal/submucosal suction or punch biopsy or deep surgical biopsy of the rectal wall of the narrowed segment. Treatment includes surgical resection of the aganglionic segment.

Acquired Motility Disorders

Constipation

Constipation, with or without colonic enlargement, is a common symptom; it is more frequent in women than in men and its incidence rises with advancing age. A widely used definition is less than two bowel movements weekly, but the primary symptom may be hard, pellet-like stools or difficult emptying with excess straining at stool.

■ Etiology

Several medications impair bowel transit, including opiates, anticholinergics (including tricyclic antidepressants), calcium channel blockers, and ganglionic blockers. Endocrine-metabolic causes are hypothyroidism, hypercalcemia, and uremia. Neurogenic and myogenic constipation may follow heavy metal intoxication, spinal cord lesions, Hirschsprung's disease, Parkinson's disease, muscular dystrophy, multiple sclerosis, and autonomic neuropathy. Finally, any stenotic lesion of the colorectum and anus, including rectal prolapse, may cause constipation of recent onset. When no underlying cause is found, idiopathic constipation is diagnosed.

Idiopathic Constipation

In adults, etiology of idiopathic constipation is obscure and treatment remains a challenge; eventual success depends on step-wise treatment (Table 87.1), the aims of which are to evoke artificial bowel regularity, reduce symptoms and prevent fecal impaction. The

merits of increasing stool weight by a high-fiber diet are unclear. Bulk laxatives (methylcellulose, polycarbophil, psyllium) or stool softeners (docusate) are useful, as are hyperosmotic cathartics given periodically (orally or rectally) including saline cathartics (Mg^+ salts) PEG-electrolyte solution (GoLYTELY™), lactulose or sorbitol syrup, and hypertonic phosphate solutions (Fleets™). Cisapride, a prokinetic drug, 10–20 mg t.i.d., may be used. Stimulant laxatives (phenolphthalein, danthron, bisacodyl, and cascara) should be used sparingly.

■ Fecal Impaction

Symptoms and findings of bowel obstruction may be caused by the accumulation of firm, immovable fecal masses, 70% of which form in the rectum. This condition occurs mainly in chronically debilitated and immobile patients. Potential complications are dehydration, the formation of stercoral pressure ulcers, and colonic perforation. Treatment consists of hydration and careful disimpaction by digital means and/or repeated retrograde irrigation and suction.

■ Overuse of Laxatives

Known or surreptitious laxative use may cause the following conditions. **Melanosis coli** is marked by a reticular, brown-black discoloration of the colonic mucosa. Lipofuscin-laden macrophages accumulate in the lamina propria. While specific for long-term use of

TABLE 87.1. Treatment of Idiopathic Constipation

Step 1:
  Rule out metabolic and medication causes
  Reassure and educate patient
  Regular physical exercise
  Attempt daily defecation
  Stool softeners
  If small, hard stool: bulk laxatives; add bran
    (20g/d); mineral oil
  Try cisapride, 10-20 mg q.i.d.
Step 2:
  Osmotic cathartics
  Nonabsorbed sugars (sorbitol, lactulose)
  PEG-electrolyte solution
  Enemas: saline; hypertonic phosphate
  Psychologic evaluation?
Step 3
  Stimulant laxatives
Special situations:
  • Pelvic outlet obstruction
    Biofeedback therapy: coordinate pelvic floor relax-
    ation with defecation act.
  • Normal transit constipation: reassurance/psycho-
    logic evaluation
  • Delayed colonic transit (colonic inertia) with massive
    fecal retention: consider colectomy with
    ileoproctostomy.

anthracene-type laxatives (senna, cascara, aloe, dan-thron), the condition has no functional significance. **Cathartic colon** is a featureless, moderately dilated colon rarely found on barium enema examination. Mild, nonspecific abdominal symptoms may occur. Damage to the myenteric plexus of the colon reportedly follows chronic stimulant laxative use. **Factitious diarrhea** is an underdiagnosed cause of chronic watery diarrhea. By definition, the patient does not confess to using laxatives. The condition frequently is reflective of a complex psychiatric disorder, including the so-called Münch-hausen syndrome. (See p. 403).

Colonic Pseudo-obstruction

Acute pseudo-obstruction of the entire colon (**Ogilvie's syndrome**) is a transient motor abnormality associated with systemic illnesses, such as congestive heart failure, myocardial infarction, sepsis, and assisted ventilation. Stool output ceases and abdominal distention may develop; the bowel sounds are reduced but not absent. The condition is diagnosed by plain abdominal x-rays after excluding mechanical obstruction by proctosigmoi-doscopy or a limited barium enema. Opiates and anticholinergic agents must be stopped. Nasogastric suction, parenteral fluids, and colonoscopic decompres-sion are often successful. Surgery is necessary for impending perforation.

Irritable Bowel Syndrome

■ Definition and Epidemiology

Irritable bowel syndrome (IBS) is defined as abdomi-nal pain with changes in bowel habits, without detectable organic causes. Two or more of the following symptoms are present in most patients: (1) intermittent abdominal distention; (2) more frequent and loose bowel movements with the onset of pain; (3) pain relief after bowel movements; (4) difficult and/or painful defecation. Nearly 15% of adults have symptoms that qualify for this diagnosis, but only 20% of these consult a physician. The prevalence is twice as high in women as it is in men. Symptoms commonly begin in the second or third decade and rarely after the sixth. IBS is a major cause of time lost from work and is the most common diagnosis among patients with abdominal complaints. The terms "spastic colon" and "mucous colitis" should no longer be used.

■ Pathophysiology

IBS is a symptom complex likely to comprise several disorders and pathophysiologic mechanisms. Several abnormalities in colonic motor activity have been observed. Compared with control subjects, these patients experience a delayed but increased colonic motor response after eating (gastrocolic reflex), possibly related to abnormal sensitivity to postprandial release of chole-cystokinin. The patients have a lower pain threshold to balloon distention and gas insufflation throughout the GI tract, from esophagus to rectum, indicating increased visceral pain perception. Abnormal psychologic features are found in 70–90% of patients, predominantly depres-sion, anxiety, and somatization disorders. Such person-ality disorders are more common in patients with IBS symptoms who consult a physician than in those who do not. The prevalence of a history of sexual and physical abuse in IBS patients of either gender is quite high.

■ Clinical Features

The symptoms are quite variable, but alternating constipation and diarrhea, often with lower abdominal pain, are the most common. Flatulence and a sense of abdominal distention are frequent. The pain is rarely localized to one specific site. A common bowel pattern is the passage of a formed stool, followed by two or three loose, watery stools with mucus, soon after waking. Symptoms tend to be worsened by environmental stresses, by depression, and by eating a variety of foods. The bowel movements are small in volume and the daily stool weight is usually normal (<200g), rarely exceeding

300g/day. Features that should suggest a cause other than IBS include weight loss, nocturnal stools, soiling, progressive severity of symptoms, blood in the stool, and onset after the age of 50. The diagnosis is based on a careful medical history, physical examination, complete blood count, flexible sigmoidoscopy, stool test for occult blood, and, when indicated, a lactose tolerance test. Extensive and repeated diagnostic testing should be avoided. IBS does not predispose to diverticular disease, inflammatory bowel disease, or to cancer.

■ Management

The patient should be reassured about the absence of organic disease and the good prognosis of the disorder.

Counseling regarding changing from or adapting to a stressful environment may be needed, and perhaps, formal psychological counseling. Biofeedback therapy and relaxation training may help. Foods that evoke symptoms should be avoided, especially gas-forming items (e.g., legumes, dark bread, and high sorbitol and fructose products). Despite little evidence that a high-fiber diet is helpful in IBS, psyllium and polycarbophil may be tried. Antidiarrheal drugs (loperamide and diphenoxylate) are safe and should be taken before diarrhea tends to occur. Similarly, anticholinergics (dicyclomine, propantheline, hyoscyamine) may help with painful colonic spasms if taken before their expected onset. Some may benefit from carefully monitored, low-dose antidepressants (e.g., amitriptyline).

CHAPTER **88**   # INFLAMMATORY BOWEL DISEASE

This term embraces two diseases, chronic ulcerative colitis and Crohn's disease. Sometimes their separation is difficult. Crohn's disease of the small intestine is discussed in chapter 84. Only Crohn's colitis and ulcerative colitis are reviewed here.

Chronic Ulcerative Colitis

■ Definition and Epidemiology

Chronic ulcerative colitis (CUC), an idiopathic inflammatory disease of the colonic mucosal surface, is most prevalent among Caucasians, particularly Ashkenazi Jews. With an annual incidence of 5–10/100,000, its prevalence in the United States is 45–80/100,000. Two incidence peaks seem to occur, one at ages 20–30 and another at around age 60. A minority of patients offer a family history of inflammatory bowel disease (IBD), but the concordance rate among identical twins is low and no genetic pattern of inheritance has yet emerged.

■ Etiology

No evidence favoring an infectious, allergic, immunologic, genetic, or psychosomatic cause has held up to scrutiny. The incidence is higher in nonsmokers and ex-smokers and perhaps in oral contraceptive users. Appendectomy seems to be protective. The number of IgG_1- and IgG_2-producing plasma cells in the lamina propria is increased and the mucosal synthesis of the Interleukin (IL)-1 receptor antagonist is reportedly lower than normal. Auto-antibodies have been noted against a

colonocyte-associated protein (also present in skin and bile ducts). The ability of the colonocytes to metabolize n-butyrate is markedly decreased. The role of these epidemiologic and laboratory observations in causing CUC remains uncertain.

■ Pathology

The disease invariably begins at the anal verge with varying degrees of proximal extension. It involves only the rectosigmoid in 40–50%, large areas of the colon in 30–40%, and the entire colon (pancolitis) in about 20–40% of patients. The disease spreads proximally in 20–30% of patients with only distal involvement initially. The inflammation is confined to the colonic mucosa and submucosa with mononuclear cell infiltration at the base of the lamina propria. In the acute stages, neutrophils and eosinophils invade the surface and crypt epithelium with crypt abscess formation. Changes in crypt architecture (crypt branching and atrophy) are a constant feature that separates IBD from acute infectious colitis. As the crypts are destroyed, the mucosa thins but often, foci of regenerating mucosa develop into inflammatory pseudopolyps. The chronic and recurrent inflammation often leads to shortening and strictures of the colon. The rectum may contract. The ulceration and inflammation in severe, fulminant cases extend into the muscle layers with intramural plexus damage, causing dilatation, impaired motor function and, ultimately, perforation—the so-called **toxic megacolon.**

Clinical Features and Course

The symptoms of CUC vary from mild and frequent bloody rectal discharges with tenesmus (a painful spasm of the rectum with an urge to defecate, and passage of little fecal matter), to a fulminating form with severe systemic and abdominal symptoms. The onset of CUC is most commonly gradual with small, bloody stools, and tenesmus. Abdominal pain preceding urgent defecation is due to frequent, giant migrating colonic contractions. Fever, weight loss, anemia, and hypoproteinemia occur in more severe cases. Fecal losses of water, sodium, and potassium are not severe, given that bowel movements are small-volume and contain only blood and mucus. While 80% of patients have intermittent exacerbations with total remissions, 10–15% remain continuously active without a remission. Nearly 5% remit permanently after the first episode; however, some of these may actually represent infectious colitis—a misdiagnosis, in other words.

Extracolonic manifestations occur in about 10% of patients and may precede the bowel symptoms occasionally. Oral aphthous ulcers, episcleritis, uveitis, pyoderma gangrenosum, erythema nodosum and an asymmetric nondeforming arthropathy of large joints tend to parallel the course of the colitis; sacroiliitis, **primary sclerosing cholangitis (PSC),** ankylosing spondylitis, and secondary amyloidosis, however, may progress even without active colitis and even after proctocolectomy. Most patients with PSC have associated CUC. PSC features chronic inflammation, fibrosis, and stricture formation of the intra- and extra-hepatic bile ducts. Cholestatic jaundice, pruritus, and bouts of suppurative cholangitis follow in the ensuing years, causing secondary biliary cirrhosis and liver failure. A raised serum alkaline phosphatase is the earliest laboratory finding; endoscopic retrograde cholangiography is required for diagnosis. While ursodeoxycholic acid can slow the worsening of liver tests, the only effective treatment is liver transplantation. Cholangiocarcinoma ultimately develops in 10% or more of patients with PSC.

Diagnosis

The physical examination may be normal, but often patients look ill and pale and have a moderate fever. Abdominal examination commonly shows tenderness over the colon. Abdominal distention, tympany, and increased tenderness in acutely ill patients suggest a toxic megacolon. A slightly granular texture is noted on digital rectal examination; bloody mucus is often seen on the glove.

There are no diagnostic laboratory abnormalities. All patients with a dysenteric syndrome (tenesmus and frequent, bloody stools) should undergo fiberoptic sigmoidoscopy without patient preparation by enemas or laxatives. Beginning at the dentate line, the mucosa is uniformly friable, hyperemic, finely ulcerated, and granular. Edema obscures the usual fine tracery of blood vessels beneath the mucosa. With limited distal disease, these gross changes are demarcated proximally by normal mucosa within the viewing range of the sigmoidoscope.

A plain abdominal x-ray can assess the colonic diameter in suspected toxic megacolon (Figure 88.1) and an upright view can detect free intra-abdominal air. In extensive CUC, the gas-filled, dilated transverse colon will show a shaggy, thickened mucosal profile with few or no haustrations. Barium enema can determine the extent of the disease and better define its nature. It may be nearly normal in early or mild disease. In the acute stage, spasm and irritability are more prominent. Ulcerations, usually tiny and difficult to see, often appear as

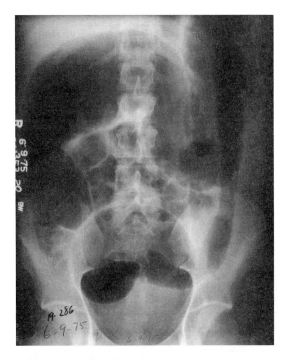

FIGURE 88.1. Toxic megacolon. Pronounced distension of the cecum and ascending colon are noted. Note the absence of haustrations in the air-filled descending colon.

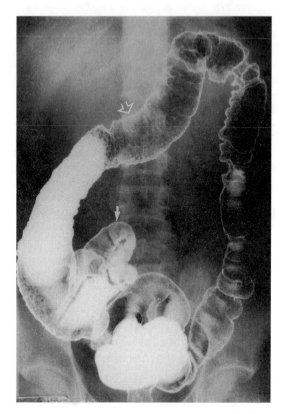

FIGURE 88.2. Acute ulcerative colitis. The colon and rectum are diffusely involved. Normal haustral pattern is lacking in the proximal and transverse colon segments. Note superficial ulcerations, causing the spiculated contours of the transverse colon (open arrow). The terminal ileum (solid arrow) is normal.
(Courtesy of Edward Stewart, MD, Milwaukee, Wisconsin.)

fuzzy serrations or fine spiculations (Figure 88.2). Large ulcerations resemble a collar button. In less active stages, the mucosal surface may be nodular and finely polypoid, reflecting inflammatory pseudopolyps. Air-contrast study makes these details clearer. In chronic disease, the colon is shortened and the lumen is tubular and narrowed with absent haustra (i.e., the "lead pipe" colon). When the entire colon is involved, "backwash ileitis" is not uncommon, with a dilated ileal segment showing a smooth mucosa. Full colonoscopy with inspection and biopsy of the terminal ileum can supplant barium enema, but neither should be done in acute, severe colitis for risk of perforation or precipitating toxic megacolon.

The differential diagnosis includes infectious, Crohn's, indeterminate, ischemic, and radiation colitis. Acute infectious colitis due to *Entameba histolytica*, Salmonella, Shigella, Yersinia, Campylobacter, and enterohemorrhagic *E. coli* O157:H7 may mimic IBD at sigmoidoscopy but their onset is more abrupt than CUC and Crohn's colitis. On endoscopy, the hallmark of CUC is the uniformity of inflammatory changes in the circumferential and longitudinal direction, beginning at the anal verge and ending at a clear demarcation to normal-appearing mucosa located within the colon or at the ileocecal valve.

■ Medical Management

Medical management aims to terminate the acute attack, prevent recurrences, and correct nutritional, fluid, and electrolyte deficits. While both corticosteroids and 5-aminosalicylate (5-ASA) compounds shorten acute attacks, corticosteroids act faster, are more effective than 5-ASA, but have cumulative side effects that are more serious. Patients whose CUC ends distal to the splenic flexure can generally be managed by self-administered hydrocortisone as enemas or rectal foam and 5-ASA as enemas or suppositories. Patients with mild to moderate, extensive colitis may be given sulfasalazine (4–6g/d), or oral prednisone (30–60 mg/d) if the clinical severity requires it. A severe attack is one with more than six bloody stools daily with systemic signs (fever, tachycardia, anemia, or ESR >30 mm/hr). Despite the lack of precision, this definition remains useful when applied with clinical common sense. Such patients are hospitalized and closely watched for abdominal distention, increasing tenderness, fever, tachycardia, and rectal bleeding; hydrocortisone (100 mg q6h) is given IV and by rectal drip. Most patients tolerate only clear liquids and require parenteral nutrition. Early surgical consultation is mandatory; emergency proctocolectomy is indicated in the 20–30% of patients who fail to improve within 1 week.

Because 5-ASA is absorbed in the small intestine, sulfasalazine was developed to ensure targeted 5-ASA delivery to the colon. The sulfonamide is a mere carrier, with no therapeutic effect in CUC; colonic bacteria split the azo-bond that links 5-ASA and sulfapyridine. Side effects, which are common, are mostly due to sulfapyridine. Dose-related effects are nausea, vomiting, headaches, and folate malabsorption. Other side effects are skin rash, fever, hemolytic anemia, alveolitis, hepatitis, and reversible male infertility. Once remission occurs, patients are maintained indefinitely on a 5-ASA drug (e.g., sulfasalazine, 1 g b.i.d), so as to reduce the risk of clinical relapse. Patients intolerant of sulfasalazine and men concerned about fertility impairment may use one of the newer 5-ASA drugs, such as 5-ASA enclosed in a pH-sensitive membrane (Asacol®, Pentasa®) and olsalazine (Dipentum®), which has two 5-ASA molecules linked by an azo-bond. Olsalazine causes watery diarrhea in 10–15% of patients.

Surgical Management

Indications for surgery are a severe attack unresponsive to medications, toxic megacolon, chronic disease activity uncontrolled by medical therapy, or unacceptable side effects from drugs. Total proctocolectomy cures CUC. Less extensive surgical resections or temporary colon bypass are not appropriate. A standard, right lower quadrant end-ileostomy works well, but has cosmetic ramifications and requires self-care of the ileostomy. An increasingly utilized alternative is the creation of an ileal pouch that is anastomosed to the preserved anal sphincter. Fecal continence is attained in most cases when this two-step operation is done by experienced surgeons.

Risk of Colorectal Cancer

CUC carries a 0.8–1% annual risk for developing colorectal cancer (CRC), beginning 10 years after initial presentation. Patients with pancolitis are at the highest risk, but the risk is increased also in patients with left-sided involvement. The diagnosis of cancer in CUC is difficult since the symptoms mimic those of the underlying colitis and x-ray and endoscopy are less accurate than in the normal colon. Dysplastic changes of the colonic mucosa occur in many patients before CRC develops and are nearly universal when a cancer is diagnosed. Yearly surveillance colonoscopy with multiple biopsies obtained at 10 cm intervals, beginning 10 years after diagnosis, is currently recommended for all CUC patients, regardless of the disease activity. High-grade dysplasia requires prompt colectomy; low-grade dysplasia warrants a repeat colonoscopy in 2–3 months. When adjusted for tumor stage at diagnosis, CRC complicating CUC has the same prognosis as CRC in general. The surveillance colonoscopy confers a survival advantage due to the early detection of CRC.

Crohn's Colitis

In 20% of patients, Crohn's colitis (Crohn's disease of the colon) involves only the colon, with similar pathological features as that of small bowel. The rectum is affected in 60%, pancolitis occurs in 30%, and "skip areas" develop in 20% of patients. Fistulas with adjacent organs and colonic obstruction, as well as perforation with abscess formation (Figure 88.3), may follow. Mucosal biopsies contain granulomas in only 25% of cases.

Clinical Features

Most patients have diarrhea, abdominal pain, and weight loss, often with an insidious onset. Painful defecation is a harbinger of anal and perianal disease. While pneumaturia and fecal matter in the urinary sediment suggest an ileovesical or colovesical fistula, dyspareunia and a brownish, malodorous vaginal discharge are clues to a rectovaginal fistula. Physical examination may reveal a tender, inflammatory abdominal mass. The anal canal is often narrowed, with dusky skin tags, representing inflamed anal papillae, and perianal openings of fistulous tracts. Digital rectal examination may cause exquisite pain, especially when there are anal canal ulcers and perianal abscesses. Such anal disease may precede the intestinal and colitis symptoms by months or years. The terminal ileum should be evaluated by imaging or by colonoscopy in patients presenting de novo with such lesions. While extraintestinal complications usually parallel those of CUC, erythema nodosum is more common and PSC and pyoderma gangrenosum are less common in Crohn's colitis than in CUC.

Diagnosis and Management

When proctosigmoidoscopy shows mucosal inflammation, other types of colitis, including infectious, need to excluded, as for CUC. The distinction from CUC is important but challenging; helpful features are listed in Table 88.1. Even so, in 5–10% of patients with IBD, CUC cannot be separated from Crohn's colitis— the so-called "indeterminate colitis."

The management principles are much the same as for Crohn's disease of the small bowel. Drugs of established effectiveness are corticosteroids, azathioprine/6MP, and 5-ASA. Bowel rest and total parenteral nutrition do not influence the disease, but may provide short term rehabilitation. High-dose metronidazole, given for many months, may help temporary fistula closure, although the drug may induce a neuropathy. Once remission is attained, maintenance therapy lowers the frequency of recurrent attacks somewhat. Oral mesalamine, (2.4g/d) and low-dose azathioprine/6-MP (50–100 mg/d) are effective in this regard. However, azathioprine/6-MP may cause pancreatitis early on and bone marrow suppression at any time.

Surgery by an experienced surgeon is reserved for treating intractable disease and local complications. The implications of proctocolectomy for Crohn's colitis differ from those for CUC. The disease may not be eradicated;

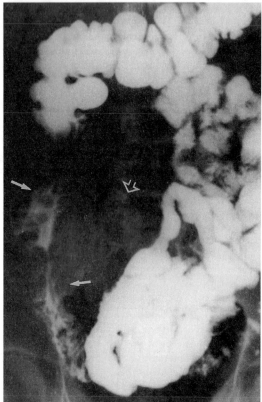

FIGURE 88.3. Crohn's ileocolitis. Small bowel x-ray shows ulcero-nodular Crohn's disease of terminal ileum and ascending colon (solid arrows). The x-ray distinction between terminal ileum and colon is no longer possible. Note the large area in the right hemiabdomen without bowel. The bowel is displaced by extramural inflammation. The open arrow shows the collection of contrast material in this area, which is an abscess communicating with the diseased bowel. A palpable, tender mass was noted clinically.
(Courtesy of Edward Stewart, MD, Milwaukee, Wisconsin.)

20–50% of patients develop Crohn's disease later in the remaining terminal ileum. An ileoanal pouch anastomosis is not indicated, given the risk of ileal recurrence. In contrast to CUC, an ileo-rectal anastomosis and segmental colectomy are options, depending on the location of severe involvement. Severe perirectal and anal disease require definitive surgery.

■ Risk of Colorectal Carcinoma

The risk of colorectal carcinoma in extensive Crohn's colitis approaches that in CUC. As in CUC, surveillance colonoscopy with multiple biopsies is widely practiced. A number of cases of adenocarcinoma of the ileum have been reported in patients with ileal Crohn's disease; no guidelines exist for regular surveillance of the small bowel for premalignant changes or early cancer.

TABLE 88.1.   Differential Diagnosis of Ulcerative vs. Crohn's Colitis

	CUC	Crohn's Colitis
Distribution	Continuous	Segmental
Ileal involvement	0	Diagnostic, if present
Histology:		
Inflammation	Diffuse	Focal
Granulomas	0	++ (~30%)
Transmural	0	4+
Clinical:		
Perianal lesions	1+	3+
Fistulae	(+)	2+
Strictures	1+	3+
Hemorrhage	2+	(+)
Endoscopy:		
Friability	3+	1+
Aphthoid lesions	0	4+
Granularity	3+	1+
Cobblestone	(+)	3+
Linear, deep ulcers	1+	3+
Involvement	Uniform	Non-uniform

CUC = ulcerative colitis.
The scale of 0–4+ indicates the frequency of a finding in each of the two diseases.

CHAPTER 89   # DIVERTICULAR DISEASE OF THE COLON

True colonic diverticula, with all bowel wall layers, are rare. Most are pseudodiverticula, with only mucosal herniations through the muscular layer of the colonic wall, commonly occurring at points of penetration of the circular muscle by intramural blood vessels, located between the mesenteric and the two anti-mesenteric taenia. Diverticula most commonly involve the sigmoid. Nearly unknown in developing countries, the high incidence of diverticulosis in the West is felt to be due to life-long, low dietary fiber intake. High intraluminal pressure is a postulated mechanism. The incidence rises with age, and two-thirds of individuals have diverticula by age 85. No association exists between irritable bowel syndrome and colonic diverticulosis. Complications, mainly diverticulitis and hemorrhage, arise in about 12% of patients.

Uncomplicated Diverticulosis

While readily apparent during colonoscopy, diverticula are often diagnosed incidentally on barium enema examination (Figure 89.1). In the early, prediverticular state, the x-rays suggest muscular thickening of the sigmoid with an irregular, sawtooth appearance of the mucosal outline. While most patients are asymptomatic, a minority report episodic, often left lower-quadrant abdominal pain, lasting several days and often temporarily relieved by bowel movements. On palpation, the area of reported pain, usually the left lower abdominal quadrant, may be tender. Anticholinergics, including hyoscyamine, rarely relieve this type of abdominal pain. Increased dietary intake of fiber, such as unprocessed wheat bran, is often helpful. An amount of up to 20 g/d is reached over several weeks, thus allowing the patient to adjust to the initial fullness and flatulence associated with high fiber intake. Methylcellulose or psyllium are also useful and better tolerated, albeit more expensive.

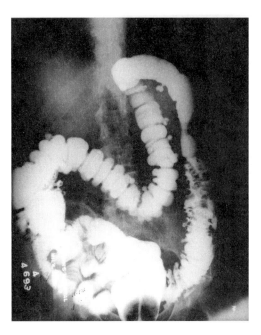

FIGURE 89.1. Barium enema showing diverticulosis of the colon.

Diverticulitis

Diverticulitis occurs in perhaps 10% of patients with diverticulosis, and follows perforation of one or more diverticula, causing extracolonic inflammation, which may be complicated by abscess, sinus tracts running parallel to the lumen, colo-vesical or colo-vaginal fistulae, and, rarely, by free perforation and peritonitis. Extraluminal compression by an inflammatory mass may cause obstruction and closely mimic an obstructing cancer. The features are severe pain, a tender and palpable mass, usually in the left lower quadrant, fever, and rarely, rectal bleeding. Rebound tenderness and involuntary abdominal rigidity are unusual and indicate perforation of a diverticulum or a retroperitoneal abscess into the peritoneal cavity. The differential diagnosis includes colonic infarction, acute infectious colitis, an attack of ulcerative or Crohn's colitis, and an obstructing or perforating colon cancer. The diagnosis is confirmed by abdominal CT or ultrasound (US). Colonoscopy and barium enema should be avoided during the active stage. Most episodes are mild and can be managed medically. Oral intake is restricted to clear liquids. Antibiotic treatment is empirical; metronidazole and a third-generation cephalosporin, or imipenem/cilastatin, are frequently used. Recurrent and complicated attacks mandate resection of the involved segment, usually the sigmoid. Abscesses require drainage (surgically or under US or CT guidance), followed by bowel resection when the inflammation has subsided.

Diverticular Bleeding

Almost 3% of the patients, often elderly, develop sudden, potentially severe, but rarely fatal, painless rectal bleeding. Up to 70% of these arise from proximal colonic diverticula. Selective angiography, ^{99m}Tc-labeled RBC scans, and colonoscopy are helpful diagnostic tests, but none of them is useful once active bleeding stops. The major differential diagnosis is bleeding from angiodysplasia, which also tends to occur in the proximal colon. Selective arterial infusion of vasopressin can control bleeding, but rebleeding is common. Repetitive, severe bleeding requires partial colectomy; its success depends on correct preoperative localization of the bleeding site.

CHAPTER 90 APPENDICITIS

ppendicitis is the most common abdominal disease requiring surgical intervention. While no age is exempt, its incidence is highest in young adults. Rare below the age of 2, it is not uncommon in the elderly. The life-time risk of acute appendicitis is nearly 10%, with a preponderance of men being affected.

Obstruction of the lumen by a fecalith, causing stasis, followed by ischemia, mucosal ulceration, infection, vascular thrombosis, infarction, and occasional perforation, is a commonly outlined sequence. In many cases, however, no obstruction, foreign body, or precipitating event is found. Some acute attacks reverse spontaneously and the process subsides. Usually, the symptoms evolve over 24 hours; the appendix perforates in 15–20% of cases.

Classically, the patient reports periumbilical pain, followed by anorexia, nausea, and low-grade fever. Pain in the early stages is visceral and, thus, felt in the midline. As the serosa and adjacent peritoneum are involved, the pain shifts and becomes somatic in the right lower quadrant. Localized, rebound tenderness and muscle spasm are apparent at McBurney's point, which is about

halfway between the anterior superior iliac spine and the umbilicus. With a retrocecal inflamed appendix, abdominal signs may be absent but pain my be elicited by iliopsoas muscle stretching.

Many conditions mimic acute appendicitis, including mesenteric lymphadenitis, acute gastroenteritis, referred abdominal pain from pneumonia, pelvic inflammatory disease, acute Crohn's disease, ureteric colic, ruptured ovarian follicle or tubal pregnancy, and right-sided diverticulitis. The diagnosis rests mainly on the history and physical findings, including a rectal and pelvic examination. Abdominal or transvaginal ultrasound may demonstrate an enlarged, thick-walled appendix in around 85% of cases and can effectively exclude other conditions like ectopic pregnancy, ovarian cysts, and other adnexal diseases. CT scan may be required to diagnose periappendiceal abscess in those suspected to have appendiceal perforation. Diagnostic uncertainty should not delay surgical exploration. Surgery confirms the diagnosis in about 70% of patients and another diagnosis or no diagnosis are found in 15% each.

CHAPTER 91 ACUTE INFECTIOUS COLITIS

cute inflammatory diseases of the colon, such as shigellosis, amebic colitis, salmonellosis, pseudomembranous colitis, and *Campylobacter* and *E. coli* O157:H7 infection lead to cramps and tenesmus, watery or bloody stools, fever, and, at times, nausea and vomiting, which most often reflect tissue invasion.

Both stool examination for ova and parasites, and bacterial culture, should precede other GI diagnostic studies. Sigmoidoscopy can then follow to inspect the mucosa for hyperemia, edema, friability, exudate (pseudomembranes), and ulceration. Wet smears should be examined for amebae and biopsies from ulcerated areas should be stained for amebic trophozoites. Serology (indirect hemagglutination) testing can also reliably diagnose amebiasis. *Campylobacter fetus ssp jejuni,* an organism that exists widely in the animal kingdom and has

been isolated in water, unpasteurized milk, and poultry, has recently emerged as an important pathogen causing a dysenteric syndrome. It often produces a prodrome of malaise followed by abdominal cramps, diarrhea (often grossly bloody), anorexia, fever, nausea, and vomiting. Proctoscopic findings may mimic pseudomembranous colitis or inflammatory bowel disease. Laboratory evaluation of all acute diarrheas should include tests to identify this organism. Erythromycin therapy, while commonly used, may not alter the natural course of the disease if begun several days after the onset of illness.

Sometimes acute colitis occurs without apparent etiology; thus the term "acute self-limited colitis." The central dilemma is to separate this transient condition (2–4 weeks) from the first attack of idiopathic IBD—that is, ulcerative colitis or Crohn's disease. Gross and histologic morphology can be useful.

Pseudomembranous Colitis

This disease, caused by strains of *Clostridium difficile*, a sporulating anaerobe, may occur during or following a

course of broad-spectrum antibiotics, most commonly penicillins, cephalosporins, and clindamycin. Watery diarrhea, abdominal cramps, and fever are extremely common; rebound tenderness, bloody diarrhea, and leukocytosis are less frequent. Erythema, edema, erosions, and cream-colored pseudomembranes are usually seen on sigmoidoscopy. Occasionally, only the proximal colon is involved. *C. difficile* produces two toxins concurrently: toxin A, an enterotoxin causing the mucosal damage, and toxin B, a cytotoxin. The diagnosis requires a combination of listed symptoms *and* finding toxin A and/or B in the stool. Very few healthy adults and 10–15% of hospitalized patients are carriers of *C. difficile*. Isolation of patients with this disease and enteric

precautions are essential, given its transmissibility by the fecal-oral route. Only symptomatic cases with toxin-positive stools require therapy. Metronidazole, 250 mg q.i.d., and Vancomycin, 125 mg q.i.d., for 10 days are equally effective. Metronidazole is preferred, given its lower cost. Clinical response is prompt, but relapses occur in 25% of cases, which usually abate after a second course of therapy. Half of those retreated may relapse again, requiring metronidazole or vancomycin for a further 4–6 weeks. Clostridial toxins may be bound by cholestyramine. Carriers need not be treated.

Enterohemorrhagic E. coli Infection

Enterohemorrhagic *E. coli* (EHEC) infection is caused by verotoxin (Shigella toxin I and II)-producing *E. coli,* predominantly the O157:H7 strain. Transmitted via undercooked beef, unpasteurized milk, apple cider, drinking water, and possibly person-to-person, the infection leads to severe abdominal cramps, diarrhea (may become bloody after 1–2 days), and in 50% of cases, fever. Because the right colon is principally involved, sigmoidoscopy may be normal. The disease,

which usually lasts 5–7 days, occurs as local outbreaks. The diagnosis requires bacteriologic confirmation. The hemolytic-uremic syndrome (acute renal failure, hemolytic anemia, and thrombocytopenia) develops in about 5% of those affected, particularly in the very young and the very old. Antibiotic therapy has not been effective, possibly because of delays in the diagnosis.

CHAPTER 92 OTHER COLORECTAL DISORDERS

Ischemia of the Colon

Colonic ischemia, most commonly seen in patients over 50 years of age with atherosclerotic disease elsewhere, may be part of the syndrome of mesenteric insufficiency (chapter 81). Mostly an isolated event, it may follow acute interruption of the inferior mesenteric artery during intra-abdominal aneurysm surgery or bowel surgery. Its association with vasculitis, amyloidosis, or oral contraceptive use is rare.

The usual features are acute lower abdominal pain and cramps, rectal bleeding, and, perhaps, fever and vomiting. Tenderness, guarding, and leukocytosis are common and may mimic acute diverticulitis. Life-threatening infarction and perforation may follow, requiring urgent laparotomy. More often, the blood supply to that segment of the colon remains sufficient to ensure viability, but with tissue changes termed *ischemic colitis.* Characteristically segmental, these particularly affect the splenic flexure and the rectosigmoid, the "watershed" areas with respect to blood supply. Sometimes, patients are seen after the acute episode, or may give a history suggestive of prior ischemic events. Colonoscopy has

been useful in early diagnosis. Barium enema (Figure 92.1) shows "thumbprinting"; it reflects intramural edema and bleeding, causing some segmental narrowing. There is no specific therapy; usually the process subsides, restoring a normal-appearing colon. The sporadic, residual stricture or ulceration that follows may mimic Crohn's disease or even adenocarcinoma.

Radiation proctocolitis

Acute radiation colitis frequently seen in patients during or soon after radiotherapy for cervical, ovarian, uterine, rectal, or prostatic cancers. Usual symptoms are nausea, vomiting, cramping, tenesmus, diarrhea, and rectal bleeding. Sigmoidoscopy often shows a hyperemic, edematous mucosa with variable friability and, occasionally, ulcerations. **Chronic radiation colitis** may occur months or years after therapy, due to progressive occlusive changes in small mural arteries, leading to ischemic necrosis, **mucosal ulceration, and stricture formation.** Crampy abdominal pain, tenesmus, and stool with blood and mucus are the usual symptoms; occa-

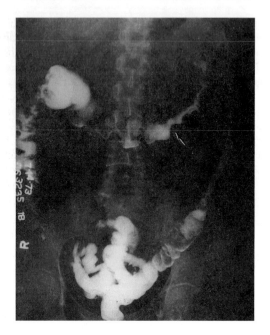

FIGURE 92.1. Ischemia of the colon. Barium enema examination showing thumbprinting (arrow).

sionally obstruction may develop. Sigmoidoscopy usually shows a granular, friable membrane, variable-sized ulcers, and prominent telangiectases (neovascularization). Surgery is rarely necessary and laser therapy may control bleeding if it is severe enough to require attention.

Pneumatosis Cystoides Intestinalis

This rare condition is characterized by multiple gas-filled mural cysts with surrounding chronic inflammation in the small and/or large intestine (Figure 92.2), encountered incidentally on abdominal x-rays. In most cases, an underlying condition can be identified that allows gas to dissect into the intestinal wall. Treatment consists of a formula diet free of complex carbohydrates and providing high O_2 supplements, to promote the diffusion of N_2 and H_2 out of the gas-filled cysts.

The distal ileum may be involved as well due to its location within the pelvis. Consequently, malabsorption of vitamin B_{12}, and of bile salts may result. In the latter case, diarrhea will respond to cholestyramine therapy.

Collagenous and lymphocytic colitis

Patients with these two diseases present with chronic watery diarrhea; abdominal pain is minor or absent. Most are in their fifth or sixth decade with a striking predominance of women. The colon is normal on endoscopic and radiologic examination and there are no consistent laboratory abnormalities. The daily stool volume may be as high as 1.5L, although dehydration and weight loss are rare. The diarrhea tends to wax and wane without any therapy. There is an unexplained association with autoimmune disorders, such as rheumatoid arthritis, scleroderma, and the sicca syndrome. The diagnosis is established by mucosal biopsies obtained proximal to the rectum. These show increased intraepithelial lymphocytes, accumulations of mononuclear cells in the lamina propria and a disarray of the surface epithelium; the crypt architecture remains intact. Patients with marked thickening of the collagen plate beneath the surface epithelium are designated as having collagenous colitis; those without this thickening are called lymphocytic colitis. Both probably represent a single disease entity, sometimes termed microscopic colitis. The prognosis is excellent. Initial treatment consists of antidiarrheal drugs. Patients who do not respond receive a trial of sulfasalazine or one of the newer 5-ASA formulations. A few patients require short courses of systemic corticosteroids.

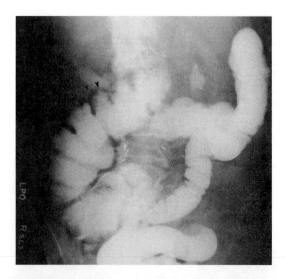

FIGURE 92.2. Pneumatosis intestinalis. Barium enema examination showing accumulation of air (arrows) in the colonic walls.

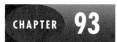

COLORECTAL NEOPLASMS

■ Incidence

Adenomas and cancers arising from the colorectal epithelium form a sequential development from benign to malignant neoplasms. Their incidence, linked to dietary factors, has great geographic variation. Strong epidemiological data link colorectal neoplasia with consumption of a high-fat, red meat, low-fiber diet. In the United States, the lifetime risk of colorectal cancer (CRC) is 5–6%, with 160,000 new cases and 60,000 deaths yearly. The incidence of both adenoma and carcinoma rises with age. About 40–60% of persons over 60 years of age harbor one or more colon adenomas.

■ Pathogenesis

The adenoma-carcinoma sequence

Most, if not all, CRCs are thought to arise within benign adenomas; the probability of such malignant transformation depends on the size, histology, and degree of epithelial dysplasia of an adenoma. The progression from normal epithelium through adenoma to cancer is determined by accumulated genetic alterations that manifest as hypomethylation of DNA and aneuploidy, signifying an abnormal DNA content. Specific genetic changes involve somatic mutations of proto-oncogenes and of tumor suppressor genes; the latter include adenomatous polyposis coli (APC) and

mutated in colon cancer (MCC), both located on chromosome 5q; deleted in colon cancer (DCC) on 18q; and p53, located on 17p. Inactivation of one allele has no effect on cell proliferation. Abnormal growth occurs only when the second allele mutates or is deleted (loss of heterozygosity, LOH). Proto-oncogenes, such as K-ras (12p) and C-myc, may be activated or amplified by a point mutation and then act as mitogenic signals. Mutation or allelic loss of APC and MCC result in a hyperproliferating epithelium; the progression to adenoma formation is associated with K-ras mutations and DCC inactivation and the appearance of carcinoma with the loss or mutation of the tumor suppressor gene, p53. Over 90% of CRC exhibit two or more of these gene alterations (Table 93.1).

TABLE 93.1. DNA Alterations Commonly Present During the Evolution of Colorectal Carcinoma

Tumor Suppressor Gene: Deletion and/or Mutation	Oncogene: Activation	Result
APC, MCC		hyperproliferation
DCC	K ras	adenoma
p53	C-myc	carcinoma

The sequence and numbers of genetic alterations are variable. Mutations and deletions of additional genes are likely to be discovered in the future.

Neoplastic Polyps

Tubular adenomas are characterized by branching adenomatous glands and epithelial dysplasia. When the glands elongate to the center of the polyp, finger-like projections result; the polyp is termed **villous adenoma.** About 85% of all neoplastic colorectal polyps are tubular and 5% are villous adenomas. The remaining 10% are of the mixed type. Polyps grow either pedunculated (on a stalk) or sessile (broad-based). Approximately 90% of neoplastic polyps are below 1 cm in size. Among patients with one identified polyp, one-half harbor multiple lesions. Approximately 70% of all polyps detected during colonoscopy occur distal to the splenic flexure—that is, within reach of a fiberoptic sigmoidoscope. In only 5–10% of patients are neoplastic polyps solely located in the proximal colon. The degree of epithelial dysplasia ranges from mild to moderate to severe or high-grade. In high-grade dysplasia (carcinoma-in-situ), the neoplastic

cells do not extend beyond the basement membrane. Intramucosal carcinoma, the next step in the progression to overt malignancy, invades the lamina propria, but not the muscularis mucosae. Because lymphatics are absent above the muscularis mucosae, these malignancies are not invasive. Neoplastic polyps with foci of carcinoma in situ or intramucosal carcinoma are often called "malignant polyps." High-grade dysplasia and noninvasive carcinoma are more common in larger polyps, particularly the villous type. Diminutive polyps, below 5 mm in size, do not pose an increased risk of developing future cancer.

Colorectal polyps generally are asymptomatic and rarely bleed; fecal occult blood testing (FOBT) is positive in only 20–30% of affected patients. In general, only polyps over 2 cm in size tend to bleed intermittently. Patients with large rectosigmoid villous adenomas occasionally present with all the sequels of secretory diarrhea, including dehydration and hypokalemia, owing to rectal discharge of copious amounts of mucoid fluid.

Colorectal polyps should be removed completely, usually by endoscopy. The entire polyp is studied histologically in order to establish its nature (neoplastic or not) and the degree of dysplasia. Polypectomy is efficient therapy of malignant polyps when extension beyond the muscularis mucosa is absent. Diminutive polyps (<5mm) may be simply fulgurated without biopsy in view of the very low risk of subsequent cancer associated with them. If neoplastic polyps are found during sigmoidoscopy, complete colonoscopy is required

with removal of all lesions. Follow-up surveillance involves colonoscopy in 3 years and then every 5 years.

■ Surveillance and Screening for Colorectal Neoplasia

Surveillance is aimed at individuals with increased risk (Table 197.1) for colorectal carcinoma. Individuals with an affected first-degree relative have a fourfoldincreased risk for CRC at a relatively young age—that is, less than 60 years old. Surveillance colonoscopy is needed every 3–5 years, starting at age 35. Screening is discussed in chapter 197, with suggestions in Table 93.2 and Figure 197.2.

TABLE 93.2.	Screening and Surveillance for Colorectal Polyps and Carcinoma: Provisional Recommendations		
	Group	Start	Procedure
Screening	General population	Age 40	Annual FOBT
		Age 50	FFS. When negative, repeat once after 5 years
Surveillance	≥1-First-degree relative with CRC	Age 35	C every 3–5 years
	Ulcerative colitis	10 yrs. after onset	Annual C with biopsies
	Extensive Crohn's colitis	10 yrs. after onset	Annual C with biopsies
	Family history of FAP, Turcot's syndrome	Age 12	Annual FFS
	Family history of HNPCC	Age 25	C every 2 years
	Patients with Peutz-Jeghers syndrome; juvenile polyposis	?	C in kindreds with associated CRC; frequency ?

FOBT = fecal occult blood test; FFS = flexible fiberoptic sigmoidoscopy; C = colonoscopy; FAP = familial adenomatous polyposis; HNPCC = hereditary nonpolyposis colorectal carcinoma.

Familial Adenomatous Polyposis

Familial adenomatous polyposis (FAP) inherited in an autosomal dominant mode accounts for approximately 1% of all cases of CRC. An estimated 20% of affected patients represent new mutations. The genetic basis is a germline mutation in one allele of the APC gene on chromosome 5q21; cancer develops as additional mutations occur, including deletion or mutation of the second allele of the APC gene (see Table 93.1). Myriad small adenomatous polyps develop throughout the colon; 50% of patients develop this by age 25. Nearly all patients progress to CRC, on average by age 42. Retinal pigment epithelium hypertrophies and polyps develop in the upper GI tract. The incidence of duodenal and ampullary carcinoma is increased. Approximately 15% of FAP families additionally develop mesodermal abnormalities, including osteomas, dental abnormalities,

and desmoid tumors (**Gardner's syndrome**). A rare association of FAP with malignant brain tumors is called **Turcot's syndrome.**

Potentially affected family members should undergo annual surveillance sigmoidoscopy starting at age 12. Those with established FAP should also have upper endoscopy performed every 1–3 years. Proctocolectomy is mandatory when colonic polyps are detected. Ileoanal anastomosis with creation of an ileal pouch obviates the need for a permanent ileostomy in these young persons. If an ileorectal anastomosis is done, frequent follow-up is required for rectal cancer. Sulindac causes polyps to regress in this syndrome, but it is not a substitute for colectomy, nor for regular surveillance of a remaining rectum.

Hereditary nonpolyposis colorectal carcinoma

Previously called the Lynch Syndrome, hereditary nonpolyposis colorectal carcinoma (HNPCC) is an autosomal dominant disorder, characterized by 100 or less adenomas in the proximal colon and the development of predominantly right-sided CRC by approximately age 45. The rather stringent so-called **Amsterdam criteria** form the current basis for the diagnosis of HNPCC: 1) three or more blood relatives of the proband have CRC, one of whom is a first-degree relative of the other two; 2) the relatives with CRC belong to more than one generation; 3) at least one relative with CRC is diagnosed prior to age 50. Type I HNPCC affects only the colon.

Type II presents with additional non-colonic cancers of the endometrium, breast, ovary, stomach, and other organs. The genetic defect consists of germline mutations in several genes involved in DNA repair. Approximately 5% of all CRC patients are currently estimated to have HNPCC. Diagnostic molecular biology testing for the presence of the implicated germline mutations is expected to become available in the near future. Such testing will probably establish the diagnosis of HNPCC in many patients who do not meet the current, family history-based criteria. Patients at risk should undergo screening colonoscopy every 2 years, beginning at age 25.

Colorectal Carcinoma

CRC is the end-stage of the evolution from normal mucosa through adenoma, and severe dysplasia, to noninvasive and then to invasive adenocarcinoma. Inflammatory bowel disease and HNPCC are the only conditions where adenoma formation is omitted from this sequence. The risk and the time interval for adenoma to evolve into carcinoma correlate with the size and histologic featuresof the adenoma; on average, this process takes nearly 10–12 years. A 50-year-old person has a 5% chance of developing CRC and a 2.5% risk of dying from it. Approximately 4% of patients have a second CRC at the time of diagnosis (synchronous) and 3% develop it subsequently (metachronous). Rectal carcinoma represents nearly one-third of all cases of CRC.

■ Clinical Features, Diagnosis, and Management

The clinical presentation depends on the site and size of the tumor. Right-sided lesions commonly present with anemia from chronic blood loss, palpable right lower quadrant mass, and enlarged liver with an irregular surface due to metastases; colonic obstruction, tenesmus, decreased stool caliber, pencil stools, and visible blood separate from the stool are more common with left-sided lesions. Rectal bleeding should not be ascribed to co-existing hemorrhoids without further evaluation.

Digital rectal examination may show blood in the stool and/or a tumor in the lower rectum. Barium enema may reveal a polypoid or annular filling defect (Figure 197.1), or wall infiltration with mucosal destruction; this radiologic approach can miss *rectal* tumors. The diagnostic procedure of choice is full colonoscopy with biopsy. The entire colon needs to be inspected preoperatively in order to exclude a synchronous carcinoma and

to remove adenomas beyond the area of planned resection. Carcinoembryonic antigen (CEA), a cell surface glycoconjugate, is elevated in one-third of patients with early CRC and in three-fourths of those with advanced CRC. Cancers of other organs, colitis, and smoking may also elevate CEA, which seriously limits its use as a diagnostic or screening tool for CRC. Serial postoperative CEA monitoring can help detect local and distant recurrences following surgical resection.

Management of colorectal cancers is discussed in chapter 197. Briefly, surgical resection in the form of partial colectomy or low anterior resection of the rectum remains the standard treatment of CRC. Palliative resection is often needed for relief of symptoms (bleeding, obstruction) even when all tumor tissue cannot be removed. Prognosis and further management decisions depend on the operative tumor staging. (Table 93.3 shows a widely used system and Table 197.3 shows the TNM staging.)

Non-neoplastic Colorectal Tumors

Hyperplastic colon polyps are small and usually sessile. Their incidence approaches that of adenomatous polyps; most occur in the distal colon and rectum. These polyps are not premalignant; their detection in the rectosigmoid does not call for colonoscopy or regular surveillance.

Peutz-Jeghers syndrome consists of autosomal, dominantly inherited hamartomatous polyps throughout the GI tract, especially the small bowel, and mucocutaneous pigmentation of the lips, oral mucosa, and fingers. The polyps may cause intussusception, obstruction, and bleeding. An increased incidence of colonic and upper gastrointestinal carcinomas has been noted in several affected families.

TABLE 93.3.	Staging of Colorectal Carcinoma Astler-Coller Modification of the Dukes' Classification		
Stage	**Extent**	**Incidence at Time of Diagnosis**	**5-Year Survival**
A	Limited to mucosa	14%	90–100%
B_1	Into muscularis propria	38%	65%
B_2	Through muscularis propria (and serosa)		45%
C_1	Same as B_1, plus regional node metastases		43%
C_2	Same as B_2, plus regional node metastases	25%	15%
D	Distant metastases	23%	0–5%

CHAPTER 94 ANATOMY AND PHYSIOLOGY OF THE PANCREAS

■ Anatomy

The pancreas is entirely retroperitoneal and lacks a capsule. It is 12–15 cm long and weighs 70–100 g. The head and the uncinate process lie within the curve of the duodenum; body and tail extend obliquely to the splenic hilus. Its blood supply is from branches of the celiac and superior mesenteric arteries; the splenic artery branches mainly supply the body and tail. The venous drainage is to the splenic and the portal vein. Nonunion of the dorsal (Santorini) and the ventral (Wirsung) ducts occurs in 7% of individuals. In **pancreas divisum** the dorsal duct drains all but the uncinate process through the minor papilla. It has both parasympathetic and sympathetic innervation. The pancreas has proximity to the inferior vena cava, the common bile duct, the diaphragmatic crura, the spleen, both kidneys, the celiac and superior mesenteric ganglia, the mesocolon, small bowel mesentery, and the lesser omental sac.

The exocrine tissue is arranged as a tubuloacinar gland consisting of acini and intercalated intra- and inter-lobular ducts, which converge on the main pancreatic duct. Acinar cells synthesize and export proteins, while ductal cells secrete bicarbonate in exchange for chloride.

■ Physiology

The pancreatic acinar cells synthesize nearly 20 digestive enzymes, the pancreatic secretory trypsin inhibitor (PSTI), and colipase. While some of the digestive enzymes are released in the active form (amylase, lipase, ribonuclease), the proteases (trypsin, chymotrypsin, carboxypeptidases, elastase) and phospholipase are released as proenzymes or zymogens. Enterokinase, released from the duodenal mucosa, converts trypsinogen to active trypsin, which activates all

other proenzymes within the duodenal lumen. The PSTI protects against the digestive action of small amounts of trypsin that may be prematurely liberated from trypsinogen in acinar cells and the pancreatic duct system.

Enzyme synthesis and secretion (Figure 94.1) are stimulated by circulating cholecystokinin (CCK), by central vagal pathways and by gastro- and entero-

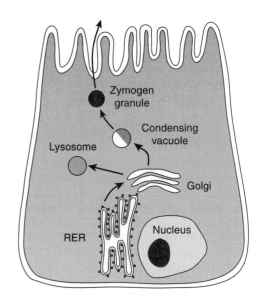

FIGURE 94.1. Synthesis, sorting, and secretion of zymogens and hydrolytic enzymes in the pancreatic acinar cell. Post-translational processing occurs in the Golgi apparatus. The subsequent sorting step separates lysosomes from condensing vacuoles. Without this separation, the acid pH and the hydrolases within lysosomes will activate trypsinogen to trypsin. The content of zymogen granules is discharged into the acinar lumen by exocytosis.
(Reprinted from Soergel KH. Acute pancreatitis. In: Sleisenger MH, Fordtran JS (eds.). Gastrointestinal Disease. 5th ed. Philadelphia: W.B. Saunders Co., 1993: 1630. Used with permission.)

pancreatic reflexes. CCK is released from the proximal small intestine by the products of protein and fat digestion; this release is inhibited by free intraduodenal trypsin (feedback inhibition). In patients with low duodenal protease activity due to pancreatic insufficiency, plasma CCK levels rise; feeding trypsin-containing pancreatic extracts lowers them. At the intracellular level, lysosomal enzymes are segregated from proteins destined for export into the acinar lumen, a process that is believed to be disturbed in the pathogenesis of acute pancreatitis.

The pancreatic ductal cells are stimulated by secretin to add a bicarbonate-rich fluid to the acinar proteinaceous secretion. The action of secretin is potentiated by CCK and acetylcholine. The cystic fibrosis transmembrane regulator (CFTR), which functions as an apical Cl^- channel, and the Cl^-/HCO_3^- anion exchanger participate in this process. Secretin is released from the duodenal mucosa when the luminal pH decreases to 4.5 or less. This mechanism, plus direct duodenal HCO_3^- secretion, account for the continued neutralization of gastric acid leaving the stomach. Pancreatic secretions are supersaturated with Ca^{++} ions; their precipitation in the form of $CaCO_3$ is prevented by lithostathine, a protein produced and secreted by the acinar cells.

| CHAPTER | 95 | PANCREATITIS |

Acute Pancreatitis

■ Definition and Incidence

Acute pancreatitis is a process of autodigestion by prematurely activated zymogens and enzymes escaping from acinar cells and pancreatic ducts into periacinar and periductal connective tissue. The course is determined by the degree and extent of digestion and inflammation within the gland and by variable involvement of adjacent and remote organs. In contrast to chronic pancreatitis, the pancreas eventually regains normal structure and function. Unless the precipitating cause is removed, the risk of recurrence is nearly 50%. The annual incidence is close to 10/100,000 population.

■ Etiology and Pathogenesis

In animal models, the rate of exocytosis of the content of zymogen granules is decreased, leading to accumulation of zymogens within the acinar cells. The isolation of zymogens from lysosomal enzymes fails, with the consequent activation and misdirected exit of active enzymes across the basolateral cell wall. The factor initiating this chain of events is unknown, but obstruction of the pancreatic duct at or near the ampulla of Vater may explain some, though not all, episodes of acute pancreatitis. Reflux of duodenal contents or bile into the pancreatic duct does not play a role. Certain causes of acute pancreatitis (hypercalcemia, ethanol, hypoperfusion) increase pancreatic duct permeability, allowing pancreatic enzymes and zymogens to escape into the periductal tissue. Circulating trypsin inhibitors partly inactivate pancreatic proteases released into the blood; the remaining active trypsin liberates several kinin peptides from their inactive blood precursors. These peptides exert harmful systemic effects—vasodilatation, excessive vascular permeability, and lowered pain threshold.

Several conditions and drugs lead to acute pancreatitis in humans (Table 95.1). Gallstones cause acute

TABLE 95.1.	Conditions Frequently Associated with Acute Pancreatitis
Obstruction	*Trauma*
Choledocholithiasis*	Blunt abdominal trauma
Tumors	Abdominal operations
Sphincter of Oddi	ERCP procedure
stenosis	
Metabolic	*Vascular*
Hypertriglyceridemia	Shock
Acute hypercalcemia	Vasculitis
Toxins	*Drugs*
Ethanol*	Valproic acid
Methanol	Azathioprine (6-MP)
Scorpion venom	Metronidazole
	Sulfonamides
	Most diuretics
	Pentamidine
	Tetracycline
	Mesalamine
	ACE inhibitors
	DDI (2′ 3′ dideoxyinosine)
	Cocaine abuse

*Common cause.
ACE = angiotensin converting enzyme.

pancreatitis when they impact in the ampulla of Vater; these stones are rarely greater than 5 mm in diameter because they must first pass through the cystic duct. Viruses and bacteria (e.g., mumps, and *C. jejuni*) are very rare causes.

■ Pathology

Initially, there is periacinar and periductal fat necrosis, which progresses to inflammation involving the secretory cells in the acinar periphery, pancreatic ductules and duct, and local blood vessels. The process frequently spreads to peripancreatic tissue and adjacent organs. Fatty acids liberated from lipid-containing cells combine with Ca^{++} to form calcium soaps. Local complications include (1) fluid collections, frequently multiple and lacking a defined wall; (2) patchy pancreatic necrosis, which may remain sterile or become infected by enteric bacteria transmigrating across the colonic wall, and, rarely, (3) pancreatic abscess, representing an area of liquefied pancreatic necrosis that is infected.

■ Clinical Features

Steady midepigastric pain is the key feature. It rapidly peaks in intensity (15–60 min), frequently radiates straight to the back, and is often relieved by sitting and leaning forward. Nausea, vomiting, and low-grade fever are common. Hypotension occurs in about 30% of patients, owing to retroperitoneal fluid sequestration, generalized excessive vascular permeability, and low peripheral vascular resistance. The abdomen is tender, but without rigidity and rebound tenderness (i.e., no peritoneal irritation). Bowel sounds are sparse or absent (possible onset of paralytic ileus). Painless ecchymoses may develop later in the flanks (Grey-Turner's sign) or periumbilical area (Cullen's sign). No complications arise in 80% of cases with a mild course and brief hospitalization

(<1 week); the 6–10% overall mortality occurs in the remaining 20%.

■ Diagnosis

Acute pancreatitis is diagnosed by a combination of clinical, laboratory, and, in some cases, radiologic findings. Serum amylase activity, the most frequently used test, rises within 2–12 hours after the onset of pain and is normal within 3–5 days. The probability of acute pancreatitis rises with the degree of rise in serum amylase; it is nearly 100% with values over five times the upper limit of normal. With lipemic serum, results may be false-negative. Determining pancreatic (P) and salivary (S) isozymes of amylase, or measuring urine amylase, or estimating the amylase-creatinine clearance ratio serve no added benefit. Many other conditions may elevate serum amylase—for example, gastric-, duodenal-, or jejunal perforation, mesenteric infarction, chronic pancreatitis, salivary adenitis, ovarian neoplasms, renal failure, ethanol intoxication, upper GI endoscopy (including ERCP), and critical illness. Serum lipase has a similar diagnostic value; it tends to remain high longer than amylase. Together, these two tests are 95% sensitive and 90% specific for diagnosing pancreatitis.

Other laboratory features include leukocytosis (75%), mild hypocalcemia (30%) with normal ionized calcium (which explains the rarity of tetany), transient hyperglycemia which requires no therapy, and, regardless of the etiology of the attack, moderate increase in serum aspartate transaminase (AST). High serum C-reactive protein (>120 mg/L) can reliably predict pancreatic necrosis. Together, many tests obtained during the first 48 hours of illness may help predict prognosis. However, the Ranson and the Glasgow criteria and the APACHE II (Acute Physiology and Chronic Health Evaluation) score can reliably predict a mild versus a complicated course only in 70–80% of cases (Table 95.2).

TABLE 95.2. Prognostic Signs in Acute Pancreatitis (Ranson Criteria)			
On Admission		**During Initial 48 Hours of Therapy**	
Age	>55 yrs	Hematocrit	>10% decrease
WBC	>16,000/mm³	BUN	>5 mg/dl increase
Serum glucose	>200 mg/dl	Serum calcium	<8 mg/dl
Serum LDH	>350 IU/l	PaO₂	<60 mm Hg
ALT	>250 SFU	Base deficit	>4 mEq/l
		Fluid sequestration	>6 liters

Fewer than three signs present: benign clinical course.
Three or more signs present: serious clinical illness/death in up to 67% of patients.
ALT = serum alanine-aminotransferase; BUN = blood urea nitrogen; LDH = lactate dehydrogenase; PaO_2 = arterial oxygen tension; SFU = sigma Frankel units.
(Modified from: Ranson JH, Rifkind KM, Turner JW. Surg Gyn Obstet 1976;143:210. Used with permission.)

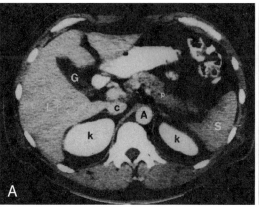 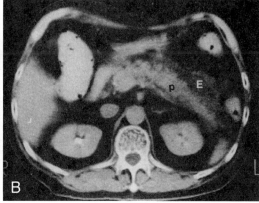

FIGURE 95.1. A. Normal pancreas. B. Mild acute pancreatitis with thickening of the pancreas and peripancreatic edema. CT scans at the head of the pancreatic body and tail after IV contrast administration. G = gallbladder; k = kidney; S = spleen; A = aorta; c = inferior vena cava; p = pancreas; E = peripancreatic edema.

(Reprinted from Soergel KH. Acute pancreatitis. In Sleisenger MH, Fordtran JS (eds.). Gastrointestinal Disease. 5th ed. Philadelphia: W.B. Saunders Co., 1993: 1641, Fig. 80-6. Used with permission.)

Imaging studies

Plain abdominal x-rays should always be obtained; they may show free air due to a perforated viscus, pancreatic calcifications of chronic pancreatitis, radio-opaque gallstones, and paralytic ileus. Chest x-rays often show pleural effusions and basilar atelectasis due to the subphrenic inflammation. Abdominal ultrasound is the preferred method for detecting gallstones and bile duct dilatation. The latter findings combined with elevation of more than three laboratory tests (bilirubin, GGT, ALT, ALT/AST ratio >1.0, alkaline phosphatase) indicate gallstone-related pancreatitis. Abdominal CT (Figure 95.1), while abnormal in 90% of cases of acute pancreatitis, is not required routinely.

■ Management

Mild pancreatitis, (i.e., uncomplicated illness), requires only supportive care. The goals are prompt rehydration to achieve euvolemia, full pain relief with opiates, and to rest the intestines by avoiding all oral intake. Nasogastric suction is employed for vomiting or evolving paralytic ileus. Routine antibiotic use is of no benefit. Small feedings of a diet low in fat and protein are started once the pain subsides and the bowel sounds resume. The patient must be watched closely for early signs of complications. Persistent shock, increasing abdominal tenderness, fever, and dyspnea require prompt evaluation.

Complications

Systemic complications tend to occur during the first week of illness, while local complications and involve-

ment of adjacent organs follow during the next two weeks (see Table 95.3). About 20% of patients develop one or more complications.

Early **circulatory shock**, an ominous sign, often signals pancreatic necrosis; admission to ICU, aggressive hydration, and vasopressors are indicated. Shock later in the course may reflect gram-negative sepsis. **Acute renal failure** due to acute tubular necrosis may arise from the combination of shock and high renovascular resistance. The **adult respiratory distress syndrome** (ARDS) often complicates severe, acute pancreatitis, and is ascribed to alveolar surfactant damage by phospholipases and circulating free fatty acids; hypoxemia unrelated to other causes is an early clue. Treatment consists of oxygen, and in severe cases, ventilatory support with positive end-expiratory pressure (PEEP). **Sepsis** may follow ascending cholangitis and infected pancreatic necrosis. Hyperglycemia and hypocalcemia, while common, rarely need therapy. Distinguishing toxic psychosis from delirium tremens and opiate effects may be a challenge in diagnosis and therapy.

Persistent impaction of a gallstone in the ampulla of Vater delays the resolution of pancreatitis. Progressive jaundice and spiking fevers follow, reflecting ascending cholangitis. Besides prompt endoscopic or surgical disimpaction of the stone, antibiotics are also indicated. **Pancreatic necrosis** (PN) occurs in 80% of patients with a clinically severe course during the second or third week of illness. Prognosis and management critically depend on whether the necrotic tissue is infected. A dynamic CT with rapid IV contrast injection is performed and necrotic areas, defined by the lack of contrast enhancement, are aspirated using a CT-guided fine-needle. Gram-stain of

TABLE 95.3.	Complications During Acute Pancreatitis	
Systemic	**Local**	**Adjacent Organs**
Shock	Impacted common bile duct stone	Splenic vein occlusion
Acute renal failure	Pancreatic necrosis	Splenic infarct
ARDS*	Sterile	Bleeding
Sepsis	Infected	Colonic necrosis
Miscellaneous	Fluid collection	Pleural effusion
DIC**	Sterile	Pancreatic fistula
Hyperglycemia	Infected	
Hypocalcemia	Pancreatic abscess	
	Bleeding	

*Adult respiratory distress syndrome.
**Disseminated intravascular coagulation.

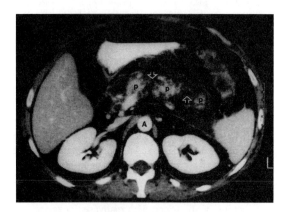

FIGURE 95.2. Necrotizing pancreatitis. CT scan during rapid IV bolus injection of contrast material. P: normally perfused areas of the pancreas. Open arrows: nonperfused necrotic areas. A. Aorta. The pancreas is surrounded by fluid that extends into the small bowel mesentery.
(Reprinted from Soergel KH. Acute pancreatitis. In Sleisenger MH, Fordtran JS (eds). Gastrointestinal Disease. 5th ed. Philadelphia: W.B. Saunders Co., 1993:1642, fig. 80-10. Used with permission.)

the aspirate diagnoses or excludes infection. Patients with sterile PN are treated conservatively. In infected PN, unless the affected tissue is promptly excised surgically, the mortality exceeds 60%. Combined excision and antibiotics (fluoroquinolones or imipenem/cilastatin, plus metronidazole) lowers the mortality to 10–20%. **Fluid collections** form in up to 50% of patients with severe pancreatitis. Most resolve spontaneously; persistent col-

lections over 6 weeks old evolve into pseudocysts. For enlarging or infected collections (pancreatic abscess) percutaneous aspiration and drainage can be employed.

Splenic vein thrombosis may later result in gastric fundic varices. *Splenic infarcts and necrosis* result from thrombosis of the splenic artery or vein or from direct extension of the inflammation to the splenic hilum. Extension of the inflammatory process into the mesocolon may cause bleeding and **perforation of the transverse colon.** *Bleeding* may have several sources, including antral and duodenal erosions and from erosion of splenic or pancreatic vessels, in which case blood may enter a disrupted pancreatic duct and empty into the duodenum. *Pleural effusions* are common and arise from a variety of mechanisms, and tend to resolve spontaneously.

Preventing recurrence

The care of the patient with acute pancreatitis mandates a thorough search for the cause (Table 95.1). If abdominal US shows gallstones, cholecystectomy should follow, with surgical or endoscopic exploration of the common bile duct as soon as pancreatitis subsides. Hypertriglyceridemia and hypercalcemia should be ruled out. At this point, nearly 20% of patients would remain in whom a cause is elusive. These patients, after experiencing one severe or two mild attacks, should undergo an elective ERCP, which will reveal a variety of correctable causes. A systematic search, as shown in Figure 95.3, will identify only 5–10% of patients as "idiopathic pancreatitis."

Chronic Pancreatitis

■ Definition and Pathogenesis

Chronic pancreatitis is marked by irreversible, usually progressive, fibrosis of the gland, along with decreased exocrine and endocrine function. Episodes

clinically resembling acute pancreatitis may occur, especially during the early years of alcoholic pancreatitis. The 10-year mortality approaches 25%. The disease occurs in two major categories, **chronic calcifying**

pancreatitis being the most common. The initial event is the precipitation of proteins in pancreatic duct radicles and, later, in the main duct. An abnormal lithostathine metabolism is said to be responsible—that is, either its decreased acinar secretion or its proteolysis within the ducts, yielding a fibrillar, insoluble peptide. These protein plugs eventually calcify and cause irregularly distributed obstruction of the small and large ducts, leading to duct dilatation, acinar atrophy, chronic inflammation and fibrosis. The islets of Langerhans are progressively destroyed late in the disease. **Chronic obstructive pancreatitis** follows tumors or duct strictures obstructing the flow of pancreatic juice. A special form is **pancreas divisum,** where a narrow dorsal duct and small-caliber minor papilla may initiate chronic pancreatitis.

▪ Etiology

Most cases of chronic pancreatitis arise from alcohol abuse. Pancreatitis in an alcoholic is really chronic pancreatitis from the start. Subsequent alcohol abstinence does not alter the progression to pancreatic exocrine insufficiency, but may decrease pain and delay the onset of diabetes mellitus. The onset of symptoms is typically between the ages of 35 and 45. **Senile pancreatitis/ atrophy** seen in older (>60 yrs) nonalcoholics occurs mainly as malabsorption along with pancreatic calcification; pain is either mild or absent. **Familial pancreatitis,** an autosomal dominant disorder, accounts for about 2% of the patients. Episodic abdominal pain begins at ages 10–14, with pancreatic calcifications on x-rays; pancreatic adenocarcinoma is reportedly frequent.

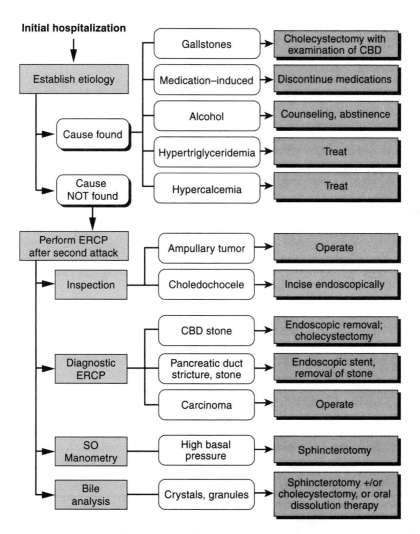

FIGURE 95.3. Suggested approach to identifying the cause of acute pancreatitis. CBD = common bile duct; Dissolution therapy = therapy with chenodeoxycholic acid or ursode- oxycholic acid; ERCP = endoscopic retrograde cholangiopancreatography; SO = sphincter of Oddi.

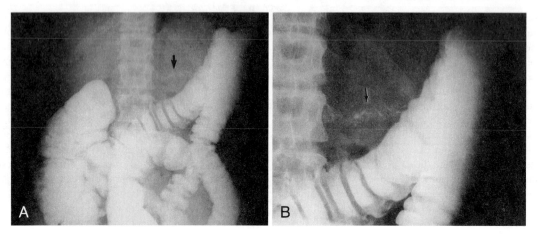

FIGURE 95.4. A. Pancreatic calcification. (A barium enema was being performed for other reasons.) B. Magnified view.

Chronic pancreatitis seen with *primary hyperparathyroidism* and *hyperlipidemia*, and after *renal transplantation*, has an elusive mechanism and frequency. In **obstructive pancreatitis,** removing the obstructing lesion can halt the course of chronic pancreatitis. No cause is found in one-fifth of cases; however, bouts of recurrent acute pancreatitis, regardless of cause, do not cause chronic pancreatitis. **Tropical pancreatitis,** presenting mainly with calcifications, pain and diabetes mellitus, is common in teenagers and young adults in southeast Asia and Central Africa.

■ Clinical Features and Diagnosis

The leading symptom is intermittent or chronic epigastric pain that frequently radiates straight through to the back and may be aggravated after eating and on the morning after a drinking bout. The pain may be due to raised intrapancreatic tissue and duct pressure from ductal obstruction by fibrosis or stones, and perineural fibrosis. Weight loss, diabetes mellitus due to progressive destruction of islets of Langerhans, steatorrhea, and local complications tend to develop 5–15 years after the pain onset.

The diagnosis of chronic pancreatitis rests on symptoms, radiological studies, and, rarely, tests of exocrine pancreatic function (see chapter 70). Blood tests add little to the diagnosis. Serum amylase and lipase may be normal or rise during episodes of pain. Plain abdominal x-rays may reveal intraductal pancreatic calcifications (Figure 95.4); this finding, along with a typical pain pattern, is diagnostic. Abdominal CT and ERCP (Figure 95.5) frequently show ductal dilatation;

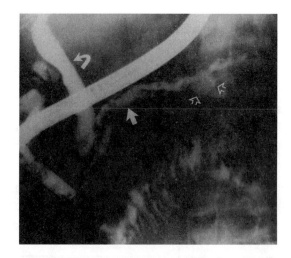

FIGURE 95.5. ERCP in chronic pancreatitis. The pancreatic duct (straight solid arrow) is irregularly dilated and contains several round filling defects (stones). Contrast material extravasates into a small pseudocyst (open arrows). The common bile duct (CBD), indicated by the curved arrow, is moderately dilated (11 mm diameter). The terminal portion of the CBD is narrowed by pancreatic fibrosis.

their main value lies in revealing potentially correctable lesions (tumors, stones, and pseudocysts).

■ Management and Complications

Chronic, often disabling, **upper abdominal pain** is the main therapeutic challenge. Acute exacerbation of the pain may warrant brief hospitalization, cessation of oral feeding, and parenteral analgesics. Opiate analgesics are eventually required in most; they should not be withheld or curtailed because of concomitant alcoholism or concerns about addiction. The pain resolves spontaneously in about 60% of patients after 5–10 years. Orally administered pancreatic extract (6 tablets/meal of Viokase™, Cotazym™, or Isozyme™) reduces pancreatic secretion by feedback inhibition of CCK release; an H2-receptor antagonist should be co-administered so as to prevent their inactivation at low gastric pH. This approach lessens pain in a minority of patients with idiopathic chronic pancreatitis. Percutaneous injection of the celiac ganglion with alcohol or phenol transiently relieves pain in about 50% of patients. Patients with intractable pain and a dilated main pancreatic duct should be considered for surgical decompression. A longitudinal pancreaticojejunostomy relieves pain in almost 70% of patients, provided they abstain from alcohol.

Malabsorption occurs late in the course, when pancreatic enzymes secretion is reduced by 90% or more. Deficiencies of vitamins, including B_{12}, and of iron and calcium generally do not develop owing to intact intestinal absorptive function. Treatment is indicated only when weight loss continues despite attempts at increasing caloric intake. Pancreatic extracts as described above, or enteric-coated preparations that dissolve only at the alkaline pH of the duodenum and upper jejunum, may be tried (e.g., Pancrease™ or Creon™, 2–3 capsules/meal).

Diabetes mellitus eventually develops in about 70% of patients, and one-half of those require insulin. In contrast with the usual diabetic, the risk of iatrogenic hypoglycemia is even greater, given the combined deficiency of insulin and glucagon, erratic dietary habits, and alcohol-induced hypoglycemia. **Pancreatic pseudocysts** appear in about 60% of patients, representing a type of retention cyst from pancreatic duct destruction or disruption. Surrounded by a rim of chronic inflammation and fibrosis, and located within or adjacent to the pancreas, they may compress the distal common bile duct. Enlarging (>5 cm in diameter) pseudocysts or those complicated by internal or percutaneous drainage warrant surgical treatment.

External compression of the common bile duct by a pseudocyst or by pancreatic fibrosis with resulting jaundice calls for surgical correction so as to prevent secondary biliary cirrhosis. **Pancreatic ascites,** a form of chemical peritonitis caused by leakage of pancreatic juice from a disrupted ductal structure, is rare; the levels of amylase and lipase in the fluid are far greater than those in the serum. The treatment is surgical—that is, a partial pancreatectomy or drainage of the leaking duct into a loop of jejunum.

CHAPTER 96 ## CYSTIC FIBROSIS

General aspects of cystic fibrosis (CF) and its respiratory manifestations are discussed in chapter 223. Malabsorption and intestinal obstruction from cystic fibrosis are discussed here. *Malabsorption*, with steatorrhea, occurs in about 85% of affected persons, starting in early childhood, and is caused by pancreatic exocrine insufficiency due to painless obstruction of the pancreatic duct system by proteinaceous, inspissated secretions. The resulting growth failure and malnutrition can be ameliorated by administering high doses of pancreatic extracts. Partial substitution of dietary fat by medium-chain triglyceride may produce additional weight gain.

Colicky abdominal pain and distention signaling acute or **chronic intestinal obstruction** occur frequently in these patients. This complication, due to accumulation of masses of tenacious, putty-like material in the ileum or proximal colon, is treated acutely by 20% N-acetylcysteine (30 ml in 120 ml of water) given orally or rectally as a retention enema. Chronic cases may be given less expensive agents, including diatrizoate (Gastrografin) or 1–2L of a polyethylene glycol-electrolyte solution (GoLYTELY) orally. The dosage of pancreatic extract should be increased and poorly digestible, stringy cellulose materials (e.g., the pulp of citrus fruit) should be avoided. Patients with CF cannot respond to bacterial enterotoxins with Cl^- secretion given the absence of CFTR gene product from the apical cell membrane throughout the bowel. Thus they are protected against secretory diarrhea mediated by increases in intracellular cAMP or calcium concentration.

CHAPTER 97

NEOPLASMS OF THE PANCREAS

ancreatic neoplasms with endocrine manifestations originate in the islet cells. Examples of these rare neoplasms are insulinomas (chapter 65) and gastrinomas (chapter 76).

The great majority of non-endocrine pancreatic neoplasms are malignant. Their etiology remains unknown except for some rare types of familial endocrine tumors. Pancreatic cancer is the fifth most common carcinoma as a cause of death; it accounts for more than 20% of all gastrointestinal cancers. Its incidence has increased steadily during the past 40 years; it now causes almost 25,000 yearly deaths in the United States.

Adenocarcinoma

About 90% of pancreatic tumors are mucinous adenocarcinoma of ductal origin, predominating among men (2:1) and associated with cigarette smoking, beer drinking, certain industrial carcinogens, and, probably, chronic pancreatitis. It affects all age groups, but is most common in the seventh and eighth decades of life.

■ Clinical Features

Pain and weight loss, lasting several months, occur in up to 75% of patients. The pain is upper abdominal, vague, dull, and constant; it implies retroperitoneal extension or perineural infiltration by tumor. Anorexia due to pain or liver metastases, pancreatic exocrine insufficiency, onset of diabetes mellitus, all lead to weight loss. Obstructive jaundice occurs in over 50% of cases, particularly with a tumor located in the pancreatic head and compressing the intrapancreatic common bile duct. Rarely, it presents with an episode of otherwise unexplained acute pancreatitis. Anorexia, loss of weight, and vague abdominal pain in the face of negative diagnostic studies may mimic depression. Duodenal or gastric wall invasion may cause vomiting, bleeding, or obstruction. The tumor is usually not palpable. The liver may be enlarged, firm, and irregular due to metastases. Jaundice along with a palpably enlarged gallbladder (Courvoisier's sign) signals common bile duct obstruction by a pancreatic or ampullary cancer. Most patients are surgically incurable by the time of diagnosis.

■ Diagnosis

Early diagnosis of pancreatic cancer is a clinical challenge, with no practical screening test for early pancreatic cancer being available. The emphasis should be on the detection of small tumors, less than 2–3 cm in diameter, that might be resectable for cure. Such small lesions, however, tend to be subclinical and frequently beyond the limits of abdominal US and CT. Positive findings on current diagnostic testing imply a tumor that has less than a 2% chance for cure. Finally, the presenting complaints are shared by many other abdominal disorders; thus, the tests for this tumor must be highly specific. Clues for pancreatic cancer include upper abdominal or back pain suggesting a retroperitoneal origin, unexplained dyspepsia and weight loss with negative conventional work-up, recent onset of mild diabetes in the elderly without predisposing factors, and acute pancreatitis with no obvious cause in the sixth decade and beyond.

Routine blood tests have limited use. Mild anemia or hyperglycemia may be present. Serum amylase and lipase are moderately high in only 10–20% of patients. Hyperbilirubinemia and cholestatic liver tests are found with common bile duct encroachment and with extensive liver metastases. A raised plasma carcinoembryonic antigen level (CEA) occurs in one third of cases. The level of carbohydrate antigen CA 19-9, the sialylated blood group Lewis A, is high in 70% of patients, with the degree of elevation correlating with the tumor size. However, CA 19-9 levels are moderately high in 20–30% of patients with acute and chronic pancreatitis.

Several imaging tests can yield findings suggestive of, but not completely diagnostic of, pancreatic cancer. Transabdominal US may suggest the disease in 60% of cases, CT in 80%, and ERCP in 93%. MRI scan is a useful adjunct to CT and can also be used as an alternative to CT in those who cannot be given iodinated contrast. Although MRI has a greater contrast resolution, at present it is still a secondary imaging modality with CT being the examination of choice. In experienced hands, endoscopic US can demonstrate lesions that are beyond the resolution of the other techniques. With evidence of unresectability, CT- or US-guided fine-needle aspiration for cytology can confirm the diagnosis with a high degree of accuracy. When a small, potentially resectable tumor is found, its resectability can be confirmed preoperatively by selective visceral arteriography and by diagnostic laparoscopy. Tumor invasion of stomach or duodenum can be demonstrated by upper GI series or by endoscopy.

■ Management

The objectives are palliation or an attempt to cure. If the need for palliation is obvious, excessive testing should be avoided in favor of confirming the diagnosis at surgery. Gastric and duodenal obstruction can be by-passed by a gastrojejunostomy without any resection. Obstructive jaundice with pruritus, anorexia, or bacterial cholangitis is palliated by endoscopic insertion of plastic or expandable metal stents into the obstructed common bile duct. When this attempt fails, surgical or percutaneous decompression can be attempted.

Approximately 15–20% of patients with carcinoma of the head of the pancreas have an apparently resectable lesion at operation, with only a few cures. Essentially, all carcinomas of the body and tail have progressed beyond the curative resection stage. Choice of the operative procedure lies between resection of the duodenum and head of the pancreas (**Whipple operation**) and total pancreatectomy, both with regional node removal. The results of the Whipple operation for ampullary carcinoma are considerably better. Irradiation therapy by high-dose external beam techniques or by intraoperative radiation may provide limited palliation of symptoms and minor prolongation of survival. Debilitating abdominal and back pain in advanced pancreatic carcinoma may be relieved or significantly improved by percutaneous block and chemical neurolysis of the celiac and superior mesenteric sympathetic ganglia. This procedure should be more widely employed. Chemotherapy, so far, has been unable to provide measurable benefits to patients with this disease.

■ Questions

INSTRUCTIONS: For each question below, select only **one** lettered answer that is the **best** for that question.

1. A 53-year-old man, who was diagnosed to have a gastric ulcer on upper GI x-rays, was given Ranitidine (300 mg daily) for 12 weeks. On follow-up, his epigastric pain persists. The next step in his management should be to:
   A. Continue Ranitidine for another 4 weeks.
   B. Increase the dose of Ranitidine until patient responds.
   C. Repeat barium upper GI examination.
   D. Evaluate the gastric ulcer by endoscopy.
   E. Treat patient for H. pylori infection.

2. A 58-year-old man has a 15-year history of recurrent duodenal ulcer disease. His ulcer heals promptly with H2-receptor antagonists, but recurs within 2–6 months after stopping treatment. There is no history of NSAID use. Management of this patient should include which of the folllowing?

A. Long-term treatment with H2-receptor antagonists
B. Treating patient with Omeprazole instead of H2-receptor antagonist
C. Consideration of treatment for H. pylori infection
D. CT scan of abdomen to rule out gastrinoma
E. Referring the patient for duodenal ulcer surgery

3. A 72-year-old man has a 6-month history of dysphagia, mainly for solids, and a 15 lb. weight loss. He is a heavy smoker but claims to have stopped smoking 4 months ago. The most likely diagnosis is:
   A. Esophageal carcinoma
   B. Gastric carcinoma
   C. Achalasia
   D. Peptic esophageal stricture
   E. Pill injury of the esophagus

4. A 28-year-old woman has a 1-hour history of passing maroon stools. The pulse is 120/min and blood pressure is 100/60 mm Hg. She feels dizzy on standing. The hematocrit is 44%, hemoglobin 13 is g/dl, and MCV is 88 fl. This patient has which of the following?
   A. Acute, significant blood loss
   B. Acute, minimal blood loss
   C. Acute and chronic blood loss
   D. Chronic blood loss
   E. None of the above

5. A 45-year-old patient has history of recurrent vomiting. Upper GI examination shows evidence of gastric outlet obstruction. Which of the following could be expected?
   A. Projectile and bilious vomiting
   B. Gastric volvulus
   C. Paraesophageal hernia
   D. Hypokalemic acidosis
   E. Hypokalemic alkalosis

6. In Barrett's esophagus:
   A. Gastroesophageal reflux should be aggressively treated in order to make the metaplastic epithelium disappear.
   B. Periodic endoscopic evaluation should be done with biopsy.
   C. Anti-reflux surgery is the treatment of choice.
   D. Patients have a higher incidence of esophageal infection.
   E. Squamous epithelium extends below the gastro-esophageal junction.

7. All of the following are true about Helicobacter pylori, EXCEPT:
   A. Over 90% of patients with duodenal ulcer are positive for H. pylori.

B. Eradication of H. pylori lowers duodenal ulcer recurrence rate.

C. Prior infection predisposes to gastric adenocarcinoma.

D. Prior infection predisposes to gastric MALT lymphoma.

E. Infected patients have a higher incidence of Achalasia.

8. A 42-year-old woman has watery diarrhea and mild lower abdominal cramping distress for 4 months. She lost 4 kg through attempts at weight reduction. Systemic symptoms, blood in stool, and recent foreign travel are absent. All the following considerations are appropriate, EXCEPT:

A. Laxative abuse.

B. Idiopathic ulcerative colitis.

C. Consumption of sorbitol-containing diet foods.

D. Functional diarrhea.

E. Microscopic colitis.

9. Based on the above information, the following are indicated, EXCEPT:

A. Proctosigmoidoscopy with biopsies.

B. Esophagogastroduodenoscopy (EGD) with duodenal biopsies.

C. Urine laxative screen.

D. Thorough dietary history.

E. Stool testing for occult blood.

10. A 28-year-old married man with a 12-year history of ulcerative colitis suffers his eighth relapse, with tenesmus, frequent bloody stools, abdominal cramps, and a fever of 100.5°F. Each previous attack responded to a 2-month course of corticosteroids; he took no medications during remissions. The serum alkaline phosphatase is 2.5 times the upper limit of normal. ERCP shows caliber irregularities of intra- and extra-hepatic bile ducts. All of the following issues are relevant, EXCEPT:

A. Proctocolectomy should be considered in order to prevent progression of primary sclerosing cholangitis.

B. The patient should have received maintenance therapy with a 5-ASA-containing medication.

C. The couple's plans to have children need to be considered in choosing the type of 5-ASA-containing medication.

D. The patient needs surveillance colonoscopy with biopsies in the near future.

E. The patient may have osteoporosis.

11. A 32-year-old nonalcoholic man has recovered from an initial episode of acute pancreatitis. Abdominal ultrasonography showed no gallstones, and serum triglyceride and calcium levels were normal. All of the following may help determine the etiology of pancreatitis, EXCEPT:

A. Endoscopic retrograde cholangio-pancreatography (ERCP)

B. Review of pre-illness medication intake

C. Bile analysis for cholesterol crystals

D. Inquiries about possible cocaine abuse

E. Upper gastrointestinal series

12. The following conditions are associated with, or may be a consequence of, celiac sprue, EXCEPT:

A. Diabetes mellitus

B. Lymphoma of the small intestine

C. Carcinoma of the colon

D. Ulcerative jejunitis

E. Squamous carcinoma of the oropharynx

13. A 1.2 cm tubular adenoma was removed from the sigmoid colon of a 65-year-old man. Colonoscopy shows no additional lesions. He has no symptoms and his family history is unremarkable. A fecal occult blood test (FOBT) is negative. Which of the following statements is correct?

A. He should undergo fiberoptic proctosigmoidoscopy in 6 months.

B. Further follow-up depends on the results of serial FOBT.

C. An abdominal CT scan should be ordered.

D. He should undergo colonoscopy in 3 years.

E. His risk of developing colorectal carcinoma remains high despite regular colonoscopic surveillance and removal of any new polyps.

14. A 45-year-old man with well-established alcoholic chronic pancreatitis has lost 5 kg during the past 4 months. Possible direct causes of this weight loss include all of the following, EXCEPT:

A. Excessive consumption of ethanol

B. Newly developed diabetes mellitus

C. Malabsorption with diarrhea

D. Decreased food intake due to constant pain

E. Lack of funds to purchase food

15. If a 3-day stool collection obtained from the above patient yielded a daily stool weight of 360 g and 38 g of fat/day, which of the following tests is expected to be abnormal?

A. A serum iron level

B. A glucose breath H_2 test

C. The blood folate concentration

D. A test of vitamin B_{12} absorption

E. The serum vitamin D concentration

■ Answers

1. D	2. C	3. A	4. A	5. E
6. B	7. E	8. B	9. B	10. A
11. E	12. C	13. D	14. A	15. D

SUGGESTED READING

Textbooks and Monographs

Arias IM, Boyer JL, Fausto N, et al (eds.). The Liver: Biology and Pathology. 3rd ed. New York: Raven Press, 1994.

Blaser MJ, Smith PD, Ravdin JI, et al (eds.). Infections of the Gastrointestinal Tract. New York: Raven Press, 1995.

DeDombal FT. Diagnosis of Acute Abdominal Pain. 2nd ed. Edinburgh. Churchill Livingstone, 1991.

Feldman M, Scharschmidt B, Sleisenger MH (eds.). Sleisenger & Fordtran's Gastrointestinal and Liver Disease. 6th ed. Philadelphia: WB Saunders Co., 1997.

Go VLW, DiMagno E, Gardner JD, et al (eds.). The Pancreas, Biology, Pathobiology and Disease. 2nd ed. New York: Raven Press, 1993.

Gollan JL, Kalser SC, Pitt HA, et al (eds.). Proceedings of the NIH Consensus Development Conference on gallstones and laparoscopic cholecystectomy. Am J Surg 1993;165: 388–548.

Sherlock S, Dooley J (eds.). Diseases of the Liver and Biliary System. 10th ed. Oxford, England/Boston: Blackwell Scientific Publications, 1997.

Targan SR, Shanahan F (eds.). Inflammatory Bowel Disease. From Bench to Bedside. Baltimore: Williams & Wilkins, 1994.

Yamada T (ed.). Textbook of Gastroenterology. 2nd ed. Philadelphia: Lippincott, 1995.

Articles

Esophageal Disorders

Anonymous. Continuous ambulatory esophageal pH monitoring in the evaluation of patients with gastroesophageal reflux. Diagnostic and Therapeutic Technology Assessment. JAMA 1995;274(8):662–668.

Brewer TG. Treatment of acute gastroesophageal variceal hemorrhage. Med Clin North Am 1993;77(5):993–1014.

Ellis P, Cunningham D. Management of carcinomas of the upper gastrointestinal tract. *BMJ*. 1994;308(6932):834–838.

Jalan R, Redhead DN, Hayes PC. Transjugular intrahepatic portasystemic stent-shunt in the treatment of variceal haemorrhage. Br J Surg 1995;82(9):1158–1164.

Pope II CE. Acid-reflux disorders. N Engl J Med 1994;331: 656–660.

Schroeder PL, Filler SJ, Ramirez B, Lazarchik DA, Vaezi MF, Richter JE. Dental erosion and acid reflux disease. Ann Intern Med 1995;122(11):809–815.

Stein C, Korula J. Variceal bleeding. What are the treatment options? Postgrad Med 1995;98(6):143–146.

Trate DM, Parkman HP, Fisher RS. Dysphagia. Evaluation, diagnosis, and treatment. Primary Care 1996;23(3):417–432.

Gastrointestinal Hemorrhage

Cook DJ, Fuller HD, Guyatt GH, et al. Risk factors for gastrointestinal bleeding in critically ill patients. N Engl J Med 1994;330:377–381.

Cook CJ, Cuyatt GH, Salena BJ, et al. Endoscopic therapy of acute nonvariceal upper gastrointestinal hemorrhage: a meta analysis. Gastroenterology 1992;102:139–148.

Laine L, Peterson WL. Bleeding peptic ulcer. N Engl J Med 1994;331;717–727.

Moses PL, Smith RE. Endoscopic evaluation of iron deficiency anemia. A guide to diagnostic strategy in older patients. Postgrad Med 1995;98(2):213–216.

Manten HD, Green JA. Acute lower gastrointestinal bleeding. A guide to initial management. Postgrad Med 1995;97(4): 154–157.

Sharma R, Gorbien MJ. Angiodysplasia and lower gastrointestinal tract bleeding in elderly patients. Arch Intern Med 1995;155(8):807–812.

Diseases of the Stomach and Duodenum

Fennerty MB. Helicobacter pylori. Arch Intern Med 1994;154: 721–727.

Laine L. The long-term management of patients with bleeding ulcers: Helicobacter pylori eradication instead of maintenance antisecretory therapy. Gastrointest Endosc 1995;41: 77–79.

Parsonnet J, Hansen S, Rodriguez L et al. Helicobacter pylori and gastric lymphoma. N Engl J Med 1994; 330: 1267–1271.

Diseases of the Small Intestine

Avery ME, Snyder JD. Oral therapy for acute diarrhea. The underused simple solution. New Engl J Med 1990;323:891–894.

Cook GC. Persisting diarrhoea and malabsorption. Gut 1994; 35(5):582–586.

Donowitz M, Kokke FT, Saidi R. Evaluation of patients with chronic diarrhea. N Engl J Med 1995;332(11):725–729.

DuPont HL, Ericsson CD. Prevention and treatment of traveler's diarrhea. N Engl J Med 1993;328(25):1821–1827.

Elson CO. The basis of current and future therapy for inflammatory bowel disease. Am J Med 1996;100:656–662.

Fantry GT, James SP. Whipple's disease. Dig Dis 1995;13(2): 108–118.

Farthing MJ. Travellers' diarrhoea. BMJ 1993;306(6890):1425–1426.

Hodgson HJF, Mazlam MZ. Assessment of drug therapy in inflammatory bowel disease. Alim Pharmacol Therap 1991; 5:555–584.

Stanghellini V, Camilleri M, Malagelada JR. Chronic idiopathic intestinal pseudo-obstruction: clinical and intestinal manometric findings. Gut 1987;28:5–12.

Trier JS. Celiac sprue. N Engl J Med 1991;325:1709–1719.

Diseases of the Colon

Almounajed G, Drossman DA. Newer aspects of the irritable bowel syndrome. Primary Care 1996;23(3):477–495.

Cohen LB. Colorectal cancer: a primary care approach to screening. *Geriatrics*. 1996;51(12):45–49.

Connell WR, Lennard-Jones JE, Williams CB, et al. Factors affecting the outcome of endoscopic surveillance for cancer in ulcerative colitis. Gastroenterology 1994;107:934–944.

Deckmann RC, Cheskin LJ. Diverticular disease in the elderly. J Am Ger Soc 1993;41(9):986–993.

Kelly CP, Pothoulakis C, LaMont JT. Clostridium difficile colitis. New Engl J Med 1994;330:257–262.

Locke GR III. The epidemiology of functional gastrointestinal disorders in North America. Gastroenterol Clin North Am 1996;25(1):1–19.

McGuire HH Jr. Bleeding colonic diverticula. A reappraisal of natural history and management. Ann Surg 1994;220(5): 653–656.

Rustgi AK. Hereditary gastrointestinal polyposis and nonpolyposis syndromes. N Engl J Med 1994;331:1694–1702.

Scott N, Quirke P. Molecular biology of colorectal neoplasia. Gut 1993;34:289–292.

Tempero M, Anderson J. Progress in colon cancer: do molecular markers matter? N Engl J Med 1994;331(4):267–268.

Winawer SJ, Zauber AG, Ho MN, et al. Prevention of colorectal cancer by colonoscopic polypectomy. N Engl J Med 1993; 329:1977–1981.

Diseases of the Pancreas

Beger HG, Büchler M, Bittner R, et al. Necrosectomy and postoperative local lavage in necrotizing pancreatitis. Br J Surg 1988;75:207–212.

Lankisch PG, Löhr-Happe A, Otto J, et al. Natural course in chronic pancreatitis. Pain, exocrine and endocrine pancreatic insufficiency and prognosis of the disease. Digestion 1993; 54:148–155.

Lee SP, Nicholls JF, Park HZ. Biliary sludge as a cause of acute pancreatitis. N Engl J Med 1992;326:589–593.

Warshaw AL, Fernández-Del Castillo C. Pancreatic carcinoma. N Engl J Med 1992;326:455–465.

Wilson C, Heath DI, Imrie CW. Prediction of outcome in acute pancreatitis: a comparative study of APACHE II, clinical assessment and multiple factor scoring systems. Br J Surg 1990;77:1260–1264.

CHAPTER 98 ANATOMY AND PHYSIOLOGY OF THE LIVER AND LABORATORY EVALUATION OF LIVER FUNCTION

■ Anatomy

Based on its blood supply and biliary branching, the liver is divided into right and left lobes of nearly equal weight. Each lobe receives a separate blood supply with essentially no collateral circulation between them. The **hepatic artery** from the celiac axis supplies 30% of the liver's resting blood flow; the **portal vein** provides the remainder. The caudate lobe and the rest of the liver separately drain into the inferior vena cava.

Hepatocytes (liver cells) are arranged in a continuum of single-cell plates separated by sinusoids; in the sinusoids, the blood flows from hepatic artery and portal vein to the terminal hepatic or central venule. Each hepatocyte is bathed by sinusoidal blood on two surfaces. The sinusoids are lined with a fenestrated network of endothelial cells and phagocytic **Kupffer cells.** The **space of Disse** between the sinusoidal endothelial lining and the hepatocyte surfaces contains, besides the lipid-storing Ito cells, interstitial lymph fluid that drains via the lymphatics through the porta hepatis and, finally, into the thoracic duct.

The hepatic microvasculature has two structural subunits. The **classic lobule** has several portal tracts surrounding a central vein. The other, the **hepatic acinus,** is more functionally relevant, since it centers on the portal tract. Blood flows from the portal vein and hepatic artery toward either of two terminal hepatic venules located at the apices of an acinus (Figure 98.1). The acinus is divided into three zones; zone 1 is closest to the portal tracts and zone 3 is closest to the terminal hepatic venules. Zone 1 hepatocytes have abundant mitochondria and are rich in enzymes of the citric acid cycle. Cells in zone 3, being more remote from nutrient and oxygen input, are more vulnerable to ischemia than those near the point of blood inflow. They are also the site of protein, triglyceride, and lipoprotein formation.

The parenchymal cell surfaces facing the sinusoids are lined with microvilli that lie in the space of Disse just beneath the sinusoidal endothelium. Interspersed between nonsinusoidal surfaces of adjoining liver cells are bile canaliculi, the terminal radicles of the biliary system. Lysosomes adjacent to bile canaliculi contain hydrolytic enzymes and act as an intracellular digestive system for the disposal of worn-out organelles and other intracellular substances via **biliary secretion.** The **Golgi apparatus,** also lying near bile canaliculi, is regarded as a packaging apparatus for preparing materials for biliary secretion. Bile canalicular flow is toward the portal tracts, where it drains into interlobular bile ducts.

■ Physiology

Bilirubin metabolism

Bilirubin, a lipid-soluble linear tetrapyrrole, is a waste product with no known physiologic function. Its metabolism is schematically shown in Figure 98.2. The accumulation of bilirubin produces jaundice.

Protein synthesis and metabolism of carbohydrate and fat

Hepatocytes synthesize many proteins, the major one being **albumin.** The average daily albumin synthesis of 12 to 14 g/day can be increased several-fold by a normal liver to offset excessive losses. The amino acids necessary for albumin synthesis are derived from a healthy diet, although in the case of starvation, the liver uses its own protein. Osmotic pressure in hepatic interstitial fluid is a sensitive regulator of albumin synthesis, and in healthy persons, the rate of albumin degradation equals its rate of synthesis. In chronic liver disease, albumin synthesis may be impaired and **hypoalbuminemia** and **hypergammaglobulinemia** may commonly follow.

The liver also synthesizes plasma transport proteins, clotting factors, enzymes, and storage proteins. It can utilize endogenous and exogenous amino acids for fat metabolism and excrete nitrogenous waste by converting ammonia into urea and purines into uric acid.

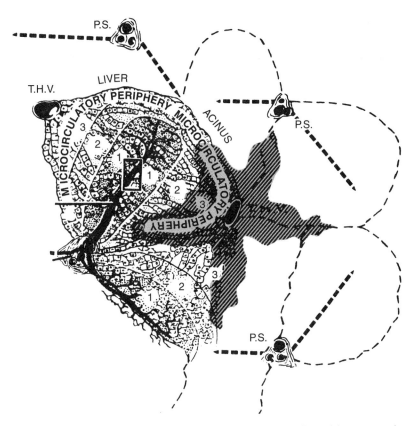

FIGURE 98.1. Blood supply of the simple liver acinus, the zonal arrangement of cells, and the microcirculatory periphery.
(From: Farber and Fisher (eds.). Toxic Injury of the Liver. (New York: Marcel Decker, Inc., 1979. Used with permission.)

Liver is the linchpin of **carbohydrate homeostasis:** under hormonal control, the liver maintains a stable serum glucose level; provides a continuous fuel supply for itself and other vital organs; converts excess dietary monosaccharides into triglycerides, or polymerizes them to glycogen or phosphorylates them; supplies glucose on demand from glycogen by **glycogenolysis;** and converts amino acids, lactate, and glycerol to glucose via **gluconeogenesis.** Liver disease, however, rarely perturbs carbohydrate metabolism. Hypoglycemia— which, along with excess liver glycogen stores, occurs in genetic deficiencies of glycogenolytic enzymes—may complicate acute fulminant hepatitis or acute alcohol intoxication.

Dietary sources, fatty tissue, and synthesis within the liver from acetate and the coenzyme, nicotinamide-adenine dinucleotide phosphate (NADPH) all generate liver lipid, which normally constitutes 5% of total liver weight. After uptake into the liver, fatty acids are oxidized, or exported as lipoproteins after con- version into triglycerides. The liver utilizes large amounts of hepatic fatty acids as a major energy source or partially metabolizes them to ketones, thus pro- viding an energy substitute for skeletal and cardiac muscle.

Immunologic function

The liver is pivotal in the defense against infections, which are often lethal in acute or chronic liver failure. Susceptibility to bacterial and opportunistic fungal infections is increased in severe liver disease.

The **reticuloendothelial (RE) system,** a mass of fixed phagocytes, remove bacteria, endotoxins, and particulate debris from the blood. The Kupffer cells lining the hepatic sinusoids constitute approximately 85% of the functioning RE cell mass. In addition, the hepatocytes synthesize complement factors and other **opsonins.** Severe liver disease predisposes to bacterial and oppor- tunistic fungal infections, which are frequently lethal in this setting.

■ Blood Tests of Liver Function

Available blood tests that assess the integrity of the liver are listed in Table 98.1. Although individual blood tests reflect specific processes of the liver (e.g., liver injury, cholestasis, or liver function), in clinical parlance, all are collectively called **"liver function tests"** (LFTs or **liver tests**).

Serum bilirubin

Serum bilirubin is a liver function test and a marker of cholestasis. Most often, direct-reacting (conjugated) and total bilirubin levels are measured through a **diazo reaction;** subtracting the direct from the total yields the indirect (unconjugated) fraction. Normally, up to 1.5 mg total bilirubin/dl is present, essentially all conjugated. Unconjugated hyperbilirubinemia may follow overpro-duction (as in hemolysis) or signify a genetic defect in hepatic uptake or conjugation. Conjugated hyperbilirubinemia is most often caused by liver or biliary tract disease. Isolated, chronic hyperbilirubinemia of the *unconjugated* type is almost always from **Gilbert's syndrome,** while the *conjugated* type is characteristically from defects of hepatic storage or excretion (e.g., **Dubin-Johnson syndrome** and **Rotor syndrome**). Excess urine urobilinogen indicates conjugated hyperbilirubinemia.

Serum alkaline phosphatase

Serum alkaline phosphatase represents the sum of its fractions from bone, liver, and intestine; the fractions are measured as isoenzymes or by heat sensitivity (bone-derived fraction is heat-labile). A marker of cholestasis, serum alkaline phosphatase may rise in biliary obstruction and in infiltrative and malignant diseases of the liver.

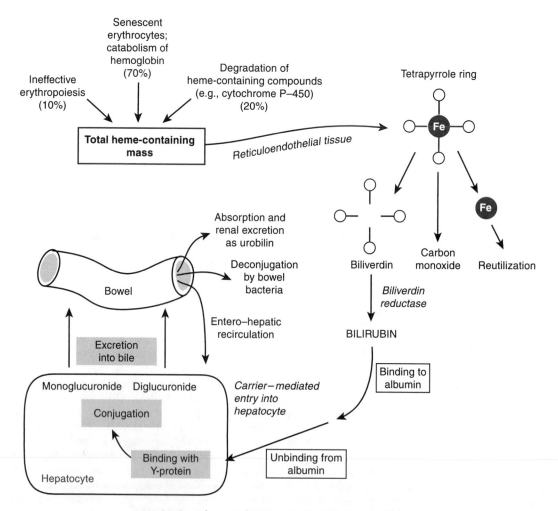

FIGURE 98.2. Schematic diagram showing bilirubin metabolism.

TABLE 98.1.	Blood Tests of Liver Function		
Test	Liver Injury	Cholestasis	Liver Function
Bilirubin	(−)	+	+
Alkaline phosphatase	(−)	+	(−)
Aspartate amino-transferase (AST)	+	(−)	(−)
Alanine amino-transferase (ALT)	+	(−)	(−)
Gamma glutamyl transpeptidase	(−)	+	(−)
Prothrombin time (PT)	(−)	(−)	+
Albumin	(−)	(−)	+

(−) = Normal/not elevated; + = Elevated.

Gamma-glutamyl transpeptidase

Gamma-glutamyl transpeptidase (GGTP or GGT) is derived from the canalicular membranes of the hepatocyte and from the microsomal fraction. GGT is, perhaps, the most sensitive marker of liver dysfunction. It rises in biliary obstruction, and is a more sensitive marker for cholestasis than alkaline phosphatase. Drugs or other substances that induce microsomal enzyme activity may elevate GGT; a prime example is alcohol.

Serum aminotransferases

Serum aminotransferases, also known as transaminases, are tests for liver injury and necrosis. **Alanine aminotransferase (ALT)** is uniquely derived from hepatocytes. While hepatocyte necrosis may elevate serum levels of **aspartate aminotransferase (AST),** muscle injury or hemolysis may produce the same result. ALT is the best measure of liver injury; however, both enzymes are simultaneously measured in most "panels." A high ratio of AST:ALT (>1.5) is typical of alcoholic liver disease and may help identify this form of liver injury, although other forms of liver disease may also manifest a high ratio. Transaminase levels rise strikingly in various forms of acute hepatic necrosis (caused, e.g., by drug abuse or viral hepatitis) and in severe ischemic hepatitis, but more modestly in alcoholic hepatitis and cholestasis. Transaminase levels usually rise only mildly in metastatic liver cancer. Elevated aminotransferases can be seen in asymptomatic persons; alcohol and obesity account for most cases (70%), followed by hepatitis C (almost one-fifth).

Serum protein levels

The **serum albumin** level is the most common serum protein test to be clinically utilized as a liver function test. Given its rather long (14–20d) half-life, serum albumin is commonly quite low in chronic liver failure and may be normal or only slightly reduced in severe, acute liver failure. The **prothrombin time (PT)** is a simple and useful marker of liver function. Factor V level may be used to assess liver function and prognosis in acute fulminant liver failure. Since many clotting factors (II, VII, IX, and X) are vitamin K–dependent, impaired blood coagulation in chronic cholestatic jaundice may be due to vitamin K malabsorption rather than to liver disease. When jaundice and a high PT co-exist, prompt correction of the PT by IV vitamin K supports obstructive jaundice rather than liver failure.

■ Imaging of the Liver

Computed tomography and magnetic resonance imaging

Computed tomography (CT) of the liver accurately evaluates the size, shape, density, and mass of the liver, which enables it to reliably detect and characterize solid and cystic lesions, abscesses, and hemangiomas in the liver. It can suggest fatty liver and hemochromatosis by lesser and greater liver densities. Detection of dilated bile ducts is less accurate by CT than with ultrasound, but CT defines extrahepatic structures and lesions causing biliary obstruction. Although magnetic resonance imaging (MRI) and CT share many advantages (ability to identify liver density, solid and cystic lesions, etc.), MRI can also assess the blood flow, thus enabling it to diagnose thrombosis of hepatic veins. MRI is particularly useful for detecting small, cavernous liver hemangiomas.

Radionuclide scintiscanning

Technetium-99m-sulfur colloid is most frequently used for this purpose. It is taken up by the Kupffer cells of the liver and on external scanning, yields an image of the liver. Primary liver cancer, metastases, cysts, hemangiomas, and abscesses appear as filling defects since these lesions lack Kupffer cells. In cirrhosis, fatty liver, and hepatitis, the uptake is generally low and inhomogeneous. In chronic liver disease, an increased uptake by the spleen and bone marrow is also noted.

Scintiscanning lacks the resolution and specificity of ultrasound, CT scanning, or MRI scanning in demonstrating primary and metastatic tumors.

Ultrasound

Hepatobiliary ultrasound (US) can image solid and cystic liver lesions as small as 1 to 2 cm, bile ducts, gallbladder, portal and hepatic veins, hepatic artery, and the vena cava. Its cost is relatively low, it is noninvasive, and involves no radiation. US detection of dilation of the biliary tree is an essential first step in the work-up of cholestasis. Combined with Doppler flow analysis, it can noninvasively assess portal vein and portosystemic shunt patency and the direction of blood flow.

■ **Invasive Tests**

Liver biopsy

Indications for **needle biopsy** are listed in Table 98.2. Coagulation status must be tested through PT and platelet counts prior to biopsy; the hemoglobin level must be adequate. Patients must be alert and cooperative. Contraindications include coagulation disorders capable of causing hemorrhage, defined as PT exceeding 15 sec and/or platelet count below 100,00/mm^3. Performed mostly on an outpatient basis, biopsy is followed by close observation. A right flank approach through an intercostal space is most commonly used to enter the liver. Evanescent pain commonly follows biopsy, at the needle site or in the right shoulder. Hemorrhage, bile leak, and hypotension are infrequent and, when encountered, usually occur within 3 hours of the biopsy. Space-occupying lesions are often safely and accurately approached by CT- or US-guided fine needle aspiration and biopsy.

In patients with severe and uncorrectable coagulopathy, a **transvenous liver biopsy** may be appropriate. After cannulating the subclavian or femoral vein, liver tissue may be obtained through the hepatic veins using biopsy forceps or a biopsy needle. Bleeding at the biopsy site enters the venous circulation and it is of no clinical concern. **Peritoneoscopy,** often combined with directed biopsy, is occasionally valuable in diagnosing liver disease or malignancy, but is more invasive than percutaneous liver biopsy.

TABLE 98.2. Indications for Liver Biopsy
Chronic viral hepatitis
Chronic liver enzyme elevation
Liver mass
Unexplained hepatomegaly
Suspicion of the following entities:
Cirrhosis
Hemochromatosis
Alcoholic liver disease
Wilson's disease
To monitor drug toxicity (e.g., methotrexate)
To diagnose systemic infection:
Viral
Fungal
Mycobacterial
To diagnose infiltrating liver disease:
Sarcoidosis
Amyloidosis

CHAPTER **99** CLINICAL PRESENTATIONS OF LIVER DISEASE

Jaundice

In most clinical instances, jaundice implies hepatobiliary or hematologic disorders. Jaundice due to hepatobiliary disease may be associated with pruritus, biliary colic, fatigue, anorexia, nausea, vomiting, or diffuse right upper quadrant pain. Conceptually, jaundice may be **prehepatic** (i.e., disturbances of bilirubin metabolism before bilirubin enters the liver); **hepatic,** which refers to diseases of the liver; and **posthepatic,** where the bile flow is impeded within the liver or in the extrahepatic biliary channels (Table 99.1).

In the pathogenesis of jaundice associated with liver diseases, more than one mechanism may operate simultaneously, making any classification artificial;

TABLE 99.1. Etiology of Jaundice		
Prehepatic	**Hepatic**	**Posthepatic**
Hemolytic anemia	Acute hepatitis	Biliary stricture
Resolving hematoma	Chronic hepatitis	Gallstones
Sickle cell disease	Cirrhosis	Primary sclerosing cholangitis
Massive blood transfusions	Alcoholic liver disease	Biliary cancer
		Pancreatic cancer

nevertheless, this classification fosters understanding and a logical diagnostic approach. Hematological disorders as the etiology of jaundice may be readily obvious (i.e., evidence for hemolytic anemia). Once hemolysis is excluded, the pivotal issue is whether the jaundice is intra- or extrahepatic. The next step is to determine whether the biliary tree caliber is normal or dilated. Ultrasound (US) is the most useful test for this purpose. If necessary, US may be followed by cholangiography, through either an endoscopic retrograde (ERCP) or percutaneous transhepatic (PTC) approach. Although the local expertise available guides the choice, ERCP is usually preferred since it offers expanded therapeutic options, such as the ability to extract gallstones, to dilate strictures, or to place stents.

Elevated Liver Enzymes

Asymptomatic abnormalities in liver blood tests most often involving serum aminotransferases—may be the first presentation of liver disease (Table 99.2). Symptoms, when present, are usually vague: fatigue, abdominal discomfort, nausea, and anorexia being the most common. Important historical data include ingestion of alcohol and medications, exposure to solvents, and history of blood transfusions, tattoos, or IV drug abuse. Physical signs of chronic liver disease, such as gynecomastia, palmar erythema, spider angiomata, testicular atrophy, or right upper abdominal tenderness may or may not be present. Further studies include testing for chronic viral hepatitis, autoimmune disease, and metabolic liver disease (alpha-1-antitrypsin deficiency and hemochromatosis), and liver imaging. In a young person, screening for Wilson's disease is imperative; while rare, this disease is devastating if left untreated.

TABLE 99.2. Causes of Elevated Liver Enzymes
Viral hepatitis
Acute
Chronic
Drug-induced hepatotoxicity
Alcoholic liver disease
Gallstone disease
Autoimmune hepatitis
Metabolic liver disease
Hemochromatosis
Wilson's disease
Steatohepatitis[a]
Passive hepatic congestion (biventricular or right heart failure)

[a]See Table 105.1.

Hepatomegaly

Hepatomegaly may be noted on physical examination or by liver imaging. Its etiology includes many entities (Table 99.3), some of which are diagnosed only by imaging. Alcoholic hepatitis is an important and common cause of hepatomegaly in North America. Often, a patient acknowledges alcohol abuse only after alcoholic liver disease is diagnosed. Primary biliary cirrhosis and autoimmune hepatitis may present with hepatomegaly. Presence of systemic disease elsewhere (sarcoidosis), metabolic tests (hemochromatosis), and liver biopsy (amyloidosis) may all be involved in making a diagnosis.

TABLE 99.3. Etiology of Hepatomegaly	
Hepatic tumors	Infiltrative liver disease
Primary	Hemochromatosis
Benign	Amyloidosis
Malignant	Sarcoidosis
Secondary	Vascular
Hepatic cysts	Passive hepatic congestion
Benign	Hepatic vein thrombosis
Malignant	Inflammatory
Alcoholic hepatitis	Primary biliary cirrhosis
	Primary sclerosing cholangitis
	Autoimmune hepatitis

F ive distinct hepatitis viruses have been identified and isolated, duly classified as A, B, C, D, and E. Acute hepatitis may also be caused by infection with Epstein-Barr virus, herpes simplex virus, cytomegalovirus, and adenovirus.

Hepatitis A

Hepatitis A (syn., infectious hepatitis, HAV) is caused by an RNA enterovirus, 27 nm in diameter, and transmitted by the fecal-oral route. Most common in the first two decades of life, the disease has a variable geographic, but worldwide distribution. Its incidence is falling with improved hygiene and sanitation. Sporadic cases follow person-to-person transmission, but epidemics are usually from a point source (e.g., contaminated food or water). The incubation period is 14 to 50 days. The time course of HAV viremia, viral shedding in stool, and antibody response are shown in Figure 100.1. The initial antibody

is of the IgM class. The IgM antibody peaks in 1–2 weeks and then gradually wanes. IgG anti-HAV peaks in 1–2 months and persists for years. Thus, IgM-specific anti-HAV connotes recent acute infection, whereas IgG anti-HAV alone signifies remote (earlier) infection.

Hepatitis A is usually benign; histologic damage is mild and does not lead to a carrier state or any chronic sequelae. Given the transient viremia, it is rarely transmitted by blood transfusion. Stool and blood become non-infectious after the first 1–2 weeks of illness.

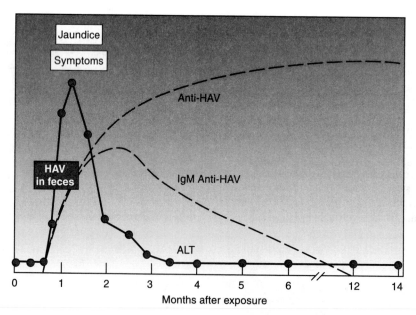

FIGURE 100.1. Typical course of acute hepatitis A. ALT = alanine aminotransferase; HAV = hepatitis A virus; Anti-HAV = antibody to HAV.

(From: Hoofnagle JH, DiBisceglie AM. Sem Liver Dis 1991;11:73-83. Used with permission.)

Hepatitis B

The hepatitis B virus (HBV) belongs to a group of unique DNA viruses with retrovirus characteristics and reverse transcriptase—conferring replication capability of viral DNA through an RNA intermediate. The complete hepatitis B (HB) virion, a 42 nm diameter infectious particle **(Dane particle),** has an inner core of hepatitis B core antigen (HBcAg), double-stranded DNA, and DNA polymerase surrounded by an outer envelope of hepatitis B surface antigen (HBsAg) (see Figure 100.2 and Table 100.1). The infected hepatocytes synthesize surplus

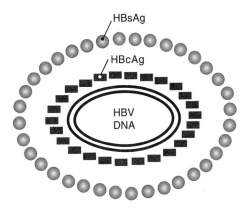

amounts of HBsAg, which appear in the serum in several forms: tubules, round particles, and tadpole-shaped pieces. Another antigenic component of HBV, hepatitis B e antigen (HBeAg), is a fragment of the HBcAg. Virtually all hepatitis B patients become transiently seropositive for HBeAg. HBcAg itself is not measured in routine laboratories as it does not appear in serum in free form.

■ Infectiousness and Antibody Response

Hepatitis B virus DNA (HBV DNA) measurement is used as a marker for viral particles. It has been demonstrated in numerous body fluids and secretions—sweat, semen, vaginal secretions, bile, pancreatic juice, and saliva. Despite the highly variable transmissibility of each, it is prudent to treat all biological fluids as potentially infectious; blood, owing to the highest viral concentration, is the most infectious. IgM class hepatitis B core antibody (HBcAbIgM) develops early in acute infection, and reliably indicates recent infection. HBcAbIgG supersedes the IgM class over several months and persists for years, both in patients who recover from acute hepatitis B and in those with chronic disease. In chronically infected patients, HBcAg elicits IgM and IgG antibodies. In chronic hepatitis B, the presence of HBeAg implies a greater level of infectivity, and HBeAb suggests a lesser level. Hepatitis B surface antibody (HBsAb) protects against HBV infection.

FIGURE 100.2. Structure of hepatitis B virus. HBcAg = hepatitis B core antigen; HBsAg = hepatitis B surface antigen; HBV = hepatitis B virus.

TABLE 100.1.	Hepatitis B Virus Markers						
	HBs Ag	HBsAb	HBcAb	HBcAb IgM	HBeAg	HBeAb	HBV DNA
Acute hepatitis B	+	(−)	+	+	+	(−)	+
Convalescent hepatitis B	(−)	+	+	(−)	(−)	+/(−)	(−)
Chronic hepatitis B replicating phase	+	(−)	+	(−)	+	(−)	+
Chronic hepatitis B integrated phase	+	(−)	+	(−)	(−)	+	+/(−)
Hepatitis B vaccination	(−)	+	(−)	(−)	(−)	(−)	(−)

TABLE 100.2.	Prevalence of Serologic Markers for Hepatitis B Virus in Various Populations in the United States	
	Prevalence of HBV Markers (%)	
Population	**HBsAg**	**Any Marker**
Immigrants from endemic areas	13	70–85
Institutionalized persons	10–20	35–80
Intravenous drug abusers	7	60–80
Male homosexuals	6	35–80
Household contacts of HBV carrier	3-6	30–60

HBsAg = Hepatitis B surface antigen; HBV = Hepatitis B virus.
(Adapted from: Dindzans V. Postgrad Med 1992;92:43–52. Used with permission.)

Populations at high risk for HBV infection are listed in Table 100.2, based on prevalence of serum markers. Viremia occurs 1–4 weeks after exposure, well before and persisting for some time after the onset of symptoms

(Figure 100.3). The appearance of HBsAg is the first sign of HBV infection; the incubation period and the appearance time of the HBsAg depend on the route of infection and the size of the inoculum—as early as 2 weeks after

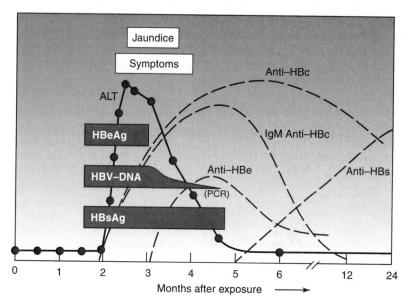

FIGURE 100.3. Typical course of acute hepatitis B. ALT = alanine aminotransferase; HBsAg = hepatitis B surface antigen; HBeAg = hepatitis B e antigen; HBV-DNA = hepatitis B viral deoxyribonucleic acid; anti-HBc = antibody to hepatitis B core antigen; anti-HBe = antibody to HBeAg; Anti-HBs = antibody to HBsAg; PCR = polymerase chain reaction.
(From: Hoofnagle JH, DiBisceglie AM. Sem Liver Dis 1991;11:73–83. Used with permission.)

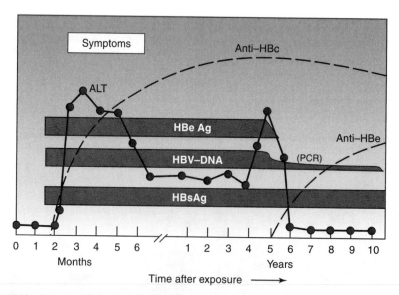

FIGURE 100.4. Typical course of chronic hepatitis B, with acute infection followed by chronic disease. Disease remits when seroconversion occurs from HBeAg to AntiBe. Abbreviations same as in Figure 100.3.
From: Hoofnagle JH, DiBisceglie AM. Sem Liver Dis 1991;11:73–83. Used with permission.)

infected blood transfusion, and longer—perhaps 3 months—after personal contact. HBsAg declines progressively during the acute clinical illness and disappears within weeks of onset of laboratory abnormalities; persistence beyond 6 months defines chronic hepatitis B (Figure 100.4). Persistence of HBeAg, as the acute hepatitis resolves, increases the risk for chronic infection.

Chronic hepatitis B occurs in 5–10% of infected adults. Chronic infection occurs in up to 90% of infected neonates and up to 30% of infected children. Up to 30% of immunosuppressed persons (e.g., organ transplant recipients, hemodialysis patients) will develop chronic hepatitis B. Chronic hepatitis has an initial replicating phase, with intensive viral replication and presence of HBeAg. With the passage of years, and with the loss of HBeAg and attainment of HBeAb, spontaneous seroconversion (marked reduction in viral replication) follows, to the integrated phase. The intensity of hepatitis generally lessens in the integrated phase. Patterns of liver disease vary, ranging from minimal histological changes in the so-called chronic carriers to significant chronic active hepatitis, fibrosis, and cirrhosis.

Hepatitis C

The hepatitis C virus (HCV) is an RNA virus that is the predominant cause of post-transfusion hepatitis in the United States. It is transmitted predominantly by parenteral routes. However, epidemiological studies show HCV infection in patients without any history of percutaneous exposures; obviously, other forms of person-to-person contact are important. Hepatitis C is diagnosed by the detection of antibody to HCV by enzyme immunoassay (EIA). HCV RNA can be detected by polymerase chain reaction (PCR) at a high level of sensitivity. Acute hepatitis C is generally anicteric and less severe than acute hepatitis B. There is a high rate (85%) of chronic infection; fluctuating ALT levels attest to chronicity. Chronic hepatitis C results in cirrhosis in up to 40% of cases.

Hepatitis D

Hepatitis D virus (HDV) is a defective RNA virus with a unique genome and inner core antigen (HDAg) that are encapsulated by a coat of HBsAg. HDV depends on HBV infection for its replication and infects only HBsAg-positive persons. While acute HDV infection may occur simultaneously with acute HBV infection, it is more commonly an acute infection superimposed on chronic HBV infection. Superinfection with HDV in chronic hepatitis B may be subclinical or present as an acute, even fulminant, hepatitis. Worldwide, HDV infection appears to be parenterally transmitted; it is seen predominantly in IV drug abusers and recipients of multiple transfusions. Hepatitis D is diagnosed by detection of HDVAb in patients who are also positive for HBsAg.

Hepatitis E

Hepatitis E virus (HEV, formerly epidemic non-A, non-B hepatitis virus) has a RNA genome, and is transmitted by the fecal-oral route. Clinically, it occurs as a water-borne epidemic in areas with crowding and poor sanitation (e.g., refugee camps). All HEV cases in the United States appear to have been contracted outside, through foreign travel. HEV causes acute hepatitis but not chronic liver disease. It leads to an unusually high mortality in pregnant women.

■ Pathology

Regardless of the type of infecting virus, the liver histology is similar. The characteristic features are acinar disarray, increased cellularity of Kupffer cells, and hepatocyte pleomorphism. This appearance results from combinations of (1) hepatocyte ballooning, acidophilic degeneration, and necrosis occurring in foci throughout the acini; (2) hepatocyte regeneration; and (3) an inflammatory response with mononuclear cells in the acini and portal and periportal areas. Cholestasis is variable but usually mild.

■ Clinical Features

Symptoms frequently associated with acute viral hepatitis include anorexia, nausea, vomiting, dyspepsia, abdominal pain, and aversion to cigarette smoking. More than 50% of individuals with all forms of acute viral hepatitis remain anicteric. Jaundice and a flu-like illness develop in 30–40%, and fulminant hepatitis occurs in 1–3% of patients. No major clinical distinctions exist between types of acute viral hepatitis with regard to symptoms, laboratory and other tests, pathology, major aspects of diagnosis, and treatment. However, when groups of serologically confirmed cases are considered together, distinct clinical patterns of viral hepatitis emerge. The onset of hepatitis A tends to be abrupt and associated with nonspecific viral symptoms such as fever, headache, coryza, and cough. The onset of hepatitis B and C is more protracted and insidious. Toward the end of the incubation period, in 10–20% of patients with acute hepatitis B, a prodromal syndrome evolves, with erythematous, macular-papular rash, urticaria, or angioedema and polyarthralgias or arthritis. This transient serum sickness–like syndrome is felt to be related to immune complex formation with HBsAg, HBsAb, and complement in the setting of HBsAg excess. These complexes are deposited in vessels of the skin and joints as well as in glomerular basement membranes. Extrahepatic immune complex-mediated manifestations (e.g., arthritis, skin rash, cryoglobulins, and glomerulonephritis) have also been described in acute hepatitis A and C. The symptoms of chronic viral hepatitis are often mild, with many patients even being asymptomatic. Common symptoms are fatigue and discomfort in the right upper abdominal quadrant. In more chronic HBV infections, immune complex formation may cause other syndromes, including forms of necrotizing vasculitis, polyarteritis nodosa and a syndrome of mixed cryoglobulinemia. With advanced chronic hepatitis, symptoms and signs of cirrhosis may predominate.

■ Immunoprophylaxis of Viral Hepatitis

See table 100.3.

Hepatitis A

Passive immunization with immune serum globulin (ISG, 0.01 ml/kg) can effectively prevent hepatitis A or suppress its clinical manifestations. Household contacts who are at high risk of secondary attack rates (children, 45%; adults, 5–20%) should be given prophylaxis. It is not indicated for casual contacts at school or in the workplace. The period of passive immunity is 6 months. Vaccination against hepatitis A is recommended for child care workers, military personnel and travelers to endemic areas.

Hepatitis B

Postexposure prophylaxis of hepatitis B is recommended in health care workers and others, employing both the vaccine and hepatitis B immune globulin (HBIG). The latter does not impair the response to the vaccine, and the combination gives prompt, sustained high antibody levels to HBsAg. Sexual contacts of persons with acute hepatitis B or carriers should receive HBIG soon after contact and should be vaccinated. The vaccine is efficacious and safe. Perinatal hepatitis B risk is managed by routine screening of all pregnant women for HBsAg. On delivery, prompt administration of HBIG and vaccine to the newborn is highly efficacious for preventing hepatitis B infection.

Despite the availability of the hepatitis B vaccine since the early 1980s, the overall incidence of hepatitis B remains unchanged in the United States. Therefore, universal hepatitis B vaccination of children has been recommended as a cost-efficient method to control hepatitis B in this country.

Hepatitis C, D, and E

Attempts are ongoing to develop a vaccine for hepatitis C. Although not proven effective, postexposure administration of ISG is recommended after needle stick injuries to prevent acute hepatitis C. Hepatitis D infection can only occur in the presence of concurrent hepatitis B infection. Therefore, all strategies for prevention of hepatitis B are effective for hepatitis D as well. There are

TABLE 100.3. Immunoprophylaxis of Viral Hepatitis				
Virus	**Preexposure Prophylaxis**	**Vaccine Available**	**Postexposure Prophylaxis**	**Perinatal Prophylaxis**
Hepatitis A	IG[a], Hepatitis A vaccine	Yes	IG[b]	IG[c]
Hepatitis B	Hepatitis B vaccine	Yes, for all high-risk persons	HBIG within 24h, Vaccine in 1 wk	HBIG, vaccine
Hepatitis C	No	No	IG	IG[c]
Hepatitis D	Hepatitis B vaccine	Hepatitis B vaccine	IG	IG[c]
Hepatitis E	IG[c]	No	IG[c]	IG[c]

[a]For persons planning to reside or work in endemic areas.
[b]Best given soon after exposure; efficacy reduced if delayed for more than 2 weeks.
[c]Often used in practice, but of questionable value.
HBIG = Hepatitis B immune globulin; IG = Immune globulin.
(Adapted From: Dindzans V. Postgrad Med 1992; 92:43–52. Used with permission.)

no definite recommendations for specific immunoprophylaxis of hepatitis E. The administration of ISG to prevent hepatitis A in international travelers may prevent hepatitis E as well.

■ Management

Supportive care for the patient with acute hepatitis consists of rest, bland diet, H2-receptor antagonists for dyspeptic symptoms, and anti-emetics for control of nausea and vomiting. When administering drug therapy to these patients, it is important to remember that many drugs are metabolized in the liver and their clearances are impaired owing to hepatitis, especially in the active phase. Since H2-blockers affect hepatic metabolism of many other drugs, concurrent drug therapy with H2 blockers should be administered with caution. No therapy is available that specifically accelerates the recovery from acute hepatitis.

Chronic hepatitis B (with positive HBeAg) can be treated with recombinant interferon alpha. A remission rate up to 50% has been found for termination of viral replication and seroconversion from HBeAg to HBeAb. Long-term follow up of patients with successful seroconversion indicates that HBsAg disappears within 5 years. Chronic hepatitis C treated with recombinant interferon alpha produces a long-term conversion rate of only 10–15%. Combination treatment with recombinant interferon and ribavirin (a nucleoside analogue) improves the response rate to 35–40%.

CHAPTER 101 AUTOIMMUNE AND CHRONIC HEPATITIS

Chronic hepatitis is a clinical syndrome, with chronic liver inflammation leading to necrosis and possibly progressing to fibrosis, cirrhosis, and liver failure. The liver enzymes should remain high for a minimum period of 6 months to exclude most self-limited hepatitis. Liver biopsy is essential for diagnosis and classification. Both chronic persistent hepatitis and chronic active hepatitis feature mononuclear cell infiltration and minimal fibrosis of the portal tracts, but chronic active hepatitis requires necrosis of the limiting plate as well ("piecemeal necrosis"). The new histological classification is shown in Table 101.1. Chronic hepatitis has a diverse etiology, including chronic viral hepatitis B, C, and D, drug toxicity, autoimmune hepatitis, and Wilson's disease. While other determinants of liver disease (hemochromatosis and alcohol abuse) cause chronic liver enzyme elevations, they do not cause the characteristic histology; thus, they are not included as causes of chronic hepatitis.

TABLE 101.1. Histological Classification of Chronic Hepatitis

Old Classification	New Classification
Chronic Active Hepatitis	Chronic hepatitis
Mild	Mild activity, mild or moderate fibrosis
Moderate	Moderate activity; mild, moderate, or severe fibrosis
Severe	Severe activity; mild, moderate, or severe fibrosis
Chronic persistent hepatitis	Chronic hepatitis Minimal or mild activity, mild fibrosis
Chronic lobular hepatitis	Chronic hepatitis Mild, moderate or severe activity; no fibrosis

Autoimmune Chronic Hepatitis

Defined as hepatitis that occurs by autoimmune mechanisms, autoimmune chronic hepatitis (ACH) is diagnosed when chronic hepatitis occurs in the setting of serum autoimmune markers (antinuclear antibody, anti-smooth muscle antibody, antimicrosomal antibody) and associated extrahepatic autoimmune diseases (e.g., autoimmune thyroiditis, rheumatoid arthritis, and Sjögren's syndrome), and without evidence of viral hepatitis. It has a wide range of presentations—i.e., asymptomatic, severe acute hepatitis, fulminant hepatic failure, or complications of cirrhosis. The onset may be insidious with fatigue, malaise, vague abdominal discomfort, arthritis, arthralgias, low-grade fever, and, in women, amenorrhea. Laboratory tests show a variable rise in bilirubin, aminotransferases, gamma globulin, and alkaline phosphatase. Although autoimmune chronic hepatitis responds well to therapy, cirrhosis and liver failure follow in many patients.

■ Management

On a regimen of prednisone (10 mg/d) and azathioprine (50 mg/d), nearly 80% of ACH patients show ameliorated symptoms, improved biochemical tests, and partial to complete histological remission. Unfortunately, relapse follows when therapy is stopped. Because no controlled treatment trials have been conducted for mild autoimmune chronic active hepatitis, the decision to treat such patients is difficult; in many instances, several months of mere observation may suffice. Liver biopsy is essential in making treatment decisions—patients with chronic hepatitis with moderate activity or fibrosis clearly require therapy whereas those with lesser degrees of activity or fibrosis do not.

CHAPTER **102** ALCOHOLIC AND DRUG-INDUCED LIVER DISEASE

Alcohol is metabolized almost entirely in the hepatocytes. Some of the metabolic effects of alcohol include type IV hyperlipidemia, direct inhibition of mitochondrial function, microsomal P-450 enzyme induction, and alcoholic ketoacidosis. Major stages of alcoholic liver injury are fatty liver, alcoholic hepatitis, and cirrhosis.

Alcoholic Fatty Liver

Fatty liver (**hepatic steatosis**), the most common alcohol-related liver disease, has multiple mechanisms: increased mobilization of free fatty acids from peripheral fat stores, increased triglyceride formation, decreased fatty acid oxidation, and reduced lipoprotein release by the liver. Fat, mostly triglyceride, which displaces the nucleus to one side, is termed "macrovesicular fat." Such fat cells may coalesce to produce fat cysts. Aside from liver enlargement, there may be no symptoms or physical findings. The gamma-glutamyl transpeptidase is markedly high, AST only mildly so. The fat clears slowly after alcohol is stopped.

Alcoholic Hepatitis

Histologically, alcoholic hepatitis features fatty infiltration, neutrophil infiltration around clusters of necrotic hepatocytes, and clumps of intracellular eosinophilic material (Mallory bodies) within some hepatocytes. New collagen forms in pericellular and perisinusoidal locations. Fibrosis is often seen around terminal hepatic

---

TABLE 102.1. Drug-Induced Hepatotoxicity

Mechanism	Histopathology	Examples
Direct hepatotoxicity	Zonal necrosis	Carbon tetrachloride
Indirect hepatotoxicity	Zonal necrosis	Acetaminophen
Acute hepatitis	Acute hepatitis	Isoniazid, phenytoin
Immune mediated		
Chronic hepatitis	Chronic hepatitis	Alpha methyl dopa
Granulomatous hepatitis	Granulomas	Allopurinol
Bland cholestasis	Bile plugs	Estrogens
Inflammatory cholestasis	Acute hepatitis	Erythromycin
Fibrosis	Fibrosis/fat	Methotrexate
Fatty Liver		
Macrovesicular	Macrovesicular fat	Steroids, chemotherapy
Microvesicular	Microvesicular fat	Valproic acid
Phospholipidosis	Resembles alcoholic hepatitis	Amiodarone

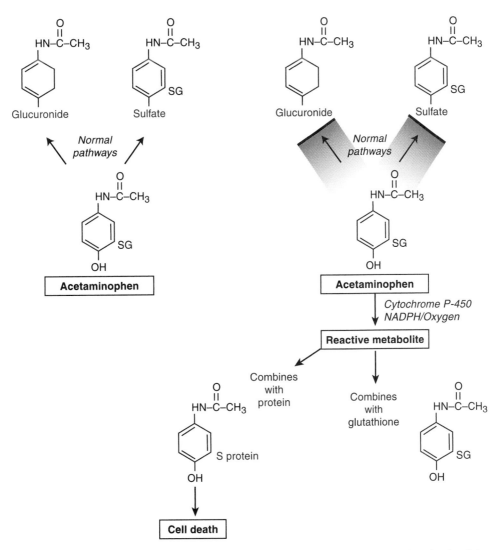

FIGURE 102.1. Acetaminophen toxicity. Normal acetaminophen metabolism is shown in left panel. With these pathways saturated in an overdose, the metabolism yields a reactive agent, which, when combined with cellular protein, causes cell-death; combination with glutathione renders an inoffensive product.

venules. Some regard this perivenular fibrosis in fatty livers without full-blown alcoholic hepatitis to be a precursor lesion of cirrhosis.

Clinically, patients with alcoholic hepatitis may be asymptomatic to severely ill. An enlarged tender liver is an important finding. In the more acute or "florid" cases, jaundice, fever, right upper quadrant tenderness with guarding and mild rebound may mimic acute cholecystitis. Cholestasis may be severe, with bilirubin climbing to 25 mg/dl. Encephalopathy and signs of chronic liver disease, such as spider angiomas, edema, and ascites may be noted. Hyperlipidemia, leukocytosis, and macrocytosis are associated, occasionally with hemolytic anemia. Modest elevations of alkaline phosphatase and AST (<5 to 8 times normal), are common, with a high (>2) AST:ALT ratio and a prolonged prothrombin time that responds poorly to vitamin K. Oliguria, raised serum creatinine, hyponatremia, and hypokalemia are other findings.

If the clinical picture and setting do not yield the

diagnosis, histologic confirmation is desirable. However, a refractory hypoprothrombinemia may preclude biopsy. Distinction from acute cholecystitis is made possible by ultrasound examination. These patients are at risk for serious infection, GI bleeding, and coma.

■ Management

Seriously ill patients are best hospitalized. A low-sodium diet, diuretics, and supplemental nutrition

may be necessary. Jaundice, hypoprothrombinemia, and encephalopathy carry a mortality risk of 40–50%. Corticosteroids have improved survival in some patients with severe alcoholic hepatitis. Some physicians base steroid use on a calculated discriminant score: 4.6 x (prothrombin time) + serum bilirubin (mg/dl). A value over 93 defines candidates for corticosteroid therapy.

Drug-induced Liver Disease

The liver, aided by the numerous enzymes in the endoplasmic reticulum and the cytoplasm of hepatocytes, is a major site for biotransformation and metabolism of drugs. Lipophilic drugs are transformed into polar metabolites, which can be excreted more easily. The more highly charged metabolites are transported into the bile; the increased aqueous solubility of metabolites enhances elimination in the stool or urine. Drugs are metabolized in two main phases: first, they are oxidized or reduced by reactions catalyzed by the cytochromes P450; second, a charged molecule is added or conjugated, in order to increase the water solubility of the metabolite produced by phase I. Phase I reactions often produce highly toxic intermediates, whereas phase II, through covalent bonding by glucuronic acid or sulfate, generally results in nontoxic agents. Drug-related hepatotoxicity arises from interaction of these products within hepatocytes.

The spectrum of clinical drug-induced hepatotoxicity is shown in Table 102.1. Many chemicals are direct hepatotoxins, which implies a toxic effect caused by the agent itself. Very few drugs are of this type; most drug toxicity arises via chemical reactions of the drug's phase I products. An example is the toxicity of phase I product in **acetaminophen poisoning** (see Figure 102.1), to which chronic alcoholics are especially prone. Because acetaminophen is metabolized via cytochrome P450, and since zone 3 hepatocytes are richest in cytochrome P450 enzymes, the cell injury is striking in zone 3. Acetylcysteine increases synthesis of glutathione, the liver's most important endogenous reducing agent, thus detoxifying reactive acetaminophen intermediates. Ethanol induces cytochrome P450 enzymes and facilitates the production of reactive intermediates. Chronic alcoholism also causes malnutrition and, thus, glutathione deficiency.

CHAPTER 103 CIRRHOSIS

■ Definition and Classification

Cirrhosis is the final common pathway for many chronic liver diseases that share the typical ongoing destruction and regeneration of hepatic parenchymal cells. Associated inflammatory cell infiltration and fibrosis may be present. The liver architecture is distorted and the parenchyma is organized in nodules of regenerated hepatocytes, duly surrounded by scars. The microvasculature is also severely distorted; the sizable portion of hepatic blood flow that traverses these vascular scars of the liver bypasses the parenchymal cells within the regenerating nodules. Portal hypertension, portosystemic shunting, and impaired excretory and synthetic liver function follow.

A popular classification of cirrhosis is morphologic, based solely on the size of regenerative nodules.

Micronodular cirrhosis, in which nodules are less than 3 mm in diameter, classically results from alcohol and hemochromatosis. **Macronodular cirrhosis,** in which nodules exceed 3 mm in diameter (generally considered "postnecrotic"), classically results from multiacinar destruction in chronic viral hepatitis. Morphologic classification has limited use, since the diseases causing either morphological pattern overlap widely and both patterns occur in the same liver. An etiological classification is shown in Table 103.1.

■ Clinical and Laboratory Features

Cirrhosis and liver failure share common clinical and biochemical features. Well-established cirrhosis may be clinically silent or patients may experience fatigue, weakness, ankle swelling **(edema),** or abdominal disten-

TABLE 103.1.	Etiology of Cirrhosis

Viral
  Hepatitis B, C, D
Drugs
  Ethanol, methotrexate
Chronic hepatitis
  Autoimmune chronic hepatitis
Biliary
  Primary biliary cirrhosis
  Primary sclerosing cholangitis
  Secondary biliary cirrhosis
  Cystic fibrosis
Metabolic
  Hemochromatosis
  Wilson's disease
  Alpha 1 antitrypsin deficiency
  Tyrosinemia
  Galactosemia
  Glycogen storage disease
Vascular
  Hepatic vein thrombosis
  Veno-occlusive disease
  Right ventricular failure
  Constrictive pericarditis
Other
  Sarcoidosis
  Cryptogenic

tion (**ascites**). There may be abdominal wall **venous collaterals, splenomegaly, reduced muscle mass,** and **Dupuytren's contractures.** Abdominal and inguinal herniae may be worsened by ascites. Stigmata of cirrhosis include **palmar erythema, spider angiomata, gynecomastia,** and **testicular atrophy.** Patients with cirrhosis are predisposed to bacterial infections; **spontaneous bacterial peritonitis** portends a particularly poor prognosis.

Anemia, frequently macrocytic, is common. Splenic sequestration causes **leukopenia** and **thrombocytopenia. Hypoprothrombinemia** is usually refractory to vitamin K. **Hypoalbuminemia** is due to decreased albumin synthesis and/or hemodilution. Serum bilirubin and aminotransferases may be normal or may rise slightly. Renal failure with oliguria, azotemia, and avid Na+ retention is ominous. Prothrombin time and platelet count permitting, and ascites not massive, it is desirable (but not essential) to confirm the diagnosis of cirrhosis by biopsy. Prognosis and life expectancy can be estimated by assessing Child's class (Table 103.2). Focal abnormalities on abdominal ultrasound or CT may raise the question of hepatocellular carcinoma, a useful marker of which is serum a-fetoprotein (AFP) level, despite its sensitivity of only 75% for this diagnosis.

■ Complications

Portal Hypertension

Some of the most important clinical manifestations and complications of cirrhosis arise from the deranged hepatic vascular architecture that disturbs the hepatic blood flow. A useful classification of portal hypertension is based on the location of the flow resistance (Table 103.3). Clinically, patients with extrahepatic portal hypertension have well-preserved liver function without the clinical problems seen in cirrhosis.

Cirrhosis is the most common example of sinusoidal portal hypertension. Portal hypertension and the ensuing anastomotic flow cause the following **portosystemic collaterals:** (1) from the left gastric and short gastric veins to the esophageal and azygous veins; (2) from the liver via the umbilical vein remnant to the abdominal wall; (3) from the superior hemorrhoidal vein to the inferior hemorrhoidal veins and then to the inferior vena cava; and (4) via mesenteric and visceral veins through the retroperitoneal spaces and abdominal wall. Given the high flow resistance in the liver, the majority of portal blood may bypass the liver via these collaterals.

Clinical features and ancillary studies

Symptoms of portal hypertension are often inseparable from those of the associated liver disease. There may be **prominent abdominal wall veins** radiating from the umbilicus, **ascites,** and **congestive splenomegaly.** The portal-systemic collaterals predispose to variceal or hemorrhoidal bleeding. Splenomegaly may cause left upper abdominal discomfort. Signs of chronic liver disease are usually seen in portal hypertension due to cirrhosis.

With portal hypertension and congestive splenomegaly, leukopenia and thrombocytopenia are often noted. The associated cirrhosis, depending on its etiology, may or may not produce additional laboratory findings. Esophageal varices may be demonstrated either by endoscopy or barium examination of the esophagus. The

TABLE 103.2.	Child-Turcotte Classification		
Criterion	**A**	**B**	**C**
Bilirubin (mg/dl)	<2	2-3	>3
Albumin (gm/dl)	>3.5	2.8–3.5	<2.8
Ascites	Absent	Slight	Moderate
Encephalopathy	None	1–2	3-4
Nutrition	Good	Moderate	Poor
Prothrombin time (seconds prolonged)	<4	4–6	>6

TABLE 103.3. Classification of Portal Hypertension

Pre-sinusoidal	Sinusoidal	Post-sinusoidal
Portal vein thrombosis	Cirrhosis	Hepatic vein thrombosis
Schistosomiasis		Veno-occlusive disease
Sarcoidosis		Chronic pericarditis
Congenital hepatic fibrosis		Chronic right ventricular failure

TABLE 103.4. Variceal Bleeding: Summary of Therapeutic Options

Option	Limitation(s)
Endoscopic sclerotherapy or band ligation	Multiple sessions may be needed; does not influence long term survival; small or controlled bleeds only.
Vasopressin	Effective therapy for 3--4 days only; tachyphylaxis.
Balloon tamponade	Temporary use only, effective in 90% of cases in arresting/controlling acute hemorrhage.
Surgical portal-systemic shunting	Reduced hepatic blood flow causing encephalopathy.
TIPS[a]	Stents thrombose and occlude within a year.
Propranolol	Ineffective in preventing recurrent bleeding, but can prevent first bleed.

[a]TIPS = Transjugular intrahepatic porto-systemic shunting.

patency and direction of flow in the portal venous system are assessed by ultrasound with Doppler studies. The portal venous system may be imaged by venous phase mesenteric arteriography. These latter studies may not be needed in the usual patient with portal hypertension, but may be performed in suspected portal vein thrombosis or hepatic vein thrombosis.

Bleeding Esophageal Varices

Variceal hemorrhage, due to rupture of thin-walled varices into the esophageal lumen, is the most common acute emergency in cirrhotics with portal hypertension, and a major cause of death in cirrhotics. Hemorrhage is usually unprovoked, but a history of aspirin- or nonsteroidal anti-inflammatory drug ingestion may be noted. Upper GI endoscopy, by assessing the size of these veins and their surface irregularities due to thinning of the mucosa, best estimates their bleeding risk. Bleeding may be slow and gradual or abrupt and massive with hematemesis, melena, or both. GI bleeding in patients with cirrhosis may also be due to other causes. Urgent endoscopy is thus needed in a cirrhotic with an upper GI bleed, in order to determine its source.

Patients with bleeding esophageal varices should be promptly hospitalized. Transfusion with blood products is urgent. Coagulopathy due to hypoprothrombinemia responds well to transfusion with fresh frozen plasma. Usual treatments for variceal hemorrhage and their limitations are shown in Table 103.4. The primary treatment is **endoscopic injection sclerotherapy,** in which the varices are directly injected endoscopically with caustic liquids (sodium morrhuate), causing their thrombosis, local ulceration, and ultimately, fibrosis to prevent variceal recurrence and bleeding. **Band ligation** of varices has also been shown to be as efficacious as sclerotherapy in attaining the same objectives. While these methods preserve liver blood flow and are as effective as surgery in controlling bleeding, they do not increase survival. Sclerotherapy sessions are repeated until all varices are obliterated. Annual follow-up endoscopy is then indicated in order to screen for variceal recurrence.

Acute and massive variceal hemorrhage may not be amenable to endoscopy and sclerotherapy. **Vasopressin** can then be used to temporize the bleeding. It vasoconstricts the splanchnic arterioles and reduces the portal venous inflow and portal pressure. Concomitant **IV nitroglycerin** may also be given in order to offset systemic vasoconstriction. Variceal hemorrhage can thus be effectively controlled for up to 3–4 days, beyond which tachyphylaxis develops to vasopressin. However, it helps stabilize the patient sufficiently so that more definitive treatment can be administered for the esophageal varices.

Other options (Figure 103.1) include esophageal **balloon tamponade** and **surgical portal-systemic shunting.** The surgical shunt decompresses the portal venous system, but it also decreases hepatic blood flow, thus drastically worsening liver function and predisposing to hepatic encephalopathy. Thus, this procedure is usually performed in persons with excellent liver function in whom liver transplantation would not be anticipated for several years.

Transjugular intrahepatic porto-systemic shunting (TIPS) is the fluoroscopic placement of an expandable intrahepatic stent to create an intrahepatic portacaval shunt. It effectively controls variceal bleeding and ascites by reducing portal hypertension. The proclivity to encephalopathy is less than that in a surgical shunt, as TIP shunts do not unduly divert hepatic blood flow. They also have a high rate of thrombotic occlusion within 1 year. The exact role of TIPS in managing patients with cirrhosis and its complications still needs further definition.

Propranolol also lowers portal hypertension. While it effectively prevents the first variceal bleed, it is ineffective in preventing recurrent bleeding. The dosage is titrated to reduce the resting pulse rate by 25%.

Ascites

Ascites is the intraperitoneal collection of fluid, most often from cirrhosis. Portal hypertension increases portal

TABLE 103.5.	Serum-Ascites Albumin Gradient[a] in Diagnosis of Ascites
High (>1.1)	**Low (<1.1)**
Cirrhosis	Peritoneal carcinomatosis
Alcoholic hepatitis	Pancreatic ascites
Right ventricular failure	Biliary ascites
Hepatic vein thrombosis	Nephrotic ascites
Fulminant liver failure	Peritoneal tuberculosis

[a] = SAAG; difference between albumin levels in the serum and ascitic fluid.

capillary pressure and the formation of hepatic lymph that escapes into the abdominal cavity as ascites. Despite an expanded blood volume, there is avid renal retention and low urinary Na^+ output. Renal Na^+ retention in patients with cirrhosis is highly complex; excess renin and aldosterone play a key role. Albumin synthesis is often low, thus lowering plasma oncotic pressure.

Ascites may develop insidiously or it may follow worsening liver function during an episode of hemorrhage, an alcoholic spree, or surgery. Physical examination, which generally detects only larger amounts of ascites, may show a fluid thrill or shifting dullness. Pleural effusions may be associated. Tense ascites may cause respiratory distress. Stigmata of liver disease may be observed. Ventral, inguinal, and umbilical hernias may be induced or worsened. Ascites is readily demonstrated by abdominal ultrasound.

All patients with ascites should have an initial diagnostic paracentesis, with examination of protein, albumin, amylase, total and differential cell count, and culture (collected in blood culture bottle), as well as cytology. The fluid protein level is usually low, with a wide range of values. A high serum-ascites albumin gradient (SAAG) confirms that ascites is related to portal hypertension (Table 103.5).

Spontaneous Bacterial Peritonitis

Spontaneous bacterial peritonitis (SBP) frequently complicates advanced liver disease and low protein ascites. Clear signs of infection are often lacking, and SBP should be considered in any patient with cirrhosis who demonstrates clinical deterioration, fever, abdominal pain, or a sudden decrease in liver function. The most common organisms are gram-negative coliforms, streptococci, and staphylococci, in that order of frequency. Paracentesis and ascitic fluid analysis with culture are key to diagnosis. Ascitic fluid neutrophils exceeding $250/mm^3$ strongly suggest SBP. At paracentesis, the ascitic fluid should be collected directly into blood culture bottles for microbiologic studies. Cirrhotic ascites clearly predis-

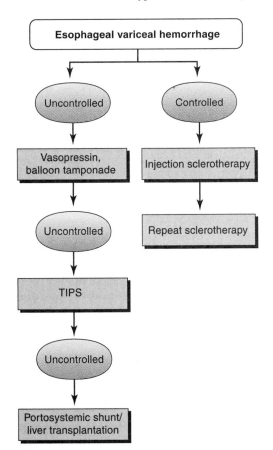

FIGURE 103.1. Management of esophageal variceal hemorrhage.

* = Or band ligation.

poses to **peritoneal tuberculosis;** the largest cross-section of patients with tuberculous peritonitis have prior cirrhotic ascites.

Management of ascites

Patients with ascites should be started on a low Na^+ diet and oral spironolactone (50 mg daily); Na^+ restriction alone is rarely successful. Since the net loss from the peritoneal compartment through mobilization and urinary excretion is limited to 900 ml/day, the aim should be to ensure a net fluid loss of 900 ml/day or a weight loss of 1 kg/day. Conversely, losses exceeding these in a nonedematous patient with ascites may cause hypovolemia and acute renal failure. For ascites resistant to maximal spironolactone dose (200–300 mg/day), a loop diuretic—e.g., furosemide (40–80 mg/day)—may be added. Large-volume paracentesis (up to 5 L) is also safe and effective for diuretic-resistant ascites. However, diuretic-resistant ascites, which portends worsening liver function, indicate a possible need for liver transplantation. The peritoneal-venous shunt (the LeVeen shunt), a surgically placed catheter between the peritoneum and the superior vena cava, may be useful in a minority of cirrhotics with medically intractable ascites but good liver function. TIPS is another consideration (Figure 103.2).

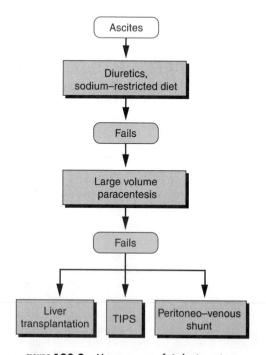

FIGURE 103.2. Management of cirrhotic ascites.

Hepatorenal Syndrome

Oliguria and **azotemia** without organic renal abnormalities, complicating severe liver disease, define this syndrome. It is usually precipitated by sepsis, GI bleed, overzealous diuretic use, and, sometimes, large-volume paracentesis. Signs of liver decompensation, such as ascites, jaundice, and encephalopathy are obvious. Characteristically, the blood creatinine and urea nitrogen (BUN) rise, with a disproportionate BUN/Creatinine ratio and very low urinary sodium (<10 mEq/L). The fractional urinary Na^+ is below 1 (see chapter 162). The pathogenesis is related to reduced effective renal blood flow and redistribution of renal circulation to the point of decreased cortical blood flow. GI bleeding, superimposed infection, or electrolyte disturbances should be appropriately managed. This highly lethal condition has no satisfactory therapy. When recovery of liver function is anticipated, hemodialysis may be useful.

Hepatic Encephalopathy

Also known as portosystemic encephalopathy (PSE), this neuropsychiatric syndrome occurs in acute and chronic liver failure. Its pathogenesis is elusive, and many factors—including ammonia, fatty acids, gamma aminobutyric acid, mercaptans, and false neurotransmitters—have been implicated. Likewise, no critical protective substance normally elaborated by the healthy liver has been found remiss in patients with PSE. The current hypothesis is that PSE results from the combined effect of various cerebral toxins whose individual contributions in any one patient may differ.

Clinical features of hepatic encephalopathy

Features of PSE, besides those shown in Table 103.6, include **fetor hepaticus** (a fishy, ammoniacal odor on the breath) and **asterixis** (syn., flapping tremor), in which the hand momentarily falls forward and then suddenly resumes the hyperextended position. Asterixis is best demonstrated when the patient's hands are outstretched, wrists hyperextended, and fingers separated. Being the hallmark of a metabolic encephalopathy (uremia, respiratory failure, or sedative overdose), it lacks specificity for hepatic encephalopathy. Other neurological abnormalities may also be seen in advanced PSE, especially spasticity, hyperreflexia, and extensor plantar responses. Simple bedside tests of cerebral function (tests of handwriting, the Reitan trailmaking test, and drawing 5-pointed stars) help diagnose early encephalopathy and monitor its response to therapy. While venous blood ammonia is elevated in the majority of patients, it correlates poorly with the degree of coma. However, sequential measurements in the same patient can help

TABLE 103.6.	Staging of Hepatic Encephalopathy
Stage	**Features**
I.	Mental slowing, confusion, or altered motor behavior. Psychometric defects are detectable.
II.	Agitation, greater confusion, inappropriate behavior.
III.	Stupor but arousable.
IV.	Coma, without response to pain; possible seizure activity.

follow the course of the encephalopathy. Cerebrospinal fluid examination, which is normal in PSE, may help to distinguish PSE from intracranial infection; however, the distinction may not be clinically possible in all cases.

Management

General treatment measures in hepatic encephalopathy are prevention-oriented. The diet should be high in fiber and moderate in protein. A reasonable protein intake is 100 g/day. Anorexia and malnutrition are common in liver failure and, therefore, protein restriction below 100 g/day is often detrimental. Careful maintenance of electrolyte and volume status is critical, especially if diuretics are used. Medications with sedative

properties must be used with caution to avoid exacerbating encephalopathy. Constipation enhances the absorption of toxins from the GI tract, and should be treated by dietary measures and with lactulose. Where encephalopathy is the presenting feature, infection and gastrointestinal hemorrhage must be excluded by appropriate workup.

Oral lactulose, a nonabsorbable disaccharide, is the main treatment for hepatic encephalopathy. In the colon, it is metabolized to short-chain organic acids, which acidify the colonic contents and cause an osmotic diarrhea. Some postulate that toxic byproducts are "trapped" within the acidic colonic lumen. The dose of lactulose is titrated to cause at least three loose stools per day, but severe diarrhea must be avoided. Oral metronidazole, which improves hepatic encephalopathy by killing the anaerobic colonic bacteria, is a useful adjunct when response to lactulose alone is inadequate. Many enteral and parenteral nutritional products enriched in branched chain amino acids are available for use in PSE. While their benefit in hepatic encephalopathy is controversial and their efficacy unproven, their use is nonetheless reasonable in hospitalized patients requiring nutritional supplements. Significant hepatic encephalopathy in cirrhosis indicates far advanced liver disease and liver failure; timely liver transplantation must, therefore, be considered.

CHAPTER 104 METABOLIC LIVER DISEASES

Hemochromatosis

This disorder is characterized by a generalized and progressive increase in total body iron stores with resultant cellular damage and dysfunction of the liver, heart, pancreas, and other organs. The majority of patients with gross iron overload have genetic hemochromatosis inherited as an autosomal recessive trait, the iron-loading gene being situated on chromosome 6 in association with HLA-A3 and HLA-B7 and 14 phenotypes. Genetic hemochromatosis is among the more common genetic disorders in adults, with a point prevalence of 0.5% and gene frequency of 6%–7%. Heterozygotes may show a mild increase in hepatic iron concentration without gross iron overload. The etiology is excessive intestinal iron absorption inappropriate to the level of body iron stores. Secondary hemochromatosis

follows iron loading from repeated blood transfusions for chronic anemia.

■ Pathology

Early cases are marked by portal fibrosis and iron deposition in periportal hepatocytes and Kupffer cells. Ultimately, cirrhosis develops without fat and little inflammation. Iron accumulates progressively in the hepatocytes, Kupffer cells, and bile duct epithelium, as well as pancreatic acinar cells, gut epithelium, kidneys, and heart muscle. Iron deposition and fibrosis occur in many endocrine tissues, including the pituitary, adrenal cortex, and thyroid. In secondary hemochromatosis, liver biopsies show excess iron deposition, although it may be difficult to distinguish the secondary form of the disease from genetic or primary hemochromatosis.

■ Clinical and Laboratory Features

The disease is more common in men. Characteristically, there is a gray skin pigmentation, and many patients eventually develop cardiac dysfunction. Other features are shown in Table 104.1. **Arthropathy** complicates two-thirds of the cases, usually beginning in the interphalangeal joints and progressing to larger joints. Not uncommonly, acute arthritis involves the knees, due to

TABLE 104.1. Clinical Features of Hemochromatosis
Weakness
Apathy
Decreased libido, impotence
Diabetes mellitus
Increased skin pigmentation
Hepatomegaly
Cardiomegaly
Testicular atrophy
Reduced body hair
Decreased muscle mass
Arthropathy

calcium pyrophosphate-related acute synovitis. Often x-rays show calcification of the joint cartilage (chondrocalcinosis). The enlargement and abnormal histology of the liver are without parallel abnormalities in liver tests. However, serum measurements of iron metabolism are high (Table 104.2). The *fasting* transferrin saturation exceeds 62% and often may be as high as 100%. Ferritin levels are markedly elevated. Definite diagnosis depends on liver biopsy with analysis of hepatic iron concentration, which is further corrected for the patient's age to yield a hepatic iron index.

■ Management

Weekly phlebotomies (500 ml) are performed, each removing 250 mg of iron at a time. Patients tolerate many phlebotomies before hemoglobin declines. However, patients with chronic anemia and secondary hemochromatosis do not tolerate phlebotomy well. Desferrioxamine, which chelates iron and facilitates its urinary excretion, is much less efficient than phlebotomy for depleting iron. With iron depletion, hepatic, cardiac, and endocrine functions improve, while arthritis may not. Cirrhosis is not irreversible and, despite iron depletion, hepatocellular carcinoma occurs in one-fifth of cases. Family screening is also indicated for early detection of homozygotes. HLA-typing is performed along with measurements of serum ferritin, iron, and total iron binding capacity.

TABLE 104.2. Hemochromatosis: Measurements of Iron Indices		
Index (Criterion)	Normal Range	Hemochromatosis
Transferrin saturation (%)	20–50	>62
Ferritin (ng/ml)	15–300	>500
Hepatic iron concentration (µg/gm dry wt)	300–1800	10,000–30,000

Wilson's Disease

Wilson's disease is an inherited autosomal recessive disorder of copper metabolism. A mutated copper transporting enzyme prevents the excretion of copper detached from the copper-transporting ceruloplasmin into the bile. Rising copper levels inhibit ceruloplasmin formation from apo-ceruloplasmin. Excess copper in the brain, liver, kidneys, and corneas lead to degeneration of the frontal lobes and basal ganglia of the brain, cirrhosis, renal tubular lesions, and corneal Kayser-Fleischer rings, respectively. A marker for Wilson's disease is deficient ceruloplasmin, which transports copper in plasma. Deficient ceruloplasmin, however, does not play a pathogenetic role in Wilson's disease. Although ceruloplasmin

level is significantly depressed in most patients with Wilson's disease, cases with normal levels have been reported.

■ Pathology

Liver changes vary widely from mild portal and periportal inflammation and fibrosis to acute massive necrosis and chronic active hepatitis to cirrhosis. The histologic picture may mimic chronic hepatitis with considerable fatty infiltration, parenchymal cell necrosis and alcoholic hyalin but usually with less neutrophil and inflammatory infiltrate. Special stains for copper dem-

TABLE 104.3.	Clinical Features of Wilson's Disease
System	**Manifestations**
Hepatic	Chronic active hepatitis, cirrhosis, fulminant liver failure, unexplained hepatitis
Neurologic	Incoordination, dysarthria, gait disorder, rigidity, tremor, ataxia, dysphagia, decline in intellect
Psychiatric	Psychoneurosis, schizophrenic psychosis, dementia
Ophthalmic	Kayser-Fleischer ring, cataracts
Hematologic	Coombs-negative hemolytic anemia
Renal	Renal tubular acidosis (aminoaciduria, phosphaturia, glycosuria, and full-fledged Fanconi syndrome in some cases)
Skeletal	Osteoporosis/osteomalacia

onstrate excess copper deposition in the liver, albeit inconsistently so.

■ **Clinical Features**

Wilson's disease is known for its great variability of clinical expression, with manifestations in the blood, joints, kidneys, eyes, liver, and brain (Table 104.3). It may present with acute or chronic liver disease. Most often, the liver disease begins insidiously and runs a chronic, advancing course with fatigue, anorexia, weakness, mild jaundice, and hepatosplenomegaly. Wilson's disease, however, merits consideration in fulminant hepatitis, chronic active hepatitis, cirrhosis, or unexplained liver disease in persons below 35 years of age. Other presentations are hemolytic anemia, declining intellectual skills, personality or behavioral changes, and neurological illness with extrapyramidal signs (movement disorders). **Kayser-Fleischer rings,** a subtle yellow-brown corneal discoloration close to the limbus, may also be present.

■ **Diagnosis and Management**

Early diagnosis is critical. Liver test abnormalities with elevated serum bilirubin and aminotransferase val-

ues, are nonspecific. Serum ceruloplasmin and copper levels are usually low, and urinary copper excretion is high. Slit-lamp examination is advisable, as it is the only way to detect Kayser-Fleischer rings. Liver biopsy is mandatory for both histology and measurement of copper content. Treatment consists of oral penicillamine to chelate body copper and to promote urinary copper excretion. Chronic liver disease and neuropsychiatric features respond to penicillamine. Platelets, leukocyte count, and urine protein must be monitored to detect penicillamine toxicity. If penicillamine is not tolerated, triethylene-tetramine may be substituted as a chelating agent. Chronic zinc acetate is another potential therapeutic agent, since zinc inhibits intestinal absorption of copper and thus induces a negative body balance of copper.

Because of autosomal recessive inheritance, a patient with this disease is the offspring of two heterozygotes. Approximately 25% of the children of two heterozygotes will have the disease, 50% are carriers, and 25% are normal. Thus, all siblings of established cases should be screened with determinations of serum ceruloplasmin and 24-hour urinary copper excretion. Those with abnormal results should undergo liver biopsy with analysis of copper content.

CHAPTER **105** **OTHER LIVER DISEASES**

Fatty Liver Syndromes

While fat in the liver is clinically unimportant by itself, the inflammatory reaction that macrovesicular fat may sometimes elicit resembles alcoholic hepatitis. Histologic features include macrovesicular fat, focal necrosis,

mixed inflammatory infiltrates, and, in a few instances, Mallory's bodies. These features are termed **nonalcoholic steatohepatitis,** the frequent causes of which are listed in Table 105.1. The natural history of

TABLE 105.1.	Causes of Nonalcoholic Steatohepatitis

Diabetes mellitus
Hyperlipidemia
Obesity
Jejuno-ileal bypass
Medications
Amiodarone
Corticosteroids
Perhexilene maleate
Total parenteral nutrition

steatohepatitis is variable, but most patients manifest little progression. However, in a minority of patients, it may progress to cirrhosis. Treatment consists of weight reduction; total resolution has been shown to follow weight loss of 15% of body weight.

Vascular Liver Disease

Cardiac Failure

Hypoperfusion, as in prolonged shock or acute heart failure, results in reduced hepatic arterial and portal venous blood flow. The resultant liver injury consists of acinar zone 3 necrosis with high transaminases, jaundice, and hypoprothrombinemia. In right ventricular failure, particularly with tricuspid disease, raised right-sided pressures are transmitted to the liver, causing sinusoidal dilatation and congestion, perivenular hemorrhage, and centrilobular liver cell necrosis. With chronicity, collagen formation and fibrosis evolve from the perivenular region, producing cardiac cirrhosis. Findings include jaundice, tender hepatomegaly, and ascites. There are no unique laboratory findings; however, alkaline phosphatase, unconjugated bilirubin, and prothrombin time are elevated. Constrictive pericarditis with or without cirrhosis should always be considered in patients with ascites of obscure etiology.

Hepatic Vein Occlusion

Obstruction of the major hepatic veins, with occlusion of hepatic venous outflow, also known as **Budd-Chiari**

Microvesicular fatty liver, associated with fulminant hepatic failure, is seen in acute fatty liver of pregnancy and Reye's syndrome. Acute fatty liver of pregnancy typically occurs with the first pregnancy in a young woman in her third trimester and presents as acute liver failure with associated renal failure. Vomiting, epigastric discomfort, jaundice, encephalopathy, hypoglycemia, and renal failure make up the usual clinical picture. Histologically, the liver shows multiple intracellular fat droplets with little necrosis or inflammation. This form of liver failure is highly lethal, and urgent liver biopsy may be indicated to establish the diagnosis. The only treatment is to induce labor rapidly and to deliver the baby swiftly.

syndrome, results in right upper quadrant pain, hepatomegaly, and high protein content-ascites. Occlusion may be due to malignancy, accelerated clotting, as in polycythemia vera or oral contraceptive use, and, rarely, a "web" or malformation of the vena cava. Clinically, upper abdominal pain, hepatomegaly, and ascites occur with variable abruptness in a patient with one of the above underlying predisposing diseases. The course is commonly one of relentless progression with ascites, portal hypertension, and liver failure.

The transaminases are elevated and the prothrombin time prolonged. Radionuclide scanning shows reduced and inhomogeneous liver uptake, but excessive uptake in the caudate lobe owing to its separate drainage into the inferior vena cava. Ultrasonography with Doppler flow imaging is diagnostic and is the recommended diagnostic test. Hepatic venography shows occluded vessels; usually the major hepatic veins cannot be fully visualized or may show partial recanalization. Treatment of the acute syndrome with anticoagulants or thrombolytic agents is rarely successful. Portocaval shunts, if performed early, have successfully decompressed the congested liver. If there is prior liver failure, then the only recourse is liver transplantation.

CHAPTER 106

TUMORS OF THE LIVER

Benign Tumors

Cavernous hemangioma is the most common benign liver tumor. It may be any size, single or multiple, and is often detected incidentally while imaging the abdomen for other reasons. These tumors are more common in women and more often occur in the right lobe. Only a minority of patients with lesions exceeding 4 cm in diameter are symptomatic, with mild to moderate abdominal fullness or discomfort. Spontaneous bleeding is extremely rare. Physical examination may reveal a soft bruit over the liver. Labeled RBC radionuclide scanning, dynamic CT, and MRI can all be diagnostic. Selective hepatic arteriography is invasive and rarely used. Needle biopsy should be avoided if hemangioma is suspected, because diagnostic tissue samples are often not obtained and severe hemorrhage may result. Surgical resection is seldom necessary.

Hepatic adenomas occur in a very small percentage of women using oral contraceptives for more than 7 years. Single or multiple, the adenomas consist of thickened trabeculae or sheets of hepatocytes without bile ducts, portal tracts, or terminal hepatic venules. The lesions may be asymptomatic and detected incidentally. Large adenomas may cause discomfort or they may rupture or bleed spontaneously. Ruptured hepatic adenomas present with sudden acute right upper quadrant pain and shock. These estrogen-sensitive lesions may grow rapidly during pregnancy or oral contraceptive therapy; they may wane with cessation of oral contraceptives and recur with their resumption. Transformation to hepatocellular carcinoma has been reported. Ultrasound, CT, radionuclide scanning, and angiography are not diagnostic. If acute symptoms are absent, and the diagnosis is certain, it is best to stop the oral contraceptives and follow the patient with CT or ultrasound every few months. If hemorrhage or other symptoms occur, or if it is not possible to distinguish these adenomas from focal nodular hyperplasia, laparotomy and resection are indicated.

Focal nodular hyperplasia is a congenital malformation in which the connective tissue elements of the liver are contained within a stellate scar. It is not a true neoplasm. Oral contraceptive use is not implicated in its pathogenesis. Focal nodular hyperplasia appears as one or more lobulated discrete masses, which consist histologically of liver cell cords and sinusoids look normal but disorganized. Typically, there is a stellate scar near the center of the lesion from which fibrous septa radiate into the mass. There are bile ducts and some inflammatory cells within the lesion. Patients with focal nodular hyperplasia are seldom symptomatic. Thus, it is usually discovered incidentally. Often a wedge biopsy is necessary to make the diagnosis. Surgical excision is not indicated.

Hepatocellular Carcinoma

Hepatocellular carcinoma (HCC), the most common primary liver cancer, accounts for 75–85% of all primary liver tumors. Geographic area of residence, gender, and environment have emerged as important determinants of its etiology and prevalence. In the United States, HCC is relatively uncommon, whereas in most of Africa and Asia, it is the most common malignancy. It is almost always associated with cirrhosis (Table 106.1). Prospective studies in Japan and Taiwan have shown that chronic hepatitis B infection increases the risk of hepatocellular carcinoma by a factor of 250. In areas where HCC is common, hepatitis B virus infection is endemic and often vertically transmitted at the time of birth. Using molecular biological means, HBV DNA is found to be integrated into the genome of the tumor cells.

■ Clinical Features

There is a 4:1 predominance in men. Abdominal pain, anorexia, and weight loss are common early symptoms. In a cirrhotic, abrupt deterioration in liver function or a change in the size or configuration of the liver should suggest HCC. Sometimes, if hemorrhage occurs in the tumor, acute pain and tenderness may follow. Erythrocytosis, hypercalcemia, hypoglycemia, and other paraneoplastic syndromes are well recognized but rare.

Usual liver tests are of little or no diagnostic help. Alpha fetoprotein (AFP), a normal fetal serum protein, is produced by HCC cells. Serum AFP rises significantly in approximately 50% of patients with HCC in North America. A level above 400 ng/ml is regarded more

TABLE 106.1.	Risk Factors for Hepatocellular Carcinoma
Cirrhosis	
Chronic hepatitis B	
Chronic hepatitis C	
Hemochromatosis	
Alpha-1-antitrypsin deficiency	
Dietary aflatoxins	
Chronic anabolic steroid use	
Industrial carcinogens	

diagnostic of HCC, but concurrent chronic liver disease lowers its specificity. Ultrasound (US) may be more sensitive than AFP for early detection of HCC. Current screening protocols include serial 6-monthly to yearly AFP tests and liver US. While any patient with cirrhosis may be screened thus, those with chronic hepatitis B or C are particular candidates, given their particular predis-

position to HCC. Despite a lack of proven efficacy or cost-effectiveness, such protocols have been embodied into routine clinical practice. CT provides supplementary information over US. When a tumor is found, liver biopsy should follow, to obtain tissue. In a patient who has significant coagulopathy and hepatic decompensation, a markedly elevated AFP is deemed diagnostic and liver biopsy can be avoided.

Management

Surgery offers the only possibility of cure for HCC, but less than 15% of tumors are resectable, and coexistent cirrhosis limits resectability even further. Both radiation therapy and systemic chemotherapy are ineffective. Most current therapy for unresectable HCC is directed at local measures, including Gelfoam embolization of the tumor and direct injection of tumor masses with caustic agents (e.g., absolute ethanol). A better outcome of treatment of HCC clearly depends on screening for and early detection of HCC.

Metastatic Cancer of the Liver

The liver is more frequently invaded by cancer metastases than is any other organ. Primary neoplasms of the alimentary tract, pancreas, breast, and lung most commonly metastasize to the liver. Most metastases are hematogenous. When seen on the liver surface, metastases are characteristically round and white and often show umbilicated centers. The size and number of metastases vary greatly.

Typically, the patient reports gradual, but progressive, dull, right upper quadrant abdominal ache, abdominal fullness, anorexia, malaise, and nausea. Fever or severe pain is rarely reported. The liver size may be normal, but late liver metastases present with hepatomegaly and a hard liver. With advanced disease, ascites and lower extremity edema may occur from hepatic vein and inferior vena cava compression by the tumor. Elevation of serum alkaline phosphatase is the predominant abnormality, but its sensitivity is low. There may be mild hyperbilirubinemia, leukocytosis, and slight elevation of serum aminotransferases. The diagnosis is most often suggested by abnormalities on imaging. Needle biopsy is diagnostic and it may be done with or without the guidance of an imaging procedure.

Generally, liver metastases are treated by whatever systemic chemotherapy is indicated for the type of cancer

involved. Liver metastases portend a poor prognosis regardless of the primary site. There has been interest and growing experience in surgical resection of hepatic metastases in a small subgroup of patients with colorectal cancer without other evidence of residual disease. The 5-year survival rate after resection of metastatic cancer is nearly 25%.

Liver transplantation

Since the early 1980s, liver transplantation has developed into a standard and effective treatment for patients with advanced liver disease of any etiology, owing largely to improvements in immunosuppression and surgical technique. By definition, candidates for liver transplantation are victims of severe liver disease who have experienced many of the medical complications of cirrhosis and liver failure, and in whom liver transplantation restores normal liver function. Patients who have undergone liver transplantation experience excellent quality of life, and are often able to return to work and a productive lifestyle. One-year survival is in the range of 80% and five-year survival, approximately 65%. Significant controversy surrounds the applicability of liver transplantation for reformed alcoholics and substance abusers, or patients with chronic hepatitis B infection and hepatic cancer.

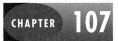

THE GALLBLADDER AND BILIARY TRACT

■ Physiology of Bile

Formation and secretion

The gallbladder, which serves as a reservoir for bile, can hold 20–40 ml when full. It concentrates hepatic bile with an 80–90% reduction of volume. Along with **Oddi's sphincter,** it also regulates the pressure within the biliary system. Contraction of the gallbladder occurs in response to cholecystokinin (CCK) as well as to vagal stimuli. With absorption of sodium and water, concentrations of bile, cholesterol, and bile acids increase in proportion, but cholesterol saturation does not change. Bile acid micelles (Figure 107.1) permit the solution that contains high concentrations of electrolytes, bile acids, phospholipids, and cholesterol to be isotonic. Little bile enters the duodenum between meals. Soon after food intake, CCK released from the duodenal mucosa stimulates gallbladder contraction. Bile flow via the common duct is influenced by Oddi's sphincter.

Bile acids

Normal bile acid physiology is schematically shown in Figure 107.2. The liver synthesizes from cholesterol approximately 0.5 grams of two primary bile acids,

cholic acid and chenodeoxycholic acid daily. They are conjugated and excreted into the bile; more than 95% of the bile acids are absorbed by an active transport mechanism and returned via the portal blood to the liver for re-excretion into the bile. The small unabsorbed fraction undergoes bacterial deconjugation and 7-dehydroxylation, thus forming secondary bile acids (deoxycholic acid and lithocholic acid), which are excreted in the feces or reabsorbed. Further sulfation and re-excretion into the bile follow. Thus, the total body pool of bile acids is a composite of primary (cholic and chenodeoxycholic) and secondary (deoxycholic and small amounts of lithocholic) bile acids that total 2–3 grams. It is essentially constant in size because fecal loss is balanced by hepatic synthesis. The pool has been shown to cycle twice with each meal; thus, the enterohepatic circulation carries 12 to 13 grams of bile acids per day.

Bile acid synthesis is governed by its own negative feedback. Bile acids returning to the liver suppress HMGCoA reductase, the rate-limiting enzyme for synthesis of cholesterol, and 7-alpha-hydroxylase, the rate-limiting enzyme for bile acid synthesis. If the return of bile acids to the liver is eliminated, hepatic synthesis of bile acids can increase five–tenfold. Feeding bile acids reduces hepatic synthesis.

Bile formation and secretion

Hepatic bile secretion totals 0.5–1.0 L/24 hours, 96% of which is water. Bile solids consist of bile acids, lecithin, cholesterol, bilirubin, calcium, sodium, potassium, and chloride. Bile also serves as the main route of excretion of numerous endogenous substances, such as cholesterol, bilirubin, porphyrins, and steroid hormones, as well as many exogenous organic ions, including radiopaque media, conjugated drugs, copper, and iron. Bile formation and secretion have been divided into components dependent on and independent of bile acids. The primary controlling factor of bile volume and flow rate is the active secretion of bile acids into the canalicular lumen, thus producing osmotic and electrical gradients with resulting movement of solutes, water, bile pigments, and organic ions. The bile acid-independent component of bile flow is thought to be driven by active sodium transport. Ductular bile secretion is less well understood, but appears at least partly under hormonal control in that secretin stimulates active secretion of bicarbonate by duct epithelium.

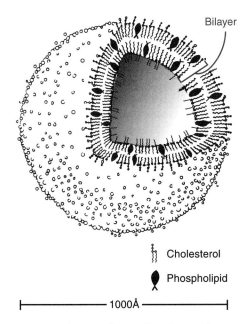

Bilayer

🦴 Cholesterol

🎋 Phospholipid

├─────── 1000Å ───────┤

FIGURE 107.1. Biliary unilamellar vesicle.
(From: Sleisenger M, Fordtran J. Gastrointestinal Disease. Pathophysiology, Diagnosis, Management. 4th ed. Philadelphia: W.B. Saunders, 1989. Used with permission.)

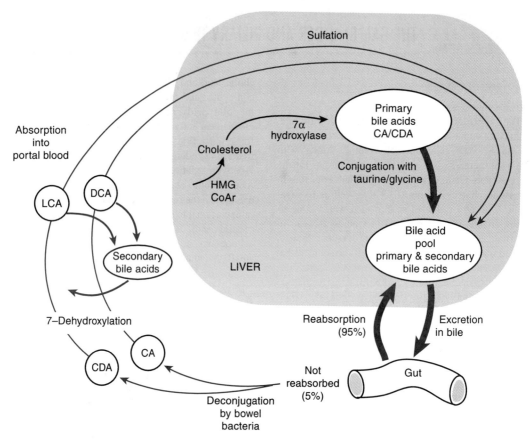

FIGURE 107.2. Normal bile acid metabolism. CA = cholic acid; CDA = chenodeoxycholic acid; DCA = deoxy- cholic acid; HMG CoAr = HMG CoA reductase; LCA = lithocholic acid.

CHAPTER 108

DISEASES OF THE GALLBLADDER AND BILIARY TRACT

Cholestasis

Cholestasis is defined as impaired bile formation and flow. The anatomic location of the abnormality resulting in cholestasis varies from the interior of the liver cell to the duodenum. Mechanical obstruction is a common cause of cholestasis; however, cholestasis does not necessarily mean mechanical obstruction. Isolated hy- perbilirubinemia in the absence of liver dysfunction results from interference with the transport and metabo- lism of bilirubin within hepatocytes (Table 108.1).

Cholestasis is classically divided into intra- and extrahepatic forms based on the anatomic location of impairment of bile flow (Table 108.2). A more detailed conceptual scheme classifies cholestasis according to

more specific sites as follows: (1) *intrahepatic cholesta- sis* at the hepatocellular level (e.g., cholestatic forms of alcoholic hepatitis and viral hepatitis, cholestasis caused by drugs such as chlorpromazine and sulfonamides); (2) *cholestasis due to lesions at the bile canalicular membrane* (e.g., cholestasis caused by sex hormones, cholestasis occasionally seen with Hodgkin's disease, the cholestatic jaundice of pregnancy in the third trimester, and the unusual syndrome known as benign recurrent intrahepatic cholestasis); (3) *cholestasis due to lesions of the interlobular bile ducts*, which includes that due to primary biliary cirrhosis, primary sclerosing cholangitis, sarcoidosis of the liver, allograft rejection, and graft-

TABLE 108.1.	Hyperbilirubinemic Syndromes			
Characteristic	Gilbert's		Crigler-Najjar	Dubin-Johnson
Prevalence	5% of population		Very rare	Rare
Bilirubin type	Unconjugated		Unconjugated	Conjugated
Age of onset	Young adult		Infant	Adult
Inheritance	Autosomal dominant		Autosomal recessive	Autosomal dominant
Mechanism	Uptake, conjugation		Conjugation	Canalicular secretion
Outcome	Harmless		Kernicterus/death	Harmless
			Liver transplant	

TABLE 108.2.	Etiology of Cholestasis

Intrahepatic
   Primary biliary cirrhosis
   Primary sclerosing cholangitis
   Drug-induced
   Pregnancy
   Sarcoidosis
   Sepsis
Extrahepatic
   Common bile duct obstruction
      Stone
      Stricture
      Carcinoma
      Choledochal cyst
      Primary sclerosing cholangitis
   Pancreas
      Pancreatitis
      Pseudocyst
      Carcinoma

versus-host disease; and (4) *cholestasis due to obstructing lesions of the extrahepatic bile ducts*, including that caused by choledocholithiasis, cholangiocarcinoma, benign strictures, primary sclerosing cholangitis, choledochal cysts, and stenosis of the distal common bile duct due to pancreatic tumor or inflammation.

■ **Histopathology of the Liver**

Many histologic features in the liver are common to cholestasis regardless of the cause. Bile stasis is most prominent in the centrilobular regions with only minimal cellular necrosis and foci of mononuclear cells. In prolonged cholestasis, portal fibrosis and round cell infiltration develop with fibrous strands connecting adjacent portal tracts, plus ductal proliferation. With further prolonged cholestasis, portal fibrosis becomes more extensive, with septa developing between portal tracts and hepatic veins, then nodular regeneration and the picture of secondary biliary cirrhosis. Grossly, the liver is enlarged, green, and nodular.

■ **Clinical Features**

Common symptoms are jaundice and pruritus, which may precede jaundice. Hyperlipidemia, xanthomas, and xanthelasmas may follow long-standing cholestasis. Other features of cholestasis include *acholic stools*, owing to the lack of bile reaching the duodenum; *steatorrhea* due to the absence of bile acids in the small bowel; *dark urine* due to bilirubinuria; *osteomalacia* and *osteoporosis*, probably due to several factors, such as impaired vitamin D and calcium absorption from the gut; *easy bruising* or hemorrhage due to vitamin K malabsorption in the liver; and *excoriations* from scratching.

■ **Laboratory Features**

Some degree of conjugated hyperbilirubinemia is usually present in cholestasis (Table 108.3). With complete bile duct obstruction, serum bilirubin rises to 15–20 mg/dl but then stabilizes due to extrahepatic bilirubin disposal mechanisms. Serum alkaline phosphatase usually rises more than threefold, due to increased synthesis in the obstructed liver. Often a unique lipoprotein X, thought to be a low-density lipoprotein, appears in the serum. Serum bile acids are the most sensitive indicator of cholestasis, since their concentration rises in all forms of cholestasis even before jaundice appears.

■ **Diagnosis and Management**

Important elements in the history include fever, chills, pain, and colic, suggesting mechanical obstruction and cholangitis, current and recent drug use (oral contraceptives, phenothiazines), weight loss, prior abdominal or biliary tract surgery, prior diseases clinically associated with cholestasis, and family history. The examination should include careful palpation of the liver and spleen, and a search for an enlarged, palpable gallbladder (Courvoisier's sign), lymph nodes, and xanthomas. The first imaging procedure in cholestasis is usually an ultrasound or CT, performed to answer the critical question: *Is there dilation of the intra- or extrahepatic bile ducts?* The advantages of these imaging

TABLE 108.3.   Laboratory Values in Cholestasis

Test	Range of Values
Bilirubin	↑-↑↑↑
Transaminases	Normal-↑
Alkaline phosphatase	↑↑
Gamma glutamyl transpeptidase	↑↑↑
Cholesterol	↑
Albumin	Normal
Prothrombin time	Normal
Serum protein electrophoresis	Normal

↑ = mildly increased; ↑↑ = moderately increased; ↑↑↑ = quite increased.

methods are shown in Table 108.4. If the biliary tree appears dilated, then direct cholangiography is indicated, usually through endoscopic retrograde cholangiopancreatography (ERCP), since it offers expanded therapeutic options, such as the ability to do sphincterotomy (severing the muscle fibers of the sphincter of Oddi in order to enlarge the outlet of the biliary tree into the duodenum), extract gallstones, or dilate strictures or place stents over mechanically obstructing mass lesions.

If the initial imaging examinations fail to demonstrate bile duct dilation, then a needle biopsy of the liver needs to be considered. Biopsy is indicated if the clinical picture strongly supports alcoholic hepatitis, drug-induced cholestasis, or autoimmune disease of the liver.

TABLE 108.4.   Diagnosis of Cholestasis: Computed Tomography vs. Ultrasound Examination

Procedure	Advantages	Disadvantages
Ultrasound	Better at detecting gallstones in the gallbladder	Only uncommonly detects gallstones in the common bile duct
	Accurately measures diameter of common bile duct	Less than optimal visualization of pancreatic tumor, cyst, etc.
Computed tomography	Better visualization of pancreas	Poor sensitivity for detecting gallstones within gallbladder or common bile duct

---

CHAPTER 109   GALLSTONES

Bile contains three lipid polar amphipaths: cholesterol, lecithin, and bile acids. Cholesterol, with only one hydroxyl group, is practically water-insoluble; lecithin can interact with water and forms liquid crystalline complexes; bile acids have a major hydrophilic side and thus have detergent properties and form micelles (Figure 107.1). Bile acids in water form micelles and incorporate lecithin, greatly increasing the capacity to incorporate cholesterol in the hydrophobic interior of the micelle.

Several methods for expressing the solubility relationships of the three biliary lipids have been devised. They illustrate that the solubility of cholesterol is finite and that bile with insufficient bile acids and lecithin to dissolve all the cholesterol in micellar solution is supersaturated with cholesterol. Such bile is termed lithogenic, in that it fosters cholesterol nucleation and crystal formation, leading to crystal growth and gallstone formation. Patients with cholesterol gallstones have been shown to have lithogenic bile. Either the

biliary level of solubilizing lipids is decreased (diminished hepatic bile acid secretion, a smaller bile acid pool, excess loss of bile acids in stool due to terminal ileal disease or use of bile acid binders) or there is increased secretion of cholesterol (from increased activity of HMGCoA reductase, or diminished activity of 7α-hydroxylase).

Gallstone disease afflicts 10% of Americans; its incidence increases with age, with nearly one-third of the elderly having gallstones. They are more prevalent in women (Table 109.1). In the United States and most Western countries, cholesterol gallstones predominate; bile pigment stones account for about 20% of all gallstones. Pigment stones contain less than 25% cholesterol, appear as dark or black calculi, are radiopaque, and are seen in chronic hemolytic states, cirrhosis, and chronically obstructed bile ducts, such as those due to benign strictures. Pigment stones predominate in the tropics and the Orient. The association of gallstones with pregnancy remains inconclusive.

Natural History of Gallstones

Most gallstones are asymptomatic; most are incidentally detected during ultrasound examination of the abdomen. During the natural history of asymptomatic gallstones, the cumulative probability of symptoms developing is about 10% at 5 years and no greater than 20% at 15–20 years. In most patients, biliary symptoms precede the onset of complications. Thus, cholecystectomy is not indicated in the asymptomatic patient. Some gallstones become symptomatic, but the mechanisms are unclear (Figure 109.1). Abdominal pain usually follows impaction of gallstone(s) at the cystic duct (acute cholecystitis and chronic cholecystitis) or their migration through the cystic duct and impaction within the common bile duct (choledocholithiasis). Common bile duct stones are particularly dangerous because they may evoke gallstone pancreatitis and

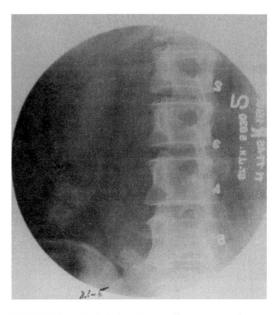

FIGURE **109.2.** Oral cholecystogram showing opacification of the gallbladder, which contains gallstones.

bacterial cholangitis. Symptoms from gallstones, albeit episodic, have a high rate of recurrence. Thus, once gallstones evoke symptoms, cholecystectomy is recommended even though symptoms may be absent at the time of surgery. Finally, in a small group of patients, the gallstones disease is "complicated" by pancreatitis, fistula formation, gallstone ileus, cholangitis, or liver abscess. These patients clearly mandate therapy for ongoing active disease.

TABLE 109.1.	Risk Factors for Gallstones

Age
Feminine gender
Caucasian race
Obesity
Diabetes mellitus
Rapid weight loss
Chronic oral contraceptive or estrogen use
Terminal ileal disease (e.g., Crohn's disease)
Bile salt sequestrants (e.g., Cholestyramine)

Diagnosis

Only 10% of gallstones, mostly pigment stones, are radiopaque. Some are lucent but have calcium rings near the surface. Oral cholecystography (Figure 109.2) identifies most gallstones, but a successful study requires reliable ingestion and normal absorption of the contrast medium, a healthy liver, and a patent cystic duct. Ultrasound (Figure 109.3), a highly reliable and accurate imaging technique for identifying gallstones, has replaced oral cholecystography for this purpose. ERCP also identifies common duct and gallbladder stones, but is not routinely employed for this purpose.

Management

The patient's age and concomitant health problems bear heavily in deciding on appropriate therapy. Cholecystectomy remains the most effective treatment for

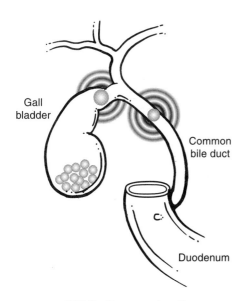

FIGURE **109.1.** Symptomatic gallstone.

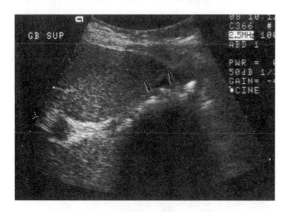

FIGURE 109.3. Ultrasonogram showing gallstones (arrow).

cholelithiasis. The most significant advance in surgical techniques in recent years has been the revolutionary development of the laparoscopic technique for cholecystectomy. This technique, which has become the preferred method for cholecystectomy worldwide, permits a cholecystectomy to be performed safely and effectively using instruments that are introduced into the abdomen through a few stab punctures. Consequently, a formal laparotomy is avoided and the recovery time is greatly curtailed.

A great deal of research has gone into the use of oral medications to dissolve gallstones, which is based on the premise that patients with cholesterol gallstones who have a small bile acid pool could expand it with oral use of bile acids to produce unsaturated bile. Two agents, chenodeoxycholic acid and ursodeoxycholic acid, have been approved for this indication. A functioning gallbladder, radiolucent stones, and a patent biliary tract are prerequisites for their use. With optimum dosages, only 30%–50% of this select group will show complete stone dissolution; even after dissolution, there is significant recurrence.

Acute cholecystitis

Most instances of **acute cholecystitis** result from a **gallstone impaction** in the cystic duct. The classical attack is discrete, comes on rather suddenly, often at night and lasts hours to days. There may be history of similar episodes in the past. The patient usually reports epigastric pain, generally unrelated to movements or respiration, and often, nausea and vomiting. Later, the pain com-

monly shifts and localizes in the right upper quadrant; it may radiate to the shoulder and the right scapular area. Tenderness to palpation (Murphy's sign) and signs of peritoneal irritation are noted. Fever or leukocytosis are common. There may be the impression of a tender mass in the right subcostal area.

The diagnosis depends largely on the history and physical findings. Cholecystitis may simulate perforation or penetration of peptic ulcer, myocardial infarction, acute pancreatitis, pneumonia, hepatitis and acute right-sided pyelonephritis. **Ultrasonography** accurately detects cholelithiasis and gallbladder wall edema. The **HIDA scan** (following IV administration, the radiopharmaceutical is taken up by hepatocytes and excreted into the biliary tree, which may be imaged) is also useful in this setting. With an obstructed cystic duct, no radioactivity is noted in the gallbladder (positive HIDA scan).

Hospitalization is required for pain relief and IV fluids, and surgical consultation. **Cholecystectomy** is usually performed on the same admission. Cultures of the gallbladder and bile will be positive in at least one-half of patients with acute cholecystitis at surgery. The most common organisms are aerobic coliforms, streptococci, clostridium and bacteroides. Therefore, fever or leukocytosis mandates antibiotics.

Other types of cholecystitis

Some patients have recurrent attacks of mild to severe acute cholecystitis. Almost all have gallstones and require cholecystectomy. Many others with gallstones may experience vague symptoms without such attacks. **Chronic cholecystitis** could be present in such a setting, and cholecystectomy should be given careful consideration.

Acalculous cholecystitis occurs in the absence of gallstones. Gallbladder ischemia is felt to be responsible, causing inflammation and secondary infection. It is seen largely in older persons with recent trauma or recent surgery or with vasculitis on corticosteroid therapy. It has been reported in patients with AIDS and Cryptosporidium infection of the biliary tract. The clinical presentation is the same as for acute cholecystitis. Ultrasound examination often shows an inflamed gallbladder wall with sludge but no stones. The HIDA scan is positive and these patients require urgent surgery.

Choledocholithiasis

In Asian and African countries, calcium bilirubinate stones predominate; these appear to arise, not only in the gallbladder, but also primarily in intra- and extrahepatic portions of the biliary tract. Bile duct stones produce biliary colic with nausea and vomiting. A common bile

duct stone may acutely obstruct the common bile duct with jaundice and liver enzyme elevations or acute pancreatitis. However, 20% of patients with bile duct stones have no pain and 25–30% of patients have no jaundice.

■ Diagnosis and Management

Elevated serum alkaline phosphatase and mild hyperbilirubinemia are the most characteristic abnormalities. The former may occur without pain, jaundice, or other symptoms. Common bile duct stones with acute bacterial cholangitis cause spiking fever and a picture of sepsis. With acute pancreatitis, abdominal pain is more epigastric and radiates to the back. Leukocytosis is common; bacteremia due to enteric organisms may occur. Plain abdominal x-rays may show an ileus and, uncommonly, gallbladder stones. Ultrasonography usually shows biliary tract dilation, but this finding is often absent.

Symptomatic common duct stones should be treated with antibiotics, analgesics, and IV fluids. As soon as the patient has been stabilized, ERCP should follow, to establish a diagnosis and to extract the gallstones. Following recovery, these patients should also undergo a laparoscopic cholecystectomy. If the common bile duct stones cannot be removed by endoscopy, then open cholecystectomy and common bile duct exploration are required.

Internal Biliary Fistulae

Biliary-enteric fistulae may form due to chronic inflammation from long-standing cholelithiasis, adhesions of the duodenum, or hepatic flexure at the gallbladder. This condition has no characteristic clinical picture, but patients may report symptoms of biliary colic or chronic cholecystitis and sometimes have associated cholangitis. A plain abdominal x-ray may reveal air in the biliary tree (pneumobilia). Gallstone ileus may follow erosion of a gallstone into the intestinal tract with mechanical obstruction, most commonly in the terminal ileum.

Benign Stricture of the Bile Ducts

Benign strictures arise in the common bile duct from operative trauma at the time of biliary tract surgery, choledocholithiasis, or chronic pancreatitis. Jaundice insidiously develops a few weeks or months following surgery, often with abdominal pain, fever, chills, and pruritus. Bile pigment stones may form above the stricture in more chronic cases. Unrelieved obstruction leads to secondary biliary cirrhosis and bacteremia and hepatic abscess. Liver tests show variable but chronic cholestasis. Ultrasonography shows dilation of the bile ducts above the stricture, and ERCP accurately defines the biliary anatomy. Until recently, surgery to bypass the stricture was the only treatment available. Recent advances allow the passage of stents, and balloon dilation of strictures to relieve obstruction and cholestasis without surgery.

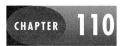 **110** CHRONIC CHOLESTATIC LIVER DISEASE

Primary Biliary Cirrhosis

Primary biliary cirrhosis (PBC), a chronic cholestatic liver disease, results from **autoimmune chronic cholangitis;** its etiology is unknown. An immune attack on small bile ducts results in portal inflammation and destruction of interlobular bile ducts. Cholestasis, liver cell necrosis, fibrosis, cirrhosis, and eventually liver failure evolve. Genetic factors are implicated by family clustering and positive autoimmune markers in relatives.

■ Clinical and Laboratory Features

PBC, which predominantly afflicts women (80%), most commonly presents in the fourth and fifth decades. Fatigue and pruritus without jaundice are the most common initial symptoms. Mild pigmentation and hepatosplenomegaly are noted. A long, anicteric, and mildly symptomatic period eventually culminates in xanthomas, steatorrhea, bone pain, osteomalacia, portal hypertension, and liver failure. Notable clinical associations are CREST (see chapter 259) syndrome, the sicca or dry eye syndrome and other autoimmune disorders, autoimmune thyroiditis, pigmented gallstones, and arthritis.

Laboratory studies show a cholestatic pattern; serum alkaline phosphatase is raised more than threefold. Serum bilirubin is normal or elevated in the later stages. A positive antimitochondrial antibody, the most typical and sensitive finding, occurs in 95% of cases. It is not absolutely specific, because it is noted in 10–15% cases of chronic active hepatitis. PBC-associated mitochondrial antibodies have recently been described.

■ Diagnosis and Management

Jaundice from chronic drug use, primary sclerosing cholangitis, and mechanical common bile duct obstruction should be excluded in all cases by ultrasound examination; cholangiography is rarely indicated. Long-term use of ursodeoxycholic acid evokes clinical improvement. Pruritus may be controlled or lessened with cholestyramine or rifampin. Vitamin D and supplemental calcium help prevent metabolic bone disease. In patients with end-stage liver failure, liver transplantation is life-saving and highly successful. To date, PBC does not seem to recur in the transplanted liver.

Sclerosing Cholangitis

Sclerosing cholangitis is defined as chronic inflammation and fibrosis of intrahepatic and extrahepatic bile ducts. It is diagnosed by cholangiography, which shows irregular bile ducts with numerous saccular dilatations and strictures. It may follow autoimmune mechanisms (primary). Biliary infections, such as *Clonorchis sinensis* (which is seen in Southeast Asia), recurrent bacterial infection associated with biliary strictures, and Cryptosporidium infection (which is seen in patients with AIDS) may lead to sclerosing cholangitis. Vascular causes of sclerosing cholangitis include artery ligation, usually used to treat hepatic cancer; intra-arterial chemotherapy; and hepatic artery strictures and thrombosis following liver transplantation.

Primary sclerosing cholangitis (PSC) is characterized by obliterative inflammatory fibrosis of the intrahepatic and extrahepatic bile ducts without any secondary cause. The etiology is not known; it occurs primarily in young men. The mean age at onset of clinical features is about 40. In two-thirds of cases, it is associated with inflammatory bowel disease (usually ulcerative colitis), which may precede the primary sclerosing cholangitis.

Intermittent pruritus, fatigue, jaundice, and pain are the usual presenting symptoms. The disease is generally slowly progressive and eventually leads to cirrhosis, portal hypertension, and death from liver failure. Biochemical evidence of cholestasis is present. The diagnosis is established by cholangiography. The differential diagnosis includes causes of secondary sclerosing cholangitis and bile duct cancer. Cholangiocarcinoma is found in 15% of persons with PSC undergoing liver transplantation.

No medical treatment has been proven effective; however, pruritus and jaundice can be improved by treatment with ursodeoxycholic acid. In patients with dominant strictures of the common bile duct, improvement in symptoms and jaundice can be obtained by endoscopic dilation of the strictures. In patients with liver failure, liver transplantation is life-saving and highly successful.

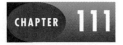

CHAPTER 111 **CYSTIC DISEASES OF THE LIVER AND BILIARY TREE**

This term embraces a group of conditions associated with liver cysts, which may or may not communicate with the biliary tree. Often, the kidneys are involved. Despite the considerable overlap of clinical features, the classification presented in Table 111.1 is useful.

TABLE 111.1. Classification of Hepatic Cysts

Type of Cyst	Heredity	Biliary Communication	Other Organs	Prognosis
Solitary cyst	None	No	None	Good
Adult polycystic disease	Autosomal dominant	No	Kidney cysts	Good
Congenital hepatic fibrosis	+/−	Yes	Medullary sponge kidney	Poor
Choledochal cysts	+/−	Yes	None	Good
Carroli's disease	+/−	Yes	Medullary sponge kidney	Poor
Liver abscess	−	May occur	None	Good

+/− = may or may not be hereditary.

CHAPTER 112

NEOPLASMS OF THE BILIARY TREE

Carcinoma of the Bile Ducts

Carcinoma arising from the intrahepatic ducts (**cholangiocarcinoma**) may mimic hepatocellular carcinoma. Chronic biliary tract disease resulting from primary sclerosing cholangitis, sclerosing cholangitis due to chronic Clonorchis infection, and Caroli's disease are its predisposing factors. Cirrhosis itself may be a risk factor for cholangiocarcinoma, but this association is not as strong as that for hepatocellular carcinoma. The diagnosis and management are essentially the same as for hepatocellular carcinoma.

A common site for bile duct carcinoma is the junction of the right and left main hepatic ducts at the porta hepatis; it may locally extend into the liver (**Klatskin tumor**). Slow and insidious growth at this site produces a gradually evolving clinical picture of cholestasis that mimics a non-neoplastic cholestatic disorder. A collapsed gallbladder and dilation of the intrahepatic bile ducts as detected by ultrasonography and confirmed by cholangiography will usually establish a diagnosis.

Primary common bile duct cancers may be polypoid but are more commonly scirrhous and produce a stricture that may simulate a benign stricture or sclerosing cholangitis. Jaundice and pruritus are the most common presenting features. There is usually no significant pain, and secondary bacterial cholangitis is uncommon. The liver is usually enlarged and rounded. A nontender, enlarged, palpable gallbladder is a useful sign of malignant biliary obstruction (**Courvoisier's sign**). Laboratory findings are those of cholestasis; diagnosis is best established by cholangiography.

Because these cancers can rarely be cured by surgery, the nonoperative management of bile duct cancer, using endoscopically placed stents over the obstructing lesions, has become increasingly important. Relief from jaundice and pruritus, and improved quality of life follow endoscopic stenting techniques. No effective chemotherapy has evolved thus far for biliary tract cancer.

■ Questions

INSTRUCTIONS: Questions 1-4. For each question, select only **one** lettered answer that is the **best** for that question.

1. Which test is most useful for the early diagnosis of spontaneous bacterial peritonitis?
   A. Neutrophil count of ascitic fluid

B. Lactate level in ascitic fluid
C. pH of ascitic fluid
D. LDH of ascitic fluid
E. Culture of ascitic fluid
F. None of the above
G. All of the above

2. Which is the most useful feature for identifying esophageal varices with a high risk of bleeding?
   A. Diameter of varices and abnormalities in the variceal walls
   B. The prothrombin time
   C. Liver size
   D. Presence of portal hypertensive congestive gastropathy

3. The treatment of choice for a patient with cirrhosis who has sustained a recent esophageal variceal hemorrhage and is presently not bleeding is which of the following?
   A. Mesocaval portosystemic shunt
   B. Distal splenorenal Warren shunt
   C. Transhepatic Gelfoam embolization of esophageal varices
   D. Endoscopic sclerosis or banding of varices
   E. Transjugular intrahepatic portosystemic shunt (TIPS)

4. A 56-year-old woman is referred for evaluation of ascites of 4 months' duration. She is a former intravenous drug abuser and has a known diagnosis of chronic hepatitis C. Physical examination shows abdominal distention with shifting dullness. The ALT is 67 U/l; AST, 31U/l and serum albumin, 4.0 g/dl. Ascitic fluid shows 1000 WBC/mm^3 with 70% lymphocytes, 25% macrophages, and 5% neutrophils; the albumin in the fluid is 3.5 g/dl. Which of the following is true?
   A. Cefotaxime should be started for probable spontaneous bacterial peritonitis.
   B. This patient most likely has cirrhosis. Diuretic treatment will be effective.
   C. Large-volume paracentesis is indicated for cytology examination.
   D. Ascites should be cultured for fungi and mycobacteria.

Questions 5–10. For each laboratory abnormality grouping shown in the table, choose the most likely clinical

No.	Anti-mitochondrial antibody	Antinuclear antibody	Total protein (g/dl)	Albumin (g/dl)	Total bilirubin (mg/dl)	Alkaline phosphatase (U/l)	AST (U/l)	ALT (U/l)
5	(-)	(-)	7.2	3.8	1.2	480	52	48
6	1:40	1:320	9.0	3.8	7.0	200	1544	1852
7	(-)	(-)	7.8	3.8	9.8	180	942	1052
8	1:320	1:80	8.0	4.2	1.8	810	68	75
9	(-)	(-)	7.6	4.0	8.0	80	132	178
10	(-)	(-)	7.1	4.0	1.0	140	90	170

ALT = alanine aminotransferase; AST = aspartate aminotransferase; (-) = negative.

picture from A through F. Each choice may be used once, more than once, or not at all.

A. A 38 year old woman with a history of fatigue, arthralgias, dryness of eyes and mucous membranes, and for the last 16 months, amenorrhea. Examination shows jaundice.

B. A 40-year-old woman with history of malaise and pruritus for the last 6 months. She has been taking 125 μg of thyroxine daily as replacement therapy for the past four years.

C. A 42-year-old man with history of multiple episodes of bloody stools, diarrhea, and fever. Mild icterus was noted at the last office visit.

D. A 52-year-old obese woman with a 5-year history of diabetes mellitus. Examination shows hepatomegaly.

E. A 25-year-old man with history of anorexia and abdominal pain for the past 2 days. Urine began to look like a cola drink on the morning of the office visit. Jaundice and tender hepatomegaly are present.

F. A 56-year-old man with a 7-year history of worsening personality disorder, who has been having fatigue, anorexia, and weakness for the past several weeks. Examination shows mild jaundice and hepatomegaly. Laboratory studies show a moderate hemolytic anemia.

■ **Answers**

1. A	2. C	3. D	4. C	5. C
6. A	7. E	8. B	9. F	10. D

SUGGESTED READING

Textbooks and Monographs

Schiff E. Management of difficult problems in hepatology. Semin Liver Dis 1993;13:319–435.

Zakim D, Boyer T. Hepatology. A Textbook of Liver Disease. 2nd ed. Philadelphia: W.B. Saunders Co., 1997.

Articles

Laboratory Evaluation of Liver Function

Rosalki SB, Dooley JS. Liver function profiles and their interpretation. Br J Hosp Med 1994;51:181–186.

Saini S. Imaging of the hepatobiliary tract. N Engl J Med 1997;336:1889–1894.

Theal RM, Scott K. Evaluating asymptomatic patients with abnormal liver function test results. Am Fam Phys 1996;53:2111–2119.

Clinical Presentations

Herrera JL. Abnormal liver enzyme levels. Clinical evaluation in asymptomatic patients. Postgrad Med 1993;93:119–120.

Katkov WN, Friedman LS, Cody H, et al. Elevated serum aminotransferase levels in blood donors: The contribution of hepatitis C virus. Ann Intern Med 1991;115:882–884.

Levinson MJ. Jaundice in the intensive care unit. Hosp Pract 1993;28:51–54.

Rossi RL, Traverso LW, Pimentel F. Malignant obstructive jaundice. Evaluation and management. Surg Clin North Am 1996;76:63–70.

Viral Hepatitis

Bhandari BN, Wright TL. Hepatitis C: an overview. Annu Rev Med 1995;46:309–317.

Dindzans VJ. Viral hepatitis. Pre-exposure and postexposure prophylaxis. Postgrad Med 1992;92:43–46.

Fried MW, Hoofnagle JH. Therapy of hepatitis C. Semin Liver Dis 1995;15:82–91.

Hoofnagle JH, Di Bisceglie AM. Serologic diagnosis of acute and chronic viral hepatitis. Semin Liver Dis 1991;11:73–83.

Regenstein F. New approaches to the treatment of chronic viral hepatitis B and C. Am J Med 1994;96:47S–51S.

Chronic Hepatitis

Czaja AJ. Chronic active hepatitis: the challenge for a new nomenclature. Ann Intern Med 1993;119:510–517.

Sherlock DS. Chronic hepatitis C. Dis Mon 1994;40:117–196.

Alcoholic and Drug-induced Liver Disease

el-Newihi HM, Mihas AA. Alcoholic hepatitis. Recent advances in pathogenesis and therapy. Postgrad Med 1994;96:61–64.

Wrona SA, Tankanow RM. Corticosteroids in the management of alcoholic hepatitis. Am J Hosp Pharm 1994;51:347–353.

Cirrhosis

Ferenci P. Treatment of hepatic encephalopathy in patients with cirrhosis of the liver. Dig Dis 1996;14 Suppl 1:40–52.

Habeeb KS, Herrera JL. Management of ascites. Paracentesis as a guide. Postgrad Med 1997;101:191–2, 195–200.

Lipsky MS, Sternbach MR. Evaluation and initial management of patients with ascites. Am Fam Phys 1996;54:1327–1333.

Longmire-Cook SJ. Pathophysiologic factors and management of ascites. Surg Gynecol Obstet 1993;176:191–202.

Mammen EF. Coagulation defects in liver disease. Med Clin North Am 1994;78:545–554.

Parsons SL, Watson SA, Steele RJ. Malignant ascites. Br J Surg 1996;83:6–14.

Roberts LR, Kamath PS. Ascites and hepatorenal syndrome: pathophysiology and management. Mayo Clin Proc 1996;71:874–881.

Roberts LR, Kamath PS. Pathophysiology and treatment of variceal hemorrhage. Mayo Clin Proc 1996;71:973–983.

Metabolic Liver Disease

Kumar A, Riely CA. Inherited liver diseases in adults. West J Med 1995;163:382–386.

Little DR. Hemochromatosis: diagnosis and management. Am Fam Phys 1996;53:2623–2628.

Jackson GH, Meyer A, Lippmann S. Wilson's disease. Psychiatric manifestations may be the clinical presentation. Postgrad Med 1994;95:135–138.

Cox DW. Molecular advances in Wilson disease. Prog Liver Dis 1996;14:245–264.

Tumors of the Liver

Khakoo SI, Grellier LF, Soni PN, et al. Etiology, screening, and treatment of hepatocellular carcinoma. Med Clin North Am 1996;80:1121–1145.

Sherlock S. Viruses and hepatocellular carcinoma. Gut 1994;35:828–832.

Smith CS, Paauw DS. Hepatocellular carcinoma. Identifying and screening populations at increased risk. Postgrad Med 1993;94:71–74.

Gallstones

Aucott JN, Cooper GS, Bloom AD, Aron DC. Management of gallstones in diabetic patients. Arch Intern Med 1993;153:1053–1058.

Johnston DE, Kaplan MM. Pathogenesis and treatment of gallstones. N Engl J Med 1993;328:412–421.

Kadakia SC. Biliary tract emergencies. Acute cholecystitis, acute cholangitis, and acute pancreatitis. Med Clin North Am 1993;77:1015–1036.

Ransohoff DF, Gracie WA. Treatment of gallstones. Ann Intern Med 1993;119:606–619.

Schwesinger WH, Diehl AK. Changing indications for laparoscopic cholecystectomy. Stones without symptoms and symptoms without stones. Surg Clin North Am 1996;76:493–504.

Cholestasis

Balan V, LaRusso NF. Hepatobiliary disease in inflammatory bowel disease. Gastroenterol Clin North Am 1995;24:647–669.

Harnois DM, Lindor KD. Primary sclerosing cholangitis: evolving concepts in diagnosis and treatment. Dig Dis 1997;15:23–41.

Khandelwal M, Malet PF. Pruritus associated with cholestasis. A review of pathogenesis and management. Dig Dis Sci 1994;39:1–8.

Neoplasms of the Biliary Tree

Farmer DG, Rosove MH, Shaked A, Busuttil RW. Current treatment modalities for hepatocellular carcinoma. Ann Surg 1994;219:236–247.

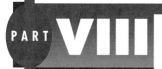

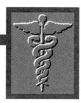

PART VIII

Mary E. Cohan
Edmund H. Duthie Jr.

GERIATRIC MEDICINE

CHAPTER 113 AGING PROCESS

ging refers to the physiological changes that occur in living beings with the passing of time. The aging process, a subject of a number of theories based on empirical evidence, is not yet completely understood. Programmed cellular senescence, free radicals, and random gene mutation have all been proposed as causes of aging. To recognize and distinguish aging processes from disease processes is important in the clinical treatment of older patients.

The U.S. population older than age 65 has increased dramatically since the beginning of the twentieth century. Life expectancy is the average number of years of expected life remaining from birth or a stated age. Since 1900, life expectancy at birth has dramatically increased in the United States for both genders and all races. During the same period—most remarkably in the past two decades—mortality rates have declined among older persons. Death rates from both cardiovascular disease and cerebrovascular disease—two of the foremost killers of the aged—have also been declining. As a result, the number of elderly people has increased dramatically, creating challenges in health care, the political arena, and the economy that have yet to be met.

A thorough knowledge of gerontology and geriatric medicine is essential for the physician of the future. Older persons currently occupy approximately one-third of U.S. hospital beds and more than 90% of nursing home beds. The latter now outnumber acute care hospital beds. Although they constitute only 12% of the U.S. population, elderly persons account for one-third to one-half of an internist's encounter time with patients. Public expenditures for the elderly—Social Security, Medicare, and Medicaid—are rising, and major changes in reimbursement systems and practice styles have occurred as a consequence. Certainly, these costs will escalate as the number of older persons steadily increases through the next century.

Age itself is less important than the influence of concomitant disease processes and physiologic parameters in predicting outcomes in older patients. Careful attention to physiologic organ reserve and the principles of functional assessment and multidisciplinary care will enhance the treatment of older patients and optimize outcomes.

CHAPTER 114 CLINICAL APPROACH TO THE ELDERLY PATIENT

■ Bedside Techniques

The fundamental skills of history taking—with some modification—are basic to accurate diagnosis and promotion of well-being in the elderly. Traditional teaching requires assessment of the patient's reliability as a historian; this assessment is especially necessary with older patients owing to the increased prevalence of delirium and dementia in this population. Thus, some type of mental status examination should be administered formally to elderly patients. Questionnaires and aids help the practitioner perform a complete assessment within a reasonable period of time (e.g., Folstein Mini-Mental State Exam, Table 114.1). Sensory deficits, pain, illiteracy, nonorganic mental illness, poor motivation, and aphasia may all interfere with the interpretation of such test results.

Multiplicity of problems is almost the rule in elderly persons. It is estimated that 85% of persons age 65 and older are afflicted with at least one chronic illness; among nursing home patients an average of five or six illnesses is quite common. The physician must consider these factors and expect multiple and complex problems, especially in the frail or dependent elderly person. The principle of economy of diagnosis (i.e., attempting to explain a patient's signs and symptoms with one unifying hypothesis) has little applicability in the aged. Identifying problems and addressing each with an appropriate treatment plan are challenging clinical activities. The clinician must give highest priority to conditions that most adversely affect the patient's functioning.

The elderly patient may have communication difficulties; the physician must allow more time to take a history and also develop strategies to deal with common communication problems. Patients with hearing and eyesight impairments should be urged to bring their hearing aids and eyeglasses to the visit. Patients with obvious hearing difficulties should be given an otoscopic examination and cerumen disimpaction if needed. Hearing-impaired persons function much better in quiet surroundings. The physician should face the patient at

TABLE 114.1.	Mini-Mental State Examination

If a patient's answer is incorrect, record response.
If a patient's answer is accurate, circle the score.
Add up the circled numbers to get the total score

ORIENTATION

1 What is the today's date?	1 What is the name of this state?
1 What is the month of the year?	1 What is the name of this county?
1 What is the current year?	1 What is the name of this city/town?
1 What is the day of the week?	1 What is the name of this hospital or building?
1 What is the season?	1 What floor or room are we in now?

REGISTRATION

Instruct the patient to try and remember the three objects you are going to name.
With 1 second to say each, name three unrelated objects (horse, chair, apple).
Ask the patient repeat all three. On the first repitition, give 1 point to each correct answer. Record score. Repeat them until all three are learned. Count number of trials to learn and record.

1 _____   Number of trials _____ (up to 6)
1 _____
1 _____

CALCULATION AND ATTENTION

Count backward from 100 by 7's (down to 65) **OR** Spell "WORLD" backwards

1 93 _____	1 D _____
1 86 _____	1 L _____
1 79 _____	1 R _____
1 72 _____	1 O _____
1 65 _____	1 W _____

(Assign score for each item in correct order)

RECALL

What are the three objects I asked you to remember?

1 _____
1 _____
1 _____

LANGUAGE

Show the patient the following and ask him or her to name them.	Ask the patient to repeat the following (one trial only):	Say to the patient as a 3-step command:
1 Wristwatch	1 "No ifs, ands, or buts."	1 "Take this paper in your right hand
1 Pen		1 Fold it in half
		1 Put it on the floor"

1 Ask the patient to read and obey the following instruction: **CLOSE YOUR EYES.**
1 Ask the patient to write a sentence of his or her own choosing in the space below.
1 Ask the patient to copy the following design (pentagons) in the space provided.

RECORD TOTAL SCORE (MAXIMUM 30)
Normal   24–30
Cognitive Impairment 23 or less

Adapted from Folstein MF, et al. J Psych Research 1975; 12:189–198.

eye level in a well-lit room. Speech should be at a reasonable pace. Yelling into the patient's ear is ineffective and should be avoided. Hearing-impaired patients depend on visual cues; their eyeglasses must be worn before the interview begins and throughout the interview. Aphasic persons sometimes can be interviewed best using questions that require a simple yes or no response.

Taking a history of the present illness proceeds as it might for any other patient. However, presentations of acute illnesses or exacerbations of chronic conditions differ in the elderly patient compared to the young. For example, myocardial infarction may be painless and present with signs or symptoms of heart failure; dyspnea caused by exertion may represent an anginal equivalent; a fall may presage a serious infection or represent a cardiac arrhythmia or stroke. Such lists of atypical presentations are almost endless, and texts of geriatric medicine are replete with them.

Obtaining a history of medication use in the aged person is critically important. Significant morbidity in this population results from drug side effects and interactions. Patients must be instructed to bring all their medications to the interview. Many elderly patients see more than one physician (e.g., internist, ophthalmologist, urologist, or dermatologist), with each prescribing a drug or two, and often not mindful of some of the other agents being prescribed. The elderly also commonly use over-the-counter preparations (e.g., vitamins, antacids, laxatives, and aspirin), which may cause side effects that necessitate medical attention. Over-the-counter agents may also complicate an established treatment plan.

The review of systems in the elderly should highlight a few areas, as listed in Table 114.2.

■ Functional Assessment and the Team

Determining functional ability is a critical element in the assessment of the aged patient. In contrast to the younger patient, disability in the elderly patient may be multifactorial, owing to multiple illnesses. In the frail or dependent elderly person, the interplay of multiple and complex illnesses creates the need for teamwork. The goal of the geriatric health care team is to provide the elderly patient with the highest level of function in the least restrictive environment. For elderly patients, the

TABLE 114.2. Geriatric System Review: Special Issues	
Sensory function	Falls
Sexuality	Constipation
Incontinence	Nutrition
Dental health	Depression

TABLE 114.3. The CADET Functional Assessment
C: Communication
A: Ambulation
D: Dressing
E: Eating
T: Toileting

emphasis is often on quality of life rather than on life prolongation. Dependent elderly persons are not only stressed biologically but also psychologically and socially as well. For optimal patient care, the physician must work closely with colleagues in nursing, social work, dietetics, dentistry, pharmacy, rehabilitation, psychology-psychiatry, podiatry, and chaplaincy. It is important that such interdisciplinary teams be able to clearly identify groups of patients who will benefit maximally from a team approach so that resources are expended optimally. Discharge planning teams in many hospitals also involve the physician in optimizing the disposition and treatment plan.

The **activities of daily living** (ADL) describe those practical dimensions required for patients to function daily. In the elderly, the decline and recovery of physical function in response to diseases occur in a sequential manner, regardless of their cause. Bathing, dressing, using the toilet, transferring, and feeding abilities are lost in that order during decline and regained in the reverse order during recovery. Many scales and instruments are available to help assess the ADL domains. One popular scale helps describe components by a simple mnemonic, "CADET" (Table 114.3). ADL may also be measured by many other tools; the Eastern Cooperative Oncology Group (ECOG) scale or the Karnofsky scale (Table 114.4), both widely used in oncology, can be applied in the elderly to assess the global disability caused by multiple, chronic illnesses.

Higher functioning levels have been described as the **instrumental activities of daily living** (IADL). The IADL include cooking, cleaning, doing laundry, shopping, using the telephone, handling finances, and managing transportation. Function is best assessed by directly observing the patient performing the tasks. Because direct observation is not always possible, obtaining the information from the patient or a caregiver is often necessary. The physician should assess these domains in each elderly patient evaluated. If screening reveals deficits, a physiatrist, occupational therapist, speech therapist, audiologist, or physical therapist can assist in defining the problem more accurately and instituting treatment.

■ Clinical Pharmacology

Adverse effects of drugs are common in the elderly, some of which result from physicians' prescribing habits and lack of insight regarding geriatric physiology. The pharmacokinetic and pharmacodynamic factors altered by age are listed in Table 114.5.

The following practical suggestions should be kept in mind when prescribing for the elderly:

TABLE 114.4. Performance Status Scale: Eastern Co-operative Oncology Group (ECOG) Compared to Karnofsky Scale

ECOG Scale	Karnofsky Scale
0 Asymptomatic	100 Asymptomatic
1 Symptomatic, fully ambulatory	90 Normal activity, minor signs or symptoms
	80 Normal activity with effort
2 Less than fully ambulatory, but in bed less than 50% of each day	70 Cares for self, unable to carry on normal activity or work
	60 Requires occasional assistance but self-care for most needs
3 In bed more than 50% of each day	50 Requires considerable assistance
	40 Disabled, requires special care and assistance
4 Bedridden	30 Severely disabled, hospitalization indicated
	20 Very sick, hospitalization needed
	10 Moribund
	0 Dead

TABLE 114.5. Clinical Pharmacology in the Elderly Patient

Variable	Mechanism	Clinical Example	Clinical Correlates
1. Drug absorption			No important clinical effect
2. Drug distribution	Total body water decreases	Water soluble drugs have a high initial concentration	Alcohol has a higher concentration for a given dose
	Total body fat increases	Lipid soluble drugs have prolonged $t_{1/2}$	Diazepam has a prolonged $t_{1/2}$ in elderly
3. Hepatic metabolism	Decreased rate of Phase I hepatic metabolism	Diazepam, quinidine have prolonged biotransformation	These medications needed in smaller doses; more opportunities arise for drug interaction; when possible, monitor drug levels
4. Renal excretion	Decreased creatinine clearance	Renally excreted drugs will have a prolonged clearance	Adjust dose and timing of administration of aminoglycoside and other renally excreted drugs based on creatinine clearance*; measure serum levels whenever possible
5. Pharmacodynamic changes	Change in target organ sensitivity to drugs	β agonists have decreased cardiostimulatory effect; benzodiazepines cause more sedation	Drug dose may need to be adjusted depending on pharmacodynamic effect

*Creatinine clearance (Cockcroft-Gault equation):
$$Cr.Cl = \frac{(140 - age) \times wt~(kg)}{72 \times serum~creatinine~(mg/dl)}$$
0.85 (Cr.Cl) = Cr.Cl for women

1. Establish whether drug therapy is really required. The need for constant and critical review of the older patient's drug regimens cannot be overemphasized.

2. Start low and go slowly.

3. Educate the patient about his or her drugs, their importance to well-being, and their possible side effects.

4. Simplify dosing schedules as much as possible.

5. Consider the cost of agents and, whenever possible, choose less expensive products that have equal efficacy.

6. Consider the type of container to be used. It should display the name of the drug and easy-to-read instructions; it should also be easy to open.

CHAPTER 115 AGE-RELATED CHANGES IN ORGAN SYSTEMS

The physician must understand the changes that occur in the body as a result of age and be able to differentiate these changes from disease. This section will delineate some of the age-related changes that occur in different organ systems (Table 115.1). At times, reference will be made to common pathology. More detailed discussions of pathology can be found in other chapters.

■ **Cardiovascular System**

Arteriosclerosis affects the media of blood vessels and causes them to become less distensible or more "stiff." This change, which appears to be a physiologic result of aging, contributes to a progressive rise in systolic blood pressure throughout life. Diastolic blood pressure, however, rises steadily into middle age, and then it plateaus; it may actually decline in late life. Hypertension has been arbitrarily defined as a systolic blood pressure greater than 160 mm Hg and diastolic greater than 95 mm Hg. As many as 30–40% of the elderly may be classified as hypertensive using these criteria. **Isolated systolic hypertension** (systolic >160 mm Hg and diastolic <90 mm Hg) is a condition found almost exclusively in the aged. Older adults have no change in cardiac output—either at rest or with exercise—when compared to younger adults. It is noteworthy, however, that the aged have a lower heart rate response to stress than the young. It appears, therefore, that cardiac output with stress is maintained in the aged by increased diastolic filling and reliance on the Frank-Starling mechanism.

Echocardiography of healthy elderly subjects reveals that left ventricular wall thickness increases with advancing age, possibly from increasing afterload. Ambulatory electrocardiographic monitoring in healthy aged subjects shows that 88% of subjects have supraventricular ectopic beats and 80% have ventricular ectopic beats. Holter monitor results in aged patients must be interpreted cautiously.

Systolic heart murmurs are not a normal consequence of aging, but they can be heard frequently (a prevalence as high as 50–60%) in aged patients.

■ **Neurologic, Sensory, and Psychologic Systems**

Older people maintain intellectual performance when measured by tests of verbal abilities, such as vocabulary, information, and comprehension. However, their performance on timed tasks indicates a progressive decline throughout adult life. Experimental measurements reveal that learning occurs in late life, but that it takes longer than in youth or middle age. Immediate recall and long-term memory are preserved into late life, but short-term memory shows impairment when tested experimentally. The clinical significance of these findings is not obvious. In general, healthy elderly people should score well on the bedside mental status examinations used by most clinicians; thus, deficits in performance require an explanation.

Even the untrained observer recognizes differences in the gaits of the young and the old. When ambulating, elderly persons have a shorter stride; they flex more at their elbows, trunk, and knees and lift their heels and toes less. Tests of balance show that older persons are less able to control sway when standing still as compared with younger persons. Even healthy older persons have problems balancing on one leg for more than a few seconds.

The pupils of the eye become smaller and less able to dilate maximally with advancing age. The lens undergoes degeneration, becoming less pliable; it develops a yellow hue and frequently becomes opaci-

TABLE 115.1. Clinically Relevant Age-related Organ System Changes	
System and Pattern of Change	**Clinical Significance**
Cardiovascular	
Decreased distensibility of blood vessels	Senile purpura, bounding arterial pulse
Increased peripheral vascular resistance	Systolic hypertension
Unchanged cardiac output	
Increased left ventricular wall thickness	Diastolic dysfunction
Impaired baroreceptor function	Orthostatic hypotension
Decreased heart-rate response to stress	Modification of maximum predicted heart rate with exercise stress testing
Nervous System	
Impaired temperature regulation	Hypothermia and hyperthermia
Impaired baroreceptor response	Orthostatic hypotension
Brain atrophy	Predisposition to delirium
Decreased neurotransmitter concentration	Predisposition to delirium
Altered gait and balance	Propensity for falls
Short-term memory loss	More time required to learn new material
Special senses	
Presbyopia	Visual difficulties (see text)
Presbycusis	Hearing difficulties (see text)
Increased threshold for taste	Potential for altered dietary intake (e.g., sodium)
Arcus senilis	
Decreased pupil size	Difficulty seeing in dim light
Decreased color sensitivity	
Pulmonary	
Decreased lung elasticity	
Decreased vital capacity, increased residual volume	
Decreased PaO$_2$	
Decreased mucus clearance	? Higher incidence of bronchitis and pneumonia
Renal/Genitourinary	
Decreased creatinine clearance	Alterations in drug clearance
Decreased capacity to concentrate urine	Potential for dehydration
Prostatic hypertrophy	Nocturia, hesitancy, and hematuria
Musculoskeletal	
Degeneration of intervertebral discs	Loss of height
Decreased bone mass	Predisposition to osteoporosis
Articular cartilage degeneration	Propensity for osteoarthritis
Increased fat to lean body mass ratio	May reduce serum creatinine
Endocrine	
Menopause	Acclerated bone loss and athereosclerosis; vaginal mucosal atrophy
Impaired glucose tolerance	Can cause misdiagnosis of diabetes mellitus
Selected impaired hormonal responses to stimulation	May affect endocrine function tests
Hematologic/Immunologic	
Mild elevation of sedimentation rate	
Impaired cell-mediated immunity	May enhance risk of reactivation of tuberculosis or Varicella
Skin	
Gray hair	Change in appearance
Decreased dermal thickness	Makes assessment of skin turgor unreliable
Increased wrinkling	Change in appearance; scars may be difficult to detect
Atrophy of sweat glands	Decreased sweating and tendency for hyperthermia

fied. These age-related changes in the eye lead to several vision problems: difficulty seeing in low light or in areas with significant glare, problems with depth perception, decreased perception of blues and greens, and difficulty focusing on nearby objects (accommodation). This constellation of changes is often referred to as **presbyopia.**

Hearing decline, referred to as **presbycusis,** also

accompanies aging. Characterized by a loss of ability to hear consonants and some high-frequency sounds, presbycusis is also coupled with difficulty screening out background noise.

■ Oral System

Tooth loss is not a normal part of the aging process. Until recently, however, most people older than 65 were **edentulous** (without teeth). Salivary flow is unchanged from youth. **Xerostomia** (dry mouth), although not attributable to old age, may be due most commonly to drugs (i.e., agents with anticholinergic side effects), connective tissue diseases, or radiation therapy. It can cause discomfort, diminished food intake, and impaired taste, and can also accelerate caries. Alterations in pain perception may keep older patients from promptly seeking the dental treatment they require.

Flavor perception, a product of both taste and olfaction, declines with advancing years. The thresholds for salty taste and bitter taste increase in older subjects; data for sweet and sour tastes are conflicting. Changes in taste may cause a decrease in eating pleasure and an increased reliance on salt and other spices to improve palatability.

■ Pulmonary System

Changes in the connective tissue of the lung and chest wall reduce the elasticity of the lung and increase the stiffness of the chest wall in aged patients, and pulmonary function declines. Total lung capacity remains unchanged; however, vital capacity drops and residual volume rises. A decline in the **forced expiratory volume in the first second** ($FEV_{1.0}$) has been noted in numerous studies. Arterial blood gas measurements indicate that the PaO_2 declines with advancing years. The following formula is used to calculate the PaO_2 of patients at different ages:

$$104 - (0.27 \times age).$$

■ Gastrointestinal System

An increased frequency of atrophic changes of the gastric mucosa has been noted with advancing age. Gastric secretion diminishes, and frank **achlorhydria** is five to seven times more prevalent in the aged than in the young.

Nutrient absorption is not changed significantly, but a decrease in metabolism and absorption of sugars, calcium, and iron may occur. Colonic diverticula are common but by no means universal in old people. A low-residue diet throughout life has been implicated as one potential pathogenetic factor for this problem.

■ Renal and Genitourinary Systems

Studies of renal function demonstrate a steady fall in creatinine clearance with advancing age. This change may not be readily apparent to the clinician, however, because older people do not demonstrate a dramatic rise in serum creatinine (because of reduced production of creatinine due to loss of lean muscle mass from aging). In a given elderly patient, creatinine clearance is difficult to predict. When the patient is undergoing drug therapy, checking blood levels and close monitoring are required to predict the precise dose and interval for agents renally excreted.

The urine concentrating ability declines with advancing age. This decrease, combined with an altered thirst mechanism, may easily predispose elderly patients to dehydration during periods of stress. Lower values for renin and aldosterone are found in either the basal or stimulated state in the elderly.

In men, benign hyperplasia of the prostate represents a common aging phenomenon. Bladder physiology has not been completely elucidated in the aged. Nocturia is reported by large numbers (60–70%) of nonselected elderly persons. Incomplete bladder emptying may occur in subjects who have no urinary symptoms, and residual volumes of 75–100 milliliters of urine may be acceptable. Bacteriuria is relatively common in elderly men and women (10–30%). The prevalence rises in frail, institutionalized populations. Usually, treatment of asymptomatic bacteriuria is not warranted in older patients. The cause for the bacteriuria should be considered; the extent of evaluation will vary with the individual clinical circumstance.

In elderly women, atrophic changes of the introitus and vagina follow estrogen loss. However, sexual activity remains possible into late life and should continue to be pleasurable—despite decreases in vaginal barrel elasticity, vaginal lubrication with sexual arousal, and the intensity and duration of orgasm. In older men, erections require more genital stimulation. In addition, seminal fluid volume is reduced, with less expulsive pressure and less need to ejaculate with orgasm. Orgasm shortens and penile flaccidity may quickly follow. The time from orgasm to achievement of next erection (**refractory period**) lengthens with age and may last 12–24 hours. Impotence or symptoms of sexual dysfunction should be pursued and never be attributed to age per se.

■ Musculoskeletal System

From adolescence through middle age (30–50 years of age), body weight steadily increases and then plateaus. (Although weight loss may occur in the later years, it is not predictable.) Body composition changes simultaneously. As a percentage of body weight, the total body water decreases, as does lean body mass; total body fat, however, increases.

Although loss of bone mass is normal in men and women throughout adult life, it does not produce clinical sequelae in all people. Thus, osteoporosis is not part of normal aging. Population studies of nonselected elderly show up to 50% of people have x-ray or clinical evidence of degenerative joint disease.

■ Endocrine System

Sex hormones

Menopause is characterized by declining serum estrogen and rising gonadotropin levels. As estrogen-sensitive tissues, subcutaneous vulvar fat is lost and the vaginal mucosa become atrophic, with loss of rugae. Estrogen loss also accelerates age-related bone loss. Testosterone levels in elderly men decline, but studies are conflicting. The normal range for testosterone levels is wide; subnormal values in elderly men should prompt determining whether the hypogonadism is primary or central and whether a specific disease mechanism exists for the hypogonadism. Depressed testosterone levels should not be attributed to old age.

Thyroid hormone

Similarities between normal aging and hypothyroidism are so striking that, at times, the diagnosis of hypothyroidism can easily be missed in older patients. Serum levels of thyroid hormone and thyroid-stimulating hormone remain constant into later life. The elderly hypothyroid patient requires a lower dose of thyroid replacement than a young counterpart; changes in body weight and loss of metabolically active lean body mass in later life may be responsible.

Glucose metabolism

Glucose tolerance gradually declines in older persons as the result of age-related relative insulin resistance. Standard criteria for the diagnosis of diabetes incorporate this age-related change and should prevent misdiagnosis of diabetes mellitus. Nomograms are available to assist with the interpretation of glucose tolerance tests. Fasting blood sugar is not significantly influenced by age.

■ Hematologic and Immunologic Systems

An apparent age-related decline in hemoglobin reported in some studies is mostly due to diseases or conditions that influence hemoglobin concentration. The adult norms for hemoglobin also apply to the elderly person.

Erythrocyte sedimentation rate (ESR) increases slightly in older subjects. The meaning of this increase remains unclear. However, marked elevations of ESR (such as those seen in polymyalgia rheumatica) should never be interpreted as related to old age. Leukocyte count and function remain stable into late life. The increased prevalence of bacterial infection in the aged may be explained by diseases that alter leukocyte function or by changes in organ systems that alter barrier function or impede leukocyte response to pathogens. Both the number and function of T and B lymphocytes decline. Impaired cell-mediated immunity may enhance the risk of reactivation of tuberculosis or Varicella.

The prevalence of autoantibodies (e.g., rheumatoid factor and antinuclear antibodies) in low titer increases in elderly patients. Although the clinical significance of this increase is unclear, the clinician should correlate such results carefully with the clinical findings to avoid misdiagnosis of rheumatoid arthritis or systemic lupus in the elderly patient.

■ Skin

To the patient and physician alike, aging is most obvious on the skin and hair. Pigment production within hair follicles declines; thus, graying of the hair occurs. Hair loss occurs both in men and women. Scalp hair loss is usually androgen-dependent, and a male pattern of baldness in a woman should raise suspicion of androgen production, possibly as the result of a neoplasm.

The skin becomes dry, wrinkled, and lax with age. Loss of dermal thickness gives the skin a transparent quality. Skin turgor is a notoriously unreliable key to assessing hydration in the elderly. Flat, pigmented lesions over sun-exposed areas are called **lentigo senilis** (liver spots or age spots); their incidence increases in the elderly. Interestingly, the prevalence of melanocytic nevi (moles) decreases in older patients; they are rarely seen in those over 80. Ecchymoses on the forearms and dorsum of the hands are frequent in older people; in the absence of any coagulopathy, they can be termed **senile purpura.** Changes in the connective tissues of the blood vessels and their surrounding skin may account for the leakage of blood into the skin with incidental trauma. Benign neoplastic proliferation of blood vessel components results in the frequently observed **capillary hemangiomas** (cherry red spots); these punctate, raised, bright red lesions are of no pathologic consequence.

Although not part of normal aging, a number of other dermatologic conditions are noted in the elderly; these include seborrheic keratoses and seborrheic dermatitis. The physician should assess the skin of the older patient for actinic keratoses and malignant neoplasms (such as basal cell carcinoma or squamous cell carcinoma) because their prevalence increases with age. The clinical features of these conditions are fully outlined in chapters 47 and 48 in part V, Dermatology.

Xerosis (dry skin) with or without pruritus is probably the most common dermatological symptom among older patients. The physician should consider and exclude conditions known to cause pruritus (e.g., renal disease, liver disease, hypothyroidism, diabetes, malignancies, and myeloproliferative disorders). Symptomatic treatment should include avoidance of excessive hydration by reducing the frequency of bathing or showering; using soaps such as Basis, Dove, or Tone; and using topical emollients immediately after wetting the skin.

CHAPTER 116 DELIRIUM AND DEMENTIA

Delirium and dementia are significant geriatric concerns. The physician should approach dementia and delirium as brain failure. Just as with any other major organ failure (cardiac, renal, or hepatic), the physician must determine whether the problem is acute or chronic and whether it is reversible—fully or partially.

■ Delirium

Acute reversible brain failure, referred to as **delirium,** is present in about 30% of elderly patients admitted to general medical and surgical wards. The search for a cause can be painstaking in view of the many possibilities; a partial list of possible causes is provided in Table 116.1. Drugs notorious for precipitating delirium are the sedative-hypnotics, minor tranquilizers, major tranquilizers, and tricyclic antidepressants. Other agents are listed in Table 116.2.

Patients with delirium are difficult to evaluate. History must be obtained from family, friends, and/or the nursing staff. The physical examination is hindered by patient uncooperativeness. The cardinal features of de-

TABLE 116.2.	Drugs Reported to Cause Delirium in the Aged

Amantadine
Antiadrenergic agents (e.g., β-blockers and central alpha-blockers)
Anticholinergic agents
Cimetidine
Digoxin
Lithium
Nonsteroidal antiinflammatory agents
Psychotropics (e.g., hypnotics, major and minor tranquilizers, and antidepressants)
Corticosteroids
Theophylline

lirium are a decreased awareness of the environment and impaired attention span (clouding of consciousness), perceptual disturbance (e.g., visual hallucinations and illusions), incoherent speech, sleep-wake disturbance, increased or decreased psychomotor activity (e.g., tachycardia, diaphoresis, mydriatic pupils, and fever), disorientation and memory impairment, rapid onset with fluctuating course, and the presence of some underlying organic factors. The foremost consideration in differential diagnosis should be a drug-induced delirium.

The prognosis of delirium depends on the underlying cause. Given a mortality risk as high as 25%, delirium is a true medical emergency, requiring skillful evaluation to define the underlying cause.

Therapy requires a gentle approach that optimizes sensory function, diminishes extraneous environmental stimuli, and incorporates familiar people, such as family members. Restraints should be used sparingly and caution exercised to avoid decubitus ulcers, peripheral nerve damage, and aspiration. Restraints are potentially injurious to agitated patients. Sedation should be used sparingly, especially in cases in which a drug is the suspected cause. Adding a second agent may only further complicate matters because many of the agents

TABLE 116.1.	Common Causes of Delirium

Drug toxicity (see table 116.2)
Infections
Fluid and electrolyte abnormalities
Acid-base disturbances
Hypoxemia/hypercarbia
Hypoglycemia or hyperglycemia
Hypotension
Intoxication (alcohol, other)
Hypothermia or hyperthermia
Sensory deprivation (ICU psychosis)
Fecal impaction
Urinary retention
Congestive heart failure
Primary CNS disturbance

TABLE 116.3.	Clinical Features Differentiating Delirium From Dementia	
Characteristic	**Delirium**	**Dementia**
Onset	Sudden	Insidious
Course over 24 hours	Fluctuating, with nocturnal exacerbation	Stable
Consciousness	Reduced	Clear
Attention	Globally disordered	Normal, except in severe cases
Cognition	Globally disordered	Globally impaired
Hallucinations	Usually visual or visual and auditory	Often absent
Delusions	Fleeting, poorly systematized	Often absent
Orientation	Usually impaired, at least for a time	Often impaired
Psychomotor activity	Increased, reduced, or shifting unpredictably	Often normal
Speech	Often incoherent, slow or rapid	Difficulty finding words, perseveration
Involuntary movements	Often asterixis or coarse tremor	Often absent
Physical illness or drug toxicity	One or both are present	Often absent, especially in senile dementia of the Alzheimer's type

(Adapted from: Lipowski ZJ. New Engl J Med 1989; 320(9):580.)

used to treat delirium may also produce it. However, in instances in which the patient is a danger to self or others and cannot be managed with nonmedical measures alone, drug therapy may be necessary. One approach in using drug therapy is to use a major tranquilizer, such as haloperidol, in low doses (0.5 to 1.0 mg) every 1 to 2 hours until the patient is sedated. The patient should then be gradually weaned off the drug. Management of such patients is further complicated by the possibility that delirium may be superimposed on dementia, with the premorbid mental status abnormal as well (see Table 116.3).

■ Dementia

Dementia is the chronic form of brain failure, afflicting roughly 10% of the population older than 65 and almost half of those older than 85. The major causes of dementia are **primary degenerative dementia** (Alzheimer's disease or senile dementia of the Alzheimer's type), **vascular dementia,** and a combination of these two. Together, these causes account for three-fourths or more of all cases of dementia. Other causes are listed in Table 116.4.

Dementia has several main features: loss of intellectual abilities of sufficient severity to interfere with social or occupational functioning, memory impairment, impairment of abstract thinking (e.g., concrete proverb interpretation or the inability to find similarities and differences between related words), impaired judgment, disturbances of higher cortical function (e.g., aphasia, apraxia, agnosia, and an inability to copy three-dimensional figures), personality change, normal level of consciousness, and an organic factor judged to

TABLE 116.4.	Causes of Dementia
Alzheimer's disease	
Vascular (cerebrovascular accident)	
Drugs (alcohol, others)	
Posttraumatic	
Degenerative diseases of central nervous system (Creutzfeld-Jakob, Parkinson's, Huntington's, Pick's)	
Space-occupying lesion (tumor, infection)	
Normal pressure hydrocephalus	
Vitamin deficiencies (vitamin B_{12}, thiamine)	
Metabolic disorders	
Major organ dysfunction (cardiac, renal, hepatic)	
Depression (pseudodementia)	
Infectious (HIV, syphilis)	
Vasculitis	

be causative. Isolated memory loss, especially short-term memory, differs from dementia and is termed **benign senescent forgetfulness** or age-related memory impairment.

The distinction between dementia and **pseudodementia** (depression masquerading as dementia) is important because depression is usually treatable. Depression is suggested when the patient is actively seeking medical attention; the onset is more rapid and is known with precision; the patient is aware of cognitive loss; depressed affect is present with vegetative signs; "don't know" answers are given to questions on the mental status examination; and behavior is observed that is not congruent with the severity of the cognitive loss. Neuropsychological testing, referral to a psychiatrist, and/or an empiric trial of antidepressant therapy may help

TABLE 116.5. Workup for Treatable Causes of Dementia

History
  Characterize symptoms (nature, onset, progression)
  Associated symptoms (urinary incontinence, behavioral
    abnormalities)
  Medications
  Alcohol use
  Past medical history (neurologic disorders, cardiovas-
    cular disorders, depression)
  Family history
Physical examination
  Blood pressure
  Mental status
  Sensory exam
  Neurologic examination
Psychological examination
  Depression screen
Laboratory
  CBC
  Glucose
  Electrolytes
  Renal function
  Hepatic function
  Thyroid function
  Chest X-ray
  Vitamin B_{12}, folate
  Syphilis serology
  Calcium, phosphate
  Electrocardiogram
Other**
  Neuroimaging (CT scan, MRI, PET, SPECT)
  HIV
  EEG
  Formal psychiatric evaluation
  Neuropsychological evaluation
  Speech/language evaluation
  Lumbar puncture
Abbreviations
  CBC   Complete blood count
  CT   Computed tomography
  EEG   Electroencephalogram
  HIV   Human immunodeficiency virus
  MRI   Magnetic resonance imaging
  PET   Positron emission tomography
  SPECT   Single photon emission computed tomography

**Studies may be appropriate in certain clinical situations.
(Adapted from: Anonymous. JAMA 1987;258(23):3411–3416.)

differentiate depression from dementia in cases when the diagnosis is in doubt.

The evaluation of dementia includes history, physical examination, and adjunct laboratory testing (Table 116.5). A history of hypertension, transient ischemic attack, stroke, abrupt onset, and stepwise deterioration indicates vascular dementia. Focal neurologic findings on physical examination suggest a localized central nervous system (CNS) pathology. Usually, a reversible or treatable condition is uncovered through evaluation in only a small number of cases. Yet, the human suffering that could be alleviated and cost savings achieved by reducing needless institutionalization through such an evaluation cannot be discounted. As with many areas of medicine, the evaluation should be tailored to the individual clinical circumstance.

As noted, **Alzheimer's disease** (primary degenerative dementia) is the most common cause of dementia, but its cause remains obscure. Genetic factors may play a role, but no clear-cut pattern of genetic transmissibility has been identified. A few families have shown an autosomal dominant pattern of transmission. Evidence suggests that the gene for familial Alzheimer's disease is located on chromosome 21. Data from twin studies indicate the importance of both genetic and nongenetic factors in the development of this illness. Putative nongenetic factors include slow-acting viral agents, environmental toxins and trace metals, chromosomal

TABLE 116.6. Managing Patients with Dementia

Optimize function
  Treat medical conditions/provide ongoing medi-
    cal care
  Optimize sensory function—glasses, hearing aids
  Avoid medications with CNS side effects
  Encourage physical and social activity
  Educate about good nutrition
  Assess the environment and recommend adaptations,
    e.g., OT home safety evaluation (see text)
Identify and manage complications
  Psychosis
  Agitation and aggression
  Depression
  Wandering
  Incontinence
Educate patients and families
  Nature of the disease
  Prognosis
  Advance directives
  New treatments and research protocols
Provide social service and legal information
  Community resources
  Legal and financial counseling
  Respite or institutional care
  Ethical issues
Abbreviations
  CNS Central nervous system
  OT Occupational therapy

(Adapted from: Kane RL, Ouslander JG, Abrass IB. Essentials of Clinical Geriatrics. 3rd ed. New York: McGraw-Hill, 1994.)

abnormalities, and deficiencies of neurotropic hormones. Neurotransmitter deficits in the CNS have been noted, especially concerning acetylcholine. However, attempts to modulate neurotransmitter levels have had limited success. Microscopic hallmarks of the illness include selective neuronal death, neurofibrillary tangles, and neuritic plaques.

In order to diagnose Alzheimer's disease, the patient must first meet the clinical criteria for dementia. Next, other known causes of dementia should be considered, using history, physical examination, and laboratory tests (see Table 116.5).

Alzheimer's disease progresses through mild, moderate, and severe stages. Patients with mild disease exhibit mild changes in memory and language. In the moderate stage, many behavioral domains are involved, and the classic syndrome is identifiable. Severe Alzheimer's is characterized by marked impairment of all intellectual abilities. Motor dysfunction may emerge. Death may be caused by aspiration pneumonia, sepsis from decubitus ulcers or urinary tract infection, or concomitant medical illnesses.

No cure currently exists for Alzheimer's disease. Physicians caring for these patients should help patients and their family try to cope with the illness. A comprehensive approach is needed in the management of patients with dementia, who often require the coordination of many resources. Some key management principles are outlined in Table 116.6.

Medications are being developed to ameliorate signs and symptoms of dementia. One agent (Donepezil) is a central acetylcholinesterase inhibitor that has shown some effect. Its use has been recommended in patients with mild to moderate degenerative dementia.

CHAPTER 117 URINARY INCONTINENCE

The involuntary voiding of urine is common in the elderly and is underreported to physicians. An estimated 15–20% of elderly community dwellers and up to 50% of institutionalized geriatric patients suffer from this condition. Transient incontinence should be excluded before evaluating this problem in depth. The mnemonic DIAPPERS (Table 117.1) is helpful in recalling causes of transient incontinence. Correction of these conditions may rectify the incontinence, thus obviating any further exploration.

Chronic persistent incontinence can be evaluated in the ambulatory setting. Important elements of the history, physical examination, and initial investigation are outlined in Table 117.2. Patients with large residual volumes (>150 ml) need evaluation for anatomic obstruction or detrusor dysfunction. A small residual volume can mean a normally functioning bladder (**functional incontinence**) or **detrusor instability** (small spastic bladder or uninhibited neurogenic bladder). It also occurs in patients (primarily women) with stress incontinence. Urologic consultation for cystoscopy and urodynamic evaluation may be required in some instances.

The main types of urinary incontinence are listed in Table 117.3. Therapy depends on the cause. Stress incontinence is managed by weight loss for obese patients, pelvic floor exercises, α-adrenergic agents to promote internal sphincter competence, and systemically or topically administered estrogens in women. Failure of conservative measures and demonstration of improper urethral anatomy may warrant surgical correction of the anatomic problem. Pads and diapers are adjuncts for refractory nonoperative patients or patients with a poor surgical result.

Treatment of detrusor instability consists of providing easy access to toilet facilities. Habit training (sched-

TABLE 117.1. Common Causes of Transient Incontinence
Delirium or confusional state
Infection, urinary (symptomatic)
Atrophic urethritis or vaginitis
Pharmaceuticals
Sedatives or hypnotics, especially long-acting agents
Loop diuretics
Anticholinergic agents (antipsychotic agents, antidepressants, antihistamines, anti-Parkinsonian agents, antiarrhythmics (disopyramide), antispasmodics, opiates, and antidiarrheal agents)
Alpha-adrenoceptor agonists and antagonists
Calcium-channel-entry blockers
Vincristine
Psychological disorder, especially depression
Endocrine disorder (hypercalcemia or hyperglycemia)
Restricted mobility
Stool impaction

(Adapted from: Resnick NM. Medical Grand Rounds 1984;3:284. Used with permission.)

TABLE 117.2.	Clinical Evaluation of the Incontinent Patient

History
   Type (urge, reflex, stress, overflow, or mixed)
   Frequency, severity, duration
   Pattern (diurnal, nocturnal, or both; temporal relationship to medication administration)
   Associated symptoms (straining to void, incomplete emptying, dysuria)
   Alteration in bowel habit/sexual function
   Other relevant factors (e.g., cancer, diabetes, acute illness, neurologic disease, pelvic or lower urinary tract surgery)
   Medications, including nonprescription agents (diuretics, anticholinergics, sedative-hypnotics, and adrenergic agents)
   Incontinence chart (frequency, timing, and amount of continent and incontinent voids)
Functional assessment (CADET)
Physical examination
   General medical examination
   Test for stress-induced leakage when bladder is full
   Observe/listen to voiding
   Palpate for bladder distension after voiding
   Pelvic examination (atrophic vaginitis/urethritis; pelvic muscle laxity; pelvic mass)
   Rectal examination (resulting tone and voluntary control of anal sphincter; prostate nodules; fecal impaction)
   Neurologic examination (mental status and elemental examination, including sacral reflexes and perineal sensation)
Initial workup
   Metabolic survey (measurement of electrolytes, calcium, glucose, and urea nitrogen)
   Measurement of postvoid residual volume (straight catheterization or ultrasound)
   Urine analysis and culture

(Reprinted with permission from: Kane RL, Ouslander JG, Abrass IB. Essentials of Clinical Geriatrics. 3rd ed. New York: McGraw-Hill, 1994.)

TABLE 117.3.	Basic Types and Causes of Persistent Urinary Incontinence	
Type	**Definition**	**Common Causes**
Stress	Involuntary loss of urine (usually small amounts) with increases in intraabdominal pressure (e.g., cough, laugh, or exercise)	Weakness and laxity of pelvic floor musculature, bladder outlet or urethral sphincter weakness
Urge	Leakage of urine (usually larger volumes) because of inability to delay voiding after perceiving sensation of bladder fullness	Detrusor motor and/or sensory instability, isolated or associated with one or more of the following: Local genitourinary condition (cystitis, urethritis, tumors, stones, diverticula, and outflow obstruction) CNS disorders (stroke, dementia, Parkinsonism, suprasacral spinal cord injury or disease*)
Overflow	Leakage of urine (usually small amounts) resulting from mechanical forces on an overdistended bladder or from other effects of urinary retention on bladder and sphincter function	Anatomic obstruction by prostate, stricture, cystocele Non-contractile bladder associated with diabetes mellitus or spinal cord injury Neurogenic (detrusor-sphincter dyssynergy), associated with multiple sclerosis and other suprasacral spinal cord lesions
Functional	Urinary leakage associated with inability to toilet because of impairment of cognitive and/or physical functioning, psychological unwillingness, or environmental barriers	Severe dementia and other neurological disorders Psychological factors such as depression, regression, anger, and hostility

*When detrusor motor instability is associated with a neurological disorder, it is termed "detrusor hyperreflexia" by the International Continence Society.
(Reprinted with permission from: Kane RL, Ouslander JG, Abrass IB. Essentials of Clinical Geriatrics. 3rd ed. New York: McGraw-Hill, 1994.)

uled voiding) and biofeedback are also beneficial. Drug therapy using flavoxate, anticholinergic agents (imipramine), oxybutynin, and calcium channel blockers have been used with varying clinical results. Although pads, undergarments, or condom catheters can be used in men, these measures should be deferred until other measures have been tried.

Whenever possible, urinary catheterization with an indwelling Foley catheter should be avoided because of the high risk of infectious complications. However, such catheterization may be necessary in patients with ana-tomic obstruction who cannot be surgically managed or patients with an underactive detrusor who cannot be intermittently catheterized. Patients with indwelling catheters should receive antibiotics only for symptomatic urinary tract infections because they may rapidly develop resistant organisms. The frequency of catheter change is empirical. Although monthly changes have been advocated, little data supports this practice. It may only be necessary to change the catheter when the flow becomes obstructed. Catheterization can precipitate meatal damage, stones, and urosepsis.

<h1>CHAPTER 118 DISTURBANCES OF TEMPERATURE REGULATION</h1>

Despite the association of heat illness with athletes or military recruits who perform in high ambient temperatures, and of hypothermia with winter sports or alcohol debauch, the fact remains that both conditions are most prevalent in the elderly.

The body maintains a constant temperature through a balance between heat generation and heat dissipation (see chapter 146, Temperature Homeostasis, in the part on Infectious Diseases). Aging alters the body's ability both to generate and to dissipate heat. Older adults experience impaired temperature perception, sweating, vasoconstriction, vasodilatation, chemical thermogenesis, and shivering, all of which place them at an increased risk of developing hypothermia and/or hyperthermia.

■ Hyperthermia

Hyperthermia (heat illness) includes a spectrum of conditions marked by heat cramps, heat exhaustion, and heat stroke. Whenever the environmental temperature exceeds the body's ability to dissipate heat, the possibility of heat stroke arises. Body temperature of 105–106°F in the setting of abnormal mental status, anhidrosis, and warm skin suggest the diagnosis. Some investigators found the elderly to show many differences from the young when exposed experimentally to a heat stress; older subjects may have a delayed return of core temperature to baseline levels, sweat less, and vasodilate less efficiently than the young. Factors other than age that are associated with heat illness include reduced activity; alcoholism; the use of major tranquilizers, anticholinergics, or diuretics; and the inability of persons to care for themselves.

Full-blown heat stroke is a serious medical condition, involving multiple organ systems. The manifestations of heat stroke include the following: altered mental status, volume depletion, acid-base disorders (mixed picture of metabolic acidosis and respiratory alkalosis), renal dysfunction, disseminated intravascular coagulation, rhabdomyolysis, and hepatic dysfunction.

Immersion in cold water is the most widely used therapy. Close monitoring of the temperature and other vital signs is an important adjunct as is supportive therapy for any damaged organ system (e.g., dialysis for renal failure). Use of salicylates is not considered beneficial.

Physicians should identify susceptible patients in their practice, especially frail elderly who live in inner-city urban areas and use the previously listed drugs. During periods of prolonged high environmental heat, these patients should be advised to wear loose-fitting clothing, ingest adequate amounts of fluid and salt (diuretic therapy may have to be suspended for a few days), take cool tub or sponge baths, and spend some time in air-conditioned environments, if possible.

■ Hypothermia

Hypothermia is defined as a core body temperature less than 95°F. Studies of the elderly suggest problems with both heat production and heat conservation when subjects are exposed to a cold stress. Environmental temperatures need not be extreme to precipitate this condition; even temperatures in the 60s (°F) may be sufficient to overwhelm certain patients. As with heat illness, certain elderly persons are predisposed to this condition. Risk factors include living alone, low income that causes inability to maintain adequate heating, the use of phenothiazines or alcohol, hypothyroidism, CNS disease (stroke or Parkinson's disease), overwhelming sepsis, and malnutrition.

Patients will present with mental obtundation; cool skin (especially over the abdomen or low back) that may be edematous; bradycardia (sometimes irregular); and hypotension. Muscles may be rigid from attempts at shivering. Neurologic findings, such as miotic pupils and upgoing plantar responses, can be noted. The key to diagnosis is suspecting the condition and checking the core body temperature.

Laboratory evaluation can show evidence of volume depletion, (e.g., high hemoglobin and elevated serum proteins), acid-base disorders (e.g., metabolic acidosis), disseminated intravascular coagulation, and hyperamylasemia. The electrocardiogram frequently will show atrial fibrillation with a slow ventricular response; the Osborn wave, or J-wave, may be seen in the terminal portion of the QRS complex.

Controversy surrounds most aspects of therapy. However, good supportive care and close monitoring and restoration of normal body temperature are essential. Predisposing conditions should be sought for and treated. In cases in which vital signs are stable and the temperature is 90°F or higher, performing **passive rewarming** by removing the patient from the cold, wrapping the patient in blankets, and administering warm IV fluids with or without warm humidified oxygen is a sufficient treatment course. Temperatures of 85–90°F require **active rewarming**. In addition to the previously mentioned measures, warm blankets should be applied. (Some physicians believe that active external rewarming with warm blankets or heating pads may be detrimental: the process may induce cardiovascular stress through

peripheral vasodilatation and return cool peripheral blood to the core, causing a drop in core temperature. These theoretical disadvantages for the use of active external rewarming are reported periodically in clinical practice.)

Patients with a core temperature below 85°F or with cardiovascular instability should receive **core rewarming**. Numerous methods have been described, including peritoneal dialysis, mediastinal irrigation, hemodialysis, extracorporeal blood warming, gastric lavage with warmed fluids, or colonic irrigation with warmed fluids. Each medical center or hospital will generally have at least one of these techniques available, with personnel trained to carry it out efficiently. However, where facilities exist, extracorporeal blood warming using cardiopulmonary bypass is the preferred method.

Ventricular tachycardia is the most feared complication of hypothermia. Patients with a temperature in the 80s°F or less may be refractory to the usual measures used to treat this arrhythmia. The outcome in hypothermia frequently depends on the underlying or associated illnesses rather than on the patient's age or the degree of temperature depression.

As with heat illness, patients who are at risk for hypothermia should adopt preventive measures. Sick or frail elderly should not keep room temperatures too low. Although 65°F may be adequate for healthy elderly people, 70°F may be required for the sick or frail elderly.

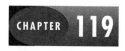

CHAPTER 119 MISCELLANEOUS SYNDROMES WITH INCREASED PREVALENCE IN THE ELDERLY

■ Accidents and Falls

Injuries rank as the fifth leading cause of death in aged persons. The elderly, who constitute 12% of the general population in the United States, sustain 75% of all fatal falls. Prevalence surveys indicate falls among one-half of all elderly women and one-third of elderly men.

In addition to death, sequelae to falls include fractures of the hip, spine, skull, or radius; disabling soft-tissue injuries; subdural hematoma; and accidental hypothermia if the patient is in a cool environment and is unable to get up. The loss of confidence and family anxiety that these episodes cause are more difficult to quantify, but they have significant impact. Falls are an indication of poor functional status and a contributing reason for nursing home placement.

The differential diagnosis for falls is lengthy (Table 119.1). The majority of falls are caused by neurologic

factors, not cardiac abnormalities. In addition, many falls are multifactorial.

Obtaining a careful history is essential. Observers of the event should be closely queried about whether loss of consciousness ensued and exactly how the fall occurred. Drug and alcohol history is important. The physical examination should be comprehensive and include a survey for serious injury. No standard laboratory evaluation is recommended for these patients. Instead, laboratory tests should be selective, based on the history and physical examination.

Most falls in the elderly are multifactorial. Patients can compensate for a single disability, but a number of problems can cause decompensation with stress. Corrective action in multiple areas simultaneously may improve the situation. Therapy depends entirely on the cause identified. The temptation to immobilize or restrain the "faller" must be balanced against the patient's wishes

TABLE 119.1. Causes of Falls		
	Nursing Home (4 Studies; 1076 Falls)	**Community Living (7 Studies; 2312 Falls)**
Cause	**% Range**	
Gait and balance disorder or weakness	26 (20–39)	13 (2–29)
Dizziness or vertigo	25 (0–30)	8 (0–19)
"Accident" or environment-related	16 (6–27)	41 (23–53)
Confusion	10 (0–14)	2 (0–7)
Visual disorder	4 (0–5)	0.8 (0–4)
Postural hypotension	2 (0–16)	1 (0–6)
Drop attack	0.3 (0–3)	13 (0–25)
Syncope	0.2 (0–3)	0.4 (0–3)
Other specified causes	12 (10–34)	17 (2–39)
Unknown	4 (0–34)	6 (0–16)

(Reprinted with permission from: Rubenstein LZ, Josephson KR, Robbins AS. Ann Intern Med 1994;121(6):443.)

and the risks from immobility. Patients may decide that the risk of a fall outweighs the isolation and depression that accompany impaired mobility.

Osteoporosis

A significant proportion of elderly people are prone to fractures of the hip, wrist, and vertebrae, which result in a serious burden of morbidity and cause a major economic drain on medical resources. Based on observed fracture rates, osteoporosis afflicts approximately one-third of elderly persons, primarily women. The approach to patients with fractures often emphasizes operative therapy and perioperative management; however, diagnostic studies to assess the etiology of the bone disease receive little emphasis. The usual x-rays employed to diagnose fractures cannot distinguish between various causes. (Osteoporosis is fully discussed in chapter 60 in part VI, Endocrinology and Metabolism.) Assessing and treating older patients for risk factors for osteoporosis is important.

Macular Degeneration

The leading cause of irreversible blindness in the elderly is macular degeneration. It presents with a loss of central vision. Examination of the fundus may reveal drusen and retinal pigmented epithelial changes. Advanced cases can show disciform scars, neovascularization, and retinal detachments. Therapy with laser photocoagulation has proved beneficial in selected cases; concurrent management with an experienced ophthalmologist is critical for success. Patients with irreversible poor visual acuity should be referred to a low-vision clinic. Local agencies are present in most large communities to help the visually impaired.

Pressure Sores

Pressure sores are localized areas of tissue injury that occur after prolonged exposure to pressure. Four factors contribute to the development of tissue injury: pressure, shearing forces, friction, and moisture. The National Pressure Sore Advisory Panel has developed the staging system in Table 119.2.

Two-thirds of pressure sores develop in the hospital setting and more than one-half of all persons with pressure sores are 70 years old or older. Pressure sores increase hospital costs, prolong length of hospital stay, and increase mortality. Risk factors for the development of pressure sores include immobility, poor nutrition, advanced age, urinary or fecal incontinence, and impaired level of consciousness.

The key element in pressure sore management is prevention, particularly in high-risk individuals. Preventive strategies relieve pressure and minimize the effects of risk factors (including immobility, incontinence, and poor nutrition). Pressure relief can be achieved with repositioning and the use of specialized cushions or mattresses.

The treatment of stage I pressure sores is pressure relief. Treatment of stage II sores involves both pressure relief and maintenance of a moist physiologic environment. Occlusive, vapor-permeable dressings (Op-site, Tegaderm) and hydrocolloid dressings (DuoDerm, Intra-Site) are often used for stage II ulcers. Stage III and IV ulcers take months to heal and require pressure relief, cleansing, and debridement of necrotic tissue. Debridement can be accomplished surgically, with wet to dry saline gauze, with irrigation, or with enzymatic debriding agents. Patients with a compromised vascular supply who have ulcers on their feet and legs should be referred to a vascular surgeon for debridement. The use of topical

TABLE 119.2.	Pressure Sores: Staging and Treatment	
Stage	**Description**	**Treatment**
Stage I	Nonblanchable erythema of intact skin, the harbinger of skin ulceration	Pressure relief
Stage II	Partial thickness skin loss involving epidermis and/or dermis; superficial ulcer that presents clinically as an abrasion, blister, or shallow crater	Pressure relief and maintenance of a moist physiologic environment
Stage III	Full thickness skin loss involving damage or necrosis of subcutaneous tissue that may extend down to, but not through, underlying fascia. The ulcer presents clinically as a deep crater with or without undermining of adjacent tissue.	Pressure relief Cleansing Debridement
Stage IV	Full thickness skin loss with extensive destruction, tissue necrosis, or damage to muscle, bone, or supporting structures (for example, tendon or joint capsule). Note: Undermining and sinus tracts may also be associated with Stage IV pressure ulcers.	Pressure relief Cleansing Debridement Skin grafts and myocutaneous flaps in special cases

(Reprinted from: Clinical Practice Guideline, No 3. AHCPR Publication No. 92-0047. Rockville, MD: Agency for Health Care Policy and Research, Public Health Service, U.S. Dept. of Health and Human Services. May 1992.)

antibiotics is controversial. Systemic antibiotics are indicated for cellulitis, sepsis, or osteomyelitis but not for routine pressure sore treatment. Surgical treatments (such as skin grafts or myocutaneous flaps) are reserved for special circumstances such as non-healing stage III or IV pressure sores.

■ Preventive Geriatric Health Care

The concept of prevention applies to the treatment of the elderly as well as to younger patients. Certain measures can stave off morbidity with its attendant suffering and consequent loss of independence. For example, diet or lifestyle modifications that affect the risk for osteoporosis or falls can improve the patient's chances for a better quality of life. Immunization schedules, cancer screening, and treatment recommendations for hypertension are discussed in other sections of the text. The reader is referred to chapter 5 for recommendations on immunizations and cancer screening. Treatment recommendations for hypertension are considered in chapter 176 in part XI, Kidney Diseases and Hypertension.

Nutrition

In general, the vast majority of community-dwelling elderly persons are adequately nourished. Obesity may be a more prevalent problem than malnutrition in the aged population in the United States. Studies vary in their findings of nutrients that tend to be deficient in the diets of the aged. Calcium, iron, and total caloric intake have been found deficient in the diets of some elderly subjects surveyed. Several vitamin and mineral deficiencies are more common in older adults: calcium, vitamin D, vitamin B_{12}, folate, thiamine, and zinc. Reliable serum levels are readily available for vitamin B_{12} and folate, but screening for the others should be guided by the history and physical examination.

A clinical assessment should include a history of weight loss or gain, edema, anorexia, vomiting, diarrhea, or chronic illness. Other factors that contribute to poor nutrition include poor dentition, sensory loss, disability that impairs food preparation or shopping, loss of taste or smell, alcoholism, mental deterioration, certain drugs (especially those used to treat malignancies), and low socioeconomic status. The physician should evaluate the patient's height and weight and look for signs of cachexia (e.g., muscle wasting and loss of subcutaneous fat), cheilosis (B vitamins), glossitis (vitamin B_{12}, folate, iron), edema (protein), or jaundice.

These simple measures should suffice for a screening evaluation when coupled with laboratory tests (such as hemoglobin, white cell count with differential, red cell indices, and serum protein and albumin). If undernutrition is suspected, performing a more detailed dietary history, physical assessment, and, possibly, further laboratory evaluation is necessary; a dietician may conduct these procedures. A plan for treatment will require identifying the reasons for the poor nutrition. (Clinical nutritional assessment is discussed in chapter 66 in Part VI, Endocrinology and Metabolism.) A careful assessment of dietary calcium intake should be made for patients with osteoporosis. At present, the Recommended

Daily Allowance (RDA) is similar for middle-aged adults and the elderly, with the exception of caloric intake, which has been modified downward for the older patient.

Physical activity

The value of physical activity in the elderly cannot be overemphasized. Exercise has been demonstrated to yield a training effect in populations studied into their ninth decade. Thus, improved cardiovascular function can be achieved with a regular program of exercise even in the elderly. Although there is as yet no proof, several other benefits are believed to accrue due to physical activity in the elderly. Retaining muscle strength and joint flexibility may allow the elderly individual to maintain better agility and thereby lessen the propensity to fall. As mentioned earlier, bone mass appears to increase with activity. Finally, from a psychologic standpoint, a program of regular physical activity may contribute to the individual's sense of well-being and improve the overall quality of life.

■ Questions

Instructions: For each question below, select only **one** lettered answer that is the **best** for that question.

1. The usual decline in function in the elderly follows a hierarchical pattern. Which one of the following is the correct order of the decline in functioning?
   A. Dressing, feeding, bathing, toileting, transferring
   B. Toileting, bathing, dressing, transferring, feeding
   C. Bathing, transferring, toileting, feeding, dressing
   D. Transferring, bathing, feeding, dressing, toileting
   E. Bathing, dressing, toileting, transferring, feeding
   F. None of the above

2. A 74-year-old woman has urinary incontinence. It was previously sporadic, but in the last two months it has worsened, much more so in the last week. At this point in her care, each of the following measures might have a potential role EXCEPT:
   A. The topical use of estrogen-containing creams in the vulvovaginal areas
   B. A 10-day course of trimethoprim-sulfamethoxazole if evaluation suggests a urinary tract infection
   C. A careful review of medication use
   D. The prescribed use of pads/diapers
   E. An inquiry about her loss of interest in her surroundings, disturbance in sleep patterns, and weight loss

3. An 80-year-old man is brought to the emergency department with somnolence, confusion, and combativeness for 12 hours. He has no history of psychiatric illness. His medications are ibuprofen, propranolol, and diazepam. He is febrile (101.5°F), and his lungs are clear. Serum sodium is 154 mEq/L and BUN is 50 mg/dL. Urinalysis shows 3+ bacteria, and leukocyte esterase is positive. Likely contributing causes of the confusion include all of the following EXCEPT:
   A. Drug toxicity
   B. Underlying dementia
   C. Dehydration
   D. Urosepsis

4. An elderly woman was found on the floor in her apartment by a vigilant neighbor. In the emergency department, her pulse was 98/min, temperature 91.5°F, blood pressure 100/60 mm Hg, and respirations 19/min. There is alcohol on her breath. She apparently takes 400 mg of ibuprofen 3 times per day. Which of the following is LEAST likely to cause her hypothermia?
   A. Pneumococcal septicemia
   B. Ibuprofen
   C. Undiagnosed hypothyroidism
   D. Alcohol use and inadvertent exposure
   E. Impaired shivering and decreased temperature perception

5. A 70-year-old man has fallen several times in the past month. He has no associated symptoms or dizziness. He takes digoxin 0.25 mg daily and warfarin 2.0 mg daily for atrial fibrillation and nortriptyline 20 mg at bedtime for depression. Supine BP is 140/80 mm Hg, pulse 70/min, standing BP is 110/70 mm Hg, pulse 78/min. Initial management will include which of the following?
   A. Discontinue nortriptyline.
   B. Discontinue warfarin.
   C. Prescribe full-length elastic stockings to promote venous return.
   D. Prescribe fludrocortisone 0.1 mg qd.

6. The most important factor when selecting a benzodiazepine for an older patient is which of the following?
   A. Antidepressant effect
   B. Half-life
   C. Potency
   D. Rate of absorption
   E. Sedative effect

7. Which of the following is true regarding dementia?
   A. Dementia is a normal part of aging.
   B. Patients have an alteration in their sensorium (i.e., there is clouding of consciousness).
   C. Most cases are reversible.
   D. Alzheimer's disease is the most frequent cause.

■ Answers

1. E	2. D	3. B	4. B	5. A
6. B	7. D			

SUGGESTED READING

Textbooks and Monographs

Hazzard WR, Bierman EL, Blass JP, et al (eds.). Principles of Geriatric Medicine and Gerontology. 3rd ed. New York: McGraw-Hill, 1994.

Kane RL, Ouslander JG, Abrass IB (eds.). Essentials of Clinical Geriatrics. 3rd ed. New York: McGraw-Hill, 1994.

Stewart, CE. Environmental Emergencies. Baltimore: Williams & Wilkins, 1990.

Articles

Clinical Pharmacology

Greenblatt DJ, Sellers FM, Shader RI. Drug disposition in old age. N Engl J Med 1982;306:1081–1088.

Delirium and Dementia

Francis J. Delirium in older patients. J Am Geriatrics Soc 1992;40:829–838.

Geldmacher DS, Whitehouse PJ. Evaluation of dementia. N Engl J Med 1996;335:330–336.

Falls

Rubenstein LZ, Josephson KR, Robbins AS. Falls in the nursing home. Ann Intern Med 1994;121:442–451.

Tinetti ME, Speechley M. Geriatrics. Prevention of falls among the elderly. N Engl J Med 1989;320:1055–1059.

Urinary Incontinence

Urinary Incontinence Guideline Panel. Urinary Incontinence in Adults: Clinical Practice Guidelines, 2 1996 Update. AHCPR Pub NP 96-0682. Rockville, MD: U.S. Dept. of Health and Human Services. March 1996.

Hyperthermia and Hypothermia

Weinberg AD. Hypothermia. Ann Emerg Med 1993;22:370–377.

Danzl DF, Pozos RS. Accidental hypothermia N Engl J Med 1994;331:1756–1760.

Simon HB. Hyperthermia. N Engl J Med 1993;329:483–487. Senile Macular Degeneration

Ferris FL. Senile macular degeneration: Review of epidemiologic features. Am J Epidemiol 1983;118:132–151.

Pressure Sores

Panel for the Prediction and Prevention of Pressure Ulcers in Adults: Prediction and Prevention. Clinical Practice Guideline, No 3. AHCPR Publication No. 92-0047. Rockville, MD: Agency for Health Care Policy and Research, Public Health Service, U.S. Dept. of Health and Human Services. May 1992.

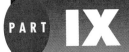

PART IX

Anthony V. Pisciotta
Janet R. Hosenpud
Tom Anderson
Kevin S. Madigan
Jerome L. Gottschall

HEMATOLOGICAL DISORDERS

CHAPTER 120

PROLIFERATION AND DIFFERENTIATION OF CIRCULATING BLOOD CELLS

Peripheral blood cells originate from uncommitted **multipotential stem cells,** which are essential for self-renewal of bone marrow lines. These cells also give rise to the precursors of each of the committed cell lines morphologically recognizable in the bone marrow, and whose mature products appear in the peripheral blood as the normal elements—leukocytes (including neutrophils, eosinophils, basophils, and monocytes), erythrocytes, and platelets. Each of these committed cell lines proliferates under the influence of growth factors, now cloned and generally available in clinical practice for supportive care. Figure 120.1 demonstrates the conceptual development of these cell lines. Operationally referred to as "Colony Forming Units" because of their historical identification in the spleens of irradiated mice, these **committed** stem cells are also referred to as CFU or Burst-Forming-Units (BFUs); an accompanying suffix delineates lineage. Thus, CFU-G refers to CFU of granulocytic lineage, that is, giving rise to granulocytes; CFU-E refers to CFU of erythrocytic lineage giving rise to red blood cells, and so forth. In the milieu of a healthy bone marrow, and under the appropriate "hormonal" stimulation (erythropoietin—erythrocyte stimulation; thrombopoietin—megakaryocyte proliferation; G-CSF—granulocyte colony forming factor, etc.) these colonies proceed to produce a large but limited number of mature progeny resulting in a normal blood profile. These committed colonies, however, lack self-renewal capability. Therefore, the uncommitted stem cell replenishes these clones of cells, as it responds to various feedback stimuli that are still being intensively studied.

The morphological identification of each clone of committed cells in the bone marrow is critical to sophisticated hematological diagnostic consultation. Each cell lineage is recognizable; aberrations of individual morphology, absolute number, and proportion in relationship to other marrow elements allows the hematologist and/or pathologist to render a diagnosis. The earliest recognizable granulocytic precursor is the myeloblast; during subsequent divisions and morphological maturation succeeding generations of cells evolve into progranulocytes [with their unique primary granules], then sequentially into **metamyelocytes, myelocytes, band** and ultimately **granulocytes** (neutrophil) forms. Unique variants of these intermediary stages of maturation are also recognizable for the eosinophilic, basophilic, and monocytic cell clones. During this process, the cells transform their appearance as their intracellular organelles shift from replication imperatives to that required for physiological function (e.g., granulocytes and monocytes require critical recognition and phagocytic abilities for defense against infections).

A similar process occurs in erythrocytic proliferation and maturation. The earliest recognizable erythroid cell is the **pronormoblast,** which evolves into a **normoblast.** During this maturation process, the intracellular cytoplasm changes from supporting replication to the synthesis of hemoglobin; this latter function is under exquisite, precise control, aberrations of which lead to significant consequences (e.g., thalassemia syndromes). Morphologically the cell cytoplasm transforms from an RNA-rich appearance (basophilic) to a hemoglobin-rich appearance (eosinophilic). The maturing erythrocyte's nucleus becomes progressively involuted and is ultimately extruded from the cell. Imprecise retention of nuclear fragments are morphologically recognizable in the peripheral circulation as **Howell-Jolly bodies, "nucleated red cells,"** and so forth.

Megakaryocyte precursors are converted from a mononuclear precursor to clones of cells with 4, 8, and even 16 individual nuclei, which undergo secondary fusion. The resulting characteristic bone marrow element, the megakaryocyte, is volumetrically 10–50 times larger than most other marrow elements and contains characteristic azurophilic granules and the serpiginous cytoplasmic boundaries. Through a unique "budding" process, each megakaryocyte, during its finite life-span, gives rise to thousands of individual platelets. Its unique appearance allows the experienced morphologist to recognize otherwise subtle underlying bone marrow dysfunctional states, as many dysplastic conditions produce smaller cells lacking characteristic granules, paradoxically termed **micro-megakaryocytes.**

During fetal development, hematopoiesis is widely distributed throughout the marrow cavity of most bones. Hematopoiesis in the fully matured adult occurs only in the medulla of the flat bones, ribs, the sternum, and pelvis (the latter two sites allow marrow aspiration and biopsy). Proliferating cells in marrow normally constitute 30–50% of marrow volume in adults; the rest is fat. At times of need (such as blood loss or infection), the marrow cellular area expands to fill the fatty sites and even replaces the fat in the long bones. Presence of active marrow replication in long bones of adults is always a manifestation of an underlying disease state.

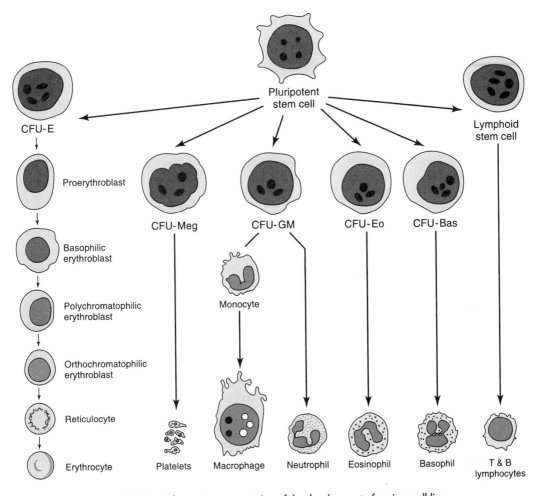

FIGURE 120.1. Schematic representation of the development of various cell lines.

| CHAPTER 121 | GENERAL ASPECTS OF ANEMIA |

In anemia, the hemoglobin, and volume of packed RBC (**hematocrit**) are reduced; with the exception of some thalassemias the number of RBC is reduced as well. Most anemias are secondary to other diseases and/or conditions; therefore it is imperative that the physician attempt to identify and correct the underlying etiology whenever possible. Symptomatic/supportive therapy of anemias is important, even critical in many circumstances, but one should avoid immediate intervention unless the patient is critically ill and/or a diagnostic evaluation has been initiated. While most underlying causes can ultimately be identified, indiscriminate use of

transfusions before obtaining simple straightforward tests should be discouraged.

The pattern and severity of anemia, coupled with the patient's history, provides many clues; patients with profound degrees of anemia with minimal symptoms usually have conditions which produce anemia over prolonged periods of time wherein the body can adapt to a lower oxygen-carrying capacity in the blood (e.g., pernicious anemia, slow chronic GI or menstrual blood loss, etc). In contrast, sudden significant anemia in a previously healthy person causes significant symptoms (e.g., dyspnea on exertion, easy fatigability, etc). The physician should inquire about diet, alcohol consumption, and blood loss. Because all patients do take notice of and usually seek medical attention for bright red blood per rectum, such rectal bleeding often does not cause severe anemias; conversely many patients fail to notice chronic melenic stools or the chronic GI bleeding may be inapparent, and severe anemia follows insidiously. Many women underestimate the degree of their menstrual blood losses. In those with consistently excessive menses, the mere reproducibility of it may cause a false sense of "normalcy." The number of pregnancies gives a clue regarding prior stress on a women's baseline iron stores which may severely compound other iron losses. Besides information about occupational or environmental exposure to potentially toxic chemicals, solvents, or medications, other useful data include family history of anemia, icterus, splenectomy, or gallstones at an early age.

Examination may show pallor. Although not always a reliable finding, pallor may give clues, especially when coupled with other findings of atrophic glossitis and/or neurological abnormalities (pernicious anemia—B_{12} deficiency), cutaneous and retinal hemorrhages (iron deficiency secondary to a bleeding diathesis, etc.). Cardiovascular examination may disclose tachycardia, cardiac dilatation, or flow murmurs; high output heart failure may be present with prolonged or severe anemia. Pelvic or rectal examination may show bleeding or its causative lesion (e.g., uterine fibroids with menometrorrhagia, hemorrhoids, cancer). Hypothyroidism is suggested by the facial appearance, slowly relaxing reflexes, and body alopecia. (Some other physical findings and their significance are shown in Table 121.1, categories of anemia in Table 121.2, and laboratory studies required in anemia in Figure 121.2.)

The RBC morphology in anemia has diagnostic significance. Because the normal erythrocyte population has characteristic features, deviations from the normal give insightful clues as to the general categories of anemias, suggest possible causes, and thus guide the clinician regarding prioritization of diagnostic testing. While examination of the peripheral smear is ideal, it is becoming a "lost art" among physicians; however, the clinician should at least be able to interpret the laboratory technician's report of the smear and/or the newer computerized values, including nomograms, etc., which calculate parameters with diagnostic implications. Variations from normalcy result from imbalances in nuclear or cytoplasmic development. Persistence of normal parameters in the face of significant anemia usually implicates that the anemia is secondary to multiple causes or syndromes, which also must be identified and assessed. Based on cell morphology and calculated red cell indices, anemia occurs in three categories: hypochromic microcytic anemia, macrocytic anemia, and normocytic normochromic anemia (Figure 121.2). Normocytic anemias have two subtypes: those with normal or low reticulocyte count (<2% or <0.085 × 10^6/mm^3) and those with elevated reticulocytes (>2% or >0.1 × 10^6/mm^3). Variations in the size of RBC are indicated by **red cell distribution width** (RDW), normally 11 to 15%.

Normocytic, normochromic anemias are those anemias wherein the indices suggest that the RBC production has not been perturbed by serious disorders in nuclear or cytoplasmic maturation, but the production rate is simply inadequate, either because the marrow is suppressed, or because there is an increased destruction rate or loss of cells. Most often this is due to a concomitant clinically active disease that is readily apparent. Depending upon the identification of such entities these anemias are historically characterized as the

TABLE 121.1. Anemia: Some General Physical Findings and Their Significance	
Finding(s)	**Significance**
Pallor + icterus + splenomegaly	Hemolytic anemia, pernicious anemia, or liver disease
Neck, axillary, or inguinal lymphadenopathy	Lymphoma, leukemia, or infection
Hepatosplenomegaly	Myeloproliferative or lymphoproliferative disorders, chronic liver disease
Sternal tenderness	Acute leukemia
Absent vibration/position sense and a positive Romberg test	Subacute combined degeneration of the spinal cord in pernicious anemia
Transient, focal neurologic disturbances + obtundation/ coma + hemolytic anemia and thrombocytopenic purpura	Thrombotic thrombocytopenic purpura (TTP) or hemolytic uremic syndrome (HUS)
Spooning of the finger nails (koilonychia, Figure 121.1), + dry coarse hair	Severe iron deficiency
Small (1 mm) well circumscribed red lesions on the lips or nasal mucosa	Hereditary hemorrhagic telangiectasia (HHT) causing severe iron deficiency.

TABLE 121.2.	Required Basic Laboratory Studies In Anemia		
		Normal Values	
Test(s)		**Men**	**Women**
Hemoglobin (g/dl)		13–16	11–15.5
Hematocrit (%)		38–50	36–48
RBC count (×10^{12}/L)		4.5–6	4–5.6
Mean cell hemoglobin (MCH [pg])		28–34	1
Mean cell volume (MCV) (fl)		80–95	
WBC count (×10^{12}/L)			4–11
Platelet count (×10^{12}/L)		150–450	
Reticulocyte count (%)			0.5–1.5

Calculation of red cell indices

$$MCV = \frac{\text{Hematocrit (L/L)}}{\text{Red cell count } (\times 10^{12}/L)}$$
In Femtoliters (fl: 10^{15}/L)

$$MCH = \frac{\text{Hemoglobin (g/L)}}{\text{RBC } (\times 10^{12}/L)}$$
In picograms

$$MCHC = \frac{\text{Hemoglobin (g/dl)}}{\text{Hematocrit (L/L)}}$$

anemia of "chronic renal failure", "hepatic disease", "inflammation" and so forth. In essence, if one identifies a clinically active co-morbid condition requiring intervention, and especially if there is clinical or laboratory evidence of other organ dysfunction, a mild anemia with relatively normal indices is most likely a secondary anemia and need not be aggressively evaluated unless its severity is out of proportion to the co-morbid condition, does not correlate with subsequent changes in the co-morbid condition, or is of such severity that treatment is required. In any of these situations one is obligated to test for other concomitant forms of anemia which might also be present, and whose treatment can be readily effected (Table 121.3). Normocytic anemias with low reticulocytes and a normal morphology occur in systemic disorders, whereas those with elevated reticulocyte counts accompany active hemorrhage, hemolytic anemia, or removal of a myelotoxic factor. Causes of elevated reticulocyte count are shown in Figure 121.3. The anemias mentioned above will be discussed subsequently in greater detail.

The clinician should be alert to the presence or absence of abnormal numbers or forms of other blood elements as additional clues. Immature leukocyte precursors such as metamyelocytes may suggest infections, myeloblasts suggest underlying malignancies including leukemias; if accompanied by abnormal platelet forms this picture of **"leukoerythroblastosis"** suggests an underlying myelophthisic condition due to metastatic cancer. RBC rouleaux suggests a circulating paraproteinemia consistent with an inflammatory state if polyclonal, and multiple myeloma if monoclonal.

Macrocytic anemias are associated with disease states where nuclear maturation is delayed relative to the cytoplasmic production of hemoglobin. While the list of specific causes is extensive (see subsequent discussion) the clinician should consider disorders in cobalamin (B_{12}) or folate metabolism (e.g., pernicious anemia [an autoimmune disorder], malabsorption states, GI diseases). Many drugs are responsible for iatrogenic macrocytic anemias, including all the anti-cancer antimetabolites such as 5-fluorouracil and methotrexate (which is also used in many patients with rheumatoid arthritis), imuran (used in systemic lupus erythematosus and solid organ transplant recipients), and alkylating agents for cancers. An interesting syndrome, common among members of the dental profession, is nitrous oxide abuse which interferes with B_{12} metabolism causing macrocytosis and ultimately, anemia and other effects of B_{12} deprivation.

Microcytic anemias are associated with disease states where cytoplasmic production of hemoglobin is delayed relative to nuclear maturation. If the patient can be documented to have had a normal CBC within the past few years, this implies a diagnosis of iron deficiency in adults; testing must be done to confirm or refute this possibility; if documented, iron deficiency must prompt a diagnostic search for the cause of blood loss. If there is previous evidence of a microcytic anemia, especially dating back to childhood, an inherited congenital form of hemoglobin synthesis dysfunction—a hemoglobinopathy state such as thalassemia—should be suspected.

■ Etiologic Factors for Anemia

Anemias can be conceptualized in many ways. One straightforward way is to realize that anemias are due to

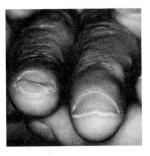

FIGURE 121.1. Nails of a patient with severe iron deficiency anemia showing koilonychia.

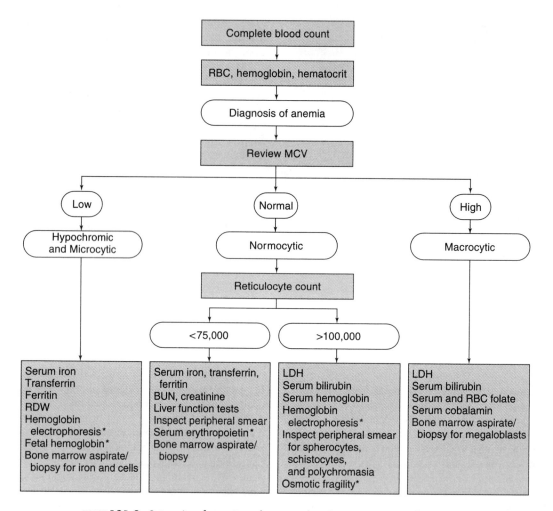

FIGURE 121.2 Categories of anemia and suggested studies. * = not routinely required.

TABLE 121.3. Causes of Normochromic Normocytic Anemia with Normal or Low Reticulocyte Count	
Abnormal Morphology	**Normal Morphology**
Aplastic anemia	Chronic disease
Metastatic malignancy	Renal insufficiency
Leukemia/lymphoma	Endocrine disorders
Myeloma/macroglobulinemia	HIV infection
Myelodysplastic anemia	Hepatocellular disorders

one or more of the following conditions: (1) inadequate production; (2) excessive loss; (3) excessive destruction.

(1) Inadequate production. Several substances are essential for the manufacture of hemoglobin or RBC: iron, B_{12}, folic acid, and certain hormones (such as thyroxine, testosterone, or hematopoietic growth factors, e.g. erythropoietin). Iron deficiency in the adult almost invariably is due to chronic blood loss caused by localized lesion(s) or from an inability to absorb iron following certain surgical procedures. The list of causes of iron deficiency is extensive; however, one should think in terms of anatomical causes, e.g., diverticula or angiodysplasia (bowel), peptic ulcer (stomach), and menstrual losses, excessive reproductive losses and fibroids (uterus). Iron absorption may be defective in malabsorption due to iatrogenic or other causes in the proximal small intestine (e.g., gastric bypass surgery), or disorders affecting gastric acidification (e.g., atrophic gastritis). Parasitic infections are uncommon in the United States, but still a major health problem worldwide.

Vitamin B_{12} requires **intrinsic factor** (IF), produced by gastric parietal cells to enable its systemic absorption from the gut. Without adequate intrinsic factor, B_{12} can not be absorbed in the terminal ileum, the site of its most efficient absorption. Thus atrophic gastritis, or pernicious anemia can cause inadequate IF production, and thereby cause B_{12} malabsorption. Similarly, diseases which cause inflammation or injury to the mucosa of the terminal ileum interfere with absorption, e.g.—Crohn's disease; surgical resection for such conditions produces a permanent iatrogenic mechanism for B_{12} malabsorption. Anemia from folic acid deficiency may follow nutritional deprivation or enhanced demand (late pregnancy) in the face of prior nutritional deficiency. It is exacerbated in hematological conditions that cause a constant excessive stress on folate metabolism (e.g., hemoglobinopathies, such as sickle cell disease or immunological states, such as autoimmune hemolytic anemia with markedly reduced RBC lifespan), requiring a more rapid production rate. In the United States, folate deficiency is only rarely an isolated problem unless the patient's lifestyle produces a constant behavior of nutritional deficiency (e.g., chronic alcoholism).

Important, potentially life-threatening conditions associated with inadequate production include bone marrow failure states such as aplastic anemia, myelodysplastic syndromes, myelofibrosis, or myelophthisic anemias (bone marrow infiltration by diseases, including cancer). Anemia of chronic infection, inflammation, or renal failure all represent dysfunctional inadequate production due to concomitant illnesses. These conditions should be identified and if possible, corrected; failure or inability to do so will lead to a chronic condition which may expose the patient to otherwise unnecessary expense, discomfort and/or blood replacement therapy.

(2) Excessive blood loss. Chronic blood loss is complicated by the resultant iron deficiency so that the patient's anemia is secondary to both excessive losses and compromised production. Blood loss should be relatively easily identified by performing a careful history, physical examination, and selected diagnostic tests. Durations of signs and symptoms are important, as are inquiries regarding whether the patient is aware of previous medical encounters which can retrospectively document the presence or absence of anemia. (Has this mother of five children, still menstruating heavily at age 45, *had* a normal hemoglobin/hematocrit, mean cell volume (MCV), or iron studies? Has the patient ever been prescribed iron therapy? At the time of elective surgery in the recent past was the patient anemic? Has there been use of aspirin or other nonsteroidal medications for chronic arthritic problems? Does the patient (and family) have a history of easy bruisability, irregular menses, etc.? Is there a family history of anemias?) Laboratory tests will quickly identify many sources of blood loss, e.g., repetitive examination of stool or urine for blood. The CBC findings, especially the RBC numbers and the MCV, will give clues to the underlying mechanisms of anemia.

(3) Excessive destruction. This usually results from immune challenges (e.g., autoimmune hemolytic anemia alone or as a manifestation of a more general immunological disorder such as SLE), a pharmacological stress (certain antibiotics in patients with underlying G6PD deficiency), or a congenital hereditary hemoglobinopathy such as sickle cell disease. Pernicious anemia exemplifies how physiologically complex anemias can be: while pernicious anemia follows nutritional B_{12} deficiency leading to inadequate production, technically, the failure to produce erythrocytes is due to intramedullary destruction of defective RBC owing to the B_{12} deficiency. The component of hemolysis in severe pernicious anemia exceeds all but the most severe, and unusual immune hemolytic states.

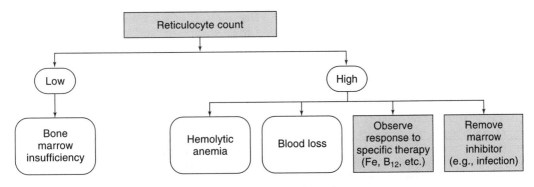

FIGURE 121.3. Causes of elevated reticulocyte count.

CHAPTER 122 HYPOCHROMIC, MICROCYTIC ANEMIAS

Hypochromic microcytic anemias result from a failure to synthesize normal amounts of hemoglobin. Iron deficiency anemia is the most common form of this type of anemia in adults; thalassemias are most common in children, and less common in adults, as are the sideroblastic anemias, a subcategory of myelodysplastic syndromes. Their laboratory differentiation is shown in Figure 122.1.

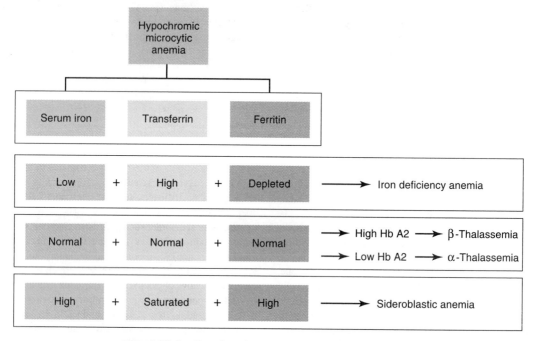

FIGURE 122.1. Hypochromic, microcytic anemias—an overview.

Iron Deficiency Anemia

Most functioning iron is included as constituents of porphyrin compounds (hemoglobin and myoglobin) and as trace elements of respiratory enzymes (e.g., cytochrome C and catalase). The balance of the total body iron is nonporphyrin, set aside for transport and storage. Iron is a highly reactive substance with the potential to cause serious oxidative damage to cells, especially as a cofactor with other oxidative stresses. Hence it can only safely be transported when bound to specialized proteins such as **transferrin.** Normally, 100 ml plasma contains about 300 to 400 mg of transferrin, which binds 50 to 150 µg of iron. About 1/3 of the plasma transferrin is normally saturated with iron. Iron is stored in the liver, spleen, and marrow as ferritin or hemosiderin. **Ferritin,** a composite of iron-containing micelles, is water-soluble, and is leached from cells during staining procedures, and is, thus, invisible in marrow on ordinary microscopy. **Hemosiderin,** an insoluble product made of multiple ferritin micelles (molecular aggregates) bound to insoluble proteins, is seen microscopically with the Prussian blue stain.

▪ The Iron Cycle

The iron cycle is depicted in Figure 122.2. About 10% of dietary ferrous iron is absorbed into the bloodstream from the duodenum. Bound to transferrin, it is taken to the marrow for storage or use in erythropoiesis. In the normoblastic mitochondria, ferrous iron joins with protoporphyrin to assemble heme (Figure 122.3). Heme is transported to the ribosomes. It then combines with two of each alpha and beta polypeptide chains to create the intact hemoglobin molecule consisting of four heme moieties integrated into the four discrete polypeptide chains creating the intact hemoglobin structure with its intricate tertiary structure and intermolecular charges which facilitate oxygen binding. Hemoglobin synthesis abates as the RBC matures, manifested by extrusion of the nucleus and cessation of ribosomal RNA-directed protein and heme synthesis. Once this occurs the human RBC has a discrete lifespan as there is no mechanism to further synthesize the proteins necessary to maintain the functional and structural components of the RBC. After a life span of 120 days, the enzymatically depleted RBC is phagocytosed by macrophages (Figure 122.2). Some of the iron is recycled via transferrin back to the marrow for new hemoglobin synthesis. Unused iron is deposited in reticuloendothelial cells as ferritin and hemosiderin (Figure 122.4). Excess ferritin is released into plasma; its measurement serves as an index of iron deficiency or overload because its serum level reflects tissue iron turnover.

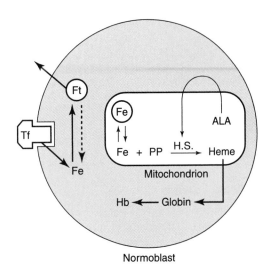

FIGURE 122.3. Heme synthesis in the mitochondria of normoblast. ALA = aminolevulinic acid; Fe = iron; H.S. = heme synthetase; Hb = hemoglobin; PP = protoporphyrin; Ft = ferritin; Tf = transferrin.

■ Iron Absorption and Distribution

The infant starts life with an adequate supply of iron at the expense of its mother's own iron stores. During the early years of growth, the demand for iron is met through diet. At the time of puberty, body iron stores are established. Adult men lose about 1 mg of iron daily (through desquamation, minor bleeding, hair loss, etc.); this loss is readily offset by a normal diet that provides over 10 mg of iron daily. Women, during their menstruating years, require about 2 mg of iron daily, depending

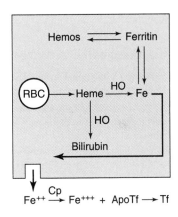

FIGURE 122.4. Iron disposition in the reticuloendothelial cell. ApoTf = apotransferrin; Cp = ceruloplasmin; Hemos = hemosiderin; HO = heme oxygenase; Tf = transferrin.

upon menstrual frequency, flow and duration. Iron loss is further exacerbated during pregnancy; each pregnancy entails a net transfer to the infant, and loss to the mother, of 700 mg iron, even before the continued increased losses caused by lactation and resumption of menses. After the menopause, iron requirements in men and women equalize at 1 mg per day, but many women enter menopause iron deficient, or at least iron depleted.

Iron exchange is almost entirely endogenous. Physiologically designed to avidly retain iron, the body lacks a mechanism to secrete or otherwise eliminate excess iron. Hence, any evidence of iron deficiency in the adult

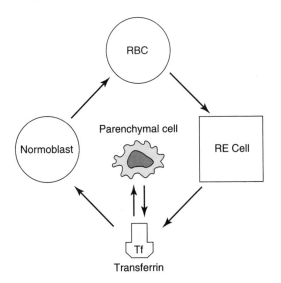

FIGURE 122.2. The iron cycle.

requires a careful search for the site of chronic bleeding. The major sources of bleeding are the gastrointestinal tract (peptic ulcers, reflux esophagitis, carcinoma, polyps, hemorrhoids), menstruation and pregnancy. Less common sites of blood loss include the nasal cavity, the oral cavity, and lungs (e.g., hemoptysis due to hereditary hemorrhagic telangiectasia or pulmonary hemosiderosis); urinary blood loss, as hemosiderin, occurs in intravascular hemolysis from paroxysmal nocturnal hemoglobinuria (PNH).

■ Clinical Features

Both the degree of anemia and the rapidity of its development influence the clinical picture. Symptoms may be completely absent or the patient may report variable weakness, light-headedness, and palpitations. Muscular weakness may occur, because iron is an integral component of myoglobin. Dyspnea may be caused by a diminished oxygen carrying capacity, although a deficiency in respiratory enzymes may also be responsible. The hair may be coarse and lusterless and the fingernails, brittle. In far advanced iron deficiency, fingernails show spooning (**koilonychia,** Figure 121.1).

■ Laboratory Features

Normal values for iron studies in the adult and their aberrations in iron deficiency are shown in Table 122.1. Iron deficiency anemia evolves through several stages. Early in the development of iron deficiency, storage iron is greatly diminished as observed by low ferritin values and depleted stainable marrow iron. The peripheral blood smear may be normal. As the disorder progresses, RDW increases, followed by hypochromia and microcytosis (Color Plate 22), then by anemia. Simultaneously, serum iron gradually declines, with a corresponding increase in transferrin and a progressive drop in the percent of saturation of transferrin. With the cessation of blood loss and initiation of iron therapy, these values gradually

become normal in the reverse order. The ferritin level and the bone marrow storage iron are the last to be restored to normal.

■ Management

The management of iron deficiency is twofold: to give therapeutic iron and to locate and correct the site of blood loss. **Therapeutic iron** is administered in the form of simple iron salts, such as ferrous sulfate or gluconate; composite capsules are best avoided. Oral iron, 325 mg daily provides 30 mg of elemental iron, far in excess of what the normal GI tract is capable of absorbing, even in the iron-depleted state where the mucosal cell receptors are upregulated to increase iron absorption. Thus the practice of increasing the daily iron dosage to 2–3 tablets should be discouraged unless there is a reason to assume underlying iron malabsorption. Higher iron doses causes

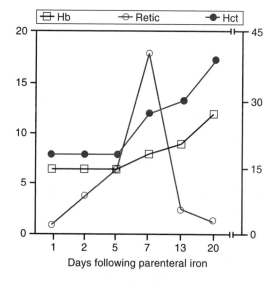

FIGURE 122.5. Response of blood elements to Iron therapy.

TABLE **122.1.** Laboratory Studies in Various Stages of Iron Deficiency			
Laboratory Test	**Early**	**Advanced**	**Iron Deficiency Anemia**
Peripheral smear	Normal	Slight hypochromia	Marked hypochromia and microcytosis
MCV (fl)	>80	75–85	<80
MCH (pg)	>32	28–32	<27
RDW	14–18	14–18	>18
Serum iron (μg/dl)	>35	<30	<10
Transferrin (μg/dl)	250–350	300–450	>450
% Saturation	35	15–30	<10
Ferritin (μg/mL)	15–20	10–20	<10
Bone marrow iron			Completely depleted

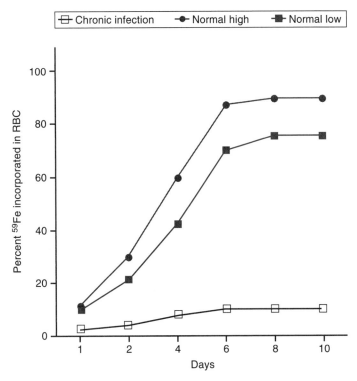

⊟ Chronic infection   ● Normal high   ■ Normal low

FIGURE 122.6. Incorporation of radiolabeled iron into RBCs in healthy individuals and those with anemia of chronic infection.

GI side effects and tends to promote noncompliance. Many experienced physicians prefer to use only one tablet daily to enhance patient compliance for longer periods of time. Adequate replacement will produce a recovery of hemoglobin of 1 g/dl/week (Figure 122.5). Oral iron should be continued for at least 6 months after hemoglobin level is normal, assuming the cause of blood loss can be corrected; if it cannot be corrected, life-long replacement may be necessary. If anemia is not corrected by an adequate trial of oral iron in a compliant patient, then an α or ß thalassemia trait must be suspected, although malabsorption remains a possibility.

Transfusions are not necessary for most types of anemia for which effective medications are available. Furthermore, transfusions are sometimes hazardous, and they may lead to a false security by ignoring the basic cause of the infirmity. While transfusions should be given for an exsanguinating hemorrhage or to prepare for impending major surgery, most patients with iron deficiency adequately respond to oral iron. Parenteral iron, despite its perceived risks is normally well tolerated and can very effectively reverse serious iron deficiency. However, it should be administered carefully under the supervision of a hematologist.

Anemia of Chronic Inflammation

■ Pathogenesis and Pathophysiology

Anemia of chronic inflammation (also called anemia of chronic disease) is a common form of anemia. It is grouped with the iron deficiencies because it is associated with a major aberration in the way iron is handled and not because of any morphologic similarity. Normally, when ^{59}Fe is intravenously administered, half of the plasma radioactive ^{59}Fe (T1/2) disappears in 90

minutes; it reappears in RBC in 24 hours and peaks in 7 days with 80–90% accumulation. In contrast, in chronic inflammation, plasma T1/2 of ^{59}Fe occurs in less than 30 minutes, and only a small fraction (<20%) of the dose reappears in the RBC (Figure 122.6). Most of the cleared iron is sequestered in the spleen, suggesting that reticuloendothelial tissues play a role in iron clearance during infection. Iron compounds are required to promote bacterial proliferation as well as hematopoiesis. Thus, iron sequestration may, in a manner of defense, help deprive invading bacteria of a required growth factor. Anemia of chronic inflammation appears to be mediated by negative regulatory cytokines, such as IL-1, TNFα, and TGFß, all of which inhibit erythropoietin production and produce hypoproliferative anemia with defective RBC life span.

■ Clinical and Laboratory Features

Many chronic inflammatory disorders cause anemia —pyelonephritis, osteomyelitis, bacterial endocarditis, tuberculosis, HIV, pleuritis, and rheumatoid arthritis, to name a few. Each dominates the clinical picture; the anemia is incidental to or part of the clinical picture. A low serum iron (frequently <10 μg/dl) and a low transferrin (as low as 100 mg/dl) indicate aberrations in iron metabolism. In contrast to iron deficiency, because both the serum iron and transferrin levels are low, the transferrin saturation is normal. An elevated serum ferritin (Figure 122.7) and abundant iron deposition in bone marrow macrophages attest to increased iron storage. The iron, iron binding capacity [transferrin], and serum ferritin levels in various clinical disorders are shown in Figure 122.8.

The anemias of chronic inflammation are usually normocytic and normochromic, although they may become hypochromic in later stages. The RBC or platelets lack a distinctive morphology, but an underlying infection may cause leukocytosis. Reticulocytes are less than 1.5% (75,000/cµm). The granulocytes and their precursors often display exaggerated ("toxic") granulation, which is an index of accelerated granulocytopoiesis. Dohle inclusion bodies in the WBC are an important indicator of pyogenic infection. The bone marrow shows granulocytic hyperplasia. Prussian blue staining of marrow aspirates confirms excess stainable iron, much of which is contained in the cytoplasm of the macrophages. The anemia and abnormal iron values all normalize if the infection is overcome. Erythropoiesis may be accelerated by using recombinant erythropoietin. Transfusions are rarely indicated because the anemia is not severe, but they may be necessary to prepare for, or recover from, intercurrent surgery.

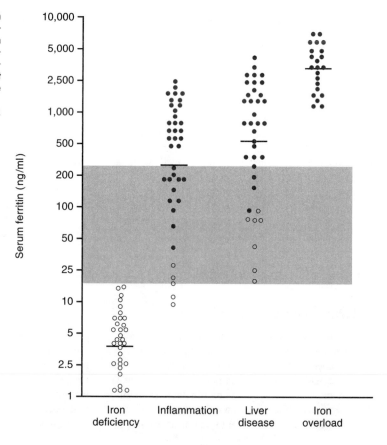

FIGURE 122.7. Serum ferritin in various clinical disorders. Horizontal lines indicate geometric means. Open circles show iron deficiency (total iron-binding capacity <400 mg /dl and transferrin saturation <16% and/or absent marrow iron). Shaded area shows the normal range.

(Redrawn from: Lipshitz DA et al. N Engl J Med 1974;290:1214. Used with permission.)

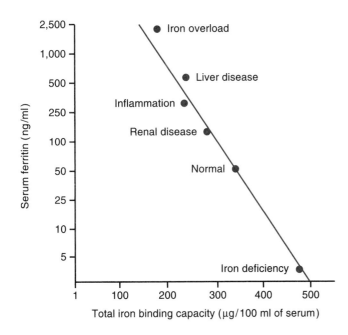

FIGURE 122.8. Serum ferritin and total iron binding capacity in various clinical disorders.
(Redrawn from: Lipshitz DA et al. N Engl J Med 1974;290:1215. Used with permission of publisher.)

Anemia of Chronic Renal Insufficiency

Anemia of chronic renal insufficiency is similar in morphology to that of chronic inflammation, but with some notable differences. While ^{59}Fe is rapidly cleared during inflammation (T1/2 = <30 min), its plasma T1/2 is prolonged (>120 min) in renal failure. The RBC lifespan is reduced by half when measured in the patient's body, but it is normalized if introduced into a normal person. This diminished survival is attributed to chemical damage from azotemia, oxidation by free radicals, and mechanical damage due to RBC fragmentation and membrane loss; this is often manifested morphologically in the peripheral smear by the presence of "burr cells." Erythropoiesis is somewhat suppressed by abnormal amounts of inactivated cytokines (IL-1, TNF-γ, and interferon-γ), but the major cause of anemia is due to inadequate production of **erythropoietin,** a glycoprotein hormone made in the kidney; patients with advanced renal failure have a defect in erythropoietin production. Because of this combination of a shortened RBC lifespan (nearly 50 days), and inadequate production due to erythropoietin deprivation, RBC transfusions were common in the past, often leading to iatrogenic iron overload states. The development of synthetic erythropoietin has somewhat ameliorated this problem.

Sideroblastic Anemia

Sideroblastic anemia is caused by a defect of iron incorporation into the heme molecule. The iron is retained in the mitochondria, where it accumulates, leading to a functional blockade of iron incorporation in RBC, and deposition of excess iron in reticuloendothelial cells in the marrow and liver. As a result, iron rises in plasma and eventually saturates all of the transferrin. The peripheral RBC display a biphasic distribution curve; some are large, but others are small with low hemoglobin content. Ringed sideroblasts, representing RBC precursors with excess iron retained in the perinuclear mito-chondria are easily seen in marrow (Color Plate 23), and are diagnostic.

Several clinical types of sideroblastic anemia are known. One is a rare hereditary sex-linked disorder involving only men; it responds to a degree to pharmacological doses of pyridoxine, which partly corrects an enzymatic defect in the first stage of heme synthesis. **Acquired sideroblastic anemia** may follow exposure to certain drugs or chemicals that interfere with various enzymes required in heme synthesis; possible environmental or medical causes include alcohol (inhibits heme synthetase), lead exposure (inhibits multiple enzyme steps), chloramphenicol (an antibiotic which inhibited mitochondrial protein synthesis, once the most frequent cause of sideroblastic anemia but rarely used anymore), and isoniazid (interferes with pyridoxine utilization, jeopardizing early

stages of heme synthesis). Another type, without obvious cause (**"idiopathic" sideroblastic anemia),** occurs most frequently in the elderly; it is included among myelodysplastic anemias. Presently, sideroblastic anemias are not curable unless an offending drug can be identified and removed.

CHAPTER 123   THE MACROCYTIC ANEMIAS

n **macrocytosis,** erythrocytes appear large upon visual evaluation, with an increase in both MCV and RDW. RBCs in normal newborns normally exhibit macrocytosis. In liver disease and alcohol ingestion, cholesterol may be adsorbed onto RBC membranes producing increased distensibility with resulting unusual morphology. Frequently, plasma cholesterol is decreased correspondingly in this type of macrocytosis. An unusually large proportion of reticulocytes may elevate the MCV, because reticulocytes are larger than mature RBC. Finally, RBCs may agglutinate when hyperglobulinemia or cold agglutinins are present, causing falsely high indices as the automated machine inad-

vertently counts clusters of cells. As a result, the MCV is falsely elevated.

Macrocytic anemias are disparate entities. In megaloblastic anemias, functional proliferation fails, because defective DNA synthesis leads to effective diminished mitosis; the result is large RBCs. Megaloblastic anemias are caused by a deficiency of B_{12} or folic acid or the failure to incorporate folate because of iatrogenic factors such as antimetabolite drugs used in treating malignancy or autoimmune diseases. Occasionally, myelodysplastic syndromes such as idiopathic sideroblastic anemia may demonstrate macrocytosis associated with ineffective erythropoiesis.

The Megaloblastic Anemias

■ Definition and Pathophysiology

Megaloblastic anemias are characterized by accumulations of large cells with disordered maturation. In cobalamin (B_{12}) and folate deficiency, all dividing cells show a similar abnormality: large size, inadequate chromatin due to deficient DNA content, and profuse cytoplasm with excessive RNA. B_{12} is an important cofactor in converting homocysteine to methionine to produce methyl groups. Folic acid transports these methyl groups (as $N^{5,10}$-methylene THF) to the site of cellular proliferation in order to convert uridylate (RNA base) to thymidylic acid (DNA base). Without B_{12}, methyl groups are not formed; without folic acid, they are not transported to sites of activity. However, with either deficiency, DNA synthesis becomes defective and cytoplasmic RNA accumulates. The marrow and blood pictures associated with B_{12} and with folate deficiencies are indistinguishable from each other. However, serious, even irreversible, neurological disturbances may follow cobalamin deficiency because of its unique role in providing fatty acids to protect the spinal cord. While folic acid may correct the abnormal blood picture of B_{12} deficiency, it offers no protection from neurological disease. Thus, it is essential to distinguish between these

two deficiencies and to correct a B_{12} deficiency. Incorrect presumption of folate deficiency with repletion may precipitate an irreversible neurological injury in patients with significant underlying B_{12} deficiency.

■ Etiology and Pathogenesis

Cobalamin is available only from diet. The adult daily requirement is 1.0–2.0 μg. In the gastrointestinal tract, cobalamin binds first to R-proteins and then to intrinsic factor (IF), a glycoprotein from gastric parietal cells (see Malabsorption syndrome, Chapter 70; and Figure 70.2). Cobalamin is released from the cobalamin-IF complex in the ileum, where it is absorbed. B_{12} is transported by several transcobalamins. Dietary B_{12} deprivation is exceedingly rare because of its ubiquitous distribution, its minuscule daily requirement, and its long biological half life; vegans (strict vegetarians), exceptions to this rule, sometimes manifest B_{12} deficiency after many years of adapting this dietary lifestyle. However the normally repleted patient will not manifest megaloblastic anemia for many months, often years after discontinuation of B_{12} replacement or the development of malabsorption.

In **pernicious anemia** (PA), intrinsic factor (IF)

deficiency causes B_{12} malabsorption. Autoantibodies are directed against gastric parietal cells, more specifically, the gastric H^+/K^+-ATPase. The gastritis that follows impairs IF secretion; ultimately IF deficiency develops. Also, antibodies to IF that occur in the gastric juice bind to the B_{12}-binding sites in the IF, thus preventing formation of B_{12}-IF complex. Partial gastrectomy severely impairs B_{12} absorption by removing parietal cells. B_{12} absorption may also be curtailed by ileal disease or resection; more unusually, this effect may result from competition for B_{12} from bacterial overgrowth in blind

intestinal loops or infestation with the fish tapeworm, *Diphyllobothrium latum*. Rarely, the cause may be exposure to nitrous oxide (either during anesthesia or by illicit use). B_{12} malabsorption ultimately causes B_{12} depletion.

■ Clinical Features

Anemia due to cobalamin deficiency develops very slowly, thus allowing ample cardiovascular compensation. Patients whose cobalamia deficiency is due to PA are

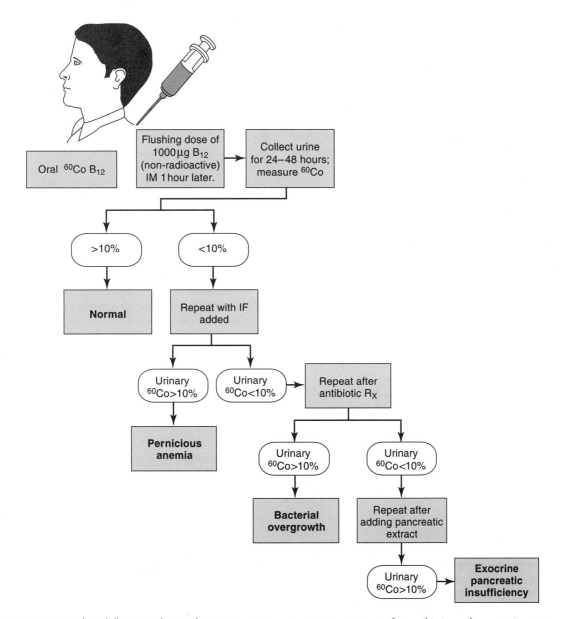

FIGURE 123.1. The Schilling test. The initial test is Stage I; Stage I + IF is Stage II. Tests after antibiotics and pancreatic extracts are Stages III and IV.

usually elderly. Pernicious anemia, an autoimmune disorder, is rarely seen in younger patients. Full-fledged cases exhibit severe anemia and pallor. An acquired intracorpuscular defect and ineffective erythropoiesis cause hemolysis, and, thus, mild icterus. Characteristic signs include papillary atrophy and an extremely pallid appearance of the tongue and buccal mucosa (resembling boiled veal). Angina, dyspnea, and eventually, high-output heart failure follow. Palpitations, vertigo, and syncope are reported. Because of cobalamin's unique role in myelin metabolism, its deficiency predisposes to several neurological changes: subacute combined degeneration of the spinal cord (impaired vibration and position senses, hyporeflexia, and a positive Romberg test), bizarre behavior (paranoia), and "megaloblastic madness" (psychosis). Because pernicious anemia is an autoimmune disease it is frequently associated with concomitant autoantibodies directed against other glands as well. Thus all pernicious anemia patients should be evaluated for hypothyroidism and the presence of antithyroid antibodies. Gastric cancer develops in 8% of cases of patients with pernicious anemia, a rate still greater than expected in the population cohort.

■ Diagnosis

In PA, there is complete achylia and achlorhydria (gastric juice). The serum B_{12} level is usually diminished. The diagnostic findings of PA are severe anemia, macrocytosis, leukopenia, and thrombocytopenia. RDW is increased; the RBC show great **anisocytosis** and **poikilocytosis** (vary in size and shape) often with large oval-shaped RBC dubbed "macro-ovalocytosis." The neutrophils are also large, with increased nuclear lobulations (hypersegmented cells, Color Plate 24) and "giant" metamyelocytes. The bone marrow is megaloblastic— large cells (large nuclei) due to disordered maturation (Color Plate 25). These changes quickly disappear when B_{12}, folate, or transfusions are given;

thus if a bone marrow biopsy is delayed even a few days the morphology may have reverted to normal leading to a misconception regarding the diagnosis. Patients should always have serum B_{12}, and folate levels drawn prior to replacement therapy. In emergent situations a bone marrow aspiration should be performed to confirm the diagnosis.

The Schilling test (Figure 123.1) is definitive for pernicious anemia even after the blood picture is completely reversed by treatment; it also distinguishes pernicious anemia from other megaloblastic anemias (e.g., malabsorption or bacterial overgrowth, Table 123.1). Normally, more than 10% of the oral ^{60}Co-cobalamin will appear in the urine. The diagnosis of pernicious anemia is confirmed by the Schilling test and corroborated by a subsequent transient reticulocytosis (10–40%) which appears 5–10 days after the first injection. Antibodies to parietal cells occur in 90% of patients with PA and antibodies to IF occur in 60%; neither of these findings is specific or as definitive as the Schilling test. Serum or urine methylmalonic acid level, which is 10 times higher in B_{12} deficiency than in folate deficiency or normal patients, can be used to confirm subtle, ambiguous cases wherein the B_{12} level is normal, but the bone marrow suggests pernicious anemia. If the bone marrow is not examined, then these tests should be done prior to an empirical trial of B_{12} replacement.

■ Management

Pernicious anemia is treated by daily injection of B_{12}, 1000 μg for 1 week with careful observation of the reticulocyte and RBC response. A lack of improvement means that a disorder other than B_{12} deficiency is present, and a search for the etiology must be continued. After 1 week, the injections may be continued at weekly intervals for 1 month, then once a month for the rest of the patient's life. Transfusions are not necessary as long as the patient responds promptly to cobalamin.

TABLE 123.1.	Radioactive Cobalamin Absorption (Schilling) Tests			
	Materials Given			
Condition	**Stage I: B_{12}**	**Stage II: B_{12} + IF**	**Stage III: B_{12} After Antibiotics**	**Stage IV: B_{12} + Pancreatic Extract**
Normal	Normal	Normal	Normal	Normal
Pernicious anemia	Low	Normal	Low	Low
Blind loop syndrome	Low	Low	Normal	N.A.
Pancreatic insufficiency	Low	Low	Low	Normal
Malabsorption syndrome, bowel resection	Low	Low	Low	Low

N.A. = Not applicable.

Folic Acid Deficiency

■ Pathogenesis

Folic acid, as it occurs in natural foodstuffs (e.g., fresh leafy vegetables), is a complex macromolecule—polyglutamic folic acid. Before it can be absorbed, it must be converted to monoglutamic folic acid (pteroylglutamic acid) by enzymes in the intestinal wall. Following absorption and blood-stream transport, folic acid passively diffuses into the cell, where it is restored to a polyglutamate storage form which prevents counterdiffusion out of the cell. The average daily requirement is 50 μg/day; its biological half-life is 3 weeks. The total folate body stores are small. After total dietary deprivation, serum folate levels decline rapidly. Sequential morphologic features of folic acid deficiency consist of hypersegmented PMN, macro-ovalocytosis, and megaloblastic changes in bone marrow. Four to five months of total dietary deprivation culminate in macrocytic anemia, in contrast to 4–5 years for B_{12} deficiency.

The blood picture in folic acid deficiency is identical to that of cobalamin deficiency, but it is often seen in younger subjects. Truly nutritional folic acid deficiency occurs toward the end of pregnancy, during anticonvulsant therapy, in alcoholism, and in malabsorption syndrome (tropical sprue, gluten sensitivity, or ileal resec-

tion). Increased folate requirements in pregnancy (or in sickle cell and other hemolytic anemias) may hasten its depletion. Anticonvulsants are believed to inhibit the enzymes that convert polyglutamates, causing a failure to absorb folate.

■ Management

The treatment of folic acid deficiency first requires recognition of the possible causes. In simple nutritional deficiencies or late-stage pregnancy, folic acid (1 mg/day) may be followed by reticulocytosis, and, later, by restoration of normal hematological values. The treatment of folate and other nutritional deficiencies in alcoholism is complicated by the many psychosocial issues of alcoholism. However, the nutritionally deprived alcoholic will usually show a reticulocyte surge soon after folate replacement, either through diet or as folate tablets, assuming cessation of direct alcoholic toxicity to the marrow. Folate deficiency caused by anticonvulsant therapy may be treated by the concurrent use of folic acid. In malabsorption syndromes due to intestinal disease or inflammation, folate and other nutrients may require parenteral restoration.

CHAPTER 124 APLASTIC ANEMIAS

Aplastic anemias result from bone marrow failure, which may be total or selective for RBC, WBC, or platelets. The hallmark of aplastic anemia is **pancytopenia**: anemia, leukopenia, thrombocytopenia, and reticulocytopenia; the precursors of these cells—normoblasts, granulocytes, or megakaryocytes—are absent in the bone marrow. Pancytopenia occurring with a hyperplastic marrow is not aplastic anemia; megaloblastic anemias, PNH, aleukemic leukemia, or related malignancies and myelodysplastic states warrant consideration. **Hypoplastic anemia** differs in degree, and usually there is some degree of persistence of neutrophil and megakaryocytic proliferation.

■ Etiology

Ionizing radiation (accidental, therapeutic, or military) damages proliferating cells or stem cells. Some anti-cancer drugs produce dose-dependent marrow depression, damaging committed stem cells or hemato-

logical cell lines in sufficient dosage. Cis-platinum toxicity also includes renal failure with its concomitant erythropoietin deficiency. Unless uncontrolled hemorrhage or infection proves lethal, the cytopenia is often self-limited: the unharmed, committed stem cells will repopulate the marrow when the drug is stopped. A few drugs (chloramphenicol, phenylbutazone, mephenytoin, etc.) produce marrow suppression only in rare, susceptible individuals. Benzene and its derivatives, which cause aplastic anemia or leukemia, are classic examples of chemicals or solvents that can enter the body by ingestion, inhalation, or through the skin.

Almost half of the cases of aplastic anemia have no discernible etiology ("idiopathic"). An immunological attack on uncommitted stem cells has been postulated in some cases, because studies have shown that lymphocytes from some patients with aplastic anemia can suppress granulocytopoiesis (CFU-GM) or erythropoiesis (CFU-E) in normal marrows in culture. Adding anti-thymocyte globulin to cultures of aplastic marrows may help annul such suppression. Similar cell-bound antibodies are noted in the lymphocytes or serum of congenital hypoplastic anemia of the Blackfan-Diamond variety. In some cases immunosuppressive therapy (using anti-thymocyte globulin, cyclosporin, or doses of chemotherapy drugs in preparation for a subsequently aborted bone marrow transplantation) has led to restoration of marrow function. Marrow aplasia may be due to a defect in the marrow microenvironment. Bone marrow transplantation, either by ablating the endogenous immune system and/or replacing a pool of stem cells, is an effective strategy to treat aplastic anemia regardless of whether the aplastic anemia follows immunosuppression of stem cells, injured stem cells or damaged microenvironment.

Pancytopenia with an empty bone marrow has been found to occur before or after paroxysmal nocturnal hemoglobinuria (PNH). In fact, if reticulocytosis suddenly develops during the course of treating a patient for aplastic anemia, it is worthwhile to do an acid hemolysis test to help distinguish between PNH and recovery from aplasia.

■ **Management**

Effective treatment of aplastic anemia is difficult, calling for interaction with a well-trained hematologist. It is extremely important to confirm the diagnosis of aplastic anemia, and to identify its etiology if possible, as the therapy is extremely expensive and potentially toxic, even lethal. Aplastic anemia should be distinguished from acute leukemia, myelodysplastic syndromes, PNH, and acute or chronic granulomatous infection. Potentially toxic substances must be removed from the patient's environment. This step is not curative, but continuing exposure to the toxic agent could otherwise protract the course of the anemia, and might prove lethal. The patient and all siblings should be typed for HLA-compatibility.

Once the diagnosis is established, a comprehensive program of blood component support, and concomitant therapy should follow. Transfusions are life-supporting, but may cause subsequent bone marrow transplantation (BMT) failure. Thus the physician must provide support, but begin an evaluation for possible BMT as soon as supportive care, and immunosuppression has begun. Initial therapy is designed to stimulate any residual clones of marrow precursors using androgens, and to oppose the offending immunosuppression by using anti-thymocyte globulin and cyclosporin. A limited number of patients will respond to this therapy, but rarely is complete hematopoietic restoration achieved. Unless the patient responds to therapy in the first few weeks, a search for a BMT donor must follow via family or national registry programs. While inherently dangerous, BMT is also highly effective, and for practical purposes, is the only cure for patients who fail to respond to initial therapy within weeks. If an HLA-matched sibling is available as a donor, and the patient not subjected to excessive blood component therapy, BMT is curative in 85% of cases.

If a suitable donor is absent, packed RBC should be transfused, as for any severe anemia. Platelets are transfused only as an emergency stopgap measure in limited circumstances: if the platelet count is below 10,000, if active hemorrhage is present, or if surgery is planned. A platelet count should be done 1 hour after the platelet transfusion to detect an acceptable rise in the count. If such a rise is absent, anti-platelet antibodies are suspect; HLA-matched platelets are then the only possible way to provide platelets for emergencies. Infections should be promptly treated. CMV, candida, and Aspergillus are frequently the causative agents. Broad-spectrum antibiotics are required if specific microbes are not found.

Testosterone with or without prednisone, while no longer recommended as initial therapy, may be used to augment the therapy with cyclosporin and anti-thymocyte globulin. Thymectomy is beneficial in the rare thymoma-associated pure red cell aplasia, but is not effective in true aplastic anemia.

CHAPTER **125** GENERAL ASPECTS OF HEMOLYTIC ANEMIAS

■ **Definition**

Hemolytic anemia is characterized by a diminished red cell survival time, which will be followed by anemia unless compensated by increased marrow production. An RBC survival time between 20–100 days may be offset by increased bone marrow activity. Anemia, if any, is mild, demonstrating that the normal marrow can sustain an increased RBC production of 2–5-fold. However, the limit of compensatory bone marrow activity is reached when the red cell survival time is less than 20 days. Any intercurrent illness which partially suppresses marrow production, even transiently, will exacerbate a previous borderline, compensated anemia. Successful management of hemolytic anemia requires careful confirmation of the diagnosis and then identification of the specific cause.

■ Diagnosis and Differential Diagnosis

General features of hemolytic anemias are summarized in Table 125.1. Several general clues suggest hemolytic anemia: an unexplained, abrupt drop in hemoglobin/hematocrit, sustained reticulocytosis, and elevated serum LDH. Leukocytosis often occurs, as does thrombocytosis; if the marrow is otherwise healthy, it will compensate by developing hyperplasia of marrow precursors, granulocytes, megakaryocytes, and especially normoblasts. More specific signs include elevated serum hemoglobin if hemolysis is acute and of significant magnitude, and a predictable decline in unbound haptoglobin (see caveats in Table 125.1), and the appearance of blood pigments in the urine. The classification of hemolytic anemias is shown in Table 125.2. Other conditions in which anemia develops rapidly may mimic hemolytic anemia, but careful clinical correlations can avoid this confusion (Table 125.3).

TABLE 125.2. Classification of Hemolytic Anemias
A. According to duration or length of course
1. Acute
2. Chronic
B. According to RBC abnormality
1. Intracorpuscular defects
a. Hereditary
i) Spherocytosis
ii) Non-spherocytic
a. Abnormalities in Embden-Meyerhof pathway
b. Deficiency of G-6PD
iii) The hemoglobinopathies
a. Sickle cell anemia
b. Hemoglobin-C disease
c. Unstable hemoglobin—the Heinz body anemias
b. Non-hereditary
i) Paroxysmal nocturnal hemoglobinuria
2. Extracorpuscular—all acquired
a. Immune
b. Non immune
c. Drug-induced
d. Mechanical fragmentation

TABLE 125.1. General Features of Hemolytic Anemias Feature

Feature	Finding/Observation	Comment
Degree of anemia	Highly variable	Hb ranges from 11–12 g when well compensated to <2 grams when severe
Pattern of anemia	Normocytic and normochromic	May be macrocytic with reticulocytosis
Morphologic abnormalities	Not specific	
	None	In PNH
	Spherocytes	Hereditary spherocytosis/certain immune hemolytic anemias
	Peculiar RBC structures (sickle cells, target cells, or RBC inclusion bodies	The hemoglobinopathies
	Schistocytes	Microangiopathy
Serum lactate dehydrogenase (LDH)	Increased from release of contents of hemolyzed cells into plasma	Non-specific for hemolytic anemia
Serum hemoglobin	Rises in intravascular hemolytic anemias	Must be drawn and interpreted with care (normal RBC may disintegrate on venipuncture)
Serum haptoglobin	Disappears	Haptoglobin depleted in severe liver disease; interpret test carefully if there is decompensated liver disease.
Urinary hemoglobin, hemosiderin, and methemalbumin	Present in and confirms intravascular hemolysis	Hemoglobin not bound by haptoglobin spills into the urine
Splenomegaly	Frequent in hemolysis primarily by phagocytosis in reticuloendothelial sinusoids	
Sustained reticulocytosis	Often indirectly identifies hemolytic anemia	Highly sensitive, but not specific
Normoblasts in peripheral blood	Present with brisk hemolysis	Nonspecific

TABLE 125.3. Disorders That May Be Confused With Hemolytic Anemias

Disorder/Condition	Cause for Confusion
Rapid hydration in severe dehydration	Sudden drop in hemoglobin and hematocrit
Anemia with severe hemorrhage	Reticulocytosis
Folate, iron, or B_{12} replacement in anemias due to their deficiencies	Reticulocytosis
Nutrition and alcohol cessation in alcohol-related marrow failure	Reticulocytosis
Anemia + jaundice, but no bilirubinuria	Unconjugated hyperbilirubinemia
Myoglobinuria (traumatic/exertional)	Positive test for urine hemoglobin
Bleeding into muscle or a body cavity (e.g., ruptured ectopic gestation)	Anemia, icterus and reticulocytosis

■ Pigment Metabolism in Hemolytic Anemia

RBC senescence occurs when their supply of energy-related enzymes is depleted with resultant ATP depletion. Once this occurs, the RBC can no longer actively pump sodium and water back out of the cell, leading to engorgement, relative membrane rigidity and fragility; such cells get trapped in the splenic macrophages and undergo hemolysis. Their components are then recycled or excreted. Iron is returned to the iron pool for hemoglobin synthesis and amino acids are reused for protein synthesis. Heme is recycled but may be converted to bilirubin faster than it can be conjugated and/or excreted by the normal mechanisms demonstrated in Figure 98.3, leading to jaundice. In the intestine, bilirubin is converted to the fecal pigments known as **stercobilin,** and to **urobilinogen,** a soluble, colorless product.

Part of the hemoglobin discharged to the plasma during intravascular hemolysis is oxidized to **methemoglobin,** which binds to plasma albumin to form **methemalbumin,** an elevated level of which indicates intravascular hemolysis. The remaining (90%) hemoglobin from hemolyzed RBC is conjugated by haptoglobin and recycled to the bone marrow and other iron storage sites. Although haptoglobin is an acute phase reactant, its production can increase. When hemolysis shortens RBC survival below 30 days, free haptoglobin disappears from the plasma, and serum free hemoglobin begins to rise. Serum free hemoglobin above 100 mg/ml is freely filtered by the kidney and enters the urine as methemoglobin and hemosiderin. The presence of any or all of these pigments in urine is *prima facie* evidence for significant intravascular hemolysis.

CHAPTER 126 HEMOLYTIC ANEMIAS DUE TO INTRACORPUSCULAR DEFECTS

The RBC membrane is a complex structure providing important structural integrity to the cell, but even more importantly providing the matrix for a complex series of enzymatic and metabolic activities pivotal for cell integrity. The cell membrane retains critical intracellular elements from leaking out of the cell and depleting it of metabolic support prematurely. It functions to anchor critical intracellular processes to the submembrane region of the cell, maintaining cation and water transport. Besides being a barrier to exogenous and often dangerous compounds, it maintains the basic structure of RBC as a biconcave disc. It must maintain its

normal plasticity and distensibility to allow RBCs to traverse the extensive capillary structures in all organs. Protein comprises 50% of the RBC membrane; it consists of spectrin, actin, ankyrin, and protein 4.1. About 10% of the RBC membrane is carbohydrate, organized as glycophorin and sialic acid; it produces a negative charge, enabling RBC to repel each other to remain in discrete suspension. Thus aberrations of RBC membrane structure and function lead to a complex and diverse spectrum of hemolytic anemias referred to as (inherent) intracorpuscular defects.

Hereditary Spherocytosis

Hereditary spherocytosis (HS) is an autosomal dominant disorder with mild hemolytic anemia in which RBC maintain a normal mean volume but a smaller surface area. The RBCs are small, with a dense, globular appearance, and lack central pallor.

Pathophysiology

The RBC membrane is very permeable to sodium and water, which require active ejection by an energy-consuming ATP pump. HS is characterized by a deficiency of spectrin, ankyrin band 3, or protein 4.2 in the RBC membrane; this abnormal protein structure results in dysfunctional changes in membrane distensibility which in turn confer a spherical appearance and peculiar thickness to the RBC. These cells are also poorly deformable and thus undergo retention and stasis in the narrow splenic sinusoids. The erythrocyte suffers a relative depletion of plasma and glucose, compromising the ATP pump function; the entrapped, now rigid spherocytes are then phagocytized by splenic macrophages. Transfused normal RBC survive normally in the HS patient, and the HS RBC survive normally when transfused into a splenectomized individual (normal T1/2 using ^{51}Cr tagged RBC, 25–35 days). However, the HS RBC survival is considerably shortened in HS patients with an intact spleen (T1/2 <10 days).

Clinical Features

Patients with HS adapt so well to their mild anemia present since birth that they are often asymptomatic. The medical interview may elicit a history of gallstones at an early age in the patient, a sibling, or a parent; frequently there is a family history of "yellow eyes" and splenectomy. The icterus is mild and frequently overlooked. Obvious splenomegaly is invariable, unless there has been prior splenectomy; intractable leg ulcers are seen at times over bony prominences.

Severe crises may occur, frequently preceded by brief fever, myalgia, and malaise ("viral syndrome"); these are caused by a parvovirus B-19 infection, which inhibits cellular proliferation. Cluster cases of aplastic crisis may affect multiple members of the same family, if in close proximity. The crises display a life-threatening, precipitous drop in RBC due to inhibition of RBC production and a persistently shortened RBC lifespan. The previous compensatory recticulocytosis is aborted. Consistent with the theory of an intercurrent viral infection, mild leukopenia and thrombocytopenia are also noted. Chronic hemolysis creates an increased demand for folate, and unless a higher folate intake is maintained, such patients can develop a concomitant megaloblastic anemia; such a superimposed ineffective erythropoiesis may greatly intensify anemia in the setting of chronic increased hemolysis.

Laboratory Features

The characteristic blood picture consists of well-compensated anemia and a double erythrocyte population (also indicated by a high RDW), consisting of spherocytes (small diameter, a globular shape, and a dense appearance with no central pallor) and reticulocytes (bluish-gray, "polychromatophilic" cells). Reticulocytosis is a constant, invariable compensatory phenomenon, unless there is aplastic crisis and/or splenectomy. Spherocytosis is indirectly determined by **increased osmotic fragility** wherein these cells demonstrate increased hemolysis to hypotonic solution because of the aforementioned membrane deficiency. Thus the HS patient's RBCs begin to undergo lysis at saline concentrations of 0.64% and are virtually completely hemolyzed in saline concentrations as low as 0.5%, the level at which normal RBCs just begin to hemolyze. Unless there is a viral infection or marked folate depletion, the bone marrow shows pronounced normoblastic hyperplasia. In an aplastic crisis, no RBC precursors are present.

Management

With an established diagnosis of HS, the only treatment is splenectomy. Splenectomy produces a normal RBC life span, restores the erythrocyte count to normal, dispels the risk of future aplastic crises, and removes the risk of further bilirubin gallstone formation. However, the spherocytic defect and the increased osmotic fragility remain and can be confirmed by laboratory testing. Because of the risks of overwhelming sepsis from encapsulated bacteria, all afflicted teenagers should receive pneumococcal vaccination and splenectomy delayed until adulthood if possible.

Other Hereditary Intracorpuscular Defects

The mature erythrocyte consumes glucose as its chief source of energy; each step is controlled by a different enzyme. The glycolytic process consists of two major components: the anaerobic (Embden-Meyerhof) pathway and the aerobic hexose monophosphate shunt (Figure 126.1). Hereditary defects at certain stages of each component can lead to nonspherocytic hemolytic anemia.

The Anaerobic Pathway

In the RBC, 90% of glucose undergoes anaerobic glycolysis; this process generates ATP in order to maintain active transport. The key enzymes involved are phosphoglycerate kinase (which produces two moles of ATP per mole of glucose) and pyruvate kinase (which produces two more moles of ATP later in the sequence). The end product of the Embden-Meyerhof pathway is

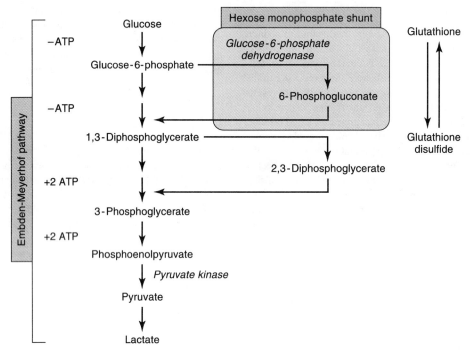

FIGURE 126.1. Embden-Meyerhof pathway and the hexose monophosphate shunt.

lactate (Figure 126.1), but there is also a net gain of four moles of ATP. Without ATP generation at each of these loci, less ATP is produced and active transport is lost. Notably, the resulting hemolysis from accumulation of cations and water in the RBC mostly affects the older cells, which have diminished concentrations of ATP and enzymes.

Laboratory tests to affirm red cell enzymopathies and intracorpuscular hemolytic anemias require direct assays for pyruvate kinase or other key enzymes. These assays are expensive, tedious, and not generally available. Indirect evidence for glycolytic defects is provided by an estimate of increased autohemolysis that is corrected entirely by ATP, or by glucose and ATP.

■ The Hexose Monophosphate Shunt

When malaria prophylaxis was instituted in the military, almost 10% of black men receiving primaquine suffered severe intravascular hemolysis; the outcome was attributed to an inherent defect in their RBC that remained subclinical until exposure to an oxidant drug (e.g., primaquine). It was accompanied by an accumulation of **Heinz-Ehrlich bodies** and unstable glutathione

of RBC subjected to oxidants. Later, disordered glycolysis within the hexose monophosphate shunt (HMS) was identified as the cause.

Glucose-6 phosphate dehydrogenase (G-6PD) is a vital component of the HMS; it keeps triphosphopyridine nucleotide (TPN) in a functional or reduced state (TPNH). This system continually provides hydrogen ions, which maintain glutathione in the reduced state (GSH) to maintain methemoglobin reductase and eventually to protect hemoglobin from oxidation. Diminished HMS activities generate H_2O_2. This oxidant denatures hemoglobin to produce Heinz bodies and compromises the RBC membrane integrity. RBC life span is believed to be limited by G-6PD activity. A mutant enzyme with a life span less than that of normal RBC correspondingly diminishes the RBC survival. G-6PD deficiency is an X-linked recessive trait. Hemolysis from exposure to various oxidant drugs (Table 126.1), vegetables (fava beans, henna, senna), diabetic ketoacidosis, and infections affects only RBC. Platelets and WBC, however, turn over more rapidly than the T 1/2 of G-6PD and never grow old enough to undergo lysis due to G-6PD deficiency.

The Hemoglobinopathies

Hemoglobinopathies are summarized in Table 126.2. Many of these mutations have been found in single individuals or families. The most common hemoglobinopathies are more widely dispersed, and will be described further.

Sickle Cell Anemia

Sickle cell anemia is a hereditary disorder of hemoglobin structure produced by a mutant replacement of valine for glutamic acid in position 6 of the ß polypeptide chain (Table 126.2). The hemoglobin polymerizes to an elongated fibrocrystalline structure, especially during hypoxia, dehydration, or infection. These rigid crystals force the RBC membrane to elongate; the intertwined, affected RBCs occlude small blood vessels. Areas supplied by the occluded blood vessels undergo necrosis. Hemolytic anemia is a constant feature, arising from shortened RBC lifespan due to these relatively rigid cells and is confirmed by evidence of anemia, with accompanying reticulocytosis, decreased haptoglobin, elevated LDH, and sickle cells (Color Plate 26).

■ Clinical Features

Symptoms of sickle cell anemia develop around 4 to 6 months of age, concomitant with the physiological change from fetal to adult hemoglobin synthesis. Recurrent vascular occlusion can occur in almost any organ. Repeated, painful bone infarcts with malformation and avascular necrosis commonly occur. Pulmonary fibrosis and progressive pulmonary hypertension also evolve from repeated infarcts. Myocardial infarcts cause ventricular dysfunction. Cerebral infarcts produce stroke-like syndromes. Recurrent renal infarctions lead to an inability to concentrate urine (isosthenuria) which further exacerbates sickle crisis during periods of pyrexia. Functional asplenism resulting from splenic infarcts leads to encapsulated bacterial sepsis. The presence of a palpable spleen is a *priori* evidence that an adult patient does not have SS disease, but rather has sickle trait combined with another hemoglobinopathy. Persistent GI mucosal infarcts can lead to achlorhydria. The chronic hemolysis in this disorder produces bilirubin gall stones in virtually all adults.

These organ injuries are compounded by the risk of **thromboembolism.** A particularly life-threatening and painful condition is known as the **acute chest syndrome** wherein the patient suffers a major infarct of the lung with severe pain, and a potentially vicious cycle of severe hypoxia and intravascular sickling throughout the circulation. In men, sickle crisis in penile veins produces protracted painful priapism often requiring surgical

TABLE 126.1. Drugs That Cause G-6 PD Deficiency-Related Hemolysis

Analgesics	Antimalarials	Nitrofurans	Sulfonamides	Sulfones
Acetanilid	Chloroquine	Nitrofurantoin	Sulfamethoxazole	Dapsone
Acetylsalicylic acid (in large doses)	Primaquine		Sulfapyridine	Thiazolesulfone
Phenacetin			Sulfacetamide	

TABLE 126.2. Some Hemoglobinopathies

Example	Amino Acid Substitution	Clinical Abnormality	Functional Abnormality
Hb.G Philadelphia	α 68 (E17) ASN Lys	None	None
Sickle cell anemia	β 6 (A3) Glu Val	Hemolytic anemia Painful crises	Reduced solubility with O_2 tension
Hb. Koln	β 98 (FGS) Val Met	Heinz body hemolytic anemia	Unstable
Hb. Chesapeake	α 92 (FG4) Arg Len	Erythrocytosis	Increased O_2 affinity
Hb. M-Milwaukee	β 67 (E11) Val gln	Cyanosis	Decreased O_2 affinity; methemoglobinemia
α-Thalassemia trait Hb. Bart's disease Hb. H disease	α Chain gene Deleted	Hypochromic anemia	Rate of α chain synthesis diminished or absent
β Thalassemia	β Chain gene deleted	Hypochromic anemia	β chain synthesis suppressed or deleted

intervention. Because of the severe obligatory hemolysis in SS disease, these patients' cells often have a lifespan of only 10–15 days; hence these patients are dependent on a compensatory reticulocytosis. They also are susceptible to aplastic crises produced by intercurrent viral infections and/or folate depletion. Frequent acute illness leads to days lost at school and work; repeated tissue injury threatens normal organ function throughout the life of such patients. Prompt symptomatic therapy and intervention are highly desirable.

■ Diagnosis

The diagnosis of sickle cell anemia requires that the heterozygous sickle cell trait be differentiated from homozygous sickle cell anemia. The trait patient, who usually has a normal or borderline hemoglobin level, is rarely anemic except during an intercurrent disease, and does not exhibit a significant baseline reticulocytosis. Because these cells "sickle" only with profound hypoxic stresses (e.g., reduced oxygen tension such as in military exposures), the lifespan of these heterozygous RBCs is relatively normal. By exposure to extreme hypoxic states during laboratory testing, in vitro sickling can be induced, thus enabling a simple way to screen for sickle cell trait. As shown in Figure 126.2, only one of the two sets of hemoglobin molecules has the mutant valine amino acid substitution, whereas the other is normal unless another aberrant mutation occurs from another hemoglobinopathy, such as thalassemia. In contrast, the homozygous patient manifests anemia, reticulocytosis, icterus, and virtually absent haptoglobin. The diagnosis is suspected by the appearance of sickle cells on the routine peripheral smear, and confirmed by hemoglobin electrophoresis. Identification of true sickle cell disease versus sickle cell trait is important, as is the presence of additional concomitant hemoglobinopathies such as Hemoglobin C, thalassemias, etc. whose presence modulates disease behavior, thus altering prognosis.

■ Management

The goal of management is to maintain an adequate proportion of normal hemoglobin and conversely a relatively low proportion of hemoglobin S. Since spontaneous sickling crises are rare unless the concentration of hemoglobin S exceeds 50–60% of total circulating hemoglobin, systematic transfusion may be sufficient to maintain this proportion and a total hemoglobin of about 10 g/dl. Such an aggressive transfusion approach includes limited exchange (e.g. 5 units packed RBC transfused with concomitant phlebotomy of 4 units of whole blood sufficient to maintain S Hg below 30%). Sickle cell crises are exquisitely painful. Affected people are usually started on analgesics at an early age; consequently, there is a risk that addiction will develop, especially if the patient is noncompliant or has inadequate access to supportive care and early intervention. Simple analgesics (salicylates, ibuprofen, etc.) are adequate for pain control of minor infarcts, but narcotics are often required for more severe episodes. Need for narcotic analgesia can be minimized by strict attention to support care, such as hydration, oxygen administration during crises, and the judicious use of transfusions.

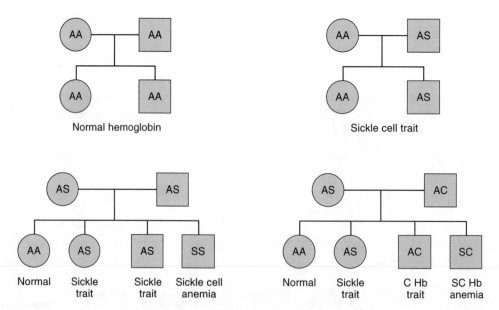

FIGURE 126.2. Inheritance of the sickle cell trait.

Since infants with high levels of fetal hemoglobin (Hgb F) do not have sickling phenomena, and occasional adults with sickle cell disease who have endogenously elevated Hgb F production have fewer crises, pharmacological approaches have been made to increase Hgb F production. Judicious doses of hydroxyurea, usually 500–1500 mg/day, may paradoxically induce Hgb F production; HgF levels above 5% often significantly decreases frequency, duration, and severity of sickle crises. In higher doses, hydroxyurea suppresses bone marrow production of all cell lines. Its use must be carefully and frequently monitored by an experienced hematologist. The importance of careful compliance, and the potential need for repetitive dose modification by the treating physician must be emphasized to the patient.

■ Complications

Iron overload (nonhereditary hemochromatosis or hemosiderosis) may develop in sickle cell patients as a result of ongoing hemolysis and repeated blood transfusions. Its hallmarks are a high serum ferritin, high serum iron and a high transferrin saturation, even as high as 100%. Stainable iron is abundant in the bone marrow; it is deposited in the macrophages or in the interstitium. Excess iron is deposited in the liver (causing liver dysfunction, hepatomegaly and ultimately, cirrhosis), myocardium (leading to cardiomegaly, cardiac dysfunction, and congestive heart failure), pancreas (causing diabetes mellitus) and testicles (producing testicular atrophy, gynecomastia, and feminization). This type of iron overload, which closely mimics hereditary hemochromatosis, is also treated by chelation with desferrioxamine.

Hemoglobin C Disease

Hemoglobin C disease results when leucine is substituted for glutamic acid in the 6th position of the ß chain. The resulting mutant hemoglobin precipitates to form crystals within the RBC, producing RBCs with relatively rigid cell membranes which cause the cells to be trapped and phagocytized by the reticuloendothelial cells. Clinical features include splenomegaly, mild anemia, reticulocytosis, and the presence of many target cells in the peripheral blood (Color Plate 27). The diagnosis is established by hemoglobin electrophoresis. The characteristic crystals may be noted on a Wright-stained smear.

Hemoglobin C disease is moderately severe, but the association of hemoglobin C with S hemoglobin (**SC disease**) causes even more problems, because of the added risk of intravascular sickling events. Pregnancy poses a significant physiological challenge to the patients with SC disease. Besides the risk to the fetus because of injury to the placenta, such patients are at extremely high risk of thromboembolism or aseptic necrosis.

The Unstable Hemoglobins

Amino acid substitutions in the vicinity of the heme pocket may make the hemoglobin molecule unstable, which causes the hemoglobin to precipitate and form **Heinz-Ehrlich bodies**—the harbinger of unstable hemoglobins (Color Plate 28). RBCs with Heinz bodies are trapped in the spleen or destroyed as they circulate. **Heme fragments** (dipyrrholes), which are diagnostic, escape into the urine as a mahogany brown pigment.

Affected patients develop hemolytic anemia and splenomegaly. Viral infections or therapy with sulfonamides or oxidants may worsen the hemolysis. Paradoxically, some of the mutant hemoglobins have a higher oxygen affinity causing slight erythrocytosis rather than anemia. Hemoglobin electrophoresis is not helpful in these cases because the location of these mutations fail to significantly alter the conformational shape or molecular charge of the hemoglobin molecules. A reliable diagnosis is made only by determining the amino acid sequence of the hemoglobin molecule or by finding Heinz-Ehrlich bodies. (Unstable hemoglobins are "heat labile" because the hemoglobin comes out of solution if hemolysates are heated to 50°C for 1–2 h.)

The Thalassemias

The thalassemias are characterized by absent or diminished production of alpha chains (α-thalassemia) or beta chains (ß-thalassemia). Varying degrees of hemolysis occur because of the intracellular deposition of excessive amounts of the opposite form of hemoglobin chains, leading to shortened RBC lifespan. However, the major defect is the diminished hemoglobin production causing a hypochromic microcytic anemia, which is frequently confused with iron deficiency. The ensuing individual molecules of hemoglobin are normal, but the disrupted regulation of intact hemoglobin chains causes an imbalance in hemoglobin production. The functional result is a lowered hemoglobin concentration within the cell.

■ Alpha-Thalassemia

Alpha chain synthesis is controlled by four separate genetic loci on chromosome 16. The position of the affected alleles determines the resulting abnormality. A deletion of one or two genes, typical of patients with an African heritage, leads to the α-thalassemia trait, a mild form of anemia with hypochromic, microcytic erythrocytosis, mimicking iron deficiency. A three-gene deletion, as in some Asiatic patients, causes a chronic, severe, debilitating homozygous hemolytic anemia, which is associated with intracellular inclusions (Hemoglobin H disease). With deletion of all four genes, the fetus has no α chains, becomes severely anemic, and dies at birth of **"hydrops fetalis"** (Figure 126.3).

Affected persons display a hypochromic, microcytic anemia; it is usually mild and may even feature a high RBC count **(hypochromic erythrocytosis),** an important, essentially pathognomonic clue since the RBC count is invariably low in iron deficiency. Unless this is recognized, since the MCV and MCH are low, such patients are frequently and mistakenly treated with iron for years without improvement. Serum iron, transferrin, and ferritin are normal, and are also clues that this is an underlying hemoglobinopathy rather than iron deficiency. The bone marrow shows normal stainable iron. The hemoglobin electrophoresis pattern is normal, as these mutations rarely alter the electrophoretic charge on the hemoglobin molecule. Often, this is a diagnosis of exclusion by ruling out iron deficiency and other hemoglobinopathies; evaluation of other family members can often be helpful.

■ Beta-Thalassemia

Beta-thalassemia is more frequent in people of Mediterranean origin. However, the mutant gene has been introduced into the non-Mediterranean population through migrations, military incursions into northern Europe, and intermarriages.

Beta polypeptide chains are controlled by two genes, located on chromosome 11. Deletion of one gene with a normal second gene results in the ß-thalassemia trait, which is characterized by mild anemia with low MCV and MCH. Hemoglobin electrophoresis shows a compensatory elevation of minor component A_2 or increased hemoglobin F. If both ß genes are deleted, the offspring will have a markedly diminished β chain production rate leading to imbalanced production of α and ß chains. The excess α chains then precipitate, leading to hemolysis.

Clinically, homozygous ß-thalassemia features severe hypochromic microcytic anemia, with increased serum bilirubin and hemoglobin F and a hyperplastic bone marrow with marked erythroid hyperplasia; physical examination reveals splenomegaly, resorption of bone due to expansion of the medullary compartment within, and characteristic facies. Pathologic fractures are common. Peripheral blood smear shows many misshaped target cells.

Through analysis of DNA isolated from circulating peripheral nucleated cells (a common finding in these patients), it is possible to identify specific mutations using restriction fragment length polymorphism analysis. These, and similar tests can be used to identify the specific genetic defect and assess its otherwise occult

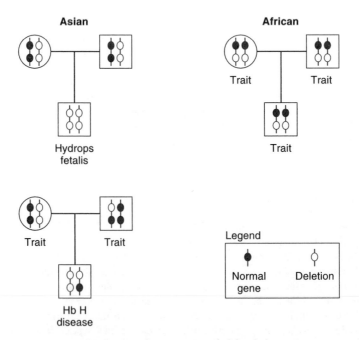

FIGURE 126.3. Hereditary patterns of alpha-thalassemia.

presence in family members. With the potential of gene insertion technologies such biological probes will gain practical importance.

■ Management

Beta-thalassemia trait requires no treatment, but it is important to distinguish it from iron deficiency to avoid needless iron therapy. Homozygous ß-thalassemia should be regularly and frequently treated with packed RBC transfusions to keep hemoglobin values at about 10 gm/dl in order to minimize bone resorption and skeletal deformities. Frequent transfusions in these

patients and their inability to use iron in hemoglobin synthesis lead to severe iron overload. As a result, these individuals assume a peculiar grayish-brown pallor with deposition of iron into the skin and parenchymal organs. Since many patients will require frequent lifelong transfusions serial ferritin determinations should be performed. Chelation therapy with desferrioxamine should be begun early in life, and comprehensively administered in order to reduce the intracellular iron stores, and resulting parenchymal damage. Splenectomy may be helpful in controlling severe hemolytic anemia. Bone marrow transplantation remains the only curative procedure at this time.

CHAPTER 127 HEMOLYTIC ANEMIAS DUE TO EXTRACORPUSCULAR DEFECTS

Autoimmune Hemolytic Anemia

First described in 1907, autoimmune hemolytic anemia (AIHA) is characterized by a hemolytic antibody capable of causing both intravascular and in vitro hemolysis of the individual's own RBCs. The breakthrough that led to the discovery of thousands more cases of AIHA was the demonstration of an antibody—through Coombs test, named after its discoverer— that directly adheres to the surface of RBC, inducing hemolysis by fixing complement and damaging the cell membrane. Antibodies that can cause hemolysis are themselves immunogenic and antigenic; thus antibodies known as Coombs sera (or antiglobulins) can be developed against either broad-spectrum classes of naturally occurring antibodies (e.g., IgG classes), or specifically identified antibodies.

The immune hemolytic anemias vary widely in their clinical presentation and treatment. Warm antibodies, produced in limited amounts, do not generally occur free in serum, but are demonstrable by the Coombs' reaction, using a rodent antihuman polyclonal antibody directed against human autoantibodies adherent to RBC surface antigens. It is possible to elute this immunoglobulin from the RBC surface in order to study its characteristics in the laboratory at physiological temperatures, hence the historical term "warm antibody". The specificity of the antibody, and its agglutination or hemolytic capabilities can be defined through transfer to various RBCs in blood banks. Warm antibodies are generally polyclonal, and contain both IgG and IgM components, commonly directed against typical RBC antigens. Hemolysis varies depending upon the classes and subclasses of the

antibody present; for example, IgG1 fixes complement poorly, IgG3 avidly; hence patients with a high IgG3 autoantibody titer would be more prone to severe hemolysis than those with IgG1 autoantibodies.

Warm hemolytic anemia is mediated by reticuloendothelial macrophages that have membrane receptors for IgG; they phagocytize any particulate matter to which IgG adheres. As the RBC with its adherent antibody, with or without complement, is exposed to macrophages, that component of the cell membrane is phagocytized by excising the cell membrane (antigen)-antibody complex. This occurs repetitively such that the original morphology of the cell is gradually transformed from a cell with maximal surface area per unit volume (biconcave disc) to a cell with the minimal surface area per unit volume (a spherocyte). As this process evolves, the spherocyte becomes progressively smaller, until its ultimate demise in the spleen. Immune-mediated hemolytic anemias produce spherocytes (Color Plate 29), unlike mechanical hemolysis, which confers blatant microangiopathic changes on the RBC, and yields schistocytes (typical of DIC, endocarditis, etc).

Warm hemolytic anemias have diverse causes. Approximately one-half of all cases are idiopathic, and the remaining have an underlying spontaneous or iatrogenic autoimmune disease, or a lymphoproliferative disorder. The diagnosis of AIHA mandates a workup to exclude the presence of one or more of the associated conditions noted in Table 127.1; conversely, hematological parameters should be monitored in patients with a

TABLE 127.1.	Disorders Associated With Warm Autoimmune Hemolytic Anemia

1. Lymphoproliferative disease
  Chronic lymphocytic leukemia
  Non-Hodgkin's lymphoma
  Hodgkin's disease
  Thymoma
  Myeloma
2. Collagen disease
  Systemic lupus erythematosus (SLE)
  Scleroderma
  Rheumatoid arthritis

3. Other immunologic disorders
  Hypogammaglobulinemia
  Dysglobulinemia
4. Gastrointestinal disease
  Ulcerative colitis
5. Ovarian tumors
  Dermoid cysts

TABLE 127.2.	Antiglobulin Sensitization Patterns	
Adhering Immunoglobulin	Characteristics	Serologic Specificity
IgG alone	Reacts at 37°C non-agglutinating except with Coombs serum non-hemolyzing	"Rh" antigen
IgG + C'	Same but may hemolyze	Same
IgM + C'	Cold agglutinins (3°C)	Anti-I
	Mycoplasma (polyclonal)	Anti-i
	Infectious mononucleosis Lymphoma (monoclonal)	Anti-i
C' alone	Donath-Landsteiner	Anti-P
C' alone	SLE	Polyclonal

SLE = Systemic lupus erythematosus.

previous diagnosis of these conditions so as to identify the development of an associated autoimmune hemolysis.

The classification of Coombs reactivity according to immunological criteria is found on Table 127.2. In some circumstances autoantibodies are also directed against other blood elements, e.g., platelets, and can be associated with autoimmune insults against solid organs such as seen in SLE.

AIHA is treated initially by immunosuppression, with prednisone, 1–2 mg/kg body weight. Side effects include glucose intolerance, hyperkalemia, gastritis, insomnia, and so forth; patients must be monitored closely for the first few weeks to manage possible side effects as well as to assess response. Signs of a favorable response include a rising hemoglobin/hematocrit and RBC numbers, as well as a decreasing reticulocyte count and antibody titer. Steroids should be used aggressively initially, and once a response is documented, tapered weekly over a period of months. In many cases, successful discontinuation of steroids may not be possible; in such cases, the physician must evaluate the benefit of long-term use of steroids against the complications, such as immunosuppression, cataracts, and osteoporosis, or consider other alternatives (e.g., splenectomy and/or alternative immunosuppressive, such as cyclophosphamide, Imuran, etc). Packed cell transfusion is limited to severe or critical situations since the transfused cells share the same target membrane antigens recognized by the autoantibody and will thus be rapidly destroyed.

Cold Agglutinin-Associated Hemolytic Anemia

The presentation and treatment of cold agglutinin-associated hemolytic anemias differ entirely from those with the warm agglutinins. Patients are often more symptomatic, although the degree of anemia may not be as severe as that seen in the warm antibody type. The cold agglutinin syndrome is dominated by the clinical features not only of hemolysis, but of compromised microcirculation, especially in anatomical areas exposed to ambient temperatures significantly below physiological tempera-

tures. Thus, patients invariably have features similar to Raynaud's phenomenon and/or characteristic acrocyanosis, with recurrent capillary thrombosis in the malar areas of the face and ears. An early avascular pale appearance results with later progression to a livedo reticularis syndrome of violaceous and ultimately permanent disfigurement.

In contrast to warm hemolytic anemias, cold-agglutinin disease produces a monoclonal autoantibody, which almost always targets the "I"-antigen system. (This system has an adult type "I" antigen which develops after birth, and a downregulated but present fetal type "i" antigen; the clinicians refer to "anti-big I" or "anti-little I" respectively.) The idiopathic form of the disease, which usually occurs in the elderly, as well as those associated with underlying autoimmune or lymphoproliferative diseases, feature an anti-I antibody. In contrast, infections such as **Mycoplasma pneuomoniae,** which usually occur in younger persons, produce an anti-i antibody.

The natural history of this condition relates to the possible underlying etiology. If determined to be "anti-i", and especially if temporally associated with a known or suspected infectious episode, the syndrome will probably be self-limiting. Conversely "anti-I" is usually chronic and will necessitate protracted therapy analogous to that used in warm antibody syndromes. Similarly, diagnosis of an "anti-I" syndrome mandates a workup for the same spectrum of associated conditions. Careful analysis of the complement-fixing capability of the antibody, and its thermal amplitude can be helpful. Besides educating the patient regarding the need to avoid cold exposure, the physician should recognize that transfusions, especially if not warmed to the physiological temperature, may provoke a clinical crisis by aggregating in the microcirculation, and that immunosuppression and splenectomy, although fortunately not often needed, are also less effective.

CHAPTER 128 DISORDERS OF PHAGOCYTIC CELLS

The sequential proliferation, maturation, and differentiation of the white blood cells (WBC) are discussed in Chapter 120. Table 128.1 presents normal total and differential WBC counts; the distribution of WBC appears in Tables 128.2 and 128.3.

■ Morphology

The granulocytes are characterized functionally and morphologically by cytoplasmic granules. Early granulocyte precursors (i.e., progranulocytes) bear only primary granules (primary granules consist of lysosomal membranes that encase hydrolytic enzymes, myeloperoxidase, and cationic proteins, all of which have bactericidal properties). As maturation proceeds, primary granules are replaced by secondary granules; secondary granules have specific staining features that identify them as neutrophils, eosinophils, and basophils (e.g., neutrophils: diffusely dispersed, fine lavender–staining cyto-

TABLE 128.2.	Distribution of Phagocytes
Total Number of WBC × 10¹²/L - 4.5–11.0	
Type of Phagocyte	**Predominant Location**
Polymorphonuclear leukocyte	Blood & tissues
Monocyte	Blood & tissues
Tissue macrophage	Spleen lymph nodes & bone marrow
Kupffer cells	Liver sinusoids
Alveolar macrophages	Lungs

plasmic granules; eosinophils: bright red, acidic (eosin) staining, large and round granules that are fewer per cell than neutrophilic granules; basophils: large, irregular granules that are even fewer and attracting basic (black) dyes).

Mature PMN granules consist of lactoferrin and proteolytic enzymes. Quantitative fluctuations of alkaline phosphatase play a diagnostic role in certain myeloproliferative disorders. Granulocyte precursors derive energy through mitochondrial respiration. As the PMN mature, mitochondria disappear; energy is then derived from glycolysis.

■ Phagocytic Properties

The major function of polymorphonuclear cells is phagocytosis. The particle (e.g., bacteria) is identified by appropriate immunoglobulin markers so as to be recognizable to membrane receptors. The external membranes of both PMN and macrophages contain receptors for both complement and immunoglobulins, which is necessary

TABLE 128.1.	Numbers of White Blood Cells in Normal Blood	
A. Total white blood cells:		4.5–11.0 × 10¹²/L
B. Types and proportion of WBC:		%
	Band form—neutrophils	<3
	Segmented—neutrophilic PMNs	40–70
	Lymphocytes	25–45
	Eosinophilic PMNs	3
	Basophils	0.5
	Monocytes	4

TABLE 128.3.	Distribution of Granulocyte Compartments	

1. Proliferative pool—capable of mitosis, 10-20 × circulating pool

Stage	Characteristic	Frequency %
a) Myeloblast	No granules 1-3 nucleoli	0.2–1.5
b) Promyelocyte	Primary granules 0-1 nucleoli	2–4
c) Myelocyte	Secondary granules, oval nucleus	8–16

2. Non-proliferative (reserve) pool

a) Metamyelocyte	Progressively indented nucleus	10–25
b) Band cell	Elongated nucleus	10–15
c) PMN	Segmented nucleus	6–12

Seem to have defective bactericidal property. Mature polymorphonuclear leukocyte (PMN) deformable because of lobed nucleus. May change shape to penetrate between endothelial cells and enter circulation or tissues.

3. Peripheral blood pool
   a) Circulating pool
   b) Marginating pool

for their physiological phagocytic function. PMN motility, also critical to phagocytosis, is directed by chemotaxis to a specific target so that PMN are attracted to the site of the bacterial invasion. Complement components 3a and 5a and fibrinopeptide B are important chemotactic stimuli. Products of tissue damage (such as denatured proteins) and arachidonic acid metabolites share in this function. Energy for phagocytosis is driven by glycolysis; lactate and CO_2 are released as final products.

Once a bacterial particle is engulfed, the leukocyte granules deploy around the phagosome; the lysosomal and vacuolar membrane eventually fuse. As the lysosomal contents are discharged into the vacuole, the granules disappear. For cell protection, the proteolytic contents of lysosomes cannot come in contact with PMN interior structures. With the appropriate enzymes, bacteria may be killed or digested. Bacterial killing is mediated by membrane oxidase enzymes that obtain electrons from reduced pyridine nucleotides (NADPH). These enzymes convert oxygen (O_2) to superoxide anion (O_2^-) and hydrogen peroxide (H_2O_2) which, together with myeloperoxidase, are highly bactericidal. H_2O_2 is detoxified by glutathione derived from the hexose monophosphate shunt (Figure 126.1). The entire process of phagocytosis is accompanied by a short respiratory burst resulting in CO_2 release (see neutrophil kinetics and function, Chapter 141).

Reactive Leukocytosis

Leukocytosis may arise from infectious or noninfectious causes. It is caused physiologically during parturition, exercise, and stress, probably mediated by the effect of endogenous epinephrine on marginated PMN. Neutrophilia (high neutrophil count) is primarily due to infection. Absolute neutrophilia, a normal response to infection, consists of a "left shift" in myeloid elements, a term meaning the increased number of mature and immature neutrophils and precursors thereof which have been released from the marginated pool of cells in the circulation, as well as from the marrow cavity as a stress response. The presence of myelocytes, metamyelocytes, and even promyelocytes or myeloblasts can be transiently observed if the infectious stress is severe and the patient's marrow is capable of responding. Absolute or relative lymphocytopenia is often present in severe infection; the former is due to acute lysis or apoptosis of circulating lymphocytes by the endogenous corticosteroids secreted physiologically; the latter is the artifact of the laboratory reporting system. Clinicians are encouraged to critically assess the lymphocyte count in such laboratory reports. An absence of lymphopenia is unexpected and raises the possibility of concurrent viral infections and/or lymphoproliferative diseases.

Polymorphonuclear cells in mild infections show "toxic" granules (i.e., azurophilic granules from accelerated granulocytopoiesis). In more severe infections, neutrophils (polymorphonuclear cells) contain Dohle bodies (grayish blue membrane-attached inclusions). Leukocyte alkaline phosphatase (LAP) content rises. Fever follows pyrogen release from damaged leukocytes. These changes dissipate as the infection resolves.

Noninfectious factors also cause leukocytosis (e.g., uremia, gout, acidosis, burns, eclampsia, severe dehydration and hemoconcentration, acute hemorrhage, or hemolysis). Tissue necrosis in major surgery, myocardial infarction, and malignancies are other causes.

Neutrophilia may be due to certain physiological substances and medications. Corticosteroids and epinephrine enhance delivery of neutrophils from reserve marrow pools. Lithium promotes granulocytopoiesis.

Overwhelming infection by invading micro-organisms or infections in "closed" serosal cavities may engender overwhelming leukocytosis ($>100 \times 10^9$/L). This leukemoid reaction may seemingly resemble chronic myelocytic leukemia (CML). Leukemoid reactions occur only in acutely ill patients with a serious infection. In recently diagnosed CML, patients are asymptomatic and fully ambulatory. LAP score is high in infectious leukocytosis; it is depleted in CML.

Leukopenia

Leukopenia occasionally follows overwhelming infections, including bacterial infections, when the bone marrow fails to provide neutrophils in sufficient numbers. In leukopenia, total WBC declines, the ratio of neutrophils and bands to lymphocytes increases, and small numbers of metamyelocytes and myelocytes appear. The polymorphonuclear cells display heavy toxic granulation or degranulation, Dohle bodies, and cytoplasmic vacuolization. The usual setting is an immunocompromised host, an alcoholic, or a patient with metastatic malignancy. Leukopenia in these settings suggests a limited leukocyte response to infection. Thus, it is a poor prognostic sign.

Leukopenia also accompanies other disparate clinical states besides infection (Table 128.4). In pseudoleukopenia, an enhanced leukocyte response to epinephrine is characteristic. Leukopenia is regularly noted in systemic lupus erythematosus and autoimmune leukopenia. Increased peripheral destruction or sequestration in large spleens gives rise to leukopenia (3,000–4,000) and thrombocytopenia (60,000–90,000). Leukoerythroblastosis (normoblasts appear together with immature granulocytes in periphery) accompanies leukopenia due to malignancies. In "aleukemic" leukemia, replacement of granulocyte precursors in the marrow leads to leukopenia. Because blasts are not always present peripherally, the diagnosis is confirmed by bone marrow biopsy.

TABLE 128.4.	Causes of Leukopenia

Physiologic
  Otherwise normal blacks and middle eastern people
Pseudoneutropenia—increase in marginating pool
Chronic benign neutropenia
Systemic lupus erythematosus
Aplastic anemia
  Drugs and chemicals—e.g., chloramphenicol
  Virus disease
  Congenital—Fanconi's Syndrome
  Idiopathic acquired
Infections
  Gram negative bacteria—e.g., typhoid, brucella virus and rickettsial disease
  Protozoa—malaria, kala-azar
  Overwhelming infection—e.g., septicemia, miliary tuberculosis
Splenomegaly (hypersplenism): cirrhosis, Felty's syndrome, Gaucher's disease, sarcoidosis, etc.
Aleukemic and preleukemic leukemia, metastatic carcinoma, myelofibrosis
Megaloblastic anemia–e.g., folate and B_{12} deficiency
Paroxysmal nocturnal hemoglobinuria (PNH)
Congenital neutropenia—Kostmann's syndrome
Drug-induced agranulocytosis
  Immune mediated, e.g., aminopyrine.
  Toxic suppression, e.g., chlorpromazine.

Drug-Induced Leukopenia and Agranulocytosis

Some drugs (e.g., antineoplastic agents) given in a sufficiently high dosage regularly and universally suppress hematopoiesis. Agranulocytosis is a rare complication of drug therapy in which affected individuals develop precipitous leukopenia in response to doses of the drug that are ordinarily not toxic to the population at large. Usually a latent period of 30–50 days of therapy with the offending drug precedes the sudden drop in neutrophils. These events occur selectively in persons with specific characteristics.

■ Basic Mechanisms of Agranulocytosis

Although the clinical and hematological expression of drug sensitivity is remarkably similar for most offending drugs, the mechanisms differ profoundly for different medications. The basic abnormality exists in the host rather than the drug. Despite overlap and specific differences, two basic mechanisms are proposed:

1. **Nonimmunological**
   a. Direct chemical suppression in a host with a pre-existing proliferative defect.
   b. Accumulation of toxic metabolic end-products in a host who is constitutionally unable to detoxify or excrete them.
2. **Immunological**
   Immune destruction by drug-related antibodies (or their precursors) that destroy peripheral polymorphonuclear cells.

Causes of drug-induced agranulocytosis are listed in Table 128.5. **Immunologically related agranulocytosis** is ushered in by abrupt symptoms, such as chills, fever, and collapse. The symptoms are explained by the peripheral lysis of WBC with the release of toxic pyrogens. Rapidly escalating sepsis is almost inevitable when patients are suddenly deprived of the protection afforded by polymorphonuclear cells. The usual incubation period (time from drug exposure to the development of symptoms) is 40 days.

Nonimmune toxic marrow suppression is dose-dependent, and develops concomitantly with treatment. Hence the clinical history is important because the interval between drug exposure and development of neutropenia is usually shorter than that seen in immunologically mediated types, is usually precipitous, but fortunately rapidly reversible if the offending agent is withdrawn promptly. If not recognized, this syndrome may progress to involve other cell lines, producing an aplastic anemia which may or may not be reversible.

■ Etiology

While no longer used, the immunogenic drug aminopyrine is the prototype of all drug-induced neutropenia, or agranulocytosis syndromes, and the first drug identified that causes immunological suppression of granulocytes. Consistent with known attributes of immunological reactions, the initial aberrant response is the development of an IgM class immunoglobulin that can attach to the neutrophil, binding complement, and inducing cell lysis. A secondary IgG response follows; while this may less avidly fix complement, it can recognize granulocyte precursors, and inhibit committed stem cells once they acquire typical granulocytic membrane antigens. This can be documented by assessing in vitro growth of precursor clones of cells known as CFU-Gs. Addition of patients' sera will inhibit the growth of CFU-G clones obtained from normal volunteers; adsorption of these antibodies from patients' sera before exposure to normal marrow cells abrogates its inhibitory effects. Presence of the antibody is self-limiting unless the patient is rechallenged with the offending agent. In the case of phenothiazine derivatives, the neutropenia may be self-limiting and relatively mild, and unless monitored for, not recognized. However, any intercurrent challenge to granulocytopoiesis may be catastrophic.

■ Management

Identification and discontinuation of the offending drug is critical to the successful treatment of drug-induced agranulocytosis. The serious risk of infection dictates the use of reverse isolation and broad spectrum antibiotics (see Chapter 157). Recovery from agranulocytosis may be hastened by the prompt injection of GM-CSF or G-CSF for the duration of the leukopenia. Once the offending drug is identified, it must never be readministered.

TABLE 128.5. Drug-Induced Agranulocytosis

I. *Immune*
  A. *Mediated by WBC antibodies*
    Aminopyrine
    Thiouracil
    Methimazole
    Chlorpropamide
    Sulfanilamides
    Levamisole
    Clozapine
  B. *Immune lupus reaction*
    Procainamide
    Hydralazine
  C. *Antibiotics*
    Penicillin-nafcillin
    Cephalosporins
    Stibophen
II. *Toxic chemical depression*
    Chlorpromazine
    Depression by accumulation of toxic metabolites
    Carbamazepine
    Phenytoin

Monocytosis, Eosinophilia, and Basophilia

Monocytosis

Monocytosis is present if the number of monocytes exceeds 900/µl (9–10%). Monocytes divide and transform into other phagocytic cells, release cytokines (CSF and IL-1), and process and present antigen to lymphocytes. Thus, they modulate immune and lymphocyte function.

TABLE 128.6. Conditions Associated With Monocytosis

Infections
  Brucellosis
  Fever of unknown origin
  Infective endocarditis
  Recovery phase from infection (transient)
  Syphilis
  Tuberculosis
Inflammatory conditions
  Autoimmune diseases
    Polyarteritis
    Rheumatoid arthritis
    Systemic lupus erythematosus
  Granulomatous diseases
    Crohn's disease
    Sarcoidosis
    Ulcerative colitis
Neoplastic disorders
  Acute myeloid leukemia
  Hodgkin's disease
  Monocytic leukemia
  Myelomonocytic leukemia
  Preleukemia
  Solid tumors (malignant)
Others
  Histiocytoses
  Postsplenectomy
  Recovery phase of agranulocytosis (transient)

Clinically, monocytes rise transiently during **recovery from infection** or from agranulocytosis, where they play a role in clearing debris from the inflammatory sites (Table 128.6). With **chronic infection** (bacterial endocarditis, tuberculosis, syphilis, and brucellosis), they persist longer in the peripheral blood. Monocytes are harbingers of **chronic granulomatous disorders** (sarcoidosis, SLE, rheumatoid arthritis). In **hematological malignancies**—notably monocytic leukemia, myelomonocytic leukemia and Hodgkin's disease,—persistent monocytosis frequently exceeds 25×10^9/L.

Infectious Mononucleosis

Infectious mononucleosis is an acute viral disorder caused by **Epstein-Barr** virus (EBV), affecting young adults and characterized by fever, pharyngitis, lymphadenopathy, splenomegaly, and absolute lymphocytosis with many atypical cells (Color Plate 30). Palatal exanthem in the form of red petechiae at the junction of the hard and soft palates, although not diagnostic, is quite characteristic. Patients treated with ampicillin experience an increased incidence of macular skin rash. Develop-

Eosinophilia and Basophilia

Eosinophilia is present when the absolute or the proportional count of eosinophils exceed 700/μl or 10% respectively. It occurs in conditions shown in Table 128.7, most of which represent **allergic or atopic diseases** or inflammatory skin diseases. Eosinophilia is an important finding in **parasitic infestations** associated with tissue invasion (e.g., trichinosis, schistosomiasis, hookworm, echinococcosis or filariasis). **Hypereosinophilic syndrome,** defined as eosinophilia exceeding 1500/μl, is a progressive disorder with tissue necrosis and multiple organ damage. It can be controlled with corticosteroids or hydroxyurea. **Eosinophilia-myalgia syndrome,** which followed the use of contaminated L-tryptophan, is characterized by skin rashes, dyspnea, peripheral neuropathy, eosinophilia, and myositis. Characterized now as **eosinophilic fasciitis,** this syndrome may occur episodically without an apparent inciting event, presumably due to some unrecognized environmental insult. Specific inquiry regarding drug or chemical exposures is important, since it may progress to irreversible bone marrow aplasia.

Basophils are the least numerous of the granulocytes and rarely exceed 150/μl. While transient increases may occur in allergic or inflammatory states, chronic progressive basophilia is related to chronic myelocytic leukemia. Late-stage basophilia is a harbinger of impending blast transformation.

TABLE 128.7. Causes of Eosinophilia

1. Allergy (asthma, hayfever, atopy)
2. Dermatitis
3. Parasitic infestations
4. Malignant disease, e.g. Hodgkin's disease
5. Pulmonary infiltrates with eosinophilia
6. Irradiation
7. Hypereosinophilic syndrome
8. Eosinophilic leukemia
9. Miscellaneous disorders (polyarteritis, eosinophilia-myalgia syndrome)

ment of transient heterophil antibodies (HA) and persistent EBV antibodies are characteristic. With a typical clinical and hematological picture, a high HA titer is diagnostic. HA are antibodies to sheep RBC that can be absorbed by beef RBC, but not by guinea pig kidney cells.

HA have been replaced by a highly sensitive and specific commercial "Monospot" test, which depends upon the rapid development of an IgM antibody, but only 85–95% cases are positive in the first week of the illness. If infectious mononucleosis is strongly suspected but the test results are negative in the first week, retesting is useful in the second or third week of illness. Detection of antibodies against specific components of EBV is useful making the diagnosis in the rare situation where the Monospot test is negative, or when the presence of chronic infections is of concern. IgM antibodies to the viral capsid antigen (VCA) are diagnostic of a primary EBV infection. IgG anti-VCA antibodies almost universally occur in all cases at first presentation and persist for life, but they cannot reliably diagnose primary infection. Abnormal liver tests are not uncommon. Cold agglutinins are frequently elevated; clinical hemolysis is rare. Because the clinical syndrome of "mononucleosis" is occasionally due to cytomegalovirus (CMV) rather than EBV, when Monospot test is negative, CMV titers should be performed.

Treatment is symptomatic in uncomplicated cases. Recovery is almost universal. Complications are extremely rare; Coombs-positive hemolytic anemia has been reported. Splenic rupture, severe hepatitis, and toxic encephalopathy may be lethal in a few cases. Corticosteroids are indicated for hemolytic anemia, thrombocytopenia, neurological complications, and respiratory problems.

Myeloproliferative Disorders

The myeloproliferative disorders represent a diverse group of clinical disorders caused by the uncontrolled clonal proliferation and expansion of an identifiable marrow cell line. Interestingly, while each of these entities has a predominant clonal expansion, often the other marrow and blood elements are also increased, indicating that the mutational event occurred prior to the discrete differentiation into a selected cell line. Thus while **polycythemia vera** (P. vera) is an entity dominated by marked erythrocytosis, most patients have at least mild elevation of neutrophils and/or platelets. **Chronic myelogenous leukemia** (CML) often shows thrombocytosis at presentation, and in fact the platelet count in CML has some prognostic significance. In **essential thromb-** **ocythemia,** abnormalities of other elements may rarely be noted. Thus the differential diagnosis of these conditions is often difficult and requires careful clinical and laboratory evaluation. Since the mutational event precedes true selective differentiation, one form of disease can later evolve into another (e.g., from P. vera into essential thrombocythemia, or myeloid metaplasia, etc.); therefore, diagnosis of any of these conditions calls for careful follow-up and monitoring. Such morphological and pathological transformations also alter disease behavior mandating changes in treatment, and alter prognosis. The clinical and laboratory features of the myeloproliferative disorders and their therapy are reviewed in Chapters 134 through 138.

CHAPTER 129 EVALUATION OF THE PATIENT WITH A BLEEDING DISORDER

The approach to the patient with a suspected bleeding or thrombotic disorder begins with a complete history, a physical examination, and basic screening tests of the hemostatic system. Thorough, careful questioning in patients with hereditary bleeding disorders will often yield a history of excessive bleeding. While the family history can be very helpful in diagnosis in younger patients, mild congenital coagulation factor deficiencies may not surface until adulthood, when excessive bleeding follows a surgical procedure or trauma.

The clinical profile of the bleeding may offer diagnostic clues. While localized, excessive, postoperative bleeding may require only local therapy, such bleeding from multiple sites calls for consideration and confirmation of a more generalized hemostatic defect.

Delayed bleeding after surgery or trauma may follow certain factor deficiencies, drugs, or blood vessel factors. Prolonged bleeding after superficial trauma often indicates platelet function defects, whereas hemarthrosis and deep hematomas often suggest a coagulation disorder.

■ Coagulation Cascade

The normal hemostatic system is often described as a "cascade" of chemical reactions occurring after the system is activated, and continuing until an irreversible hemostatic plug is formed (Figure 129.1). The system consists of three intertwined and interdependent parts, designed to produce effective hemostasis yet prevent excessive thrombosis. The first of these is the coagulation system, consisting of coagulation factor proenzymes

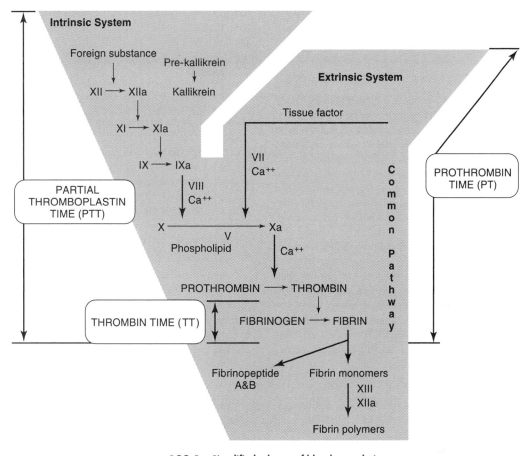

FIGURE 129.1. Simplified schema of blood coagulation.

(XII, XI, VII, IX, X, prothrombin) and nonenzymatic cofactors (VIII, V). When activated, these generate thrombin from prothrombin. The platelets that form a reversible platelet plug are the second part of the system. They also provide the phospholipid surface necessary for coagulation factor activation. The fibrinolytic and anti-thrombin systems complete the picture, limiting the "cascade", and thus preventing unwanted and excessive thrombus generation.

The central event in the coagulation system is the generation of activated Factor Xa, the only known enzyme that can activate prothrombin. This event follows either the exposure of inactive factor VII to tissue factor on fibroblasts, or an altered endothelial surface or exposed subendothelial proteins. The commonly used terminology reflects the underlying concept that when exposed to negatively charged protein surfaces, the coagulation factors become activated, and the "cascade" proceeds. As hemostasis proceeds, this activation of X to Xa is inhibited, and the direct VIIa-tissue factor effect on X must be supplemented by the complex of IXa-

phospholipid-VIIIa. Once Xa is generated, it can link up with Va, phospholipid, and prothrombin to produce thrombin.

Thrombin is the linchpin of coagulation. It breaks down fibrinogen to form fibrin monomers and it activates Factor XIII, promoting the cross-linking of fibrin polymers into an insoluble fibrin meshwork. It can activate Factor V and Factor VIII to promote its own formation, and it can activate platelets and induce the platelet release and platelet aggregation reactions. Fibrin monomers ultimately congeal into fibrin polymers that create a stable, hemostatic thrombus. The entire coagulation system is a sequence of amplified reactions. Interestingly the concentrations of coagulation factors in the early portion of the cascade are markedly less (often by a factor of several hundred) compared to fibrinogen, or even prothrombin. Thus most bleeding disorders are due to deficiencies of these factors. Only some nutritional deficiencies, liver disease, and/or consumption of coagulation factors affect Factors I and II. Hemophiliacs can survive on only fractions of normal plasma factor levels (about 5%, or only 10–20µg/dl), compared to 4,000 µg/dl for fibrinogen. However, depletion of Factor VIII below a critical threshold is catastrophic.

■ The Fibrinolytic and Antithrombin Systems

The coagulation cascade is inhibited both by "natural" anticoagulants and by the fibrinolytic system. The most important natural anticoagulant is antithrombin (AT) III. ATIII inhibits thrombin and several other activated proteins (VIIa, Xa, IXa, XIa, kallikrein, and plasmin) by forming stable bonds to these factors. Heparin accelerates the reaction. Thrombomodulin, a component of the endothelial cell membrane, is another important anticoagulant. When bound to thrombin, thrombomodulin can activate protein C. Activated protein C can join with protein S and phospholipid to break down factors Va and VIIIa.

The fibrinolytic system is a series of proteins that, when activated, can degrade cross-linked fibrin. Plasminogen requires activators to convert into plasmin, the enzyme able to degrade fibrin. Some natural plasminogen activators are factor XII and prekallikrein. Several drugs are capable of plasminogen activation (streptokinase, urokinase, and recombinant tissue plasminogen activator, tPA). Like all parts of the coagulation system, this system also has inhibitors.

■ Platelets

Endothelial injury also results in the activation of platelets. In response to such injury, platelets will adhere to one another and release their granules into the microenvironment of the injury. This release reaction will generate the formation of a reversible platelet plug, capable of combining with the fibrin polymers to create a stable, irreversible platelet thrombus. The platelet release reaction is affected by many drugs, of which aspirin is the most studied and potentially therapeutic. Aspirin decreases cyclooxygenase and thus prevents thromboxane A2 synthesis, thereby inhibiting the release reaction (Figure 129.2).

■ Laboratory Evaluation

While there is no substitute for a complete clinical history in the diagnosis of bleeding disorders, laboratory screening tests are the key to their diagnosis. (See Table 129.1.)

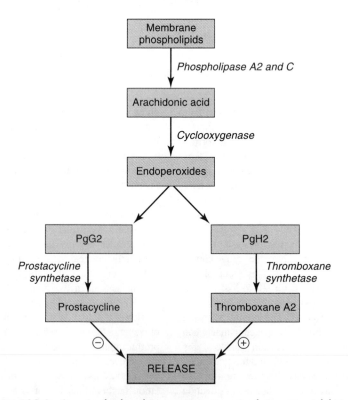

FIGURE 129.2. Steps in platelet release reaction. ⊕ = stimulation; ⊖ = inhibition.

TABLE 129.1. Laboratory Evaluation of Bleeding Disorders: Causes of Abnormal Screening Tests			
Condition/Cause	↑ PTT	↑ PT	↑ TT
Deficiency of:			
HMW kininogen	+		
Prekallikrein	+		
XII	+		
XI	+		
IX	+		
VIII	+		
VII		+	
V	+	+	
X	+	+	
Dysfibrinogenemia		+	+
Afibrinogenemia	+	+	+
Hypofibrinogenemia		+	+
Lupus anticoagulant	+	+	
Oral anticoagulant	+	+	
Liver disease	+	+	
Polycythemia	+	+	
Heparin	+		+

Prothrombin time

The prothrombin time (PT) measures the function of the proteins of the "extrinsic" and the common (fibrinogen, II, V, X) pathways. The vitamin K–dependent proteins (II, VII, IX, X) are measured by the PT, and levels are affected by warfarin. The PT is most sensitive to deficiencies of factors V, VII, X, or prothrombin, but it may also be prolonged when the fibrinogen is low, or when heparin or fibrin split products are present. An elevated hematocrit prolongs the PT as it affects the relative amount of anticoagulant and plasma in the test. Because the responsiveness of the test varies with thromboplastins of varying sensitivity, the test results have been standardized and the results are reported as the **international normalized ratio (INR).**

Partial thromboplastin time

The partial thromboplastin time (PTT) measures the "intrinsic" (factors XII, XI, IX, VIII, prekallikrein) and the common pathway factors (fibrinogen, II, V, X), and detects circulating anticoagulants. Heparin inhibits many of the same factors in its role as a antithrombin III cofactor. Thus, the PTT is also used to monitor heparin dose. Because the PTT is more sensitive to deficiencies of the early intrinsic pathway factors and less sensitive to deficiencies of the common pathway (later) factors, occasionally, fibrinogen deficiency will prolong only the PT and not the PTT. In general, the PTT is prolonged when XII, XI, X, IX, VIII, V, or prothrombin is low or in

the presence of an inhibitor to any of these factors, a high fibrinogen level, fibrin split products, heparin, or DIC.

The PT and PTT are the basic screening tests of the coagulation system. If one of them is abnormal, a mixing study is the next step. Normal plasma and the patient's plasma are mixed in a 1 : 1 ratio. Normal plasma has such a surplus of factors that the test should become normal if a factor is simply deficient. If the test is abnormal due to the presence of an inhibitor, the test will remain abnormal, and further studies are necessary to locate the specific inhibitor. In rare coagulation disorders with a strong history of bleeding (e.g., factor XIII deficiency) PT and PTT may be normal, necessitating additional tests.

Thrombin time

The thrombin time indicates the time for plasma to clot when thrombin is added to the mixture. It can screen for decreases in fibrinogen, abnormal fibrinogens, the presence of fibrin split products, or the presence of heparin.

Fibrin or fibrinogen degradation products

The **fibrin or fibrinogen degradation products** (FDP) test detects breakdown products of fibrin or fibrinogen and can confirm the diagnosis of **disseminated intravascular coagulation** (DIC). These tests determine the highest dilution of plasma at which the specimen agglutinates; they are usually reported semiquantitatively. The d-dimer test uses monoclonal antibody very specific for cross-linked FDP only. Both tests will be positive in DIC, often in acute venous or arterial thrombosis, in late pregnancy and often, immediately postoperatively.

Euglobulin clot lysis time

This test evaluates the presence of systemic fibrinolysis. The plasma fraction used is free of the lytic system inhibitor. If the fibrinogen is normal, the clot formed should be rapidly dissolved. If the test clot dissolves more rapidly than the control clot, it is evidence of activation of the fibrinolytic system.

Reptilase time

This test is used to evaluate fibrinogen. It measures fibrin formation after the snake venom cleaves fibrinopeptide A from the fibrinogen molecule.

Platelet studies

The peripheral smear should be examined to exclude thrombocytopenia as a cause of bleeding. Abnormal platelet morphology may suggest abnormal platelet function in thrombotic disorders, in the storage pool diseases, or in the myelodysplastic/myeloproliferative diseases. If the count is normal and the history suggests a bleeding disorder due to abnormal platelet function, a qualitative abnormality may be suspected. The bleeding time (BT) is the basic test of the ability of the platelets to form a hemostatic plug. A small cut is made in the skin and the time until bleeding stops is measured. A prolonged BT may indicate either abnormal platelet function or abnormal skin and blood vessel fragility. It is a difficult test to standardize and perform, and its unreliability limits its usefulness. Because of the difficulties in interpretation and the lack of predictive value, it is used as a screening test for the evaluation of bleeding disorders but not as a preoperative screening test. A normal test does not exclude a significant platelet function abnormality.

Platelet aggregation tests can be performed to further define the functional characteristics of platelets. Platelet-rich plasma is added to various known aggregating agents (ADP, epinephrine, ristocetin, thrombin), and the solution is placed in an aggregometer. If the platelets aggregate, increasing amounts of light are able to pass through the specimen. The patterns of aggregation after each agent may often suggest whether the platelet function abnormalities are congenital or due to drugs.

Factor assays

Specific functional assays have been developed for all of the factors listed in Table 129.2. Generally, levels of 50–150% are considered normal. For many of the factors, antigenic assays are also available. An abnormal functional assay coupled with a normal antigenic assay suggests a structurally abnormal protein. More recently, using the polymerase chain reaction (PCR), amino acid substitutions causing functionally abnormal factors have been identified. An example is the guanine-to-adenine substitution at nucleotide position 1691 of the factor V gene, leading to the substitution of arginine (R) by glutamine (Q) at position 506 of the polypeptide chain of factor V (Factor V Leiden). The resulting inability of activated protein C to inactivate factor V—**"activated protein C (APC) resistance"**—leads to a thrombotic tendency. The most common manifestations are deep vein thrombosis and superficial thrombophlebitis. This allele (factor $V:Q^{506}$) is highly prevalent among Caucasians, with a frequency between 2–15%. Conversely, in patients with venous thrombosis, studies show a prevalence of 10–40% for factor $V:Q^{506}$ allele. Retrospective studies show a very high prevalence of factor $V:Q^{506}$ in

TABLE 129.2. Coagulation Factors and Their Kinetics

Factor Number	Coagulation Factor	Biologic Half-Life (h)
I	Fibrinogen	90
II	Prothrombin	72
III	Tissue thromboplastin	—
IV	Calcium	—
V	Labile factor	16
VII	Stable	5
VIII	Antihemophilic A (AHF)	12
IX	Antihemophilic B (AHB) (Christmas factor)	24
X	Stuart-Prower factor	48
XI	Plasma thromboplastin antecedent (PTA)	60
XII	Hageman factor	60
XIII	Fibrin stabilizing factor	120
	Prekallikrein (Fletcher factor)*	
	High-molecular-weight kininogen (Fitzgerald, Williams, or Flaujeac factor)*	
	von Willebrand factor*	
	Protein C*	
	Protein S*	

*Not usually referred to by a Roman numeral or has not been assigned a number.

pregnancy-associated deep vein thrombosis and deep vein thrombosis associated with oral contraceptive use. It is not uncommon for it to coexist with other genetic thrombotic disorders, which may alter the severity, pattern and frequency of thrombotic events.

Factor VIII, the protein involved in the coagulation cascade, is attached to the much larger, von Willebrand carrier protein, which is also responsible for platelet aggregation and adhesion to the endothelium. Functional assays of Factor VIII protein are designated VIII:C, and antigenic assays, VIII:Ag. The **von Willebrand factor** (vWF) is a large multimeric protein composed of vWF monomers joined by polymerization to form the large multimers of plasma vWF. Functional assays for vWF are the Ristocetin Cofactor assay, and the antigenic assay is the vWF:Ag. These multimers can be measured in the plasma, and results are important to define the various types of von Willebrand's disease.

CHAPTER 130

BLEEDING DISORDERS DUE TO FACTOR DEFICIENCIES

The diagnostic approach to a bleeding disorder varies depending on the clinical circumstance, as well as on the results of a careful drug, family, and overall medical history. Most severe congenital bleeding disorders become apparent very early in childhood, but the less severe factor deficiencies may escape recognition until adulthood or until the system is unable to cope with the stress of either surgery or trauma.

Hereditary Bleeding Disorders

Hemophilia A

Hemophilia A is an X-linked bleeding disorder (incidence, 1:10,000 men) due to a deficiency of factor VIII. Since spontaneous mutations may cause up to 30% of cases, the family history may be negative. Chromosome changes consist of frameshift, deletions, inversions, and point mutations within the factor VIII gene. A true deficiency of the protein occurs in up to 90% of severe cases. The severity of the bleeding usually correlates with factor VIII levels. Severe hemophilia (VIII <1%) presents in childhood with spontaneous hemarthroses and internal hematomas. The risk of long-term complications (e.g., joint fibrosis and intracranial hemorrhage) has been dramatically decreased by prophylactic infusions of factor VIII concentrates. While the risk for spontaneous bleeding is proportionately less in moderate (VIII 2–5%) and mild (VIII 5–30%) hemophilia, the risk for bleeding after even "minor" surgical procedures or trauma persists (Table 130.1).

The PTT is variably prolonged, depending on the severity of the factor deficiency. The VIII:C is decreased but the PT, bleeding time, and vWF:Ag are normal. Women who are carriers have low VIII:C levels (20–50%) and normal vWF:Ag levels, and usually present as a mild bleeding disorder.

■ Management

Mild deficiency often requires prophylaxis before dental or surgical procedures, but prophylactic factor VIII concentrate infusions are usually not needed. **IV desmopressin** (DDAVP) induces the release of stored factor VIII and vWF from endothelial cells. While mild or moderate cases often respond to DDAVP, severe cases do not, as they have no stored VIII. These individuals require both prophylactic and therapeutic infusions of factor VIII concentrates.

One unit of VIII/kilogram will raise the VIII level by 2%. The dose of concentrate required to achieve a desired VIII level is calculated by the following formula: Units VIII = desired level (%) × weight (kg) × 0.5. The type of bleeding to be stopped settles the dose required—a level of 15–20% is required to control spontaneous joint or muscle bleeding, 30–40% for more severe bleeding, 50–100% for major surgery and 30–50% for prophylaxis between 10–14 days postoperatively. Factor VIII has a half life of nearly 12 hours. Thus, it should be infused every 12 hours, or as indicated by the VIII levels, to achieve the levels mentioned. Mild hemophilia A patients undergoing dental procedures may also be adequately treated with oral epsilon-aminocaproic acid or tranexamic acid, inhibitors of fibrinolysis.

The management of hemophilia A has been complicated by the transmission of contaminating viruses. Since 1985, all factor VIII concentrates in the U.S. have undergone some type of viral inactivation procedure, so that the risk of transmitting hepatitis, HIV, and other viruses has declined substantially. Unfortunately, more than 70% of hemophiliacs exposed to concentrates have acquired HIV, and immune suppression in HIV-negative hemophiliacs with hepatitis is a continuing problem as a result of prior exposure to contaminated concentrates.

TABLE 130.1. Clinical Bleeding in Relation to Coagulant Factor Levels in Hemophilia

Severity	Coagulant Factor Activity (%)	Type of Bleeding
Severe	<1	Spontaneous bleeding
Moderate	1–5	Severe bleeding after minor injury, occasional spontaneous bleeding
Mild	5–20	Severe bleeding after major hemostatic stress, no spontaneous bleeding

Inhibitor-related resistance to factor concentrates occurs in nearly 15% of severe hemophiliacs on replacement therapy; it is usually apparent when the infusions no longer raise the factor level in a previously responsive patient, or when the PTT fails to normalize in a 1:1 mix of patient's and pooled plasma. Inhibitors, measured in **Bethesda units** (BU), are IgG antibodies. An inhibitor below 5 BU ("low responder") may be overcome by high doses of factor VIII concentrate. Most inhibitors are species-specific, so that inhibitors to human VIII may be evaded by infusing porcine factor VIII, thus still attaining an increase in VIII level. Cross reactivity of the inhibitor to the porcine VIII should be excluded. With higher inhibitor activity (>10 BU; "high responder"), anamnestic response is likely on factor infusion. Options are porcine factor VIII, factor IX complex concentrates, or recombinant VIIIa concentrates. Immunosuppression of the inhibitor output is not always successful. Inhibitors cause management problems and a 20% mortality.

Hemophilia B

Hemophilia B (also known as factor IX deficiency or Christmas disease) is also an X-linked recessive trait (1:50,000 male births). Its clinical features and correlation of bleeding to factor levels resemble hemophilia A. The PTT is prolonged; the PT, BT, and platelet count are normal. The liver produces factor IX; thus severe liver disease may lower factor IX level. Required factor IX levels for treatment or prophylaxis are similar to those for hemophilia A. However, factor IX diffuses extravascularly, so that to attain similar factor levels to those in hemophilia A, it takes twice as much factor infusion (Units IX = desired level (%) × weight (kg) × 1.0).

The half-life of factor IX exceeds 24 hours, so that once daily (twice on the day of surgical procedures) infusions usually suffice. Factor IX complex concentrates contain varying amounts of factors II, VII, and X, and may cause thrombotic complications (**disseminated intravascular coagulation** [DIC], deep venous thrombosis, and pulmonary embolism). These patients also develop inhibitors, with outcomes and management similar to Hemophilia A.

Von Willebrand's disease

Von Willebrand's disease (vWD), an autosomal dominant and variably expressed illness, is the most common (1 in 125 persons) heritable coagulation disorder. The **vW protein** (vWF), a very large, multimeric protein produced by endothelial cells and megakaryocytes, is stored in the platelet α granules and the Weibel-Palade bodies of the endothelial cells. A carrier of factor VIII, it helps the platelets aggregate among themselves and adhere to the endothelium, leading to a platelet plug. Thus, loss of vWF resembles decreased platelet function (easy bruising, menorrhagia, and mucosal and gastrointestinal bleeding). Severe vWF deficiency may occasionally cause a bleeding pattern resembling a coagulation factor deficiency (bleeding after surgery or trauma, spontaneous hemarthrosis, etc.). The diagnosis of mild vWD can be difficult in stressed patients, as the stored vWF in the endothelial cells is released as an acute phase reactant, and vWF levels may become normal.

Using the multimeric pattern on plasma electrophoresis (Table 130.2) several subtypes of vWD may be identified. Type I is the commonest. In Type IIB, vW molecule has an abnormal affinity for the platelet surface. The large multimers are intravascularly bound and vWF levels are low. Platelet aggregates form and are removed, causing thrombocytopenia. Use of DDAVP in these patents may worsen the thrombocytopenia by increasing the release of abnormal vWF; it is thus contraindicated. **Pseudo-von-Willebrand disease** (or "platelet type")

TABLE 130.2.	Laboratory Abnormalities in von Willebrand's Disease by Type				
	Type I	Type IIA	Type IIB	Pseudo	Type III
PT	N	N	N	N	N
PTT	Mild ↑	Mild ↑	↑	↑	↑
BT	↑	↑	↑	↑	↑↑
Platelet count	N	N	N or ↓	N or ↓	N
VIII: C	SI ↓	N or SI ↓	N or ↓	N or ↓	↓↓
VWR: Ag	SI ↓	↓	↓ or N	N or ↓	↓↓ <5
Multimer	N distribution ↓ numbers	↓ large & intermediate; ↑ small	No large multimers	↓ large	None
RCvWFA	↓	↓	↓ or N	↓ or N	↓↓ <1
Comments	Most common	10–15% of cases	Autosomal dominant	Really a platelet disorder	Often homozygous

RCvWFA = Ristocetin Co factor VWF; Activity: ↓ = Decreased; ↑ = Increased; N = normal; For others, see text.

mimics type IIB. The vWF is normal, but the platelet receptor has an abnormally high affinity for the large vW multimers, causing platelet aggregation as the protein is released. Circulating large multimers are low. Cryoprecipitate induces spontaneous platelet aggregation in the pseudo-vW type, thus differentiating it from type IIB. In type III, the vWF and VIII:C severely decline and all multimers are completely absent; the severe bleeding here resembles severe hemophilia A or B (hemarthrosis/soft tissue bleeding). Screening studies may also be normal in a significant number of patients, thus making the diagnosis difficult.

■ Management

The treatment of von Willebrand's disease depends on the type (Table 130.2). At the time of diagnosis,

DDAVP is often infused to document response and to help anticipate therapy if a bleeding emergency arises. Thirty minutes after infusion, the platelet count, factor VIII, and vWF/ristocetin cofactor levels are drawn. DDAVP often suffices in less severe deficiencies or for minor surgery (e.g., tooth extractions). It is usually quite effective in type I, but responses are variable in type IIA. Since it only releases stored vWF and factor VIII:C, DDAVP will not be useful in severe deficiencies or in those not producing these factors, nor should it be given in type IIB and platelet-type vWD. Either cryoprecipitate or vWF concentrate is used in severe deficiency and type IIB. Oral antifibrinolytic agents are often used in mild or moderate deficiency to prevent bleeding after dental surgery or for arduous mucosal bleeding (e.g., epistaxis) or menorrhagia.

CHAPTER 131 BLEEDING ASSOCIATED WITH PLATELET DISORDERS

Platelets, fragments of the megakaryocyte cytoplasm, have a normal life span of ten days in the circulation. Their surfaces provide the phospholipid base for many of the coagulation factors to function, and their storage granules provide procoagulant and vasoactive proteins that are key to the ability to form a hemostatic plug. Young platelets appear to be more hemostatically active. Disorders in platelet numbers and/or function, therefore, often cause bleeding disorders, whether hereditary or acquired. The normal blood has 140,000 to 400,000 circulating platelets per mm^3. Roughly one-third of the circulating platelets are pooled in the spleen.

Thrombocytopenia

■ Definition and Etiology

Thrombocytopenia is a decrease in the number of circulating platelets in the blood. Due to poor platelet plug formation, a bleeding diathesis results, the severity of which correlates with the degree of thrombocytopenia. No significant hemostatic abnormalities follow thrombocytopenia when the platelet count exceeds 100,000/mm^3. In uncomplicated thrombocytopenia, spontaneous bleeding is unusual when platelet count exceeds 40,000/mm^3. An inverse linear correlation is noted between bleeding time and a platelet count below 100,000/mm^3.

Thrombocytopenia may result from **decreased production, increased destruction,** or **increased pooling** of platelets (Table 131.1). Decreased production of megakaryocytes and platelets follows damage to the marrow or as a part of aplastic anemia. Megaloblastic anemias, myeloproliferative disorders and certain hereditary disorders (e.g., Wiskott-Aldrich syndrome, and May-Hegglin anomaly) are frequently associated with ineffective thrombopoiesis. Accelerated platelet destruction, caused by an autoantibody, frequently causes thrombocytopenia or the platelets may be consumed by intravascular thrombosis (e.g., disseminated intravascular coagulation and microangiopathic processes). The bone marrow in these instances usually shows an increase in megakaryocytes. It is important to obtain a history of drug ingestion in any patient with thrombocytopenia, because drugs may directly suppress the bone marrow or they may act as antigens and stimulate antibody formation.

TABLE 131.1.	Pathogenesis and Frequent Causes of Thrombocytopenia

Decreased Production	Aplastic anemia
	    Radiation, cytotoxic drug therapy
	Pancytopenia
	Marrow infiltration
	    Myelofibrosis, cancer
	Ineffective megakaryopoiesis
	    Vitamin B$_{12}$ or folate deficiency
	Drug-induced
	    Ethanol, gold, sulfonamides, trimethoprim-sulfamethoxazole, quinine ("cocktail purpura")

Increased destruction	Immune destruction
	    Immune thrombocytopenic purpura (ITP), lymphomas, SLE
	    ITP with Coomb's positive hemolytic anemia (Evan's syndrome)
	    Drug-induced (some involving anti-platelet antibody)
	        Thiazides, acetaminophen, phenytoin, heparin, quinidine, quinine
	Nonimmune destruction
	    Infections
	        Infectious mononucleosis, septicemia
	    Disseminated intravascular coagulation (DIC), microangiopathic hemolytic anemia,
	        thrombotic thrombocytopenic purpura (TTP), hemolytic uremic syndrome (HUS)

Normal production	Peripheral pooling Splenic sequestration

Immune Thrombocytopenic Purpura

■ Clinical Features and Diagnosis

Immune thrombocytopenia may be either primary (idiopathic) or secondary (Table 131.2). Acute **Idiopathic immune thrombocytopenia** most commonly affects children between 2–6 years of age, and the chronic form most frequently affects young women. Autoantibody coated platelets are rapidly sequestered in the spleen, causing thrombocytopenia.

Patients usually report petechiae or mucosal bleeding. Blood-filled blisters may be seen in the oral cavity. Neither lymphadenopathy nor splenomegaly occurs in **idiopathic thrombocytopenic purpura** (ITP). Clinical features of the associated disease are seen in secondary types. The platelet count is low and the bleeding time is prolonged; the blood smear shows a reduced number of platelets, some of which may be large. Bone marrow examination reveals an increased or normal number of megakaryocytes. The platelet antibody test is positive in a majority of the patients.

ITP is a diagnosis of exclusion. In some patients with ITP, especially if associated with autoimmune hemolytic anemia (Evans' syndrome), SLE develops eventually. The history of any drug ingestion should be noted. In a thrombocytopenic patient, all but the very essential drugs should be stopped. Drug-related immune thrombocytopenia usually resolves rapidly after stopping the offend-

TABLE 131.2.	Principal Causes of Immune Thrombocytopenia

Idiopathic
  Acute
  Chronic
Secondary
  Lymphoproliferative disorders
  Systemic lupus erythematosus
Drug-related

ing drug. ITP in children may exhibit spontaneous remissions.

■ Management

Adults with ITP or children without spontaneous remission are treated with corticosteroids. In some patients with ITP, platelet counts may transiently rise following a transfusion, but the majority of cases do not exhibit this feature. High dose prednisone is initiated (1–2 mg/kg/d). If thrombocytopenia resolves, prednisone is slowly tapered and eventually stopped. Patients not responding to or requiring large maintenance doses of prednisone (>10 mg/d) require splenectomy, which can induce a remission in about 70% of patients. Patients with a prior response to prednisone are more likely to respond to splenectomy. If splenectomy fails, immunosuppression is begun with cyclophosphamide, vincristine, or azathioprine. The following agents may be useful in resistant cases: high-dose IV IgG, plasmapheresis, and danazol, an androgen with reduced virilizing ability. IV IgG, which transiently increases platelet count, has been more effective in children than in adults with ITP; it is useful in certain situations (e.g., prior to splenectomy or suspected CNS bleed). Danazol has recently been added to the long-term management of refractory ITP.

Patients with secondary thrombocytopenia are treated in the same manner; additional treatment may be needed for the primary disorder.

Acquired Platelet Function Defects

Acquired platelet function defects, the most common cause of bleeding (see Table 131.3), are most commonly caused by drugs; but underlying diseases may also be responsible. While the cause of the defect is unclear in uremia, uremic platelets appear to bind the von Willebrand factor defectively, interfering with aggregation and with the subendothelial adhesion of platelets. Dialysis will sometimes correct the abnormality partially, and life-threatening bleeding may be treated with platelet concentrates. Lesser bleeding episodes often respond to either cryoprecipitate, DDAVP, and /or estrogen.

In myeloproliferative and myelodysplastic syndromes, the platelets are commonly abnormal; however, the pattern of aggregation and adhesion abnormalities is not usually characteristic or diagnostic. Most commonly, aggregation and release to epinephrine, ADP, and/or collagen are abnormal. The bleeding time, while often abnormal, does not reliably gauge the risk of bleeding. Paraproteinemias often cause platelet defects, apparently by abnormal protein coating of the platelet surface. The abnormality is independent of the type of paraprotein, and it usually improves with either treatment of the underlying disorder or plasmapheresis.

A variety of drugs adversely affect platelet function, a feature with therapeutic merit in some (e.g., aspirin) and adverse sequelae in others (Table 131.4). A significant bleeding diathesis may arise during cardiopulmonary bypass (CPB), partly due to platelet dysfunction; platelets seem to degranulate while circulating in the CPB and often appear as "ghosts" in the peripheral smear. While therapeutic doses of antiplatelet drugs prior to CPB may enhance the bleeding risk, platelet transfusions usually promptly correct the defect.

TABLE 131.3. Acquired Platelet Function Defects

Uremia
Myeloproliferative diseases
Myelodysplastic syndromes
Paraproteinemia
Autoimmune
  Collagen vascular disease
  Antiplatelet antibodies
  Immune thrombocytopenia
Liver disease
Cardiac surgery
Drugs
  Alcohol
  Ampicillin
  Aspirin
  Cephalothin
  Chlorpromazine
  Clofibrate
  Cocaine
  Cyclosporin A
  Dipyridamole
  Vincristine, vinblastine
  Nitrofurantoin
  NSAIDs
  Penicillins
  Phenylbutazone
  Sulfinpyrazone
  Tricyclic antidepressants

TABLE 131.4. Drugs Affecting Platelet Function

Antihistamine
Aspirin
β-blockers
Cephalosporin antibiotics
Dextran
Diltiazem
Nifedipine
Nitroglycerin
Nitroprusside
NSAIDs
Penicillin
Prostacyclin
Quinidine
Tricyclic antidepressants
Verapamil

Hereditary Platelet Disorders

Bernard-Soulier Syndrome

In this autosomal dominant disorder, the platelets lack the membrane glycoproteins necessary for binding vWF to the platelet surface. Clinical features include easy and sometimes spontaneous bruising, epistaxis, menorrhagia, petechiae and purpura. The peripheral blood smear shows giant platelets. VIII:C and VIII:RAg are normal, but bleeding time and ristocetin aggregation tests are abnormal, differentiating this disorder from von Willebrand's disease. Severe, life-threatening hemorrhage requires the transfusion of normal donor platelets. Heterozygotes are often asymptomatic.

Glanzmann's Thrombasthenia

This autosomal recessive disorder, the lack of glycoprotein IIb/IIIa complex on the platelets surfaces render the platelets unable to bind fibrinogen to their surface. Mucosal bleeding, spontaneous bruising, petechiae, and, rarely, hemarthrosis are the features. Platelet-to-platelet interaction is abnormal, and the bleeding time is prolonged. The disorder tends to improve with age. Severe hemorrhage requires platelet concentrates, but because antibodies might develop to glycoprotein IIb/IIIa, platelets should be transfused in only severe bleeding episodes. Epsilon-aminocaproic acid may be used for relatively minor mucosal bleeding.

Hereditary Storage Pool Diseases

These secondary aggregation disorders are more common than primary aggregation defects. Other congenital abnormalities such as Wiskott-Aldrich syndrome, thrombocytopenia with absent radii (TAR) syndrome, Chediak-Higashi syndrome may be occasionally associated, but inheritance is variable and most patients are otherwise normal. Mucosal bleeding, epistaxis, easy bruising, and hematuria are reported. The bleeding time is prolonged, and platelet adhesion and aggregation are abnormal in the presence of collagen. Severe hemorrhage requires platelet concentrates.

CHAPTER 132 ACQUIRED BLEEDING DISORDERS

■ Etiology

Acquired coagulation disorders may be caused by a panoply of medical conditions. As a cause of bleeding diathesis, they are much more common than hereditary coagulation or platelet disorders. Some major clinical issues include acquired bleeding problems due to liver disease, disseminated intravascular coagulation (DIC), drugs, malignancies, massive transfusions, thrombotic thrombocytopenic purpura, and hemolytic-uremic syndrome.

Liver Disease

Liver disease, through multiple mechanisms (Table 132.1), is probably the most common cause of coagulation abnormalities in a general hospital population. Deficiencies of coagulation factors synthesized in the liver may lead to life-threatening bleeding, while profound thrombocytopenia may arise from cirrhosis and splenic sequestration. The spectrum of abnormalities is wide, from normal coagulation profile in a patient with mild liver disease to life-threatening severe hemorrhage with DIC or fibrinolysis.

TABLE 132.1.   Hemostatic Abnormalities in Liver Disease

Mechanism	Result
Decreased synthesis of Vit K–dependent factors	Elevated PT
Splenic sequestration	Thrombocytopenia
Circulating platelet inhibitors	Platelet dysfunction
Synthesis of abnormal coagulation factors	Dysfibrinogenemia ↓ Protein C function
Increased factor consumption	Primary fibrinolysis DIC
Decreased clearance of factors	DIC Fibrinolysis
Decreased AT-III and protein C production	DIC

AT-III = Anti-thrombin III; DIC = Disseminated intravascular coagulation.

Disseminated Intravascular Coagulation

Disseminated intravascular coagulation (DIC) is a pathologic process that activates the coagulation, fibrinolytic, and platelet systems. Many underlying disorders seem to cause the expression of tissue factor to initiate the process. Coagulation factors and platelets are consumed as the coagulation cascade is continuously activated; despite the initial event being thrombin generation, excessive bleeding usually dominates the clinical picture. Thrombin converts fibrinogen to fibrin, elevates the fibrin degradation products, activates platelets, and initiates fibrinolysis (Figure 132.1). DIC may occur as a fulminant bleeding event with end-organ

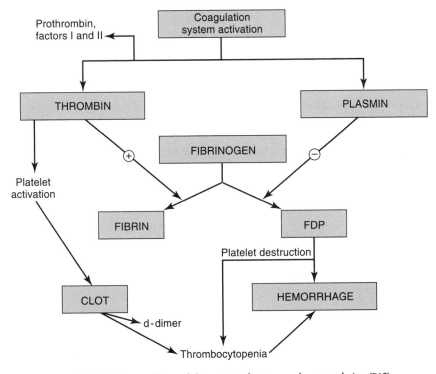

FIGURE 132.1. The evolution of disseminated Intravascular coagulation (DIC).

TABLE 132.2. Causes of Disseminated Intravascular Coagulation (DIC)
Infection
Gram (–) and gram (+) bacteremia, viruses (herpes, Lassa, dengue), Rocky Mountain spotted fever, fungi (candida, aspergillus) and others (clostridia, toxic shock syndrome, malaria)
Trauma
Crush injuries, brain injuries, thermal injuries
Vascular injuries
Giant hemangioma, aortic aneurysm, vasculitis, aortic balloon pump, acute myocardial infarction, pulmonary embolism, malignant hypertension
Obstetric complications
Abruptio placentae, eclampsia, amniotic fluid embolism, hydatidiform mole, uterine rupture, retained dead fetus/missed abortion
Malignancies
Adenocarcinomas, tumor lysis syndrome, acute leukemia
Other
ARDS, amyloidosis, inflammatory bowel disease, cirrhosis, fulminant hepatic necrosis, pancreatitis, snake bites, Reyes syndrome, hypovolemic/hemorrhagic shock

TABLE 132.3. Laboratory Abnormalities in Disseminated Intravascular Coagulation (DIC)

Test	Reliability (% abnormal)
d-dimer	93
Antithrombin III	89
Fibrinopeptide A	88
FDP titer	75

and erythrocyte fragments). In severe DIC, virtually all coagulation tests are abnormal. FDP rises in 80–100% of patients with DIC, and the protamine sulfate or ethanol gel tests (indicating circulating soluble fibrin monomers) are usually positive. The d-dimer assay is specific for FDP, and it is the most reliable test for diagnosing DIC. Some other tests for diagnosing DIC are listed in Table 132.3.

Treatment of DIC is primarily that of the underlying cause, thus removing the stimulus for the coagulation activation. In addition, the replacement of factors, individualized to fit the pace of the patient's consumption and guided by repeated laboratory monitoring, is usually necessary to prevent fulminant hemorrhage. Low dose heparin (5–10 U/kg/h) is occasionally used if the cause of the DIC is ongoing. It is also used to try to lower the rate of factor consumption so that replacement therapy can keep up with the demand. Heparin resistance occasionally develops due to low antithrombin III levels; ATIII concentrates may be helpful. Cryoprecipitate is used for severe hypofibrinogenemia and as a source of VIII:C, and platelets are transfused to maintain counts of 20,000/μL.

ischemia related to intravascular microthrombi, or as a chronic complication of malignancy featuring recurrent thrombosis and compensated factor consumption. Table 132.2 represents a partial list of causes of DIC.

Diagnosis of acute, fulminant DIC is usually easy in an actively bleeding patient. However, the diagnosis of chronic DIC may be difficult, especially if the underlying disease remains elusive. Laboratory results indicate coagulation factor consumption, evidence of fibrin and fibrinogen degradation, fibrinolytic activity, and evidence of microangiopathy on a peripheral smear (schistocytes

Thrombotic Thrombocytopenic Purpura

Thrombotic thrombocytopenic purpura (TTP) and the closely related hemolytic-uremic syndrome (HUS) are of uncertain etiology, and until recently, uniformly fatal. TTP and HUS are compared in Table 132.4. They accompany pregnancy, malignancies, rheumatoid arthritis, HIV infection, and the use of certain chemotherapy agents (mitomycin C). A high-molecular-weight form of von Willebrand's protein as well as a platelet-aggregating protein have been noted in TTP plasma, which may be play a pathogenetic role. Most often, the blood vessel lumen throughout the body show a PAS-positive, hyaline material deposition. Besides general supportive mea-

TABLE 132.4. Comparative Features of Thrombotic Thrombocytopenic Purpura (TTP) and Hemolytic-Uremic Syndrome (HUS)

	TTP	HUS
Age group	Mostly adults	Mostly children
Etiology	Unknown	Illness often follows gastroenteritis by Escherichia coli O157:H7
Prodrome	Less common	Bloody diarrheal illness
Clinical Features	Hemolytic anemia, thrombocytopenia, renal failure, fever, and neurologic symptoms	Hemolytic anemia, thrombocytopenia, and acute renal failure; either hemoglobinuria or anuria in most
Renal involvement	Occurs, but renal failure is usually less severe	Integral part of illness, very severe.
CNS involvement	Profound; headache, blurred vision, seizures and/or coma	Unlikely
Recurrences	Common (up to 20%)	Rare
Coombs Test	Negative	Negative
Therapy	Steroids, plasmapheresis, splenectomy	Dialysis and transfusions
Peripheral smear	Schistocytes	Schistocytes
LDH	High	High

sures, the management of TTP usually includes emergent, daily plasmapheresis along with relatively large doses of corticosteroids. If plasmapheresis cannot be started rapidly, fresh frozen plasma may be infused in large volumes as a temporary measure. Rarely, splenectomy may be effective in TTP unresponsive to these measures. With aggressive plasmapheresis, up to 80–90% of patients with TTP recover.

Drugs

Drugs are a major cause of bleeding disorders, commonly as a therapeutic effect in patients with thrombosis and sometimes as an unwanted secondary effect on the function of platelets (Table 131.4). Aspirin and the nonsteroidal anti-inflammatory agents inhibit platelet cyclooxygenase and thereby decrease platelet aggregation. Unless the hemostatic system is otherwise compromised, few drugs with antiplatelet effects cause clinically significant bleeding. Heparin is widely used in the treatment of thrombotic disorders. Serious bleeding during carefully monitored heparin therapy is unusual; however, the risk is higher in older patients, after recent surgery, in hypertensives, or in patients with other bleeding diatheses.

A modest thrombocytopenia develops in nearly 5% of patients undergoing heparin therapy; it is noted within 4 days of beginning heparin and usually requires no intervention (type I). However, a more severe, progressive and heparin-dependent IgG antiplatelet autoantibody-mediated form may occur generally within 4–6 days of beginning heparin. The antibody leads to extensive platelet aggregation in the presence of heparin (type II). The thrombocytopenia is associated with thromboembolism. The antibodies may also react with the heparin bound to the endothelial cells, thereby causing an immune-mediated endothelial cell injury. This, in conjunction with the platelet aggregation, may predispose to arterial or venous thrombosis.

Heparin-induced thrombocytopenia (HIT) may be managed by changing the type of heparin (e.g., bovine to porcine). If this does not suffice, heparin is discontinued. Diagnostic studies include heparin-induced platelet aggregation, platelet factor-4 immunoglobulin (PF4-Ig) by ELISA, and serotonin release assay. Low molecular weight heparin, warfarin, platelet transfusions, and inferior vena caval filters should be avoided, but antithrombotic therapy continued, using alternative agents such as danaparoid. Plasma exchange may be beneficial in selected cases. In most cases, the course of the HIT may be truncated by beginning warfarin and heparin simultaneously, and discontinuing heparin as soon as thrombocytopenia develops. By 4–6 days of such combined therapy, warfarin would have usually attained a therapeutic level, thus assuring adequate anticoagulation despite withdrawal of heparin. Patients who develop HIT should not be given heparin subsequently.

Warfarin is the most widely used long-term oral anticoagulant. It blocks the regeneration of vitamin K, thereby blocking synthesis of factors II, VII, IX, X, protein C, and protein S. The risk of bleeding in patients on warfarin is directly proportional to the intensity of anticoagulation, as determined by the **international normalized ratio** (INR). Various drugs profoundly affect warfarin clearance and, therefore, the risk of bleeding (Table 132.5). In unselected patients, the risk of bleeding while on warfarin varies from 0.1–3% per year. Warfarin overdose is treated with oral or IV vitamin K, or infusions of fresh frozen plasma; the choice depends on the severity of the anticoagulation and whether or not there is active bleeding. Because of the prolonged half-life of warfarin, a bleeding patient may require repeated plasma infusions.

Massive transfusions, usually following trauma, cause bleeding from multiple mechanisms; these include dilution of clotting factors from replacement fluids lacking factors, consumption of available factors in a bleeding patient, DIC due to hypovolemia, acidosis, or sepsis, dilutional thrombocytopenia, and acquired platelet dysfunction, possibly due to degranulation by traumatized platelets. Patients are treated with infusions of fresh frozen plasma, platelets, red blood cells, and cryoprecipitate, with repeated laboratory monitoring.

TABLE 132.5. Drugs Influencing Warfarin Effect[#]	
Intensify Warfarin Effect	**Decrease Warfarin Effect**
Phenylbutazone	Barbiturates
Metronidazole	Penicillin
Sulfinpyrazone	Rifampin
Trimethoprim-sulfamethoxazole	Cholestyramine
Amiodarone	Quinidine
Tamoxifen	
Isoniazid	
Ketoconazole	
Thyroxine	
Cimetidine	
Erythromycin	
Phenytoin (Dilantin)	

[#] = not a complete list.

CHAPTER 133

THROMBOTIC DISORDERS

Disturbances in the balance of the coagulation system may result in a hypercoagulable state. It may result from either a congenital lack of one of the natural anticoagulants, congenital defects in the fibrinolytic system, or a variety of acquired defects in the coagulation system. The term "hypercoagulable state" in general refers to an abnormality in the coagulation system predisposing to recurrent thrombotic events.

Antithrombin III Deficiency

Antithrombin III (AT-III), a glycoprotein, inactivates factors XIa, Xa, IXa, and thrombin by forming a 1:1 insoluble complex with each of these activated factors. AT-III is produced by the liver, and its deficiency is inherited in an autosomal dominant mode, with an incidence of 1 per 2500–5000 persons. The homozygous state is felt to be incompatible with life. Heterozygotes may have either low levels (50–70%) of functionally normal protein (type I), or normal levels of abnormal protein (type II). Acquired deficiency may occur in nephrotic syndrome. Typical initial thrombotic events, which usually occur by age 35, are pulmonary emboli, Budd-Chiari syndrome, or thrombosis of deep veins, renal veins, or mesenteric or iliofemoral vessels. Other factors (e.g., surgery, pregnancy, oral contraceptives, or trauma) may precipitate these events.

Other tests of the coagulation system are typically normal. Because AT-III levels normally decrease with acute thrombosis or after heparin therapy, the diagnosis of AT-III deficiency should be confirmed by checking levels when the patient is off anticoagulation (except warfarin) and not experiencing an acute thrombotic event. Prophylactic heparin treatment is given during pregnancy, and AT-III concentrates may be given to all others at risk (surgery, delivery, or trauma). Replacement is given to maintain AT-III levels above 80%.

Protein C Deficiency

Protein C, a vitamin K dependent protein, is produced in the liver. It exerts its anticoagulant effect by inactivating factors Va, VIIIa, and inhibition of tissue plasminogen activator. Its deficiency is inherited as autosomal dominant, albeit with incomplete penetrance. The homozygous state was fatal prior to the advent of concentrates. A heterozygous protein C deficiency state (30–50% of normal) causing thrombosis occurs in fewer than 1 in 1000 persons. A deficiency leads to recurrent thromboembolism, often in early life, and usually precipitated by some other event. Protein C concentrates or antithrombotic therapy with warfarin are appropriate treatments. Initiating warfarin in these persons causes the already low protein C levels to decline even further and faster than the procoagulant factors, owing to the shorter half-life of circulating protein C. The initial result is a net *prothrombotic* state. Thrombosis of the dermal vessels and skin necrosis follow. Full heparinization concurrent with initial warfarin doses prevents this complication. Activated protein C resistance is discussed in chapter 129.

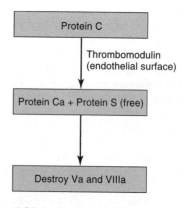

FIGURE 133.1. Protein C and Protein S system.

Protein S Deficiency

Protein S, a vitamin K-dependent factor produced by the liver, circulates both free and protein-bound. Free protein S is a cofactor of protein C in its inhibition of factors Va and VIIIa (Figure 133.1). Its deficiency is inherited as an autosomal dominant trait. Its clinical features are similar to protein C deficiency. Acquired deficiency occurs in nephrotic syndrome. Warfarin decreases protein S levels, and should be stopped for at least one week before testing protein S levels. Heparin does not lower protein S level, but acute thrombosis does. The treatment is long-term warfarin to prevent spontaneous thrombosis.

Fibrinolytic Defects

The fibrinolytic system is schematically shown in Figure 133.2. Nearly 30% of patients with thrombosis might have abnormalities of their fibrinolytic systems. **Tissue plasminogen activator** (tPA) is made by endothelial cells; its deficiency, an autosomal dominant trait, manifests with venous and/or arterial thrombosis. Acquired tPA deficiency may contribute to cancer-related hypercoagulability. Plasminogen abnormalities and dysfibrinogenemias (both inherited and rare) lead to thrombosis. Homocystinuria, an autosomal recessive disease, is also rare and manifests with vascular abnormalities and thrombosis.

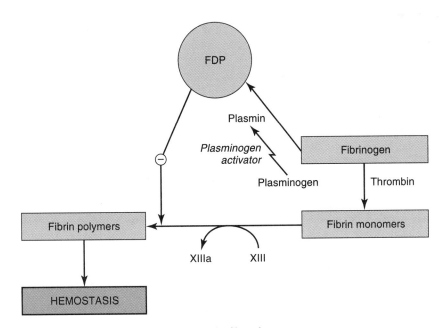

FIGURE 133.2. The fibrinolytic system.

Acquired Thrombotic Defects

The **lupus anticoagulant** (LA), which is frequently implicated in recurrent thromboses, is a heterogeneous group of anti-phospholipid immunoglobulins that interfere with prothrombin activation, and exert procoagulant activity by increasing platelet adhesiveness and activation, interfering with protein C activation, and causing abnormal AT-III activity. LA occur in infections, systemic lupus erythematosus, and lymphoproliferative disorders. Venous thrombosis and pulmonary embolism are the major features; however, other major arterial and/or venous thromboses occur as well. An autoimmune thrombocytopenia coexists in some patients because of LA's autoimmune basis; however, the usual clinical features are thrombotic. LA is usually recognized when thrombosis is evaluated in the young or when a prolonged PTT is seen in asymptomatic persons. The type of phospholipid reagents used and the antiphospholipid antibody interference prolong the PTT, but the clinical picture is clotting, not bleeding.

Patients without lupus or other autoimmune diseases may have **anticardiolipin antibodies,** an antiphospho-

lipid antibody syndrome also causing venous and arterial thrombosis. These antibodies have been implicated in coronary artery disease, recurrent coronary bypass graft occlusion, retinal artery occlusion, and stroke. Drugs associated with this syndrome include phenytoin, quinine, phenothiazines, alpha-interferon, cocaine, and hydralazine. Assays are available to detect IgG, IgM, idiotype and IgA anticardiolipin antibodies. Treatment is with long-term oral anticoagulation to prevent recurrent thrombosis.

Other Diseases Associated With Hypercoagulability

The myeloproliferative disorders have all been associated with both bleeding and thrombosis, but most of these disorders tend to exhibit only one or the other. **Polycythemia vera** leads to thrombosis, whereas patients with essential thrombocytosis and myeloid metaplasia tend to bleed. Hyperviscosity, platelet dysfunction, and hyperaggregability, and/or acquired storage pool disease may all cause excessive clotting. All types of thrombosis are seen: usual types include pulmonary embolism, deep venous thrombosis, and coronary or cerebrovascular occlusions; unusual types include Budd-Chiari syndrome and microvascular thrombosis. **Paroxysmal nocturnal hemoglobinuria** may present with thrombosis as the first symptom. Here, the hypercoagulability results from increased sensitivity and aggregation of platelets to the complement, accompanied by an increased sensitivity to thrombin.

Malignancy, by unclear mechanisms, also leads to a hypercoagulable state. Solid tumors may activate factor VII by the tissue factor pathway, while mucin-

secreting tumors may directly activate factor X. Some anticancer agents (cyclophosphamide, methotrexate, fluorouracil) confer an increased risk of thrombosis. Migratory thrombophlebitis in malignancies (Trousseau's syndrome) usually occurs with adenocarcinomas of the stomach, pancreas, or prostate. The apparent intrinsic hypercoagulable state in any cancer may be augmented by the immobility, advanced age, and increased tissue trauma also common to these patients. Tumor impingement on vessels increases the turbulence of flow and predisposes to local hypercoagulable conditions (e.g., superior vena cava syndrome or pelvic thrombosis).

The laboratory evaluation in these patients may show high fibrinogen, thrombocytosis, a short PTT, and, occasionally, d-dimers. The risk of thrombosis may be lessened by treating the primary condition. Acute thrombotic events are treated in the usual way with heparin. Many of these may be refractory to oral anticoagulation, requiring heparin therapy on an ambulatory basis.

CHAPTER 134 **ERYTHROCYTOSIS**

Erythrocytosis represents a significantly elevated RBC, Hgb, and Hct. Its classification is shown in Table 134.1. In dehydration, burns and shock, erythrocytosis is considered *relative*, since the plasma volume is diminished and the total red cell

volume is normal. Chronic hypoxia increases erythropoietin (EPO) secretion, leading to erythrocytosis. Carbon monoxide from heavy cigarette smoking stimulates RBC production. Smoking may also cause airflow obstruction; the resulting hypoxemia leads to excessive

EPO secretion. A similar hypoxia-mediated mechanism operates in erythrocytosis of high altitude and other cardiopulmonary diseases since any condition which effectively lowers O_2 saturation will elicit release of EPO as a normal physiological response. In high-affinity hemoglobinopathies, mutant hemoglobins yield oxygen less readily to the tissues, thus stimulating RBC production. A hormonally mediated mechanism occurs in Cushing's syndrome and with androgen-secreting tumors.

TABLE 134.1.   Causes of Erythrocytosis

A. Primary erythremia—polycythemia vera
B. Secondary
  1. Relative (reduced plasma volume and normal RBC volume)
    Burns
    Dehydration
    Shock
  2. With elevated erythropoiesis
    Cigarette smoking ↑ CO
    Hypoxia—cardiopulmonary, high altitude living
    Renal cysts or masses
    Infratentorial tumors
    Cushing's syndrome
    Androgens
      (i) Therapeutic
      (ii) Androgen secreting tumors
    High O_2 affinity hemoglobinopathy

Polycythemia Vera

Primary erythremia or **polycythemia vera** (P. vera) derives from increased or hyperproliferative stem cells that proliferate independently of EPO. The resulting peripheral picture is one of erythrocytosis, leukocytosis, and thrombocythemia.

■ Pathophysiology

Among the physiopathologic alterations in P. vera (Table 134.2), the risk of hemorrhage is an important issue, attributed to stasis, vascular distension, and increased blood viscosity. The platelets also function abnormally; these, in conjunction with a relatively low plasma volume and limited total fibrinogen, cause **frequent, fragile blood clots,** followed by **hemorrhage.** The chief morbidity of leukocytosis is histamine release from the PMN, which causes **pruritus** and peptic ulcer. Excessive hematopoiesis leads to overproduction of purine substrates for nucleic acid synthesis; **hyperuricemia** and **gout** follow. Megakaryocytes and platelets stimulate fibroblastic proliferation via platelet derived growth factor; myelofibrosis and myeloid metaplasia of the spleen result eventually . The cellular proliferation in P. vera is monoclonal. The stem cells of P. vera are capable of independent growth and do not require the addition of EPO to ensure in vitro proliferation of CFU-E.

■ Clinical Features

P. vera is relatively rare and usually affects older individuals, with a slight preponderance in men. Because of its insidious onset, years go by before patients realize that anything is wrong with them. Symptoms, if present, are caused by the large RBC mass, including **headache, tinnitus, vertigo, visual disturbances, paresthesias,** and **erythromelalgia.** Severe pruritus, especially after a hot bath, results from histamine release from the neutrophils. The excess blood viscosity causes thrombosis, and, paradoxically, hemorrhage. **Venous thromboembolism** and intermittent claudication are very common. Other sites of thrombosis are the myocardium, spleen, brain, mesentery, and gastrointestinal tract. **Peptic ulcers** that develop in about 10% of patients are attributed to increased histamine release. The patient with fully expressed P. vera is plethoric, with marked conjunctival injection and **splenomegaly.** Central cyanosis is absent, a helpful distinction from hypoxic disorders that cause erythrocytosis.

■ Laboratory Features

The differentiation between various causes of erythrocytosis depends on three major findings (Table 134.3). The first and most important is an elevated total RBC volume as shown by ^{51}Cr-RBC with normal plasma volume (Normal RBC volume: 32–34 ml/kg in men and 30–32 ml/kg in women). In P. vera, the figure is significantly greater, unless there has been recent major hemorrhage or repeated phlebotomies. Secondly, the arterial oxygen saturation (SaO_2) must exceed 92% in P. vera, in contrast to hypoxia-mediated erythrocytosis, where SaO_2 is below 87%. Blood samples removed for

TABLE 134.2. Pathophysiology of Polycythemia Vera

Predominating Marrow Cell	Pathophysiology	Complication
Erythroblast	Blood viscosity	Vascular stasis, hemorrhage, thrombosis, impaired cerebral blood flow
Megakaryocytes	Platelets	Hemorrhage
	Hypercoagulable	Thrombosis
	Ineffective platelets	
Granulocytes	Cobalamin Binding	Pruritus
	Histamine	Peptic ulcer
		Gout
Fibroblasts	Platelets	Leukoerythroblastosis
	Myelofibrosis	Massive spleen
	Myeloid metaplasia	Anemia
Primary Mechanism	Proliferation of a single clone which grows independently of EPO	

EPO = Erythropoietin.

TABLE 134.3. Differentiating Between Various Causes of Erythrocytosis

Condition	Arterial O_2 Saturation	Total RBC Volume	Splenomegaly	EPO Value
Cigarette Smoking	↑ CO	Slightly ↑	0	N
Hypoxia	↓	Normal	0	↑
Renal Disease	Normal	↑	0	↑
P. Vera	Normal	↑	↑	↓

CO = Carbon monoxide; EPO = Erythropoietin.

SaO_2 should also be examined for CO content (normally <2%) and for P50 (which is 27 mm Hg in normals and lower [left-shifted] in high-affinity hemoglobins). When these findings are present, splenomegaly confirms P. vera. If not, two of the three may be considered diagnostic when one minor criterion is present. Minor criteria include leukocytosis (>20,000/10^{12}/L) or thrombocytosis (>800,000/10^{12}/L) in the presence of greatly increased marrow cellularity (>80–90%). With early myelofibrosis, reticulin fiber deposition may be increased.

In P. vera as well as other members of the myeloproliferative group, the leukocyte alkaline phosphatase (LAP) score exceeds 190 (normal: generally 80–100). In contrast, its is depleted in CML. Leukocytes play a role in B_{12} transport through their transcobalamin II content. With high WBC turnover, excess transcobalamin II is released into the plasma. Cobalamin binding capacity is thus enhanced in P. vera. Frequently, serum iron is diminished, transferrin is increased, and ferritin is very low, a pattern suggesting iron deficiency from repeated phlebotomies. Besides, most available iron is preferentially used for erythropoiesis, leading to diminished iron stores. With increased RBC, endogenous EPO synthesis should cease, and serum EPO levels are low. In contrast, in secondary polycythemia from hypoxia, the serum EPO level increases.

■ **Management**

Once the diagnosis of P. vera is established, the RBC volume should be rapidly reduced through weekly phlebotomy. As the hematocrit declines to 45–48%, the choice must be made between phlebotomy alone, or myelosuppressives (hydroxyurea [HU]), or ^{32}P. While phlebotomy rapidly regulates hematocrit, it does not control the splenomegaly, pruritus, or thrombosis. Myelosuppressives should be limited to those over 50 years of age. (With HU, the dose is adjusted to maintain WBC at 10×10^9/L, and platelets at 500×10^9/L) However, phlebotomies must continue for hematocrit above 45–48%. Probably the most convenient treatment is ^{32}P. The initial dose is frequently effective for more than one year, but an aggressive disease may recur sooner. If the platelet count increases to more than 800×10^9/L, ^{32}P is readministered. Even with ^{32}P, or HU, phlebotomy should be employed when the hematocrit exceeds 45%.

Within 10 years following ^{32}P therapy, about 10% of patients develop burned-out P. vera, myelofibrosis, or leukemic transformation. The oncogenic properties of HU remain a hazard, but its leukemogenic potential remains unknown. Surgery in patients with P. vera must be undertaken with the greatest of caution because of the severe risk of hemorrhage and thrombosis in these patients immediately postoperatively; each patient about to undergo surgery should be warned of the profound hazards. Surgery should be done only if the platelet count and hematocrit are sufficiently regulated.

■ **Course and Prognosis**

P. vera eventually stabilizes, as RBC no longer increase. During this spent phase, therapy is no longer required. Hematopoiesis shifts from a bone marrow that becomes fibrotic to myeloid metaplasia of the liver and spleen. These organs massively enlarge within 10 years of onset. Paradoxically, erythrocytosis transforms to anemia; transfusion, and not phlebotomy, may now become necessary. The most limiting prognostic factor is the transformation to acute leukemia, which is terminal and rapidly fatal.

CHAPTER 135 CHRONIC MYELOCYTIC LEUKEMIA AND MYELOFIBROSIS

Chronic Myelocytic Leukemia

■ **Definition**

Chronic myelocytic leukemia (CML) results from massive clonal expansion of granulocyte marrow precursors. The resulting extreme and progressive peripheral leukocytosis manifests all of the various morphologic stages of developing granulocytes. The characteristic marker is the Philadelphia chromosome (Ph), found in all the bone marrow-derived cells; it establishes CML as a clonal disorder derived from a disordered proliferation of uncommitted stem cells. Ph appears as a minute structure derived from chromosome 22, in which part of the long (p) arm is broken off and adheres to the short (q) arm of chromosome 9 in a rearrangement known as (t 9:22) (q 34:11). Genetic material (C-abl) is thus transposed from chromosome 22 to chromosome 9, creating a new fusion gene between 5'-bcr and C-abl. Uncontrolled cellular proliferation follows the production of a new hybrid messenger RNA and a new product —tyrosine kinase. The abnormal RNA transcript can be noted on a northern blot. Using polymerase chain reaction (PCR), the bcr-abl fusion RNA may be amplified by 100,000 fold, thus allowing detection of the genetic abnormality, even when the disease is in remission. Ph is found in 90% of cases of CML. The 10% of CML patients who lack Ph are more refractory to treatment. However, even in these cases, the bcr-abl fusion RNA can be detected by amplification using PCR.

■ **Clinical Features**

The onset of typical Ph positive CML is asymptomatic. CML is frequently found during an incidental examination for unrelated reasons. Weight loss may develop later in the course, despite a good appetite; hyperthyroidism may be suspected. Slowly developing mild anemia leads to fatigue, loss of vigor, and exercise intolerance. Early satiation, a feeling of abdominal fullness, and left upper quadrant or left shoulder pain are related to splenomegaly. As in P. vera, serum histamine levels may rise with leukocytosis and cause pruritus. With high granulocyte turnover urate production increases, leading to gout. Splenomegaly, frequently massive, is the outstanding clinical sign. Hepatomegaly and bony pain and tenderness (from increased intramedullary pressure causing pressure on nerve-rich endosteum) may be noted. Pallor, fever, and lymphadenopathy are late manifestations. Splenic infarction occurs as the spleen enlarges and outstrips its blood supply.

Late in the course of disease, the number or function of the platelets may be compromised. Bleeding into the skin or from the mucous membranes may then follow. Infection is rarely a problem because the PMN retain their normal phagocytic function. However, if PMN are eventually replaced by nonfunctioning blast cells, uncontrolled infection may result.

■ **Laboratory Features**

The total WBC count almost invariably exceeds 50×10^9/L. The WBCs are distributed in the peripheral smear in all developmental stages in descending proportions (segmented PMN [60–70%], band forms, metamyelocytes, myelocytes, promyelocytes, and blasts). The total aggregate of granulocyte precursors frequently exceeds 20–25%. Notably, the basophils increase to 3–4% or more during remission. Monocytosis, while variable, may be 20% or higher in Ph negative CML or CMML. The RBCs are usually normal or slightly elevated early in the course of the disease, but decline later. Similarly, the platelet count is elevated at first but may diminish preterminally.

A major objective manifestation of CML is the low or suppressed leukocyte alkaline phosphatase (LAP) score, which distinguishes CML from other myeloproliferative disorders (P. vera, myelofibrosis, or essential thrombocythemia) where it is high. A low LAP score occurs in very few conditions besides CML; exceptions are paroxysmal nocturnal hemoglobinuria, gout, or chronic liver disease, conditions readily separable from CML clinically or by laboratory means. Serum uric acid is elevated and there may be evidence of urate deposition. Increased B_{12} binding capacity results from increased granulocyte turnover. A bone marrow biopsy, while rarely needed for diagnosis, may differentiate CML from myelofibrosis, or help detect the Ph chromosome, especially if nonproliferating cells are present in the peripheral blood.

Philadelphia Chromosome-Negative CML

About 10% of patients with CML are Philadelphia-chromosome negative. Their WBC count is elevated, but not to the same level as in the Ph positive type. The monocyte count is elevated more characteristically, leading to the designation as **chronic myelomonocytic leukemia** (CMML). Serum and urine muramidase (lysozyme) values are elevated. More important, this group fails to respond to conventional chemotherapy, thus indicating a worse prognosis.

■ Course

The clinical course of CML is determined by the presence or absence of the Ph chromosome. The initial phase of Ph (+) CML is asymptomatic, indolent, and fully responsive to chemotherapy. In the accelerated phase that develops eventually, mature and immature granulocytes as well as basophils increase in number and previously effective chemotherapeutic agents become ineffective. Abnormal forms of PMN also emerge, with two nuclear lobes (**Pelger-Huët cells).** The bone marrow may become difficult to aspirate. The spleen enlarges

massively; anemia and thrombocytopenia worsen. In the blast phase that follows, nucleated blast cells replace the peripheral PMNs. Some blasts harbor a pathologic enzyme, **terminal deoxyribonucleotide transferase** (TdT), which is normally manifested by thymus-derived cells. Despite an occasional, transitory response to vincristine and prednisone, the ensuing course inexorably deteriorates and is rapidly lethal.

■ Management

Truly effective therapy for CML is the elimination of the Ph chromosome and the restoration of normal hematopoiesis, which are presently possible only through bone marrow transplantation. The recipient must be young enough to withstand the rigors of transplantation and there must be a donor exactly matched to his or her HLA type. The recipient's marrow is completely ablated with total body irradiation and high-dose chemotherapy, a process that would be fatal unless the donor's marrow cells were completely engraft. If there is no suitable sibling donor, a nonrelated donor may suffice if a suitable match can be found through a marrow registry. Another alternative is autotransplantation of the patient's own marrow harvested during periods of remission.

Chemotherapy must be employed if conditions for successful marrow transplant cannot be achieved. Hydroxyurea is the safest and most effective agent for achieving prolonged remission. Successful treatment restores the spleen size and WBC to normal. However, the Ph chromosome remains, as does a slowly increasing LAP score. Most physicians prefer to maintain the patient on a small dose of HU, but a few prefer its intermittent use. Recombinant human α-interferon, an alternative agent is also effective. Given alone or in combination with chemotherapy drugs, it can produce prolonged remissions with disappearance of Ph(+) cells from the bone marrow. Blast transformation must be aggressively treated with daunorubicin and cytosine arabinoside. Patients with TDT positive blasts may respond temporarily to vincristine plus prednisone.

Myelofibrosis

Myelofibrosis is the conversion of the aspiratable, semi-fluid bone marrow to a nonaspiratable, solid collection of fibrous tissue. The spleen enlarges, sometimes massively, because it engages in erythropoiesis in order to compensate for the loss of marrow. The disease arises from a single clone of pluripotent stem cells. Because megakaryocytes and platelets persist in marrow, the fibrosis appears to be stimulated by platelet-derived growth factor.

■ Clinical Features

Characteristically, myelofibrosis affects older individuals and is more frequent in men. Often, it develops late or preterminally in P. vera or CML. Its clinical hallmark is splenomegaly and, often, gout. Its symptoms include those of anemia, as well as an enlarging left upper abdominal (LUQ) fullness and early satiation. Splenic infarction, a distressing complication, manifests with pain in the LUQ and left shoulder. Ascites and pleural effusions are apt to occur if the extramedullary hematopoiesis involves pleural and peritoneal sites. Weight loss, progressive splenomegaly, and increasing anemia are prominent events with preterminal infections, hemorrhage, or leukemic transformation.

■ Laboratory Features

Anemia may be moderate or severe, with variable WBC and platelet counts. The RBC resemble "tear-drops," with a small projection at one end. The peripheral smear is "leukoerythroblastic" (immature WBC and normoblasts seen simultaneously). A simple distinction from CML is that the sum total of WBC precursors rarely exceeds 20%. Many large platelets are present peripherally; some of them are megakaryocytic fragments. Bone marrow is usually not aspiratable (**dry tap**). Diagnosis requires biopsy (with Jamshidi-type needle), which shows bundles of fibrous tissue and many residual megakaryocytes. The Ph chromosome is absent unless the myelofibrosis has evolved from CML.

■ Management

Myelofibrosis has no treatment; its course being indolent, the disease smolders for five years or longer. Anemia may require occasional blood transfusions. Hydroxyurea is given sometimes to control the size of the spleen, and its dosage carefully regulated by titration of WBC and platelets. Oxymetholone (a form of testosterone) may be helpful, but it requires careful monitoring for the development of icterus or edema. Splenectomy, while not recommended, may be necessary to relieve pain, or occasionally, to allay severe cytopenias arising from sequestration and hemolysis.

CHAPTER 136 ESSENTIAL THROMBOCYTHEMIA

■ Etiology

The platelet count may rise in a variety of clinical situations (specific stimulatory disorders, post-splenectomy, chronic blood loss, hemolytic anemia, and iron deficiency). If all of these causes are excluded, what remains is **essential thrombocythemia** (ET). ET is comparable to P. vera, because it represents an uncontrolled clonal proliferation of stem cells that produces too many platelets.

■ Clinical Features

ET occurs predominantly in persons over the age of 50. It is usually asymptomatic. When symptoms develop, they are usually of a thromboembolic nature. However, ET also causes hemorrhage, since the platelets, despite being abundant, are abnormal and nonfunctional. The thrombosis may occur at various sites: the cerebrum, myocardium, mesentery, and peripheral veins or arteries. Splenomegaly is the only outstanding physical sign. Patients with exceptionally large spleens may develop painful splenic infarctions. Eventual transformation to acute leukemia is rare.

■ Laboratory Features

Serial platelet counts are very high (they must exceed 800,000/mm^3). Hematocrit and RBC are usually normal in ET (but if Hct >48% or RBC >6.0 × 10^{12}/l confirmation is required by a ^{51}Cr RBC red cell volume; red cell volume is >34 ml/kg in P. vera, but <30 ml/kg in ET). The bone marrow is hypercellular in ET, with clumps of megakaryocytes. Marrow iron stores are normal. Absent stainable iron suggests iron deficiency as the cause of thrombocytosis; iron should then be given continuously for one month and hematologic tests reexamined thereafter. Bone marrow biopsy readily shows myelofibrosis and excess reticulin. The Ph chromosome is present in chronic myelocytic leukemia (CML), but absent in ET. The **leukocyte alkaline phosphatase** (LAP) score is very high, but is low or absent in CML.

■ Management

No consensus exists as to whether all patients with ET, especially young women, should be given myelosuppressives. In young women, especially if the menses are heavy, a month's trial of oral iron may help lower the platelet count. However, older persons with persistent thrombocytosis and splenomegaly are better treated with myelosuppression. The elderly (age >70) who are unable to visit their physician frequently, are best treated with ^{32}P, which may be required about once a year, and which carries a risk of leukemic transformation.

Most physicians prefer to treat ET with hydroxyurea. Other agents include busulfan, chlorambucil, and 6-thioguanine, but their leukemogenicity or toxicity makes HU preferable. Recently, anagrelide has been approved by the FDA.

CHAPTER 137 THE MYELODYSPLASTIC SYNDROMES

The myelodysplastic syndromes (MDS) are examples of irreversible, disordered proliferation of clonal growth, that feature profoundly atypical hematopoiesis (usually with cytopenias), increased bone marrow cellularity, malfunctioning peripheral blood cells, and eventual conversion to leukemia.

■ Classification and Subtypes

The MDS represent a collection of dissimilar cytopenias grouped by predominant features. **Refractory anemia** consists of normocytic to macrocytic anemia, accompanied by leukopenia and a small number of blasts (<5%) in the bone marrow (the term is a misnomer, as it was used to describe an anemia unresponsive to common hematinic drugs—B_{12}, folic acid, and iron). The marrow is frequently hypercellular, with increased iron content.

Refractory Anemia with Ringed Sideroblasts

Refractory anemia with ringed sideroblasts (RARS) shows increased numbers of dysplastic erythroblasts, many of which resemble megaloblasts. The key finding is an increased number of ringed sideroblasts where stainable iron is present in mitochondria disposed around the nucleus (Color Plate 23). Ringed sideroblasts may occur in younger persons as a sex-linked hereditary abnormality or after toxicity (by alcohol, INH, etc.). The myelodysplastic syndrome with ringed sideroblasts (MDS-RS) is most frequent in older age groups (>60 years) and is characterized by macrocytic anemia and varying degrees of leukopenia and thrombocytopenia. While the marrow is megaloblastic, RARS fails to respond to B_{12}, folic acid, pyridoxine, and other hematinics. About 15% of patients succumb to total marrow failure or leukemia.

Refractory Anemia with Excess of Blasts

Refractory anemia with excess of blasts (RAEB) features anemia and leukopenia, sometimes with peripheral (usually <5%) blasts. Bone marrow is inappropriately hyperplastic; the presence of less than 20% blasts provides arbitrary distinction from leukemia. Commonly, megakaryocytes are represented by micromegakaryocytes and giant platelets with bizarre granulation. The peripheral PMN are hypogranular and show bilobed structures (**Pelger-Huët cells**) or a peculiar ropy nucleus with clumped chromatin.

Chronic Myelomonocytic Leukemia

Chronic myelomonocytic leukemia (CMML) has a number of features atypical for MDS. Some argue that this entity does not even belong to this group. Such patients present with chronic anemia, leukocytosis, and thrombocytopenia. The leukocytosis suggests chronic myelocytic leukemia, but the Ph chromosome is absent and the peripheral blood shows monocytosis and monoblasts. The monocytes contain excess muramidase (lysozyme), which is detected in the serum and urine. The LAP score may or may not be low.

Refractory Anemia with Excess of Blasts-in-Transition

Sooner or later, refractory anemia with excess of blasts-in-transition (RAEB) will progress to the point that blasts exceed 25%. While many blasts contain Auer rods, they do not fulfill the criteria for acute leukemia. Certain cytogenetic abnormalities may be seen in MDS, especially deletions of all or part of chromosome 5 that do not necessarily correlate with the morphologic subtype.

Management

Therapy is usually discouraging, but, fortunately, most of the MDS disorders are indolent. RBC and platelet transfusions are frequently required. Hematopoietic growth factors (G-CSF and EPO) may temporarily improve peripheral blood counts. Small doses of cytosine arabinoside, 13 cis-retinoic acid, and 5-azacitidine may produce a therapeutic response. If a suitable HLA-matched donor is found, allogeneic bone marrow transplantation may be "curative", especially in recipients below 40 years of age.

CHAPTER **138 CHRONIC LYMPHOCYTIC LEUKEMIA (CLL)**

Definition

Chronic lymphocytic leukemia (CLL) is a clonal expansion of mature-appearing, nonfunctioning, and exceptionally long-lived lymphocytes. There is no specific cytogenetic marker, but its monoclonality may be shown by a uniform surface immunoglobulin expression. Some regard it as an overaccumulation and not overproduction of indolent, nonfunctioning lymphocytes.

Clinical Features

At its onset, CLL is insidious and found incidentally during routine laboratory testing or during the course of other disorders. In many, the initial finding in CLL is an absolute lymphocytosis exceeding 10,000/µl. The Rai system of classification (Table 138.1) effectively stages clinical and prognostic indices. Only infrequently do new patients present with lymphadenopathy or hepatosplenomegaly. With progressive disease, the lymphocytosis increases slowly. A doubling time less than one year carries the most serious prognosis. Lymphadenopathy or hepatosplenomegaly during observation has prognostic and therapeutic significance.

Because lymphocytes synthesize and transport immunoglobulins, the effect of CLL on the immune system has clinical implications. The failure of nonfunctional lymphocytes to secrete immunoglobulins leads to a slow decline in serum IgG, IgM, and IgA levels, and, consequently, to an increased susceptibility to infection, especially pneumonia and viruses. In addition, an increased sensitivity to insect antigens causes an exaggerated response (huge welts) to mosquito and other insect bites. Patients with CLL frequently lose their ability to distinguish between native and foreign cells. As a result, autoimmune diseases evolve, e.g., autoimmune hemolytic anemia and/or immune thrombocytopenia. Immune neutropenia and pure red cell aplasia also occur, although they are more difficult to prove, because of the preponderance of lymphocytes in the marrow.

Management

Most patients with Rai stage 0-1 CLL require only periodic clinical, hematologic, and immunologic documentation. Treatment may be started if the lymphocytes double in less than 1 year (or if they exceed 150,000/µL). Most patients in stages 3 or 4 need treatment. Anemia or thrombocytopenia requires therapy once the cause is established. Recurrent infections, progressive weight loss, or immunologic abnormalities also call for treatment. CLL predisposes to other neoplasias, so a regular and diligent search for malignancies is needed. Treatment, when indicated, is usually begun with an alkylating agent (e.g., chlorambucil or cyclophosphamide given alone or with prednisone). Lymphadenopathy and splenomegaly plus systemic symptoms require aggressive treatment either with traditional multi-drug regimens developed for lymphoma, e.g., "CHOP" or more recently, fludarabine–based regimens. Infections associated with hypogammaglobulinemia require IV human IgG. Autoimmune hemolytic anemia or immune thrombocytopenia is treated with prednisone therapy, and with splenectomy, if refractory to medical management.

TABLE 138.1.	The RAI Staging System	
Stage	Characteristic Feature	Median Survival–Yrs
0	Lymphocytosis	12.5
1	Lymphocytosis and lymphadenopathy	8–10
2	Lymphocytosis and splenomegaly	6
3	Lymphocytosis and anemia	1.5
4	Lymphocytosis and thrombocytopenia	0

CHAPTER 139 ACUTE LEUKEMIA

Definition

Acute leukemia is a clonal malignancy of immature hematopoietic cells in which the malignant clone proliferates, but fails to mature. The immature cells accumulate in the bone marrow and suppress normal hematopoiesis. Diagnosis requires at least 30% immature cells or blasts in the bone marrow.

Classification

Acute leukemias are usually classified by both the histologic and the immunologic appearance of the malignant cells. The **French-American-British** (FAB) classification, the standard nomenclature used to subtype the leukemias, relies on morphology and the results of cytochemical stains to differentiate the various leukemias (Table 139.1 and Table 139.2). However, some leukemic blasts lack morphologic features to indicate whether their lineage is myeloid or lymphoid. A variety of specialized stains are then used to clarify the lineage. For instance, peroxidase-positive granules indicate myeloid lineage, while PAS (**Periodic-acid Schiff**)-positive cytoplasm indicates erythroid or occasionally lymphoid differentiation.

Unfortunately, leukemic blasts do not always follow rules. Blasts may be negative or give equivocal results on stains, making it necessary to focus on the results of leukemic blast reactivity with monoclonal antibodies, rather than on histochemistry. The monoclonal antibodies react to antigens found on cells only at specific times in their maturation; they are specific for leukemic blasts that have undergone maturation arrest. Classification schemes are available based on the surface antigenic "appearance" and the cytogenetic make-up of leukemia cells (Table 139.3).

In approximately 70% of acute leukemics, nonran-

dom, specific genetic rearrangements can be observed, many of which are not only diagnostic of a myeloid or lymphoid lineage, but also have prognostic significance. These rearrangements or translocations appear only in the neoplastic clone, and not in the patient's normal hematopoietic cells. For instance, **acute myelomonocytic leukemia with an inverted chromosome 16** (M4Eo) and eosinophilia in the bone marrow is a specific AML subtype (Table 139.1). It carries a high rate of complete remission (>90%) and a 40–50% chance of remaining in complete remission after treatment. The best prognosis for response to therapy and remission duration is in inv(16), t(8;21), and t(15;17). A poorer prognosis is associated with 11q, +8, 20q-, and -5q, and -7q, and 9;22. Leukemias with normal karyotypes have an intermediate prognosis.

Clinical Features

The clinical features of acute leukemia are related to the depression of normal blood counts. Fatigue, weakness, mucosal bleeding, and recurrent infection are all common presenting symptoms; despite the term "acute", they may be present for weeks or months beforehand. Occasionally, more acute symptoms will prompt a diagnostic evaluation (e.g., serious bleeding due to **disseminated intravascular coagulation** (DIC), sepsis, pyoderma gangrenosum, or neurologic symptoms due to leukemic CNS involvement or leukocytosis). Some leukemias (e.g., the monocytic variants) tend to infiltrate tissues, and may present with respiratory compromise.

Acute leukemia is usually not a diagnostic problem, but rather, one of management. **Hyperleukocytosis** (blood blast counts of 100,000 per mm^3) predisposes to **leukostasis syndrome,** in which aggregates of blast cells occlude small arteries in multiple organs. The

TABLE 139.1. FAB Classification of Adult Acute Lymphoblastic Leukemia

Subtype	Morphology	Cytochemistry	Immunophenotype	CR%	3-Yr Remission %
L1 (Childhood)	Small uniform blasts Small nucleoli	Myeloperoxidase PAS (++)	CD 10+ (CALLA+)	85	40
L2 (Adult)	Larger blasts, irregular nucleoli	Myeloperoxidase PAS (+)	Same as L1	35	
L3 (Burkitt-like)	Large blasts, basophilic cytoplasm and vacuolated large nucleoli	Myeloperoxidase PAS (−)	CD 10− CD 19, 20+	10	

CR = Complete remission.

TABLE 139.2. Subtypes of Acute Myeloid Leukemia			
FAB		**Monoclonals**	**Cytogenetics**
M0	Undifferentiated	CD13+ CD14+ CD33+ CD34+	
M1	AML with minimal differentiation	CD13+ CD14+ CD33+ CD34+	Various, includes +8, del7
M2	AML with differentiation (granules, Auer rods)		t(8;21)
M3	Acute promyelocytic leukemia		t(15;17)
M4	Acute myelomonocytic		11q
	M4EO—with eosinophils		inv(16) t(16;16)
M5	Acute monocytic leukemia		t(9;11)
M6	Erythroleukemia		del(7a) del(5a)
M7	Megakaryocytic leukemia	Antiplatelet GP11b/111a	

TABLE 139.3. Cytochemical Stains	
Stain	**Significance**
Myeloperoxidase (MPO)	Myeloid cells containing peroxidase
Nonspecific esterase (NSE)	Monocytes and precursors Some ALL weakly + Some APL
Periodic acid-Schiff (PAS)	+ when glycogen present, especially erythroid precursors, occasional myeloid or lymphoid
Terminal deoxyribonucleotide transferase (TdT)	Nuclear enzyme present in immature lymphoid neoplasms

ALL = Acute lymphocytic leukemia; APL = acute promyelocytic leukemia.

features of this rapidly fatal syndrome include coma, obtundation, confusion, intracranial hemorrhage, massive hemoptysis, respiratory failure, or myocardial infarction. Emergent leukopheresis and initiation of antileukemic therapy are required. Extramedullary presentations of acute leukemias occasionally occur, more commonly in AML than ALL. While these chloromas usually occur concurrently with the bone marrow leukemia, they also arise independently thereof.

Acute Myelogenous Leukemia

Acute myelogenous leukemia (AML; synonyms include "acute nonlymphocytic leukemia", "acute myeloblastic leukemia", "acute myelocytic leukemia," and "granulomatous leukemia") is a disease of advancing age, with a slightly higher incidence in men. More than 50% of all cases occur in patients over 60 years of age. The etiology of AML is unknown, but heredity, radiation exposure, and exposure to certain chemicals and drugs exposure are implicated. Patients with Down's syndrome are twenty times more prone to acute leukemia (ALL and AML) than normal. Increased risk prevails in other diseases also (Wiskott-Aldrich, Bloom's syndrome, ataxia-telangiectasia). Despite the implication of viruses in animal leukemias, conclusive evidence of a viral etiology in human leukemia is lacking.

Following treatment with almost every antineoplastic agent, whether used to treat cancer or autoimmune disease, there is a small but finite risk of

TABLE 139.4.	Useful Monoclonal Antibodies
Lymphoid (B)	CALLA (Common ALL antigen) (CD10)
	B4, Lev 12:CD1
	B1, Lev 16:CD20, CD 22
	Surface immunoglobulin
Lymphoid (T)	T6, Lev 6:CD1
	Lev 1 T 1:CD5, CD7
Monocytes/ myelocytes	CD33
	CD13
	CD14
Progenitor cells	CD34
Platelets/ megakaryocytes	CD41
	CD42

developing myelodysplastic syndrome and/or AML. The alkylating agents, nitrosoureas, and etoposide are particularly known for this fatal complication. The use of radiation with chemotherapy appears to confer an additive risk in this context. These secondary leukemias tend to be resistant to standard treatment and frequently involve cytogenetic abnormalities of chromosomes 5, 7, and 8.

In the standard FAB classification system, AML has seven subtypes. Monoclonal antibody phenotyping and cytogenetics are listed in Table 139.2. This subclassification is increasingly important, as treatment and prognosis vary depending on the FAB type and the cytogenetic findings.

Acute Leukemias, M0 through M2

In **acute undifferentiated leukemia** (M0), the abnormal blasts do not resemble either myeloblasts or lymphoblasts, and there are no Auer rods. The blasts are not lineage-specific. The group probably includes true AML, some mixed lineage leukemias, and some stem cell malignancies. In **acute myeloblastic** (M1) **leukemia** (Color Plate 31), the blasts are mainly undifferentiated, but some will have Auer rods. The cells usually show clear myeloid differentiation on monoclonal antibody staining. In **acute myeloid leukemia with differentiation** (M2), leukemic cells show a more clearly myeloid lineage. They are typically positive for myeloperoxidase staining and have Auer rods; the 8:21 translocation has been associated with the phenotype.

Acute Promyelocytic Leukemia, (M3)

These leukemias show dramatic granularity and multiple Auer rods. The coagulation system is virtually always activated, with DIC either at diagnosis or with the initiation of treatment; patients require aggressive blood and platelet support besides consumed factor replacement. Overall, patients are younger, and the survival ranges between 40–50%. Recognition of this subtype is important before the initiation of induction therapy, so that the coagulopathy is treated early and serious bleeding prevented. In addition, M3 is uniquely sensitive to treatment with **all-trans-retinoic acid** (ATRA), which appears to induce maturation of the leukemic cells.

Acute Leukemias, (M4 through M7)

M4 leukemic cells, while still mainly myeloid, show some monocytic features. A variant is the M4Eo subtype with the inverted chromosome 16, as described previously. **Acute monocytic leukemia** (M5) is "pure" monocytic leukemia, in which the leukemic cells are either **monoblasts** (M5a) or **promonoblasts** (M5b). Tissue infiltration is common, with hypertrophy of the gums (Figure 139.1) or pulmonary infiltrates due to leukemic blasts. In **acute erythroleukemia** (M6), the blasts show clear erythroid features with dysplastic, megaloblastic erythroid maturation. Typical cytogenetic abnormalities include -7 and -5. The malignant cells are erythroid lineage, and the criteria require that at least 30% of the cells be proerythroblasts. Finally, in **acute megakaryocytic leukemia** (M7), the blasts are relatively undifferentiated; small "microblasts" are often seen in the blood. The bone marrow may show extensive fibrosis. The blasts must have surface glycoprotein IIb-IIIa, von Willebrand protein in the cytoplasm, or stain positive for factor VIII to confirm megakaryocytic lineage. Acute megakaryocytic leukemia is the most common leukemia in Down's syndrome (trisomy 21).

■ Management

Therapy of AML, with the exception of M3, initially involves induction therapy and some postinduction

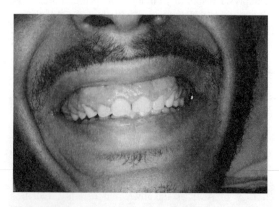

FIGURE 139.1. Gum hypertrophy in M5; the patient had swollen, bleeding gums and febrile episodes.

"consolidation." Induction attains a complete remission: normal bone marrow with fewer than 5% blasts, plus adequate bone marrow function to attain normal peripheral blood counts. Usually, profound bone marrow hypoplasia is produced by treatment with an anthracycline (e.g., idarubicin, mitoxantrone, or daunorubicin) plus a 7-day infusion of cytosine arabinoside; the hypoplasia usually lasts 3–6 weeks, until the patient's normal bone marrow can recover hematopoiesis.

Blood products are transfused in the interim to maintain hemostasis, and antibiotics are given for fevers and infections. By 21–36 days after the initiation of therapy, the marrow produces sufficient normal cells, thus lessening the need for transfusions and antibiotics. Complete remission occurs when the marrow turns normal (<5% blasts and normal morphology) and the peripheral counts have recovered. The incidence of mortality during induction—usually due to infection or uncontrolled bleeding—is nearly 10%, although it may be 60–80% in older (>65) persons. Reducing the dosage of chemotherapy in the elderly to lessen toxicity also lowers the antileukemic effect. It is more promising to attenuate the duration of cytopenias in these patients by using G-CSF and/or GM-CSF. Many patients will require a second, usually lesser dose of therapy during induction to attain a remission. About 10% of patients are primarily resistant to chemotherapy; they usually have secondary leukemias, prior myelodysplasia, abnormalities of chromosomes 5, 7, 8, and 13, and blasts positive for CD34.

Some postinduction treatment is necessary. Without it, the leukemia invariably recurs within 4–18 months.

Consolidation therapy improves both remission duration and overall survival. It is usually chemotherapy, given soon after recovery from induction, in doses that produce bone marrow hypoplasia. It may be given 2–4 times as the marrow recovers from each cycle of therapy. Late intensification treatment is intensive chemotherapy given after a delay of 6–12 months from the time of induction. While some form of postinduction therapy is needed, its duration and intensity after a documented remission are not yet clearly standardized. The median survival is 18–24 months. Approximately 15–20% of patients appear to achieve long-term remission and, possibly, cure.

Bone marrow transplant (BMT) is conceptually a late intensification therapy. High-dose chemotherapy and, usually, radiation are given to destroy completely native leukemic bone marrow, in the process also destroying normal bone marrow; it is followed by transplantation of donor marrow to restore the hematopoietic abilities. BMT appears to be most effective in the first remission, with approximately 50% surviving at 10 years. For BMT done during either the first relapse or second remission, survival drops to 15–20%. Leukemia relapse is the major cause of failure in these patients. Highly lethal and morbid complications of BMT are graft-versus-host disease, infection, bleeding, interstitial pneumonia and respiratory failure, and veno-occlusive disease of the liver. The rigors of BMT make it an option only in younger patients and those with good performance status. Innovations in "standard" treatment and improvements in long-term survival in some leukemias (APL, inv16) demonstrate that BMT should be used selectively.

Acute Lymphoblastic Leukemia

Acute lymphoblastic leukemia is most common in the pediatric population, with a peak incidence between 2–6 years. Adult ALL usually refers to patients older than 15–18 years, and it is biologically different from childhood ALL. The disease has a second peak incidence in adults over the age of 60. The diagnosis of ALL is based on the morphology of the malignant blasts, plus their immunophenotypic and cytochemical characteristics. Three subtypes of ALL are recognized by the FAB, and their characteristics are given in Table 139.1.

■ Clinical Features and Diagnosis

In general, the diagnosis of acute leukemia is not difficult, with the signs and symptoms of bone marrow failure, including fatigue, bleeding and/or fever, depending on the degree of cytopenias at the time of the diagnosis. As a result of tissue infiltration by malignant

lymphoblasts, ALL manifests testicular enlargement, skin nodules, lymphadenopathy, splenomegaly, and cranial nerve palsies. The peripheral blood may show dramatically high WBC with circulating lymphoblasts, or it may show neutropenia and few abnormal cells. The bone marrow is usually hypercellular because of the lymphoblastic infiltration, and normal marrow elements may appear to be completely absent. While the morphology of the blasts distinguish ALL from AML, occasionally in very undifferentiated cells the diagnosis must rely on the results of either special stains or monoclonal immunocytochemistry stains.

The lineage of 75% all adult ALL is B-cell, including leukemic cells with a more mature B-cell phenotype (expressing surface immunoglobulin) and others with a "pre-B-cell" phenotype (only a rearrangement of the immunoglobulin genes, but no surface immunoglobulin). The remaining adult ALL are of T-cell lineage, with either mature T-cells or pre-T-cells. Cytogenetic findings are occasionally needed to pinpoint the exact lineage of the malignant cells. Up to 20% of adult ALL will have some myeloid antigens. Rarely, the leukemic cells—otherwise typical blasts—will show both myeloid and lymphoid antigens on their surface. Some of these cells appear to be best classified as M0-AML, and may best be treated using an AML regimen. Others are truly ALL with myeloid antigens, and it is controversial whether or not this confers a poor prognosis.

■ Management

Conventional treatment of ALL in general, involves a sequence of induction (3 drugs), consolidation/intensification (given several times in sequence), and maintenance chemotherapy (for 1–2 years). Induction usually involves some combination of vincristine and prednisone, plus anthracyclines. The complete remission rate is 65–85%, with a mortality of 3–20%. The value of consolidation/intensification treatments in adult ALL is controversial; however, the more intensive, multiple-drug programs seem to confer longer remissions and survival. Likewise, the benefit and necessary duration of maintenance therapy in adult ALL is

unknown. Most maintenance therapies include methotrexate, 6-mercaptopurine, and possibly vincristine, L-asparaginase, and/or prednisone. All therapy regimens in ALL include some type of prophylactic treatment of the CNS. Leukemia recurs in the CNS in 30% of untreated cases, and 5% of adults will present with CNS disease. CNS prophylaxis, historically done with craniospinal radiation, has more recently been accomplished by intrathecal drugs and/or high dose methotrexate or cytosine arabinoside systemically.

Twenty-five percent of adults with ALL will be cured with conventional chemotherapy. Efforts have been undertaken to improve these results with bone marrow transplantation (BMT). Allogeneic BMT is currently reserved for patients following their first relapse, after they have attained a second remission, But it may also be used in the first remission in patients in a poor risk group, patients presenting with high WBC, patients with unfavorable translocations (4;11, 1;19), or L3 patients. Autologous BMT may be used in older patients, in poor prognosis patients as a intensification maneuver, or in patients without tissue matched donors. Current treatment programs in adult ALL lead to 70–80% remission rates and cure rates of 20–30%.

CHAPTER 140 CLINICAL USES OF BLOOD AND BLOOD COMPONENTS

■ Blood Processing

Blood and blood products are a limited resource. Following collection, the donated blood is routinely tested for the ABO and Rh (D) antigen and for antibodies and infectious disease markers associated with hepatitis B, hepatitis C, HIV-1/2, HTLV-I, and syphilis. Units with any of these infectious disease markers are discarded and the donors are deferred from future blood donation. The availability of anticoagulant-preservative solution and plastic materials has enhanced blood storage capability, permitted the easy separation of blood into its components, and allowed the use of specific component therapy instead of whole blood transfusions when appropriate.

■ Transfusion Orders

After carefully assessing the patient's transfusion needs, the physician orders the appropriate blood product. The transfusion order should include the type of blood component to be transfused, its amount (in ml. or units), the urgency of the need for the product (i.e., routine, STAT, specific date, etc.), the time of adminis-

tration and duration of the transfusion, and any special needs (i.e., irradiation, leukocyte reduction, CMV-antibody negative).

■ Compatibility Testing

Upon the physician's order, the patient's blood sample is obtained by careful phlebotomy and correctly labeled. The need to meticulously follow hospital policy concerning these procedures cannot be overemphasized. The patient's blood is typed for ABO and Rh (D) (RBC transfusions must be ABO Rh compatible) and screened for alloantibodies (from prior transfusion or pregnancy and directed against an RBC antigen in the donor unit). Through a crossmatch, compatibility is confirmed between the patient's plasma and the actual donor unit to be transfused. Finally, at the bedside, the unit to be transfused is carefully identified and matched with the appropriate patient before transfusion is begun.

The **maximum surgical blood ordering schedule** (MSBOS) is a list based and compiled on a broad experience with transfusion needs according to procedures. It ensures the proper preoperative blood order (i.e., order for blood, type and screen, or type and crossmatch). One MSBOS option, called the type and screen (T & S), is utilized when there is only a small chance (<10%), that a patient undergoing a particular surgical procedure will require a blood transfusion. No blood will be cross-matched and set aside for the patient's surgery, unless an unexpected need for transfusion develops during surgery. The MSBOS and T & S effectively employ blood resources without increasing the risk to the patient.

■ Blood Product Therapy

Whole blood

Whole blood transfusions must be ABO identical to the patient. They are indicated for patients who require both oxygen-carrying capacity and volume expansion (usually an actively bleeding patient). Whole blood contains a satisfactory amount of all coagulation factors except V and VIII (labile coagulation factors), and it may diminish the effects of dilutional coagulopathy in massively transfused patients. Importantly, whole blood generally does not contain viable platelets.

Packed red blood cells

The vast majority of RBC transfusions are given as packed red blood cells (PRBC) They are meant to increase the oxygen carrying capacity in patients with symptomatic anemia or to prevent the symptoms of anemia in patients at risk. Transfusions should be given only after appropriate alternatives have been considered (e.g., iron, B_{12}, folate, and erythropoietin). There is no specific hemoglobin or hematocrit "trigger" at which patients should be transfused. It has been established that many patients can tolerate a hemoglobin level of 8 gm/dL or a hematocrit of 24% without significant risk. Anemic patients with a normal intravascular volume can tolerate a lower hematocrit than those with a similar hematocrit and a contracted intravascular volume. Comorbid conditions (e.g., cardiac, vascular, and lung disease, and states of excessive oxygen consumption) may require that a patient's hemoglobin and hematocrit be kept at higher levels than noted above. One unit of RBC generally raises the hematocrit by about 3% and the hemoglobin by about 1 gm/dl.

RBC transfusions must be ABO compatible. In emergencies where the blood type of the recipient is not known, group O Rh-negative RBC are the safest alternative. Patients requiring massive fluid and blood replacement are commonly resuscitated using crystalloid and/or colloid solutions in conjunction with PRBC transfusions. One consequence of this combination may be dilutional thrombocytopenia and dilutional coagulopathy, which may require the transfusion of fresh frozen plasma and platelets to correct the hemostatic defects if microvascular bleeding is associated.

Fresh frozen plasma

Fresh frozen plasma (FFP) is the plasma separated from whole blood and frozen at -18°C or below within 8 hours of blood collection. It contains all the coagulation factors and anticoagulant proteins—proteins C, S, and AT III. FFP does not contain viable platelets. It is indicated in several instances: (1) acquired or congenital deficiency of coagulation factors for which a specific, safe clotting factor concentrate is not available, (2) massively transfused patients (exceeding 1 blood volume within several hours) with a dilutional coagulopathy and microvascular bleeding, (3) serious bleeding or emergency surgery requiring rapid reversal of warfarin, (4) acquired coagulopathy in an actively bleeding patient or one who is to undergo an invasive procedure, and (5) thrombotic thrombocytopenic purpura (TTP) for plasma exchange.

FFP is transfused as ABO compatible and does not require a crossmatch. It should not be used routinely as a volume expander. Patients receiving it should have their coagulopathy properly documented with coagulation tests; follow-up studies should be done to document the effectiveness of the transfusion. Risks of FFP include blood-borne infections, allergic reactions, alloimmunization, and increased intravascular volume.

■ Platelet Transfusions

Platelet concentrates are prepared from units of donated blood (each unit provides a minimum of 0.55×10^{11} platelets) and can be stored at room temperature (20–24°C) for up to 5 days. Each platelet concentrate should raise the platelet count 5,000–10,000/μl in an average size adult. The standard order of platelet concentrate for an adult is 1 unit/10 kilograms. To obviate the number of donor exposures, approximately 6–8 units (4–6×10^{11} platelets) may be obtained from a single donor who undergoes plateletpheresis; the product is labeled as "platelets- pheresed" (random donor platelet concentrates).

Specific indications for platelet transfusions include (1) active bleeding and a platelet count less than 50,000/μl or platelet function defect, (2) thrombocytopenia resulting from temporary myelosuppression (for a platelet count of 10,000/μl, a prophylactic transfusion is given), (3) surgical procedures in thrombocytopenic patients (transfusions are often given to keep a platelet count of 50,000–100,000/μl, depending upon the procedure and the risk of bleeding), (4) bleeding due to thrombocytopenia or platelet function abnormalities following cardiopulmonary bypass for open heart surgery, and (5) thrombocytopenia and microvascular bleeding following massive blood transfusions (replacement exceeding one blood volume in several hours).

Prophylactic platelet transfusions are not generally indicated for stable patients with chronic aplastic anemia or myelodysplasia. Platelet transfusion for symptomatic thrombocytopenia is more rational in such patients. Except in the presence of life-threatening hemorrhage, platelet transfusions are generally contraindicated in TTP and immune-mediated thrombocytopenic purpura, including heparin-induced thrombocytopenia.

The platelet count may fail to rise as expected in patients with fever, sepsis, splenomegaly, or disseminated intravascular coagulation, or in patients with antibodies to HLA or platelet-specific antigens. Refractoriness to platelet transfusions is most commonly—but not always—due to the development of antibodies against Class I HLA antigens on transfused platelets. HLA-matched or platelet crossmatched platelet transfusions are the solution. If at all possible, ABO compatible platelets should be transfused, since ABO incompatibility seems to impair the survival of transfused platelets.

Cryoprecipitate

Cryoprecipitate (cryo) is the cold precipitated protein fraction derived from fresh frozen plasma when it is thawed at 1–6°C. It contains ample fibrinogen, factor VIII, von Willebrand factor, and factor XIII and fibronectin. Cryoprecipitate was previously used heavily in hemophilia A and von Willebrand disease, but it has now been replaced by significantly safer commercial concentrates. Cryoprecipitate is specifically indicated for the treatment of hypofibrinogenemia and for use as a fibrin sealant (fibrin glue, a surgical adhesive). In an average-sized adult with significant hypofibrinogenemia, an appropriate dose is 8–12 units.

Special blood products

Some patients require manipulations in the transfused products to meet special transfusion needs (e.g., cytomegalovirus [CMV] antibody testing of the donor units, gamma irradiation, and leukocyte reduction of blood products). CMV transmission is a known complication of blood transfusions since the 1960s, especially in immunosuppressed patients. Prevention of CMV transmission by blood products is most beneficial in this patient group. Obtaining blood from voluntary, CMV seronegative blood donors is one method of prevention; another is the removal of WBC in blood products by specialized filters (CMV resides in the WBC of asymptomatic seropositive persons). CMV seronegative blood products are indicated in the following CMV seronega-

tive patient groups: pregnant women and their fetuses, premature infants (<1,200 gm) of CMV seronegative mothers, recipients of allogeneic bone marrow transplants, patients with HIV infection and/or AIDS, organ transplant recipients (kidney, heart, liver, lung), and patients undergoing splenectomy or autologous bone marrow transplant.

Posttransfusion graft versus host (PGVH) disease is mediated by lymphocytes in the blood product that recognize the transfusion recipient as foreign and mount an immune response. Immunocompromised patients are at greatest risk. PGVH, which is characterized by fever, skin rash, diarrhea, liver abnormalities and pancytopenia, is nearly always fatal. It can be prevented by gamma irradiation of blood products, which prevents the T-lymphocyte from undergoing the proliferation necessary to mount an immune response. Gamma irradiation of cellular blood products is indicated in known or suspected congenital T-cell immunodeficiency, bone marrow transplant recipients, Hodgkin's disease, and immunocompetent patients receiving directed donations from blood relatives and HLA-matched cellular blood components. Many hospital blood banks routinely irradiate all blood products for neonates, and many physicians prefer that their patients with malignancy receive irradiated blood products.

"Passenger" WBC in blood products cause posttransfusion adverse effects (e.g., febrile transfusion reactions, alloimmunization, transmission of CMV, transfusion-induced immunosuppression, and reperfusion injury following cardiopulmonary bypass procedures). Therefore, many investigators believe in removing leukocytes from blood products through the use of specialized blood filters. Leukocyte-reduced blood products are used to prevent 1) febrile, non-hemolytic transfusion reactions, 2) alloimmunization to HLA antigens in recipients of multiple transfusions, and 3) CMV infection in at-risk patients.

Autologous blood transfusion

The advent of AIDS and increasing public awareness of blood-borne infections have kindled both physician and patient interest in autologous blood transfusions. The safest blood to receive is one's own blood. Autologous blood transfusion methods include preoperative (days or weeks before) autologous donation, preoperative hemodilution (collecting 1–2 units with saline volume replacement immediately preoperatively and subsequent transfusion of blood), and intraoperative and postoperative blood salvage (recovery of shed blood and reinfusion into the patient). Physicians should ensure that all patients who may benefit from autologous blood transfusion are given the opportunity to do so.

Complications of Blood Transfusion Therapy

Transfusion of blood products is followed by a number of adverse consequences (Tables 140.1 and 140.2). Any decision to transfuse a blood product must follow careful reflection of the risks and benefits. Physicians must also be familiar with these adverse consequences to inform their patients of the risks and benefits.

Immediate Complications—Immunologic

Acute hemolytic transfusion reaction

The most severe, life-threatening, hemolytic transfusion reaction results from the inadvertent administration of ABO-incompatible blood to a recipient who has an antibody directed against the A and/or B antigen of the transfused RBC. The ABO-incompatible transfusion causes an antigen-antibody interaction with ensuing complement activation, causing RBC lysis. Signs and symptoms include fever, chills, generalized flushing, nausea, dyspnea, chest pain, back pain, and hypotension. The resulting severe complications include shock, acute renal failure, and disseminated intravascular coagulation. ABO incompatible blood transfusion may be lethal.

Nonhemolytic febrile transfusion reaction

Nonhemolytic febrile transfusion reaction is defined as a febrile response of at least 1°C shortly after a blood

TABLE 140.1. Classification of Transfusion Reactions

Immediate—Immunologic
  Acute hemolytic transfusion reaction
  Non-hemolytic febrile transfusion reaction
  Allergic reaction, anaphylactic reaction
  Transfusion related acute lung injury (TRALI)
Immediate—Nonimmunologic
  Hypervolemia
  Complications of massive transfusion
  Bacterially contaminated blood product
Delayed—Immunologic
  Delayed hemolytic transfusion reaction
  Post-transfusion graft vs. host disease
  Post-transfusion purpura
Delayed—Nonimmunologic
  Iron overload
  Infections
    Hepatitis B, Hepatitis C
    HIV, HTLV-I
    Cytomegalovirus
    Malaria, Chagas' disease, Babesiosis
    Syphilis

transfusion. It generally results when the recipient has antibodies to WBC antigens present in the transfusion. Such antibodies might be attributable to a previous pregnancy or transfusion. Common symptoms include fever, chills, and, occasionally, shortness of breath. The fever usually responds to antipyretics. Some nonhemolytic, febrile transfusion reactions are associated with cytokine release by WBCs during storage of the blood product, particularly the WBCs present in platelet concentrates. Using special filters to remove the leukocytes from the blood products can prevent many nonhemolytic febrile transfusion reactions; reactions associated with cytokine production require pre-storage filtration.

Allergic reactions

Allergic reactions are some of the most common transfusion reactions, but, fortunately, they are usually mild. Symptoms generally include urticaria (hives) and itching. They usually result when the patient has an antibody to a plasma protein present in the transfused blood product. These reactions can be treated easily with antihistamines or perhaps even prevented by premedication with antihistamines prior to the transfusion. Occasionally, life-threatening anaphylaxis occurs with blood transfusions. The classic occurrence is in patients who are IgA deficient and who have developed antibodies to the IgA molecule; these patients require transfusion with IgA-deficient blood, washed red cells, frozen deglycerolized blood, or IgA-deficient plasma. These reactions are treated in a similar manner to other types of anaphylaxis.

Immediate Complications—Nonimmunologic

Volume overload

One of the most under-reported complications of transfusions is the development of mild to moderate congestive heart failure or its worsening after blood transfusion. Patients at risk for heart failure following a blood transfusion should be carefully monitored and may require diuretics. RBC transfusion—**not** whole blood— should be used for patients with euvolemic anemia.

Adverse effects of massive blood transfusion

Massive blood transfusion may be associated with a number of adverse effects, including dilutional thrombocytopenia, dilutional coagulopathy, hypothermia (if massive amounts of cold blood are rapidly infused), and citrate reaction (development of hypocalcemia). Physicians administering massive blood transfusions must be

TABLE 140.2.	Estimated Risk of Infectious and Noninfectious Complications of Blood Transfusion	

Complication	Instance(s) per Million Component Units Transfused
Infections	
Virus	
HIV	4
Hepatitis B	5
Hepatitis C	333
HTLV-I	14
Bacterial	
Bacterial contamination red cell unit	2
Bacterial contamination of platelet concentrate	83
Noninfectious	
Acute hemolytic transfusion reaction	40
Delayed hemolytic transfusion reaction	400
Acute lung disease	100
Anaphylaxis	7

\# Not a complete list.
(Modified from: Dodd R. AABB publication, 1993.)

aware of these complications and carefully monitor the patient.

Bacterial contamination

Rarely, units of blood may contain bacteria that can cause a severe septic transfusion reaction. Bacterial contamination has been reported in red cell units, but more commonly with platelet concentrates (Table 140.2). Many bacteria have been implicated, including Pseudomonas, *E. coli*, *Yersinia enterocolitica*, and *Staphylococcus aureus*. This issue has recently taken on an even greater prominence as a significant adverse event of blood transfusion.

■ Delayed Complications—Immunologic

Delayed hemolytic transfusion reaction

Delayed hemolytic transfusion reaction is usually manifested by a fall in the hemoglobin and hematocrit. This reaction occurs several days to weeks following a transfusion. It is caused by the development of an alloantibody to a red blood cell antigen, either by primary immunization or by a secondary anamnestic response. Signs and symptoms include unexplained anemia, fever, jaundice, and, occasionally, hemoglobinuria. Such reactions are usually not life-threatening; future transfusions will require blood that lacks the antigen to which the antibody in the patient's plasma is directed.

■ Delayed Complications—Nonimmunologic

Infectious complications

HIV transmission as an adverse consequence of blood transfusion has brought the infectious complications of blood transfusion into public focus. With the development of highly accurate tests for HIV and hepatitis C, blood is safer today than it has ever been from an infectious risk. However, significant infectious risks continue to be associated with blood transfusion. It is important for physicians to be mindful of these risks and of their extent.

■ Questions

Instructions: For each question below, select only **one** lettered answer that is the **best** for that question.

1. Pernicious anemia is characterized by which of the following?
   A. Abnormal serum transport of Vitamin B_{12}
   B. Increased degradation of Vitamin B_{12}
   C. Impaired DNA synthesis of all dividing cells
   D. Erythroid hypoplasia of bone marrow
   E. Development of antibodies against Vitamin B_{12}

2. Which of the following is characterized by decreased serum iron concentration, increased serum transferrin, diminished serum ferritin, and hypochromic microcytic erythrocyte indices?
   A. Iron-deficiency anemia
   B. Sex-linked hereditary pyridoxine responsive anemia
   C. The third trimester of pregnancy
   D. Thalassemia minor
   E. Osteomyelitis

3. Which is the most important safeguard against iron overload?
   A. Urinary excretion of iron if a serum concentration is exceeded
   B. Chronic blood loss from gastrointestinal tract
   C. Selective absorption of dietary iron; saturation of lining gastrointestinal. epithelium with iron, followed by desquamation of saturated cells
   D. Retention of iron by phagocytic macrophages
   E. Oxidation of ferrous iron to nonabsorbable ferric iron

4. The anemia associated with total gastrectomy is caused by:
   A. Folic acid deficiency due to anorexia.
   B. Iron deficiency due to achlorhydria.
   C. Antiparietal cell antibodies.
   D. Malabsorption of B_{12} due to diminished intrinsic factor.

E. Failure to generate erythropoietin.

Questions 5–9: Match the items in column I with those in column II

I Substance		II Function	
5.	Transferrin	A.	Tissue respiration
6.	Ferritin	B.	Oxidation of iron
7.	Cytochrome	C.	Oxygen transport
8.	Hemoglobin	D.	Iron transport
9.	Ceruloplasmin	E.	Iron storage

Questions 10–17. Select only **one** lettered answer that is the **best** for that question.

10. Release of mature polymorphonuclear leukocytes from the bone marrow into the circulating blood is in part dependent upon:
    A. Microtubular ultrastructure.
    B. Function of actin and myosin.
    C. Glycolysis.
    D. Replacement of primary granules by secondary granules.
    E. Cellular deformability.

11. The presence of toxic granulation in a mature polymorphonuclear leukocyte is indicative of which of the following?
    A. Accelerated granulocytopoiesis
    B. An abnormal serum factor that causes coagulation of leukocyte granules
    C. Residual ribosomal RNA that persists after cellular maturation
    D. The effect of endotoxin on lysosomal membranes
    E. Accelerated leukocyte destruction

12. Leukocytes that adhere to endothelial surfaces may be mobilized and identified by which of the following?
    A. Injection of endotoxin
    B. The skin window test
    C. Activation of C'_3 and C'_5 to C'_{3A} and C'_{5A}
    D. Injection of epinephrine
    E. The phagocytic index

13. The chief function of folic acid is to:
    A. Transport Vitamin B_{12} to reactive site.
    B. Protect against oxidation of iron compounds.
    C. Enhance production of erythropoietin.
    D. Provide methyl groups to convert uridylic to thymidylic acid.
    E. Protect against proliferation of malignant (leukemic) cells.

14. A stimulus that promotes production of erythropoietin is known to be:
    A. Colony-stimulation factor.

B. Hypoxia.
C. Plethora.
D. Decompensated renal disease.
E. IL-3.

15. A 65-year-old man is admitted for severe epistaxis. History reveals a recent transient ischemic attack complicating atrial fibrillation; he receives daily warfarin. The patient states that his eyesight has been less than satisfactory lately. His vital signs are a pulse of 92/min; BP, 120/68 mm Hg, and respirations, 22/min. Physical examination is otherwise normal, except for continuing nasal bleeding. His hemoglobin is 13.1 g/dl and hematocrit, 36%. The INR is 6.5. Besides cessation of warfarin therapy, the management of this patient includes which one of the following?
    A. Cryoprecipitate
    B. Fresh frozen plasma
    C. Type and cross-match for 2 units of PRBC; transfuse one unit as soon as available
    D. DDAVP infusion
    E. Aquamephyton, 10 mg IV now

16. A 61-year-old man of Greek ancestry is admitted to the hospital for left lower extremity swelling. The patient had a history of blurring of vision approximately 5 years ago; a retinal vein thrombosis was found. He reports complete recovery after some laser photocoagulation. Examination now reveals a swollen, edematous left lower extremity. Real-time ultrasound shows a clot involving the left calf veins, extending into the popliteal vein. Which one of the following best explains the reason for his thrombotic disorder?
    A. Protein C deficiency
    B. Antithrombin III deficiency
    C. Activated protein C resistance
    D. Homocystinuria

17. A 74-year-old asymptomatic man is noted to have a normal physical examination, but his WBC count is 26,000/mm³. The peripheral smear shows 23% PMNs, 62% lymphocytes, 8% monocytes, 5% basophils and 2% eosinophils. The lymphocytes are mature-appearing. The most appropriate management for this patient is which of the following?
    A. Fludarabine with prednisone
    B. Cyclophosphamide with prednisone
    C. Chlorambucil with Prednisone
    D. Consider splenectomy
    E. Observation with periodic documentation of clinical and hematologic data

■ Answers

1. C	2. A	3. C	4. D	5. D
6. E	7. A	8. C	9. B	10. E
11. A	12. D	13. D	14. B	15. B
16. D	17. E			

SUGGESTED READING
Books and Monographs

Gross S, Roath S (eds.). Hematology: A Problem-Oriented Approach. Baltimore: Williams & Wilkins, 1996.

Lee GR, Bilhell TC, Foerster J et al. (eds.). Wintrobe's Clinical Hematology. 9th ed. Philadelphia: Lea and Febiger, 1993.

Petz LD, Swisher SN (eds.). Principles of Transfusion Medicine. 3rd ed. New York: Churchill Livingstone, 1996.

Petz L. Platelet Transfusions. In Pisciotto PT (ed.). Blood Transfusion Therapy: A Physician's Handbook. 3rd ed. Arlington, VA: American Association of Blood Banks, 1996.

Articles
Proliferation and Differentiation of Circulating Blood Cells

Brugger W, Kanz L, Mertelsmann R. Cell proliferation and differentiation and clinical applications of hematopoietic growth factors. Curr Opin Hematol 1993;1:214–220.

Microcytic and Macrocytic Anemias

Kazazian HH Jr. The thalassemia syndromes: molecular basis and prenatal diagnosis in 1990. Semin Hematol 1990;27:209–228.

Sahay R, Scott BB. Iron deficiency anemia—how far to investigate? Gut 1993;34:1427–1428.

Sears DA: Anemia of chronic disease. Med Clin North Am 1992;76:567–579.

Stabler SP, Allen RH, Savage DG, Lindenbaum J: Clinical spectrum and diagnosis of cobalamin deficiency. Blood 1990;76:871–881.

Toh BH, van Driel IR, Gleeson PA. Pernicious anemia. N Engl J Med 1997;337:1441–1448.

Aplastic Anemias

Gordon-Smith EC: Aplastic anemia and allied disorders. Curr Opin Hematol 1993;1:45–51.

Hemolytic Anemias and Hemoglobinopathies

Ballas SK. The pathophysiology of hemolytic anemias. Transf Med Rev 1990;4:236–256.

Lubran MM. Hematologic side effects of drugs. Ann Clin Lab Sci 1989; 19:114–121.

Rosenwasser LJ, Joseph BZ. Immunohematologic diseases. JAMA 1992;268:2940–2945.

Shapiro BS. The management of pain in sickle cell disease. Pediatr Clin North Am 1989;36:1029–1045.

Stamatoyannopoulos JA. Future prospects for treatment of hemoglobinopathies. West J Med 1992;157:631–636.

Steingart R. Management of patients with sickle cell disease. Med Clin North Am 1992;76:669–682.

Tabbara IA. Hemolytic anemias. Diagnosis and management. Med Clin North Am 1992;76:649–668.

Wayne AS, Kevy SV, Nathan DG. Transfusion management of sickle cell disease. Blood 1993;81:1109–1123.

Bleeding Disorders

Kitchens CS. Approach to the bleeding patient. Hem Onc Clin North Am 1992;6:983–989

Wallerstein RO Jr. Laboratory evaluation of a bleeding patient. West J Med 1989;150:51–58.

Thrombotic Disorders

Furie B, Furie BC. Molecular and cellular biology of blood coagulation. N Engl J Med 1992;326:800–806.

Hillarp A, Zöller B, Dählback B. Activated Protein C Resistance as a basis for venous thrombosis. Am J Med 1996;101:534–540.

Warkentin T, Kelton JG. A 14-year study of heparin-induced thrombocytopenia. Am J Med 1996;101:502–507.

Harenberg J, Huhle G, Piazolo L, Wang LU, Heene DL. Anticoagulation in patients with heparin-induced thrombocytopenia type II. Semin Thromb Hemost 1997;23:189–196.

Myeloproliferative Disorders

Hocking WG, Golde DW. Polycythemia: evaluation and management. Blood Rev 1989;3:59–65.

Schafer AI. Essential thrombocythemia. Prog Hemost Thromb 1991;10:69–96.

Silver RT. Chronic myeloid leukemia. A perspective on the clinical and biologic issues of the chronic phase. Hematol Oncol Clin North Am 1990;4:319–335.

Weinstein IM. Idiopathic myelofibrosis: historical review, diagnosis and management. Blood Rev 1991;5:98–104.

The Myelodysplastic Syndrome

Zuckerman KS. Myelodysplasia. Curr Opin Hematol 1993;1:183–188.

Leukemias

Armitage JO. Bone marrow transplantation. N Engl J Med 1994;330:827–838.

Bloomfield CD, Herzig GF (eds). Management of acute leukemia. Hematol Oncol Clin North Am 1993;7:1.

Champlin R, Gale RP. Acute lymphoblastic leukemia: Recent advances in biology and therapy. Blood 1989;73:2051–2066.

Foon KA, Rai KR, Gale RP. Chronic lymphocytic leukemia: new insights into biology and therapy. Ann Intern Med 1990;113:525–539.

Oeffler HP. Syndromes of acute nonlymphocytic leukemia. Ann Intern Med 1987;107:748–758.

Clinical Uses of Blood and Blood Products

Fresh Frozen Plasma — Indications and Risks; NIH Consensus Conference. JAMA 1985;253(4):551–553.

Lundberg G. Practice parameters for the use of fresh frozen plasma, cryoprecipitate, and platelets. JAMA 1994;271(10): 277–278.

NIH Consensus Conference. Perioperative red cell transfusion. JAMA 1988;260:2700–2703.

Sayers MH, Anderson KC, Goodnough LT, et al. Reducing the risks for transfusion-transmitted cytomegalovirus infection. Ann Intern Med 1992;116:55–62.

Simon TL, Stehling L. Indications for autologous transfusions. JAMA 1992;267:2669.

Linden JV, Pisciotto PT. Transfusion-associated graft vs. host disease and blood irradiation. Trans Med Rev 1992;2:116–123.

PART X

David K. Wagner
David Letzer

INFECTIOUS DISEASES

An individual is protected against invading microorganisms in a variety of ways (Table 141.1). These protective mechanisms involve **nonspecific host defenses,** including the skin and mucosal membranes and components of the immune system, such as the complement system and granulocytic phagocytes. The cellular and humoral immune systems are categorized as **specific host defenses** because they respond to specific antigens and because there is a memory of a preceding encounter with that same organism in the immune response. In the following sections, the function of the normal host defenses is described, followed by clinical examples of infections that occur in immunocompetent individuals. Chapter 14, Immunodeficiency, in the Allergy and Immunology part, and Chapter 157, Infections in Immunocompromised Patients, later in this part, discuss the types of infections seen in immunocompromised persons.

■ Nonspecific Host Defenses

Intact skin and normal flora

Intact skin and mucous membranes form a physical barrier to external microbes. These surfaces, especially the mucous membranes, are normally colonized by bacterial species, which vary according to the site (Table 141.2). The resident microorganisms perform a protective function primarily by competing with nonresident flora for cutaneous or mucosal attachment sites. In addition, certain bacteria, such as the viridans streptococci, produce a high molecular weight antibiotic, called bacteriocin, which may inhibit pathogenic bacteria. Others may stimulate phagocytosis and production of natural antibodies at mucosal sites. Natural antibodies, found in previously healthy persons without a history of

TABLE 141.2.	Common Bacteria Colonizing at Various Sites
Site	**Organisms**
Skin	Staphylococci (usually *S. epidermidis*) Corynebacteria Propionibacteria
Intestinal tract	Anaerobes and gram-negative bacilli
Oropharynx	Streptococci and anaerobes
Female genital tract	Anaerobes and gram-positive bacilli

specific infection, are believed to be important in immunity to certain encapsulated organisms (e.g., *Haemophilus influenzae, Neisseria meningitidis*).

The barrier defense provided by normal skin or mucous membranes breaks down with traumatic injuries, surgical incisions, burns, vascular insufficiency, radiation injury, chemotherapy, and various inflammatory conditions. Such breakdown allows for the invasion of bacteria, leading to cutaneous or mucocutaneous infection. For instance, *Streptococcus pyogenes,* which usually dies on intact skin, requires a breakdown in the epidermis to cause cellulitis. In certain other cutaneous infections, which occur in the presence of epidermal trauma, the microbiologic cause is suggested by the mechanism of injury (Table 141.3).

Breakdown of the normal microbial flora can result in colonization by potentially pathogenic and invasive bacteria. Chronic diseases (diabetes mellitus and alcoholism) as well as severe illness that leads to general debilitation favor the adherence of gram-negative bacilli to oropharyngeal mucosal cells, predisposing to pneumonia. However, antibiotic use is the biggest factor leading to altered microbial flora. The frequent use of "broad-spectrum" antibiotics can cause the depletion of normal flora and lead to colonization and infection by more pathogenic organisms.

Local antimicrobial factors

Factors that locally inhibit invading microorganisms include excretory secretions, ciliary movement, local production of antimicrobial substances (e.g., lysozyme), and gastric or urinary acidity (Table 141.4).

Complement system

The complement system contains a number of plasma proteins which are important mediators in host

TABLE 141.1.	Host Defenses: An Overview	
Nonspecific		**Specific**
Intact skin and normal flora		Cellular immune system
Local antimicrobial factors		T lymphocytes
Nutrition		Humoral immune system
Stress and exercise		B lymphocytes
Hormonal factors		
Immune system • Complement • Phagocytic cells		

defense to a variety of organisms. These proteins cooperate in a series of interactions via either the **classical** or **alternate pathway** (Figure 141.1).

Complement-deficient states may be acquired or inherited (Table 141.5). Acquired deficiencies include severe burns, where the deficiency follows a loss of all serum proteins or nephrotic syndrome, where only some

factors (B) are reduced, with the other complement components remaining normal. Some autoimmune diseases, such as systemic lupus erythematosus, may be associated with consumption of complement or with development of serum inhibitors to specific complement components. Inherited complement deficiencies are uncommon.

TABLE 141.3.	Relationship of Setting of Epidermal Trauma to the Type of Cutaneous Infection
Setting	**Organism**
Dog or cat bite	*Pasteurella multocida;* oral aerobes and anaerobes
Wound contamination by freshwater	*Aeromonas hydrophila*
Burn wounds	*Staphylococcus aureus* (commonly), Candida, *Pseudomonas aeruginosa, Klebsiella pneumoniae, Escherichia coli*
Lower extremity ulcers in diabetic persons	Mixture of gram positive, gram negative and anaerobic organisms
Radiation and chemotherapy	Usual residents of intact skin or mucosa
Secondary infection complicating atopic dermatitis or eczema	Usual residents of intact skin

TABLE 141.4.	Local Antimicrobial Factors		
Site	**Factor**	**Normal Mechanism**	**Mechanism Interfered By**
Respiratory tract	Turbulent airflow	Deposition of large particles	Endotracheal intubation/tracheostomy
			Clearance of aspirated material impeded by diminished cough during altered states of consciousness
	Lysozyme	Antibacterial activity	Phagocytic cell dysfunction
Gastrointestinal tract	Gastric pH	Mucosal barrier for ingested organisms	Decreased acidity fosters bacterial overgrowth - Salmonella enteritis more common in achlorhydric patients; use of antacids in critically ill patients leads to colonization of the upper GI tract with gram (−) bacilli
	Pancreatic enzymes, bile and intestinal secretions	Antimicrobial action	Obstruction
	Peristaltic action	Propels and removes microbes	Antimotility agents
Genitourinary tract	Urinary flow	Stimulates a flushing mechanism	Obstruction to urinary flow predisposes to infection which may ascend into the kidney.
	Hypertonicity of renal medulla, urine pH and urea	Inhibitory for bacteria	
	Acidic pH of vagina	Maintained by the commensal flora	Antibiotic use
Eyes	Tears	Exerts bathing action; expels bacteria mechanically	Obstruction or decreased production of tears
	Lysozyme	Antibacterial action	

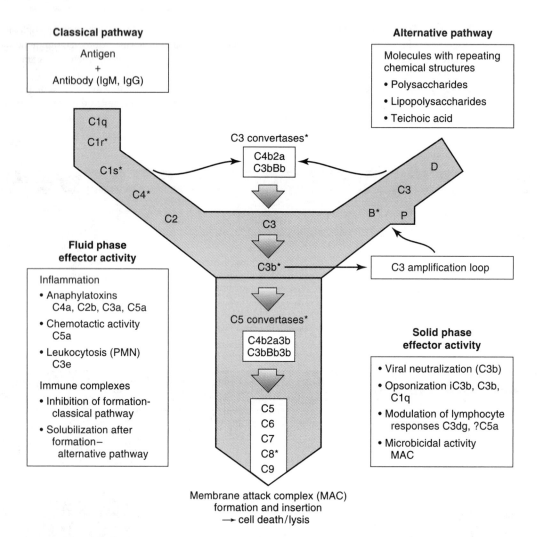

FIGURE 141.1. The **complement cascade,** showing both classical and alternate pathways, with the components arranged in order of their activation. Sites of down-regulation of complement activity are indicated by asterisks.
(From: Densen P. Complement, Ch. 6, Fig. 1, p. 60. In Mandell GL, Bennett JE, Dolin R (eds). Principles and Practice of Infectious Diseases. 4th ed., New York: Churchill Livingstone, 1995, Figure 1, p. 60. Used with permission.)

TABLE 141.5.	Major Complement Deficiencies
Acquired	**Inherited**
Severe burns	Classical pathway
Nephrotic syndrome	Alternative pathway
Sickle cell disease	Terminal complement com-
Autoimmune diseases	ponents

Phagocytic cells

Neutrophil kinetics and function

Neutrophil precursors are the major cell type in the bone marrow. It takes about 10 days for myeloblast to develop into mature neutrophils, which then are released into the circulation. Circulating neutrophils normally survive 6–10 hours, but during severe infections, their survival may be reduced to even less than 1 hour.

The neutrophil's function involves migration to a site of infection, followed by killing the invading organism. The first step in activating neutrophils is through **chemoattractants** (e.g., complement C5a), which are produced at sites of inflammation. The neutrophil moves toward the chemoattractant and adheres to the vascular endothelial cells. It then enters the extravascular space and migrates toward the infection, where it engulfs the offending organisms in a process known as **phagocytosis.** Complement component C3b may aid in the phagocytosis process. The ingested microorganisms are killed by either oxidative ("respiratory burst," see Figure 141.2) or oxygen-independent mechanisms.

Quantitative and qualitative neutrophil defects

Defects in neutrophil function may be due to inadequate cell numbers (quantitative) or because of defective cell function (qualitative) (Table 141.6).

Peripheral neutrophil counts normally range from 1500 to 8000 cells/μl. The risk of infection increases as counts decrease below 1000/μl, and it increases dramatically at counts below 100/μl. The most common infecting organisms in patients with low neutrophil counts (neutropenia) include enteric gram-negative organisms *(Escherichia coli,* Enterobacter, *Pseudomonas), Staphylococcus aureus,* and fungi (e.g., *C. albicans, Aspergillus).* The most common quantitative defect is due to bone marrow toxicity resulting from drugs or infection. Myelotoxicity is most frequently associated with cytotoxic chemotherapy but also may be due to other drugs, such as chloramphenicol, trimethoprim-sulfamethoxazole, and zidovudine.

Qualitative neutrophil defects are mostly hereditary and usually diagnosed in childhood. However, some disorders of neutrophil motility may be associated with autoimmune disorders, diabetes mellitus, alcoholism, or corticosteroid use. Alcohol also causes neutropenia, in addition to other negative effects, including depressed barrier defenses (depressed glottic reflex, aspiration) and decreased cell-mediated immunity. Corticosteroids, on the other hand, raise the neutrophil count (neutrophilia) due to demargination. They also can affect cell-mediated and humoral immunity (antibody formation).

■ Specific Host Defenses

The specific host defenses consist of the cellular and humoral immune systems. These systems respond to specific antigens that are recalled through an immunologic memory of a preceding encounter with a specific organism.

Cellular immunity

T-lymphocyte development and function

The cellular immune system is the linchpin of specific host responses. T-lymphocytes mature in the fetal thymus where they develop distinct surface receptors, including those for antigens. The T-cell receptor is a heterodimeric protein containing four parts (the variable, diversity, joining, and constant regions) that recognizes a foreign antigen with its variable region structure. The variable region of the T cell, which is expressed in conjunction with the CD3 molecule, is capable of changes to match the multitude of antigens, although each T-lymphocyte will have only one variable region structure specific for only one antigen.

T-lymphocytes do not respond to foreign antigens by themselves, but do so in conjunction with **antigen-presenting cells** (Figure 141.3). Antigen-presenting cells are primarily macrophages or dendritic cells. After a foreign antigen (microbe) is engulfed by a macrophage, the antigen is processed and expressed on the surface of the macrophage in conjunction with **major histocompatibility complex (MHC) class II** molecules. The T-lymphocyte receptor recognizes the antigen–MHC complex with the help of the accessory molecules CD4 or CD8. After attachment of the receptor to the antigen–

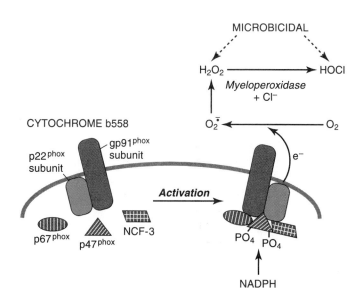

FIGURE 141.2. Components of the phagocytic cell respiratory burst. The cytochrome b558 is an integral membrane protein and the p47phox, p67phox, and neutrophil cytosol factor 3 (NCF-3) are cytoplasmic proteins. When activated, the p47phox is phosphorylated and translocates to the membrane together with the other cytoplasmic factors; NADPH oxidase is formed following interaction with the cytochrome. When electrons are transferred from NADPH to molecular oxygen, superoxide is formed, which breaks down into H_2O_2. Interaction with myeloperoxidase in the presence of chloride generates hypochlorous acid. The H_2O_2 and hypochlorous acid are extremely microbicidal.

(From: Gorbach SL, Bartlett JG, Blacklow NR (eds.). Infectious Diseases. Philadelphia: WB Saunders Company, 1992, Figure 7–3, p. 49. Used with permission.)

TABLE 141.6.   Major Quantitative and Qualitative Neutrophil Defects

Quantitative Defects	Qualitative Defects
Marrow toxicity from drugs or infection	Chronic granulomatous disease
Autoimmune disorders	Chediak-Higashi syndrome
Acquired cyclic neutropenia	Myeloperoxidase deficiency
Inherited cyclic neutropenia	Specific granule deficiency
	Leukocyte adhesion deficiency
	Motility disorders

CD4 T Cell

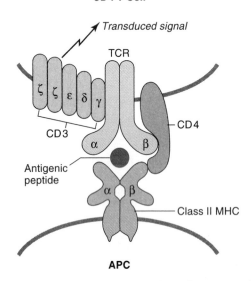

FIGURE 141.3. Antigen recognition by and activation of T cells. Antigen is presented by an antigen-presenting cell (APC) in the form of peptide bound to MHC molecules on the APC surface, which in turn is recognized by the α/ß-T-cell receptor (TCR). Most CD4-positive T cells recognize peptides bound to class II MHC, whereas most CD8-positive T cells recognize peptides bound to class I MHC. Following recognition of antigen, the CD3 complex of proteins, which is associated with the α/ß-TCR, produces an intracellular signal that causes T cell activation.)

(From: Lewis DB, Wilson CB. In Remington JS, Klein JO (eds.). Infectious Diseases of the Fetus and Newborn Infant. 4th ed. Philadelphia: WB Saunders, 1995, p. 22. Used with permission.)

MHC complex, a **cytokine** signal (usually interleukin-1 [IL-1] produced by the macrophage) initiates a clonal expansion of the T-lymphocyte population.

T-lymphocytes respond usually by differentiating into one of three types:

- T-lymphocytes that express CD4 molecules are called **helper T cells.** These cells respond to foreign antigens by producing other cytokines, which regulate the immune response by other cells, including T-lymphocytes and B lymphocytes.
- T-lymphocytes that express CD8 molecules are called **suppressor T cells.** These cells downregulate the immune response once the offending organism is controlled. These CD8 expressing cells are also able to mature, through cytokine stimulation, into cytotoxic T-lymphocytes. Cytotoxic T-lymphocytes recognize antigen in conjunction with MHC class I antigens and are important in killing virus-infected cells.
- The third cell type, termed the **natural killer cell,** are lymphocytes with the ability to lyse target cells in a non–HLA-directed manner. They are important in resistance to tumors and viruses.

Cellular immune defects

Cellular immune defects may be either acquired or congenital (Table 141.7). The most widely recognized example of an acquired defect is infection with the human immunodeficiency virus (HIV). Other viruses (e.g., influenza, Epstein-Barr virus [infectious mononucleosis], and cytomegalovirus), fungi (e.g., coccidioidomycosis), tuberculosis, and parasites (e.g., Toxoplasma) also have been associated with depressed cellular immunity. Malignancies that suppress cellular immunity include Hodgkin's disease and certain other lymphomas. Cellular immunity may also be depressed by pharmacologic agents (cytotoxic agents, [e.g., cyclophosphamide and methotrexate] corticosteroids, and cyclosporin). Radiation therapy used for malignancies affects cellular immunity in a way similar to cytotoxic agents, by reducing lymphoid populations. Both nutrition and alcohol can inhibit cellular immune responses.

Humoral immunity

B-lymphocyte development and function

Antibodies are antigen-specific immunoglobulins produced by B lymphocytes and play several roles in

TABLE 141.7.   Defects in Cellular Immunity

Acquired Defects	Congenital Defects
Infections	DiGeorge syndrome
Malignancies	Severe combined immuno-deficiency
Pharmacologic agents	
Radiation	
Nutrition	
Alcohol	

protection against infection. At mucosal sites, in conjunction with nonspecific host defenses, local IgA antibody may inhibit attachment of pathogenic organisms. Systemically, antibody may interact with complement to enhance phagocytosis (opsonization) or to achieve complement-mediated cytolysis. Other cytolytic processes involving antibody include **antibody-dependent cellular cytotoxicity** (ADCC) and IgE-mediated parasitic immunity. In these respective processes, lymphocytes or eosinophils, with the aid of antibodies, kill antigen-bearing target cells. Antibodies also act in neutralization processes, either with cell-free bacterial products (toxins) or cell-free viruses.

Immunoglobulin-deficient states

Several major causes of immunoglobulin-deficient states are listed in Table 141.8. In some malignancies, such as multiple myeloma and chronic lymphocytic leukemia, expansion of malignant cells occurs at the expense of normal immunoglobulin production. Primary

TABLE **141.8.** Immunoglobulin-Deficient States	
Acquired Defects	**Primary Deficiencies**
Multiple myeloma	X-linked hypogammaglobulinemia
Chronic lymphocytic leukemia	Ataxia-telangiectasia
Severe burns	Wiskott-Aldrich syndrome
Nephrotic syndrome	Common variable hypogammaglobulinemia
Splenectomy	Selective IgA deficiency
HIV infection	

B-cell deficiencies usually have an X-linked inheritance pattern and are discovered in infancy or early childhood, although common variable hypogammaglobulinemia and selective IgA deficiency are more likely to be discovered or treated in adulthood.

CHAPTER **142** # MANIFESTATIONS OF INFECTION

Whereas some infectious diseases are classically localized to an organ system with a textbook list of symptoms, their severity can vary greatly, depending on the resistance pattern of the organism and the sensitivity of the host. For instance, herpes zoster presents classically in a dermatomal pattern (Figure 142.1), but it may present in a widely disseminated form in an immunosuppressed host.

Infections also may involve one or several organ systems. The clinician must therefore be aware of not only the range of symptoms that might suggest a particular organ system infection, but also the combination of symptoms and signs that are consistent with a multisystemic infectious disorder. Certain simple **historical features** may suggest an infection. For example, acute rhinorrhea and a sore throat in the winter months might be consistent with a rhinovirus-associated rhinitis. Dysuria and frequency in a non-sexually active woman would be consistent with *Escherichia coli*-associated cystitis. Abrupt onset of fever above 103°F with cough, purulent sputum and pleuritic pain are characteristic of pneumococcal pneumonia.

On the other hand, many other infectious diseases are more difficult to diagnose, and the diagnosis rests on a compilation of historical factors, physical findings, and clues from the laboratory. In some cases, despite all the information, there still may be confusion as to whether the particular clinical presentation is consistent with an infectious disorder, connective tissue disease, or neoplasm.

■ **Patient History**

In all diseases, the history is important in establishing a list of possible entities for the differential diagnosis; this is particularly true in infectious diseases. Important historical considerations include geographic factors, which determine the range of potential infectious exposure, and several host factors, which determine the susceptibility of an individual to a particular infection.

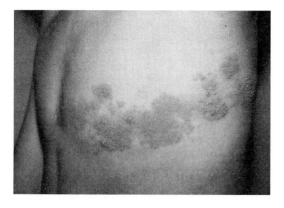

FIGURE 142.1. Herpes zoster (shingles) showing a dermatomal distribution.

Geographic and environmental factors

Geographic factors can be divided roughly into travel considerations and local geographic or environmental concerns. **Travel** is an ever-increasing concern, given the ease and frequency of international travel and immigration. Many infectious disorders, especially parasitic infections, are endemic outside the United States. For example, a lifelong resident of Wisconsin with new onset of seizures would not likely have neurocysticercosis as the cause. However, this etiology would be considered in a patient from, or with an appropriate travel history to, Mexico, Africa, or South America. Similarly, febrile episodes in a patient from Wisconsin would not warrant a consideration of malaria in the differential diagnosis, unless that person had recently returned from places endemic for malaria (e.g., Africa, South America, Southeast Asia).

One must next consider **local geographic or environmental factors,** which include place of residence, place of work, and other environmental factors, such as contact with a person having a transmissible infection. **Place of residence** includes both the geographic region and dwelling where the person resides. Local geography is an important consideration for certain infections. For example, a febrile pulmonary process in a patient in the southwestern United States could represent coccidioidomycosis, whereas the same in the Mississippi river valley could be blastomycosis.

The other important consideration in place of residence is the type of dwelling in which a person resides or is housed at the time the infection occurs. In the etiology for a pneumonia, for example, the differential diagnosis differs for a community-acquired versus hospital-acquired or nursing home–acquired (nosocomial) pneumonia. In general, patients who are institutionalized have a greater risk for exposure to more resistant pathogens, and those pathogens may cause a more severe illness. Other examples involving the place of residence would include a building with a contaminated air-conditioning system, leading to legionellosis, or incarceration, predisposing to tuberculosis or penicillin-resistant pneumococcal infection.

The **place of employment** sometimes may hold important clues as to the nature of the infection. The differential diagnosis of a systemic febrile illness in abattoir workers (slaughterhouse-workers), for example, includes brucellosis, a diagnosis that is unusual in most other occupations. A febrile illness with nausea and right-upper-quadrant tenderness might represent acute hepatitis or cholecystitis with cholangitis in a typical patient, but if the individual were a day-care worker, acute hepatitis A would be more likely, especially if other cases have recently occurred in such a facility. Attendance at a school or day-care center and **avocational activities** (hobbies) should also be considered.

Other **environmental concerns** might include sporadic exposures to infectious diseases that should be pursued in the history. Certain diseases, especially common respiratory illnesses, can spread easily among family members. Therefore, eliciting a history of illnesses, such as streptococcal pharyngitis or mycoplasmal pneumonia, in another family member is an important finding and underscores the importance of known contacts in evaluating many infectious disorders. Although many infectious diseases are sporadic, in others, contact tracing is important in the workup (e.g., sexually transmitted diseases, hepatitis, influenza, and tuberculosis).

Host-specific factors

The type of host is of utmost importance in assessing the manifestations of infection, both in terms of the entities to be considered and the potential severity of the infection. **Age** (e.g., hepatitis A is generally seen in younger persons), **coexisting disease** processes (e.g., cirrhosis is a major risk factor for tuberculous peritonitis), and **immune status** (e.g., HIV infection or immunosuppressive drug therapy) are key considerations.

Infections in immunocompromised patients are outlined in more detail in other chapters of this section. Suffice it to say that the **type of defect in host defense** affects the differential diagnosis, certain conditions being more likely depending on the defect. A patient with a pulmonary infiltrate will arouse certain considerations, such as *Streptococcus pneumoniae* or *Haemophilus influenzae* pneumonia, but if the same patient is receiving high-dose corticosteroids for some period of time, other pathogens may need to be considered, including *Aspergillus* or *Mycobacterium tuberculosis.*

Certain infections also may be much more fulminant in an immunocompromised host. For example, a pneumococcal pneumonia may assume a lobar configuration in many instances, but the splenectomized patient may manifest bacteremic pneumococcal disease with severe septic shock and disseminated intravascular coagulation.

■ Physical Signs

Organisms encountered by the host from the environment either are killed, colonize the skin or mucosal surfaces and become part of the normal flora, or are pathogenic. Pathogenic microorganisms either cause a local inflammatory response or invade the tissues. However, even bacteria that are part of the normal flora may, in the right circumstances, cause infection (e.g., cystitis or pyelonephritis due to *Escherichia coli*). It is the inflammatory response in the tissues that leads to the physical signs or manifestations of infection.

Manifestations due to inflammatory responses

Particular pathogenic microorganisms may be fairly organ-specific, having **tropism** to certain tissues, whereas other pathogens have a more varied effect. Some organisms, in fact, are named for their target organ. For example, the family of hepatitis viruses all have tropism for the liver. Hepatitis viruses, therefore, predictably cause an inflammatory reaction in the liver with the attendant physical signs of hepatic enlargement and tenderness.

Other organisms also may affect one organ system most commonly but, not uncommonly, will affect other organ systems, too. For example, *Streptococcus pneumoniae* most commonly causes pneumonia (with bronchial breath sounds, or rales, egophony; *lobar* consolidation may or may not be present) although it may also cause meningitis (with signs of meningeal irritation, such as nuchal rigidity), and infection of other organs.

Infectious disorders are not always simple to categorize in terms of etiology and may manifest with constellations of findings that do not immediately suggest the diagnosis. For instance, endocarditis, which may be due to a number of organisms, can manifest acutely with fever and a new murmur, or the physical manifestations may be more subacute, with fever, malaise, and weight loss. The acute presentation is most likely associated with *Staphylococcus aureus,* whereas the subacute process is often due to the viridans streptococci. The findings with the subacute presentation, however, may or may not immediately suggest endocarditis, and they might initially suggest a malignancy or a collagen vascular disorder.

Both the microbe and host influence the physical manifestations of an infection. Compared to the normal host, the immunocompromised patient not only tends to have more severe physical manifestations of infection in the involved organ system, but also suffers an enhanced risk of disseminated infection. A striking example mentioned earlier is pneumococcal sepsis and disseminated intravascular coagulation seen in the splenectomized patient. The clinician must be especially diligent, careful, and complete when examining these patients so that no clues are overlooked.

General signs: fever

Fever is one of the first physical clues to a potential infectious disease. Although some localized infections, such as rhinitis, urethritis, or vaginitis, are usually not accompanied by fever, most patients with a significant infection of an organ system will be febrile. Fever, by no means, is specific to infection, as patients with malignancy or connective tissue disorders can also be febrile. The clinician should also be aware that hypothermia can occasionally accompany a significant infection, such as gram-negative sepsis, and portends a poor prognosis (see Chapter 146).

■ Laboratory Findings

A complete blood count is frequently obtained to support the possible diagnosis of infection. Bacterial infections commonly, but not invariably, manifest with an elevation of the total leukocyte count with an increase in immature forms (bands) — "a shift to the left." Similarly, a lymphocytosis may correlate with a viral infection (e.g., influenza), and eosinophilia, with helminthic infections (e.g., strongyloidiasis). Anemia of chronic disease may be related to an underlying subacute or chronic infection. Numerous other laboratory tests are also used to support the diagnosis of infection, as described in more detail in subsequent chapters.

CHAPTER 143 **LABORATORY DIAGNOSIS OF INFECTIOUS DISEASES**

Although knowledge of the patterns of infections in different clinical settings is essential in the diagnosis and differential diagnosis of specific infections, the laboratory is vital in helping make specific therapeutic decisions. The laboratory diagnosis of infectious diseases first involves proper collection and processing of specimens, so that the results can be interpreted appropriately. The importance of good communication with the microbiology laboratory cannot be overemphasized. Information about the suspected disease process helps the laboratory personnel to process the specimens properly.

Once in the laboratory, the specimen is subjected to various types of direct visualization (e.g., microscopy) and culture, as directed by the clinician. Some organisms are fastidious or grow poorly on culture, but they may elicit certain types of immunologic responses in the host that can be assayed. The clinician needs a clinical understanding of the possible tests in order to know which tests will give the best information in a particular clinical setting.

■ Collection of Specimens

Before specimens are collected from a patient with a suspected infection, it is important to remember that the body has a normal microbial flora on all its mucocutaneous surfaces. In sampling most normally sterile sites (e.g., blood, cerebrospinal fluid), one must traverse this normally nonsterile skin or mucosal surface to access the sites of collection. Avoiding contamination by normal flora requires that special attention be given to maintaining a sterile procedure.

When specimen collection is contemplated, there also should be a reason for obtaining a particular specimen. The practice of "pan-culturing" or culturing all potentially available sites, is appropriate in some, but not all, settings. Especially with cultures of nonsterile sites, one must always anticipate what potential culture results the microbiology laboratory may return so that interpretation can be made in view of the clinical setting.

Culture of blood and other normally sterile sites

1. A disinfectant is applied to the skin for at least 30 seconds before blood cultures are drawn.

2. The samples should be obtained percutaneously. Because skin contaminants may interfere with the results of blood cultures, at least two separate blood cultures should be obtained for adequate interpretation.

3. When preparing blood cultures, microbiology laboratories routinely use systems that allow for the detection of both aerobes and anaerobes. Thus, it is necessary to inoculate blood into two separate bottles or devices.

4. For suspected peritonitis, peritoneal fluid should be inoculated directly into blood culture bottles at the bedside.

5. In evaluating catheter-related sepsis, some housestaff routinely obtain one culture through the catheter and one percutaneously. However, catheters are often colonized, and these colonizing organisms will grow on the culture. When catheter-related sepsis is suspected, the catheter should be removed; its distal two inches aseptically clipped into a sterile container, it then should sent to the laboratory for quantitative culture. In addition, blood cultures should be obtained.

6. After the samples have been obtained, they should be properly labeled and expeditiously transported to the laboratory. Repeating the test, especially from sterile sites (e.g., lumbar puncture), may not be easily accomplished.

Culture of normally nonsterile sites

The practice of "pan-culturing" is especially problematic when obtaining cultures from nonsterile sites. The clinician must anticipate what potential culture results the microbiology laboratory may return and order tests as dictated by the clinical setting. For example, culturing of respiratory secretions frequently yields numerous organisms; deciphering the finding of organisms in the sputum (i.e., which is pathogenic versus simply colonizing) then rests with the clinician.

To make optimum use of culture results from nonsterile sites, the physician should exercise care in collecting specimens. Laboratories often screen samples from nonsterile sites, and samples that do not meet certain requirements for appropriate culture may be rejected.

1. Because the mouth cannot be sterilized to avoid contamination, the patient should be encouraged to expectorate after a deep cough. To be suitable for culturing, the sputum specimen should contain a predominance of neutrophils and, if at all, scant epithelial cells (see sputum examination, Chapter 209).

2. For urine samples obtained from women, the best sample is a midstream specimen procured after meatal cleaning. A urine specimen may need to be leukocyte esterase-positive before being processed for culture by the laboratory.

3. Sampling of open wounds, such as decubitus ulcers, is especially difficult due to the presence of numerous colonizing organisms. If a soft tissue abscess is present or suspected, the abscess material should be aspirated into a syringe through a sterile needle. The needle is then removed, the syringe is capped with a sterile cap, and the whole syringe then sent to the laboratory.

4. It is important to inform the laboratory of the suspected diagnosis.

5. Body sites that have an abundant endogenous microbial flora (e.g., oral cavity, vagina) should not be sampled for anaerobic pathogens. Sputum, because of passage through the oral cavity during expectoration, suffers from this limitation.

6. Use of appropriate transport media is important in delivery of samples to the microbiology laboratory. Pus or purulent material is best injected into anaerobic transport vials; syringes used for aspiration are best avoided for transportation of specimens, because of risk of needle-stick injury and diffusion of oxygen across the plastic syringe walls.

■ Direct Examination of Specimens

Microscopy

Pathogenic organisms can often be directly visualized through a **light microscope** in a variety of clinical specimens. A number of stains are utilized in the laboratory, the most common being the Gram stain.

Gram staining

Because the Gram stain is a common procedure, the clinician should be familiar with its performance and interpretation (Table 143.1). The Gram stain is helpful in identifying organisms through their staining characteristics but also the morphology (see Figure 148.1).

Bacterial organisms are classified as either **gram-positive** or **gram-negative,** meaning they enhance with the stain or not. Organisms are further classified by their shape, either round (**cocci**) or rod-like (**bacilli).** Gram-positive cocci, for instance, indicate staphylococcal or streptococcal species. Gram-positive organisms may be further differentiated visually by their relationship to each other. Staphylococci tend to **cluster,** while streptococci tend to form **chains.** Similarly, gram-negative organisms can be differentiated somewhat by their morphology. For example, abundant, small, gram-negative coccobacilli might indicate *Haemophilus influenzae.*

Other staining techniques

Because the Gram stain does not stain all types of organisms, other stains or visualization methods are helpful in selected circumstances.

Mycobacteria are best seen with an **acid-fast stain,** on which they appear pink and beaded. These organisms may be difficult to detect, and an experienced technologist is needed to examine the specimen. Most bacteria, except for Nocardia and some Legionella species, do not retain the pink dye of the acid-fast stain.

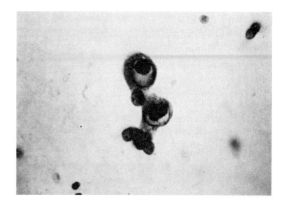

FIGURE 143.1. Intranuclear inclusion bodies of cytomegalovirus seen on hematoxylin-eosin staining.

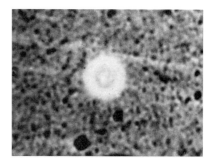

FIGURE 143.2. India ink preparation showing the capsule of *Cryptococcus neoformans.*

Viral inclusion bodies (e.g., cytomegalovirus) may be seen by direct examination of smears stained with **hematoxylin and eosin** (Figure 143.1).

A **potassium hydroxide** (KOH) preparation helps to identify fungi in selected specimens (see Figure 216.1). A drop of KOH applied to a slide containing sputum, skin, oral, or vaginal scrapings destroys bacteria and mucus but allows the fungal elements to be visualized.

Other methods of staining fungi include the **india ink** preparation which, for example, will stain the capsule of *Cryptococcus neoformans* (Figure 143.2). Fungal elements can also be seen in biopsied tissue samples with the use of other stains (Gomori or methenamine-silver stains) and can indicate invasion of these tissues by the fungus.

Direct visualization using a variety of stains is also commonly used when examining for intestinal parasites. Extensive experience is required in interpreting wet preparations of stool samples.

Dark-field microscopy

Another method of directly visualizing organisms, besides light microscopy, is with the use of a special

TABLE 143.1. Gram Stain Procedure
1. Air-dry and heat-fix specimen on a glass slide.
2. Flood the slide with crystal violet and allow to sit for 10–15 sec.
3. Rinse the slide with water.
4. Flood the slide with Gram iodine and allow to sit for 10–15 sec.
5. Rinse the slide with water.
6. Decolorize with 95% ethyl alcohol until blue color just disappears from thin portions of the smear.
7. Rinse the slide immediately with water.
8. Flood the slide with safranin for 10–15 sec.
9. Rinse the slide with water.
10. Air-dry and examine.

TABLE 143.2.	Examples of Antigenic Immunoassays	
Disease/Microbe	Sample/Specimen	Immunoassay
Meningitis		
• *Streptococcus pneumoniae*	Cerebrospinal fluid	Latex agglutination
• *Haemophilus influenzae*		
• *Neisseria meningitidis*		
• *Cryptococcus neoformans*		
Respiratory tract/pneumonia		
• Respiratory syncytial virus	Respiratory secretion	DFA
• *Bordetella pertussis*		
• *Legionella pneumophila*	Respiratory secretion/urine	DFA/RIA
Hepatitis		
• Hepatitis B virus	Serum	RIA
Sexually transmitted diseases		
• Herpes simplex virus	Vesicle fluid or exudate	ELISA
• *Chlamydia trachomatis*	Exudate	ELISA
• *Treponema pallidum*	Serum	Fluorescent assay (FTA-ABS)
Diarrhea/colitis		
• *Clostridium difficile*	Stool	Anitoxin assay

DFA = direct fluorescent antibody; ELISA = enzyme-linked immunosorbent assay; FTA-ABS = fluorescent trepoemal antibody absorption; RIA = radio immunoassay.

dark-field microscope). Spirochetes are best seen by this method. Motile spirochetes, for example, can be seen in the exudate from lesions in primary syphilis. Because these spirochetes are infectious, gloves should be worn when obtaining samples for dark-field examination.

Immunoassay techniques

For rapid diagnosis of infections, various immunoassays have been developed that rely on antibody reactions to unique antigens of the suspected organisms (Table 143.2). The immunoassay is a standard method for diagnosing several diseases (e.g., syphilis, *Treponema pallidum*) or active carrier states (e.g., hepatitis B), as these organisms are not cultivable in clinical laboratories.

■ Microbial Isolation and Identification (Culture)

Although it is helpful to visualize microorganisms directly, a definitive diagnosis of most bacterial infections resides with standard **culture** methods. Clinical specimens are cultured in appropriate media, and microbial identification is based on numerous factors, such as selective growth in media containing certain nutrients, the appearance of the colonies, presence of hemolytic properties, odor produced, and microscopic appearance. A number of biochemical tests are also employed, especially with gram-negative bacteria.

Some microbes grow slowly or have selective culture requirements (fastidious), causing delays in diagnosis (e.g., *Mycobacterium tuberculosis*). Good communication with the laboratory is critical in obtaining optimal

culture results. If the laboratory is aware that a particular pathogen is suspected (e.g., Legionella pneumonia), then appropriate selective plates will be used.

Antibiotic susceptibility of bacteria, which tests for antibiotic resistance, is pivotal in selecting or altering antibiotic selection in particular clinical settings. Susceptibility is determined by disk diffusion testing on plates or by testing serial dilutions of an antibiotic against a known inoculum of organism. A **minimum bactericidal concentration** (MBC) and **minimum inhibitory concentration** (MIC) are thus determined. If the culture medium is a broth, subcultures are made to a medium free of antimicrobial agent and reincubated to determine the MBC, which is the smallest concentration of the antimicrobial agent which on subculture fails to show growth of the microbe. The MIC is the minimum amount of the test agent that will inhibit visible growth of the microorganism. Determining mycobacterial sensitivities is limited to specialized laboratories, and fungal or viral susceptibilities, to research facilities. Molecular techniques, such as **DNA probes** and **polymerase chain reaction (PCR)** are sensitive and specific techniques for identifying pathogens. In PCR, the microbial DNA is amplified to make adequate nucleotide sequences. A specially labeled oligonucleotide ("gene probe") is then used to mark the results of the PCR, thus affording their detection. PCR/DNA probe is highly specific and extremely sensitive. Specific DNA probes and PCR assays are presently available for many infectious agents, most notably *Mycobacterium tuberculosis* and HIV. DNA probes are also quite useful in the investigation of outbreaks of infections, often enabling to identify the source.

CHAPTER **144** MICROBES THAT CAUSE INFECTION

The field of infectious diseases is ever-changing. New organisms are discovered in association with established clinical syndromes (e.g., *Helicobacter pylori* in peptic ulcer disease) but also with relatively new syndromes (e.g., HIV and AIDS, hantavirus pulmonary syndrome). In addition, familiar organisms sometimes reemerge (e.g., tuberculosis) or develop new antimicrobial resistance, making treatment more difficult (e.g., multidrug resistant tuberculosis and enterococcus).

■ Viruses

Viruses are composed of either RNA or DNA (which may be single-stranded or double-stranded). While they usually have an outer protein coat (capsid), some viruses have an outer lipid envelope as well.

Viral replication

Because viruses encode only a restricted number of proteins, they depend on the machinery of the host cell to accomplish their replication cycle. To initiate the replication cycle, viruses must first enter the host cell, via a process known as **endocytosis.** Some viruses use specific host receptors to accomplish this goal (e.g., CD4 receptors for HIV).

Inside the cell, a process of viral uncoating (a series of changes to the viral capsid) follows that allows replication of viral genetic material. **DNA viruses** enter the host nucleus, where they utilize host enzymes to produce mRNA. The mRNA encodes a DNA polymerase that is used for viral replication. **RNA viruses,** however, replicate through an RNA polymerase. (An exception to this pattern of RNA replication involves

the retroviruses, which use a virally encoded reverse transcriptase to make a DNA copy of the viral RNA. This DNA integrates into the host DNA and becomes latent. After a period of time, host machinery is used to make viral proteins.) After sufficient viral components are synthesized, they are assembled and released to infect other cells.

Pathogenic effects

Viruses may have several effects on the host cell. They may integrate into the host genome and remain dormant, or they can redirect the host genome into a malignant transformation. When activated in a replicative mode, the virus may be lytic to the host cell, or through transformed surface markers, the host cell may be damaged through self-directed immunologic mechanisms.

Viral taxonomy

There are six families of **DNA viruses,** as listed in Table 144.1. Of this group, the herpesvirus family is probably the most ubiquitous and well-recognized clinically. These viruses can become latent after a primary infection and reappear at a later time (e.g., recurrent mucocutaneous ulcers from herpes simplex or herpes zoster manifesting years after chickenpox). These recrudescent infections may be especially severe in immunocompromised patients. Examples of **RNA viruses** pathogenic for humans are shown in Table 144.2.

■ Bacteria

Bacteria are a diverse group of prokaryotic organisms, classified according to structural properties, pro-

---

TABLE **144.1.** Families of Human DNA Viruses		
Family	**Examples of Viruses**	**Examples of Clinical Manifestations**
Herpesviridae	Herpes simplex virus	Mucocutaneous ulcers
	Varicella-zoster virus	Chicken pox
	Epstein-Barr virus	Infectious mononucleosis
	Cytomegalovirus	Disseminated infections in immunocompromised hosts
	Human herpesvirus 6	Roseola
Adenoviridae	Adenovirus	Respiratory tract infection
Hepadnaviridae	Hepatitis B virus	Hepatitis
Parvoviridae	Parvovirus B19	Erythema infectiosum, red cell aplasia
Papovaviridae	Papilloma virus	Warts, genital warts
	Polyoma virus	Progressive multifocal leukoencephalopathy
Poxviridae	Molluscum contagiosum	Molluscum contagiosum

TABLE 144.2. Families of Human RNA Viruses		
Family	**Examples of Viruses**	**Examples of Clinical Manifestations**
Picornaviridae	Rhinovirus	Common cold
	Hepatitis A	Acute hepatitis
	Coxsackievirus	Aseptic meningitis
	ECHOvirus	Aseptic meningitis
	Poliovirus	Poliomyelitis
Orthomyxoviridae	Influenza virus	Respiratory tract infection
Paramyxoviridae	Parainfluenza virus	Respiratory tract infection
	Respiratory syncytial virus	Respiratory tract infection
	Mumps virus	Parotitis
	Measles virus	Rubeola (measles)
Retroviridae	Human immunodeficiency virus	AIDS
Reoviridae	Rotavirus	Diarrhea
Togaviridae	Rubella virus	Rubella (german measles)
	Alphavirus	Eastern equine encephalitis
Flaviviridae	Dengue virus	Dengue
	Yellow fever virus	Yellow fever
	St. Louis encephalitis virus	Encephalitis
Bunyaviridae	California encephalitis virus	Encephalitis
	Hantavirus	Hantavirus pulmonary syndrome
Arenaviridae	Lassa fever virus	Hemorrhagic fever
Filoviridae	Ebola virus	Hemorrhagic fever
Coronaviridae	Coronavirus	Upper respiratory tract infection
Rhabdoviridae	Rabies virus	Rabies

duction of enzymes or toxins, metabolic activities, and molecular homology. The Gram stain, which highlights differences in cell wall structure, is commonly used to separate large groups of bacteria (Table 144.3).

Gram-positive bacteria

Pathogenic **gram-positive cocci** are from the genera Staphylococcus, Streptococcus, and Enterococcus. Morphology may help to distinguish among these organisms, as staphylococci tend to form clusters whereas streptococci and enterococci tend to form chains.

Based on the coagulase test, staphylococci may be categorized as coagulase-positive or coagulase-negative. *Staphylococcus aureus* is pathogenic by tissue invasion (e.g., abscess) or by toxin production (e.g., toxic shock syndrome, food poisoning, scalded skin syndrome). Antibiotic sensitivity of *S. aureus* should be tested, as methicillin-resistant strains are becoming more common.

Streptococci, which typically appear in pairs or chains, are divided into several serogroups (A through H and K through V). Streptococcal infections in humans most often result from groups A, B, C, D, and G. Organisms in group D have been reclassified recently into enterococci, which cause genitourinary and wound infections as well as endocarditis. *Streptococcus pneumoniae,* an important member of the streptococcal group, causes pneumonia, meningitis and bacteremia.

Although most strains remain sensitive to penicillin, the incidence of resistance of *S. pneumoniae* to penicillin and other antibiotics has dramatically risen in recent times.

Of the **gram-positive bacilli,** the more common, clinically significant organisms are Corynebacterium, Bacillus species, and *Listeria monocytogenes.* Corynebacteria are club-shaped on gram stain and have a "Chinese letter" configuration on microscopic examination.

Gram-negative bacteria

Clinically significant disease due to **gram-negative cocci** most commonly involves two species of Neisseria, *N. gonorrhoeae* and *N. meningitidis.* Both are fastidious in their growth requirements and are identified biochemically. Another organism, *Moraxella (Branhamella) catarrhalis,* has become an increasingly common cause of lower respiratory tract infections in the elderly and in patients with underlying chronic bronchitis and emphysema.

The gram-negative bacilli comprise a large group of pathogens, the largest group of which is the Enterobacteriaceae family (Table 144.3). The lipopolysaccharide component of Enterobacteriaceae causes many of the major features of sepsis. *Helicobacter pylori* is an important cause of peptic ulcer disease.

Anaerobic bacteria

Anaerobic bacteria are the predominant commensal organisms at many body sites, including the oral cavity, intestine, and female genital tract. Infection may be associated with a defect in host defenses (e.g., trauma, diabetes) or with invasion by exogenous organisms (e.g., tetanus). Some common anaerobic pathogens are listed in Table 144.4.

Spirochetes

Spirochetes are spiral or coiled organisms that are best observed under a dark-field microscope. They are difficult to isolate on artificial media, and demonstration of the organism or serologic tests are usually required to confirm a diagnosis. Members of the genera Treponema, Borrelia, Leptospira, and Spirillum are known to cause human disease.

Treponema species pathogenic for humans include *T. pertenue, T. carateum,* and *T. pallidum. T. pallidum,* the agent of syphilis, is the most common treponeme encountered in this country. It should also be noted that treponemal species can be part of the normal oral flora.

Two disease processes caused by species of Borrelia include Lyme disease, caused by *B. burgdorferi,* and relapsing fever. Louse-borne relapsing fever is caused by *B. recurrentis* and *B. hermsii,* and tick-borne relapsing fever is caused by *B. turicatae, B. parkeri* and others.

Leptospirosis is due to two species of Leptospira, L. interrogans and *L. biflexa.* Humans are infected through accidental exposure to water or soil that is contaminated with urine of infected animals.

Spirillum minor causes rat bite fever.

Mycobacteria

Clinically significant mycobacteria can be divided into tuberculous (infection caused by *Mycobacterium tuberculosis,* see chapter 218) and nontuberculous mycobacteria (see chapter 219). These mycobacteria share the property of acid-fast staining. Because of a high lipid content in the cell wall, acid-fast bacilli retain dye after acid-alcohol washing.

Leprosy, due to *M. leprae,* is a common worldwide infection but is uncommon in the United States. It is a

---

TABLE 144.3.   Important Pathogenic Aerobic Bacteria and Some Typical Diseases They Produce

Gram-Positive Bacteria		Gram-Negative Bacteria	
Cocci		**Cocci**	
Staphylococcus epidermidis	UTI, bacteremia, catheter-related infections	Neisseria gonorrhoeae	Urethritis, cervicitis, PID
		Neisseria meningitidis	Meningitis
Staphylococcus aureus	Abscess, cellulitis, TSS	Moraxella catarrhalis	Bronchitis, pneumonitis
Streptococcus viridans	Endocarditis		
Streptococcus pneumoniae	Pneumonia, meningitis	**Bacilli**	
Streptococcus pyogenes	Pharyngitis, pyoderma	Enterobacteriaceae (Escherichia, Enterobacter, Klebsiella, Proteus) Serratia, Shigella, Salmonella	UTI, sepsis, respiratory infection, gastroenteritis
Enterococcus species	UTI, endocarditis		
Bacilli			
Corynebacteria species	Diphtheria, pharyngitis, endocarditis	Pseudomonas aeruginosa	Pneumonia, bacteremia, UTI
Bacillus species	Meningitis, bacteremia	Acinetobacter species	UTI, bacteremia, respiratory infection
Listeria monocytogenes	Meningitis	Haemophilus influenzae	Respiratory infection
		Legionella pneumophila	Pneumonia
		Helicobacter pylori	Peptic ulcer disease
		Vibrio species	Cholera, wound infections
		Campylobacter species	Diarrhea
		Pasteurella multocida	Infected dog/cat bites
		Bartonella species	Cat scratch disease, bacteremia
		Brucella species	Brucellosis

PID = pelvic inflammatory disease; TSS = toxic shock syndrome; UTI = urinary tract infection.

TABLE 144.4. Important Pathogenic Anaerobic Bacteria

Gram-positive cocci
Peptostreptococcus spp.
Peptococcus spp.
Gram-positive bacilli
Clostridium spp. (perfringens, septicum, difficile, tetani, botulinum)
Lactobacillus spp.
Propionibacterium spp.
Gram-negative bacilli
Bacteroides fragilis
Other Bacteroides
Prevotella spp.
Fusobacterium spp.

chronic granulomatous disease primarily involving skin and peripheral nerves.

Rickettsiae

The family Rickettsiae includes species from the genera Rickettsia, Coxiella, and Ehrlichia. All are obligate intracellular bacteria but with different replication cycles. The rickettsiae are engulfed by vascular endothelial cells (and sometimes smooth muscle cells), where they proliferate and damage the host cell. Rickettsial infections are transmitted by arthropods (tick, mite, body louse, or flea) from an animal host. The rickettsioses consist of a **spotted fever** group (e.g., Rocky Mountain spotted fever due to *R. rickettsii* and rickettsialpox due to *R. akari*) and a **typhus** group (e.g., *R. prowazekii* causing epidemic typhus and Brill-Zinsser disease and *R. typhi* causing murine typhus). Both groups have prominent fever and a rash that is mainly due to damage to small blood vessels.

Coxiella burnetii infects humans via aerosols of infected soil and dust; the clinical syndromes that result include Q fever and pneumonia.

Ehrlichiosis is a new syndrome similar to Rocky Mountain spotted fever. This febrile illness with transient leukopenia and thrombocytopenia is transmitted via a tick bite.

Chlamydiae

Chlamydiae were originally thought to be viruses, but they contain both RNA and DNA and are able to divide. They depend on the host cell primarily for energy, as they do not generate their own adenosine triphosphate (ATP). The developmental cycle of Chlamydia is fairly unique with two morphologic forms. One form, the **elementary body,** is suited for extracellular life but does not divide. Once attached to and internalized by the host cell, the elementary body transforms

into the metabolically active **reticulate body,** which is able to divide.

There are three chlamydial species that are pathogenic to humans, *C. pneumoniae, C. psittaci, and C. trachomatis. C. pneumoniae* (TWAR agent) is a cause of community-acquired pneumonia. *C. psittaci* produces a systemic disorder with prominent pulmonary findings, termed psittacosis (or ornithosis); exposure to parrots, parakeets, and several other types of birds is an important historical clue. *C. trachomatis* in adults causes primarily eye disease and genital tract disorders. Trachoma, a chronic follicular keratoconjunctivitis, is a common cause of blindness worldwide. Genital tract infection causes urethritis, epididymitis, pelvic inflammatory disease, proctitis and lymphogranuloma venereum (LGV).

Mycoplasmas

The mycoplasmas are small organisms like the chlamydiae and rickettsiae, yet they are able to replicate outside the host cell. Unlike bacteria, they lack a cell wall. Mycoplasmas are very difficult to culture.

The family Mycoplasmataceae contains several Mycoplasma species as well as *Ureaplasma urealyticum.* The ability of Ureaplasma to hydrolyze urea differentiates it from the Mycoplasma.

Most Mycoplasma species are not disease-producing and are found to colonize the upper respiratory or genital tracts. A few species are pathogenic: *M. pneumoniae, M. hominis, M. genitalium,* and *U. urealyticum.*

Mycoplasma tend not to be invasive. They produce disease by local damage to mucosal cells or by sensitizing host membranes into autoimmune reactions. *M. pneumoniae* is an important cause of upper respiratory tract infections and, sometimes, pneumonia in young individuals. *M. hominis* is a cause of vaginitis and pelvic inflammatory disease and may cause disease outside the genital tract. *U. urealyticum* is an important cause of

TABLE 144.5. Important Pathogenic Fungi

Fungi	Clinical Manifestations
Candida albicans	Esophagitis, bacteremia
Pneumocystis carinii	Pneumonia
Histoplasma capsulatum	Pneumonia, systemic dissemination (chapter 214)
Blastomyces dermatitidis	Pneumonia, systemic dissemination (chapter 216)
Cryptococcus neoformans	Pneumonia, meningitis
Coccidioides immitis	Pneumonia, meningitis (chapter 215)
Aspergillus spp.	Pulmonary syndromes (chapter 217)
Sporothrix schenckii	Cutaneous nodules

nongonococcal urethritis. *M. genitalium,* although less common, has been implicated in both nongonococcal urethritis and pelvic inflammatory disease.

The structure of these organisms necessitate therapy with antibiotics active at sites other than the cell wall, such as macrolides or tetracyclines.

Nocardia and Actinomyces

Nocardia and Actinomyces are higher bacteria in the order Actinomycetales. They are weakly gram-positive and resemble fungi with filamentous branching but lack cell walls characteristic of fungi. Nocardia is aerobic and weakly acid-fast (Kinyoun method), whereas Actinomyces are anaerobic and not acid-fast.

Nocardia is more commonly seen in patients with cellular immune defects, in whom it can produce a necrotizing pneumonia. Hematogenous dissemination to the brain is common. Actinomyces, which are not usually opportunistic, are oral saprophytes that can penetrate intact tissues after local trauma or infection. Actinomycosis is usually a chronic infection that can extend to superficial tissues and form a soft tissue swelling which will subsequently drain. Drainage material contains characteristic "sulfur granules" visible on microscopy, which consist of clumps of organisms.

■ Fungi

Fungi, unlike bacteria, have rigid cell walls composed of chitins and polysaccharides. Fungi are classified as yeasts or molds. **Yeasts** are round or oval and reproduce by a budding process, whereas **molds** are composed of tubular hyphal structures that grow by branching. Some fungi, called dimorphic fungi (e.g., *Histoplasma capsulatum, Blastomyces dermatitidis, Sporothrix schenckii, Coccidioides immitis*), grow in patients as yeasts but as molds in vitro at room temperatures.

Common pathogenic fungi and their clinical manifestations are listed in Table 144.5. However, many other presentations occur, particularly in immunosuppressed persons. *Pneumocystis carinii, Candida albicans, H. capsulatum, Cryptococcus neoformans* and *C. immitis* are prominent pathogens in AIDS.

TABLE 144.6. Important Protozoal Parasites	
Examples of Protozoa	**Clinical Manifestations**
Giardia lamblia	Diarrhea
Entamoeba histolytica	Dysentery, hepatic abscess
Toxoplasma gondii	Brain and eye lesions (very important in AIDS)
Trichomonas vaginalis	Vaginitis
Plasmodium spp.	Malaria (consider in the returning traveler)
Cryptosporidium parvum	Diarrhea (very important in AIDS)
Isospora belli	Diarrhea (very important in AIDS)
Enterocytozoon bieneusi (Microsporidium)	Diarrhea
Babesia microti	Fever, hemolysis
Trypanosoma	Chagas' disease, African sleeping sickness

TABLE 144.7. Important Helminthic Parasites	
Helminths	**Clinical Manifestations**
Nematodes (roundworms)	
Trichuris trichiura	Anemia, rectal prolapse (may be asymptomatic)
Ascaris lumbricoides	Intestinal obstruction
Enterobius vermicularis	Anal pruritus (pinworm)
Strongyloides stercoralis	Diarrhea, autoinfection (may be life-threatening in AIDS, lymphoma, or in the immunosuppressed)
Trichinella spiralis	Myositis (trichinosis)
Trematodes (flukes)	
Schistosoma mansoni	Hepatosplenomegaly
Schistosoma haematobium	Hematuria, hydronephrosis
Clonorchis sinensis	Biliary obstruction, cholangiocarcinoma
Cestodes (tapeworms)	
Echinococcus granulosus	Hepatic (hydatid) cysts
Taenia saginata	Abdominal cramps, bowel obstruction
Taenia solium	Seizure (neurocysticercosis)
Diphyllobothrium latum (fish tapeworm)	Megaloblastic anemia

■ Parasites

Table 144.6 lists the important **protozoal parasites** and their major clinical manifestations. Most of these protozoa are recognized on microscopic examination of appropriate clinical specimens; however, *Microsporidium* requires electron microscopy for detection.

The **helminths** (worms), a greater problem in the developing parts of the world and not common in the United States, are divided into three categories: the **nematodes** (round worms), **trematodes** (flukes), and **cestodes** (tapeworms) (Table 144.7). Helminths commonly pass eggs in the intestinal tract, and the characteristic morphology of eggs on stool microscopy is helpful diagnostically. Eosinophilia, an immune response that is a helpful diagnostic sign, may be seen with helminths having a tissue cycle.

CHAPTER 145   ANTIMICROBIAL THERAPY AND GENERAL PRINCIPLES OF ANTIBIOTIC USE

The past decade has witnessed the development of a plethora of antimicrobial agents. Although particularly applicable to antibiotics, this proliferation has also involved other antimicrobials, including antifungals, antimycobacterials, antivirals, and antiparasitic agents.

■ Antibiotics

Beta-lactam antibiotics

Beta-lactam antibiotics constitute a large group, comprising the penicillins, cephalosporins, monobactams, and carbapenems (Table 145.1). All these agents share the feature of the beta-lactam ring structure, and they inhibit bacterial growth through their action on cell wall synthesis (Table 145.2).

Penicillins

Despite the decline in the spectrum of activity of the natural penicillins (e.g., penicillin G) through decades of use, they are still the drug of choice for some streptococcal infections and are quite useful in other infections, including those by spirochetes and anaerobes. Through changes in various side chain structures, other types of penicillins have been developed with changed antimicrobial spectra, such as the penicillinase-resistant penicillins (e.g., methicillin or nafcillin, which have expanded coverage against *Staphylococcus aureus*) and the carboxypenicillins and ureidopenicillins (with broad-spectrum gram-negative activity). Another way to overcome bacterial resistance and expand the antimicrobial spectrum of penicillins is to use a **beta-lactamase inhibitor** together with a penicillin (e.g., amoxicillin-clavulanic acid, ampicillin-sulbactam).

The most common side effects of the penicillins are hypersensitivity reactions. Fortunately, IgE–mediated anaphylactic reactions, the most serious of these, are uncommon. The more common morbilliform rashes are felt to be IgM-mediated or IgG-mediated.

Cephalosporins

Cephalosporins have been commonly categorized into four generations (Table 145.1). **First-generation cephalosporins** are active primarily against gram-positive bacteria (*Staphylococcus aureus* and streptococci, but not enterococci). As a general rule, the later (more recent) generation cephalosporins cover gram-negative bacteria better, albeit at the loss of some of their gram-positive activity. Some of the **second-generation cephalosporins,** also called cefamycins (cefoxitin, cefotetan), also have enhanced activity against anaerobes.

TABLE 145.1.   Beta-lactam Antibiotics

Penicillins	
Natural penicillins	Penicillin G
Penicillinase-resistant penicillins	Methicillin, nafcillin
Aminopenicillins	Ampicillin, amoxicillin
Carboxypenicillins	Carbenicillin, ticarcillin
Ureidopenicillins	Mezlocillin, azlocillin, piperacillin
Beta-lactamase inhibitor combinations	Amoxicillin-clavulanic acid, ticarcillin-clavulanic acid, ampicillin-sulbactam
Cephalosporins	
First-generation	Cephalothin, cefazolin, cephalexin
Second-generation	Cefamandole, cefuroxime, cefaclor, Cefoxitin
Third-generation	Cefotaxime, ceftizoxime, ceftriaxone, ceftazidime
Fourth-generation	Cefpirome, cefepime
Other beta-lactams	
Monobactams	Aztreonam
Carbapenems	Imipenem

TABLE 145.2. Features of Commonly Used Antibiotics			
Class of Drug	Site of Action	Major Side Effects	Major Activity or Spectrum of Organisms
Beta-lactams	Cell wall	Hypersensitivity, GI, hematologic, hepatotoxicity	Gram-positive (gram-negative with extended-spectrum agents)
Vancomycin	Cell wall	Infusion-related hypersensitivity, nephrotoxicity	Gram-positive (especially methicillin-resistant *S. aureus*)
Aminoglycosides	Multiple ribosomal sites	Nephrotoxicity, ototoxicity	Gram-negative (synergistic for some gram-positive)
Macrolides (erythromycin)	50S ribosomes	GI, hepatotoxicity	Gram-positive, mycoplasma, chlamydia, legionella, campylobacter
Clindamycin	50S ribosomes	Hypersensitivity, GI	Gram-positive, anaerobes
Chloramphenicol	50S ribosomes	Hematologic	Broad spectrum rickettsia, salmonella
Tetracycline	30S ribosomes	Photosensitivity, GI	Mycoplasma, rickettsia, chlamydia, Lyme disease
Rifampin	RNA polymerase	GI, hepatotoxicity, hematologic	Gram-positive, neisseria, legionella
Trimethoprim-sulfamethoxazole	Nucleic acid synthesis	Hypersensitivity, hematologic, GI	Nocardia, listeria
Quinolones (ciprofloxacin)	DNA gyrase	GI, hypersensitivity	Gram-negative
Nitroimidazoles (metronidazole)	DNA damage	CNS, GI	Anaerobes

CNS = central nervous system; GI = gastrointestinal.

Ceftazidime, a **third-generation cephalosporin,** is particularly active against *Pseudomonas aeruginosa.*

Overall, these agents are well tolerated. Given the potential for cross-reactivity, patients with a history of an immediate hypersensitivity reaction to penicillin (or those with skin reactivity to minor penicillin determinants) should avoid cephalosporins.

Monobactams and carbapenems

Other beta-lactam antibiotics include the monobactams **(aztreonam)** and carbapenems **(imipenem).** While aztreonam is effective only against gram-negative organisms, imipenem covers gram-negatives and anaerobes. However, gram-positive bacteria. including *Corynebacterium bacillus (JK strain),* methicillin-resistant *Staphylococcus aureus,* and coagulase-negative staphylococci, should be considered as imipenem-resistant. Although imipenem is contraindicated in patients with a serious beta-lactam allergy, aztreonam is not. Seizures due to imipenem have been noted, especially in patients with underlying renal insufficiency or underlying CNS disease.

Vancomycin

Vancomycin, a glycopeptide antibiotic, is a cell-wall agent but acts at a different site from the beta-lactams. It has a narrow spectrum of activity, primarily against gram-positive bacteria. Susceptible organisms include streptococci, staphylococci (including methicillin-

resistant *S. aureus*), enterococci (usually), and *Corynebacterium* JK bacillus. Among the anaerobes, most clostridia are sensitive.

Vancomycin penetrates many tissues, but cerebrospinal fluid (CSF) levels are variable. Absorption after oral dosing is minimal. The most frequent adverse reaction is called the **"red man"** syndrome. It is due to histamine release from a rapid intravenous infusion and is reversible with slowing the infusion rate. The frequency of nephrotoxicity is low with vancomycin alone (5%) but increases (35%) with concomitant aminoglycoside use.

Aminoglycosides

Aminoglycosides, which contain an aminocyclitol ring linked to two or more amino sugar residues by glycosidic bonds, inhibit bacteria through their action on multiple ribosomal sites. Commonly used aminoglycosides include gentamicin, tobramycin, and amikacin. While their spectrum covers primarily gram-negative organisms, they (mostly gentamicin) also act in synergy with a penicillin against enterococci, streptococci, and staphylococci (e.g., for endocarditis therapy). When used in serious gram-negative infections, they are usually combined with a beta-lactam antibiotic.

The volume of distribution of aminoglycosides is similar to extracellular fluid (due to low serum protein binding). They penetrate poorly into the CSF and are excreted renally. Primary toxicities include nephrotoxicity and ototoxicity, which can be cochlear or vestibular.

Macrolides

Macrolides have macrocyclic ring structures and inhibit bacterial protein synthesis through 50S ribosomal binding. **Erythromycin** is the longest-standing macrolide, with clarithromycin and azithromycin being more recent additions. Erythromycin is active against gram-positive cocci (streptococci, *S. aureus*), certain gram-negative agents (e.g., *Neisseria gonorrhoeae, Campylobacter jejuni, Legionella pneumophila*), and others (e.g., Chlamydia and Mycoplasma). Newer macrolides have broader activity, particularly against *Haemophilus influenzae, Moraxella catarrhalis, Chlamydia trachomatis, Ureaplasma urealyticum* and some mycobacteria (e.g., *M. avium*).

Erythromycin toxicity commonly involves the gastrointestinal tract (vomiting, nausea, diarrhea) and hepatitis. These are less frequent with the newer agents.

Clindamycin

Clindamycin is a lincosamide, similar to lincomycin. Its mechanism of action is similar to that of the macrolides. The spectrum of clindamycin includes gram-positive aerobes (streptococci, *S. aureus*), gram-positive and gram-negative anaerobes, and certain other agents (e.g., *Pneumocystis carinii*). It attains high concentrations in many tissues, including neutrophils, but does not cross the blood-brain barrier. Elimination is primarily by biliary excretion, and therefore, the dose is usually unaffected by renal failure.

Toxicity includes hypersensitivity reactions, hepatotoxicity, and colitis. Although pseudomembranous (*Clostridium difficile*) colitis was originally associated with clindamycin, other antibiotics also cause this complication.

Chloramphenicol

Chloramphenicol is an older antibiotic that inhibits protein synthesis by binding to the 50S ribosome. Its spectrum of activity covers many aerobic gram-positive bacteria, some gram-negatives (e.g., Enterobacteriaceae), anaerobes, rickettsiae, chlamydiae, and spirochetes. It is lipophilic and gains access into most body fluids, including CSF and the brain.

Chloramphenicol is primarily indicated for severe rickettsial disease but may also be useful in severe salmonella or CNS infections in patients with serious penicillin allergy. Its hematologic toxicity relegates its use to these few indications. Bone marrow suppression is most commonly dose-dependent and reversible, but rarely it is idiosyncratic and irreversible.

Tetracyclines

Tetracyclines are classified into 3 groups, short-acting (tetracycline, chlortetracycline, oxytetracycline), intermediate (demeclocycline, methacycline), and long-acting (doxycycline, minocycline). They all inhibit protein synthesis through inhibition of the 30S ribosomal subunit.

The emergence of bacterial resistance has limited the use of tetracyclines to specified situations, which include spirochetal (drug of choice in early Lyme disease), rickettsial, Ehrlichia, and Chlamydia (genital) infections. Tetracyclines are considered alternate agents in atypical pneumonias (e.g., *Mycoplasma pneumoniae,* Chlamydia species, *Legionella pneumophila*) and are combined with other antibiotics for some less common infections (e.g., brucellosis, melioidosis, tularemia, and plague).

Tetracyclines accumulate in the skin and can cause phototoxicity; patients receiving them should therefore be warned to avoid direct sunlight. Because tetracyclines stain teeth, they should be avoided in pregnant women and children.

Rifampin

Rifampin, a rifamycin, inhibits DNA-dependent RNA polymerase. While its principal use has been against mycobacteria, rifampin's broader range of activity is not well emphasized. Among gram-positive organisms, rifampin is most active against staphylococci, regardless of coagulase status. Covered gram-negative bacteria include Neisseria, Haemophilus, and Legionella species. It is active against anaerobes (e.g., Clostridium species), Chlamydia, and some fungi.

Rifampin resistance develops rapidly, and therefore, it should never be used alone (except for short-term prophylaxis). Orange-red discoloration of the urine is the most common side effect. Others include gastrointestinal upset, hepatitis, interstitial nephritis, and bone marrow toxicity.

Trimethoprim-sulfamethoxazole

Trimethoprim-sulfamethoxazole (TMP-SMX) is a drug combination that acts at sequential steps in folinic acid synthesis. The fixed, 1:5 ratio of drugs in TMP-SMX gives maximum synergistic inhibition.

TMP-SMX covers numerous gram-positive and gram-negative organisms. Other susceptible organisms include *Nocardia asteroides, Chlamydia trachomatis, Listeria monocytogenes, Pneumocystis carinii,* and some mycobacteria. There are many clinical indications for TMP-SMX, including treatment of infections of the respiratory and urinary tracts, sinusitis, and gastrointestinal infections (salmonellosis and traveler's diarrhea), as well as treatment and prevention of *Pneumocystis carinii* pneumonia in immunosuppressed patients. They also appear to reduce the relapses in Wegener's granulomatosis. However, adverse reactions can be limiting and are particularly frequent in AIDS patients. Those most commonly seen include cutaneous, hematologic, and gastrointestinal reactions. Drug resistance to TMP-SMX is being encountered increasingly.

Quinolones

The quinolones have been available for more than 30 years, but over the past several years, many new agents have been introduced. They inhibit DNA gyrases that are needed to supercoil bacterial DNA during replication. With a wide volume of distribution, they attain high concentrations in neutrophils; however, CSF levels are only low to negligible. Excretion is by renal and/or hepatic mechanisms.

The new quinolones are particularly active against gram-negative bacteria. Evolving resistance and lack of reliability against gram-positives limited the early quinolones, such as ciprofloxacin. The newer fluoroquinolones, (e.g., trovafloxacin) have a better spectrum against these organisms, especially Streptococci and many anaerobes.

Quinolones are generally well tolerated. Toxicity includes cutaneous hypersensitivity, phototoxicity, gastrointestinal, and CNS reactions. Some quinolones (e.g.,

ciprofloxacin) prolong theophylline clearance. All quinolones are presently considered unsafe in pregnancy. Because of several instances of arthropathy among children treated with quinolones, their use in the pediatric age group is best avoided.

TABLE 145.3. Antimycobacterial Agents	
Antituberculosis Agents	**Drugs for Other Mycobacterial Diseases[a]**
Isoniazid	Macrolides
Rifampin	Quinolones
Pyrazinamide	Rifamycins (Rifabutin)
Ethambutol	Clofazimine
Streptomycin	Amikacin
Capreomycin	
Ethionamide	
Cycloserine	
Thiacetazone	
Quinolones	

[a]Primarily M. avium complex infections.

TABLE 145.4. Features of Commonly Used Antiviral Agents		
Agent/Class	**Major Side Effects/Toxicity**	**Major Activity**
Guanosine analogs (Inhibit DNA polymerase)		
Acyclovir	Crystallizes in renal tubules, GI	Herpes simplex, herpes zoster
Ganciclovir	Hematologic	CMV, herpes viruses
Foscarnet	Renal dysfunction	CMV, herpes viruses
Ribavirin	Bronchospasm	RSV
Valcyclovir	CNS, GI	Varicella-zoster
Famcyclovir	CNS, GI	Varicella-zoster
Reverse transcriptase inhibitors (nucleoside)		
Zidovudine (AZT)	Headache, hematologic, nausea/vomiting	HIV
Didanosine (ddI)	Dermatologic, GI, peripheral neuropathy	HIV
Zalcitabine (ddC)	Dermatologic, GI, peripheral neuropathy	HIV
Stavudine (d4T)	Hepatitis, peripheral neuropathy	HIV
Lemivudine (3TC)	Hematologic, GI	HIV
Reverse transcriptase inhibitors (non-nucleoside)		
Nevirapine	Dermatologic, GI	HIV
Delavirdine	Dermatologic, GI, CNS, hematologic	HIV
Protease Inhibitors		
Saquinavir	Nausea/vomiting, diarrhea, abdominal discomfort, rash, endocrine	HIV
Ritonavir	Nausea/vomiting, diarrhea, taste disturbance, paraesthesia, hypertriglyceridemia, drug interactions	HIV
Indinavir	Nephrolithiasis, asymptomatic hyperbilirubinemia	HIV
Nelfinavir	Diarrhea	HIV
Others (? inhibits viral uncoating/assembly)		
Amantadine	Confusion, hallucination	Influenza A

CMV = cytomegalovirus; CNS = central nervous system; GI = gastrointestinal; HIV = human immunodeficiency virus; RSV = respiratory syncytial virus.

Nitroimidazoles

Metronidazole, the most widely used nitroimidazole, undergoes intracellular reductive activation into reactive intermediates that interact with microbial DNA. The drug is widely distributed in tissues, including CSF, and is metabolized in the liver. It is primarily effective against anaerobes, especially Bacteroides species, and some parasites (e.g., *Entamoeba histolytica, Trichomonas vaginalis and Giardia lamblia*). Side effects are infrequent but seizures, cerebellar ataxia, and peripheral neuropathy are the most serious.

■ Antimycobacterial Agents

The most commonly prescribed agents against *Mycobacterium tuberculosis* are isoniazid, rifampin, pyrazinamide, and ethambutol (see chapter 218 and Table 145.3). **Isoniazid** (INH) is believed to act on the cell wall (mycolic acid) or nucleic acids. **Pyrazinamide** has an unknown mechanism of action. It enters the CSF well and is active intracellularly, where mycobacteria reside. **Ethambutol** inhibits nucleic acid synthesis. Significant CSF levels are reached only with inflamed meninges. It is excreted solely through the kidneys, a matter of importance in renal failure. Drug resistance is an important problem in the therapy of tuberculosis (see chapter 218).

The drugs used for **other mycobacterial diseases** are primarily the macrolides and quinolones, although many of the antituberculous agents are also useful (see chapter 219). **Rifabutin** is more active than rifampin against strains of *M. avium* complex. **Clofazimine** directly binds to DNA, inhibiting transcription. It is lipophilic and does not enter the CSF. Originally an antileprosy drug, its primary use now is in *M. avium* infections.

■ Antiviral Drugs

The features of commonly used antiviral agents are shown in Table 145.4. **Acyclovir** has a high affinity for

TABLE 145.5. Features of Commonly Used Antifungals			
	Site of Action	**Major Side Effects**	**Major Activity**
Amphotericin B	Binds ergosterol (disrupts fungal cytoplasmic membrane)	Azotemia, renal tubular acidosis, hypokalemia, hypomagnesemia	Serious or life-threatening fungal disease
Imidazoles:			
Ketoconazole	Interacts with C-14 alpha demethylase enzyme, affecting ergosterol synthesis. Absorption affected by gastric hypochlorhydria	GI, hepatotoxic depresses serum testosterone level and ACTH-stimulated cortisol level	Mucocutaneous candidiasis Non-meningeal blastomycosis Coccidioidomycosis Cryptococcosis Histoplasmosis
Miconazole	Same site of action as ketoconazole	Fever GI, hematologic	*Pseudallescheria boydii*
Triazoles			
Fluconazole	Same site of action as ketoconazole. Absorption less affected by gastric hypochlorhydria. Better CSF levels. Not metabolized. Renally excreted	GI, hepatotoxic	Oropharyngeal candidiasis Hepatosplenic candidiasis Cryptococcal meningitis (maintenance therapy)
Itraconazole	Same site of action as ketoconazole. Low CSF levels. Absorption needs gastric acidity	GI, hepatotoxic	Non-meningeal histoplasmosis Blastomycosis Coccidioidomycosis
Flucytosine	Cytosine analog (inhibits DNA and protein synthesis)	GI, hepatotoxic hematologic	Cryptococcal meningitis Invasive candidiasis (with Amphotericin B) Monotherapy for candiduria
Pentamidine isethionate	?Interferes with nuclear metabolism	Hypotension, renal insufficiency, hypoglycemia	*Pneumocystis carinii*

TABLE 145.6.	Features of Commonly Used Antiparasitic Drugs		
Drug	**Site of Action**	**Major Side Effects**	**Major Activity**
Metronidazole	?DNA damage	CNS, GI	Entamoeba histolytica, Giardia lamblia, Trichomonas vaginalis
Paromomycin (Humatin)	?Ribosomes	Possible renal toxicity if absorbed (with ulcerative bowel lesions)	Cryptosporidium, Entamoeba histolytica, Dientamoeba fragilis
Chloroquine phosphate	Asexual erythrocyte forms	GI CNS	Malaria
Mefloquine (Lariam)	Blocks invasion of sporozoites into red blood cells	Vomiting Dizziness	Drug-resistant malaria
Primaquine phosphate	Acts on hyphozoites in the liver	GI Headache Hemolytic anemia (in G6PD deficiency)	Malaria (Plasmodium vivax, Plasmodium ovale)
Mebendazole (Vermox)	Blocks glucose uptake by helminths	GI	Trichuriasis Ascariasis Enterobiasis
Thiabendazole (Mintezol)	Interferes with microtubule aggregation Inhibits fumarate reductase	GI Headache Dizziness	Strongyloidiasis Cutaneous and visceral larvae migrans
Praziquantel (Biltricide)	—	Dizziness Drowsiness	Schistosomiasis

herpesviruses and a low cellular toxicity. Epstein-Barr virus and cytomegalovirus (CMV) are affected somewhat (although minimally). **Foscarnet** inhibits DNA polymerase by a different mechanism and does not require activation, thus covering acyclovir-resistant, thymidine kinase mutants. Its advantage over **ganciclovir** is its lack of bone marrow toxicity; however, renal toxicity is observed with foscarnet.

Amantadine is useful both in preventing and treating influenza A infections. **Rimantadine** compares well in efficacy with amantadine but with fewer side effects. **Ribavirin,** a nucleoside analog, is used in aerosolized form.

Criteria for the appropriate use of the anti-HIV agents continues to evolve. Other anti-HIV agents are currently being developed and tested. (See chapter 158.)

Antifungal Agents

Features of commonly used antifungals are listed in Table 145.5. **Amphotericin B** is the drug of choice for serious, life-threatening, invasive fungal infections, such as those due to Aspergillus or Mucorales species (see chapter 213). **Fluconazole** is better absorbed in the presence of gastric hypochlorhydria (a common problem in AIDS patients) compared to **ketoconazole.** In cryptococcal meningitis in AIDS, fluconazole should be used instead of amphotericin B only in less severe disease.

Itraconazole is metabolized in the liver. Its bioavailability is improved when it is taken with food. Neither fluconazole or itraconazole adversely affects steroidogenesis. Toxicity of Amphotericin B is discussed in Chapter 213.

Antiparasitic Drugs

Commonly used antiparasitic drugs, including those used for protozoal and helminthic infections, are listed in Table 145.6. Most of these parasitic diseases are uncommon in the United States. However, protozoal infections (e.g., Cryptosporidium) are relatively frequent in AIDS patients.

Principles of Antimicrobial Use

Considering the management of a febrile patient as an example, it is easy to see that the treatment of infectious diseases often poses problems. Although many diverse conditions may cause fever, it is a common symptom of infection. Often, these infections are viral and lack any specific therapy. Even if the infection causing fever is bacterial, the organism and its sensitivity are unknown. Thus, antibiotics are often chosen empirically initially. Associated symptoms and signs may offer clues to the underlying process, and the setting of the infection (hospital vs community-acquired) may help.

The immunocompetence of the host adds another dimension. Because microbial resistance patterns vary, local patterns of antimicrobial susceptibility assume an important role.

An allergy or concomitant pregnancy may contraindicate an otherwise sound choice of an antibiotic. Although age, underlying disease (e.g., renal insufficiency), and concurrent medications may influence the selection, their implications for dosing and monitoring are profound. Infection in a patient who was previously on antibiotics might suggest resistance or a nonbacterial etiology. Cost may simply preclude certain agents, despite the better side effect profile and dosing interval than the cheaper agents. If home-based, outpatient parenteral therapy is chosen, the reliability and meticulousness of the patient become important considerations.

CHAPTER 146 · FEVER AND FEVER OF UNKNOWN ORIGIN

■ Body Temperature Homeostasis

Normal body temperatures

Body temperature, normally set around 37°C (98.6°F), varies greatly. The **hypothalamus,** as the thermoregulatory center, maintains the temperature of internal organs and great vessels (aortic blood) between 37°C and 38°C. Esophageal and tympanic membrane temperatures are closest to that of aortic blood, but rectal and liver temperatures are about 0.5°C higher, ostensibly due to the high metabolism at both sites (fecal bacterial metabolism in the rectum). Oral (from mouth breathing) and axillary temperatures are about 0.25°C and 1.0°C lower than core temperature, respectively. Skin temperature is even lower.

Body temperature is lowest in the early morning and highest in the late afternoon, with the amplitude of variation not usually exceeding 0.6°C (1°F). Individuals maintain body temperature at slightly above or below the so-called normal of 37°C (98.6°F). However, temperature exceeding 37.8°C (100.2°F) is considered abnormal.

Normal temperature homeostasis

The normal body temperature is a balance between heat production and heat loss. The major source of heat is internal, from the body's basal metabolism. Digestion of food and muscular activity add to this basal heat generation. Under normal circumstances, radiant external heat is not a major source of heat, except in some tropical or industrial settings (e.g., working near a furnace). Heat loss, the other half of the equation, occurs primarily from the skin into the environment by radiative losses.

In order to maintain the most efficient temperature balance, the circulatory system must be intact, and behavioral mechanisms and the autonomic nervous system must be functional. Behavioral mechanisms dictate how a person deals with ambient temperatures, both in terms of the clothing worn and the level of physical activity.

■ Fever and Hyperthermia

Mechanisms of fever and the body's response

Fever is a body temperature above that seen in normal diurnal variation and is sustained by abnormal thermoregulatory mechanisms. The evolution of a febrile response is illustrated in Figure 146.1. The primary initiating event is the release of endogenous **pyrogens** (e.g., interleukins 1 and 6, interferon, tumor necrosis factor), which cause fever and a number of other systemic changes collectively called **acute phase responses.** These involve alterations in leukocytes, liver protein synthesis, serum iron, hormone metabolism, and other phenomena. These changes and the behavioral and autonomic responses are outlined in Table 146.1.

Fever has some beneficial effects, such as enhanced stress response modulated by glucocorticoids; increased neutrophil counts, opsonins, and complement components; as well as enhanced T-lymphocyte activation and expansion of lymphocyte clones.

Hyperthermia

Whereas fever is a regulated response, **hyperthermia** is dysregulated and caused by a dysfunction of excessive heat production, decreased heat loss, malfunction of the thermoregulatory center, or a combination of these. Several causes of hyperthermia are listed in Table 146.2.

Management

Treatment of **fever** should focus more on the underlying cause and the effect(s) on the host rather than the temperature itself. For example, if a bacterial infection is the cause, the infection itself should be the focus of treatment. As antibiotics are given, the fever becomes the gauge of an appropriate response. Although fever may enhance the immunologic response, withholding antipyretics in viral respiratory infections has not yielded a clinical benefit.

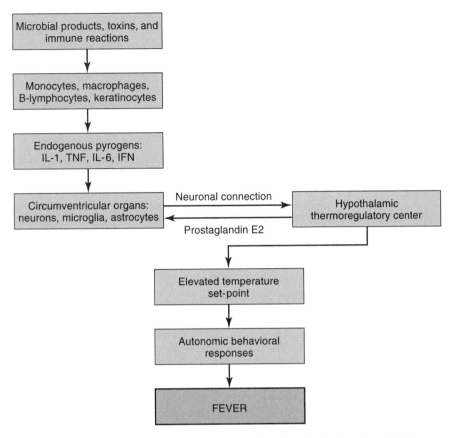

FIGURE 146.1. Pathogenesis of fever. Release of the endogenous pyrogens interleukin (IL), tumor necrosis factor (TNF), and interferon (IFN) is the primary initiating event, leading to the acute phase responses.

TABLE 146.1.	Systemic Aspects of Fever	
Behavioral Responses	**Acute Phase Responses**	**Autonomic**
Seek warmth	↑ WBC count	↓ Skin blood flow
Anorexia	Liver protein changes	↑ Pulse and blood pressure
Malaise	↓ Serum iron	
	Altered hormone metabolism (glucocorticoids, aldosterone, vasopressin, growth hormone)	↓ Sweating

TABLE 146.2.	Causes of Hyperthermia	
Excessive Heat Production	**Diminished Heat Loss**	**Hypothalamic Dysfunction**
Exertional hyperthermia	Heat stroke	Neuroleptic malignant syndrome
Status epilepticus	Neuroleptic malignant syndrome	Cerebrovascular accident
Thyrotoxicosis	Dehydration	Trauma
Pheochromocytoma	Autonomic dysfunction	Encephalitis
Malignant hyperthermia of anesthesia		
Neuroleptic malignant syndrome		

Fever enhances oxygen consumption, and thus, persons with underlying cardiac or pulmonary diseases suffer a high risk of decompensation. Fever in these individuals should therefore be treated. **Acetaminophen** and **aspirin** are equally effective in lowering the hypothalamic set point. Although usually not a consideration in adults, aspirin is contraindicated in children with influenza and varicella because of the concern about Reye's syndrome.

Hyperthermia, being an unregulated and abnormal response, generally requires treatment, especially in compromised individuals with temperatures above 39°C (102°F). The initiating event must, of course, be identified and reversed (e.g., discontinue exertion, initiate rehydration, etc.).

Fever of Unknown Origin

Whereas fever is a common manifestation of infection, sometimes the actual cause of the infection is difficult to identify. When this happens, the cause is often a transient viral illness. Occasionally, febrile states are more enduring and become difficult clinical problems. **Fever of unknown origin** (FUO) is defined as a prolonged febrile illness, lasting at least 3 weeks, with temperatures of at least 38.3°C (101°F) and no diagnosis after 1 week of evaluation in the hospital (or a similarly intensive outpatient work-up).

■ Etiology

In their classic 1961 article, Petersdorf and Beeson found that infections (36%), neoplastic disease (19%), and collagen-vascular diseases (13%) accounted for most cases of FUO. In a follow-up of this study, lasting from 1970–1980, infections accounted for 30%, neoplastic disease for 31%, and collagen-vascular diseases for 16% of cases. In these and other series, these three causes and miscellaneous entities account for 80%–90% of FUO. In 10% of cases, no diagnosis is made.

Causes of FUO are listed in Table 146.3. Although **infections** continue to cause a substantial proportion of FUO, the types of infections have changed over the years. For instance, because blood cultures are commonly obtained early in a fever work-up, bacterial endocarditis is currently a less common etiology of FUO than it was in the past.

Common infectious causes today include intra-abdominal (e.g., periappendiceal, hepatic, pericolic, perinephric, splenic) and pelvic abscesses. Dental or brain abscesses are less common. Tuberculosis is another common cause of FUO, particularly that involving extrapulmonary sites (e.g., renal, miliary, meningeal). Less common infectious causes include enteric fever, HIV infection, osteomyelitis, toxoplasmosis, endocarditis due to fastidious or nonculturable organisms, relapsing fever, leptospirosis, malaria, and others.

Despite innovations in imaging, **neoplastic disease**

TABLE 146.3. Causes of Fever of Unknown Origin

Common	Uncommon
Infections	**Collagen-vascular**
Pelvic abscess	**diseases**
Intra abdominal	Giant cell arteritis
abscesses	Periarteritis nodosa
Extrapulmonary	Adult Still's disease
tuberculosis	Systemic lupus
Miscellaneous	erythematosus
Drug fever	Rheumatoid arthritis
Alcoholic hepatitis	**Miscellaneous**
Cirrhosis	Familial Mediterranean
Neoplastic diseases	fever
Renal cell carcinoma	Hyperthyroidism
Lymphoma	Pheochromocytoma
Metastatic cancer	Subacute thyroiditis
of liver	Cyclic neutropenia
	Recurrent pulmonary
	embolism
	Factitious fever

remains a common cause of FUO. A number of primary or metastatic tumors cause fever, but some are more prone to do so than others. Occult lymphoma, particularly in the retroperitoneal area, may present with weight loss, anorexia, and fever, but usually without hepatosplenomegaly. Another common cause of FUO is renal cell carcinoma (hypernephroma), which may be difficult to localize and diagnose because hematuria may be absent. Metastatic cancer of the liver is more common than primary liver tumors, but both may cause FUO. Usually, these pose no diagnostic problems unless liver function abnormalities are absent. Other neoplasms causing FUO include leukemias, pancreatic carcinoma, atrial myxoma, and CNS tumors.

Because of improved diagnostic techniques, certain **collagen-vascular disorders** have become less common causes of FUO. For example, serologic testing has improved the detection of systemic lupus erythematosus (SLE) and rheumatoid arthritis (RA), reducing the likelihood of their presenting as an FUO. Both diseases, however, may still be rare causes of FUO. Many rheumatic and vasculitic diseases causing FUO lack specific diagnostic tests and thus require a diagnostic tissue biopsy. Examples include giant cell arteritis, periarteritis nodosa, and other vasculitides, such as Takayasu's arteritis.

Drug fever tops the list of **miscellaneous causes** of FUO. Drugs usually cause fever by acting as a foreign antigen, sensitizing T–cells, and leading to endogenous pyrogen release. Common offenders are antibiotics, particularly beta-lactams and sulfonamides, analgesics, diuretics, hypnotics, anticonvulsants, and antiarrhythmics. Intermittent eosinophilia and elevated liver enzymes may be associated. Some drugs (e.g., penicillin, isoniazid, salicylates, phenytoin, thiouracil, iodides, and methyldopa) are notable for causing fever without other clinical signs. Alcoholic and granulomatous hepatitis are liver diseases that cause FUO; these are confirmed by liver biopsy.

■ Evaluation

Almost by definition, an FUO is a diagnostic challenge, even to an astute clinician. Close attention must be paid to the **history.** Recent abdominal or pelvic surgery (abscess), exposure to tuberculosis, history of a heart murmur (consideration of endocarditis), or history of high-risk behavior (unsuspected HIV infection) are examples of historical clues that require further exploration. In addition to an examination of specific complaints, contacts, or exposures, the patient's medications should be checked. Drug fever may follow even years of use, so that the diagnosis is usually made by exclusion (i.e., withdrawing the drug and observing).

A detailed **physical examination** should follow, especially pursuing clues from the history. Of particular importance is the cardiac, abdominal, lymph node, and musculoskeletal examination. Useful findings are heart murmurs (endocarditis or atrial myxoma), hepatomegaly (some liver diseases require subsequent evaluation by liver biopsy), lymphadenopathy (infection or lymphoma), and spinal tenderness (vertebral osteomyelitis or epidural abscess).

Routine **laboratory studies,** such as a complete blood count, can give some clues. For instance, leukopenia might suggest lymphoma; eosinophilia may be consistent with lymphoma or drug fever; and a lymphocytosis might suggest infectious mononucleosis (especially if the peripheral smear shows atypical lymphocytes). Noninvasive **imaging tests** for FUO evaluation include ultrasound, computed tomography (CT), magnetic resonance imaging (MRI), and radionuclide scans. Abdominal or pelvic abscesses and retroperitoneal lymphoma are readily detected by CT or MRI.

In certain settings, **invasive tests** are required to make a specific diagnosis. Physical findings such as tenderness over the temporal arteries in the right clinical setting might suggest giant cell arteritis, but temporal artery biopsy is required for definitive diagnosis. In another setting, the finding of a liver mass on CT scan might indicate the need for a biopsy to direct definitive therapy.

CHAPTER **147** UPPER RESPIRATORY TRACT INFECTIONS

The Common Cold

The common cold is an extremely common, self-limited ailment, and caused by several viruses, including rhinoviruses, coronaviruses, parainfluenza viruses, respiratory syncytial virus, and adenoviruses. Of these, the rhinoviruses (with 100 immunotypes) are the most frequent etiologic agents.

A year-round disease, influenza is most frequent in the colder months of the year. Transmission, particularly with the rhinoviruses, is generally by close physical contact, and spread within families is common. Acquisition of new viral strains accounts for the frequency of repeat attacks (e.g., from the school or daycare setting into the family).

The incubation period of the common cold is generally 1–3 days. Usual symptoms are rhinorrhea (coryza), nasal stuffiness, sore throat, and cough. Adults are usually afebrile but a slight fever may be present (fever is more frequent in children). Nasal discharge and glassy nasal membranes are the cardinal signs. The diagnosis is usually based on these symptoms and signs, although some confusion with allergic or vasomotor rhinitis is possible. Pharyngeal erythema and exudate are not associated with rhinovirus or coronavirus infections, and these signs may implicate other respiratory viruses (e.g., adenoviruses) or streptococcal pharyngitis.

Colds due to rhinoviruses do not involve destruction of nasal mucosal membranes. Instead, many inflammatory mediators are released (e.g., bradykinin, prostaglandin, histamine, interleukin-1), and neurologic reflexes activated. Some of the other viruses may cause more destructive changes.

Pharyngitis

Pharyngitis is an inflammation of the posterior pharyngeal membranes and their draining lymphatics, including the lymphatics of Waldeyer's ring (adenoid, palatine, and lingual tonsils) and cervical lymph nodes. According to the extent of local inflammation, this condition is referred to by several terms, including **pharyngitis, tonsillitis,** or **pharyngotonsillitis.**

■ Etiology

The etiology of pharyngitis is diverse, and infectious causes are listed in Table 147.1. Most common in the colder months of the year, pharyngitis is caused by infected aerosols or direct contact with infectious materials.

The most frequent infectious causes are group A streptococci *(Streptococcus pyogenes),* various respiratory viruses (e.g., adenoviruses, influenzaviruses, rhinoviruses), and Epstein-Barr virus. Whereas rhinoviruses have little cytopathic effect (sore throat associated with them appears to be through stimulation of nerve ending by inflammatory mediators), other respiratory viruses (adenoviruses and coxsackie viruses) and *S. pyogenes* do show evidence of invasion. *S. pyogenes* also produces a number of toxins and proteases that may be important pathologically.

TABLE 147.1. Infectious Causes of Pharyngotonsillitis	
Bacteria	**Viruses**
Group A, B, C, and G	Rhinoviruses
streptococci	Influenzaviruses
Neisseria gonorrhoeae	Adenoviruses
Corynebacterium diph-	Enteroviruses
theriae	Epstein-Barr virus
Francisella tularensis	Herpes simplex virus
Mixed anaerobes	Human immunodeficiency
Chlamydia trachomatis	virus
Mycoplasma pneu-	**Fungi/Mycobacteria**
moniae	Candida species
	Mycobacterium tuberculosis

The common cold usually lasts about one week. Treatment is directed toward the control of symptoms, with decongestants, saline gargles, and cough suppressants being frequently used. Antibiotics should be avoided; however, because a small number of cases can lead to bacterial sinusitis or otitis media, the occurrence of either of these two entities following cold will require appropriate antibiotics.

■ Clinical Features

Throat discomfort, variably described as irritation, scratchiness, or pain is the cardinal symptom of pharyngitis. Pharyngeal mucosa and tonsils are usually hyperemic and edematous; there may or may not be a tonsillar exudate.

The major differential diagnosis of pharyngitis is between *S. pyogenes* and one of several other infectious causes (Table 147.2). In some of these illnesses (e.g., *S. pyogenes*), pharyngitis is the major pathologic process, whereas in others (e.g., influenza and Epstein-Barr viruses), the pharyngitis is merely part of a more systemic illness. It is usually difficult to make an etiologic diagnosis of pharyngitis on clinical grounds alone. However, S. *pyogenes* is especially important to identify because of the potential sequelae of rheumatic fever or glomerulonephritis.

■ Management

Because many of the viral causes of pharyngitis lack specific therapy, the primary diagnostic goal is to identify or exclude *S. pyogenes* through culture or a latex agglutination from a throat swab. The latex agglutination test will give results more quickly than culture; however, given its 5–30% false-negative rate, a negative latex agglutination result should be followed by a throat culture. Specific diagnostic tests for other treatable causes of pharyngitis (e.g., *Candida albicans,* herpes simplex virus) depend on the clinical setting.

Patients with a **group A streptococcal pharyngitis** should be given a 10-day course of oral penicillin or benzathine penicillin (1.2 MU IM). Penicillin-allergic patients may be given a macrolide. Depending on the circumstances, treatment may be given empirically while culture results are pending or may be started after the results are available; however, it should be instituted within one week of the onset of pharyngitis for effective prevention of rheumatic fever.

Treatment also prevents bacteremia and suppurative

TABLE 147.2.	Clinical Features of Major Causes of Pharyngitis	
Organism	**Major Associated Clinical Symptoms**	**Clinical Syndrome or Associated Diseases**
Group A streptococci (S. pyogenes)	Fever, tonsillar exudate, tender cervical nodes	May lead to rheumatic fever or glomerulonephritis
Rhinoviruses	Mild pharyngeal discomfort, rhinorrhea	Common cold
Influenzaviruses	Fever, myalgia, headache, cough	Influenza
Epstein-Barr virus	Fever, tonsillar exudate, tender cervical nodes, palatal petechiae, atypical lymphocytosis	Infectious mononucleosis
Coxsackie virus	Fever, soft palate vesicles	Herpangina
Adenoviruses	Fever, malaise, tonsillar exudate, conjunctivitis	Pharyngoconjunctival fever
Herpes simplex virus	Soft palate vesicles	Immunosuppression
Candida albicans	White plaque-like lesions	Predisposing factors include AIDS, corticosteroids, antibiotics
Mixed anaerobes and spirochetes	Membrane, tonsillar exudate, foul odor	Vincent's angina

complications, which include peritonsillar abscess and, rarely, septic thrombophlebitis of the internal jugular vein with metastatic infection (post-anginal sepsis). Suppurative complications feature prominent involvement by anaerobes.

In **recurrent tonsillitis,** poor compliance, microbial resistance, or reinfection are considerations. Amoxicillin-clavulanate, clindamycin, or metronidazole plus a macrolide may be tried.

Laryngitis

Acute laryngitis, or inflammation of the vocal cords and surrounding structures, is manifested by hoarseness. **Infections** account for a significant number of cases, but an extremely common, non-infectious disorder causing laryngitis is **gastroesophageal reflux disease.** Although all the common respiratory viruses cause hoarseness, those most frequently associated are rhinoviruses, influenzaviruses, and adenoviruses.

Acute laryngitis is diagnosed when **dysphonia** (hoarseness) occurs in the setting of a respiratory viral illness. Laryngeal examination, if performed, reveals hyperemia and edema of the vocal cords.

Treatment consists of resting the voice and inhalation of cool, moistened air. Antibiotics are generally not beneficial, except in specific circumstances (e.g., group A streptococcal or *Corynebacterium diphtheriae* infections). Usually, the disease is mild and self-limited. If symptoms persist longer than 10–14 days, laryngoscopy should be performed to rule out a tumor, granulomatous process, or other chronic laryngeal pathology.

Acute Bronchitis

■ Etiology and Pathology

Acute bronchitis is due to inflammation of the tracheobronchial tree and is typically due to a viral infection (Table 147.3). With the viruses, bronchitis may be part of the clinical spectrum of both upper (e.g., rhinovirus) and lower (e.g., influenza) respiratory tract infections.

The degree of damage to the tracheobronchial tree varies with the agent involved; while usually minimal with rhinovirus, it may be serious with influenzavirus.

TABLE 147.3.	Causes of Acute Bronchitis
Common	**Uncommon**
Influenzavirus	Mycoplasma pneumoniae
Adenovirus	Bordetella pertussis
Rhinovirus	Chlamydia psittaci
Coxsackie virus	Chlamydia pneumoniae
Respiratory syncytial virus	
Coronavirus	
Parainfluenza virus	

Hyperemia and excess bronchial secretions are generally present. Airway ciliary dysfunction and epithelial sloughing can occur in severe disease. Besides causing inflammation, some viruses (e.g., respiratory syncytial virus) may also enhance airway reactivity.

■ Clinical Features and Management

Acute bronchitis is most common during the winter months. It is characterized by **dry cough** initially, but may become productive of purulent secretions later in the illness. Other symptoms, depending on the causative agent, include rhinorrhea and sore throat. Severe disease may be associated with substernal burning with breathing or with coughing (tracheitis). Fever is unusual with mild disease but is common with illness due to some viruses (influenzavirus, adenovirus) and *Mycoplasma pneumoniae*. Chest examination may reveal rhonchi. Signs of consolidation indicate progression to pneumonia.

Most individuals with acute bronchitis probably do not seek medical care. In more severe cases with persistent cough, other causes of a persistent cough such as pneumonia, congestive heart failure, asthma and thromboembolic disease should be excluded. Cough may persist for several weeks, especially after respiratory syncytial virus or *M. pneumoniae* infection. Bacterial cultures of sputum are usually not helpful.

Treatment of acute bronchitis is generally symptomatic with over-the-counter cough remedies, although hospitalization may occasionally be needed in patients with underlying cardiac or respiratory disease. Antibiotics are not advocated routinely, as bronchitis is mostly a self-limited viral illness. However, some patients may benefit from them, particularly those with *M. pneumoniae* or *Bordetella pertussis*.

In patients with underlying chronic obstructive lung disease, acute bronchitis may exacerbate their lung disease. Clinical features and treatment of such **acute exacerbations of chronic bronchitis** are discussed in chapter 221.

CHAPTER **148** PNEUMONIAS

■ Pathogenesis and Pathology

Pneumonia is a common cause of morbidity and mortality among adults, particularly those with underlying diseases. It occurs by three possible routes: inhalation or aspiration of organisms, hematogenous spread, or contiguous spread of organisms.

Inhalation is by far the most common route. Whereas some inhaled organisms cause pneumonia because of their enhanced virulence (e.g., influenzavirus), others do so more easily following a breach in local host defenses. Aspiration pneumonia, an example of disrupted local defenses, is discussed in chapter 239. Hematogenous pneumonia most typically follows right-sided *Staphylococcus aureus* endocarditis and, less commonly, complicated oral infections. Contiguous spread to the lungs may rarely follow peritonsillar abscess (with ensuing suppurative jugular venous thrombosis and septic pulmonary emboli), complicated oral or pharyngeal infections, or even intra-abdominal infection with spread across the diaphragm.

Local mucosal defenses (chapter 141) play a pivotal protective role against respiratory infections. Microbes are abundant in the mouth, but several local pulmonary defense mechanisms usually keep the lungs sterile below the carina. Corruption or transgression of these defenses causes pneumonia (Table 148.1).

TABLE 148.1. Pulmonary Defense Mechanisms and Pneumonia	
Defense Mechanism	**Examples of Breakdown**
Trapping of particles in upper airway	Mechanical disruption (endotracheal intubation)
Mucociliary blanket	Hypoxia, cigarette smoke, viral infections, alcohol
Cough reflex and intact epiglottis	Drugs and alcohol, cerebrovascular accident, anesthesia, seizures
Phagocytic cells	Dysfunction (alcoholism), reduced numbers (neutropenia)
Humoral and cellular immunity	Hypogammaglobulinemia, multiple myeloma, AIDS

Turbulent airflow through the nasal and oral passages traps larger particles (>10 μm), and the tracheobronchial mucociliary blanket traps most smaller ones (2 or 3 μm), which are then cleared from the airway by ciliary action and coughing. The smallest particles that penetrate into the alveoli are normally tackled by phagocytosis and humoral and cellular immune mechanisms.

When one or more of these defenses breaks down or becomes overwhelmed by a large load of organisms, it sets the stage for pneumonia (Table 148.1). Such microbial invasion is met by release of inflammatory mediators (complement components and cytokines), which attract neutrophils for phagocytosis and killing of the invaders. Cell-mediated immune mechanisms play a

prime role in the defense against certain organisms (e.g., *Legionella,* mycobacteria, viruses, *Cryptococcus neoformans,* and *Pneumocystis carinii*).

Community-Acquired Pneumonia

■ Etiology

Community-acquired pneumonia (CAP) is a common clinical entity which often presents difficulties with diagnosis and treatment. Frequently encountered pathogens in the immunocompetent host are listed in Table 148.2. Nosocomial (hospital-acquired) pneumonia and pneumonia in the immunocompromised patient are discussed subsequently.

A specific etiologic diagnosis of CAP is identified in only one-half of cases. Some of these organisms (e.g., *Legionella pneumophila, Chlamydia pneumoniae*) are not easily isolated from sputum, which is an important reason that an etiologic diagnosis so often remains elusive. Other reasons contributing to the difficulty in isolating an etiology include the initiation of empiric antibiotics prior to culture, inability to raise an adequate sputum sample (especially in the obtunded or elderly patient), and the difficulty in isolating organisms such as pneumococci even with an adequate sputum sample (i.e., containing abundant neutrophils).

In the preantibiotic era, most pneumonias (>80%) were due to **Streptococcus pneumoniae.** While *S. pneumoniae* remains an important cause of CAP (20–60%), its relative role has declined in recent years, as newer pathogens have emerged.

■ Clinical Features

Given the many etiologic agents in CAP, clues from the **medical and environmental history** and host factors (e.g., underlying disease) may be helpful in suggesting the potential causative agent (Table 148.3). **Symptoms** of pneumonia include fever, chills, pleuritic chest pain, and cough, which may or may not be productive. However, pneumonia presentations are protean. Confusion, gastrointestinal symptoms and hepatic dysfunction, once felt to be peculiar for Legionella pneumonia, are no longer considered unique to it.

Traditional teaching has held that pneumonias could be separated based on their presentation into "typical" and "atypical" types. **"Typical"** pneumonias resembled the classical presentation of pneumococcal pneumonia—acute onset, high fever, rigors, pleuritic chest pain, and productive cough. **"Atypical"** pneumonias exhibited a more subacute onset, generally nonproductive cough, and less ill-appearing patient, as exemplified by pneumonias due to *Mycoplasma pneumoniae, Legionella pneumophila,* and *Chlamydia pneumoniae.* More recent analysis has shown that an etiology for pneumonia cannot be reliably determined from the clinical presentation alone.

The **physical examination** is more useful in evaluating the extent of illness than in assessing an etiology. In some cases, lobar consolidation or diffuse disease may be predicted from the physical findings (see Table 208.5), whereas in other cases (e.g., *M. pneumoniae*), the physical findings underestimate the radiographic extent of illness ("x-ray looks worse than the patient"). Other helpful physical findings may include extrathoracic inflammation (e.g., meningitis associated with pneumococcal pneumonia) or skin rashes which may be consistent with a viral etiology.

■ Diagnosis

Diagnostic evaluation beyond the history and physical examination includes a chest radiograph, analysis of pulmonary secretions (i.e., sputum), and other ancillary tests.

Roentgenographic assessment

The **chest radiograph,** the "gold standard" for diagnosing pneumonia, must be interpreted in light of clinical findings. Other inflammatory conditions (e.g.,

TABLE 148.2.	Causative Agents in Community-Acquired Pneumonia
Bacteria/bacteria-like organisms	**Viruses**
Streptococcus pneumoniae	Influenzavirus
Haemophilus influenzae	Adenovirus
Legionella pneumophila	Respiratory syncytial virus
Mycoplasma pneumoniae	**Fungi**
Chlamydia pneumoniae	Histoplasma capsulatum
Anaerobes (oral)	Coccidioides immitis
Moraxella catarrhalis	Blastomyces dermatitidis
Staphylococcus aureus	Cryptococcus neoformans
Aerobic gram-negative bacilli	
Chlamydia psittaci	
Mycobacterium tuberculosis	

TABLE 148.3. Environmental and Host Factors Suggesting a Microbial Etiology of Community-acquired Pneumonia

Clinical Feature	Potential Etiology
Environmental factors	
Residence in or travel to:	
Southwestern U.S.	Coccidiodes immitis
Mississippi, Ohio River valleys	Histoplasma capsulatum
	Blastomyces dermatitidis
Exposure to bat caves	Histoplasma capsulatum
Exposure to psittacine birds, turkeys	Chlamydia psittaci
Exposure to contaminated air-conditioning system	Legionella pneumophila
Prison, homeless shelter residence	Streptococcus pneumoniae
	Mycobacterium tuberculosis
Outbreak in winter season	Influenza virus
Cluster cases	Mycoplasma pneumoniae
	Influenza virus
Host factors	
Chronic obstructive lung disease	Streptococcus pneumoniae
	Haemophilus influenzae
	Moraxella catarrhalis
Diabetes mellitus	Streptococcus pneumoniae
	Staphylococcus aureus
Alcoholism	Streptococcus pneumoniae
	Staphylococcus aureus
	Klebsiella pneumoniae
	Oral anaerobes
Elderly age	Streptococcus pneumoniae
	Influenzavirus
Young, healthy adult	Mycoplasma pneumoniae
	Streptococcus pneumoniae
	Chlamydia

connective tissue disorders), pulmonary edema and blood, and malignancy are often indistinguishable radiographically from pneumonia.

Common radiographic patterns in pneumonias by different etiologic agents are shown in Table 148.4. **Lobar consolidation** is classically due to bacterial pathogens such as *S. pneumoniae*, while **interstitial infiltrates** are due to viruses, *M. pneumoniae*, or *Pneumocystis carinii*. *P. carinii*, usually seen in profoundly immunosuppressed hosts, may present initially with interstitial infiltrates and without a prior diagnosis of HIV disease, thus generating diagnostic confusion with pneumonias due to other pathogens. **Cavitation** features prominently, but not invariably, in anaerobic gram-negative or tuberculous causes of pneumonia.

Evaluation for **pleural fluid** is also important. Pneumonias usually associated with interstitial infiltrates (e.g., viruses, *M. pneumoniae*) rarely have significant pleural fluid. However, nearly 50% of patients with pneumococcal pneumonia show pleural effusions (frank empyema in only 1–5%).

TABLE 148.4. Community-Acquired Pneumonia: Chest X-ray Patterns

Lobar consolidation	**Interstitial**
Streptococcus pneumoniae	Viruses
Haemophilus influenzae	Pneumocystis carinii
Moraxella catarrhalis	Mycoplasma pneumoniae
Mycoplasma pneumoniae	Chlamydia psittaci
Legionella pneumophila	**Cavitation**
Chlamydia pneumoniae	Mixed aerobes/anaerobes
Multifocal opacities	Aerobic gram-negative
Streptococcus pneumoniae	bacilli
Legionella pneumophila	Mycobacterium
Staphylococcus aureus	tuberculosis

Examination of expectorated sputum

Pulmonary secretions can usually be analyzed non-invasively by examining expectorated sputum (see chapter 209). Sputum Gram stain and culture pose many problems, despite their traditional role in the diagnosis of pneumonia. Patients may produce a poor sputum sample or none at all. Cultures take time and are therefore not helpful initially. Although *S. pneumoniae* and *Haemophilus influenzae* can be pathogens, their presence on culture may reflect only oropharyngeal colonization.

Sputum Gram stains are most predictive when one adheres to strict criteria of acceptability. Only samples with over 25 neutrophils and less than 10 epithelial cells per low-power field are acceptable for analysis. On such samples, the finding of over 10 gram-positive, lancet-shaped diplococci is highly predictive of identifying pneumococci on culture (Figure 148.1). On the other hand, finding none or a few mixed organisms may suggest that organisms not easily identified on the Gram stain should be considered (e.g., *M. pneumoniae, L. pneumophila, Mycobacterium tuberculosis*).

Although the routine use of **sputum cultures** in the initial management of CAP has been questioned, cultures are helpful in certain situations. For example, cultures are necessary if antibiotic sensitivity needs to be determined or if unusual organisms (e.g., *L. pneumophila, Cryptococcus neoformans,* or *M. tuberculosis*) are suspected.

When sputum is not obtainable by expectoration or after induction, respiratory secretions may be obtained by invasive methods, such as **bronchoalveolar lavage** (BAL, see chapter 212). BAL, which has not been fully evaluated in CAP, is an expensive method and may be potentially compromised by contamination with oral flora. Samples obtained through a double-catheter brush system can be cultured quantitatively. Many consider bacterial growth exceeding 10^3 organisms/ml to be significant. Quantitative cultures, however, are expensive and not provided by all laboratories.

TABLE 148.5.	Antibiotic Treatment of Community-acquired Pneumonia
Suspected Pathogen	**Preferred Antibiotic(s)**
Streptococcus pneumoniae	Penicillin, cefuroxime, macrolide
Haemophilus influenza	Amoxicillin, TMP/SMX, macrolide (not erythromycin), cefuroxime
Mycoplasma pneumoniae	Macrolide, tetracycline
Legionella pneumophila	Macrolide, TMP/SMX, ciprofloxacin
Mixed anaerobes	Clindamycin, penicillin
Staphylococcus aureus	Nafcillin, cefazolin
Aerobic gram-negative bacilli	Second- or third-generation cephalosporin

TMP/SMX = trimethoprim-sulfamethoxazole.

Other studies

Other potentially helpful diagnostic tests include a variety of blood tests, such as a complete blood count, blood chemistries, blood cultures, cold agglutinins, and antibody titers. Tests for Legionella involve a direct fluorescent antibody assay, which can be done on sputum, pleural fluid, or other pulmonary secretions, and an antigen assay performed on urine.

Currently, none of these tests is recommended in the initial management of patients with CAP, except the complete blood count, electrolyte determinations, and renal function tests, which can help assess the prognosis and determine the need for hospitalization. However, hospitalized patients with pneumonia should routinely have blood cultures (2 sets) performed, as well as assessment of arterial oxygen saturation.

■ Management

Only occasionally do all the pieces of the diagnostic puzzle fit together easily to yield an etiology of CAP, and thus therapy is necessarily empiric most of the time (Table 148.5). In most ordinary cases of CAP, a specific etiologic diagnosis, while worthwhile, is not crucial. A few agents—*Streptococcus pneumoniae, Haemophilus influenzae, Mycoplasma pneumoniae, Chlamydia pneumoniae, Legionella pneumophila,* or viruses—cause most cases.

For **empiric outpatient therapy,** a macrolide or beta-lactam agent (e.g., cefuroxime or amoxicillin/clavulanate) would be appropriate. Erythromycin covers *S. pneumoniae, M. pneumoniae,* and *L. pneumophila* but not *H. influenzae.* It often causes gastrointestinal side effects. The newer macrolides, clarithromycin and

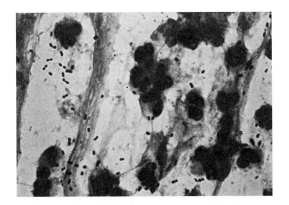

FIGURE 148.1. Sputum Gram stain in pneumococcal pneumonia showing leukocytes and gram-positive diplococci.

azithromycin, albeit more expensive than erythromycin, can cover all four agents with fewer side effects. Penicillin is still an effective, inexpensive agent for pneumococcal pneumonia when resistance is not present. For strains that show an intermediate level of resistance, high-dose penicillin or cefotaxime or ceftriaxone are appropriate; highly resistant strains mandate vancomycin.

The initial evaluation also entails determining the **need for hospitalization.** Mild pneumonias in patients without major debilitating conditions can be treated in the outpatient setting with oral antibiotics. If expectoration is problematic or IV therapy is necessary to cover more pathogens, hospitalization may be needed. Similarly, a significant abnormality in vital signs (hyperthermia,

tachycardia, hypotension, extreme tachypnea), changes in mentation, respiratory failure, inability to take medications at home, or other risk factors for complications are indications for hospitalization.

For **inpatient therapy,** if the possible causes include *S. pneumoniae, H. influenzae, L. pneumophila,* and even aerobic gram-negative bacilli, often a second-generation or third-generation cephalosporin and a macrolide may suffice. Complicated pleural effusions (chapter 243) require chest tube drainage. Antibiotics can be given orally after fever is resolved and clinical response is evident; they should be continued for a total of 7–10 days. *Legionella* pneumonia, however, requires 21 days of therapy.

Nosocomial Pneumonia

Nosocomial pneumonia is defined as pneumonia developing after a patient has been hospitalized, usually for an unrelated condition. It is a frequent problem, accounting for up to 15% of hospital-acquired infections, and ranks second only to nosocomial urinary tract infections. The most common microbial causes are listed in Table 148.6.

■ Pathogenesis and Predisposing Factors

Pneumonia develops in the hospital setting due to either aspiration of oropharyngeal flora or bacteremia. Aspiration is the most frequent mechanism. Within 2 days after hospitalization, oropharyngeal colonization occurs with a high frequency, with organisms such as *Pseudomonas aeruginosa* and enteric, gram-negative, aerobic bacilli. Daily monitoring of cultures from various sites has shown that the enteric gram-negative organisms are primarily derived from the patient's own flora,

whereas *P. aeruginosa* appears to be from an environmental source. Predisposing factors for nosocomial pneumonia are listed in Table 148.7.

■ Diagnosis

Fever, productive cough, elevated WBC count, hypoxemia, and a new infiltrate in chest radiographs of a hospitalized patient strongly suggest nosocomial pneumonia. However, the diagnosis is not always straightforward. Fever and cough may not always be present, or alternatively, fever and a high WBC count may be explainable by other entities, such as possible catheter-associated infections and antibiotic-associated colitis.

Pulmonary infiltrates in hospitalized persons are not specific for pneumonia, as other disease states also may cause a chest infiltrate and hypoxemia (e.g., a mucus plug with atelectasis, aspirated tube feeding, pulmonary embolus, congestive heart failure, pleural effusion, tumor, hemorrhage).

■ Management and Prevention

Treatment of nosocomial pneumonia is usually empiric, but special attention should be paid to underlying host factors that may predispose to specific pathogens, prior antibiotic use, and pathogens unique to specific institutions or units.

Traditionally, broad-spectrum antibiotic combinations (e.g., an antipseudomonal penicillin or cephalosporin, combined with an aminoglycoside) are utilized to cover the common gram-negative pathogens. Single agents, especially those with antipseudomonal activity (e.g., aztreonam, quinolones, and antipseudomonal penicillins or cephalosporins) have demonstrated comparable efficacy. Combination therapy should be used, however,

TABLE 148.6.	Common Causative Microbes in Nosocomial Pneumonia
Agent	**Approximate Frequency (%)**
Pseudomonas aeruginosa	17
Staphylococcus aureus	15
Klebsiella spp.	7
Escherichia coli	6
Haemophilus influenzae	6
Serratia marcescens	5
Proteus mirabilis	
Enterobacter spp.	
Acinetobacter spp.	
Legionella pneumophila	
Streptococcus pneumoniae	<3

TABLE 148.7.	Predisposing Factors Associated with Nosocomial Pneumonia
Predisposing Factor	**Comment**
Intubation, mechanical ventilation	Disruption of cough mechanism; damage to respiratory epithelium, equipment colonized by bacteria
Respiratory (aerosol-generating) equipment	Equipment colonized by bacteria; frequent handling of tubes
Advanced age	Poor cough, impaired local defenses
Underlying disease	Debilitation, increased aspiration risk
Prior antibiotics	Selection
Recent surgery	Aspiration
Antacids, H_2 blockers	Increased stomach colonization and subsequent aspiration
Poor infection control precautions (e.g., hand-washing)	Enhanced risk of transmission of gram-negative organisms from patient to patient within the same units

in certain circumstances, such as in neutropenic patients, in the presence of bacteremia, and with organisms at high risk for developing resistance.

Nosocomial pneumonia caused by some pathogens may be adequately treated with 10–14 days of therapy, but those due to gram-negative organisms (especially when associated with a necrotizing pneumonia) should be treated for 21 days. Pleural effusions meeting criteria for drainage should be drained as well.

Because nosocomial pneumonia often develops in the setting of prior gram-negative enteric colonization, the use of **prophylactic antibiotics** has received attention. Whereas antibiotic prophylaxis can decrease colonization of the oropharynx by gram-negative bacilli, it can also enhance selection of resistant organisms. Therefore, this approach does not merit widespread application. Other preventive measures include proper hand-washing, isolation, decreased manipulation of respiratory equipment, and preferential use of sucralfate for peptic ulcer prophylaxis.

Pneumonia in the Immunocompromised Host

Analysis of pneumonia that develops in the immunocompromised host must be accomplished with an awareness of the likely unique pathogens responsible for pneumonia in specific immune defects. Infections in immunocompromised hosts in general, and those in AIDS in particular, are discussed in detail in chapters 157 and 158. Common causes of pneumonia as associated with specific defects in systemic immune defenses are outlined in Table 148.8.

Pneumonias in these patients may be acquired either

TABLE 148.8.	Pneumonia in the Immunocompromised Host		
Immune Defect (Clinical Examples)		**Common Microbes Causing Pneumonia**	**Usual Chest Radiographic Patterns**
Neutropenia			
Cancer chemotherapy		Gram-negative bacilli	No infiltrate/lobar
		Staphylococcus aureus	No infiltrate/lobar
		Aspergillus spp.	Cavitary/diffuse
γ-Globulin deficiency/dysfunction			
Multiple myeloma		*Streptococcus pneumoniae*	Lobar
AIDS		*Haemophilus influenzae*	
Common variable hypogammaglobulinemia			
Lymphoma			
Cell-mediated deficiency			
AIDS		*Pneumocystis carinii*	Diffuse
Transplant		*Cryptococcus neoformans*	Nodular/cavitary/diffuse
Corticosteroid therapy		*Aspergillus* spp.	Nodular/cavitary/diffuse
		Mycobacterium spp.	Diffuse
		Legionella spp.	Lobar/diffuse
		Herpes viruses	Diffuse

at home or in the hospital, and the clinician must be aware of the possibility of one of these immune defects when taking the patient's history. One must recognize that these patients are also prone to noninfectious causes of pulmonary infiltrates, such as pulmonary emboli, radiation pneumonitis, pulmonary hemorrhage, nonspecific interstitial pneumonitis, or drug reactions (e.g., bleomycin, methotrexate). Overall, immunocompromised patients need careful attention in this often difficult diagnostic and therapeutic entity.

CHAPTER 149 URINARY TRACT INFECTIONS

■ Definitions

Infections of the urinary tract are described by many terms (Table 149.1). Patients with **bacteriuria** may be asymptomatic or symptomatic. Individuals with symptomatic bacteriuria may be divided into those with infection in the lower (**cystitis**) or upper urinary tract (**pyelonephritis**). Some patients with lower urinary tract symptoms have less than 10^5 bacteria/ml of urine, a symptom complex called the **acute urethral syndrome,** which includes early cystitis as well as other possibilities, such as nongonococcal urethritis.

Urinary tract infections (UTIs) may be **complicated** or **uncomplicated,** depending on whether or not the infection is accompanied by structural urinary tract abnormalities (e.g., congenital duplication of the collection system, vesicoureteral reflux, prostatic hypertrophy, tumors, calculi, and urinary catheterization).

Finally, UTIs may be sporadic (or infrequent) or **recurrent** events. Recurrent UTIs are further divided into relapsing infections or reinfections. **Relapsing** infections arise from a persistent focus of infection that is not eradicated, whereas **reinfections** are new infections that follow eradication of the previous episode.

■ Etiology

Differentiating uncomplicated from complicated UTIs not only helps identify urinary tract abnormalities but also helps determine the microbial etiology. Most uncomplicated episodes of either cystitis or pyelonephritis (>80%) are due to certain strains of *Escherichia coli.* Approximately 10% of cases of uncomplicated cystitis (but not pyelonephritis) result from a coagulase-negative staphylococci, *S. saprophyticus.*

Complicated UTIs, on the contrary, arise from a wider range of organisms (Table 149.2). Most are gram-negative, but gram-positive organisms and fungi are also frequent.

■ Pathogenesis and Predisposing Factors

Cystitis usually occurs by ascent of pathogenic microorganisms from the urethra to the bladder. Whereas pyelonephritis can result from further ascent of these microbes, hematogenous spread may also be causative. As mentioned, acute, uncomplicated cystitis is usually caused by a few uropathogenic *E. coli* strains, which normally colonize the bowel. The proximity of the female genitourinary tract to the anus predisposes to the **colonization** of the vagina and the urethral meatus. Following such colonization, the shorter female urethra permits an easier ascent of organisms to the bladder, a process that is facilitated by sexual activity.

A prerequisite of colonization is attachment of organisms to mucosal epithelial cells. In women with recurrent UTIs, it has been shown that bacteria increasingly bind to uroepithelial cells. Genetic susceptibility (nonsecretors of blood group antigens), hormonal factors (estrogen), and other factors (spermicide use) may all increase the attachment process and subsequent susceptibility to infection.

Protective mechanisms against UTI include the normal systemic host defenses (see Table 141.4) but also local factors, including the act of micturition, high osmolality and urea content of urine, and possibly prostatic secretions in men. As sufficient bacteria over-

TABLE 149.1.	Urinary Tract Infections: A Glossary of Terms
Bacteriuria	– Bacteria in the urine (usually ≥10^5 bacteria/ml)
Cystitis	– Infection of the lower urinary tract
Pyelonephritis	– Infection of the upper urinary tract
Acute urethral syndrome	– Symptoms of UTI with <10^5 bacteria/ml
Complicated UTI	– UTI in the presence of a structural abnormality
Recurrent UTI	– Repeated UTI which may be either a relapse or reinfection

come these barriers, an inflammatory response, primarily neutrophilic, develops. Infection of the bladder tends to be localized to the mucosa, without a prominent antibody response, whereas tissue invasion and a systemic antibody response characterize pyelonephritis.

■ Epidemiology

The prevalence of UTI by age groups in women and men is shown in Table 149.3. Except during infancy, women have a life-long higher incidence of UTIs, which peaks between ages 16–35 due to sexual activity and diaphragm use. The increased incidence in older men is primarily due to prostatic hypertrophy; incontinence and long-term urinary catheterization are other factors.

■ Clinical Features

The common "classic" symptoms of acute cystitis and pyelonephritis, as seen in young women, are shown in Table 149.4. Persons at the extremes of life, including catheterized patients, may have either nonspecific symptoms or no symptoms at all except fever. Whereas suprapubic tenderness and gross hematuria are seen in

only 10% and 30% of cystitis cases, respectively, they are fairly specific findings for cystitis. As many as one-third of patients with only symptoms of cystitis have unrecognized pyelonephritis.

Of the symptoms listed, fever and flank pain are the most specific for pyelonephritis; dysuria, frequency, and urgency may or may not be present. Clinical manifestations vary widely, with an illness ranging from mild nausea, dysuria, fever, and flank pain to fever and septic shock. Presentation with septic shock, however, tends to occur in the elderly or those with underlying disease. Patients may report low back pain or abdominal pain as opposed to flank pain.

■ Diagnosis

When UTI is clinically suspected, a urine sample should be obtained for confirmation. A **clean, midstream voided sample** is preferred in most patients, although urine can be obtained by suprapubic puncture or from a urethral catheter in those who are already catheterized. Inflammatory cells (**pyuria**) and erythrocytes (**hematuria**) in a "clean catch" urine sample support the diagnosis of a UTI.

Although **pyuria** is universally present in clinically significant UTI, it also occurs in other conditions, such as gonococcal urethritis, reducing its specificity. The presence or number of leukocytes does not differentiate a lower from an upper UTI, but the presence of leukocyte casts is consistent with pyelonephritis. Some laboratories screen urine with a leukocyte esterase dipstick method, which is somewhat less sensitive than a microscopic examination for pyuria.

Erythrocytes (**hematuria**) are not as commonly seen as WBCs. Their presence may suggest additional diagnostic possibilities, such as urinary stones or tumor, and excludes urethritis, which is not normally associated with hematuria.

Finally, an uncentrifuged urine should be **Gram-**

TABLE 149.2.	Common Microbes Causing Uncomplicated and Complicated Urinary Tract Infections
Uncomplicated	**Complicated**
Escherichia coli	Escherichia coli
Staphylococcus saprophyticus	Klebsiella spp.
	Enterobacter spp.
	Proteus spp.
	Pseudomonas spp.
	Enterococcus spp.
	Staphylococcus epidermidis
	Yeast (Candida spp.)

TABLE 149.3.	Epidemiology of UTI by Age		
	Prevalence (%)		
Age Group (yrs)	**Women**	**Men**	**Risk Factors**
<1	1	1	Anatomic or functional anomalies
1–5	4–5	0.5	Congenital anomalies, uncircumcised penis (M)
6–15	4–5	0.5	Vesicoureteral reflux (W)
16–35	20	0.5	Sexual intercourse, diaphragm use (W), homosexuality (M)
36–65	35	20	Gynecologic surgery (W), prostatic hypertrophy (M), catheterization
>65	40	35	Catheterization, incontinence

M = men; W = women.
(Adapted from: Stamm WE. In Gorbach SL, Bartlett JG, Blacklow NR (eds.). Infectious Diseases. Philadelphia: WB Saunders Co, 1992, pp. 788–798. Used with permission.)

TABLE 149.4.	Differentiating Clinical Features of Cystitis and Pyelonephritis
Cystitis	**Pyelonephritis**
Dysuria	Dysuria and frequency
Urinary frequency	Fever
Urgency	Flank pain
Suprapubic tenderness (10%)	Nausea and vomiting
Gross hematuria (30%)	Malaise

stained and examined for bacteria. The observation of *any* bacteria is consistent with a significant colony count of bacteria, but also the Gram stain findings may help guide therapy.

In patients treated as outpatients with suspected, uncomplicated, acute cystitis, a **urine culture** may not be practical or cost-effective, since the typical treatment covers the usual narrow spectrum of organisms. Any patient with suspected pyelonephritis or a complicated UTI, or any patient sick enough to require hospitalization for suspected UTI, needs to have a urine culture. To be significant, a urine culture must (classically) show $\geq 10^5$ colony-forming units (CFU) of an organism per milliliter of urine. However, more recently, it has been recognized that even $>10^2$ CFU/ml may be significant in acutely symptomatic patients.

■ Management

Successful management of a UTI is based on a clinical estimation of the site of infection, coupled with knowledge of likely pathogens and pharmacokinetics of antibiotics in the urine.

Cystitis

Because cystitis is a superficial bladder mucosal infection, choosing an antibiotic that attains good urinary concentrations against the usual pathogens is critical. A 3-day course of therapy with a variety of agents (Table 149.5) has been shown to attain a cure rate similar to that for more prolonged therapy (7–10 days). Prolonged therapy should be given to those with symptoms lasting for 7 days or more, diabetes, immunosuppression, pregnancy, or an anatomic urinary tract abnormality.

Patients with **recurrent cystitis** are divided into those with a relapsing infection (usually due to an occult

renal source) and those with reinfection. Relapsing infections are caused by the same organism as the primary infection and usually appear within 2 weeks of the primary episode, whereas reinfections usually occur after that time and are caused by a different species or strain. Management of recurrent cystitis is outlined in Figure 149.1.

Pyelonephritis

Initial management of patients with pyelonephritis is based on the need for hospitalization and parenteral therapy. Some patients, particularly younger women with only a moderate illness, can be given outpatient oral therapy. All others should be given parenteral agents.

Because patients with pyelonephritis, especially those with complicated infections, have a wider range of pathogens, initial therapy should anticipate this possibility (Table 149.5). Also, because gram-negative rods and enterococci are possibilities, the urine Gram stain can also help guide initial therapy. Further modifications can follow once the antibiotic sensitivity pattern is known. With clinical improvement and abatement of fever, one can substitute and continue a suitable oral agent for a total of 14 days.

If no improvement occurs within 48–72h on appropriate therapy, a urinary tract abnormality should be suspected. An urinary ultrasound or computed tomographic scan should be done, and possibly, a consultation with a urologist.

TABLE 149.5.	Suggested Antibiotic Regimens for Urinary Tract Infections
Cystitis	**Pyelonephritis**
Trimethoprim-sulfamethoxazole*	Trimethoprim-sulfamethoxazole*
Trimethoprim*	Third-generation cephalosporin†
Quinolone§	Quinolone§
Amoxicillin or amoxicillin-clavulanic acid†	Aminoglycoside§ plus anti-pseudomonal penicillin†
Cephalexin†	

Fetal risk: Although all drugs carry some fetal risk, the following comments apply to use of these agents in pregnancy: * = use with caution in early pregnancy; ** = avoid in late pregnancy; § = unsafe; † = appears safe.

Catheter-associated Urinary Tract Infections

In evaluating patients with urinary catheters, one must realize that bacteriuria is common and that most catheter-associated UTIs are asymptomatic. Catheterized patients with **asymptomatic bacteriuria** do not require therapy. Treatment does not reduce the chance of future infection and, in fact, may predispose to colonization with more

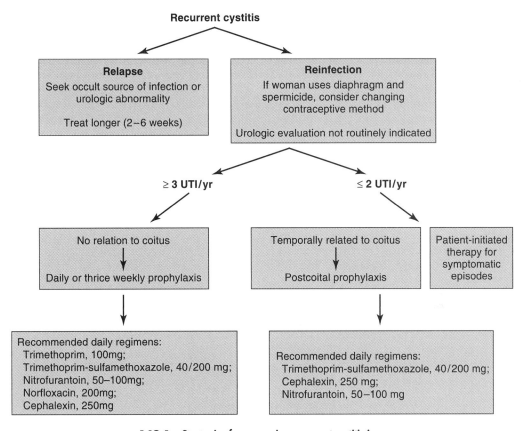

FIGURE 149.1. Strategies for managing recurrent cystitis in women.
(From: Stamm WE, Hooton TM. N Engl J Med 1993;329:1328–1334. Used with permission.)

resistant bacteria. Therefore, only symptomatic patients should be treated.

Symptoms may include fever or flank pain or patients may present more acutely with sepsis or septic shock. **Treatment** should include removal or replacement of the catheter, initiation of parenteral antibiotics, and fluid and/or pressor support as appropriate. Antibiotic selec-tion is similar to that for complicated pyelonephritis (Table 149.5), with special attention to the institutional nosocomial flora.

Reducing the risk for catheter-associated infections includes substitution of condom catheters, intermittent straight catheterization, and, if possible, removal of indwelling catheters.

Asymptomatic Bacteriuria

As described in Table 149.1, asymptomatic bacteriuria is defined as 10^5 or more bacteria per ml of urine in a patient who has no urinary symptoms. Asymptomatic bacteriuria is a common finding in certain populations, particularly catheterized patients as described above. It is also fairly common in the elderly without catheters. In general, asymptomatic bacteriuria should not be treated in adults with or without catheters. Those populations where asymptomatic bacteriuria should be treated, however, include children, pregnant women and, possibly, certain high-risk immunosuppressed patients (e.g., neutropenic or renal transplant patients).

Prostatitis

Inflammation of the prostate gland occurs in a manner similar to cystitis, with the usual mechanism being ascent of pathogens via the urethral ducts into the proximal posterior urethra. Common pathogens are similar to those listed above for UTIs, with enteric gram-negative organisms (usually *Escherichia coli*) and enterococcal species predominating.

The usual types or classifications of prostatitis include **acute bacterial prostatitis, chronic bacterial prostatitis,** and **nonbacterial prostatitis.** The symptoms of acute bacterial prostatitis include dysuria, acute urinary retention, perineal and low back pain, and sudden fever and chills. The prostate is swollen and tender on examination.

Given the similar array of pathogens, therapy for prostatitis is the same as that for other UTIs, except that prolonged therapy is needed (usually 30 days). Nonbacterial prostatitis is a relatively common inflammatory disorder of the prostate with an undefined etiology. Although the role of chlamydiae or mycoplasmas is not well-supported, a 2-week trial with erythromycin or a tetracycline may be utilized in these patients.

Epididymitis

Epididymitis occurs by ascent of pathogenic bacteria through the urethra and vas deferens and into the epididymis. Symptoms are those of a UTI, including fever and urethral discharge. Examination reveals a unilateral, tender scrotal mass, which is initially separable from the testis but may gradually involve the testis as well. Signs of prostatitis may also be noted. Conditions simulating acute epididymitis, e.g., testicular torsion or tumor, can be differentiated on ultrasound.

Epididymitis may be sexually transmitted (usually due to *Chlamydia trachomatis* or *Neisseria gonorrhoeae*) or non-sexually transmitted (usually due to enteric gram-negative organisms). It may be treated as outlined in Figure 149.2.

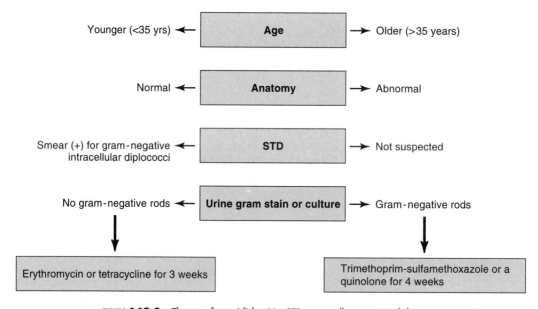

FIGURE 149.2. Therapy for epididymitis. STD = sexually transmitted disease.

A list of sexually transmitted diseases (STD) is provided in Table 150.1. In most industrialized nations, the incidence of syphilis, gonorrhea, and chancroid has steadily declined during the last two decades. However, the incidence of these disorders, particularly syphilis and chancroid, rose strikingly in the United States in the last decade. A variety of social influences brought about this rise, one of them being sex-for-drugs.

It is common to acquire more than one disorder when a person acquires an STD. Thus, the individual found to have syphilis should be screened for gonorrhea and human immunodeficiency virus (HIV), regardless of whether features of each of these diseases present or not. STDs should be viewed as a reflection of "high-risk" behavior, rather than a sporadic disease with which the individual presents.

TABLE 150.1. Sexually Transmitted Diseases

Syphilis
Gonorrhea
Chancroid
Granuloma inguinale (Donovanosis)
Non-gonococcal urethritis
Acute pelvic inflammatory disease (PID)
Vaginitis
   Trichomonas vaginalis
   Chlamydia trachomatis
Lymphogranuloma venereum (LGV)
Herpes simplex virus (HSV)
Hepatitis B
Human immunodeficiency virus (HIV)
Anorectal disease
Infections among homosexuals
   Herpes simplex, gonorrhea, syphilis
   Anorectal infection due to *Neisseria meningitidis*
   Ulcerative proctitis due to Chlamydia
   Epididymitis (from coliform organisms and *Haemophilus influenzae*)
   Enteric bacterial pathogens (Shigella, Salmonella, *Campylobacter jejuni, Entamoeba histolytica,* Giardia)
   Hepatitis
   Cytomegalovirus (CMV)

■ General Overview of Genital Lesions

The hallmark of an STD is a **genital lesion** (except in those engaging in anal receptive intercourse, who may harbor internal lesions). The morphology of genital lesions is an important clue in diagnosis. Causes of ulcerative lesions are shown in Table 150.2. In the United States, most (>50%) genital lesions are caused by HSV. Syphilis follows as the second leading cause.

Although appearance, incubation period, travel history, or mode of onset may be helpful in evaluating genital lesions, **laboratory testing** is essential for specific diagnosis (except classic herpes simplex virus [HSV] with grouped vesicles). Essential laboratory studies for ulcerated lesions include culture for HSV, a dark-field examination for syphilis, and serologic tests for syphilis. Culture for *Haemophilus ducreyi* also may be done if chancroid is suspected.

TABLE 150.2. Genital Lesions Due to Sexually Transmitted Diseases

Diagnosis/Entity	Causative Organism	Clinical Feature(s)	Confirmatory Study	Treatment
Herpes genitalis	Herpes simplex virus	Grouped vesicles	Culture	Acyclovir
Syphilis	*Treponema pallidum*	Painless ulcer, adenopathy	Dark field examination	Penicillin
Chancroid	*Haemophilus ducreyi*	Painful ulcer, adenopathy	Gram stain (?)	Erythromycin, ceftriaxone
Donovanosis (granuloma inguinale)	Calymmatobacterium	Heaped up tissue	Giemsa	Tetracycline, ampicillin, TMP/SMX
Lymphogranuloma venereum	*Chlamydia trachomatis*	Inguinal adenopathy with bubo	Serology	Tetracycline

TMP-SMX = Trimethoprim-sulfamethoxazole.

Herpes Simplex Virus

■ Epidemiology

Genital HSV causes over 400,000 episodes of primary infection each year in the United States. Up to 90% of these infections are with HSV-2, and the remainder are with HSV-1. Infection is spread by contact with infected secretions. However, recent studies have shown that viral shedding may occur without apparent lesions (subclinical infection).

■ Clinical Features and Diagnosis

The incubation period (time from infection to the first clinical manifestation) is usually 2–7 days. HSV usually starts as grouped, thin-walled vesicles which ulcerate. In heterosexual men, the vesicles present on the shaft of the penis or glans, whereas in homosexual men, they may occur perianally or present as proctitis. In women, lesions may occur on the vulva, vagina, or anus.

The lesions are usually painful. The primary infection lasts 2–3 weeks and may be accompanied by fever and tender adenopathy. Sacral radiculitis with urinary retention and aseptic meningitis are unusual presentations. Recurrent episodes are usually less severe without the systemic manifestations— fewer lesions are seen, and the duration is usually a few days. These episodes may have prodromal pain and burning. The organism lies latent within sensory ganglia between episodes.

For confirmation of the diagnosis, the base of the ulcer may be swabbed and sent for culture, direct immunofluorescence staining, antigen detection, or Tzanck preparation (Figure 42.2). The yield is highest (90%) when specimens are taken during the vesicular stage rather than the ulcerative stage (50%). There is little role for serologic diagnosis.

■ Management

Acyclovir remains the drug of choice for HSV infection. A dose of 200 mg five times a day for 7–10 days is recommended for the immunocompetent host with genital lesions or 400 mg five times per day for persons with proctitis or HIV coinfection. There is no clinical role for topical acyclovir.

Patients with primary infection benefit the most from acyclovir treatment, and those with relapses benefit only minimally. **Prophylaxis** of frequent, recurrent episodes can be done with acyclovir, 200 mg three times per day or 400 mg twice a day, which reduces the rate of recurrence in over 80% of patients. Acyclovir should be stopped after 1 year to assess further need for it; however, HIV patients usually require continuous therapy.

Acyclovir-resistant HSV has been seen among immunosuppressed persons. It should be suspected when a response is lacking, especially to IV therapy. IV foscarnet is then indicated.

Syphilis

■ Etiology and Epidemiology

Syphilis is caused by a spirochete, *Treponema pallidum*. It is a slender, coiled organism that replicates slowly and cannot be cultivated in vitro. Syphilis is primarily acquired by sexual contact, but it may be transplacentally transmitted in congenital disease. Very rarely, it is transmitted by accidental inoculation or blood transfusion. An individual with a chancre (syphilitic ulcer) or condylomata lata (flat, wartlike plaques) is most infectious.

Although no age is exempt, most cases occur in sexually active persons aged 15–30 years. In the 1980s, the incidence of syphilis began to rise in the United States, which was primarily due to increased numbers of cases among homosexual men. However, in the 1990s, there has been a rapid rise in number of heterosexual cases, due to sex-for-drugs, especially involving crack cocaine.

■ Pathogenesis

T. pallidum may penetrate intact mucous membranes or abrasions in the skin and thus enter the lymphatics and bloodstream, disseminating to almost any organ in the body. The incubation period is nearly 3 weeks, but can vary from a few days to 3 months depending on the size of the inoculum.

■ Clinical Features

Syphilis is classified into the four categories of *primary, secondary, latent* and *tertiary phases,* which differ in their clinical manifestations and treatment. It may also be divided into the two broad categories of *early* (primary and secondary stages) and *late* syphilis (tertiary stage). The skin manifestations are discussed in chapter 52.

Primary and secondary stages

The classic **primary** syphilitic lesion is the **chancre,** which begins as a single papule that erodes into a painless ulcer (Figure 150.1), along with painless inguinal lymphadenopathy. Spontaneous healing occurs in a few weeks. Multiple chancres may be seen in HIV patients.

Secondary syphilis, indicating acute dissemination, usually occurs 2–8 weeks after the chancre appears. Whereas there are no symptoms between the primary and the secondary stage, cutaneous findings are the most prominent feature in the secondary stage, occurring in 90% of cases. The classic **"coppery rash,"** that is, fleeting, rapidly progressive reddish-brown macules, precedes a generalized, symmetric polymorphous eruption of macules and papules.

Systemic features—fever, anorexia, arthralgia, and generalized adenopathy (classically epitrochlear)—occur in 70% of patients with secondary syphilis. Organs are involved less frequently but hepatitis, nephritis or meningitis may occur. Anemia, leukocytosis, significantly elevated alkaline phosphatase and a high erythrocyte sedimentation rate are the notable laboratory findings.

Latent and tertiary stages

Syphilis is considered **latent** when there is a positive test for syphilis without any manifestations of disease, including cerebrospinal fluid findings. Overall, 30% of untreated patients develop one of the forms of late-stage, **tertiary** syphilis: neurosyphilis, cardiovascular syphilis, or gumma (erosive lesions affecting organs or mucous membranes). Tertiary syphilis is now extremely rare in the United States, owing to early treatment.

◾ Diagnosis

Dark-field examination allows direct visualization of the spirochete and should be performed in patients with a chancre of primary syphilis or the condylomata

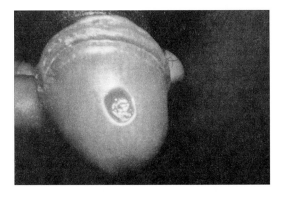

FIGURE 150.1. Chancre of primary syphilis.

TABLE 150.3.	Causes of False-Positive Results in Serologic Tests for Syphilis
Infectious Causes	**Noninfectious Causes**
Other spirochetes	Narcotic addicts
Tuberculosis	Connective tissue disorder
Leprosy	Pregnancy
Endocarditis	Old age
Mycoplasma infection	Chronic liver disease
Rickettsial infection	Laboratory error
Hepatitis	
Mononucleosis	

lata of secondary syphilis. A scraping of the lesion is placed on a slide and viewed with a phase-contrast microscope. However, the necessary expertise may not be available in all facilities.

Serologic tests for syphilis include non-treponemal tests and a specific anti-treponemal antibody test. The former tests are nonspecific and include the Venereal Disease Research Laboratory (VDRL) or the rapid plasma reagin (RPR). These tests measure IgM and IgG antibodies directed against a lipid antigen formed by interaction of *T. pallidum* and the host and are used for screening or following disease activity. A fourfold change (2 dilutions) is considered significant.

Because of frequent false-positives (Table 150.3), a confirmatory test is usually done using treponemal tests, such as the fluorescent treponemal antibody absorption (FTA-ABS) or, more recently, microhemagglutination assay for antibody to *T. pallidum* (MHA-TP).

◾ Management

Penicillin remains the drug of choice for all stages of syphilis (Table 150.4). For penicillin-allergic patients, oral tetracycline or doxycycline may be used, except in neurosyphilis because these drugs do not penetrate the CSF. Penicillin-allergic pregnant women with syphilis require penicillin desensitization regardless of the stage because tetracyclines cannot be used in pregnancy. Similarly, penicillin desensitization should be strongly considered for penicillin-allergic patients with neurosyphilis.

All patients with syphilis should be evaluated for HIV infection. Management of syphilis in patients with HIV is controversial. Questions remain as to whether all patients with HIV should undergo CSF examination regardless of stage and whether single-dose benzathine penicillin is acceptable in any stage. Regardless of the course taken, close follow-up is necessary with serological examination at 1, 2, 3, 6, 9, and 12 months. Penicillin-allergic patients should be desensitized.

TABLE 150.4. Treatment of Primary, Secondary and Latent Syphilis		
Stage	**Treatment Regimen**	**Comments**
Primary, secondary, and early latent	Benzathine penicillin 2.4 MU IM	If penicillin allergic, doxycycline
Late latent or unknown duration	As above, except benzathine penicillin weekly × 3 wks and Doxycycline 100 mg PO bid × 28 days	100 mg PO bid × 14 days for all stages; desensitize for syphilis complicating pregnancy
Tertiary syphilis (excluding neuro-syphilis)	As above	

Gonorrhea

Gonorrhea is caused by *Neisseria gonorrhoeae,* a gram-negative diplococcus. Only humans are infected by this organism, the usual route of infection being the genitourinary tract epithelium and, uncommonly, the pharynx and anal canal. Infection is usually acquired through sexual contact.

■ Epidemiology

Gonorrhea causes an estimated 1 million infections yearly in the United States. Infection may be readily recognized in symptomatic persons who seek medical attention, but a sizable number of infected men and women are asymptomatic; this reservoir may be responsible for the ongoing spread of this disease. Although no age is exempt, teenagers and young adults are most commonly infected. Its prevalence correlates with low socioeconomic status.

■ Clinical Features

A significant number of infected persons may be asymptomatic. The incubation period is typically 3–4 days but may be as long as 2 weeks.

In heterosexual men, dysuria and purulent urethral exudate are the most common presenting symptoms; pharyngitis is infrequent. Among homosexual men, besides urethritis, proctitis may be encountered in one-third to one-half of cases and pharyngitis in one-fifth of cases.

Among symptomatic women, dysuria, urethritis, pyuria, vaginal discharge, menorrhagia or menometrorrhagia (bleeding between menses), and abdominal pain are the more common features. Pharyngitis is uncommon, and anal canal infection may sometimes lead to proctitis. Other presentations are acute pelvic inflammatory disease and Bartholin's gland abscess. However, the disease may be asymptomatic, despite isolation of the organism from endocervical smears or the anal canal or the pharynx.

Disseminated infection, more common among women, results from bacteremia. Patients are febrile and generally toxic. A pustular distal skin rash, arthralgias, polyarthritis, tenosynovitis, or septic arthritis (gonococcus is the most common cause of septic arthritis in the sexually active age group) evolves as the illness progresses.

Skin lesions, more frequent in the extremities, are papular and erythematous and have a hemorrhagic or necrotic center. Typical urethral or cervical signs and symptoms may not be present. As the initial febrile episode resolves, a purulent mono- or oligoarticular arthritis may develop (see Bacterial Arthritis in chapter 256). In some, the initial febrile illness may be very transient or nonexistent, with the arthritis being the initial presentation. Endocarditis may develop as a complication.

■ Diagnosis

In a person presenting with another STD (e.g., syphilis), coexistent gonorrhea may be diagnosed even when asymptomatic if the physician is careful enough to suspect it. In such individuals as well as in symptomatic persons, urethral or endocervical smears should be submitted for Gram stain (intracellular gram-negative diplococci are diagnostic) and culture. Gram stain of the urethral discharge in men is highly sensitive (>95%) and specific. It is less sensitive in cervical (50%) and rectal infection (20%). The smears should be inoculated into selective (Thayer-Martin) medium for best results.

In patients with suspected disseminated gonorrhea, the urethra and cervix, if applicable, should be cultured. Joint fluid, if present, is often sterile initially, but with purulent arthritis, cultures are often positive. Skin lesions, sampled with a punch biopsy, may yield the organism in about half the cases. Blood cultures are positive in about one-half of cases.

■ Management

Many therapeutic options exist for gonorrhea, including ceftriaxone (125 mg IM), cefixime (400 mg orally in a single dose), or ciprofloxacin (500 mg orally in a single dose). Treatment should always cover Chlamydia. For penicillin-allergic patients, ciprofloxacin and ofloxacin are effective alternatives for uncomplicated anogenital gonorrhea in men and nonpregnant women. For disseminated gonococcal infection, hospitalization and IV antibiotics (ceftriaxone) are necessary. Purulent arthritis requires additional measures (see chapter 259).

Antibiotic resistance among gonococci has been a vexing public health problem, with resistance to penicillin, ampicillin, and tetracycline being commonplace. Strains of penicillinase-producing *N. gonorrhoeae* (PPNG) account for 7–8% of all isolates, and tetracycline-resistant *N. gonorrhoeae* (TRNG) for nearly 5%. The drug resistance develops through chromosomal mutations and plasmid-mediated penicillinase production. Whereas PPNG are encountered in high numbers on both the eastern and western U.S. coasts, TRNG are seen throughout the country. Spectinomycin-resistant gonococci are also penicillin-, cefoxitin-, and tetracycline-resistant. Fortunately, resistance has not been reported to **ceftriaxone,** making it the preferred agent for treatment of gonorrhea.

Follow-up examination is not necessary if a recommended regimen is used to treat gonorrhea. Persistent symptoms may suggest a resistant organism, associated nongonococcal urethritis, or reexposure to an infected partner. Clinical evaluation and reculturing are necessary. Notification of public health personnel is essential in the therapy for and control of gonorrhea.

Urethritis, Cervicitis, and Vaginitis

Urethritis, or inflammation of the urethra, is characterized by discharge of mucopurulent material and dysuria. It is broadly classified as gonococcal or nongonococcal, according to the etiology. **Nongonococcal urethritis** is diagnosed when neutrophils exceed 5/oil-immersion field, devoid of any organism. *Chlamydia trachomatis* is responsible for nearly 50% of cases, *Ureaplasma urealyticum* for 20–40%, and *Trichomonas vaginalis* for 2–5%; the remainder are unidentified. Complications include epididymitis and Reiter's Syndrome.

Treatment of nongonococcal urethritis is **doxycycline,** 100 mg twice daily for 7 days. Failure to respond to doxycycline may indicate resistant Ureaplasma, in which case erythromycin should be tried. Recently, azithromycin, 1.0 g as a single dose, has been approved as treatment for Chlamydia. Sexual contacts should also be treated.

Mucopurulent cervicitis is characterized by a yellow cervical discharge. Microbiology is similar to urethritis and includes *N. gonorrhoeae* and *C. trachomatis.* In women, the two organisms often occur concurrently. Treatment includes both doxycycline and therapy for gonorrhea.

Vaginitis, characterized by vulvar irritation with itching and abnormal vaginal discharge, is due to local vulvovaginal infection or to bacterial vaginosis, where the normal vaginal flora is replaced by an overgrowth of extraneous organisms. Vaginitis is commonly caused by *Trichomonas vaginalis* and *Candida albicans.*

Trichomonal vaginitis, while often asymptomatic, may cause pain on sexual intercourse (dyspareunia), dysuria, vaginal discharge and/or vulvar pruritus, often occurring during or slightly after menstruation. Abundant, frothy, foul-smelling, vaginal discharge is common. *T. vaginalis* is readily seen on Papanicolaou stain and on urinalysis, and isolated on culture of vaginal secretions. Candida overgrowth, on the other hand, causes vulvar pruritus and a thick, whitish vaginal discharge, which often precedes the menses. Dyspareunia is uncommon. Often, an underlying process such as diabetes mellitus, corticosteroid therapy, broad spectrum antibiotic therapy or pregnancy is readily identifiable in the background. Candidal vaginitis is not an STD.

Bacterial vaginosis follows replacement of the normal vaginal Lactobacillus flora with anaerobes (peptostreptococcus, peptococcus and bacteroides). Despite a correlation with heightened sexual activity and the number of sexual partners, not all forms of bacterial vaginosis are sexually transmitted. Patients report a fetid discharge, and occasionally pruritus. Dyspareunia is quite uncommon. The major diagnostic aids are the examination of the vaginal discharge for pH (>4.7) and potassium hydroxide (KOH) test. If either one of these studies does not confirm the diagnosis, then infection with *C. trachomatis* or *N. gonorrhoeae* should be pursued.

T. vaginalis is treated with metronidazole, given in a single 2.0 g dose orally or multi-dose regimen (500 mg p.o., b.i.d for 10 days). Failure of therapy is an indication for re-treatment with the longer regimen because of reported drug resistance of the organism. Patients should avoid alcohol, since a disulfiram-like reaction can occur if alcohol is consumed while taking metronidazole. In order to reduce the reinfection rate, the male sexual partner should also be treated with one single 2.0 g dose of metronidazole; the importance of this cannot be overemphasized. Candidal vaginitis is treated with nystatin or one of the topical azoles. Bacterial vaginosis is treated with metronidazole, 2.0 g daily for 5 days or clindamycin vaginal cream.

Pelvic Inflammatory Disease

Pelvic inflammatory disease is an inflammatory disorder of the upper genital tract in women and includes endometritis, salpingitis, and tubo-ovarian abscess. The causative agents are *N. gonorrhoeae, C. trachomatis,* and the anaerobic-aerobic vaginal flora.

The clinical presentation may vary from subtle with mild abdominal pain to frank peritonitis. Regrettably, clinical diagnosis is unreliable, with laparoscopy confirming the diagnosis in only two-thirds of suspected cases. Minimal diagnostic criteria include lower abdominal tenderness, adnexal tenderness, or cervical motion tenderness.

With uncertain diagnosis, abscess, pregnancy, or an HIV positive patient, inpatient therapy is recommended, cefoxitin (or cefotetan) and doxycycline being appropriate agents. Outpatient regimens include cefoxitin IM (plus probenecid) or ceftriaxone (250 mg IM) and doxycycline (100 mg twice daily) for 10–14 days.

CHAPTER **151** **INFECTIOUS DIARRHEA**

Infectious enteritis is discussed further in chapter 79. The occurrence of infectious diarrhea depends strictly on the balance between the pathogenicity of the microbe (e.g., Shigella requires an infectious dose of only 100 organisms) and predisposition of the host (intactness of defenses).

■ Etiology and Epidemiology

Agents causing infectious diarrhea are listed in 79.2 and Figure 79.1. Epidemiologic clues to the causative agent in infectious diarrhea are summarized in Table 151.1. **Noninvasive diarrhea** is enterotoxin-induced, often voluminous, and lacks inflammation. **Enterotoxigenic** *Escherichia coli,* which produces a heat-labile enterotoxin that activates mucosal adenylate cyclase, is the most common responsible organism worldwide; it also causes most instances of **traveler's diarrhea.**

TABLE 151.1.	Clinical and Epidemiological Clues in Infectious Diarrhea
Clinical Feature/ Epidemiologic Clue	**Etiology**
International travel	*Escherichia coli,* cholera
Recent antibiotic use	*Clostridium difficile*
Gay man	Enteropathogens or proctitis (STD)
Vomiting > diarrhea	Food poisoning or viral
High fever	Salmonella, shigella, or campylobacter
Bloody stool	Shigella, campylobacter, or inflammatory bowel disease

■ Clinical Features

Primarily upper gastrointestinal symptoms (i.e., nausea and vomiting, or vomiting out of proportion to diarrhea) suggest a viral illness or a preformed toxin ingested in food. Such symptoms usually present within 6 hours after ingesting food that contains a preformed bacterial toxin, such as potato salad (*Staphylococcus aureus*) or improperly re-heated fried rice (*Bacillus cereus*). Norwalk virus can cause epidemics in families and nursing homes.

Associated fever suggests **invasive organisms,** including Shigella, Campylobacter, or Salmonella. Bloody stools are more frequent with Shigella or Campylobacter.

Many parasites cause diarrhea, including *Giardia lamblia, Entamoeba histolytica* (more common in overseas travelers or travelers to Mexico), *Strongyloides stercoralis* (fulminant disease in the immunosuppressed), Cryptosporidium (recent water-borne outbreaks in several U.S. cities; also in AIDS), *Isospora belli* (acid-fast; seen in AIDS patients), and microsporidia (AIDS patients).

■ Diagnosis

The history—especially of fever, bloody stools, or weight loss—dictates the need to pursue laboratory evaluation (Table 151.2). **Stool examination** for leukocytes is the first step and, if positive, is followed by culture. Bloody stool without leukocytes suggests amebiasis (the parasite destroys leukocytes) or enterohemorrhagic *E. coli* O157:H7. The finding of stool leukocytes indicates an inflammatory process (Table 151.3). However, their absence, while not excluding an inflammatory process, usually implies a self-limited, noninflammatory process.

TABLE 151.2.	Specific Organisms Causing Infectious Enteritis		
Agent	**Transmission**	**Features**	**Treatment**
Shigella	Person-to-person	Inflammatory bloody diarrhea; bacteremia or dissemination rare; complications are HUS or Reiter's syndrome.	TMP-SMX (resistant in developing countries)
Salmonella (non-typhoid)	Contaminated water or food, esp. poultry	Nausea, vomiting, abdominal pain, fever	None unless severe
Campylobacter jejuni	Undercooked poultry	Prodrome of constitutional symptoms or a biphasic course (diarrhea-recovery-diarrhea); mimics IBD.	Erythromycin; quinolones (alternative)
Yersinia enterocolitica	Unknown	Infrequent; mesenteric adenitis or terminal ileitis may mimic appendicitis; may cause polyarthritis and erythema nodosum; patients with anemia, cirrhosis or hemochromatosis may develop septicemia.	TMP-SMX, tetracycline, quinolones or third-generation cephalosporins
Escherichia coli	Contaminated food/water. EH through poorly cooked ground beef	Travelers' diarrhea; hemorrhagic colitis occurs without fecal leukocytes; antibiotics may predispose to HUS; HUS more frequent at extremes of age.	None
Clostridium difficile		Trivial illness to toxic megacolon; prior antibiotic therapy is the predisposing factor; relapse occurs in 10%	Oral metronidazole; oral vancomycin for toxic patients

EH = enterotoxigenic strains; HUS = hemolytic-uremic syndrome; TMP-SMX = Trimethoprim-sulfamethoxazole; IBD = inflammatory bowel disease.

HIV-positivity, weight loss, and diarrhea lasting for 10 days all indicate the need for further evaluation. Appropriate use of the laboratory in this setting is summarized in Figure 79.2. General management of diarrhea and the use of oral rehydration are discussed in chapters 69 and 79. Antimicrobial agents that may be useful in acute diarrheal episodes are summarized in Table 79.3.

TABLE 151.3.	Fecal Leukocytes in Intestinal Infections	
Present	**Variable**	**Absent**
Shigella	Salmonella	Vibrio cholera
Campylobacter	Vibrio parahaemolyticus	Toxigenic E. coli
Invasive E. coli	Clostridium difficile	Viral
		Giardia
		Entamoeba histolytica

<table><tr><td>CHAPTER</td><td>152</td><td>INTRA-ABDOMINAL INFECTIONS</td></tr></table>

Intra-abdominal infection can be divided into peritonitis, visceral abscesses, and extravisceral abscesses.

Peritonitis

Patients with peritonitis usually present with steady abdominal pain, which is worsened by any movement or respiration and which may be sudden if a viscus has ruptured. Fever is usually present. Tenderness with rebound, guarding, rigidity, and diminished or absent bowel sounds are characteristic.

Spontaneous (primary) peritonitis is discussed in chapter 103. **Secondary peritonitis** arises from rupture of a part of the gastrointestinal tract (due to trauma, infarction, prior abdominal surgery, or simple perforation, such as a ruptured appendix) with leakage of its contents. The microbiology is dictated by the location of the leak. In most cases, multiple organisms are responsible. Enterobacteriaceae (*E. coli*), anaerobes (*Bacteroides fragilis,* other Bacteroides spp., Clostridia) and enterococci constitute the most frequent pathogens. Because the colon has the largest population of microorganisms, sepsis is more likely after colon perforation.

Free air below the diaphragm on a plain chest radiograph is an excellent clue to the presence of peritonitis, because it indicates the rupture of a large hollow viscus (stomach or colon). Treatment is surgical repair of the underlying defect.

Peritonitis may also be seen with peritoneal dialysis catheters. The etiology is usually *Staphylococcus aureus* or *S. epidermidis*. With antibiotic treatment, the catheter can usually be left in place unless there is a tunnel infection. Fungal infections and tuberculosis are other, infrequent causes of peritonitis.

Abscesses of Solid Organs

Thirty to 40% of **liver abscesses** are amebic, due to *Entamoeba histolytica*. The remaining pyogenic liver abscesses are usually caused by other underlying conditions, including biliary disease, infections in the drainage area of the portal vein, systemic bacteremia, trauma, or contiguous infection. Among these, the most common condition (in 30% of cases) is ascending cholangitis from biliary obstruction or procedures involving the biliary tract.

The microbiology depends on the underlying cause. Anaerobes are increasingly implicated in liver abscesses, especially *Streptococcus milleri*. Patients with neutropenia are at increased risk for fungal abscesses.

The signs and symptoms of liver abscess usually include fever and abdominal pain. The liver may be enlarged, palpable, and tender. The most consistent laboratory abnormality is elevation of alkaline phosphatase levels, although other liver tests may also be abnormal. Computed tomography is the most sensitive and specific test. Finding *E. histolytica* in the stool in the United States is considered diagnostic, but in endemic areas, this may only represent a carrier state. In a high proportion of cases (>85%), the indirect hemagglutination test is positive.

Percutaneous or open surgical drainage is usually needed. Initial antibiotic selection is guided by consideration of potential bowel pathogens until culture results become available. *E. histolytica* infection is treated with metronidazole.

Extravisceral Abscess

Extravisceral abscesses usually arise from disruption of the gastrointestinal tract with loculation of fluid from peritoneal defenses, especially the omentum (without loculation, generalized peritonitis develops). Ruptured appendix is the leading etiology. The microbiology consists of colonic flora.

Clinical features include local symptoms with fever and leukocytosis. Subphrenic and pelvic abscesses may lack any local findings, a feature shared by immunosuppressed or debilitated patients. CT scan represents the best diagnostic study.

Once the abscess is localized, surgical, or percutaneous drainage should follow. Percutaneous drainage is being applied increasingly, even for complex cases. The choice of antibiotics is guided initially by Gram stain results and later by culture. A lack of response to catheter drainage within 48 hours calls for open surgical drainage.

CHAPTER **153** CENTRAL NERVOUS SYSTEM INFECTIONS

Meningitis, encephalitis, epidural abscess, subdural empyema, and brain abscess represent the spectrum of principal intracranial infections. A variety of organisms may cause these infections. The portal of entry of infections into the intracranial cavity is generally the blood or contiguous extension from adjacent structures (e.g., bacteria may spread from infected paranasal sinuses or neurotropic viruses may penetrate via exposed endings of olfactory nerves).

The blood vessels are often involved in the inflammation, and their resulting thrombosis or occlusion produces important clinical manifestations. Cytokine-induced vascular permeability and inflammation lead to increased intracranial pressure. In leptomeningeal infections, cerebrospinal fluid (CSF), obtained by lumbar puncture, shows protein and cellular alterations and often contains the infecting organism. Antibiotics selectively cross the blood-brain barrier to penetrate the substance of the brain and meninges, which limits the choice of antibiotics in therapy for intracranial infections. Because all cranial nerves exit the skull at the base, cranial nerve involvement is an important aspect of chronic meningitis.

■ General Diagnosis and Management

Depending on the process, fever, headache, confusion, seizure, nuchal rigidity, or focal neurologic deficit may occur in varying combinations. The axiom in managing intracranial infections is to decide clinically if acute bacterial meningitis is present and to proceed accordingly.

Intracranial abscesses are space-occupying and inevitably cause increased **intracranial pressure.** With such enlarging mass lesions, lumbar puncture carries a high risk of transtentorial herniation and death. Bacterial meningitis also raises intracranial pressure, but the increase is spread diffusely across the subarachnoid space. Thus, unless the meningitis is advanced, the risk for transtentorial herniation after lumbar puncture is negligible, if any. Obtaining a computed tomographic (CT) scan in every patient prior to lumbar puncture can avoid this risk, but it is expensive and inefficient.

The **acuteness of presentation** and findings vary according to the process. Fulminant symptoms with fever, lethargy, and nuchal rigidity make bacterial meningitis likely, which calls for immediate lumbar puncture and antibiotic therapy within 1 hour. A subacute history over weeks or months, especially with focal signs and symptoms, implies a mass effect. CT is indicated first, as lumbar puncture is risky. When these distinctions are blurred and meningitis is still a consideration, blood cultures are drawn, antibiotics are given, and lumbar puncture is deferred until the CT scan.

Bacterial Meningitis

Meningitis, an inflammation of the meninges, may be acute (hours to several days) or chronic (weeks to months) according to its evolution. Acute meningitis has a variety of causes (Table 153.1).

■ Epidemiology

Three organisms together cause 80% of all cases of community-acquired bacterial meningitis: *Streptococcus pneumoniae, Neisseria meningitidis,* and *Haemophilus influenzae.* A strong relationship with age is evident, in that *H. influenzae* is usually seen in children below 1 year of age and rarely in adults unless asplenia, sinusitis, or alcoholism is present. Meningococcus is usually seen in children under age 5 but may occur in young adults sporadically or during epidemics.

Pneumococcus is seen in all ages, but is the most common organism in the adult. Predisposing factors for pneumococcal meningitis include otitis media or mastoiditis (30%), pneumonia (20%), and head trauma (10%). Sporadic bacterial meningitis cases rise in the autumn and winter months and decline during the spring, reaching a nadir during summer.

Enteric gram-negative bacillary meningitis is seen primarily in trauma, neurosurgical, or hospitalized patients. Whereas coagulase-negative staphylococcus is seen in patients with CNS shunts, *S. aureus* is usually related to trauma or endocarditis. Among adults, Listeria meningitis may occur in the elderly or those with defective cell-mediated (T-cell) immunity.

■ Pathogenesis and Pathophysiology

The portal of entry of pathogens into the meninges is not conclusively known, but mucosal colonization followed by bacteremia and penetration of the blood-brain barrier through the choroid plexus are believed to be important steps. Contiguous extension of an infected focus (sinusitis or otitis media) or entry through the cribriform plate are other possible mechanisms. The survival of the organisms in the CSF is related to the virulence of the organism (e.g., encapsuled bacteria are more virulent) and also to the general lack of defense mechanisms in the CSF (e.g., the CSF is deficient in complement concentration and immunoglobulins). Together, these two factors cause a compromised opsonizing ability.

In the subarachnoid space, the bacteria evoke an intense **leptomeningitis.** The permeability of the blood-brain barrier may increase with the evolving inflammation, causing cerebral edema. Other sequelae include increased intracranial pressure, CSF acidosis, and encephalopathy that accompanies meningitis. The subarachnoid space inflammation may also impede the CSF flow, causing hydrocephalus and increased intracranial pressure.

Thrombotic or vasculitic involvement of the blood

TABLE 153.1. Causes of Acute Meningitis	
Infectious	**Non-infectious**
Bacterial	Medications
Streptococcus pneumoniae	Nonsteroidal anti-inflammatory agents
Neisseria meningitidis	Azathioprine
Haemophilus influenzae	Carbamazepine
Group B streptococci	Connective tissue disease
Gram-negative bacilli	Systemic Lupus Erythematosus
Staphylococci	Miscellaneous
Listeria monocytogenes	Following seizures
Viral	Migraine
Enterovirus	
HIV	
Rickettsial	
Rickettsia rickettsii (Rocky Mountain spotted fever)	
Typhus (R. prowazekii, R. tsutsugamushi, R. typhi)	
Spirochetal	
Treponema pallidum (syphilis)	
Borrelia burgdorferi (Lyme disease)	
Protozoa	
Naegleria fowleri	

TABLE 153.2. Clinical Features of Bacterial Meningitis
Extremely common (80–100%)
Confusion
Fever
Headache
Neck pain and stiffness (meningismus)
Common (50–80%)
Kernig's sign
Brudzinski's sign
Sometimes (30–35%)
Seizures
Vomiting
Uncommon (<20%)
Lateralizing neurologic deficits
Rare (<1%)
Papilledema

vessels causes areas of cerebral infarction. Compromised blood supply and perhaps other factors cause the meningeal and cerebral glycolysis to shift to the anaerobic pathway, thus resulting in lactate accumulation. The resultant CSF acidosis may be partly responsible for the **encephalopathy.**

■ **Clinical Features**

One-fourth of patients have a rapid onset with headache, lethargy, and confusion within 24 hours (Table 153.2). In the others, symptoms evolve over 1–7 days. In some patients, the features of meningitis may develop as an aftermath of or in continuity with a pneumonic process.

Petechial and purpuric rash are a clue to meningococcal infection (Gram stain yields a positive result in 70% of cases) and indicate **meningococcemia.** Focal findings, consisting of cranial nerve deficits (especially cranial nerves 3, 6, and 8) may be noted in 10–20% of patients. Papilledema is rare.

■ **Laboratory Features**

The CSF classically shows an elevated WBC count that exceeds $1000/mm^3$ with a predominance of neutrophils, an elevated protein above 150 mg/dl, and a decreased glucose below 40 mg/dl (hypoglycorrhachia). On average, Gram stain of the CSF is positive in 80% (50% or so with *Listeria*) and has a 100% specificity (Table 153.3). Whereas latex agglutination tests are available for *H. influenzae, S. pneumoniae,* and *N. meningitidis,* their contribution to diagnosis beyond Gram stain has been questioned. CSF cultures are reportedly positive in 80%, with blood cultures being positive in 40–80%.

■ **Differential Diagnosis**

Occasionally, viral meningitis can resemble a bacterial process, with neutrophil counts as high as $500/mm^3$.

TABLE 153.3.	Diagnostic Value of CSF Studies in Bacterial Meningitis

Test	Sensitivity
↑CSF opening pressure	Universal
↑CSF protein	Universal
CSF latex agglutination	80–95%
CSF Gram stain	70–90%
CSF culture	80%
Blood cultures	40–80%
CSF glucose: serum glucose <0.31	70%
Gram stain of petechiae	70%
↓CSF glucose	60%
CSF glucose <34 mg/dl, glucose ratio <0.23, protein >220 mg/ml, CSF leukocytes >2000/mm³ (or >1180/mm³ of CSF polymorphs)	Each >99%

Usually, on repeat lumbar puncture within 12–36 hours, the cellular response becomes mononuclear. In the elderly and neutropenic patients, the CSF leukocyte count may not be high, and Gram stain is essential in ascertaining the presence of meningitis. If the diagnosis is in doubt, the lumbar puncture should generally be repeated within 12–36 hours.

■ Management

The initial approach to the patient with suspected meningitis is outlined in Figure 153.1. Increasing antibiotic resistance among pneumococci has prompted changes in empiric antibiotics used in adults (Table 153.4). Presently, a third-generation cephalosporin is recommended for initial community-acquired bacterial meningitis, along with vancomycin until penicillin sus-

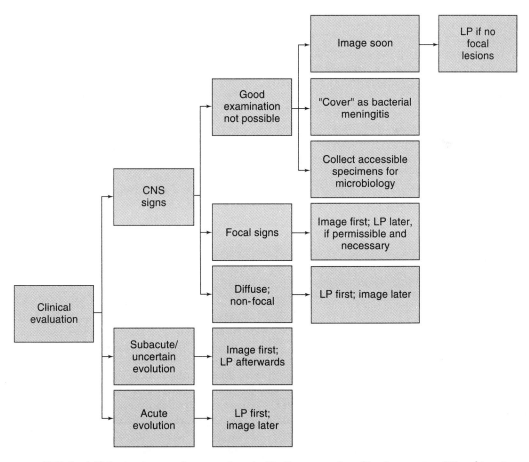

FIGURE 153.1. Initial management of suspected meningitis. The sequencing of lumbar puncture (LP) and imaging studies (CT scanning) for various presentations is outlined.

TABLE 153.4.	Bacterial Meningitis: Choice of Antibiotic Therapy		
Age	**Likely Microorganism**	**Empiric Therapy**	**Alternative Therapy**
Children <10	*Haemophilus influenzae*, pneumococcus, meningococcus	Ceftriaxone and rifampin or vancomycin until results of susceptibility testing are known	Chloramphenicol
Young Adults	Meningococcus	Ceftriaxone	Chloramphenicol
Elderly	Pneumococcus, Listeria and gram-negative bacilli	Ceftriaxone and ampicillin	

TABLE 153.5.	Causes of Aseptic Meningitis
Type	**Specific Examples**
Viral	Enterovirus or HIV
Bacterial	Listeria or parameningeal focus
Spirochete	Syphilis, Lyme, or Leptospirosis
Noninfectious	Vasculitis, sarcoid, drug, or tumor

TABLE 153.6.	Causes of Chronic Meningitis by CSF Cell Predominance	
Lymphocytic		**Neutrophilic**
Tuberculosis		Actinomyces
Syphilis		Nocardia
Lyme disease		Brucella
Cryptococcus		Candida
Coccidioides		Aspergillosis
Histoplasmosis		Blastomycosis
Cysticercosis		Drug
Sarcoid		
Vasculitis		
Behçet's		
Tumor		
Parameningeal		

ceptibility is known; ampicillin should be added for individuals at risk for Listeria infection (elderly, alcoholic, or immunosuppressed patients). Penicillin G remains the drug of choice for penicillin-sensitive pneumococci, ensuring a minimum inhibitory concentration (MIC) <0.1 mg/ml.

In general, 7 days of therapy is necessary for meningococci, 10 days for *H. influenzae* and 14 days for pneumococci. Adjunctive **corticosteroid** use in children decreases hearing loss from *H. influenzae* meningitis. Its role in adults remains controversial. Complications of meningitis include cerebral edema, brain abscess, residual neurologic deficit(s), particularly hearing deficit.

■ **Prevention**

Close contacts of patients with meningococcal meningitis, defined as household members, daycare contacts, or medical personnel performing mouth-to-mouth resuscitation, are at a 500-fold to 800-fold increased risk of developing meningococcal meningitis. Rifampin, 600 mg every 12 hours for 2 days or a single-dose quinolone, are effective prophylactic agents.

Aseptic Meningitis

Aseptic meningitis is a misnomer, since it denotes culture-negative meningitis (usually with lymphocytic predominance in the CSF), even though infectious agents are usually the cause (Table 153.5). In particular, viral agents are the most common cause, with enterovirus leading the list (coxsackievirus and ECHOvirus).

The classic clinical presentation includes headache, fever, and neck pain and stiffness (meningismus) in children or young adults during the summer months. The CSF may be neutrophilic in two-thirds of patients (usually <200 cells/mm^3), initially with mononuclear predominance occurring in 6–24 hours. The CSF glucose level is usually normal, and protein is below 100 mg/dl. Cultures of CSF and throat swabs may be positive.

Subacute (Chronic) Meningitis

The classic definition of subacute or chronic meningitis is a meningitis exceeding 4 weeks' duration. The diagnosis can further be classified into **lymphocytic** or **neutrophilic** meningitis (Table 153.6).

Routine laboratory evaluation of the CSF may include the following tests: cryptococcal antigen, VDRL, complement fixation for coccidioides and histoplasma, Lyme index, cytology, brucella and mycobacterial cultures. High-volume lumbar punctures with multiple cultures may be necessary. If no diagnosis is made and clinical status is worsening, then treatment for tuberculosis should be initiated.

Encephalitis

Encephalitis is characterized by fever, altered sensorium, seizures, and focal neurologic deficits. There may be evidence of meningeal irritation as well. Classically, encephalitis is viral in etiology, with **herpes simplex virus** (HSV) being the most common cause. However, nonviral causes may masquerade as herpes encephalitis (Table 153.7).

The pathogenesis usually involves viremia by neurotropic viruses with hematogenous seeding of the brain or ascent of viruses to the brain via peripheral nerves (e.g., HSV via the olfactory nerve or as with rabies). In HSV, the transmission is slow. Invasion of the host cell is followed by viral replication and cessation of, or interference with, cellular function. In most cases, such infections are subclinical.

Encephalitis may be epidemic or nonepidemic. Epidemic forms include **mosquito-borne arborvirus encephalitides** including St. Louis, La Crosse, and eastern and western equine encephalitis in the United States; Japanese encephalitis is common in Southeast Asia. Rarely, enteroviruses or measles virus may cause an encephalitis. The nonepidemic form is most commonly HSV. Rabies is very uncommon in the United States.

■ Clinical Features

The clinical presentation does not allow differentiation between the different causes. However, epidemiologic clues are useful. History of travel and contact with animals are important factors in the history. A history of animal bite is useful in the diagnosis of rabies.

At the onset, generally there is fever, altered sensorium, headache, vomiting, and confusion. Seizures may occur. Hyperpyrexia indicates involvement of the pontine temperature regulatory center. HSV encephalitis classically has bizarre behavior and hallucinations suggestive of a temporal lobe focus. There may be hydrophobia reported in rabies.

The course may be one of relentless progression, culminating in death (massive cortical destruction), or one of quick recovery with minimal or no sequelae (effective host response offsetting cellular damage). Progression followed by stability and slow recovery may also occur.

■ Diagnostic Tests

Specific microbiologic diagnosis is difficult in encephalitis. The CSF response is nonspecific and may be normal in HSV in 5–10% of cases. Magnetic resonance imaging and electroencephalography may be suggestive of HSV, but their specificity is unknown. **Polymerase chain reaction** of the CSF has become the best tool for diagnosing HSV, short of brain biopsy.

Acute and convalescent titers may be helpful, retrospectively, for the epidemic viruses only. Recently, an IgM antibody to the arboviruses has been developed and may be diagnostic upon presentation.

■ Management

Management of encephalitis is complicated by the nonspecific clinical picture for individual causative agents. The difficulty in making a specific microbiologic diagnosis and in ruling out HSV and the clinician's reluctance to perform a brain biopsy for HSV further compound the management dilemma. Because of these factors and because HSV is the only treatable cause, acyclovir is usually given at 10 mg/kg every 8 hours for 10–14 days whenever HSV is a possible cause. Patients whose condition progresses despite treatment should undergo brain biopsy.

TABLE 153.7.	Diseases That Mimic the Presentation of HSV Encephalitis

Bacterial abscess
Listeria
Mycoplasma
Fungal
Rickettsial
Togavirus
Mononucleosis
Tumor
Vasculitis
Subdural hematoma

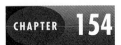

BACTEREMIA, SEPSIS, AND SEPTIC SYNDROME

Bacteremia

Bacteremia is defined as the invasion of blood by bacteria, as detected by blood cultures. Because blood circulates in a closed system, bacteremia always presupposes an infectious focus elsewhere in the body (the source), from which the blood becomes "seeded." Bacteremia also forms the quintessential diagnostic feature of infective endocarditis.

For any infection, bacterial or otherwise, the development of bloodstream invasion portends a worse prognosis and a major threat to life. Bacteremic patients have a higher rate of complications, longer hospital stay, and higher mortality. Bacteremia carries an overall mortality of 30%, which is influenced by several factors, such as the source, identity, and virulence of the organism, on one hand, and a number of host factors on the other, including the status of the specific defenses, functional status, underlying diseases, and the presence or absence of complications.

■ Epidemiology

Bacteremias may be transient, intermittent, or continuous. **Transient** bacteremia may follow dental manipulations or instrumentation of infected areas, such as dental procedures or even brushing teeth. Bacteremia that complicates undrained abscesses is generally **intermittent.** In conditions characterized by endovascular infection (endocarditis, endarteritis, or septic thrombophlebitis), the bacteremia is **continuous.**

In general medical wards, bacteremia is much more prevalent among the elderly and those with diabetes mellitus, cerebrovascular accidents, underlying neoplastic disease, or chronic renal failure.

The prevalence of bacteremia may vary, depending on the amount of blood that is obtained for individual blood cultures, since it has been shown that use of a larger volume of blood (15 ml or greater per culture) increases the rate of detection of bacteremia. The epidemiology of bacteremia differs, depending on whether it is community-acquired or nosocomial. By tradition, bacteremia detected within 72 hours of hospitalization is considered community-acquired (unless the patient was, until then, a resident of a long-term care facility). While the use of 72 hours may seem arbitrary, the separation of bacteremias into community-acquired and nosocomial has clear implications in terms of the organism(s) involved, source of the bacteremia, complication rate, and mortality.

Community-acquired bacteremia

Community-acquired bacteremia is more frequent among the elderly. The most frequent sources and most common organisms are listed in Table 154.1. In some cases, more than one organism may be detected in blood cultures. Once contamination has been excluded, polymicrobial bacteremia suggests the biliary tract, intra-abdominal sepsis, or urinary tract infection as a source.

Some organisms tend to be associated with specific underlying infections (e.g., pneumococcal bacteremia with pneumonia). It is also important to note that in some cases, the source may remain elusive after a diligent search, a feature most likely to occur with *E. coli,* Enterococcus, Pseudomonas, Bacteroides, and some polymicrobial bacteremias.

TABLE 154.1.	Community-Acquired Bacteremia: Most Frequent Source(s) and Common Organisms	
Organism	**Most Likely Primary Infectious Process/Source**	**Next Most Likely Source**
Escherichia coli	Urinary tract infection	Biliary tract (unknown in some cases)
Streptococcus pneumoniae	Pneumonia	Meningitis
Klebsiella species	Biliary tract	Urinary tract/Lower respiratory tract
Staphylococcus aureus	Lower respiratory tract	Endocarditis
Enterococcus	Urinary tract	
Proteus	Urinary tract	
Pseudomonas	Urinary tract	
Streptococcus bovis	Endocarditis	
Streptococcus viridans	Endocarditis	

(Data from: Esposito AL, Gleckman RA, Cram S, et al. Community-acquired bacteremia in the elderly: analysis of one hundred consecutive episodes. J Am Geriatr Soc 1980;18:315–319.)

TABLE 154.2.	Risk Factors for Nosocomial Bacteremia

Host factors
  Elderly patient
  Systemic antimicrobial therapy
  Multiple trauma or burns
  Life-threatening underlying illness
  Granulocytopenia
  Immunosuppression (corticosteroids or cytotoxic
    agents)
Environmental factors
  Intensive care unit
  Vascular or nonvascular invasive device
  Hemodialysis
  Infusion of large volume of parenteral fluids or blood
    products

(Adapted from: Maki DG. Am J Med 1981;70:724. Used with permission.)

Nosocomial bacteremia

Nosocomial bacteremias may be primary or secondary. A focus (source) is identifiable in the secondary and absent in the primary types. However, bacteremia occurring from an intravascular device in the absence of local purulent infection at the infusion site is also considered primary nosocomial bacteremia. Nosocomial bacteremia may also be endemic or epidemic.

Risk factors for nosocomial bacteremia are summarized in Table 154.2. Most endemic nosocomial bacteremias arise from skin (e.g., postoperative wound or intravenous catheter infections), intra-abdominal, urinary tract, pulmonary (pneumonias), or other focal infections. The most common organisms causing endemic nosocomial bacteremias are *Staphylococcus aureus, S. epidermidis,* Klebsiella, group D streptococcus, *S. pneumoniae,* and *Escherichia coli.*

■ Clinical Features

Features of bacteremia are listed in Table 154.3. **Fever** and **shaking chills** are classic symptoms, but rigors may be absent in the debilitated patient. In a significant number of patients, the fever and chills are preceded by **hyperventilation** and **changes in mental status. Hypotension** may be present in those who manifest septic shock. A **decline in urinary output** may also be noted. Patients with gram-positive bacteremias may show diffuse reddening of the skin (erythroderma), and those with Pseudomonas bacteremias may show a central vesicular lesion surrounded by a halo of erythema and induration, which becomes ulcerated (**ecthyma gangrenosum).** Hemodynamic compromise may develop when bacteremia evolves into septic shock or systemic inflammatory response syndrome (SIRS). Multiorgan failure may evolve.

Although fever is the general rule, bacteremia without fever has been well-documented. The elderly, especially those with associated renal failure or hypoalbuminemia, seem to exhibit this feature more frequently. Bacteremia may be detected incidentally in these persons from the blood cultures performed to elucidate some other disturbance. Whereas the lack of fever is a poor prognostic sign, the development of hypothermia is even more ominous.

Although further validation is necessary, five variables apparent within 24 hours of hospitalization have been proposed that may have a high predictive value for bacteremia: a low performance status prior to hospitalization, chills on admission, renal failure, low serum albumin, and presumptive admitting diagnosis of urinary tract infection.

■ Management

Major problems related to blood cultures are the false-positive (positive blood culture with no bacteremia) and false-negative cultures. The frequency of false-positive blood cultures varies widely, and most are related to contamination from the skin flora. Clues to recognize false-positive cultures are listed in Table 154.4. False-negative cultures may be due to an inadequate volume of blood sampled, inadequate number of blood cultures obtained, or the low prevalence of the bacteremia in a given condition (low pre-test probability).

Guidelines for the use of blood cultures to diagnose bacteremia are shown in Table 154.5. Use of a larger volume of blood (>15 ml/culture) increases the rate of detection of bacteremia. An underlying issue in many false-positive cultures is improper technique, which is remediable with proper education.

Patients who manifest symptoms suspicious for bacteremia should have a blood culture performed. A careful assessment is necessary to elucidate the source.

TABLE 154.3.	Manifestations of Bacteremia

Fever
Confusion, drowsiness, delirium
Lethargy
Tachycardia
Hyperventilation
Chills/rigors
Hypotension
Nausea/vomiting
Hypotension
Diarrhea
Falls†
Incontinence from altered mentation†

†In the elderly.

TABLE 154.4.	**Clues to False-Positive Blood Cultures**

Isolation of the following organisms:
  Diphtheroids
  Staphylococcus epidermidis
  Bacillus species**
Inability to isolate same organisms in subsequent cultures
Isolation of multiple organisms in the same culture
Isolation of organism after delayed bacterial growth
  (broth only)
Same species, but with varying antibiotic sensitivity
  patterns
Lack of correlation with clinical course
  No identifiable primary infection by the same organism
Lack of identifiable predisposing factors, such as
  Prosthetic devices
  Intravenous drug abuse
  Recent hospitalization
  Immunosuppression
Lack of leukocytosis or left shift

**Isolation of enteric gram-negative aerobic organisms, *Streptococcus pyogenes* or *Streptococcus pneumoniae* are seldom false-positive.
(Adapted from: Aronson MD, Bor DH. Ann Intern Med 1987;106:246–253. Used with permission.)

Once the necessary laboratory material is obtained for examination, the patient should be started on appropriate **antibiotic therapy.** Because the exact organism is not known initially, treatment is empiric, until culture results become available. The initial choice of antibiotics should cover the most likely organisms. Because gram-negative organisms are the most common in community-acquired bacteremia, an aminoglycoside and antipseudomonal penicillin would suffice. If *Staphylococcus. aureus* bacteremia is suspected, nafcillin or vancomycin should be added.

Catheter-related infections

The association of bacteremia with a catheter requires quantitative methods. In suspected cases of intravascular catheter-related infections, the catheter should be removed, and the distal two inches of the catheter should be aseptically clipped into a sterile container and sent for quantitative cultures. In addition, blood cultures should also be obtained. Others have recommended obtaining 2 sets of blood cultures, one through the intravascular line and another from a peripheral vein. Because the catheters are often colo-

nized, such colonizing organisms are isolated from the culture drawn through the catheter. Aerobic organisms (S. aureus, S. epidermidis, Klebsiella and so forth) are usually responsible, and the initial antibiotic management should take into account these possibilities.

Intravenous hyperalimentation solutions are another potential source of nosocomial bacteremia, but with a dedicated team for initiating the catheter insertion and its follow-up care, this can be minimized.

■ Complications and Prognosis

Bacteremia carries a high overall mortality of 30%. The mortality rises with increasing age and with hospital-acquired bacteremias. The mortality from pneumococcal bacteremia seems to have changed little over the decades and stands at 20%, with most deaths occurring within the first 48 hours of hospitalization.

TABLE 154.5.	**Guidelines for Blood Cultures**

1. Use strict asepsis (disinfect the skin).
2. Draw at least 10 ml of blood per culture, preferably more.
3. Draw blood through a closed collecting system or syringe and needle and transfer into the culture bottle. Disinfect the rubber stoppers of bottles before inoculating the medium.
4. Never draw blood for culture through an indwelling catheter.
5. Use universal precautions, as for handling all body fluids.
6. One blood culture is seldom enough; obtain multiple cultures.
7. If the anticipated organisms can be mistaken for a skin contaminant (e.g., *S. epidermidis* when a prosthetic valve endocarditis is suspected), then multiple sets of cultures should yield the same organism.
8. The number of cultures required depends on the anticipated organism (AO) and the pretest probability of bacteremia.
   a. If the AO is not usually a contaminant, and probability is moderate—obtain 2 sets.
   b. If continuous bacteremia is suspected—obtain 3 sets.
   c. If there has been prior antibiotic therapy—obtain 4 sets.

(Adapted from: Aronson MD, Bor DH. Ann Intern Med 1987;106: 246–253. Used with permission.)

Sepsis and Sepsis Syndrome

The terminology and nomenclature of sepsis, as prepared by the Society of Critical Care Medicine, is shown in Table 154.6.

■ Pathophysiology

Although any organism can cause sepsis, sepsis involving gram-negative organisms has been best stud-

TABLE 154.6.	Terminology for "Sepsis"
Term	**Definition**
Sepsis	Evidence of infection plus ≥2 of the following: Temperature >38°C or <36°C Heart rate >90 bpm Respiratory rate >20/min or PaCO₂ <32 mm Hg WBC >12,000/mm³ or <4000/mm³
Sepsis syndrome	Sepsis plus organ hypoperfusion: hypoxemia, oliguria, altered mentation.
Hypotension	BP <90 mm Hg or reduction >40 mm Hg from baseline
Severe sepsis	Sepsis with organ dysfunction, hypoperfusion or hypotension; including lactic acidosis, oliguria or altered mental status
Septic shock	Sepsis with hypotension despite fluids, plus above criteria for severe sepsis
Refractory septic shock	Shock lasting >1 hr despite intervention

cascade, and endothelial damage. What results are the signs and symptoms identified with sepsis (see below). The irony is that in low doses, TNF and IL-1 are protective, priming host defenses, but their massive production as in sepsis can be lethal.

■ **Clinical Features**

The earliest manifestation of sepsis is **hyperventilation,** occurring even before fever. **Fever** is typical, but hypothermia may occur and portends a poor prognosis. Mental status changes, especially lethargy, and rarely agitation may occur. Further complications may include hypotension (initially; from vasodilation or "warm shock"), characterized by decreased peripheral and pulmonary vascular resistances. The cardiac index may be elevated.

Thrombocytopenia (with or without a coagulopathy) and organ failure, including respiratory failure (hypoxia, adult respiratory distress syndrome [ARDS]), renal failure (oliguria), or liver failure (jaundice, hepatic encephalopathy), may be associated or follow. Hypoperfusion may cause lactic acidosis. The picture at this point is one of diffuse, pan-endothelial dysfunction, with enhanced capillary permeability affecting many organs, such as gut, liver, and lungs.

ied. The bacterial **endotoxin,** which is responsible for initiating sepsis, is a lipopolysaccharide making up part of the cell wall. This lipid moiety is relatively conserved among all gram-negative bacteria and is responsible for triggering sepsis via cytokines.

The **cytokines,** especially tumor necrosis factor (TNF) and interleukin-1 (IL-1), are macrophage-derived and are the primary mediators of sepsis. TNF causes the release of prostaglandins, platelet-activating factors, leukotrienes, and thromboxane, which results in excessive vascular permeability, activation of the clotting

■ **Management**

A good **history** is a key component of the clinical evaluation. Attention to underlying diseases, travel, exposures, and other factors is essential. Signs and symptoms pointing to a nidus should be sought (e.g., headache, joint pain, or diarrhea may suggest the site of focal infection). Careful, thorough **physical examination** should be completed with the realization that in

TABLE 154.7.	Empiric Antibiotic Therapy for Sepsis Syndrome		
Disease		**First Choice**	**Alternates**
Non-neutropenic	Community-acquired UTI	Third-generation cephalosporin ± aminoglycoside	Piperacillin-tazobactam/ticarcillin ± aminoglycoside
	Community-acquired infection, not UTI	Third-generation cephalosporin ± aminoglycoside	Ticarcillin-clavulanic acid ± aminoglycoside or Ampicillin-sulbactam ± aminoglycoside
	Hospital-acquired	Third-generation cephalosporin ⊕ Metronidazole ⊕ aminoglycoside	Ampicillin-sulbactam ± aminoglycoside or imipenem + aminoglycoside
Neutropenic		Ticarcillin-clavulanic acid + aminoglycoside	Imipenem + aminoglycoside or Piperacillin-tazobactam + aminoglycoside
IV Catheter-related		Same as neutropenic + vancomycin	Same as neutropenic + vancomycin

UTI = urinary tract infection.

immunosuppressed hosts, disease manifestations may be blunted. Two sets of **blood cultures** should be taken.

Further testing is dictated by the clinical setting. Usually, complete blood counts, liver function tests, and coagulation studies are performed. If no nidus is apparent, a urinalysis and chest radiograph should be done. Abdominal pain should prompt surgical consultation. Obstructing hydronephrosis should be excluded if a urinary tract infection is the nidus. One should always consider diseases that require immediate surgical intervention.

Appropriate **antibiotic selection** is extremely important in the early phases of sepsis, as mortality is reduced as much as 50% when antibiotics are chosen properly. Because microbiologic data are not available for 1–2 days, initial antibiotic selection is empiric. The clinical setting should dictate antibiotic selection (Table 154.7). The hospital's **antibiogram** (antibiotic resistance patterns) must also be considered, and recommendations may vary for individual institutions. If aminoglycosides are used, aggressive dosing is essential for sepsis, because they have concentration-dependent killing.

CHAPTER 155 NOSOCOMIAL INFECTIONS

Nosocomial infections are usually defined as infections acquired 48–72 hours after hospital admission. Approximately 5% of hospitalized patients develop a nosocomial infection, with urinary tract infection (UTI) being the most common. Other sites include the respiratory tract, surgical wounds, intravascular catheters, nonvascular prostheses, and instrumentation (e.g., endoscopy).

The microbiology varies according to site (Table

155.1), and rates for nosocomial infection vary according patient population. Hospital size influences nosocomial infection rates, with the highest incidence (8.5%) being in municipal teaching hospitals and the lowest (3.7%) in small nonteaching hospitals.

Nosocomial bacteremia is discussed in chapter 154, and nosocomial pneumonia, in chapter 148. Suggested antibiotic selection for nosocomial infections is provided in Table 155.2.

TABLE 155.1. The Microbiology of Nosocomial Infections According to Site*

Urinary tract infection	Pneumonia	IV catheter-related
Short-term catheterization	*Frequent pathogens*	*Staphylococcus aureus*
Escherichia coli	*Pseudomonas aeruginosa*	*Staphylococcus epidermidis*
Yeast	*Staphylococcus aureus*	Gram negative bacilli
Pseudomonas aeruginosa	Enterobacter spp	Candida spp.
Klebsiella spp.	Klebsiella spp.	
Coagulase negative staphylococci	*Escherichia coli*	
Other gram-negative bacilli	*Haemophilus influenzae*	
Proteus spp.	*Serratia marcescens*	
Long-term catheterization	*Streptococcus pneumoniae*	
Providencia spp.	*Infreqnent pathogens*	
Proteus spp.	*Streptococcus pneumoniae*	
Escherichia coli	Legionella spp.	
Pseudomonas aeruginosa	Influenza	
Enterococcus spp.	**Surgical wounds**	
Morganella morganii	*Staphylococcus aureus*	
Klebsiella spp.	Enterococcus spp.	
	Coagulase-negative staphylococci	
	Escherichia coli	
	Pseudomonas spp.	

*Causative organisms are arranged in the order of prevalence.

TABLE 155.2.	Suggested Antibiotic Selection for Nosocomial Infections	
Site	**Likely Organism**	**Antibiotic**
Urinary Tract	Enterobacteriaceae	Aminoglycoside, third generation cephalosporin, extended spectrum penicillin or quinolone
	Enterococcus	Ampicillin plus aminoglycoside
IV catheter	Staphylococci	Nafcillin plus aminoglycoside; vancomycin + third generation cephalosporin if MRSA is endemic, or imipenem–cilastatin
Pneumonia	S. pneumoniae	Penicillin G or vancomycin
	S. aureus	Nafcillin (vancomycin if MRSA is endemic)
	P aeruginosa	Ticarcillin plus aminoglycoside or piperacillin plus aminoglycoside
	H. influenzae	Ampicillin or cefuroxime
Site Unknown	Organism unknown, urgent empiric therapy needed	See Table 154.5

MRSA = Methicillin-resistant *Staphylococcus aureus*.

Urinary Tract Infection

Most nosocomial UTIs (80%) are catheter-associated, with an additional 10% following genitourinary manipulations. **Catheter-associated bacteremia** occurs at a rate of around 5% per day. Organisms from the patient's own colonic flora first colonize the urethra and then ascend the catheter's extraluminal surface. Intraluminal entry is much less frequent since closed systems have become standard.

Certain independent factors have been associated with the risk for **bacteriuria,** especially length of catheterization, gender (woman), diabetes, and periurethral colonization. The colonizing organism may change every 1–2 weeks. Long-term catheterized patients have complications with infected urinary stones (struvite) or periurinary infections.

Treatment is unnecessary for asymptomatic bacteriuria in catheterized patients. Bacteriuria persisting after removal of the catheter may indicate a higher likelihood of UTI and thus may warrant a short course of antibiotics. Ampicillin (for Enterococcus) and tobramycin (for gram-negative organisms) are reasonable empiric antibiotic selections for catheter-associated UTI. Changing of the catheter because of bacterial biofilm on catheters is not unreasonable.

Treatment of **candiduria** remains controversial. Bladder irrigation with amphotericin (50 mg in 1-liter sterile water) is of unknown value. Persistence of candiduria after irrigation, however, may suggest UTI. Fluconazole, being renally excreted, may be beneficial for fungal UTI, especially with *Candida albicans*. Upper urinary tract disease should be a consideration (i.e., fungus ball) in difficult-to-treat patients and may require ultrasound or CT for evaluation.

Obviously, avoidance of catheterization is the best prevention. External devices (e.g., condom catheters or intermittent catheterization) are alternative solutions. Suprapubic catheters may have lower rates of bacteriuria (less colonization of abdominal skin) and may help avoid problems of urethral strictures. The role for catheters impregnated with antimicrobials (i.e., silver-impregnated catheters) for prevention of bacteriuria is unclear. Oral antibiotics may prevent bacteriuria for a few days but may lead to selection of resistant microbes.

CHAPTER 156

SKIN, SOFT TISSUE, AND BONE INFECTIONS

Cellulitis

Cellulitis is an acute infection involving the deeper dermis and subcutaneous fatty tissues. It is most commonly caused by *Streptococcus pyogenes* and *Staphylococcus aureus*. Factors predisposing to bacterial invasion are usually present (Table 156.1).

The involved area becomes warm, swollen, and

TABLE 156.1.	Causes of Cellulitis and Associated Conditions	
Etiologic Agents	**Predisposing Conditions**	**Antimicrobial Agents**
Streptococcus pyogenes (and other streptococci)	Trauma, puncture wound, tinea pedis	Penicillin, erythromycin
Staphylococcus aureus	Trauma, puncture wound, tinea pedis	Penicillinase-resistant penicillin (e.g.. nafcillin, vancomycin)
Gram-negative bacteria (e.g., Enterobacteriaceae, Serratia, Pseudomonas, Proteus spp.)	Granulocytopenia	Third-generation cephalosporins, extended spectrum penicillins, quinolones, aminoglycosides
Vibrio spp (e.g., *Vibrio vulnificus, Vibrio parahaemolyticus*)	Traumatic wound in salt water or brackish inland water	Chloramphenicol, tetracycline, aminoglycosides
Aeromonas hydrophila	Traumatic wound in freshwater	Third-generation cephalosporins, quinolones, aztreonam, aminoglycosides
Erysipelothrix rhusiopathiae	Abrasion from handling saltwater fish, poultry, meat, hides	Penicillin
Clostridium perfringens	Contaminated traumatic or surgical wound	Penicillin
Nonclostridial anaerobic cellulitis (Bacteroides, Peptostreptococcus, Peptococcus, aerobic streptococci, gram negative bacilli)	Diabetes mellitus, local trauma	Broad spectrum therapy to cover the range of pathogens

erythematous, sometimes with lymphangitis, regional adenopathy, chills, and fever. Unlike **erysipelas,** the borders of the lesions lack distinct boundaries and are not elevated; however, like erysipelas, the diagnosis is usually clinical. Aspirating the leading edge of the cellulitis yields an etiologic diagnosis in only about 25% of cases. If the patient is febrile, blood cultures should be obtained.

Although most cases of cellulitis are due to *Streptococcus pyogenes, Staphylococcus aureus* is also covered by treatment with a penicillinase-resistant penicillin. Serious cases require parenteral therapy until clinical improvement occurs, when one may substitute oral therapy. Certain types of cellulitis with tissue necrosis (e.g., clostridial anaerobic cellulitis) require both antibiotics and surgical debridement.

Necrotizing Fasciitis

Necrotizing fasciitis is an infrequent infection of subcutaneous and fascial tissues. There are 2 types: one is due to *Streptococcus pyogenes,* and the other is caused by a mixture of anaerobes (e.g., Bacteroides or Peptostreptococcus species) and aerobes, including gram-positive cocci (e.g., staphylococci, streptococci, enterococci) and gram-negative bacilli (e.g., *Escherichia coli,* Klebsiella, Enterobacter, Proteus species). The first type tends to follow minor trauma in the extremities. Underlying diabetes mellitus, drug abuse, and alcoholism are generally present. The mixed infection tends to follow abdominal surgery or bowel perforation secondary to a gastrointestinal neoplasm or diverticulitis. In both types, patients have high fever and appear seriously ill.

A type of necrotizing fasciitis of the male genitalia, a mixed anaerobic and aerobic infection, is **Fournier's**

gangrene. The patient, generally a diabetic, has had a recent local skin, perianal, or urinary tract infection that rapidly spreads into the genital soft tissues, causing swelling, erythema, and crepitation.

In necrotizing fasciitis, the affected soft tissues display rapidly progressive and very painful erythema. Necrosis of underlying tissues and destruction of vessels and cutaneous nerves follow. Consequently, changes in the skin color, skin breakdown, and variable degrees of anesthesia result. In the mixed infection, tissue gas and a foul odor may be present, which are absent with streptococcal fasciitis. Therapy for necrotizing fasciitis includes immediate surgical debridement and antibiotics—a combination to cover the mixed flora is appropriate before definite microbiologic data are available.

Myositis with Eosinophilia

Helminthic infections with muscle involvement often manifest eosinophilia, which helps distinguish these processes. Examples that may be seen in the United States include the nematode *Trichinella spiralis* and the cestode *Taenia solium.*

Trichinosis follows the ingestion of undercooked infected pork. By the second week of infection, Trichinella larvae enter the circulation and invade skeletal muscle, where they cause muscle pain, swelling, and weakness. Extraocular muscle involvement causes a prominent periorbital edema. The diagnosis is usually made serologically. Muscle biopsy, when performed, shows encysted larvae, with muscle necrosis and a predominantly eosinophilic infiltrate (Figure 156.1).

Cysticercosis, which occurs primarily in visitors or immigrants from endemic areas (e.g., Mexico, South America, Africa) is transmitted by ingestion of food contaminated with *Taenia solium* (pork tapeworm) eggs. Widespread systemic involvement follows, including the CNS, subcutaneous tissues, and muscle (Figure 156.2). Muscle involvement is usually asymptomatic and often-

detected by the appearance of calcified cysts on radiographs. The diagnosis, as with trichinosis, is usually made serologically.

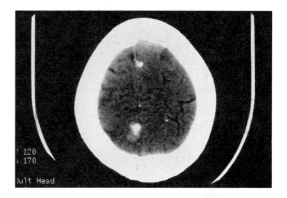

FIGURE 156.2. Cerebral cysticercosis. A CT scan first suggested this diagnosis in this patient with seizures.
(Courtesy of Katherine Slattery, MD, Medical College of Wisconsin, Milwaukee, Wisconsin.)

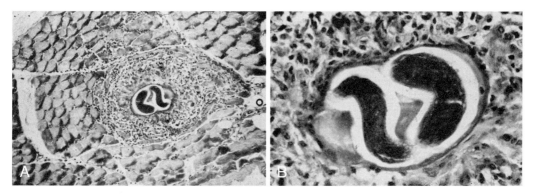

FIGURE 156.1. Trichinosis. A, Muscle biopsy showing encysted larvae of *Trichinella spiralis,* with muscle necrosis and a predominantly eosinophilic infiltrate. B, Magnified view of encysted larva.
(Courtesy of Lawrence S. Hurwitz, MD, Milwaukee, Wisconsin.)

Infected Bite Wounds

Bite wounds are common from dogs, cats, and humans, and the likelihood of infection at the site depends on the degree of tissue injury and delay in obtaining appropriate wound care. Although there is usually a localized cellulitis, there may be a deeper soft-tissue infection (including abscesses), septic arthritis, or osteomyelitis or metastatic foci from bacteremia.

Common infecting organisms and the usual therapeutic options are listed in Table 156.2. Some patients with more severe infections may need equivalent types of parenteral antibiotics and surgical debridement. The need for tetanus and/or rabies vaccines should be assessed as well.

TABLE 156.2.	Bite Wound Infections	
Type of Bite	**Usual Infecting Organisms**	**Antimicrobial Therapy**
Dog or cat	*Pasteurella multocida* *Staphylococcus aureus* Streptococcus spp. Prevotella spp. Fusobacterium spp.	Amoxicillin-clavulanic acid, penicillin, or ampicillin
Human	Streptococcus spp., *Staphylococcus aureus,* Prevotella spp. Peptostreptococcus spp. Fusobacterium spp.	Amoxicillin-clavulanic acid, penicillin, or ampicillin

Osteomyelitis

Osteomyelitis, or bone infection, is primarily bacterial, occurring either hematogenously or by contiguous extension from a soft-tissue focus of infection. Some clinical examples and typical organisms are outlined in Table 156.3. Bone infection is associated with tissue edema and vascular occlusion. With chronic infection, areas of bony necrosis, termed **sequestra,** develop.

Characteristically, the symptoms are subacute or chronic, despite the well-known acute presentation in adults with localized pain and fever (more common with the hematogenous type). Fever may or may not be present. The onset may be particularly insidious in the diabetic patient with peripheral neuropathy, owing to the lack of sensation in the extremity, and it may present with a nonhealing, chronically draining ulcer.

Bone **radiographs** may reveal nonspecific changes or the typical periosteal elevation and soft tissue swelling, but these changes lag behind the clinical disease process. Radionuclide studies or MRI can detect these inflammatory changes sooner and with more accuracy. Definitive diagnosis of osteomyelitis, however, is by culturing a biopsy or aspirate of affected bone. Except for infections involving *S. aureus,* culture of the sinus tract does not yield a good correlation with cultures of bone.

Osteomyelitis is treated using an antibiotic appropriate for the pathogen. **Antibiotics** are traditionally given parenterally for 4–6 weeks, although long-term oral antibiotics are appropriate in certain settings (e.g., oral quinolones for sensitive gram-negative organisms). Surgical debridement may be integral to successful therapy in selected cases, especially in chronic osteomyelitis where necrotic bone precludes proper penetration of antibiotics. With preexisting ulcers or prior debridement, tissue flaps may be necessary.

TABLE 156.3.	Categories and Etiology of Osteomyelitis
Underlying Disease	**Typical Organisms**
Hematogenous spread 　Endocarditis, infected 　intravascular catheter, 　urinary tract infection, 　IV drug use	*Staphylococcus aureus,* *Pseudomonas aeruginosa* (and other gram- negative bacilli), Candida spp.
Sickle cell disease	Salmonella spp., *Staphylococcus aureus*
Secondary to a contiguous focus 　Without vascular 　insufficiency	*Staphylococcus aureus,* gram-negative bacilli, anaerobes
Contamination 　from surgery or 　trauma, local soft 　tissue infection 　(e.g. decubitus 　ulcer)	
With vascular insufficiency 　　Lower-extremity 　　soft-tissue injury 　　in a patient with 　　diabetic neuropathy 　　and vascular 　　insufficiency	Staphylococci, streptococci, enterococci, gram-negative bacilli, anaerobes

Recurrences are well-known, particularly in the diabetic patient. In these patients, antibiotic therapy is termed **suppressive** and not medically eradicative. Over time, continued infection may necessitate an amputation.

Infection in Orthopedic Prosthetic Devices

Orthopedic prosthetic devices have an infection rate of 1–5%. Infection, usually initiated at the bone-cement interface, occurs by local introduction of organisms or, less commonly, hematogenously. Staphylococci (both coagulase-negative and -positive) are the most frequent pathogens, followed by streptococci and gram-negative bacilli.

Although an acute clinical presentation occurs with joint pain and fever in some patients, the typical onset is more insidious. Diagnosis rests on sampling joint fluid and isolating the pathogen. When the diagnosis is in question, more than one arthrocentesis should be performed to confirm the pathogen. Successful treatment usually involves removal of the prosthesis, followed by a 6-week course of appropriate antibiotics and then reimplantation.

CHAPTER 157 INFECTIONS IN THE IMMUNOCOMPROMISED HOST

This chapter explores infections in patients with relatively common acquired immunosuppressive conditions, such as trauma, cancer, and transplantation. Each of these conditions is associated with specific defects in host immunity (see chapter 141), with an associated set of typical pathogens. Additional information about immunodeficiencies is also given in Chapter 14. Infection with the human immunodeficiency virus is discussed in chapter 158.

Infections in Patients with Trauma

Examples of physical injury with prominent infectious complications include major burns and trauma (e.g., multiple trauma, spinal cord injury).

Major blunt or penetrating trauma, such as that from an automobile accident compromises the host defenses and increases risk of infection. Natural cutaneous barriers are violated and injured tissues made nonviable and ischemic; thus, the ability of the host to combat invading microbes is imperiled.

The nature and geographic location of the injury predisposes to certain types of microbes (e.g., injuries contaminated with freshwater may lead to wound infection with *Aeromonas hydrophila*). Although aggressive resuscitation enhances survival, it also contributes partly to the significantly increased infection-related mortality in this population. An overview of infections in trauma patients and their mechanisms is provided in Table 157.1.

TABLE 157.1. Infections in Patients with Severe Trauma		
Site	**Cause for Predisposition at This Site**	**Usual Organisms Involved**
Wound	Blunt or penetrating trauma	*Staphylococcus aureus*, Streptococci Possible mixed flora
Urinary tract	Urinary catheters	Gram-negative rods, Enterococcus spp.
Lower respiratory tract	Endotracheal intubation, sedation, aspiration, chest trauma	*Haemophilus influenzae* *Staphylococcus aureus* Gram-negative rods
IV line-associated bacteremia	Nonsterile insertion, contamination from proximate wounds, frequent manipulation	*Staphylococcus aureus* Coagulase-negative staphylococci
GI tract-associated sepsis	Penetrating trauma, shock, bacterial translocation	Gram-negative rods Enterococcus spp. Anaerobes
CNS	Basilar skull fracture, CSF leak, CSF catheters	Gram-negative rods *Staphylococcus aureus*
Pleural space	Chest tubes	Staphylococcus aureus Gram-negative rods

Infections in Spinal Cord Injury Patients

Spinal cord injury often follows traumatic injury and may occur with multiple trauma. However, the patient who is chronically or permanently disabled from spinal cord injury is also at risk for infectious complications, generally because of a breakdown of the natural defense barriers. Some of the more common causes or sites of infection, predisposing factors, and organisms are outlined in Table 157.2.

TABLE 157.2. Causes of Infection in Patients With Spinal Cord Injury		
Site	**Cause for Predisposition at This Site**	**Usual Organisms Involved**
Lower respiratory tract	Aspiration, poor cough causing inability to clear secretions	*Streptococcus pneumoniae* *Haemophilus influenzae* Gram-negative bacilli *Staphylococcus aureus*
Urinary tract	Urinary stasis, catheterization	Gram-negative bacilli *Enterococcus* spp.
Skin and soft tissue	Pressure sores, wound contamination	*Staphylococcus aureus* *Streptococcus* spp. Possible mixed flora
Bone	Pressure sores, wound contamination	*Staphylococcus aureus* Streptococcal species Gram-negative bacilli Anaerobes
Intra-abdominal Gallbladder, pancreas	Cholelithiasis	Gram-negative bacilli *Enterococcus* spp.
Colon	Antibiotics	*Clostridium difficile*

Infections in Patients with Cancer

Patients with malignant disease may be at risk for infectious complications for a variety of reasons. Host defense defects in these patients may result from impaired clearance of microbes, destruction of normal defense barriers, and tumor or treatment-related effects. Major immunodeficient states common to cancer patients, including likely infecting organisms seen with each deficiency, are listed in Table 157.3. There is very little overlap in pathogenic organisms among these three immunodeficient states, and so, once the immune deficiency is recognized, it has profound implications for an empiric therapeutic approach. Multiple defects may occur in the same patient, however, leading to a wider array of pathogens.

Neutropenia

Patients with a hematologic malignancies such as acute myelogenous leukemia are especially likely to become neutropenic, because the aggressive chemotherapy for these cancers is typically toxic to the bone marrow. Infection risk associated with neutropenia depends on the rapidity of the decline; it increases when the neutrophil count falls below 500/mm^3 and becomes especially prominent at counts <100/mm^3. The common bacteria leading to initial infection are listed in Table 157.3, with Enterobacteriaceae being *Escherichia coli* and Klebsiella species. An approach to the febrile neutropenic patient is outlined in Figure 157.1.

Humoral Immune Deficiencies

Hematologic malignancies, including multiple myeloma and chronic lymphocytic leukemia, may develop a malignancy-associated defect in normal immunoglobulin production. When serum gamma globulin levels are low, defense against encapsulated bacteria (e.g., *Streptococcus pneumoniae, Haemophilus influenzae*) is reduced, and these patients become especially prone to respiratory infections with these organisms. Clearing of encapsulated organisms is also diminished in patients with splenectomy, which may be done as therapy for advanced chronic lymphocytic leukemia. With aggressive chemotherapy, these patients also become at risk for neutropenia-related infection.

Cellular Immune Dysfunction

Malignancy-associated cellular immune dysfunction generally occurs in lymphoreticular (lymphoma, Hodgkin's disease) and hematologic (monocytic or lymphocytic leukemia) malignancies and is associated with defects along the pathway to the activated macrophage. Not only are these patients susceptible to many pathogens (Table 157.3), but they are also at risk for neutropenia-associated infections.

Therapeutic decisions are helped by focusing more on pathogens that have affinity to a certain organ system—for instance, meningitis in a patient with lymphoma or Hodgkin's disease is most likely to be due to *Listeria monocytogenes* or *Cryptococcus neoformans*. It is also helpful to know the association of pathogens

TABLE 157.3. Organisms Commonly Involved With Immunodeficient States

Class of Organism	Neutropenia	Antibody Deficiency	Cell-Mediated Immunodeficiency
Bacteria	Enterobacteriaceae Pseudomonas aeruginosa Staphylococcus aureus Staphylococcus epidermidis	Streptococcus pneumoniae Haemophilus influenzae	Salmonella spp. Listeria monocytogenes, Legionella species, Mycobacteria Nocardia asteroides
Fungi	Candida spp., Aspergillus spp. Mucor species		Cryptococcus neoformans, Coccidiodes immitis, Histoplasma capsulatum
Viruses		Enteroviruses	Herpesviridae Vaccinia virus Rubella virus
Parasites		Giardia lamblia, Pneumocystis carinii	Pneumocystis carinii, Toxoplasma gondii, Strongyloides stercoralis, Cryptosporidium parvum

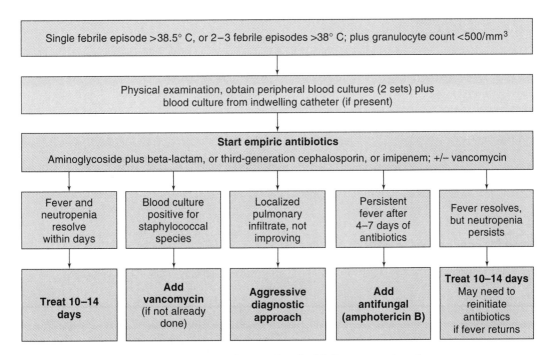

FIGURE 157.1. Suggested approach to the febrile, neutropenic patient.

with a particular malignancy—for example, patients with Hodgkin's disease (especially those following irradiation therapy) are at high-risk for Herpes zoster, and patients under treatment for acute lymphocytic leukemia are particularly at risk for *Pneumocystis carinii* pneumonia.

The many infectious possibilities in these patients generally require a search for a specific etiology. Empiric therapy is usually reserved for febrile and neutropenic patients.

Infections in Transplant Recipients

An ever-increasing number of transplantations, including those of bone marrow and solid organs (kidney, liver, heart, lung, pancreas, and small bowel), are being done for a variety of medical conditions. Just as the patient's life expectancy may be enhanced by the transplantation, so is the risk of life-threatening infection (Table 157.4).

Bone marrow transplantation is performed primarily for severe aplastic anemia, certain hematologic or lymphoreticular malignancies, and some solid tumors. Infections in patients undergoing bone marrow transplantation occur during three fairly predictable periods following marrow infusion (Figure 157.2).

Like bone marrow transplantation, transplantation of solid organs also has been an expanding field, but the infectious complications differ. Overall, patients with transplantations involving the lung (heart-lung or lung) have the highest incidence of infection and infection-related mortality, whereas infections in renal transplant

patients are least frequent. Despite these differences, some generalizations can be made regarding infections following solid organ transplantation. Table 157.5 shows a timetable of infection risk and associated types of infections in solid organ transplantation recipients.

Because of the predictability of certain types of infections, it is standard in the management of transplant recipients to use prophylactic regimens, including certain vaccines (e.g., pneumococcal and influenza vaccines) and various combinations of antibacterial, antifungal, and antiviral agents. Because prophylaxis may be difficult due to side effects (e.g., use of ganciclovir for cytomegalovirus), the approach of **preemptive therapy**—starting therapy at the time of positive cultures to prevent clinical disease from developing—has shown some success. In established infections, empiric therapy is sometimes necessary, but the clinician should be prepared to pursue a specific etiologic diagnosis aggressively so that therapy can be optimized.

TABLE 157.4.   Risk Factors for Infection and Associated Types of Infections in Transplant Recipients

Risk Factors for Infection	Types of Infections or Organisms Involved
Host factors	
Underlying medical conditions (e.g., diabetes mellitus, COPD)	Bacterial infections common to the underlying disease
Previous infection in latency	Altered host colonization and associated infection risk— infection by CMV, HSV, varicella-zoster virus, toxoplasmosis
Factors at the time of transplantation	
Length, location, and complexity of surgery	Bacterial or fungal infections at site of surgery
Infected donor organ	CMV, HSV, hepatitis bands
Infected blood products	Toxoplasmosis (cardiac), hepatitis C
Therapy for graft survival or graft vs. host disease	
Use of immunosuppressive drugs e.g., corticosteroids, cyclosporin, OKT3	Wide range of primarily cell-mediated pathogens (see Table 157.3)
New exposures	
Environmental pathogens	Legionella, Aspergillus spp.

COPD = chronic obstructive pulmonary disease; CMV = cytomegalovirus; HSV = herpes simplex virus.
(Adapted from: Ho M, Dummer JS. In Mandell GL, et al. (eds.). Principles and Practice of Infectious Diseases. 4th ed. pp. 2709–2717. New York: Churchlll Livingstone, 1995.)

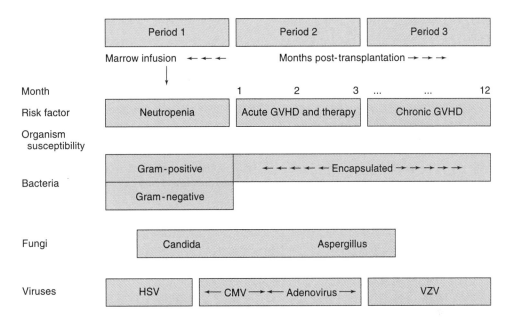

FIGURE 157.2. Timetable of infection risk following bone marrow transplantation. (GVHD = graft-vs-host disease; HSV = herpes simplex virus; CMV = cytomegalovirus; VZV = varicella-zoster virus.)

(Adapted from: Winston DJ. In Mandell GL, Bennett JE, Dolin R, et al. Principles and Practice of Infectious Diseases. 4th ed. Figure 1, p. 2718. New York: Churchill Livingstone, 1995. Used with permission.)

TABLE 157.5. Timetable of Infectious Risk and Associated Infections in Solid Organ Transplantation

Time Period Post-Transplantation	Types of Infections Seen in Each Period
0–1 mo	Wound infections, nosocomial infections
1–6 mos	Infections due to cell-mediated immunosuppression (see Table 157.3)
	Immunomodulating viruses (e.g., CMV, EBV) can worsen other infections
Over 6 mos	Graft infection; Later onset infections due to immunosuppression (e.g., cryptococcal meningitis, CMV retinitis)
	Infections common to the community in patients with minimal immunosuppression (e.g., influenza)

CMV = cytomegalovirus; EBV = Epstein-Barr virus

CHAPTER 158

HUMAN IMMUNODEFICIENCY VIRUS INFECTION AND THE ACQUIRED IMMUNODEFICIENCY SYNDROME

Infection with the human immunodeficiency virus (HIV) and the subsequent development of the acquired immunodeficiency syndrome (AIDS) have become prevalent. Although the current understanding of the disease and its treatment are summarized here, ongoing studies (particularly clinical HIV treatment trials) will require continual medical education updates.

■ **Etiology**

HIV, the etiologic agent for HIV infection and AIDS, is an RNA virus within the family of Retroviridae. Retroviruses have a wide distribution in the animal kingdom, causing related disease in several species. Retroviruses recognized to be associated with human disease include oncoviruses, HTLV-1 and HTLV-2, both being transforming viruses associated with malignancies as well as myelopathies, and lentiviruses, HIV-1 and HIV-2. The lentiviruses are celiopathic with destruction of a particular target cell being the usual pathology.

Viral infection of cells begins with attachment to a surface receptor. In HIV infection, it is the CD4 cell-surface molecule. Because **CD4-positive T cells** and **monocytes** express high levels of this receptor, they are the primary targets of HIV. However, numerous other cells (follicular dendritic cells, epidermal Langerhans cells, megakaryocytes, oligodendrocytes and epithelial or mucosal cells from the kidney, cervix, and rectum) can

express the CD4 molecule and these cells are infected as well.

The unique aspect of the retroviruses, as compared to other human RNA viruses, is the presence of the **reverse transcriptase** enzyme. After the virus enters the infected cell, the reverse transcriptase makes a DNA copy of the HIV RNA, which is then incorporated into the host DNA genome (Figure 158.1). This proviral DNA remains latent until a cellular activation event initiates proviral DNA transcription and sequential protein formation. The appropriate complement of viral genomic RNA, processed protein and enzymes are then assembled at the cell

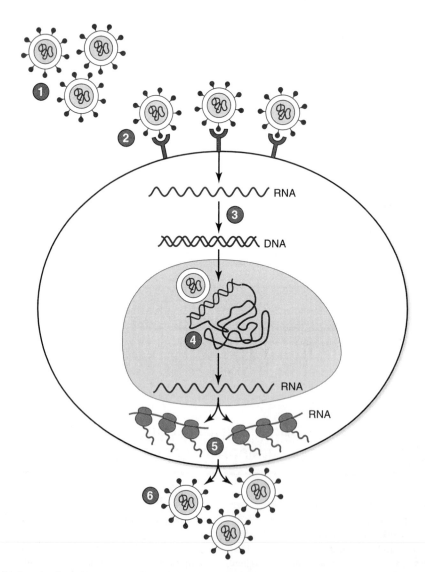

FIGURE 158.1. Lifecycle of HIV virus. 1 = virions; 2 = attachment to CD4 receptor; 3 = reverse transcriptase; 4 = incorporation of provirus into the host genome; 5 = protein coating; 6 = mature viral particle.

surface and, subsequently, bud from the cell as mature virus particles.

HIV causes a progressive dysfunction and depletion of infected cells. The exact mechanisms are not entirely clear. Interference with the host cell's functions, a virally stimulated but host-mediated cytopathic T-cell immune response which eliminates the infected cells, and programmed cell death (apoptosis) activated by the virus are all proposed mechanisms.

■ Epidemiology

The first clinical reports of AIDS were in 1981 from the east and west coasts of the United States, affecting mainly homosexual men. Since then, the disease has spread dramatically in the United States and the world.

HIV infection and AIDS occur with the highest concentration of cases being found in sub-Saharan Africa. However, in the United States, the highest concentrations are noted on the east and west coasts. It is estimated that approximately 14 million people are infected worldwide (1993 estimate) and about 1 million in the United States. These figures are ever-increasing, particularly in sub-Saharan Africa and Asia.

Of the three modes of HIV spread (Table 158.1), sexual transmission is the most prevalent. In the United States, homosexual spread is the most common form, although heterosexually contracted HIV infection is increasing. Worldwide, heterosexually transmitted HIV infection is the most common.

■ Natural History of HIV Infection

Currently, HIV infection can be divided into three general phases (Figure 158.2).

The acute retroviral syndrome

First described in 1985, the acute retroviral syndrome is believed to affect one-half to two-thirds or more of HIV-infected individuals. This syndrome, which occurs from 3–6 weeks after primary HIV infection, resembles mononucleosis and is characterized by fever, myalgias, arthralgias, malaise, nausea, vomiting, diarrhea, and headache. Frequent findings include adenopathy (usually cervical, axillary or occipital), pharyngitis, a truncal rash (macular, papular or urticarial), and, less commonly, hepatosplenomegaly.

Aseptic meningitis, encephalitis, peripheral neuropathy, or Guillain-Barré syndrome are neurologic manifestations. Abnormal blood counts (thrombocytopenia or leukopenia) or abnormal liver tests may be noted. The **differential diagnosis** of the acute retroviral syndrome includes infectious mononucleosis, other viral illness (e.g., influenza, herpes simplex, measles, rubella), as well as secondary syphilis.

TABLE 158.1.	Modes of HIV Transmission
Mode	**Examples**
Sexual	Homosexual
	Heterosexual
Blood and blood products	Contaminated needles
	Transfusions
Maternal-fetal	Intrapartum
	Perinatal
	Postnatal (breast milk)

During this symptomatic phase, there is a high level of HIV viremia (Figure 158.2), and HIV core antigen (p24) is first detected. Immunologically, there is lymphocytopenia, including both CD4 and CD8 cell populations.

The asymptomatic phase

Generally within 1 week to 3 months after the acute retroviral syndrome, there is an immune response to HIV (Figure 158.2), involving both antiviral antibodies (e.g., neutralizing antibodies and antibodies involved in antibody-dependent cellular cytotoxicity) and components of the cellular immune system. Because of this host immune response and the trapping of virus particles in lymph node germinal centers, there is reduction of viremia and p24 antigen detection.

During this immune response, a period of "clinical latency" occurs. This asymptomatic period may last up to 10 years or more but may be shorter in individuals with a higher initial viral inoculum (e.g., blood transfusion recipients, intravenous drug users). Although it was originally believed that the virus was also latent during this time, recent studies indicate that active viral replication is ongoing within lymph node germinal centers.

Despite the lack of symptoms during this period, viral replication leads to destruction of the lymph node architecture, with a subsequent decline in overall immune status. There is a progressive reduction in both the number and function of CD4 cells. Other cell-mediated immune response impairments can be seen in monocytes and natural killer cells. In addition, B-cells are abnormally activated, likely by HIV itself. This increased B-cell proliferation and immunoglobulin secretion lead to hypergammaglobulinemia. B-cells also develop a reduced capacity to respond to mitogens or antigens.

Symptomatic HIV infection

During clinical latency, HIV replication progresses and immune function worsens to the point at which individuals begin to manifest symptoms. Generally, these symptoms begin to appear as CD4 counts fall below

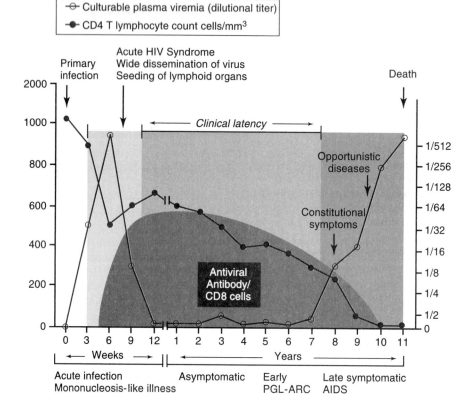

FIGURE 158.2. Timecourse of typical HIV infection. Widespread viral dissemination occurs early in the primary infection and encompasses an abrupt decline in peripheral blood CD4+ T-cell number. The ensuing immune response is accompanied by a decrease in plasma viremia (culturable virus) and a lengthy period of clinical latency. However, the CD4+ T-cell count continues to decline during this period until a critical level is reached, where the risk of opportunistic infections is markedly increased.

(ADC = AIDS dementia complex; ARC = AIDS-related complex; PGL = persistent generalized lymphadenopathy.) (Adapted from: Haase AT. In: Mandell GL, Bennett JE, Dolin R (eds.). Principles and Practice of Infectious Diseases. 4th ed. New York: Churchill Livingstone, 1995, p. 1585; and Pantaleo G, Graziosi C, Fauci AS. The immunopathogenesis of human immunodeficiency virus infection. N Engl J Med 1993;328:329. Used with permission.)

$500/mm^3$. These early symptoms of HIV disease include generalized lymphadenopathy, oral thrush (candidiasis), oral hairy leukoplakia, and herpes zoster (shingles). Thrombocytopenia, which is due to direct viral infection of megakaryocytes, can also manifest during this time.

As immune function progressively declines and CD4 counts drop below $200/mm^3$, individuals enter a stage of **late symptomatic** disease. As this disease progresses, specific antiviral immunity also declines, and there is a renewed detection of viremia (Figure 158.2). Patients become at risk for a range of opportunistic illnesses and direct effects of the virus itself.

One of the direct effects of the virus, which may occur throughout the stages of illness, is **neurologic disease.** After gaining access to the CNS possibly via infected monocytes, HIV evokes inflammatory changes (e.g., aseptic meningitis) or demyelinating or degenerative changes (myelopathy, AIDS-dementia complex). HIV may also cause CNS inflammation without obvious signs, as it has been shown that asymptomatic HIV-positive patients can have a CSF pleocytosis and positive HIV cultures.

■ Diagnosis of HIV Disease and AIDS

Within 1–3 months after primary HIV infection, circulating specific anti-HIV antibodies are detected. Determination of the presence of these antibodies by an enzyme-linked immunosorbent assay (ELISA) has become the standard screening test for HIV infection.

Serologic tests

The **ELISA test** may be negative, indeterminate, or positive. Patients with a negative result and continued high-risk behavior may be retested at intervals. Because of the possibility of a false-positive result (particularly in low-risk individuals), patients with indeterminate or positive results should have the results confirmed with a western blot.

The **western blot,** while not a good screening test, requires the presence of antibody reactivity to several HIV-specific proteins. This reactivity is determined by a banding pattern on the blot. The presence of bands to at least two major HIV gene products (p24, gp41, and gp120–160) determines a positive result. Otherwise, the test is determined to be negative or indeterminate.

If the ELISA is positive but the western blot is negative, the ELISA is considered to be false-positive. If the ELISA is positive and the western blot is positive, the patient is confirmed to be HIV-positive. If, however, the blot is indeterminate, patients may either have cross-reacting antibodies or the antibody response may be in evolution (less likely). Indeterminate western blots should be repeated in about a month. A stable, indeterminate western blot makes HIV infection less likely.

Other tests for HIV include a polymerase chain reaction (PCR) test for HIV, p24 antigen assay, and culture of HIV.

AIDS-indicator conditions

The diagnosis of AIDS has generally rested on indicator diseases, usually opportunistic infections that occur as HIV infection progresses and CD4 counts fall. As experience with this disease has accumulated, the Centers for Disease Control (CDC) has revised their case definition several times to include an increasing range of indicator diseases (Table 158.2). The latest CDC AIDS definition, revised in 1993, expanded the surveillance case definition to include a CD4 count <200/mm^3 (<14%), pulmonary tuberculosis, recurrent pneumonia, or invasive cervical cancer (Table 158.3).

■ Management of HIV Infection

Therapy for HIV infection has been an area of intense study over the past several years. Because of the unique life cycle of the retroviruses, there are several potential targets for therapy (Table 158.4). These inhibitors have been studied to various degrees; some only in vitro and others extensively in clinical trials.

Currently, the therapy for HIV consists of a combination of **nucleoside analogs** (zidovudine, didanosine, zalcitabine and lamivudine) or nucleoside analogs plus a **protease inhibitor** (usually a total of two or three drugs). Results have been promising, but therapy may be limited by toxicity, cost or the development of resistance.

■ Recognition and Management of Opportunistic Infections

Most opportunistic infections or AIDS-defining illnesses occur in late-stage disease when the CD4 count is falling and the immune system is unable to provide adequate protection. Often, these illnesses can be fatal or become chronic and, ultimately, fatal.

The CD4 counts at which common opportunistic infections usually occur are shown in Figure 158.3. Whereas tuberculosis usually occurs at a CD4 count >200/mm^3, most other infections occur <200/mm^3, and some, such as cytomegalovirus, occur at very low CD4 counts. Common opportunistic infections seen in AIDS patients and the therapeutic options are shown in Table 158.5.

Pulmonary infections

The most common cause of pneumonia in AIDS patients is **Pneumocystis carinii**. Unlike non-AIDS patients with *P. carinii* pneumonia, in whom respiratory symptoms are usually abrupt, AIDS patients have a more gradual onset of symptoms. The chest radiograph usually has an interstitial infiltrate (although it may be normal), and the differential diagnosis usually includes mycobacteria, fungi (i.e., cryptococcus, histoplasma, coccidioides), cytomegalovirus, Kaposi's sarcoma, non-Hodgkin's lymphoma, and nonspecific interstitial pneumonitis. Bacterial pneumonia may also need to be considered, but symptoms are usually more acute, with a productive cough and a lobar infiltrate. Bronchoalveolar lavage is often needed to secure the diagnosis of *P. carinii* pneumonia.

Of the treatment options for *P. carinii* pneumonia, **trimethoprim-sulfamethoxazole** is the first choice, but it may not always be tolerated. Treatment should continue for 21 days and, if the PaO$_2$ is below 70 mmHg, **adjunctive steroids** should be used. **Prophylaxis** for *P. carinii* pneumonia may be done primarily (CD4 <200/mm^3) or secondarily (after the first pneumonia episode).

Pulmonary **tuberculosis,** unlike most other AIDS-defining illnesses, tends to occur before CD4 counts fall below 200/mm^3. It has been a particular problem because of the emergence of multidrug resistant strains. In areas with this problem, a 4-drug regimen should be employed initially (Table 158.5); if the strain is sensitive, 3 drugs are continued for 2 months, with isoniazid and rifampin

TABLE 158.2. Centers for Disease Control Case Definition for AIDS (1987 Revision)

Diseases diagnosed definitively without laboratory evidence of HIV infection (in the absence of other immunodeficiency states)

Candidiasis of the esophagus, trachea, bronchi, or lungs
Cryptococcus, extrapulmonary
Cryptosporidiosis with diarrhea persisting >1 month
Cytomegalovirus disease of an organ other than liver, spleen, or lymph nodes in a patient older than 1 month of age
Herpes simplex virus infection causing a mucocutaneous ulcer that persists over 1 mo; or bronchitis, preumonitis, or esophagitis for any duration affecting a patient >1 month of age
Kaposi's sarcoma affecting a patient below 60 yrs of age
Lymphoma of the brain (primary) affecting a patient <60 years of age
Lymphoid interstitial pneumonia and/or pulmonary lymphoid hyperplasia (LIP/PLH complex) affecting a child <13 yrs of age
Mycobacterium avium complex or *M. kansasii* disease, disseminated
Pneumocystis carinii pneumonia
Progressive multifocal leukoencephalopathy
Toxoplasmosis of the brain affecting a patient >1 month of age

Diseases diagnosed definitively with laboratory evidence of HIV infection

Any disease listed above in Section A
Recurrent or multiple pyogenic bacterial infections (<13 yrs of age)
Coccidioidomycosis, disseminated
AIDS dementia
Histoplasmosis, disseminated
Isosporiasis, with diarrhea exceeding 1 mo. in duration
Kaposi's sarcoma, any age
Primary CNS lymphoma
Non-Hodgkin's lymphoma, B-cell or unknown phenotype (small, noncleaved lymphoma or immunoblastic sarcoma)
Disseminated mycobacterial disease (other than *M. tuberculosis*)
M. tuberculosis, extrapulmonary
Recurrent nontyphoid Salmonella septicemia
HIV wasting syndrome

Diseases diagnosed presumptively with laboratory evidence of HIV infection

Esophageal candidiasis
Cytomegalovirus retinitis with loss of vision
Kaposi's sarcoma
Lymphoid interstitial pneumonia and/or pulmonary lymphoid hyperplasia (<13 yrs of age)
Disseminated mycobacterial disease
Pneumocystis carinii pneumonia
Toxoplasmosis of the brain (>1 mo. of age)

Diseases diagnosed definitively with negative laboratory test results for HIV (in the absence of other immunodeficiency states)

Pneumocystis carinii pneumonia
Any other disease listed above in Section A and a CD4 count <400/mm^3

(From: MMWR 1987;36:1S-15S.)

TABLE 158.3. Expanded CDC Case Definition for AIDS (1993 Revision)

1. All HIV infected individuals with a CD4 count <200/mm^3, or a CD4 percent of less than 14%
2. Pulmonary tuberculosis
3. Recurrent pneumonia (≥2 episodes within a year)
4. Invasive cervical cancer

(From: MMWR 1992;41:1–19.)

then continued for a total of 9 months. Because of the high rate of tuberculosis reactivation, all AIDS patients with at least a 5-mm reactive tuberculin (PPD) skin test or those with a negative skin test and a suspicious history (i.e., chest radiograph consistent with previous, untreated tuberculosis; close contact with active tuberculosis; or a history of a positive skin test not adequately treated) should receive anti-tuberculosis prophylaxis with 12 months of isoniazid.

Esophageal infections

Esophagitis usually presents with symptoms of nausea, anorexia, dysphagia, or odynophagia and is most likely due to *Candida albicans,* particularly when there is the finding of oral thrush. A cobblestone appearance on an upper gastrointestinal tract radiograph (due to ulcerations and plaques) suggests the diagnosis, but most patients are treated empirically. Lacking a response to fluconazole, patients may require an upper gastrointestinal endoscopy to rule out the presence of other pathogens, such as cytomegalovirus or herpes simplex.

TABLE 158.4.	Potential Molecular Targets for HIV Therapy
Phase of HIV Replication Cycle	**Examples of Types of Inhibitors**
Viral binding and penetration	Soluble CD4 neutralizing antibodies
Reverse transcriptase	Nucleoside analogs
	Nonnucleoside analogs
Integration	Anti-integrase
Transcription	Antisense oligonucleotides
	tat antagonists
	Interferons
Assembly	Protease inhibitors
	Glycosylation inhibitors
Budding	Interferons

Gastrointestinal infections (enterocolitis)

Diarrhea is a frequent problem in patients with AIDS and includes a number of bacteria, parasites, and viruses as causative agents. Common bacterial pathogens include Salmonella, Shigella, or Campylobacter species. Although these organisms, as a cause of enterocolitis, are not associated with an AIDS diagnosis, recurrent Salmonella (nontyphoid) bacteremia is an AIDS-defining illness. Mycobacteria also may cause diarrhea, and there should also be concern about *Clostridium difficile-* associated diarrhea because of the frequent use of antibiotics in these patients.

Of the parasitic causes, cryptosporidiosis and isosporiasis are AIDS-defining illnesses. Whereas numerous therapies have been tried for cryptosporidiosis, none has been particularly successful; transient benefit has been shown with paromomycin.

Cytomegalovirus (CMV) is the most common viral etiology of enterocolitis in AIDS patients and is usually seen in late-stage disease. Stool examinations should be performed to evaluate the other possibilities, but the definitive diagnosis of CMV colitis requires colonoscopy and biopsy. HIV enteropathy also may be a cause of diarrhea in AIDS patients, but all other causes should be ruled out before assuming this diagnosis.

Central nervous system infections

The most common infection of the CNS in HIV-infected individuals is HIV itself. HIV can cause

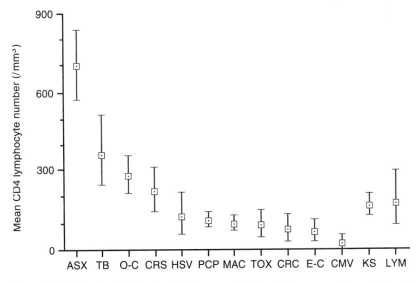

FIGURE 158.3. Mean CD4 cell levels with standard deviations *(boxes)* and 95% confidence intervals *(bars)* in 222 HIV-infected patients with opportunistic diseases and HIV-infected asymptomatic controls.
ASX = asymptomatic; CMV = cytomegalovirus retinitis; CRC = cryptococcal meningitis; CRS = cryptosporidiosis; EC = esophageal candidiasis; HSV = recurrent herpes simplex virus; KS = Kaposi=s sarcoma; LYM = lymphoma; MAC = *Mycobacterium avium* complex; O-C = oral candidiasis; PCP = *Pneumocystis carinii* pneumonia; TB = tuberculosis; TOX = toxoplasmosis. (Redrawn from: Crowe SM et al. J AIDS 1991;4:773; Figure 2. Used with permission.)

TABLE 158.5. Common Opportunistic Infections in AIDS		
Organ or Organ System	**Etiology or Type of Infection**	**Therapeutic Options**
Pulmonary	*Pneumocystis carinii*	TMP/SMX, TMP/dapsone, clindamycin/ primaquine, pentamidine
	Mycobacterium tuberculosis	Isoniazid, rifampin, pyrazinamide, +/− ethambutol (see text)
Esophagus	*Candida albicans,* Cytomegalovirus (CMV), Herpes simplex	Fluconazole, ganciclovir, foscarnet, acyclovir
GI	Cryptosporidiosis, Microsporidiosis	None, paromomycin None(?)
	Isosporiasis	TMP/SMX
	CMV colitis	Ganciclovir, foscarnet
CNS	Cryptococcal meningitis	Amphotericin B, fluconazole
	Neurosyphilis	Penicillin
	Toxoplasma encephalitis	Sulfadiazine/pyrimethamine, clindamycin/ pyrimethamine
Eye	CMV retinitis	Ganciclovir, foscarnet
Disseminated	*Mycobacterium avium* complex	Ciprofloxacin, macrolide, ethambutol, clofazimine, rifabutin (multidrug combination)
	Histoplasmosis	Amphotericin B, itraconazole

TMP = Trimethoprim; SMX = sulfamethoxazole.

asymptomatic inflammation, aseptic meningitis, or other destructive changes. **Aseptic meningitis** may be seen throughout the symptomatic phase but not in the late stages of illness, as it appears to be an immunologically mediated process.

Although there are a number of potential causes of meningitis in AIDS patients (e.g., fungal, tuberculosis, bacterial, syphilis, herpes, and other viruses), the most common opportunistic cause of meningitis is *Cryptococcus neoformans.* Most patients have nonspecific symptoms, including fever and headache, whereas a minority (≤20%) have more classic findings of meningitis (meningeal signs, photophobia, altered sensorium). CSF usually only has mild abnormalities. Tests supportive of the diagnosis include a positive india ink (50–90%), cryptococcal antigen (90–95%) and culture. Amphotericin B is the preferred treatment, particularly with severe disease, but fluconazole is the agent of choice for chronic suppression after initial therapy.

HIV disease has led to an increased recognition of **neurosyphilis** and has shortened the natural history of neurosyphilis manifestations after primary syphilis. Therefore, patients with positive serum syphilis titers and neurologic abnormalities should be considered for a spinal tap. An abnormal CSF (with or without a positive CSF VDRL) should lead to the consideration of treatment with parenteral penicillin.

With the presence of localizing neurologic findings (e.g., hemiparesis, ataxia, cranial neuropathies, seizure), intracranial mass lesions are likely, and imaging should be performed, preferably with magnetic resonance scan-

ning. **Cerebral toxoplasmosis** is the most common cause of intracranial contrast-enhancing masses, whereas other less common causes include tuberculosis, bacterial abscesses, cryptococcosis, nocardiosis, and, possibly, lymphoma. Patients are usually treated presumptively and for life. If there is no response to treatment, brain biopsy should be considered to exclude other diagnoses.

Eye infections (retinitis)

Cytomegalovirus (CMV) has an affinity for the retina and causes most of the cases of retinitis in AIDS patients. Visual symptoms include blurring, a painless vision loss, and increase in "floaters." The diagnosis is generally made by an ophthalmologist, and treatment (with ganciclovir or foscarnet) includes an induction of 14–21 days, followed by life-long maintenance therapy.

Disseminated infections

Mycobacterium avium complex usually presents as a widely disseminated illness in late-stage disease, with fever, sweats, weight loss, fatigue, abdominal pain, and diarrhea. Patients have a continuous bacteremia, and the diagnosis is usually made by blood cultures. Whereas treatment often needs to be altered due to medication intolerance, it should be with a multidrug regimen and needs to be life-long. Experts also recommend prophylaxis for this disease (e.g., rifabutin, newer macrolides) when CD4 counts fall lower than 100/mm^3.

Another common disseminated opportunistic infection is **histoplasmosis.** This illness, particularly seen in the Ohio and Mississippi River valleys, has systemic symptoms similar to those seen in *M. avium* complex disease. The diagnosis is made by blood cultures or antigen testing (urine or blood). Treatment is with amphotericin B followed by life-long itraconazole.

■ Malignancies Complicating HIV Infection

Of the malignancies complicating AIDS (Table 158.6), Kaposi's sarcoma and non-Hodgkin's lymphoma are the most frequent. These malignancies, as well as cervical cancer, are currently recognized as AIDS-defining illnesses.

Kaposi's sarcoma, a vascular (or lymphatic) endothelial neoplasm, commonly manifests as painless cutaneous lesions that appear as pigmented nodules. This clinical appearance is usually sufficient to suggest the diagnosis, but a biopsy may be required for definitive diagnosis. The disease typically is indolent but may become extensive or spread to visceral organs. Gastrointestinal Kaposi's sarcoma, for instance, may present with bowel obstruction or gastrointestinal bleeding. Pulmonary Kaposi's sarcoma may mimic *Pneumocystis carinii* pneumonia, but the chest radiograph has a more nodular pattern, often with bloody pleural effusions. Patients may also present with lymphedema (face or lower extremity), suggesting lymphatic obstruction with tumor.

Treatment of Kaposi's sarcoma is individualized, depending on the location and extent. Localized lesions are treated if they are associated with significant pain or discomfort or if they present a cosmetic problem (e.g., facial lesions). Cryotherapy, localized radiation, or intralesional vinblastine are usually employed when treatment of localized lesions is indicated. More extensive disease may require interferon or chemotherapy.

The second most common malignancy seen in AIDS patients is **non-Hodgkin's lymphoma.** Non-Hodgkin's lymphomas are of B-cell origin and include peripheral lymphoma (including immunoblastic lymphoma or Burkitt's lymphoma) or primary CNS lymphoma. Most cases (80%) are peripheral lymphomas. Presentations vary and extranodal disease is common, as are systemic symptoms (fever, sweats, weight loss). CNS lymphoma usually presents with focal neurologic findings and is in the differential diagnosis of a space-occupying brain lesion.

TABLE 158.6.	Malignancies Complicating HIV Infection
Kaposi's sarcoma	
CNS non-Hodgkin's lymphoma	
Hodgkin's disease	
Cervical cancer	
Squamous cancer of the anus	

Chemotherapy is used for peripheral lymphoma, and radiation and/or corticosteroids have been used for primary CNS lymphoma.

■ Questions

Instructions: For each question below, select only **one** lettered answer that is the **best** for that question.

1. A patient has had three documented episodes of pneumococcal pneumonia over the past 6 months. Possible underlying contributing diseases include all of the following EXCEPT:
   A. Common variable hypogammaglobulinemia
   B. Multiple myeloma
   C. Chronic lymphocytic leukemia
   D. DiGeorge syndrome

2. Corticosteroids affect the host defense through which of the following mechanisms?
   A. Affecting neutrophil kinetics
   B. Affecting antibody production
   C. Inhibiting lymphocyte and mononuclear cell function
   D. All of the above

3. *Chlamydia* organisms can cause which of the following illnesses?
   A. Pneumonia
   B. Keratoconjunctivitis
   C. Pelvic inflammatory disease
   D. All of the above

4. Tissue invasion by which of the following may cause eosinophilia?
   A. Nematodes
   B. Trematodes
   C. Cestodes
   D. All of the above

5. Of the following ß-lactam antibiotics, which is particularly noted to predispose to seizures?
   A. Cefoxitin
   B. Ceftazidine
   C. Imipenem
   D. Aztreonam

6. Of the following ß-lactam antibiotics, which can be used in a patient with a serious ß-lactam allergy?
   A. Cefoxitin
   B. Ceftazidine
   C. Imipenem
   D. Aztreonam

7. A patient is started on antituberculosis therapy with isoniazid, rifampin, ethambutol, and pyrazinamide. Several weeks later, the patient complains of a decrease in vision. Visual acuity is noted to be

decreased. Which one of the following best explains the finding?

A. Isoniazid
B. Rifampin
C. Ethambutol
D. Pyrazinamide
E. Cataract

8. Following travel to the southwestern United States, a 52-year-old Hispanic man develops a pneumonia. Which of the following organisms is a potential cause?

A. *Candida albicans*
B. *Coccidiodes immitis*
C. *Histoplasma capsulatum*
D. *Blastomyces dermatitidis*

9. In a patient presenting with pneumonia, a sputum Gram stain shows small coccobacillary gram-negative organisms. Appropriate initial choices for antibiotics include all of the following EXCEPT:

A. Amoxicillin-clavulanic acid
B. Trimethoprim-sulfamethoxazole
C. Erythromycin
D. Cefuroxime

10. If a patient presents with a sore throat, a tonsillar exudate may be seen with all of the following EXCEPT:

A. Epstein-Barr virus
B. Rhinovirus
C. Group A streptococcus
D. Adenovirus

11. Frequency, dysuria and/or urgency, and <10⁵ bacteria/ml of urine (acute urethral syndrome) are caused by which of the following?

A. Acute cystitis
B. Nongonococcal urethritis
C. Chemical sensitivity
D. All of the above

12. In which of the following settings should asymptomatic bacteruria be treated?

A. Elderly patient
B. Catheterized patient
C. Pregnant patient
D. All of the above

13. A patient presents with a painless genital ulceration as shown in the following figure.
Which of the following is the best test to determine the etiology?

A. Gram stain
B. Serology for herpes
C. Culture
D. Dark-field examination

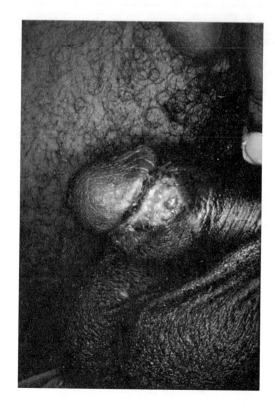

14. One of the preceding tests is performed in the patient. Additional measures should include which of the following?

A. HIV test
B. VDRL
C. Urethral swab to be inoculated into Thayer-Martin medium
D. Benzathine penicillin 2.4 MU IM
E. All of the above

15. Close contacts of which of the following causes of meningitis should receive prophylaxis to prevent disease?

A. *Streptococcus pneumoniae*
B. *Neisseria meningitidis*
C. *Listeria monocytogenes*
D. ECHO virus

16. A cause of cellulitis associated with traumatic wounds in salt water is which of the following?

A. *Staphylococcus aureus*
B. *Pseudomonas aeruginosa*
C. *Vibrio vulnificus*
D. *Aeromonas hydrophila*

17. An organism that is prominent in cat or dog bites, as opposed to human bites, is:

A. *Streptococcus pyogenes.*
B. *Staphylococcus aureus.*

C. *Pasteurella multocida.*

D. *Fusobacterium nucleatum.*

18. A patient with Hodgkin's disease is suspected of having meningitis. Of the etiologic agents listed, the most common bacterial cause is:

A. *Listeria monocytogenes.*

B. *Staphylococcus aureus.*

C. Group A streptococcus.

D. *Pseudomonas aeruginosa.*

■ Answers

1. D	2. D	3. D	4. D	5. C
6. D	7. C	8. B	9. C	10. B
11. D	12. C	13. D	14. E	15. B
16. C	17. C	18. A		

SUGGESTED READING

General

Textbooks and Monographs

Fauci AS, Lane HC. Human immunodeficiency virus (HIV) disease. In: Isselbacher, Braunwald, Wilson, Martin, Fauci AS, Kasper (eds.). AIDS and Related Disorders. New York: McGraw-Hill, Inc., 1994:1567–1618.

Gorbach SL, Bartlett JG, Blacklow NR (eds.). Infectious Diseases. 2nd ed. Philadelphia: W. B. Saunders Company, 1998.

Mandell GL, Bennett JE, Dolin R (eds.). Principles and Practice of Infectious Diseases. 4th ed. New York: Churchill Livingstone, Inc.; 1995:

Articles

Manifestations of Infection

Norman Dc, Yoshikawa TT. Fever in the elderly. Inf Dis Clin North Am 1996;10:93–99.

Laboratory Diagnosis of Infectious Diseases

Ma TS. Applications and limitations of polymerase chain reaction amplification. Chest 1995;108:1393–1404.

Whelen AC, Persing DH. The role of nucleic acid amplification and detection in the clinical microbiology laboratory. Ann Rev Microbiol 1996;50:349–373.

Wilson ML. General principles of specimen collection and transport. Clin Infect Dis 1996;22:766–777.

Antimicrobial Agents

Chao CC, Peterson PK. Exercise and the pathogenesis of infectious disease. The AIDS Reader 1993;3:77–83.

Como JA, Dismukes WE. Oral azole drugs as systemic antifungal therapy. N Engl J Med 1994;330:263–272.

Fever and Fever of Unknown Origin

Cunha BA. Fever of unknown origin. Infectious Disease Clinics of North America 1996;10:111–127.

Gordon SM. Recognizing and treating new and emerging infections encountered in everyday practice. Cleve Cl J Med 1996;63:172–178.

Knockaert DC, Vanneste LJ, Bobbaers HJ. Fever of unknown origin in elderly patients. J Am Ger Soc 1993;41:1187–1192.

Konecny P, Davidson RN. Pyrexia of unknown origin in the 1990s: time to redefine. Br J of Hosp Med 1996;56:21–24.

Larson EB, Featherstone HJ, Petersdorf RG. Fever of undetermined origin—Diagnosis and follow up of 105 cases, 1970–1980. Medicine 1982;61:269–292.

Petersdorf RG, Beeson PB. Fever of unexplained origin. Medicine 1961; 40:1–30.

Simon HB. Hyperthermia. N Engl J Med 1993;329:483–487.

Weissman AF, Fig LM, Sisson J, et al. The role of scintigraphy in the evaluation of fever of unknown origin. Am Fam Phys 1994;50:1717–1727.

Pneumonias

Bartlett JG, Mundy LM. Current concepts: Community-acquired pneumonia. N Engl J Med 1995;333:1618–1624.

Friedland IR, McCracken GH. Drug therapy: Management of infections caused by antibiotic-resistant streptococcus pneumoniae. N Engl J Med 1994;331:377–382.

Kotilainen HR. Prevention and control of nosocomial infection in the intensive care unit. In: Rippe JM, Irwin RS, Alpert JS, et al. (eds.). Intensive Care Medicine. 2nd ed. Boston: Little, Brown and Company, 1991:832–834.

Marrie TJ. Community-acquired pneumonia. Clin Infect Dis 1994;18:501–515.

Niederman MS, Bass JB, Campbell GD, et al. Guidelines for the initial management of adults with community-acquired pneumonia: Diagnosis, assessment of severity, and initial antimicrobial therapy. Am Rev Respir Dis 1993;148:1418–1426.

Bartlet JG, Breiman RF, Mandell LA, et al. Community-acquired pneumonia in adults: Guidelines for management. Clin Infect Dis 1998;26:811–838.

Urinary Tract Infections

Kunin CM. Urinary tract infections in females. Clin Infect Dis 1994;18:1–12.

Stamm WE, Hooton TM. Management of urinary tract infections in adults. N Engl J Med 1993;329:1328–1334.

Sexually Transmitted Diseases

Anonymous. Drugs for sexually transmitted diseases. Medical Letter on Drugs & Therapeutics 1995;37:117–122.

Levine WC, Brady WE, Schmid GP, et al. Sexually transmitted diseases treatment guidelines. Clin Infect Dis 1995;20:1–109.

Quinn TC, Zenilman J, Rompalo A. Sexually transmitted diseases: advances in diagnosis and treatment. Adv Intern Med 1994;39:149–196.

Infectious diarrheas

Farthing MJ. Travellers' diarrhea. Gut 1994;35:1–4.

Framm SR, Soave R. Agents of diarrhea. Med Clin North Am 1997;81:427–447.

Jacobs NF, Jr. Antibiotic-induced diarrhea and pseudomembranous colitis. Postgrad Med 1994;95:111–114.

Intraabdominal Infections

Gilbert JA, Kamath PS. Spontaneous bacterial peritonitis: an update. Mayo Clinic Proceedings 1995;70:365–370.

McClean KL, Sheehan GJ, Harding GKM. Intraabdominal infection: a review. Clin Infect Dis 1994;19:100–116.

van den Hazel SJ, Speelman P, Tytgat GNJ, et al. Role of antibiotics in the treatment and prevention of acute and recurrent cholangitis. Clin Infect Dis 1994;19:279–286.

Wittmann DH, Schein M, Condon RE. Management of secondary peritonitis. Ann Surg 1996;224:10–18.

Central Nervous System Infections

Lipton JD, Schafermeyer RW. Central nervous system infections. The usual and the unusual. Emerg Med Clin North Am 1995;13:417–443.

Nelsen S, Sealy DP, Schneider Ef. The aseptic meningitis syndrome. Am Fam Phys 1993;48:809–815.

Quagliarello VJ, Scheld WM. Treatment of bacterial meningitis. N Engl J Med 1997;336:708–716.

Segreti J, Harris AA. Acute bacterial meningitis. Inf Dis Clin North Am 1996;10:797–809.

Townsend GC, Scheld WM. The use of corticosteroids in the management of bacterial meningitis in adults. J Antimicrob Chemother 1996;37:1051–1061.

Bacteremia, Sepsis and the Sepsis Syndrome

Aronson MD, Bor DH. Blood cultures. Ann Int Med 1987;106:246–253.

Esposito AL, Gleckman RA, Cram S, et al. Community-acquired bacteremia in the elderly: analysis of one hundred consecutive episodes. J Am Geriatrics Soc 1980;28:315–319.

Leibovici L, Greenshtain S, Cohen O, et al. Bacteremia in febrile patients. A clinical model for diagnosis. Arch Intern Med 1991;151:1801–1806.

Lynn WA, Cohen J. Adjunctive therapy for septic shock: a review of experimental approaches. Clin Infect Dis 1995;20:143–158.

Maki DG. Nosocomial bacteremia. An epidemiologic overview. Am J Med 1981;70:719–732.

Richardson JP. Bacteremia in the Elderly. Journal of General Internal Medicine 1993;8:89–92.

Skin, Soft Tissue and Bone Infections

Bisno AL, Stevens DL. Streptococcal infections of skin and soft tissues. N Engl J Med. 1996;334:240–245.

Carroll JA. Common bacterial pyodermas. Taking aim against the most likely pathogens. Postgrad Med 1996;100:311–313.

Chartier C, Grosshans E. Erysipelas: an update. Int J Dermatol 1996;35:779–781.

Hacker SM. Common infections of the skin. Characteristics, causes, and cures. Postgrad Med 1994;96:43–46.

Smith JW, Piercy EA. Infectious arthritis. Clin Infect Dis 1995;20:225–231.

Infections in the Immunocompromised Host

Rubin RH, Ferraro MJ. Understanding and diagnosing infectious complications in the immunocompromised host. Current issues and trends. Hem Onc Clin North Am 1993;7:795–812.

Rubin RH, Fischman AJ. Radionuclide imaging of infection in the immunocompromised host. Clin Infect Dis 1996;22:414–423.

Thomas Cr, Jr., Wood LV, Douglas JG, et al. Common emergencies in cancer medicine: infectious and treatment-related syndromes, Part I. J Natl Med Assoc 1994;86:765–774.

HIV/AIDS

Deeks SG, Smith M, Holodniy M, et al. HIV-1 protease inhibitors. A review for clinicians. JAMA 1997; 277:145–158.

Gallant JE, Moore RD, Chaisson RE. Prophylaxis for opportunistic infections in patients with HIV infection. Ann Intern Med 1994;120:932–944.

Lane HC, Laughon BE, Falloon J, et al. Recent advances in the management of AIDS-related opportunistic infections. Ann Intern Med 1994;120:945–955.

Lipsky JJ. Antiretroviral drugs for AIDS. Lancet 1996;348:800–803.

Polsky B. Treatment of HIV infection and its complications. Clin Chest Med 1996;17:647–663.

Sullivan M, Feinberg J, Bartlett JG. Fever in patients with HIV infection. Inf Dis Clin North Am 1996;10:149–165.

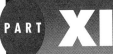

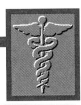

PART XI

George L. Bakris
James P. Lash
Mahendr S. Kochar

KIDNEY DISEASES, ELECTROLYTE DISORDERS, AND HYPERTENSION

he kidneys are located in the retroperitoneal space at a level between the 12th thoracic vertebra and the 2nd lumbar vertebra. Each kidney weighs about 150 grams and measures about 12 x 6 x 3 cm. The functional unit of the kidney is called the nephron, of which there are approximately 1 million in each kidney. The fundamental structure of the nephron is illustrated in Figure 159.1.

FIGURE 159.1. Functional unit of the kidney: The nephron.

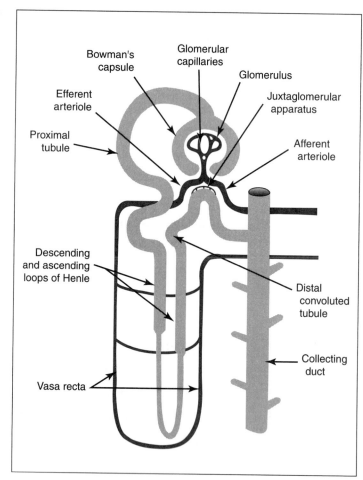

The Glomerulus

The glomerulus is about 200 micrometers in diameter and is formed by the invagination of a tuft of capillaries into the dilated blind end of the nephron (Bowman's capsule). The capillaries are supplied by an afferent arteriole and drained by a slightly smaller efferent arteriole. The two cell layers separating the blood from the glomerular filtrate in Bowman's capsule are the capillary endothelium and the tubular epithelium of the tubule. The endothelial cells that line the capillary lumen are filled with pores covered by thin diaphragms. The glomerular basement membrane is a hydrated gel of glycoproteins containing interwoven collagen fibers. Foot processes extend from the epithelial cells over the basement membrane. Their lack of tight approximation allow for the formation of a filtration slit covered by a thin semipermeable membrane. The consequent barrier formed by these three layers allows passive entry of water and low molecular weight solutes into the urinary space, but not cells and protein. Moreover, clusters of anionic bridge macromolecules on the surface of these cells and within the glomerular basement membrane, further restrict filtration of large negatively charged serum proteins such as **albumin.**

An interwoven lattice known as the mesangium serves to suspend the glomerular tufts within the urinary space. Mesangial cells are enclosed by a matrix of homogeneous fibrillary material containing mucopolysaccharides and different glycoproteins. These cells are of a contractile nature and have many properties that affect the glomerular filtration rate (GFR).

The Tubule

The tubule receives the glomerular filtrate. The tubule is composed primarily of four segments: a) the proximal convoluted tubule, b) the loop of Henle, with a thin descending limb and a thick ascending limb, c) the distal convoluted tubule and, d) the collecting duct.

The **proximal convoluted tubule** is the most metabolically active of the entire nephron, handling many substances, including creatinine, uric acid, albumin, and sodium. Over 75% of filtered sodium is reabsorbed in proximal tubule and the remainder is absorbed distally. The convoluted portion of the proximal tubule drains into the straight portion. The proximal tubule terminates in the descending limb of the loop of Henle. The loop forms a hairpin turn in the medulla and returns forward to the cortex, forming the **distal tubule.**

The tubule is finally directed again into the medullary tissues as the collecting duct empties into the renal pelvis at the ducts of Bellini located at the tips of the renal papillae.

This interesting arrangement of the tubule allows the distal tubule to come in close approximation with the vascular pole of the glomerulus. The distal tubular cells in this region are taller and more numerous. This region, called the macula densa, together with cells originating from the adjacent afferent arteriole, creates a specialized structure called the **juxtaglomerular apparatus.** The juxtaglomerular apparatus is the site of renin formation as well as endothelial derived relaxing factor or nitric oxide (NO).

Renal Physiology

The kidney not only ensures body fluid homeostasis by excreting excess solute and water in the urine, but also regulates a number of other bodily functions, summarized in Table 159.1.

■ Renal Hemodynamics

The renal plasma flow (RPF) and glomerular filtration rate (GFR) maintain a ratio of 5:1. In other words, RPF is normally about 600 ml/min and GFR is approximately 120 ml/min. These rates are maintained over a

TABLE 159.2.	Factors Affecting Afferent and/or Efferent Arteriolar Tone
Angiotensin II	
Arginine vasopressin	
Prostaglandins	
Endothelium-derived relaxing factor	
Catecholamines	
Renal nerves	
Endothelin	

TABLE 159.1.	Homeostatic Functions Performed by the Kidney
1. Electrolyte maintenance ([Na⁺], [K⁺], [Cl⁻], [PO₄], [Ca²⁺]).	
2. Urea clearance	
3. Erythropoietin production for RBC maintenance	
4. Acid-base balance	
5. Vitamin D metabolism	

wide range of mean arterial pressures, this autoregulation of renal function being secondary to efferent and afferent arteriolar regulation of pressures within the glomerular capillaries. The neurohumoral factors that influence this vascular tone are summarized in Table 159.2. Many factors affect GFR; they are listed in Table 159.3.

GFR evolves from the following equation:

$$GFR = kS \; [(P_{GC} \times P_T) \times (\Pi_{GC} \times \Pi_T)]$$

TABLE 159.3. Factors That Affect the Glomerular Filtration Rate

Decrease GFR
- Decrease in renal blood flow
- Decrease in glomerular capillary hydrostatic pressure
  a) Reduction in systemic blood pressure
  b) Afferent arteriolar constriction
  c) Efferent arteriolar dilation
- Increase in hydrostatic pressure in Bowman's capsule
  a) Ureteral obstruction
  b) Edema of kidney inside the tight renal capsule
- Decrease in concentration of plasma proteins
- Decrease in total area of glomerular capillary bed
  a) Diseases that destroy glomeruli without destroying tubules
  b) Partial nephrectomy

Increase GFR
- Opposite effects of factors that decrease GFR
- Increased permeability of glomerular filter, as seen in
  a) Diabetes mellitus
  b) Membranous nephropathy

where k is the capillary permeability, S is the size of the capillary bed, P_{GC} is the mean hydrostatic pressure in the glomerular capillaries, P_T is the mean hydrostatic pressure in the tubules, Π_{GC} is the colloid osmotic pressure of the plasma in the glomerular capillaries and Π_T is the osmotic pressure of the filtrate in the tubule.

CHAPTER 160 INITIAL EVALUATION OF KIDNEY DISEASE

The cornerstone of any evaluation is a detailed history and physical examination. In patients with renal disease, an additional vital element is to note the **time sequence** of changes in renal function. This can only be done by correlating the history with the laboratory data. The **basic laboratory tests** that should be performed on the **initial visit** in all patients with suspected renal dysfunction are summarized in Table 160.1. Urinalysis should be performed on a midstream collection in men and a "clean catch" sample in women to avoid contamination of the specimen by the external genitalia; the tests should be performed within 30–60 minutes after the specimen has been voided. Abnormal tests should be followed by additional studies, including measurement of creatinine clearance to assess GFR and/or diagnostic studies such as a renal ultrasound, radionuclide studies, arteriography or renal biopsy.

A practical method used to assess renal function in clinical practice is the creatinine clearance. However, since creatinine is also secreted as well as filtered, it can only serve as a fair estimate of GFR when renal function is normal. Moreover, this property of creatinine makes it vulnerable to change by drugs (Table 160.2).

Loss of up to half the nephron mass of both kidneys correlates with a 20–30% and not a fifty percent reduction in GFR. This is due to compensatory hyperfiltration by the remaining nephrons. The fluid and electrolyte balance may be maintained and depending on the kidney disease, urinalysis may be normal. Thus, serum creatinine and

TABLE 160.1. Initial Laboratory Screening of Renal Patients

Blood	Urine
a) Complete blood count	a) Specific gravity
b) Electrolytes, glucose, BUN, creatinine	b) Dipstick test for pH, protein, glucose, ketones, bilirubin, urobilinogen, blood, and nitrate
c) Liver function studies	c) Sulfosalicylic acid test for protein
d) Ca^{2+}, PO_4^{2-}, albumin, cholesterol	d) Micral test for microalbuminuria (only if dipstick is (–) for protein and patient has diabetes mellitus or hypertension)
	e) Microscopic analysis: urinary sediment (cells, casts, and crystals)

even creatinine clearance lack the sensitivity to detect an early decline in renal function.

Creatinine clearance may also be estimated using the Cockcroft and Gault equation:

$$Creatinine\ Clearance = ml/min + \frac{(140\text{-}age) \times body\ weight\ (kg)}{72 \times serum\ creatinine\ (mg/dl)}$$

In women, the result should be multiplied by 0.85. While this equation is useful to estimate drug dosages in acute situations, it should only be used until a 24-hour urine

collection can be obtained. It is also vitally important to ensure an adequate urine collection when obtaining a 24-hour collection. This is done by calculating the anticipated amount of creatinine in the collection. This is because creatinine is directly reflective of muscle mass. There should be about 22 mg/kg of creatinine in men and about 18 mg/kg of creatinine in women. Total urine volume should NOT be used to estimate adequacy of collection. *These formulae are not accurate in patients whose body weight or muscle mass deviates markedly from normal such as obesity, muscle wasting and muscle denervation.*

Plotting the reciprocal serum creatinine (1/Scr), which roughly indicates the residual renal function on the ordinate and months of observation on the abscissa, gives useful predictive information on the progression of renal failure in chronic kidney diseases. Extending the regression or trend line obtained from such a plot can predict with reasonable accuracy when an individual patient would reach a level of renal failure requiring dialysis or transplantation. It can also be used to monitor improvement in renal function in response to therapy (Figure 160.1).

TABLE 160.2.	Drugs That Affect Serum Creatinine

Compounds that decrease creatinine excretion by altering secretion
1. Cimetidine
2. Trimethoprim

Compounds measured as creatinine in certain assays
1. Acetoacetic acid in ketoacidosis
2. Cefoxitin
3. Flucytosine

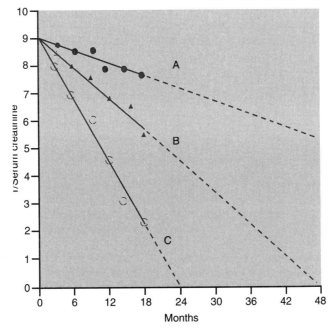

FIGURE 160.1. Plotting 1/serum creatinine against time can help predict the time of occurrence of end-stage renal disease (ESRD). Follow-up of three patients (A, B, and C) over an 18-month period is shown (solid lines). One can say with reasonable confidence that in the case of patient A, it would be several years before ESRD occurs; patient B will need dialysis in another 2 years, and patient C within the next 6 months.

Hematuria

Hematuria is defined as greater than 3 RBC per high power field on microscopic examination of the urine sediment. Gross hematuria is an insensitive indicator of the degree of blood loss, because as little as one milliliter of blood is enough to change the color of one liter of urine to red or brown. Hemoglobinuria caused by hemolysis and myoglobinuria caused by rhabdomyolysis can also cause a red/brown urine and yield a positive hemoglobin dipstick. However, in myoglobinuria, the spun specimen will have a red supernatant and no red blood cells in the urine sediment. Thus, true hematuria can only be diagnosed by microscopic examination. Causes of hematuria are shown in Table 160.3.

■ History

One should inquire regarding family and personal history of primary renal disease, hereditary nephropathies, polycystic kidney disease, sickle cell anemia, tuberculosis, or other related causes. In addition, recent infection of the upper respiratory tract should suggest the possibility of a postinfectious glomerulonephritis or IgA nephropathy. Intravenous drug use and acquired immune deficiency syndrome are also associated with glomerular disease. Flank pain radiating to the groin may indicate a kidney stone. Fever and weight loss may suggest a vasculitis, tuberculosis, or renal cell carcinoma. Rheumatic symptoms such as joint pain and rash may be present in systemic lupus erythematosus (SLE), progressive systemic sclerosis or vasculitis. Pulmonary complaints or hemoptysis may suggest Goodpasture's syndrome or Wegener's granulomatosis (Table 160.3). Passage of blood clots are not associated with glomerular disease and are more commonly seen with disorders that involve the urinary bladder. Specific risk factors for bladder cancer include heavy smoking, long-term administration of cyclophosphamide, prolonged heavy phenacetin use, and exposure to some dyes. Medication use (e.g., anticoagulants and cyclophosphamide) should be noted.

■ Laboratory Tests

Routine evaluation should include measurement of the blood urea nitrogen (BUN), serum creatinine and tests for hepatitis B surface antigen, VDRL, streptococcal serologic test, antinuclear antibody (ANA), and a hemoglobin electrophoresis. Tests such as complement levels, cryoglobulins, and other related tests should also be considered. After the screening tests, additional studies should be guided by the history, physical examination and clinical assessment. If renal tuberculosis is suspected,

PPD (tuberculin) skin test should be performed with anergy controls and at least **three** first voided morning urine specimens should be sent for acid-fast smear and mycobacterial culture. Antiglomerular basement membrane (anti-GBM) antibody titers or antineutrophilic cytoplasmic antibody (ANCA) titers should be ordered if a vasculitis is suspected.

Microscopic examination of the spun urine showing the presence of red blood cell casts is diagnostic of glomerular bleeding and disease (Figure 160.2). However, the absence of red blood cell casts does not rule out glomerular disease. Similarly, dysmorphic red blood cells and acanthocytes result from cell membranes traumatized by passage either through the glomerular capillary or by osmotic trauma as they pass through the nephron. Dysmorphic red cells correlate highly with the glomerular bleeding. Finally, dipstick results indicating 4+ proteinuria are highly suggestive of glomerular disease.

TABLE 160.3. Causes of Hematuria
Glomerular bleeding (immunologic)
Benign familial nephropathy
Progressive hereditary nephropathy (Alport's syndrome)
Mesangioproliferative glomerulonephritis
Benign form
IgA nephropathy (Berger's disease)*
Henoch-Schönlein purpura
Postinfectious glomerulonephritis
Rapidly progressive glomerulonephritis
Focal glomerular sclerosis
Membranoproliferative glomerulonephritis
Systemic diseases (e.g., systemic lupus erythematosus, Wegener's granulomatosis, Goodpasture's syndrome, hemolytic-uremic syndrome, progressive systemic sclerosis, cryoglobulinemia, thrombotic thrombocytopenic purpura, polyarteritis nodosa)
Tubulointerstitial disease
Nonglomerular bleeding (non-immunologic)
Renal tumors
Polycystic disease
Papillary necrosis (analgesic abuse, diabetes, sickle cell disease)
Renal trauma
Sickle cell disease or trait
Renal tuberculosis
Drugs (sulfonamides)
Urolithiasis

*Most common etiology, world-wide.

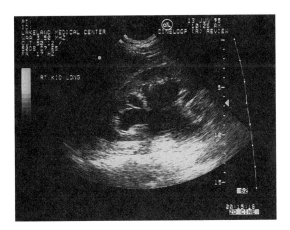

FIGURE 160.2. Hydronephrosis. The dark shadows in the center of the picture are dilated calyces.

■ Imaging

If the cause of hematuria remains elusive despite the foregoing laboratory studies, then imaging studies should be considered. Renal ultrasound is performed to evaluate renal size and calyces and to identify calculi, and renal masses. Figure 160.2 shows hydronephrosis as a result of a blocked ureter. Intravenous pyelogram requires injection of radiocontrast agents and is now seldom used except for evaluation of nephrolithiasis. If these tests are negative, a cystoscopy is recommended for evaluation of the bladder and prostate, especially in men older than 50 years of age. If a renal tumor is suspected, a CT scan and renal angiogram should be performed.

■ Renal Biopsy

A renal biopsy is performed to diagnose suspected glomerular or tubulointerstitial disease. In some circumstances, biopsy results not only provide a diagnosis, but also help guide treatment. In advanced chronic renal failure, it is of limited value. The most common complication of renal biopsy is bleeding; however, it is usually self-limited and requires no therapy. Presence of coagulopathies or poorly controlled blood pressure (>160/95 mmHg) are contraindications to renal biopsy.

Hematuria of Extra-renal Causes

Sixty-five percent of the patients with hematuria have bleeding from extra-renal sites. Common causes of extra-renal bleeding include calculi or neoplasms in the renal pelvis, ureter, bladder, and prostate. Infectious causes such as tuberculous and *Schistosoma hematobium* are common in certain parts of the world. Other causes such as trauma to the urinary tract and therapy with cyclophosphamide or anticoagulants should also be considered.

Proteinuria

Proteinuria is defined as a urinary protein excretion exceeding 150 mg in 24 hours. Healthy adults may excrete up to 30 mg of protein per day, most of it being globulin. Nephrotic range proteinuria is defined as the urinary protein excretion rate exceeding 3.5 gm/day and is often accompanied by serum lipid abnormalities and edema. In glomerular diseases due to excess glomerular capillary permeability, large amounts of albumin can leak into the urine. Conversely, in tubulointerstitial diseases most of the urinary proteins are globulins. The normal glomerulus is permeable to the light chain globulins produced by plasma cells in conditions such as multiple myeloma. These can be identified on urinary electrophoresis as monoclonal globulin peaks. Thus, proteinuria should be viewed in the clinical context. Finally, proteinuria may be the only evidence of serious underlying disease, as exemplified by the occurrence of an occult malignancy, most commonly lung, breast and colon, in 10–15% of patients with membranous nephropathy.

The approach to the patient with nonnephrotic range proteinuria should include a careful history including all medications used and a thorough physical examination. Among the numerous causes of nonnephrotic range proteinuria, (Table 160.4), prolonged, poorly controlled

TABLE 160.4.	Causes of Non-nephrotic Range Proteinuria
Hypertension causing nephrosclerosis
Primary glomerular disease
Tubulointerstitial nephritis
Cystic kidney diseases
Fanconi's syndrome
Obstructive nephropathy
Multiple myeloma
Drug-induced proteinuria (cyclosporin, amphotericin B, gold, penicillamine and others)
Benign proteinuria

TABLE 160.5.	Benign Forms of Proteinuria

Functional proteinuria: Occurs in subjects with one of the following conditions: a) high fever, b) congestive heart failure, c) strenuous exercise, and d) cold exposure.

Idiopathic proteinuria: Occurs with normal renal function and is characterized by normal microscopic urinalysis.

Orthostatic proteinuria: most commonly occurs in adolescence and is detected only when the patient is in a upright position. Total urinary protein is generally <2 gm/day.

immunoglobulin light chains. The test is performed by adding 8 drops of 20% sulfosalicylic acid to 2 ml or urine. Turbidity is proportional to the amount of protein present and ranges from visible turbidity to dense precipitation. False positive reactions occur under the following conditions: 1) alkaline urine, 2) high concentrations of penicillin or cephalosporins, 3) radiographic contrast media, 4) administration of nonsteroidal anti-inflammatory agents and 5) sulfonamide or tolbutamide metabolites. Benign proteinuria requires no treatment (Table 160.5).

A 24-hour urine collection for protein is commonly used to quantify the degree of proteinuria. Alternatively, a spot urine for protein and creatinine concentrations in mg/dl will provide a protein:creatinine ratio which compares well with the 24-hour protein quantification. With this method, a protein:creatinine ratio of 0.1 is equivalent to a normal daily protein excretion of 100 mg or less; a protein:creatinine ratio of 3 or greater is associated with a protein excretion of 3 grams per day or more consistent with nephrotic range proteinuria.

essential hypertension is perhaps the most common. Renal function should be determined in these patients by measuring serum creatinine, blood urea nitrogen, serum glucose, and electrolytes and by obtaining a creatinine clearance from a 24-hour urine collection. The urine specimen should be carefully examined for casts, cells, crystals and bacteria. If multiple myeloma is suspected, a serum and urine electrophoresis should be performed.

There are different methods used to screen for urinary protein. These include: **Dipstick method:** The dipstick detects albumin in the concentrations of 10–30 mg/dl (trace) to 2000 mg/dl (4+). Highly alkaline urine (pH >8) may yield false positive reactions. False negative reactions also occur in very dilute urine and when urine globulins and light chain immunoglobulins are present. **Sulfosalicylic acid method** detects 40–50 mg/liter of all proteins including hemoglobin and

Microalbuminuria refers to the excretion of albumin in the range of 30 to 300 mg per day (15–200 micrograms/min). Accurate quantification of albumin excretion cannot be done by the usual dipstick or quantitative protein methods but requires sensitive immunoassay techniques. In normals, urinary albumin excretion ranges from 2 to 31 mg/day. Screening for microalbuminuria is done by measuring the albumin:creatinine ratio in a first voided morning urine. The testing for microalbuminuria may have its greatest clinical value in detecting the earliest stages of diabetic nephropathy.

Leukocyturia

Normally, the urine microscopic examination contains less than 3 to 5 white blood cells per high-power field (hpf). If clean voiding techniques are carefully followed, the number of white blood cells in the urine is the same for men and women. Polymorphonuclear leukocytes contain esterases. Reagent strips detect leukocytes by the action of these esterases which causes a color change

in 1 to 2 minutes. The dipstick methodology is able to detect leukocytes in excess of 3 to 4 WBCs/hpf with a sensitivity of 92%. Leukocyturia is frequently seen in urinary tract infections, but may also occur in tubulointerstitial disease and in some patients with renal stones, even in the absence of infection.

CHAPTER 161   NEPHROTIC SYNDROME

■ Definition and Etiology

The general definition of **nephrotic syndrome** includes proteinuria exceeding 3.5 grams per day, with changes in serum lipids (increased serum cholesterol and

triglycerides) and a reduced serum albumin. Edema and hypercoagulable state are its clinical accompaniments. The hypercoagulability stems largely from urinary losses of factors that maintain clotting homeostasis such as antithrombin III. Lipiduria with epithelial cells containing fat droplets or "oval fat bodies" are also commonly seen. However, this generally occurs with massive proteinuria exceeding 5–10 gm/day. The causes of nephrotic range proteinuria are listed in Table 161.1. The most common primary renal cause of nephrotic syndrome is **minimal change disease** in children and **membranous glomerulopathy** in adults. The most common systemic disease to cause nephrotic syndrome is **diabetes mellitus.**

The **hypoalbuminemia** that occurs with nephrotic syndrome is largely due to the urinary loss of albumin, which is not compensated for by hepatic synthesis. A marked reduction in plasma oncotic pressure follows, with consequent edema, which can be generalized (generalized anasarca) and massive. Hypercholesterolemia and hypertriglyceridemia, the other components of nephrotic syndrome, occur because of increased hepatic cholesterol synthesis and decreased peripheral metabolism. Because of these changes and loss of anticlotting factors and immunoglobulins, these patients become more susceptible to atherosclerosis, thrombotic processes and infections by **encapsulated bacteria** with capsular antigens such as streptococcus, klebsiella, and others.

■ Diagnosis

In the absence of an obvious cause such as diabetes mellitus, patients with acute or new onset nephrotic syndrome within the preceding 6 months to one year should have a renal biopsy to diagnose the etiology. An acute increase in proteinuria, defined as an increase of over 2 to 3 gm/day in less than 1 year, may signify another glomerular disease or immunologic process. This is particularly important in subjects with diseases such as diabetes mellitus where as many as 20% may have another glomerular disease that accounts for the acute increase in proteinuria; renal biopsy is, therefore, important in establishing the diagnosis. Nonsteroidal anti-inflammatory agents may cause a tubulointerstitial nephritis and increased proteinuria. On physical examination, hypertension, rash, lymphadenopathy, or diabetic retinopathy may be present. Evidence for an occult malignancy (usually an adenocarcinoma) should also be sought if clinically suspected. Acute flank pain with a significant rise in proteinuria should alert one to the possibility of renal vein thrombosis, an entity to which patients with nephrotic syndrome are unusually predisposed. Venography or renal ultrasound with Doppler flow can be diagnostic.

■ Management

Treatment of the nephrotic syndrome generally depends on the underlying etiology. General principles of management, however, include the following: A sodium restricted (2–3 gm), low fat and 0.8–1.0 gm/kg/day protein diet is recommended. It is noteworthy that higher protein intake may actually exacerbate the nephrotic syndrome. Fluid intake should also be restricted if hyponatremia is present. Edema is managed generally through leg elevation and loop diuretics, although venodilating antihypertensive agents such as angiotensin converting enzyme (ACE) inhibitors are also useful. ACE inhibitors not only venodilate, but also reduce size selectivity and improve charge selectivity of the glomerular membrane to proteins. These effects are independent of their hypotensive effects. Other drug therapies that should be considered are related to the primary etiology of disease. Specifically, corticosteroids, cyclophosphamide, cyclosporine, or chlorambucil have all been found to reduce nephrotic range proteinuria associated with membranous nephropathy. However, with the exception of diabetes mellitus, there are no data to suggest that reduction in proteinuria reduces mortality.

TABLE 161.1. Causes of Nephrotic Syndrome
Primary glomerular diseases
Minimal change disease
Membranous nephropathy
Focal glomerulosclerosis
Membranoproliferative glomerulonephritis
Secondary glomerular diseases
Postinfectious: poststreptococcal, endocarditis, syphilis, hepatitis B, cytomegalovirus, AIDS, protozoa, parasitic
Metabolic: diabetes mellitus, myxedema
Connective tissue diseases and vasculitis: systemic lupus erythematosus, Sjogren's syndrome, polyarteritis nodosa, Goodpasture's syndrome, Henoch-Schönlein purpura, scleroderma, dermatomyositis
Neoplastic: solid tumors, lymphoma, leukemia
Drugs: (gold, penicillamine, mercury, probenecid, NSAIDs, captopril, lithium)
Allergens: poison ivy, insect bites
Systemic diseases: amyloidosis, malignant hypertension, sarcoidosis, severe congestive heart failure, constrictive pericarditis
Inherited diseases: sickle cell disease, hereditary nephritis, congenital nephrotic syndrome, Fabry's disease, nail-patella syndrome
Miscellaneous: renal transplant rejection, thrombotic thrombocytopenic purpura, hemolytic-uremic syndrome, preeclampsia

CHAPTER 162

ACUTE RENAL FAILURE

Acute renal failure presents as a sudden and rapid decline in kidney function, with or without oliguria, and depending on the underlying cause, hypovolemia or hypervolemia. Hyperkalemia and metabolic acidosis are commonly present, depending on the stage of evolution.

■ Etiology and Classification

The causes of **rapidly progressive renal failure** are summarized in Table 162.1. The more common ones include: volume depletion, acute tubulointerstitial nephritis, malignant hypertension, and atheroembolic renal disease. These should always be considered in situations where renal function has acutely changed. Perhaps even as common is the initiation of treatment with an ACE inhibitor in patients with hypertension secondary to subtle and unrecognized bilateral renal artery stenosis. A decrease in the effective circulating blood volume, caused either by volume depletion, a reduction in cardiovascular function (heart failure) or marked peripheral vasodilation, as in sepsis, is probably the most common etiology for acute renal failure in the United States. This is generally diagnosed by measuring the fractional excretion of sodium (FE_{Na}) in the urine. FE_{Na} is the urinary sodium excretion as a percent of filtered sodium or % excreted Na/filtered Na (% E/F_{Na}). It is calculated as follows:

$$FE_{Na} = \frac{U_{Na} \times P_{Cr}}{P_{Na} \times U_{Cr}}$$

A random or a "spot" urine specimen together with an accompanying blood sample are needed for the required measurements of plasma and urine Na and creatinine concentrations. When the kidney is underperfused, the FE_{Na} is generally far below the normal value of about 1%. Treatment of such patients is aimed at restoring renal perfusion with volume repletion, treatment of heart failure and/or blood pressure support. Prolonged periods of renal hypoperfusion may lead to acute tubular necrosis and a prolonged course of renal failure.

Acute tubular necrosis is secondary to renal ischemia or exposure to nephrotoxic drugs. Proximal renal tubular epithelial cell necrosis and sloughing of cells occurs with subsequent obstruction of the tubular lumen by casts. Some of the more common causes of intrinsic renal failure in the hospital are antibiotics (aminoglycosides, cephalosporins) or radiocontrast media. The general urinary manifestations of acute renal failure are summarized in Table 162.2. A BUN to creatinine ratio exceeding

10:1 suggests a **prerenal** cause such as volume depletion. Hyponatremia and hyperkalemia generally accompany this process and are related to the inability of the damaged kidney to excrete free water in the presence of ongoing water intake and to secrete potassium into the urine.

The most common cause of death from acute renal failure is infection. Gastrointestinal bleeding is noted in

TABLE 162.1. Causes of Acute Renal Failure

Prerenal failure
Volume depletion: poor fluid intake, diuretics, gastrointestinal losses, hemorrhage, third spacing
Peripheral vasodilation: sepsis, shock, liver failure, antihypertensive agents
Increased renal vascular resistance: anesthesia, surgery, prostaglandin inhibitors, hepatorenal syndrome
Cardiovascular disease: acute myocardial infarction, congestive heart failure, cardiac tamponade, arrhythmia, pulmonary embolism
Renal vascular occlusion: renal artery stenosis, embolism, thrombosis, vasculitis

Intrinsic renal failure
Renal vascular disorders: malignant hypertension, cholesterol emboli, vasculitides, thrombotic thrombocytopenic purpura, hemolytic-uremic syndrome, scleroderma renal crisis, toxemia of pregnancy
Glomerular diseases: acute postinfectious, diffuse proliferative, and rapidly progressive glomerulonephritis, systemic lupus erythematosus, infective endocarditis, Goodpasture's syndrome, vasculitis
Acute tubular necrosis: ischemia, nephrotoxic agents (aminoglycosides, cephalosporins, cyclosporine, amphotericin B, acyclovir, pentamidine, chemotherapeutic agents, radiographic contrast dye, heavy metals, hydrocarbons, anesthetics), rhabdomyolysis with myoglobinuria, hemolysis with hemoglobinuria, hypercalcemia, myeloma proteins, light-chain nephropathy
Tubulointerstitial diseases: allergic tubulointerstitial nephritis (antibiotics, diuretics, allopurinol, rifampin, phenytoin, cimetidine, NSAIDs), infection (staphylococcus, gram-negative bacteria, leptospirosis, brucellosis, viruses, fungi, acid-fast bacilli), infiltrative disease (leukemia, lymphoma, sarcoidosis)

Postrenal failure
Ureteral obstruction: retroperitoneal fibrosis or tumor, bilateral strictures after surgery or radiation, bilateral ureteral calculi, bilateral papillary necrosis, bilateral fungus balls, benign prostatic hypertrophy, prostatic cancer, bladder cancer, cervical cancer, neurogenic bladder

TABLE 162.2. Urinary Characteristics in Acute Renal Failure			
	Prerenal Azotemia	**Acute Tubular Necrosis (ATN)**	**Postrenal Azotemia**
Urine volume (mL/d)	<500	Oliguric <400 nonoliguric >400	Variable, from anuria to polyuria
Urine osmolality (mOsm/ kg-H$_2$O)	>500	<350	Early, resembles prerenal failure; late, more resemblance to acute tubular necrosis
U$_{osm}$/P$_{osm}$	>1.5	≤1	
Urine Na+ (mEq/L)	<20	>40	
FE$_{Na}$ %	<1	>2	
Urine sediment	Benign; few granular or hyaline casts	Renal tubular epithelial cells; hyaline and granular casts, protein "muddy brown" casts of ATN.	Normal; or hematuria pyuria, crystalluria

up to 30% of cases; cardiovascular events, such as pulmonary edema and congestive heart failure are also quite common. Lastly, there is a critical need to reduce doses of drugs that are normally excreted by the kidneys.

■ Diagnosis

The cause of acute renal failure can largely be determined by a history of recent exposure to nephrotoxic agents, hypotension during surgery or a preceding symptom(s) of an illness. Physical examination is helpful in determining the volume status of a patient, but usually does not give clues to the etiology of acute renal failure. A search for urinary tract obstruction should be made in all patients with acute renal failure. This includes: ultrasonography to examine the kidneys and ureters and a single straight catheterization of the bladder to detect urethral obstruction, especially in men. Laboratory tests begin with urinalysis. Heavy proteinuria with RBCs or hemoglobin casts are typical of severe acute glomerulonephritis. Proteinuria together with "muddy-brown" coarse granular casts are typical of tubular necrosis. Red-brown pigmented casts with no or few RBCs are typical of rhabdomyolysis. Other laboratory tests may reveal abnormalities of serum electrolytes, BUN, creatinine, calcium, phosphorus, and uric acid. Urine sodium and creatinine should be measured to estimate FE$_{Na}$ and urine and plasma osmolality should be measured to estimate the U/P osmolality ratio. A Wright or, preferably, a Hansel stain of the urine for eosinophils is quite useful to help determine the presence of drug-induced tubulointerstitial nephritis; but eosinophiluria also can be associated with bladder trauma, tuberculosis, and other causes.

Imaging of the kidney is generally unrewarding and does not aid in the diagnosis of acute renal failure except to exclude obstruction. Renal ultrasound should be performed in patients with acute renal failure to exclude this possibility. If normal, further imaging studies are not warranted. The possible exception is arteriography for diagnosis of polyarteritis nodosa or assessment of renal trauma. Renal biopsy is generally not indicated in acute renal failure, unless the history and physical examination point to a glomerular process.

■ Management

The general approach to treating these patients is to address the primary etiology. If dehydration is present, then volume repletion is required to restore effective circulating volume. Loop diuretics also have a role in converting renal failure from oliguric to nonoliguric. This conversion is associated with a better prognosis. Careful monitoring of serum electrolytes and acid-base status are obviously warranted. Care should also be taken to monitor calcium and phosphate status, especially if acute renal failure is secondary to rhabdomyolysis where hyperphosphatemia and hypocalcemia can occur quite rapidly. In these circumstances intravenous calcium gluconate, oral calcium carbonate, or acetate should be administered along with aluminum hydroxide, if necessary to control hyperphosphatemia.

Nutrition in such patients should be aimed at minimizing negative nitrogen balance while avoiding volume overload. Enteral nutrition is preferred over hyperalimentation. Specific formulations exist for patients with renal failure. These formulations have low protein content and contain little to no potassium. Calories are provided largely from carbohydrates. When enteral nutrition is not possible, hyperalimentation should be considered. Hyperalimentation should consist of 0.8–2 gm/kg/day of amino acids in nondialyzed patients, plus an added 10–20 gm/day of nonessential amino acids in the dialyzed patients.

TABLE 162.3.	Indications for Dialysis in Acute Renal Failure

Inability to control *volume* status: failure to respond to maximal doses of diuretics

Inability to control *acidosis* with intravenous therapy: pH persistently <7.2

Uremic symptoms (stupor, lethargy, pericarditis, nausea, vomiting, seizures)

Hyperkalemia: levels exceeding 7 mEq/dl unresponsive to resin binders or with ECG changes

The indications for dialysis in patients with acute renal failure are summarized in Table 162.3. In addition, patients with acute renal failure with a high catabolic rate or who are hemodynamically unstable may benefit from continuous arteriovenous hemofiltration or hemodiafiltration. This form of modified dialysis is about 20% as efficient as hemodialysis, and is useful in removing large amounts of fluid from patients who require continuous parenteral hyperalimentation. However, arterial pressure being the driving force for filtration, patients who are hypotensive i.e., systolic pressures <100 mmHg generally cannot be effectively treated with continuous arteriovenous hemofiltration.

CHAPTER 163 **CHRONIC RENAL FAILURE**

■ Definition and Etiology

Chronic renal failure is defined as a progressive and irreversible deterioration of renal function caused by a variety of diseases. The underlying primary disease is often difficult to identify when advanced renal failure is established. The two most common causes of chronic renal failure in the United States are diabetes mellitus and hypertension.

While laboratory manifestations of chronic renal failure do not occur until over 40% of renal function is lost, clinical manifestations generally do not occur until over 80% of GFR is lost. Moreover, when GFR declines below 10% of the normal value, uremia ensues and dialysis is required. The major changes that occur in chronic renal failure are summarized in Table 163.1. Causes of chronic renal failure are summarized in Table 163.2.

■ Clinical Features

Nearly all the organ systems may be affected by chronic kidney failure with resulting symptoms. These include difficult to control hypertension, cardiopulmonary abnormalities such as congestive heart failure and pulmonary edema. A bleeding diathesis occurs in these patients secondary to platelet dysfunction, manifested by an increased bleeding time. **Gastrointestinal problems** such as bleeding are common secondary to **arteriovenous malformations** or **angiodysplasia.** In addition, gastric erosions are commonly seen in patients with chronic renal disease. **Amylase** elevations to three times normal are common in dialyzed patients but pancreatitis is uncommon. Dysfunction of many organ systems

complicate chronic renal failure; the important ones are summarized below.

Bone disorders

Secondary hyperparathyroidism develops early during the course of progressive renal failure in the majority of patients. The mechanisms that cause increasing parathyroid hyperplasia and increased PTH secretion as kidney failure worsens are not completely understood but include: 1) an increase in the relative body burden of phosphate as functioning kidney mass decreases leading to hyperphosphatemia as GFR falls below 30 ml/min and 2) reduced renal synthesis of calcitriol which leads to reduced intestinal absorption of calcium. The effect of PTH to stimulate bone resorption sustains near-normal

TABLE 163.1.	Changes in Body Fluid Homeostasis in Chronic Renal Failure	
Problem	**Cause**	
Salt wasting	↓ proximal tubular function	
Hyperkalemia	↓ renal function (≥90%) and distal tubular function	
Hyperchloremic acidosis (non-anion gap)	↓ renal and tubular function	
↓ calcitriol synthesis	Hyperphosphatemia (GFR <30 ml/min)	
Normocytic normochromic anemia	↓ Erythropoietin Production (GFR <30 ml/min)	

↓ = Decreased.

plasma calcium concentrations and may cause hyperparathyroid bone disease, osteitis fibrosa cystica. As plasma phosphate concentrations rise above normal while plasma calcium concentrations are normal or only slightly reduced, the product of the two concentrations may rise above 55, potentially leading to metastatic calcification of blood vessels and joints.

Cardiovascular diseases

The most common cause of death among patients with end-stage renal disease is cardiovascular disease. The incidence of coronary artery disease markedly increases secondary to long standing hypertension and abnormal lipid metabolism.

Constrictive pericarditis and pericardial effusions are occasionally seen in dialyzed patients; however, they are confined to those who do not receive adequate dialysis or are noncompliant with dialytic therapy. Pericardial effusions seen with uremia are generally hemorrhagic.

TABLE 163.2.	Common Causes of Chronic Renal Failure

Diabetic nephropathy (most common)
Hypertensive nephrosclerosis (second most common)
Primary glomerular disease
Glomerular diseases associated with systemic illness
Tubulointerstitial diseases
Polycystic disease and other hereditary diseases
Renovascular disease
Thromboembolic disease
Chronic urinary tract obstruction (reflux)

Hematopoietic system

The anemia seen in chronic renal failure is largely due to a reduction in erythropoietin synthesis by interstitial cells in the area of the proximal tubule of the kidney. Erythropoietin is responsible for red blood cell differentiation from stem cells. While the leukocyte count in dialysis patients is generally normal, the chemotactic mechanism is generally defective. Hence, atypical immune responses result. The platelet count likewise is normal, however, platelet function is markedly defective.

■ Management

The most important maneuver to slow progression is to control blood pressure. There is ample evidence in humans that hypertension can accelerate renal damage. Control of blood pressure in a number of renal diseases slows deterioration. ACE inhibitors may have a selective advantage in preserving renal function in patients with diabetic glomerulosclerosis and a number of renal diseases including IgA nephropathy. Although many patients do not adhere strictly to a protein-restricted diet, education about its potential value and avoidance of excessive protein ingestion is recommended.

Management of patients with chronic renal failure should include: a) visible water restriction to a maximum of 1.5 liters/day; b) potassium restriction by limiting fruits (especially dried fruits), potatoes and other vegetables that have high potassium content; c) daily calcitriol and calcium supplementation with each meal, not only to provide calcium but to bind phosphate; d) recombinant erythropoietin, if hematocrit is below 25%, and in those with angina if hematocrit is below 30% with a goal to raise the level to 30%. Erythropoietin admin-

TABLE 163.3.	Dosage Adjustments of Commonly Used Medications in Renal Failure	
Use with Major Reduction in Dose	**Use with Minor or No Reduction in Dose**	**Avoid Altogether**
Antibiotics		
Aminoglycosides	Erythromycin	Tetracycline
Penicillin G	Nafcillin	Nitrofurantoin
Cephalosporins	Clindamycin	Nalidixic acid
Sulfonamides	Chloramphenicol	
Vancomycin	Isoniazid/rifampin	
Amphotericin B		
Other drugs		
Digoxin	Antihypertensives	Aspirin
Procainamide	Benzodiazepines	Sulfonylureas
H$_2$ antagonists	Quinidine	Lithium carbonate
	Lidocaine	Acetazolamide
	Codeine	Spironolactone
	Propoxyphene	Triamterene

istration, by unknown mechanisms, is followed by clinically important hypertension in approximately 20% of patients. Modifications in drug therapy may be necessary in renal failure; the common ones where this may be called for are summarized in Table 163.3.

End-stage renal disease (ESRD) is defined as permanent and almost complete (>90%) loss of kidney function, when life can be sustained only by dialysis

or kidney transplantation. Dialysis is performed using hemodialysis or peritoneal dialysis. Once the patient's condition is stabilized and there are no complications, kidney transplantation is performed. The kidney may be harvested from a matched related or unrelated live donor or a cadaver. On occasion, renal transplantation may be performed even before the patient requires dialysis.

CHAPTER 164 NEPHROLITHIASIS

Nephrolithiasis, (kidney stones) is a common disorder. Two to three percent of the population suffer at least one episode of nephrolithiasis during a lifetime. In these individuals, the risks of recurrent stones averages about 35% during the decade following the first episode.

■ Etiology

The etiologic diagnosis of nephrolithiasis depends on the history, laboratory tests and stone analysis. The history should include a family and personal history of stone disease and dietary habits, including intake of food high in calcium such as dairy products, nuts, rutabagas, spinach, beets, and chocolate. The initial evaluation of patients with this problem is summarized in Table 164.1. Laboratory tests should include: serum electrolytes, calcium, phosphate and uric acid; urine pH and microscopic examinations for crystals as well as a urine culture. Passed stones should be saved for analysis. Metabolic evaluation of kidney stones should always be performed prior to starting on a therapeutic regimen. Generally,

metabolic abnormalities are found in patients with recurrent calcium stones, rather than a single episode of a calcium stone. Moreover, calcium oxalate stone formation, which is frequent, can largely be corrected by dietary modifications. Thus, calcium stones do not deserve a full workup after the initial episode. Conversely, noncalcium stones should be investigated completely after the first episode. The general workup should include: two 24-hour urine collections for calcium, phosphate, uric acid, oxalate, citrate, creatinine, sodium, urea nitrogen, and cystine. If hypercalcemia is present, PTH level should be obtained. Despite thorough evaluation, a remediable cause of stones can be found only in 20% of patients.

Calcium stones

Calcium stones, which are radiopaque, constitute 80% of all kidney stones. If hypercalcemia is present, hyperparathyroidism is highly probable. However, other causes such as sarcoidosis, hyperthyroidism, multiple myeloma, or malignancy should also be considered. If hypercalciuria is present with normocalcemia, stones may be secondary to a distal renal tubular acidosis, renal calcium or phosphate leak or hyperthyroidism. If hyperuricosuria is present, even with a normal urinary and serum calcium, uric acid crystals may serve as the nidus for calcium stone formation. In this case, correction of the uricosuria would be useful in that it would eliminate this focus of stone formation. Hyperoxaluria with normal serum and urinary calcium levels may also be the result of acquired hyperoxaluria secondary to vitamin C abuse, excessive dietary oxalate intake, ileal resection or disease (see short bowel syndrome, Chapter 80 and regional enteritis, Chapter 84), or jejunoileal bypass surgery.

Struvite stones

Struvite stones are radiopaque and are composed of magnesium, ammonia and phosphate hydroxyapatite (also called triple phosphate stones). These stones are unique in that they form in high urinary pH, that results

TABLE 164.1.	Evaluation of the Patient with Urolithiasis	
Blood	**Urine**	**Radiography**
Calcium	pH	Plain film (KUB)
Uric acid	Crystals (oxalate, citrate)	Ultrasound
Phosphate	Gram stain (WBCs, bacteria)	IVP
Alkaline phosphatase	Culture	Serial KUBs
Parathyroid hormone	24-hour urine calcium	
1, 25(OH)$_2$ vitamin D$_3$	24-hour urine uric acid	

from urea-splitting organisms such as Proteus. These stones must be surgically removed in order to adequately treat the infection. If stones are of the appropriate size and in the proper location, lithotripsy is also an option.

Cystine stones

Cystine stones are also radiopaque, and are created by an inherited defect in the renal tubular absorption of cystine that result in cystinuria. The diagnosis is suggested by a positive urine nitroprusside test and confirmed by stone analysis.

Uric acid stones

These are the only radiolucent stones, and account for 10% of the cases. Uric acid stones are formed in hyperuricosuric states, volume depletion and acidic urine which reduces the solubility of uric acid. Fifty percent of patients with uric acid stones also have gout.

■ Clinical Features

Hematuria and/or severe colicky pain are common presentations of kidney stones. Hematuria may be gross or microscopic and the nature of pain depends on the location of the stone. Pelvic stones are usually painless unless an infection or obstruction is present. Ureteral stones, on the other hand, cause nausea, vomiting and severe abdominal flank pain radiating into the groin, urethra or genitalia or tip of the penis. Stones at the ureterovesical junction may result in dysuria, frequency and urgency. Fever and pyuria suggest associated urinary tract infection, but, if complete obstruction is present, pyuria may not occur. Chronic and complete obstruction can result in hydronephrosis.

■ Management

Acute episode

An effective analgesic must be given; however, morphine should be avoided since it aggravates the spasm of the ureter. A plain abdominal radiograph will generally show presence of stones and intravenous pyelogram can assess the size and position of the stone. A fine mesh straining device should be used to strain all urine to retrieve the stones. Water intake should be increased to maintain a daily urine output of 2 liters or more. If this is not possible, intravenous fluids should be given to increase urinary output. If large ureteral or pelvic stones cause obstruction, extracorporeal shock wave lithotripsy or surgical removal may be necessary.

Recurrent stones

For the more common type of stones such as calcium stones, hydration of at least 4–5 liters/day and reduction in calcium and oxalate intake are quite useful. Thiazide diuretics, such as 12.5 mg of hydrochlorothiazide, reduce urinary calcium excretion and are effective when administered to hypercalciuric calcium stone formers. Potassium citrate (60 mEq/day) in divided doses may also help prevent recurrence. Citrate prevents calcium oxalate and phosphate crystallization in the urine. Patients with hyperuricosuria (≤1000 mg of uric acid/24 hrs) and normal serum calcium can be benefited by 100–200 mg/day of allopurinol to reduce uric acid synthesis. Patients with acquired hyperoxaluria secondary to disease, restriction or bypass of the small intestine may benefit from oral calcium supplements to precipitate dietary oxalate within the intestine and/or by cholestyramine (4 gm three times a day) which binds oxalate in the gut. Patients with primary hyperoxaluria may be helped by pyridoxine that reduces endogenous oxalate synthesis.

Prevention of recurrent cystine stones is aimed at decreasing urinary concentration of cystine below the solubility limit of 200–300 mg/liter. Besides the methods already described, alkalinization of the urine to a pH above 7.5 is critical. This can generally be achieved with Shohl's solution which contains sodium citrate. In recalcitrant cases, sulfhydryl-containing drugs such as D-penicillamine, may be useful by increasing cystine solubility by forming mixed disulfide compounds of cystine.

Treatment of patients with uric acid stones includes increased water intake as above, and alkalinization of the urine to a pH of 7 or above with potassium citrate/ potassium bicarbonate or sodium bicarbonate in divided doses; both measures are aimed at increasing dissolution of uric acid. Additionally, acetazolamide may be used to alkalinize the nocturnal urine. Allopurinol in doses of 200 to 300 mg/day should be given for hyperuricemia to reduce the formation of uric acid. Purine-rich foods such as beef and liver should be avoided.

CHAPTER 165

GLOMERULAR DISEASES

The majority of glomerular diseases share an immunologic basis. Commonly, discrete deposition of granular deposits of immunoglobulins and complement are seen on the glomerular basement membranes of renal biopsy tissue. Alternatively, antigens can localize to this membrane and cause an antigen-antibody reaction which then initiates a cascade of reactions that results in glomerular injury.

Other glomerular diseases such as minimal change disease are also thought to have an immunologic basis; however, no deposits are found on tissue examination. Moreover, the resultant nephrotic syndrome is thought to be a disorder of the glomerular epithelial cell secondary to anti-glomerular antibodies. The terminology used in describing the pathology of the glomerular diseases is listed in Table 165.1. Some of the more common glomerular diseases are discussed next.

TABLE 165.1.	Pathologic Features of Glomerular Disease	
Focal	Less than 50% of glomeruli contain the lesion
Diffuse (global)	Most glomeruli (>50%) contain the lesion
Segmental	Only a part of the glomerulus is affected by the lesion (most focal lesions are also segmental, e.g., focal segmental glomerulosclerosis)
Proliferation	An increase in cell number of one or more of the resident glomerular cells with or without an inflammatory cell infiltration
Membranous changes	Capillary wall thickening due to deposition of immune deposits on basement membrane
Crescent formation	Epithelial cell proliferation and mononuclear cell infiltration in Bowman's space

Poststreptococcal Glomerulonephritis

This malady is manifested by sudden onset of gross hematuria, red blood cell casts in the urine and proteinuria that can occur 1–2 weeks after a pharyngeal or 3–6 weeks after a skin infection with group A β-hemolytic streptococci. Presenting symptoms include gross hematuria, edema, hypertension, back pain, oliguria, renal insufficiency and, in some cases, symptoms of heart failure secondary to volume overload. Nephrotic syndrome, while rare, occurs in 5% of newly diagnosed patients. Throat and skin culture may yield β-hemolytic streptococci if no antibiotic therapy has been given, but antibiotic treatment does not prevent glomerular disease. Serum complement levels are depressed for eight weeks and anti-DNase antibodies and ASO titers are elevated. No specific therapy is curative. Thus, treatment is supportive, with specific aims of reducing blood pressure and correcting volume overload. Diuretics are very useful in this context. It should be noted that in the majority of cases of poststreptococcal glomerulonephritis the serum creatinine generally does not exceed 4 mg/dl. If the clinical suspicion is not confirmed or if acute renal failure develops, a renal biopsy should be performed and a course of intravenous pulse steroid therapy given. The prognosis for this condition is much better in children than adults. Less than 2% of these patients die or develop end-stage renal disease and recovery is generally complete within two months. Patients over the age of 40 can develop a crescentic glomerulonephritis and generally have a poor prognosis.

IgA Nephropathy

Worldwide, IgA nephropathy is the most common glomerular disease to cause hematuria. The disease is characterized by recurrent attacks of gross hematuria frequently following a nonspecific viral illness. Hypertension and nephrotic syndrome, interestingly, are uncommon, and if present, portend a poor prognosis. The disease shows a sixfold greater predilection for men. Eighty percent of the patients with this disease are between the ages of 15 and 35 at the time of diagnosis. While gross hematuria is the most common laboratory finding, other abnormalities such as elevations in serum IgA level and skin biopsies showing deposits of IgA are generally positive. Serum complement levels are normal. Henoch-Schönlein purpura, a probably related disorder, may also be present.

Treatment is generally supportive and most patients have recurrent episodes. Interestingly, only about 25% of all patients progress to end-stage renal disease. Poor prognostic indicators include: male gender, older age, hypertension and proteinuria exceeding 2 gm/day. Lastly, impaired renal function at the time of initial presentation is a poor prognostic sign.

Rapidly Progressive Glomerulonephritis (RPGN)

This form of glomerular disease is defined as loss of renal function exceeding 50% over a period of three months associated with greater than 50% glomerular crescents on renal biopsy. This is not a specific disease but a syndrome that can occur with a severe form of primary or secondary glomerular disease, examples of which are listed in Table 165.2. A form of RPGN is anti-GBM disease. Anti-GBM antibody reacts with glomerular and alveolar basement membrane causing nephritis and Goodpasture's syndrome. This pulmonary-renal syndrome can present as an isolated pulmonary or renal disorder with the other organ affected later in the disease course. **Anti-GBM nephritis** may occur in the absence of pulmonary hemorrhage.

Clinically, anti-GBM disease accounts for 20% of all cases of rapidly progressive glomerulonephritis. Goodpasture's disease often occurs in children and young adults and is eight times more common in men than women. In contrast, anti-GBM nephritis affects middle-aged adults and has relatively equal gender distribution. Presenting symptoms can include hemoptysis, dyspnea on exertion, volume overload, uremia, fever, arthritis, and abdominal pain. Nephrotic range proteinuria is uncommon and hypertension is present in a fifth of all patients. The treatment of choice is plasma exchange combined with steroids and immuno-suppressive medications such as cyclophosphamide. Therapy is most effective when started early in the course of disease, specifically, when creatinine is less than 6 mg/dl. Prognosis for recovery of renal function is poor when the disease initially presents in the advanced stage.

■ Immune-Complex Mediated Crescentic RPGN

This disorder accounts for 30–50% of patients with RPGN. These are generally middle-aged and older patients with symptoms of anti-GBM disease. These patients, however, generally have hypocomplementemia. Treatment for this malady includes pulse steroid therapy with gradual tapering. The prognosis, however, is poor.

■ Antineutrophilic Cytoplasmic Antibody (ANCA) Glomerulonephritis

While this disease is similar to RPGN, no immune antibody (ANCA) deposits have ever been identified. Presenting features are those of systemic vasculitis and include: fever, weight loss, arthritis and abdominal pain. Therapy includes intravenous or oral cyclophosphamide, generally in combination with intravenous steroids. Therapy should be continued for a minimum of one year and at least six months after all clinical evidence of disease has disappeared.

TABLE 165.2. Causes of Rapidly Progressive Glomerulonephritis

Anti-GBM Disease
    With lung hemorrhage (Goodpasture's syndrome)
    Without hemorrhage (anti-GBM nephritis)
    Complicating membranous nephropathy
Immune complex-mediated glomerulonephritis
    Postinfectious glomerulonephritis
        Poststreptococcal
        Endocarditis
        Visceral abscess
    Collagen-vascular disease
        Systemic lupus erythematosus
        Cryoglobulinemia
        Henoch-Schönlein purpura
    Primary renal disease
        Membranoproliferative glomerulonephritis
        IgA nephropathy
ANCA-associated glomerulonephritis
    Polyarteritis nodosa (p-ANCA)
    Wegener's granulomatosis (c-ANCA)
Idiopathic crescentic glomerulonephritis

Minimal Change Disease

Minimal change disease accounts for 20% of all cases of nephrotic syndrome in adults and 75–80% of all cases in children. The peak age of onset is 2–6 years of age, however, it can be seen as late as 15–18 years of age. A second peak in incidence occurs in adults around the age of 50. This disease is characterized by the absence of hypertension. It can occur in concert with malignancy (such as Hodgkin's disease or adenocarcinoma) as well as with medications such as nonsteroidal anti-inflammatory drugs. The treatment for this disorder is oral corticosteroid therapy. In general, patients are exquisitely responsive to oral prednisone in divided doses of 1 mg/kg for a period of 1 month or continued for 1 week after remission of nephrotic syndrome. Over 90% of these patients have remission, however, 50% have a recurrence or relapse and when this occurs, low dose alternate day prednisone for 6–12 months is employed. Unresponsive patients or "steroid resistant" patients should be treated with oral cyclophosphamide 2 mg/kg per day for 2 months or oral chlorambucil 0.2 mg/kg/day for 3 months.

Focal Segmental Glomerulosclerosis

This form of glomerular disease is present in about 15–20% of all patients with nephrotic syndrome. Patients usually present with nephrotic syndrome, hypertension and mild degrees of renal insufficiency. This disease is often confused with minimal change disease, however, minimal change disease does not cause hypertension. Focal glomerulosclerosis is more common in African Americans and those with intravenous heroin, analgesic, or other drug abuse, and in those with acquired immune deficiency syndrome (AIDS), sickle cell disease, or sarcoidosis. Etiology is unknown and the prognosis is poor. There is no specific therapy, however, some reports suggest that high dose steroids for periods of four to six months may induce remission. Some of the small studies suggest that addition of plasmapheresis to steroids may slow progression of the disease.

Membranous Glomerular Disease

Membranous glomerular disease is the most common cause of nephrotic syndrome in adults, accounting for up to 50% of the cases. These people are generally between the ages of 30–50 years, men being more commonly affected than women. GFR is generally normal or slightly decreased. If history and physical examination are suggestive, malignancy should be sought, especially adenocarcinoma of the lung, colon and breast. Other secondary causes of membranous nephropathy include hepatitis B, SLE and drugs such as gold, penicillamine, captopril and nonsteroidal anti-inflammatory drugs. No definitive therapy exists for treating this disease, however, high dose alternate day steroids over a period of 2 months with gradual tapering is beneficial. In addition, cyclophosphamide and chlorambucil may induce remission but do not change the natural history with regard to progressive renal dysfunction.

Membranoproliferative Glomerulonephritis (MPGN)

This glomerulonephritis accounts for about 10% of all cases of nephrotic syndrome in adults. Usually it occurs with equal frequency between men and women and follows an upper respiratory infection in about 40% of cases. Initial presentation includes: acute glomerulonephritis, nephrotic syndrome, hematuria, hypertension, and decreased GFR associated with a low C3 level. There is no definitive therapy for MPGN. Fifty percent of patients with MPGN progress to end-stage renal disease. Aspirin at 325 mg plus dipyridamole 75 mg three times per day, has been reported to attenuate progression of this disease in some patients.

Glomerular Disorders Associated with Systemic Disease

Diabetes mellitus and systemic lupus erythematosus (SLE) are the two most common systemic diseases which are associated with glomerular injury; they are listed in Table 165.3. Renal disease due to SLE is also discussed in Chapter 258 in Rheumatic Diseases.

Sixty-seven percent of all patients with SLE have renal disease at the time of biopsy based on renal biopsy findings. Nephrotic syndrome commonly occurs in up to 60% of patients with SLE. GFR is reduced in 15–20% of the patients at the time of diagnosis. Renal biopsy is absolutely necessary in establishing the diagnosis.

People with pathologic changes associated with

TABLE 165.3.	Systemic Diseases with Renal Involvement

Diabetes mellitus (most common)
Systemic lupus erythematosus
Multiple myeloma
Polyarteritis nodosa
Wegener's granulomatosis
Scleroderma
Hemolytic-uremic syndrome
Thrombotic thrombocytopenic purpura
Amyloidosis
Cryoglobulinemia
Postpartum renal failure
Disseminated intravascular coagulation

types 1, 2, and, 5 are treated with oral prednisone, 1 mg/kg/day for two months with an 8 week tapering period. Fifty percent of these patients have proteinuria of less than 2 gm and their GFR and complement levels normalize. Those with class 3 and 4 lesions have much more extensive disease and require cyclophosphamide in addition to steroids.

■ Diabetic Nephropathy

Diabetic nephropathy is the most common cause of end-stage renal disease in the United States. Early and aggressive control of blood sugar and arterial pressure preserves renal function. Microalbuminuria, defined as albumin excretion of 30–300 mg/24 hrs is the first indication of diabetic nephropathy. Urine should be monitored for microalbuminuria every 6–12 months in all diabetic patients and those exhibiting it should be treated with an ACE inhibitor, regardless of blood pressure, to forestall renal failure. Calcium blockers such as verapamil and diltiazem, but not dihydropyridines, also reduce proteinuria. ACE inhibitors and calcium channel blockers along with a diuretic are the treatment of choice in controlling hypertension in the diabetic.

The hallmark morphologic change seen in diabetic nephropathy is mesangial matrix expansion; when nodular, it is called the nodular sclerosis or **Kimmelstiel-Wilson lesion**. Conversely, this is not seen in the early stages of hypertension without diabetes.

CHAPTER 166 TUBULOINTERSTITIAL NEPHROPATHY

This group of clinical disorders affect the renal tubules and interstitium, sparing the glomeruli and renal vasculature. Based on the temporal relationships, both acute and chronic forms of this disease exist, with the acute type resulting in a rapid decline in renal function over a period of days to weeks, and the chronic form resulting in progressive azotemia and histologic changes of interstitial scarring and fibrosis that evolve over a period of years.

Acute Tubulointerstitial Nephritis

Acute tubulointerstitial nephritis is characterized by an acute decline in renal function associated with biopsy findings of inflammatory cell infiltrates within the renal interstitium. This process accounts for approximately 15% of all cases of renal dysfunction. The two most common causes (Table 166.1) of acute tubulointerstitial nephritis are nonsteroidal anti-inflammatory drugs (NSAIDs) and antibiotics, specifically, sulfonamides or penicillins. Acute pyelonephritis is classified histologically as a form of acute tubulointerstitial nephritis, however, the mechanism for nephritis is direct bacterial invasion of the renal medulla and not an allergic reaction as is the case with other causes.

The major clinical finding in acute tubulointerstitial nephritis is the development of acute renal insufficiency. One-third of patients develop the triad of fever, skin rash and peripheral eosinophilia with arthralgias while as many as 50% have peripheral eosinophilia alone. The absence of these features does not exclude the possibility of acute tubulointerstitial nephritis. Hypertension and edema are important features of acute glomerulonephritis but generally are not seen in acute tubulointerstitial nephritis.

Generally, the first clue to the diagnosis of acute tubulointerstitial nephritis is urinary abnormalities and a rise in serum creatinine. Hematuria, often microscopic, is common with a drug-induced etiology. In addition, sterile pyuria with leukocyte casts may be seen. Presence of eosinophiluria as noted by Hansel stain or Wright stain is often diagnostic but generally present only within the first 5–7 days of the disease. Eosinophiluria is not pathognomonic for tubulointerstitial nephritis, as it is also seen in trauma and cystitis. Lastly, if red blood cell casts are found, it indicates glomerulonephritis rather than tubulointerstitial nephritis.

It is important to distinguish between tubulointerstitial nephritis induced by antibiotics and that by NSAIDs.

TABLE 166.1.	Causes of Acute Interstitial Nephritis

Drug-related	Antimicrobial drugs
	  Penicillins (esp. methicillin)
	  Rifampin
	Sulfonamides
	Nonsteroidal anti-inflammatory
	  drugs
	Allopurinol
	Loop diuretics

Systemic infections	Streptococcal infections Cytomegalovirus Infectious mononucleosis Legionnaires' disease Leptospirosis
Primary renal infections	Acute bacterial pyelonephritis
Immune disorders	Acute glomerulonephritis Systemic lupus erythematosus Transplant rejection
Idiopathic	

Corticosteroids are very effective in shortening the course of antibiotic-induced tubulointerstitial nephritis but confer no benefit in NSAID-induced type. Both improve upon stopping the drug.

Chronic Tubulointerstitial Nephropathy

There are a wide variety of diseases that cause chronic tubulointerstitial nephritis. Among the many causes of chronic interstitial nephritis (Table 166.2), chronic pyelonephritis remains one of the most prominent.

Chronic tubulointerstitial nephropathy is responsible for 25–30% of all cases of end-stage renal disease. The

clinical findings associated with chronic tubulointerstitial disease are summarized in Table 166.3. Most patients with chronic tubulointerstitial nephritis have little to no clinical evidence of active renal inflammation. Lithium therapy and disorders such as analgesic toxicity, sickle cell disease or polycystic disease affect the concentration

TABLE 166.2.	Conditions Associated with Chronic Tubulointerstitial Nephropathy		

Urinary tract obstruction
  Vesicoureteral reflux
  Mechanical
Drugs
  Analgesics
  Nitrosurea
  Cisplatin
  Cyclosporine
Vascular diseases
  Nephrosclerosis
  Atheroembolic disease
  Radiation nephritis
  Sickle hemoglobinopathies
  Vasculitis
	Heavy metals
	  Lead
	  Cadmium
	Metabolic disorders
	  Hyperuricemia/hyperuricosuria
	  Hypercalcemia/hypercalciuria
	  Hyperoxaluria
	  Potassium depletion
	  Cystinosis
	Hereditary diseases
	  Medullary cystic disease
	  Hereditary nephritis
	  Polycystic kidney disease
		Malignancies
		  Multiple myeloma
		Granulomatous diseases
		  Sarcoidosis
		  Tuberculosis
		  Wegener's granulomatosis
		Immunologic diseases
		  Systemic lupus erythematosus
		  Sjogren's syndrome
		  Cryoglobulinemia
		  Goodpasture's syndrome
		Endemic diseases
		  Balkan nephropathy

TABLE	166.3.	Findings Suggestive of Chronic Tubulointerstitial Diseases

1. Hyperchloremic metabolic acidosis (out of proportion to the degree of renal insufficiency)
2. Hyperkalemia (out of proportion to the degree of renal insufficiency)
3. Reduced maximal urinary concentrating ability (polyuria, nocturia)
4. Partial or complete Fanconi's syndrome: Phosphaturia, bicarbonaturia, aminoaciduria, uricosuria, glycosuria

mechanism of the kidney; polyuria is a common sequel. The urinalysis may show modest amounts of sterile pyuria and minimal hematuria, but in most cases, there are no cellular casts. Different diseases affect different portions of the tubule. Conditions such as multiple myeloma and heavy metal toxicity (e.g. lead), primarily affect the proximal tubule and usually result in proximal renal tubular acidosis, glycosuria, aminoaciduria and uricosuria. Conversely, chronic obstruction of the urinary tract primarily affects the distal renal tubule and can present with distal tubular acidosis, salt wasting and hyperkalemia.

CHAPTER 167 VASCULAR DISEASES OF THE KIDNEY

■ Arteriosclerosis

Disorders of the main renal vessels are usually unilateral and are discussed later in this chapter. The processes that involve the smaller vessels of the kidneys, however, are diffuse and usually affect both kidneys. Clinically, these arterial disorders are usually associated with hypertension due to activation of the renin-angiotensin system. Renal failure may occur acutely, but it is usually progressive over a period of weeks to months.

■ Thromboembolic Disease

Perhaps the most common form of arteriolar disease is secondary to atheroembolism. This process is generally seen in people with severe atherosclerotic disease who have undergone an aortogram. During or after the aortogram emboli of cholesterol crystals may shower the kidney. These waxy crystals subsequently occlude the peripheral capillary beds within the kidney and choke off circulation to that portion of the nephron. A generally diffuse process involving thousands of nephrons, hypertension and renal dysfunction are the usual sequelae. Associated eosinophilia and eosinophiluria help establish the diagnosis of atheroembolic disease, but are present in only about 25% of patients.

■ Scleroderma

This is a progressive connective tissue disease of uncertain etiology (see Chapter 259 in Rheumatic Diseases). Renal arterioles usually demonstrate intimal proliferation with progressive luminal occlusion. The

clinical course of renal involvement reflects these pathologic changes. However, the development of proteinuria or mild hypertension in this disease often heralds the onset of accelerated sclerodermal renal crises and subsequent acute renal failure. This poorly understood process is markedly improved by antihypertensive therapy with angiotensin converting enzyme inhibitors.

■ Hemolytic-Uremic Syndrome and Thrombotic Thrombocytopenic Purpura

The hemolytic-uremic syndrome (HUS) and thrombotic thrombocytopenic purpura (TTP) are two disorders characterized by microangiopathy. The renal lesion varies in severity and is characterized by fibrin thrombi in the glomerular capillary loops. HUS is generally observed in children following a bout of gastroenteritis or a flu-like syndrome. Among adults, it is seen more often in young women, in association with the use of oral contraceptives. However, some antineoplastic agents and immunosuppressive drugs have been associated with its development. The clinical syndrome of TTP, conversely, is dominated by neurologic features. The clinical course of renal involvement is acute and rapidly progressive. The prognosis is poor. Plasmapheresis is the treatment of choice.

■ Renal Arterial Occlusion

Partial obstruction of the renal arterial system by atheromatous plaques or fibromuscular dysplasia is directly linked to renovascular hypertension. Thrombosis of the renal arteries is most often seen in cases of severe blunt abdominal trauma and rarely after surgical manipulation or during angiographic study of the renal artery. Thrombosis can also occur as an embolic phenomena in patients with underlying atherosclerotic vascular disease. This may also occur following radiocontrast studies. Rarely, valvular vegetations of bacterial endocarditis embolize and obstruct renal arteries. Symptoms include severe, localized flank pain, nausea, vomiting and oliguria. Nuclear renography is useful in diagnosis.

■ Renal Vein Thrombosis

Renal vein thrombosis is generally seen in states of heavy proteinuria, with urinary loss of clotting factors and antithrombin III, such as occurs in membranous nephropathy or minimal change disease. It is generally associated with flank pain and, in rare cases, pulmonary embolism. Diagnosis can be made by Doppler renal ultrasound or renal venography. Anticoagulation is the therapy of choice and renal function generally improves with resolution of the thrombus. Prophylactic anticoagulation, however, is not recommended for patients with nephrotic syndrome who are at risk for developing thrombosis.

CHAPTER 168

CYSTIC DISEASES OF THE KIDNEY

Cysts are commonly found in the kidneys. They are characterized by epithelial lined cavities filled with fluid or semi-solid debris. The most commonly seen clinical entities associated with cystic disease are discussed here.

The finding of a solitary cyst in a middle-aged person is most compatible with a simple cyst. However, the same finding in a neonate with an abdominal mass suggests the possibility of autosomal dominant polycystic kidney disease (ADPKD) or an autosomal recessive form of the disease (ARPKD).

■ Simple Cysts

Simple renal cysts increase in frequency with age and are present in 50% of the population over the age of 50 and in over 90% of the population over the age of 75. They are generally asymptomatic and do not increase the risk of neoplastic disease. They can generally be found on renal ultrasound examination.

Polycystic Kidney Disease (PKD)

■ Clinical Features

There are both autosomal dominant and autosomal recessive forms of the disease. The autosomal dominant form is much more common and carried on chromosome 16. ADPKD is the most common hereditary disease in the United States, affecting approximately half a million people. Clinical manifestations of this disease are rare prior to the age of 20. Patients usually present either for screening because of a family history of the disease or evaluation of symptoms. While pain and hematuria are the most common clinical manifestations, a number of patients can present with vague urinary tract symptoms and presence of new onset hypertension. Thus, patients with hypertension and the presence of microscopic hematuria should receive a renal ultrasound to screen for cystic disease, especially if there is a family history of this disorder.

Hypertension can occur in up to 60% of patients before any findings of renal insufficiency are noted. Nocturia is often present at the time of diagnosis, due to a tubular urinary concentration defect. Most patients also manifest a mild salt-wasting nephropathy. Urinary tract infection and pyelonephritis are common complications. Up to one-third of patients with PKD have multiple asymptomatic hepatic cysts and 10% have cerebral "berry" aneurysms. Twenty-five percent also have mitral valve prolapse. The natural history of renal functional impairment from ADPKD is variable. The disease progresses to end-stage renal disease in about 25% of individuals by age 50 and 50% by age 70.

■ Diagnosis and Management

The diagnosis is based on radiographic evidence of multiple cysts distributed throughout the kidney and is associated with renal enlargement, increased cortical thickening and splaying of the renal calyces. A contrast

CT in adults usually defines the anatomy well. It is worth remembering that malignancies can develop in these cysts. Renal ultrasonography accurately determines whether a mass is cystic or solid. Two-thirds of renal masses fulfill all ultrasound criteria for simple cysts and require no further work-up. However, when a mass is suspected, but not confirmed by ultrasound, a CT is required. If the mass on ultrasound is solid or complex, a renal CT, both with and without contrast is the next diagnostic step. For indeterminate cases, arteriography, needle aspiration cytology or both may be needed.

It is now possible to screen patients for the presence of polycystic disease prior to their development through genetic linkage analysis. While this can predict the likelihood with a 99% certainty, it is quite expensive and requires cooperation from family members with the disease. Moreover, since there is no definitive therapy for this disease, it should be reserved for patients who can afford it and have the desire to know. The employment and insurance implications should be fully considered prior to undertaking genetic linkage analysis.

There is no definitive therapy for polycystic kidney disease; however, the results of recent studies demonstrate that aggressive control of arterial blood pressure tends to slow the disease process. A low-protein diet does not influence its natural history. Patients with ESRD secondary to ADPKD are candidates for transplantation. A unique feature of patients with ADPKD is that the coexistent anemia is only mild. This reflects the ability of the kidney to secrete some erythropoietin despite the end-stage nature of the renal disease.

■ Acquired Cystic Disease

Cysts develop in large numbers of patients with end-stage renal disease undergoing dialysis. In these cysts, much like those of the polycystic patient, the risk of developing a renal carcinoma is heightened.

■ Medullary Sponge Kidney

Medullary sponge kidney is a benign disorder that is often detected incidentally on abdominal radiographs. It is commonly associated with the development of renal stones, especially the calcium oxalate variety. It is estimated that 10% of patients who present with renal stones have medullary sponge kidney. Nephrocalcinosis occurs in about 50% of these patients, but is usually asymptomatic and noted as an incidental finding. Renal failure does not occur as part of this disease and aggressive treatment of any urinary tract infection or stone is similar to what has been previously presented in this chapter.

CHAPTER 169 HUMAN IMMUNODEFICIENCY VIRUS (HIV) NEPHROPATHY

The reader is referred to Chapter 158 for a full discussion of Human Immunodeficiency Virus (HIV) infection and HIV disease. As a systemic disease, infection with the HIV virus is associated with various forms of renal disease as well. The most common glomerular disease is a collapsing form of focal glomerular sclerosis. This process may be seen in people with active acquired immune deficiency syndrome (AIDS), AIDS related complex (ARC), or asymptomatic HIV infection. Besides this primary glomerular lesion, patients with HIV infection also can develop other forms of renal disease. These diseases may be due not only to HIV infection, but to associated infections involving CMV virus, hepatitis B, syphilis, and other related infections seen in this population.

Approximately 6% of patients with HIV infection develop a collapsing focal glomerular sclerosis. Interestingly, and for unknown reasons, most of these patients are African American men. Clinically, their presentation is similar to that of idiopathic focal glomerulosclerosis, in that they present with obstinate hypertension, substantial peripheral edema, evidence of nephrotic syndrome, hypoalbuminemia and occasional RBCs and WBCs in the urinary sediment without RBC- or WBC casts. The laboratory examination generally reveals a significant reduction in renal function as manifested by an abnormally high BUN and creatinine. Besides large echogenic kidneys compatible with renal disease, an ultrasound of the kidneys is generally unremarkable. Renal biopsy can distinguish the HIV form from the idiopathic focal glomerulosclerosis. The distinguishing features of the HIV renal disease are collapse and sclerosis of the entire glomerular tufts and microcyst formation in tubules with tubular degeneration.

Combination therapy using reverse transcriptase inhibitors such as zidovudine and didanosine and protease inhibitors such as indinavir and ritonavir as described in chapter 158 can prevent or slow the progression of renal disease.

CHAPTER 170

DISORDERS OF WATER BALANCE

Plasma osmolality is maintained within a narrow range between 285–300 mOsm. This precise degree of regulation is dependent upon the following factors: control of thirst, regulation of ADH secretion and renal concentrating and diluting mechanisms. When plasma osmolality rises, thirst is stimulated, the ADH secretion increases and a concentrated urine is excreted. As a result, plasma osmolality decreases to normal. When plasma osmolality falls, thirst and ADH secretion are inhibited. A water diuresis occurs and consequently, plasma osmolality rises to normal. A failure of these adaptive responses results in disturbances of water excretion.

Hyponatremia and hypernatremia represent the major disorders of water balance. Plasma osmolality can be measured directly using freezing point depression methodology or calculated using the following formula:

$$P_{osm} = 2 \times [Na^+] + BUN/2.8 + glucose/18$$

From the formula, it is apparent that Na^+ and Cl^-, its accompanying anion, are the most important determinants of plasma osmolality. Urea is considered an "ineffective osmole" because it readily crosses cell membranes and therefore does not result in the osmotic movement of water.

Hyponatremia

Hyponatremia, defined as a serum Na^+ below 135 mmol/L, is the most common electrolyte abnormality in hospitalized patients. Hyponatremia resulting from syndrome of inappropriate ADH secretion is further discussed in Chapter 57. Usually hyponatremia is a hypo-osmolal state and the low osmolality is responsible for the shift of water into cells. Occasionally hyponatremia may be associated with a normal or elevated plasma osmolality. It is important to recognize such situations because they are not associated with the shift of water into cells which is seen with hypo-osmolal hyponatremia. Thus, the first step in the evaluation of hyponatremia should be a determination of plasma osmolality (Table 170.1). Hyponatremia associated with an elevated plasma osmolality is usually due to hyperglycemia but may also be due to the infusion of mannitol or glycine. These solutes cause the osmotic shift of water out of cells which

can result in hyponatremia. Laboratory artifact or pseudohyponatremia should be suspected when hyponatremia is associated with a normal plasma osmolality. This can occur with elevations of lipids (usually triglycerides) or proteins (e.g., multiple myeloma or Waldenström's macroglobulinemia). In these settings, the increased quantity of lipid or protein occupies a larger portion of the plasma volume and use of standard flame photometry yields a low Na^+ concentration since it measures the concentration of Na^+ per liter of plasma. However, under the same circumstances, a Na^+ selective electrode would detect a normal Na^+ concentration since this methodology measures Na^+ concentration in the aqueous phase of plasma.

■ Classification and Etiology

Once hypotonic hyponatremia is determined to be present, a careful assessment of volume status is essential in determining the etiology of hyponatremia and choosing the most appropriate therapy (Table 170.2). Hypovolemic hyponatremia occurs when total body Na^+ is depleted in relation to total body water (TBW). This can occur with both renal and nonrenal Na^+ loss. Causes of renal Na^+ loss include diuretics and salt wasting nephropathy. Nonrenal Na^+ loss can occur with GI losses (diarrhea or vomiting), third spacing, and skin losses. In all of these settings, hypovolemia induces the release of ADH which promotes the reabsorption of water. Hyponatremia occurs as a result of the loss of Na^+ and the retention of water. Urinary electrolytes may be useful in distinguishing between renal and nonrenal losses. With renal losses, urinary Na^+ usually exceeds 20 mEq/L. In

TABLE 170.1.	Types of Hyponatremia Based on Plasma Osmolality

Elevated osmolality (hypertonic hyponatremia)
Hyperglycemia
Glycine infusion
Mannitol infusion
Normal osmolality (pseudohyponatremia)
Hyperlipidemia
Hyperproteinemia
Low osmolality (true or hypotonic hyponatremia)

contrast, urinary Na^+ is usually below 20 mEq/L with nonrenal Na^+ loss.

In euvolemic hyponatremia, volume status is normal and hyponatremia is due to a relative excess of TBW. The most common cause of euvolemic hyponatremia is the syndrome of inappropriate ADH secretion (SIADH, see Chapter 57). As shown in Table 57.4, common causes of SIADH include tumors, pulmonary conditions, intracranial conditions and medications. Urinary Na^+ typically exceeds 20 mEq/L and the urine is inappropriately concentrated (U_{osm} >100 mOsm/kg) for the degree of plasma hypoosmolality. Other causes of euvolemic hyponatremia include adrenal insufficiency and hypothyroidism (Table 170.2).

Hyponatremia may also occur in the setting of hypervolemia due to congestive heart failure, cirrhosis, and nephrotic syndrome. These settings are characterized by decreased effective circulatory volume despite the presence of an increase in TBW. The decrease in effective circulatory volume results in the secretion of ADH which in turn leads to water retention and dilutional hyponatremia. In these settings, hyponatremia generally serves as a marker of the severity of the underlying disease since it usually occurs only when advanced disease is present. In general, urine Na^+ concentrations are below 20 mEq/L because of avid Na^+ reabsorption.

■ Clinical Features

Symptoms of hyponatremia are primarily neurologic and can include lethargy, confusion, seizures, and coma. The severity of symptoms is related to the rate of development of hyponatremia. **Acute hyponatremia** is more likely to be associated with symptoms due to brain swelling. In contrast, symptoms may be mild or absent with **chronic hyponatremia** because adaptive processes (involving the cellular extrusion of electrolytes and "osmoles") minimize the degree of brain swelling.

■ Management

Before attempting to correct hyponatremia, the rate and magnitude of correction must be determined (Table 170.3). The optimal rate of correction of hyponatremia continues to be controversial. However, a consensus has emerged that acute hyponatremia should be corrected more rapidly than chronic hyponatremia. As discussed above, acute and chronic hyponatremia can usually be differentiated on the basis of symptoms. With acute hyponatremia, rapid correction is necessary in order to

TABLE 170.2. Causes of Hyponatremia		
With Decreased ECV	**Normal ECV**	**Increased ECV**
Renal Losses	SIADH (Table 57.8)	Nephrotic syndrome
Diuretics	Adrenal insufficiency	CHF
Salt losing nephropathy	Hypothyroidism	Cirrhosis
Hypoaldosteronism		
GI Losses		
Diarrhea		
Vomiting		
Skin Losses		
Fever, burns		

ECV = effective circulating volume. SIADH = Syndrome of inappropriate antidiuretic hormone secretion.

TABLE 170.3. Treatment of Hyponatremia	
I. Determine the rate of correction	
Acute hyponatremia	Rapid correction at a rate of 1–2 mEq/L/hr. until Na^+ 120 mEq/L
Chronic hyponatremia	Slow correction at a rate of 0.5 mEq/L/hr. until Na^+ 120 mEq/L
II. Determine the mode of correction	
Hypovolemic hyponatremia	Saline
Euvolemic hyponatremia	Fluid restriction; furosemide alone or with saline to replace urine Na+ losses Demeclocycline in SIADH if above is insufficient
Hypervolemic hyponatremia	Treat underlying disease Fluid restriction Furosemide alone or with saline to replace urine Na+ losses if above is unsuccessful

decrease brain swelling. In contrast, in chronic hyponatremia, since adaptive processes have normalized brain water, slower correction is indicated in order to minimize the risk of **central pontine myelinolysis**. With rapid correction, the goal of therapy is to raise the serum Na$^+$ 1–2 mEq/L/hour until the patient becomes asymptomatic, which generally corresponds to a plasma Na$^+$ of 120–125 mEq/L. The serum Na$^+$ should not be raised more than 20 mEq/L over 24 hours and overcorrection of serum Na$^+$ (>135–140 mEq/L) should be avoided. To treat chronic hyponatremia, fluid restriction (1000–1500 ml/day) may be all that is needed. Correction should occur over 48–72 hours; the rate of correction should not exceed 0.5–1.0 mEq/L/hour. In all cases of hyponatremia, underlying disease states should be treated and offending medications discontinued.

Hypernatremia

Hypernatremia is defined as a serum Na$^+$ above 150 mEq/L. It is relatively uncommon because the thirst mechanism protects against its development. As a result, most cases occur in individuals who lack access to water; hypernatremia is most likely to occur in the very young, the elderly, and in comatose patients. Occasionally, hypernatremia can occur in patients with a defective thirst mechanism secondary to a central nervous system defect.

■ Etiology

Hypernatremia, like hyponatremia, can be categorized according to the associated volume status (Table 170.4). Patients with hypervolemic hypernatremia have an increase in total body Na$^+$. This relatively uncommon form of hypernatremia is usually iatrogenic and due to administration of excessive amounts of hypertonic salt

TABLE 170.4. Causes of Hypernatremia
Hypervolemic
Administration of sodium loads
Euvolemic
Diabetes insipidus
Nephrogenic
Central
Hypovolemic
GI losses (diarrhea)
Renal losses
Osmotic diuresis (glucose, mannitol)
Loop diuretics
Insensible losses (burns, fever)

The specific mode of therapy to raise the serum Na$^+$ is best determined by the type of hyponatremia (Table 170.3). To correct hypovolemic hyponatremia, the Na$^+$ deficit must be calculated and replaced. The Na$^+$ deficit is calculated as follows:

$$Na^+ \text{ deficit} = (Desired\ plasma\ Na^+ - Actual\ plasma\ Na^+) \times TBW$$

To correct euvolemic hyponatremia, it is useful to know the free water excess, which can be derived as follows:

$$Desired\ TBW = Actual\ plasma\ Na^+/Desired\ plasma\ Na^+ \times Actual\ TBW$$
$$Free\ water\ excess\ (in\ liters) = Actual\ TBW - Desired\ TBW$$

solutions such as hypertonic saline, bicarbonate or hypertonic feedings.

Euvolemic hypernatremia is seen with diabetes insipidus (DI) and is the result of pure water loss. It is important to stress that in DI, hypernatremia is a complication seen only in patients with limited access to water or a thirst defect. Patients with diabetes insipidus can also become volume depleted with extreme water losses.

DI may be central or nephrogenic. In central DI, ADH secretion by the posterior pituitary is absent or incomplete. Central DI may occur as a result of surgery, trauma, cancer, encephalitis, granulomatous disease (sarcoidosis or eosinophilic granuloma), or may be idiopathic. In nephrogenic DI, there is an impairment in the tubular response to ADH. Nephrogenic DI occurs rarely as a congenital disease due to a gene mutation which codes for a defective ADH receptor. More commonly, it is an acquired disorder and may be due to tubulointerstitial diseases (e.g., sickle cell disease), metabolic disorders (hypokalemia, hypercalcemia), and drugs (lithium, demeclocycline). With both central and nephrogenic DI, urine osmolality is inappropriately low for the degree of hypernatremia and is lower for the complete forms of the disorders than for the incomplete ones. Water deprivation testing and the responsiveness to exogenously administered ADH is useful in distinguishing nephrogenic from central DI. If diagnostic uncertainty persists, serum ADH level should be measured.

Hypovolemic hypernatremia is due to hypotonic losses of Na$^+$ and water secondary to GI, renal, or insensible losses (Table 170.4). With nonrenal losses, urine Na is low (<20 mEq/L) and urine osmolality is high (>400 mOsm/kg).

Clinical Features

As with hyponatremia, symptoms are mostly neurological and are more severe when the disorder is acute than when it is chronic. Initially, the increase in plasma osmolality pulls water from the intracellular space and leads to cellular dehydration. As a result of brain shrinkage, symptoms can include twitching, seizures, and coma. Occasionally hemorrhage may occur as a result of ruptured cerebral veins. After 12 to 24 hours of hypernatremia, cerebral dehydration is ameliorated by adaptive processes which involve the cellular uptake of electrolytes and amino acids. Nonetheless, the mortality rate is very high for patients with serum Na^+ above 160 mEq/L.

Management

It is important to correct hypernatremia slowly with a rate of correction of no greater than 0.5–1 mEq/L/hour. Once the adaptive process has begun, overly rapid correction may lead to cerebral edema. In planning therapy, it is useful to estimate the free water deficit which can be derived as follows:

$$Actual\ TBW = Body\ weight\ (kg) \times 60\%$$

$$\frac{Actual\ plasma\ Na^+}{Desired\ plasma\ Na+} \times Actual\ TBW = Desired\ TBW$$

$$Free\ water\ deficit\ (liters) = Desired\ TBW - Actual\ TBW$$

Specific therapy for hypernatremia is dictated by the associated volume status and the underlying etiology (Table 170.5). With hypervolemic hypernatremia, administration of Na^+ should cease. If necessary, loop diuretics can be given and urinary water loss replaced with free

TABLE 170.5.	Treatment of Hypernatremia
Hypervolemic:	Discontinue administration of hypertonic load; use loop diuretics if needed and replace water loss
Euvolemic:	Free water replacement Central DI: ADH analogue (DDAVP) Nephrogenic DI: salt restriction, thiazide, +/– NSAIDs
Hypovolemic:	Saline until euvolemic; then free water

water so that there is a net loss of Na^+. If renal failure is present, dialysis may be necessary to correct the hypernatremia.

Patients with central DI are best managed using the ADH analogue, desmopressin acetate (DDAVP), which is administered by nasal insufflation (0.1–0.4 ml) once or twice daily. Nephrogenic DI is resistant to ADH. In this disorder, the goal of therapy is to induce a state of mild volume depletion which limits the volume of filtrate delivered to the diluting segment (the thick ascending limb of Henle) and thus reduce the degree of polyuria. This can be accomplished using a low Na^+ diet, Thiazide diuretics, and occasionally, nonsteroidal anti-inflammatory agents.

When hypovolemia is present, normal saline should be administered until euvolemia is restored and then fluids can be given to replace the free water deficit.

CHAPTER 171

DISORDERS OF POTASSIUM BALANCE

Whereas Na^+ is the most important extracellular cation, K^+ is the most important intracellular cation with an intracellular concentration of approximately 150 mEq/L. Extracellular K^+ accounts for only about 2% of total K^+ stores and the serum K^+ level does not always provide an accurate estimate of total K^+ stores. Potassium homeostasis is influenced by: intake, excretion, and cellular shifts. Daily intake of K^+ is usually between 50 to 100 mEq/day. Approximately 90% of dietary K^+ is excreted in the urine as a result of the distal tubular secretion of K^+. The delivery of an adequate amount of Na^+ to the distal nephron and the actions of aldosterone are key to the control of renal K^+ excretion. The distal delivery of Na^+ is important because Na^+ reabsorption by the distal nephron (which is induced by aldosterone) results in a negative luminal potential which favors K^+ secretion. Potassium enters cells via β Na^+-K^+ ATPase. Insulin, β-2 agonists, and aldosterone all enhance the activity of this enzyme system and thus can result in the cellular uptake of K^+.

Hypokalemia

Hypokalemia is defined as a serum K^+ below 3.5 mEq/L.

■ Etiology

Hypokalemia can be due to decreased K^+ intake, increased K^+ loss, and intracellular K^+ shifts (Table 171.1). Hypokalemia due to decreased intake is uncommon because K^+ is present in many foods. In addition, gastrointestinal and renal K^+ losses are minimized when the intake of K^+ is low. Eventually, however, hypokalemia does develop when intake is very low (<20–30 mEq/day) for a prolonged period as can occur in malnourished alcoholics and in elderly patients consuming a "tea and toast" diet.

■ Clinical Features

Symptoms of hypokalemia are related to changes in membrane polarization. Cardiac, neuromuscular, and renal manifestations dominate. Electrocardiographic changes of hypokalemia can include T-wave flattening, U-waves, ST segment depression, and PR prolongation. Hypokalemia can predispose patients to arrhythmias which can include sinus bradycardia, atrioventricular block, paroxysmal atrial tachycardia, and rarely, ventricular tachycardia. By increasing the sensitivity of the myocardium to digoxin, hypokalemia can also predispose patients to digoxin toxicity.

Patients with hypokalemia often complain of muscular cramps and weakness. Lower extremity weakness may occur first and then involve ascending muscle groups. In some cases, weakness can progress to paralysis. Severe hypokalemia may cause muscle ischemia and result in rhabdomyolysis. Hypokalemia may also evoke a resistance to the action ADH and result in nephrogenic DI and associated polyuria and polydipsia.

■ Management

Therapy must be directed at the underlying cause of hypokalemia and replacing the K^+ deficit. A decrement in serum K^+ from 4.0 to 3.0 mEq/L usually is indicative of a total body deficit of 200–400 mEq. K^+ levels below 2.0 mEq/L may represent a deficit exceeding 1000 mEq. When acidosis is present and the serum K^+ is low or normal, it is important to provide K^+ replacement prior to correcting the acidosis since the K^+ level will fall further as the pH rises due to intracellular shifts.

For most nonurgent situations, it is preferable to use oral K^+ replacement since it is the safest route of therapy. Oral doses can vary between 20 and 120 mEq/day. Potassium is usually administered as the chloride salt however, other available forms include potassium bicarbonate, citrate, and gluconate. However, when life-threatening hypokalemia is present or if the patient cannot tolerate oral replacement, intravenous K^+ replacement may be necessary. Administration through a peripheral line should not exceed a rate of 10 mEq/hour. However, if necessary, rates of up to 20–40 mEq/hour can be given via a central line with continuous cardiac monitoring.

TABLE 171.1. Causes of Hypokalemia
Decreased potassium intake
Alcoholism, "tea and toast" diet
Potassium losses
GI losses (diarrhea, villous adenoma)
Renal losses
Diuretics
Drugs (cisplatin, aminoglycosides, amphotericin)
Nonreabsorbed anions (ketone, carbenicillin)
Tubular disorders (RTA, Bartter's syndrome)
Intracellular potassium shifts
Alkalosis
Insulin
β_2 agonist
Hypokalemic periodic paralysis
Following treatment of megaloblastic anemia
Thyrotoxicosis

Hyperkalemia

Hyperkalemia is defined as a serum K^+ exceeding 5.0 mEq/L. In the clinical approach to hyperkalemia, spurious or pseudohyperkalemia must first be excluded. Pseudohyperkalemia is defined as hyperkalemia which occurs after the blood is drawn; it is usually due to hemolysis resulting from improper venipuncture technique (prolonged tourniquet application or excessive fist clenching). In addition, marked leukocytosis (>70,000/μL) and thrombocytosis (>1 million/μL) can lead to pseudohyperkalemia. In these settings, determination of the serum K^+ level using a heparinized tube will reflect the true K^+ level.

TABLE 171.2. Causes of Hyperkalemia
Pseudohyperkalemia
Improper venipuncture technique
Severe leukocytosis or thrombocytosis
Reduced renal K$^+$ excretion
Decreased distal delivery of Na$^+$
Volume depletion
Renal failure
Aldosterone deficiency or resistance
Hypoaldosteronism RTA
Drug-related
K$^+$ sparing diuretics
Angiotensin converting enzyme inhibitors
Redistribution of K$^+$ from cells
Insulin deficiency
β Blockers
Massive digoxin overdose
Succinylcholine

■ Classification and Etiology

Once pseudohyperkalemia is excluded, the etiology of hyperkalemia must be determined. Hyperkalemia can be due to increased K$^+$ intake, shifts of K$^+$ from the intercellular space, or decreased renal excretion of K$^+$ (Table 171.2). The presence of chronic hyperkalemia is almost always indicative of some degree of renal impairment because 90% of the daily K$^+$ load is excreted by the kidneys.

Hyperkalemia due to excessive K$^+$ loading is uncommon, but can occur with massive K$^+$ loads even in individuals with normal renal function. This can be the result of exogenous loads (oral or intravenous) or endogenous loads (as can occur with tumor lysis, crush injuries, massive hemolysis and burns).

■ Clinical Features

Symptoms of hyperkalemia usually develop when the serum K$^+$ rises above 6.5 mEq/L and are related to changes in membrane polarization. Cardiac manifestations are the most serious. On the electrocardiogram, peaked T-waves are seen earliest (Figure 25.11). Later findings can include PR prolongation, QRS widening, ventricular fibrillation, complete heart block and asystole. Weakness, paralysis, and respiratory failure may also occur as complications of hyperkalemia.

■ Management

Therapy for mild hyperkalemia should include dietary K$^+$ restriction and discontinuing any drugs which interfere with K$^+$ excretion. In addition, diuretics (loop diuretics or thiazides) may be utilized to increase renal K$^+$ excretion. In the treatment of hypoaldosteronism, mineralocorticoid replacement is useful.

Acute, life-threatening hyperkalemia requires several types of therapeutic maneuvers. When ECG changes are present, calcium should be given to antagonize the effect of hyperkalemia on the cell membrane. It can be given intravenously as 10% calcium gluconate (10 ml over 15 minutes) and the dose can be repeated in 5 to 10 minutes. Calcium has a rapid onset and the duration of efficacy is about 30 minutes.

Therapy must also be directed towards shifting K$^+$ to the intracellular space. This can be accomplished with sodium bicarbonate or insulin. Sodium bicarbonate (44 mEq) can be administered over 5 minutes and repeated every 15 minutes. Care must be taken to avoid hypernatremia and alkalosis. In nondiabetics, dextrose (25 grams) can be given to stimulate endogenous insulin secretion. Alternatively, 25 to 50% dextrose and insulin (8–10 units) may be given together intravenously.

As a third component of therapy, K$^+$ removal can be facilitated with the use of the cation exchange resin sodium polystyrene sulfonate (Kayexalate). Orally, 30 to 50 grams can be given in sorbitol (to prevent constipation) and this can be repeated every 3 to 4 hours as needed. When the oral route is not feasible, it may be given as an enema but this route is less effective. Sodium retention is a potential complication since each gram of the resin releases 1 to 2 mEq of Na$^+$ for each 1 mEq of K$^+$ which is bound. Finally, hemodialysis may be useful in certain situations, for example when volume overload, severe acidosis, or uremia is present. Peritoneal dialysis is a far less efficient method of treating hyperkalemia.

CHAPTER 172 ACID-BASE DISORDERS

rterial pH is normally maintained between 7.35 and 7.43. The following three mechanisms are important in the regulation of arterial pH: extracellular and intracellular buffering, pulmonary ventilatory exchange, and renal hydrogen (H^+) excretion. Bone, proteins, hemoglobin, and the bicarbonate-carbonic acid ($HCO_3^-- H_2CO_3$) system are among the key elements in the buffer system. The importance of the renal and respiratory components is highlighted in the Henderson-Hasselbalch equation:

$$pH = 6.1 + log \frac{[HCO_3]^-}{0.03 \ PaCO_2}$$

A primary change in the HCO_3^- is indicative of a metabolic disorder, whereas as primary change in the $PaCO_2$ is indicative of a respiratory disorder. These primary changes often evoke secondary responses in their counterparts in order to restore the pH towards, but not completely to normal—the so-called "compensation." For example, the $PaCO_2$ may decline in response to a drop in plasma HCO_3^-. For the clinician, it is useful to know the magnitude of compensation expected for a given acid-base disorder. Table 172.1 provides this information. When the observed response differs from what is expected, then a mixed acid-base disorder is present.

TABLE 172.1. Simple Acid-Base Disorders					
Acid-Base Disturbance	Primary Disorder	Compensatory Response	pH	Predicted Compensation	Limits of Compensation
Metabolic acidosis	↓HCO₃	↓PaCO₂	↓	ΔPaCO₂ = 1.0-1.5 × ΔHCO₃	10 mmHg
Metabolic alkalosis	↑HCO₃	↑PaCO₂	↑	ΔPaCO₂ = 0.5-1.0 × ΔHCO₃	60–70 mmHg
Respiratory acidosis	↑PaCO₂	↑HCO₃	↓	Acute: ΔHCO₃ = 0.1 × ΔPaCO₂	32 mEq/L
				Chronic: ΔHCO₃ = 0.4 × ΔPaCO₂	45 mEq/L
Respiratory alkalosis	↓PaCO₂	↓HCO₃	↑	Acute: ΔHCO₃ = 0.2 × PaCO₂	18–20 mEq/L
				Chronic: ΔHCO₃ = 0.5 × ΔPaCO₂	12–15 mEq/L

↓ = Decrease; ↑ = Increase; Δ = Change.

Metabolic Acidosis

Metabolic acidosis is a pathophysiologic process characterized by a primary decrease in the plasma HCO_3^- level. It is helpful to categorize metabolic acidosis according to the anion gap (Table 172.2). The anion gap is defined as follows:

$$AG = [Na^+] - [Cl^- + HCO_3^-]$$

The normal anion gap (unmeasured anion) is about 8–12 mEq/L. In general, in states of acidosis, a high anion gap indicates gain of an acid and a normal anion gap reflects loss of HCO_3^-.

■ Elevated Anion Gap Acidosis

Lactic acidosis

Lactic acidosis is a common problem in the critically ill. Usually, the rates of lactate synthesis and metabolism are closely matched and as a result lactate levels are normally less than 2 mEq/L. Lactic acidosis occurs as a result of the overproduction or impaired metabolism of lactate (Table 172.3). The overproduction of lactate is usually due to inadequate oxygen delivery as occurs with shock (septic, hypovolemic, or cardiogenic). Rarer causes of lactate overproduction include certain malignancies, diabetes mellitus, phenformin and toxic alcohol ingestion. Impaired lactate metabolism is usually due to hepatic failure.

Lactic acidosis is associated with a poor prognosis. The underlying cause of the lactic acidosis must be identified and whenever possible corrected. Bicarbonate therapy may be initiated when acidosis is severe (pH <7.1). Potential complications of bicarbonate therapy include fluid overload, hypertonicity and overshoot alkalosis.

Ketoacidosis

Ketoacidosis may be seen in the settings of diabetic ketoacidosis (DKA), alcoholic ketoacidosis and starva-

TABLE 172.2.	Metabolic Acidosis

Elevated anion gap
 Ketoacidosis
  Diabetic ketoacidosis
  Alcoholic ketoacidosis
  Starvation ketosis
 Renal failure
 Lactic acidosis
 Toxic ingestions
  Alcohols: methanol, ethylene glycol
  Salicylate
Normal anion gap
 Gain of HCl
  Hyperalimentation
  Ammonium chloride, arginine hydrochloride
 Bicarbonate loss
  Gastrointestinal
   Diarrhea
   Urinary diversions (ureterosigmoidostomy)
  Renal
   Renal tubular acidosis (proximal and distal)
   Carbonic anhydrase inhibitors

tion ketoacidosis (Table 172.2). A positive nitroprusside test may be useful in diagnosing ketoacidosis. However, a negative test does not rule out the diagnosis because it detects only acetoacetate and not β-hydroxybutyrate which can be the predominant ketone in more severe cases of ketoacidosis.

Treatment of DKA must include volume repletion and insulin. There is no evidence that bicarbonate therapy hastens the recovery from DKA and it should only be used if the pH is below 7.1. Therapy for alcoholic ketoacidosis includes discontinuation of alcohol ingestion and fluid repletion.

Renal failure

Acidosis develops when the GFR falls below 25% of normal because net acid excretion can no longer be maintained. The retention of phosphoric and sulfuric acids (which are the products of protein metabolism) elevates the anion gap. Earlier in renal failure, ammonium production may be impaired prior to the retention of anions and as a result a normal anion gap may be present. It is important to correct the acidosis of chronic renal failure to prevent bone loss due to buffering.

Toxic ingestions

The metabolism of "toxic" alcohols can lead to a high anion gap metabolic acidosis. Methanol is first metabolized to formaldehyde (by alcohol dehydrogenase) and later to formic acid. Both of these metabolites have ocular toxicity and consequently, methanol inges-

tion may result in blindness. Ethylene glycol (antifreeze) is first metabolized to glyceraldehyde (again by alcohol dehydrogenase) and later to other metabolites. Besides metabolic acidosis, it may be associated with central nervous system (CNS) changes, congestive heart failure, and oliguric renal failure (due to the precipitation of calcium oxalate in the tubules). Ethanol is useful in the treatment of toxic alcohol ingestion because it is a substrate for alcohol dehydrogenase and thus it can competitively inhibit the metabolism of both methanol and ethylene glycol.

The presence of an elevated osmolar gap may be useful in diagnosing toxic alcohol ingestion. As stated previously osmolality is calculated as follows:

$$P_{osm} = 2 \times [Na] + glucose/18 + BUN/2.8$$

The osmolar gap is calculated by subtracting the calculated osmolality from the measured osmolality. A gap less than 10 mOsm/kg is normal. A significantly elevated osmolar gap (>25 mOsm/kg H_2O) has a high specificity for the diagnosis of toxic alcohol ingestion.

Salicylate intoxication can also be associated with a high anion gap acidosis because it increases the production of endogenous acids (lactate, ketoacids and other organic acids). Metabolic acidosis alone is usually seen in children, whereas a combination of metabolic acidosis and initial respiratory alkalosis is more common in adults. Alkalinization is an important part of therapy because it favors the ionized form which is trapped in the urine and maximally excreted.

TABLE 172.3.	Causes of Lactic Acidosis

A. Excessive lactate production
 Shock*
  Hypovolemic, cardiogenic, septic
 Toxins
  Carbon monoxide, cyanide, toxic alcohols, salicylates, phenformin
 Enzyme deficiencies
  Glucose 6-phosphatase, fructose 1,6-diphosphatase
  Pyruvate carboxylase, pyruvate dehydrogenase
 Sepsis
 Hypoxemia (severe)
 Anemia (severe)
 Malignancy
 Seizure, exertional heat stroke
 D-lactic acidosis
 Mitochondrial myopathies
B. Impaired lactate metabolism
 Hepatic failure

*A component of impaired metabolism is often present due to poor hepatic perfusion.

TABLE 172.4. Causes of Metabolic Alkalosis
Bicarbonate gain
Bicarbonate or citrate administration
Metabolism of ketoacids or lactate
Milk-alkali syndrome
HCl loss
A. Gastrointestinal
Vomiting
NG suction
Villous adenoma
Congenital chloride diarrhea
B. Renal
Diuretics
Mineralocorticoid excess (primary or secondary)
Non-reabsorbable anions (such as carbenicillin)
Post-hypercapnic metabolic alkalosis
Bartter's syndrome

■ Hyperchloremic Metabolic Acidosis

Hyperchloremic metabolic acidosis may be due to the gain of hydrochloric acid (HCl) or due to the loss of bicarbonate (Table 172.2). HCl gain is far less common but it may be seen with administration of hyperalimentation when cationic amino acids are metabolized to form H^+.

Bicarbonate losses can occur renally or via gastrointestinal (GI) tract. Renal loss of bicarbonate is usually due to renal tubular acidosis (RTA), while diarrhea is the most common cause of GI loss of bicarbonate. It is usually possible to distinguish between GI and renal losses on the basis of history. However, when the history is not straightforward, a determination of the urinary anion gap is useful in distinguishing between the two. The urinary anion gap is calculated as follows:

$$Urinary\ anion\ gap = Na + K - Cl$$

The urinary anion gap is an indirect gauge of ammonium excretion. Chloride is the anion which accompanies ammonium. When the urinary ammonium concentration is high, chloride concentration is also high and consequently the urinary anion gap is negative. When the urinary ammonium concentration is low, chloride concentration is also low and consequently, the urinary anion gap is positive. A hallmark of RTA is deficient ammonium excretion and therefore RTA is associated with a positive urinary anion gap (with an average value of +20 mmol/L). Normally, ammonium excretion is greatly augmented in response to acidosis and thus acidosis due to diarrhea is associated with a negative urinary anion gap (with an average value of −20 mmol/L).

Renal tubular acidosis can be broadly categorized as being either proximal or distal. **Proximal RTA** is less common and is characterized by a defect in the proximal reabsorption of bicarbonate. This defect may be isolated or associated with the defective proximal reabsorption of other substances (including glucose, amino acids, uric acid and phosphate) which is known as the Fanconi syndrome. The urine pH in proximal RTA is variable. At very low serum bicarbonate levels, the distal nephron is able to reabsorb the filtered load of bicarbonate and, as a result, the urine pH is low (<5.2). At higher serum bicarbonate levels, the distal nephron is unable to reabsorb the filtered load. As a result, bicarbonaturia occurs and the urine pH becomes high.

Several types of defects can result in **distal RTA** (Table 172.4). A defect in the function of the distal H^+ pump (**a secretory defect**) is the most common type of distal RTA. It is associated with a low serum K^+ and a urine pH above 5.2. With a **gradient defect,** there is an abnormal increase in the permeability in the lumen and secreted H^+ leaks back into the cell. This type of defect may be caused by amphotericin. It is associated with hypokalemia and a urine pH above 5.2. A **voltage-dependent defect** occurs when distal Na^+ reabsorption is disrupted. Normally, the distal reabsorption of Na^+ leads to a negative luminal potential which potentiates the secretion of H^+ and K^+. Trimethoprim and amiloride can cause a voltage dependent defect by blocking distal Na^+ reabsorption. This kind of defect is associated with hyperkalemia and a urine pH exceeding 5.2. Finally, aldosterone is an important factor in distal acidification because it enhances distal Na^+ reabsorption, stimulates the H^+ pump and increases the synthesis of ammonia. Thus, aldosterone deficiency or resistance is associated with a distal acidification defect. Hypoaldosteronism RTA is characterized by hyperkalemia and a urine pH below 5.2 due to low urinary ammonia excretion.

The cornerstone of therapy is treatment of the underlying cause and alkali replacement. Patients with

TABLE 172.5. Urine Chloride in Metabolic Alkalosis
Low urine chloride = Saline responsive
Vomiting
NG suction
Diuretics*
High urine chloride = Saline resistant
Mineralocorticoid excess (primary/secondary)
Bartter's syndrome
Licorice (black) ingestion

*Urine chloride may be high if diuretic use is recent.

TABLE 172.6. Causes of Respiratory Alkalosis		
Site	**Mechanism**	**Specific Examples**
Stimulation of respiratory center	↑ ventilation	Salicylate intoxication
		Hyperventilation
		Psychogenic
		Hepatic cirrhosis
		Brain stem lesions
		Encephalitis
		Pregnancy
		Sepsis
Stimulation of peripheral chemoreceptors	↑ ventilation	Hypoxemia
		Hypotension
Stimulation of intrathoracic chemoreceptors	↑ ventilation	Restrictive lung disease
		Pulmonary embolus
		Pneumonia
		Pneumothorax

proximal RTA require a much higher dosage of alkali (up to 10–15 mEq/kg). Therapy for hypoaldosteronism RTA includes a low K^+ diet, loop diuretics, and, if necessary, mineralocorticoid replacement.

Metabolic Alkalosis

Metabolic alkalosis is the pathophysiologic process characterized by a primary increase in bicarbonate. Clinically, it is important to recognize the factors which are responsible for the generation and maintenance of metabolic alkalosis. Metabolic alkalosis is generated by either **bicarbonate gain** or **HCl loss** (Table 172.4). Once metabolic alkalosis is generated, it is often maintained by the presence of volume depletion and/or hypokalemia since both of these may decrease the GFR and, thereby, limit bicarbonate excretion.

The kidney has an extraordinary capacity to excrete bicarbonate so that metabolic alkalosis due to bicarbonate administration is relatively uncommon. However, it can occur when there is a limitation in the ability to excrete bicarbonate (e.g., when bicarbonate is administered to a patient with renal insufficiency). More commonly, metabolic alkalosis is generated by gastrointestinal or urinary loss of acid. Vomiting is the most common cause of the former, but it can also occur with congenital diarrhea and villous adenoma. Diuretics are the most common cause of metabolic alkalosis due to renal losses of HCl. This occurs because diuretics increase distal Na^+ delivery and may also lead to secondary hyperaldosteronism (by inducing volume depletion). The combination of these two factors results in increased distal H^+ secretion.

Clinically, it is often useful to measure the urine chloride concentration (Table 172.5). Metabolic alkalosis with a low urine chloride concentration (<15 mEq/L) is associated with volume contraction and is usually due to vomiting, nasogastric suction or diuretics. This type of alkalosis is called **"chloride-responsive"** because volume repletion with sodium chloride is an essential part of therapy. Metabolic alkalosis with a high urinary chloride is usually due to mineralocorticoid excess (primary or secondary), Bartter's syndrome, or the ingestion of imported licorice (which can have mineralocorticoid activity). This type of alkalosis is called **"chloride resistant"** because the alkalosis cannot be corrected with sodium chloride.

Treatment must be directed towards the correction of factors which are responsible for the generation of the alkalosis (for example, discontinuing diuretics or removing an adrenal adenoma). Therapy must also be directed towards the correction of volume depletion and hypokalemia which can be responsible for the maintenance of the alkalosis.

Respiratory Acidosis

Respiratory acidosis is characterized by a primary rise in $PaCO_2$ which is due to alveolar hypoventilation. This disorder can be due to diseases which affect the respiratory center, the lung tissue or chest wall muscles (See chapter 247 on respiratory failure). Intracellular buffering constitutes the initial compensatory response.

After several days, renal net acid excretion rises so compensation is more complete (Table 172.1). The treatment of respiratory acidosis should be directed at the underlying cause of hypoventilation and must include correcting hypoxia and improving pulmonary function.

Respiratory Alkalosis

Respiratory alkalosis is characterized by primary decrease in the $PaCO_2$ resulting from alveolar hyperventilation. This disorder can be due to stimulation of the central respiratory center or peripheral and intrathoracic chemoreceptors (Table 172.6). Compensatory responses to acute and chronic respiratory alkalosis are as listed in Table 172.1. Again, treatment must be directed at the underlying cause.

The Acid-base nomogram (Figure 172.1) is a useful and practical way to detect the type of acid-base disorder including mixed acid-base disturbances.

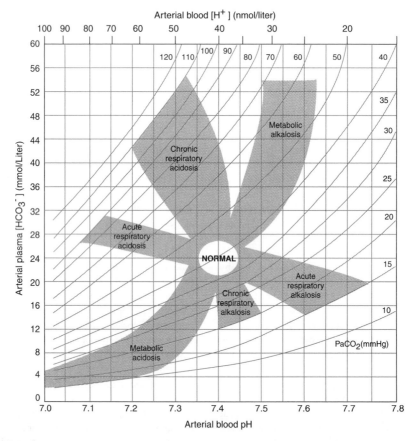

FIGURE **172.1.** Acid base nomogram. Shown are the 95% confidence limits for the normal respiratory and metabolic compensations for primary acid-base disturbances. (Reproduced with permission from: Brenner BM, Rector FC (eds.). The Kidney. Philadelphia: WB Saunders Co., 1986.)

CHAPTER 173

DEFINITION, EPIDEMIOLOGY, AND PATHOPHYSIOLOGY OF HYPERTENSION

■ Definition

Although blood pressure (BP) is a physiologic measurement similar to body temperature, heart rate, respiratory rate, height and weight, elevated blood pressure often leads to complications and, therefore, needs to be lowered. Based on the average of at least two readings on separate days, blood pressure in the adult is classified as shown in Table 173.1.

When there are elevations of systolic and diastolic BP, the severity classification is based on the higher category. Isolated systolic hypertension (ISH) is defined as systolic blood pressure (SBP) of 140 mm Hg or higher and diastolic blood pressure of 90 mm Hg or lower, and should be staged appropriately (e.g., 178/85 mmHg is stage 2 ISH). Besides classifying stages of hypertension, the physician should also specify presence or absence of target organ disease (Table 173.2) and additional risk factors for cardiovascular disease.

■ Epidemiology

Hypertension is the most common cardiovascular disease and one of the greatest public health problems of our time. In the United States, there are an estimated 60 million people with a systolic BP of 140 mm Hg or higher and/or a diastolic BP of 90 mm Hg or higher or are taking medications for hypertension. It is more common in men than women and in African Americans than Caucasians. Men and African Americans have greater morbidity and mortality. It contributes to the deaths of at least 250,000 Americans each year.

TABLE 173.2. Manifestations of Target-Organ Disease

Organ System	Manifestations
Cardiac	Clinical, electrocardiographic, or radiologic evidence of coronary artery disease
	Left ventricular hypertrophy or "strain" by electrocardiography or left ventricular hypertrophy by echocardiography
	Left ventricular dysfunction or cardiac failure
Cerebrovascular	Transient ischemic attack or stroke
Peripheral vascular	Absence of one or more major pulses in the extremities (except for dorsalis pedis) with or without intermittent claudication; aneurysm
Renal	Serum creatinine >1.5 mg/dl Proteinuria (1+ or greater) Microalbuminuria
Retinopathy	Hemorrhages or exudates, with or without papilledema

The major complications of hypertension include stroke, coronary artery disease, chronic renal failure and peripheral vascular disease. Most strokes that occur between the ages of 35 and 65 result from hypertension. Although stroke deaths have been declining in recent years largely because of early detection and better control of hypertension, it is still responsible for an estimated 150,000 deaths and 225,000 disabilities per year in the United States. Hypertension is the major risk factor for coronary artery disease, which is 3–5 times more frequent in hypertensives than in normotensives. Coronary artery disease and its complications are the most common causes of death in hypertensive patients. Target organ disease (Table 173.2) increases the risk of cardiovascular events, even if BP is controlled. Concentric **left ventricular hypertrophy** (LVH), which occurs as the left heart constantly pumps blood against a high arterial blood pressure over a long period of time, regresses as hypertension is kept under control. Sometimes, the LVH can precede severe hypertension and is probably due to an increased sympathetic tone. LVH is a powerful predictor of sudden death and myocardial infarction in hypertensive persons. Echocardiography is more sensi-

TABLE 173.1. Classification of Blood Pressure for Adults

Category	Systolic (mmHg)		Diastolic (mmHg)
Optimal	<120	and	<80
Normal	<130	and	<85
High normal	130–139	or	85–89
Hypertension			
STAGE 1 (Mild)	140–159	or	90–99
STAGE 2 (Moderate)	160–179	or	100–109
STAGE 3 (Severe)	≥180	or	≥110

tive than electrocardiography in detecting LVH. Although the incidence of kidney failure due to hypertension has declined markedly in recent years, it remains an important cause of **kidney failure** among the African Americans. Hypertension, diabetes, and increasing age lead to a higher probability of peripheral vascular disease.

The risk of complications from high blood pressure is continuous and proportionate over both systolic and diastolic blood pressure levels. Intensive antihypertensive therapy reduces, but does not normalize, both morbidity and mortality from complications of hypertension. Attention is now being directed toward preventing hypertension. Although the role of excessive sodium intake in causing hypertension remains somewhat controversial, since the average daily sodium intake is 10 to 20 times the physiologic need, a lower sodium intake is clearly indicated for most people. Obesity, particularly upper body obesity, is also a contributing factor to the development of hypertension. Every effort should be made to avoid childhood obesity as obese children often develop into obese adults. Obese patients with hypertension should be encouraged to make a vigorous effort to lose weight. Reduction in alcohol consumption can also reduce blood pressure and forestall the development of hypertension. Regular dynamic exercise and increased dietary potassium intake are also helpful in preventing hypertension.

Severe hypertension among children is usually of the secondary form. However, mild to moderate hypertension is usually the essential type. Children 3 years of age and older should have their blood pressure measured annually as part of their continuing health care.

■ Pathophysiology

Normal regulation of blood pressure

Under normal circumstances, blood pressure is maintained by the interplay of various mechanisms. It is primarily a function of cardiac output and peripheral resistance. This relationship is summarized by the following formula:

$$Blood\ pressure = cardiac\ output$$
$$\times\ peripheral\ vascular\ resistance$$

Cardiac output is the volume of blood ejected by the left ventricle into the aorta per minute. It is the major determinant of systolic blood pressure. Diastolic blood

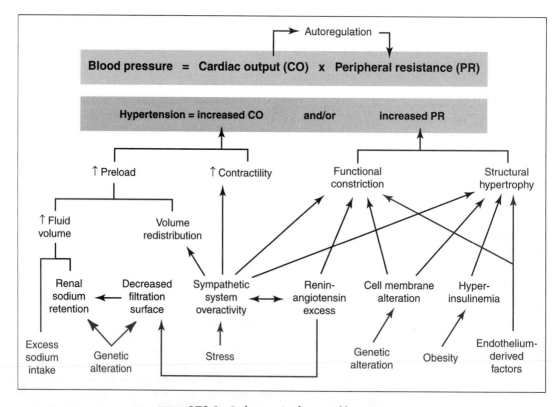

FIGURE 173.1. Pathogenesis of essential hypertension.
(From: Kaplan NM. Clinical Hypertension. 6th ed. Baltimore: Williams & Wilkins, 1994. Used with permission.)

pressure is primarily determined by the resistance in the arterioles. Cardiac output and peripheral resistance are directly and indirectly affected by such factors as blood volume, blood viscosity, sympathetic nervous system activity, the renin-angiotensin-aldosterone system, arginine vasopressin (AVP), insulin and vasodilator substances such as nitric oxide, prostaglandins, bradykinin and atrial natriuretic peptide (ANP).

Essential Hypertension

More than 95% of patients with elevated blood pressure have essential (idiopathic, primary) hypertension. These patients do not have an identifiable cause for their hypertension but have a disease of blood pressure regulation. In earlier stages with mild hypertension, the cardiac output is elevated. As the pressure rises further, cardiac output falls and the elevated blood pressure becomes a reflection of increased peripheral resistance.

The state of vasoconstriction is maintained by excess sodium content of the arteriolar smooth muscle cells, increased sympathetic nervous system activity, imbalance between endogenous vasoconstrictors and vasodilators and other unknown mechanisms. Other factors associated with hypertension include obesity, alcohol consumption, heredity, lack of regular physical activity, low dietary potassium and calcium intake, and increasing age. Significant factors involved in the control of blood pressure and possible mechanisms of hypertension are shown in Figure 173.1.

Secondary Hypertension

A specific cause of high blood pressure can be identified in less than 5% of people with hypertension. This type of hypertension, with an identifiable cause, is called secondary hypertension. It is discussed in greater length in chapter 177.

CHAPTER 174 EVALUATION OF THE HYPERTENSIVE PATIENT

Purpose of the Evaluation

The purpose of the evaluation is to answer the following questions:

1. Does the patient have hypertension? Before a patient is labeled hypertensive, at least three readings of blood pressure should be recorded. Two of the three readings and the average of the three should be elevated.

2. Is it secondary hypertension?

3. What is the extent of target organ damage?

4. Are other cardiovascular risk factors and/or alcoholism present?

5. Are certain antihypertensives contraindicated?

6. How much does the patient know about hypertension? Since hypertension is a chronic disorder requiring lifelong treatment, it is imperative that the patient understand this and participate in the medical care as much as possible.

7. Does the patient have sleep-disordered breathing? Hypoxemia and hypercapnia lead to increased sympathetic tone and can cause hypertension and, ultimately, heart failure.

History

After the patient identification information is obtained, the duration of hypertension and previous therapy should be determined. Although most patients with mild to moderate hypertension are asymptomatic and the blood pressure is elevated only to their surprise, the severely hypertensive patient may be quite symptomatic. The symptoms of hypertension are listed in Table 174.1. Review of systems may reveal symptoms suggestive of secondary hypertension. Family history in regard to hypertension, heart disease, diabetes, stroke and kidney disease must be recorded. The personal history is an extremely important part of the evaluation and includes

TABLE 174.1. Symptoms Associated with Hypertension
Occipital headache, worse on arising in the morning
Epistaxis (Nosebleeds)
Cardiovascular symptoms
Angina, dyspnea, edema, claudication
Cerebrovascular symptoms
Dizziness, blackouts, numbness, tingling, unilateral
weakness (may suggest impending stroke)

TABLE 174.2.	Drugs that May Raise BP

Estrogen
Progesterone
Steroids
NSAIDs
Nasal decongestants
Appetite suppressants
Cyclosporine
Erythropoietin
Tricyclic antidepressants
MAO inhibitors
Cocaine
Licorice

information on diet, smoking, alcohol consumption, drug abuse, exercise, sleep and sexual function.

Several medications can raise blood pressure or interfere with the effectiveness of antihypertensive drugs (Table 174.2). History of all prescribed and over-the-counter (OTC) medications should, therefore, be obtained.

■ Physical Examination

The patient's general appearance is noted, particularly in relation to gait, coordination and speech, the tell-tale signs of a past stroke. Hirsutism and truncal obesity are indicative of Cushing's syndrome. Weight and height are recorded and compared with standard charts to see if and by how much the patient is overweight. Abdominal and hip girth are measured and waist to hip ratio is calculated. Pulse rate and regularity should then be noted. Peripheral pulses, i.e., the radial, carotid, femoral, dorsalis pedis and posterior tibial pulses, are palpated. A weak pulse or a bruit indicates the presence of arteriosclerosis.

At the initial visit, the blood pressure should be recorded in both arms and a note made as to which side is higher. A discrepancy of up to 5 mmHg is not unusual. However, a larger difference may indicate the narrowing of the axillary or brachial artery on the side in which blood pressure is lower. On follow-up visits, the blood pressure is always recorded on the side with the higher blood pressure.

For measurement of BP, the patients should be seated with arm bared, supported and at heart level. They should not have smoked or ingested caffeine within 30 minutes and should have rested for five minutes prior to measurement. An appropriate cuff size, wherein the bladder encircles at least 80% of the arm and has width equal to one-third to one-half of the length of the upper arm, is necessary for accurate measurement of BP. Measurement should be taken with a mercury sphygmomanometer, a recently calibrated aneroid or a calibrated electronic device. Appearance of the Korotkoff sounds is recorded as the systolic and disappearance as the diastolic BP. Standing BP should also be recorded. Normally, the standing BP is a little higher than seated BP. If it is lower by more than 10 mmHg, it could signify orthostatic hypotension. Patients should be informed and taught the measuring of their blood pressure readings and advised of the need for periodic remeasurement.

The fundi are examined in a dark room with the patient looking straight at a distant point. The hypertensive retinopathy is graded from I to IV reflecting increasing severity (Table 174.3).

The neck is examined for a carotid bruit, goiter or any other swelling. A note is made if the jugular veins are prominent and distended.

The cardiac examination consists of palpating the point of maximal impulse (PMI or apex beat), which is shifted downward and laterally as the left ventricle enlarges. Auscultation is then performed for rhythm, heart sounds and the presence of murmurs. An S4 sound indicates a rigid left ventricle due to left ventricular hypertrophy and an S3 sound is a sign of heart failure.

The lungs are then auscultated for rales or wheezing. Basal rales are present in congestive heart failure. Wheezing may indicate heart failure, chronic bronchitis or asthma.

The abdomen is inspected and palpated to detect kidney enlargement. Polycystic kidneys and grossly enlarged, hydronephrotic kidneys are usually easily palpable. Palpable aortic pulsations may indicate aortic aneurysm. Careful auscultation over the epigastrium usually reveals a continuous (systolic and diastolic) bruit in patients with renal artery stenosis. It is not uncommon to hear a systolic bruit in the epigastrium, particularly in older patients. This is produced by the flow of blood through the celiac or hepatic artery and is of no significance.

The legs are then examined for the presence of edema and signs of peripheral vascular disease such as discoloration of the skin, loss of temperature or absence of arterial pulsations. The skin should be closely inspected for neurofibromatosis and cafe-au-lait spots, which may be seen in patients with pheochromocytoma.

TABLE 174.3.	Grades of Hypertensive Retinopathy
Grade	Finding
i/iv	Arteriolar narrowing, spasm, copper wiring, or silver wiring
ii/iv	Above changes & arterio-venous (AV) nicking
iii/iv	Above changes & hemorrhages and exudates
iv/iv	Above changes & papilledema (blurred optic disc margin)

A neurologic examination for muscle strength and deep tendon reflexes is performed to detect the presence of stroke, of which the patient may or may not be aware.

The prostate is examined in older men. An enlarged prostate and urinary retention may cause kidney damage, which can lead to or contribute to hypertension.

Laboratory Studies

Certain laboratory investigations are routinely performed as part of the evaluation of a hypertensive patient (Table 174.4). Urinalysis is necessary, since proteinuria usually indicates renal disease and hypertension may be secondary to renal parenchymal disease. However, long-standing hypertension can cause nephrosclerosis, ischemic glomerulopathy and proteinuria. Glycosuria can be easily diagnosed with dipstick urinalysis. Almost 10% of hypertensives also have diabetes mellitus. The presence of occult blood may indicate a renal or urinary tract disorder. A microscopic examination of the urine must always be undertaken, if the dipstick urinalysis is abnormal (presence of protein or blood). This helps determine the nature of renal disease. Red blood cell casts are pathognomonic of glomerulonephritis; however, granular casts simply indicate the presence of a renal disease. In diabetics, if dipstick is negative, urine should be examined for microalbuminuria to detect early glomerulosclerosis. It is a good practice to routinely record the patient's hematocrit before undertaking treatment of hypertension. Many hypertensives tend to have a somewhat higher hematocrit. If the patient is anemic, dizziness may be from anemia rather than hypertension. Fasting blood glucose or a 2-hour postprandial blood sugar measurement should be done for the diagnosis of diabetes. BUN or serum creatinine elevation indicates renal insufficiency, which may be either the cause or the result of hypertension. Serum potassium measurement is an excellent screening measure for primary aldosteronism. A normal serum potassium (3.5 to 5 mEq/L) on a normal diet excludes primary aldosteronism, for all practical purposes. Serum lipid measurements are done to detect other risk factors such as hypercholesterolemia or low levels of HDL cholesterol. After diuretic therapy, serum lipids may rise slightly. Uric acid measurement is not essential for evaluation or to determine the presence

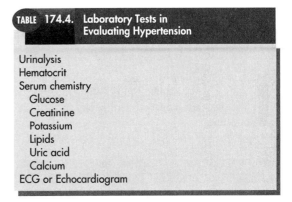

TABLE 174.4. Laboratory Tests in Evaluating Hypertension

Urinalysis
Hematocrit
Serum chemistry
  Glucose
  Creatinine
  Potassium
  Lipids
  Uric acid
  Calcium
ECG or Echocardiogram

of a risk factor; however, the uric acid level may rise with diuretic therapy, and some patients may develop clinical gout.

Serum calcium measurement is useful in uncovering hyperparathyroidism, which can cause hypertension. Also, the serum calcium level may rise with Thiazide therapy.

An electrocardiogram (ECG) should be done routinely in patients 40 years of age or older and in younger patients with severe hypertension, cardiac symptoms, arrhythmias or a strong family history of heart disease. Left ventricular hypertrophy (LVH) and myocardial ischemia are signs of hypertensive cardiovascular disease. While echocardiogram is more sensitive, the expense precludes its routine use to diagnose LVH.

Chest x-ray examination is done primarily to determine the heart size and the presence of congestive heart failure, and it is not necessary for routine evaluation of hypertension.

Special Studies

After the initial evaluation, if a patient is suspected to have secondary hypertension, appropriate laboratory and radiologic studies are undertaken to prove or disprove the suspected diagnosis. It is fruitless to investigate a patient for all possible causes of secondary hypertension. Only those investigations need be carried out that would help in the diagnosis of a specific suspected cause of secondary hypertension, discussed later in chapter 177.

CHAPTER 175 CLINICAL PHARMACOLOGY OF ANTIHYPERTENSIVE DRUGS

The antihypertensive drugs can be classified in various ways (Table 175.1). The more important ones are discussed here based on their site of action.

TABLE 175.1.   Classification of Common Antihypertensive Drugs

Diuretics
  Thiazides and related diuretics
  Loop diuretics: furosemide, bumetanide, torsemide, ethacrynic acid
  Potassium-sparing: spironolactone, triamterene, amiloride
Sympathetic inhibitors
  Centrally acting: methyldopa, clonidine
Receptor blockers
  Alpha blockers: prazosin, terazosin, doxazosin
  β-blockers
    Nonselective: nadolol, pindolol, propranolol
    Selective: acebutolol, atenolol, metoprolol
  Alpha and β blocker: labetalol, carvedilol
Angiotensin converting enzyme (ACE) inhibitors: captopril, enalapril, lisinopril, benazepril, fosinopril, quinapril, ramipril, etc.
Angiotensin II receptor blockers (ARBs): losartan, valsartan, irbesartan, telmisartan, candesartan, etc.
Vasodilators: hydralazine, minoxidil, diazoxide, sodium nitroprusside
Calcium entry blockers: verapamil, diltiazem, and dihydropyridines: amlodipine, felodipine, nicardipine, nifedipine, nitrendipine, etc.
Double calcium channel blocker: mebefradil

Diuretics

In many patients, particularly the elderly, diuretics are an appropriate first-line therapy for the treatment of essential hypertension.

■ Thiazide Diuretics

Hydrochlorothiazide is the most commonly used thiazide diuretic in the United States. The early predominant action of thiazides is to enhance sodium and water excretion, producing a mild to moderate extracellular fluid volume depletion. In addition, they mobilize sodium and chloride ions from the arteriolar smooth muscle and decrease vascular reactivity, blunting the effects of sympathetic reflexes. This results in a blood pressure drop by an average of 5–10 mm Hg. Adverse reactions of clinical importance are hypokalemia, **hyperuricemia**, hyperglycemia, hypercalcemia and hyperlipidemia. Hypokalemia is more common with long-acting diuretics such as chlorthalidone and metolazone, and may require potassium supplementation or the simultaneous use of potassium-sparing diuretics. Although hyperuricemia is not uncommon, it need not be treated unless clinical gout develops. Approximately 10% of patients develop hyperglycemia with chronic diuretic use. Hypercalcemia after thiazides is seldom of clinical importance. Fetal jaundice and thrombocytopenia have been reported after thiazide use in pregnancy. Indapamide has the same antihypertensive efficacy as hydrochlorothiazide but the biochemical alterations are somewhat less pronounced.

■ Loop Diuretics

The loop diuretics, furosemide, bumetanide and ethacrynic acid, constitute a pharmacologic rather than a chemical class. They produce diuresis far greater than thiazides over a short period of time but are not better than thiazides as antihypertensive drugs. They act at the loop of Henle. Their antihypertensive mode of action is similar to that of the thiazide diuretics. Their major use in the treatment of hypertension is in patients with renal insufficiency and fluid retention. Patients who develop hypercalcemia secondary to thiazides are candidates for a loop diuretic, since the latter increases calcium excretion. Hypokalemia can be a troublesome side effect in patients receiving loop diuretics.

■ Potassium-Sparing Diuretics

These include spironolactone, triamterene and amiloride. Spironolactone is a steroid compound with a structural formula similar to that of aldosterone; it is an aldosterone antagonist. It increases sodium and water excretion and diminishes potassium excretion. Gyneco-

mastia in men and menstrual irregularities in women are important side effects. It should be avoided in pregnancy and during lactation. Aldactazide is a combination of hydrochlorothiazide and spironolactone in a single tablet. Triamterene is used primarily to conserve potassium and prevent hypokalemia in patients treated with thiazide or loop diuretics. It is contraindicated in patients with renal insufficiency, in whom it can cause fatal hyperkalemia. Dyazide™ and Maxzide™ are proprietary combinations of hydrochlorothiazide and triamterene. Amiloride is similar to triamterene as a potassium-retaining diuretic. Moduretic™ is a combination of hydrochlorothiazide and amiloride.

Inhibitors of the Sympathetic Nervous System

This group includes drugs that interfere with sympathetic nerve impulses at different sites from the brain to target organs. The decreased arterial and venous constriction causes a fall in blood pressure. The adverse effects depend on the site of action and include orthostatic hypotension, nasal congestion, increased gastrointestinal motility, impotence, delayed ejaculation and bradycardia.

■ Centrally Acting Sympathetic Inhibitors

These include reserpine, methyldopa, clonidine, guanabenz and guanfacine. The β-adrenergic blocking agents may also have central action.

■ Receptor Blockers

Antihypertensive agents, which block α and β receptors selectively, are available.

Alpha blockers

The α-adrenergic blocking agents include prazosin, terazosin and doxazosin. They block postsynaptic α-adrenergic receptors, diminishing vascular constriction without affecting the α-adrenergic presynaptic negative feedback which inhibits norepinephrine release. Each agent can be used alone but is generally used with a diuretic. They can cause postural syncope particularly after the first dose in a small percentage of patients. The therapy is initiated with 1 mg, usually given at bedtime, and the patient instructed not to stand up for several hours. Postural dizziness and drowsiness, lethargy,

palpitations, and nausea are infrequent adverse effects. Terazosin and doxazosin have a longer duration of action. The α-blockers are also useful in treatment of prostate hypertrophy as they relax the smooth muscle in the prostate and can increase the urine flow. For this reason, they can be dually beneficial in treatment of hypertension in men with prostate hypertrophy.

Beta-blockers

Beta-adrenergic receptors are classified in two main groups: β-1 in the heart, and β-2 receptors in the bronchi and blood vessels. The chemical structures of β-blocking drugs have several features in common with the β-agonist isoproterenol. Most β-blockers such as propranolol and metoprolol are completely metabolized and are excreted by the liver. However, the longer-acting drugs, nadolol and atenolol, are poorly metabolized and are excreted by the kidney. All the β-blocking drugs are competitive antagonists of catecholamines at β-adrenergic receptor sites. They are classified as selective or nonselective according to their relative ability to antagonize the different classes of β-receptors. The selective β-1 receptor blockers such as atenolol and metoprolol, when employed in low doses, do not affect the bronchial and vascular β-2 receptors; however, in higher doses, both β-1 and β-2 receptors are blocked. Labetalol is a nonselective β-blocker which is also an α-blocker and a weak vasodilator. β-blockers are contraindicated in patients with asthma, congestive heart failure, greater than first degree heart block and bradycardia.

Blockers of the Renin-Angiotensin System

Since the renin-angiotensin system often has an important role in the maintenance of hypertension, agents that inhibit the production or action of the pressor hormone

angiotensin II are potentially useful hypotensive agents. Two classes of compounds are available: angiotensin I-converting enzyme (ACE) blockers, and angiotensin II receptor (A-II) antagonists. They are particularly useful in renin-dependent forms of hypertension such as renovascular hypertension, malignant hypertension and other conditions associated with elevated plasma renin levels. The β-receptor antagonists partially block the release of renin. Other sympatholytic agents such as methyldopa and clonidine also inhibit renin release.

■ Converting Enzyme Inhibitors

These agents competitively inhibit the angiotensin I-converting enzyme (ACE), which converts angiotensin I to angiotensin II. In addition, they inhibit the kininase enzyme responsible for the degradation of bradykinin. Thus, these drugs can lower blood pressure both by preventing the formation of the endogenous vasocon-strictor angiotensin II and by decreasing the metabolism of the endogenous vasodilator bradykinin. Captopril is a short-acting ACE inhibitor requiring 2–3 doses per day. Enalapril, lisinopril, quinapril, fosinopril and ramipril are longer-acting drugs requiring only a once a day dose. The side effects include cough, rash and taste disturbance. The contraindications include pregnancy and bilateral renal artery stenosis

■ Angiotensin Blockers

Drugs such as losartan block the angiotensin II (A-II) receptors and are useful antihypertensive drugs without causing cough, a nagging side effect of ACE inhibitors. They work particularly well in combination with a diuretic.

Calcium Entry Blockers

Verapamil, diltiazem and dihydropyridines such as amlodipine, felodipine, isradipine, nifedipine, nitren-dipine and nicardipine are coronary and peripheral vasodilators that act by interfering with the excitation-contraction coupling of smooth muscle by blocking the entrance of calcium into the cell. They are indicated in the treatment of hypertension and angina. Severe adverse reactions are rare. The side effects include hypotension, peripheral edema, headache and constipation. Asthma is not a contraindication to their use, as they have a weak bronchodilator effect and are ideal agents to use in asthmatic hypertensive patients. Short-acting dihydro-pyridines can cause myocardial infarction in patients with underlying coronary artery disease. Mibefradil blocks both L and T calcium channels and lowers heart rate without reducing myocardial contractility.

CHAPTER 176 THERAPY OF ESSENTIAL HYPERTENSION

The goal of the treatment of hypertension in the adult is to reduce the blood pressure below 140 mmHg systolic and below 90 mmHg diastolic by the least intrusive means possible. In addition, other modifiable cardiovascular risk factors must be controlled to reduce morbidity and mortality from complications of hypertension. Further reduction of BP to level of 130/85 mmHg may be pursued with due regard for cardiovascular function.

Lifestyle modifications which include weight reduction, increased physical activity, and moderation of dietary sodium and alcohol intake are useful in definitive or adjunctive therapy of hypertension. They not only help lower the blood pressure but, by ameliorating diabetes and dyslipidemia, they help lower the risk of cardiovascular disease from these disorders. If BP remains at or above 140/90 mmHg over a 3–6 month period, despite vigorous encouragement of lifestyle modifications, antihypertensive medications should be started.

Diuretics and β-blockers have been proven to reduce cardiovascular morbidity and mortality in controlled clinical trials and are, therefore, recommended for initial drug therapy (Figure 176.1) The alternative drugs, α-blockers, ACE inhibitors, A-II inhibitors, and calcium blockers are equally effective in reducing blood pressure but have not yet been shown to reduce morbidity and mortality in long-term clinical trials. These drugs, therefore, should be used when diuretics and β blockers are unacceptable or ineffective.

Drug therapy is initiated in small doses and the dose increased gradually until the desired therapeutic effect is achieved, side effects develop, or the maximal recommended dose is attained. If the first drug does not control the blood pressure or is poorly tolerated, it is replaced by another drug. If a drug is well tolerated but proves inadequate, a second drug may be added. For the convenience of patients and to facilitate compliance, several combination preparations of antihypertensive drugs are available.

Sequential monotherapy of hypertension is a newer way to manage hypertension. Four or five antihypertensive medications, one from each major class of drugs, are sequentially administered at the lowest recommended dose for one to three months. The patient is asked to maintain a record of weekly blood pressure measurements and side effects. The drug to which the patient responds best with least side effects is then chosen as the drug of choice for the long-term control of blood pressure.

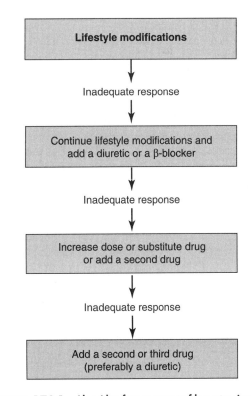

FIGURE **176.1.** Algorithm for treatment of hypertension.

Special Situations and Coexisting Conditions

It is important to individualize the therapy of hypertension to maximize the benefit and minimize risks to the patient. Hypertension among African Americans usually responds well to diuretics, as they often have an expanded plasma volume and low renin levels. Treatment of hypertension in the elderly is best initiated with half the usual dose to avoid postural hypotension and syncope. Converting enzyme inhibitors are also useful in the treatment of congestive heart failure and are, therefore, preferable in hypertensives with heart failure. β-blockers are helpful in patients with angina or migraine and may be the antihypertensive agents of choice when those conditions coexist. β-blockers should be avoided in patients with asthma. Calcium channel blockers are particularly useful in the asthmatics due to their mild bronchodilatory properties. Patients with peripheral vascular insufficiency may experience exacerbation of claudication if treated with nonselective β-blockers which should be avoided in those individuals. In patients with severe Raynaud's disease associated with collagen vascular disease such as scleroderma, treatment with ACE inhibitors, with or without calcium antagonist, may ameliorate both Raynaud's disease and the hypertension.

Patients with hypertension and diabetes mellitus are very vulnerable to cardiovascular complications and present a special challenge. Diuretics and β blockers may impair the control of diabetes. The nonselective β blockers may also interfere with catecholamine-mediated counter-regulatory responses to insulin-induced hypoglycemia. Some patients with diabetes who also have renal insufficiency may have hyporeninemic hypoaldosteronism with resultant hyperkalemia. Potassium-sparing diuretics, ACE inhibitors, and β blockers can aggravate this hyperkalemia. It is therefore imperative to monitor serum potassium and creatinine along with blood glucose in these patients. ACE inhibitors have been shown to reduce albuminuria and are considered the antihypertensives of choice in diabetic, hypertensive patients. Calcium blockers such as, verapamil, and diltiazem, but not dihydropyridines (Table 175.5), also reduce albuminuria in the diabetics.

The diuretics can induce short-term increases in levels of total plasma cholesterol, triglycerides, and LDL cholesterol. β blockers may increase levels of plasma triglycerides and reduce those of HDL cholesterol. The alpha blockers and central adrenergic agonists may decrease serum cholesterol concentration slightly, especially in the lipoprotein subfraction, and therefore, may offer an advantage in managing hypertensive patients with hyperlipidemia. ACE inhibitors and calcium antagonists have no adverse effects on serum lipids and are appropriate for these patients. Table 176.1 summarizes influence of some of the coexisting conditions on the choice of initial antihypertensive therapy.

TABLE 176.1. Choice of Initial Antihypertensive Drug Therapy

Associated Condition(s)	Drugs of Choice	Agents Not Recommended
Asthma, chronic obstructive pulmonary disease	Calcium channel blocker, thiazide diuretics	β blocker
Coronary disease	β blocker	Vasodilator
Left ventricular failure (systolic)	Angiotensin converting enzyme inhibitor, thiazide, A-II receptor blockers (ARBs)	β blocker, calcium channel blocker
Hypertrophic cardiomyopathy with severe diastolic dysfunction	β blocker, calcium channel blocker (diltiazem, verapamil)	Diuretics, vasodilators, α–1 antagonists
Diabetes mellitus	Converting enzyme inhibitor	Thiazide, β blocker
Chronic renal failure (serum creatinine >3.0 mg/dl)	Loop diuretics, calcium channel blocker	
Preeclampsia	Methyldopa, hydralazine labetalol, nifedipine	Angiotensin converting-enzyme inhibitor

CHAPTER 177 SECONDARY HYPERTENSION

Although the majority of hypertensive patients have essential hypertension, a significant number (approximately 5%) have secondary hypertension. In children, severe hypertension is almost always secondary to another process. In the evaluation of recent-onset hypertension in adults above the age of 50, one should seriously entertain the possibility of secondary hypertension. Table 177.1 lists the important causes of secondary hypertension. Following is a discussion of the major forms of secondary hypertension.

Renal Hypertension

Kidney disease of almost any nature can cause hypertension; the more important ones are listed in Table 177.1. The exact mechanism of hypertension in these renal disorders is not always clear. Fluid retention may be responsible in patients with end-stage kidney disease. This is called renoprival hypertension. In some patients with severe renal disease, plasma renin is elevated and the renin-angiotensin-aldosterone system may be responsible for hypertension. In others with renal disease and normal plasma renin activity, hypertension is presumed to be either due to accumulation of certain vasopressor substances that may be normally metabolized and excreted by the kidney, or a result of the inability of the diseased kidney to generate certain vasodilator substances such as prostaglandins and kinins.

Laboratory investigations usually reveal albuminuria, with or without hematuria, and an elevated serum creatinine. Ultrasonography is undertaken for detecting kidney size followed by intravenous pyelography, if better delineation of individual kidney function is desired. If one kidney is smaller (>2 cm) than the other, split renal vein renin studies, along with renal angiography, may be undertaken to confirm unilateral renal artery stenosis as the cause of secondary hypertension. The renal vein renin on the abnormal side is usually 1.5 to 2 times the opposite kidney. Prior administration of an ACE inhibitor augments this difference between the two kidneys in the presence of a unilateral stenosis. If parenchymal renal disease is suspected, kidney biopsy may be necessary for an accurate diagnosis.

When hypertension is a result of bilateral kidney disease, medical therapy as described for control of essential hypertension is indicated. When hypertension is due to unilateral kidney disease, such as a dysplastic or severely traumatized kidney, removal of the diseased kidney can often cure hypertension. Removal of a kidney should never be considered lightly, and a prior trial of medical therapy is always indicated. A converting enzyme inhibitor, starting with one half the usual recommended dose, can sometimes control the blood pressure. Serum potassium and creatinine should be monitored closely. Verapamil or diltiazem may be added, if ACE inhibitor alone fails to control BP. Minoxidil, when used in combination with furosemide and a β blocker, may also control BP in patients with severe, intractable hypertension. If, despite adequate antihypertensive therapy, hypertension remains uncontrolled and the kidneys have failed irreversibly requiring chronic dialysis, removal of nonfunctioning kidneys either cures the hypertension or makes it easier to manage with medical therapy.

TABLE 177.1. Causes of Secondary Hypertension

Renal diseases
  Acute glomerulonephritis
  Chronic glomerulonephritis
  Polycystic kidney disease
  Dysplastic kidney
  Diabetic nephropathy
  Hydronephrosis
  Connective tissue disorders
  Renin-producing tumors
  Renal trauma
  Analgesic nephropathy
Renal artery stenosis
  Fibromuscular hyperplasia
  Atherosclerosis
Adrenal disorders
  Cortical
    Primary aldosteronism
    Cushing's syndrome
    Congenital adrenal hyperplasia
  Medullary
    Pheochromocytoma
Medications and OTC drugs (Table 174.2)
Coarctation of the aorta
Toxemia of pregnancy
CNS disorders
Other hormonal disorders
  Hypo- and hyperthyroidism
  Hyperparathyroidism
  Acromegaly
Sleep-disordered breathing

■ Renal Artery Stenosis

Constriction of one or both renal arteries, as may happen in congenital fibromuscular hyperplasia or atherosclerotic narrowing of the renal arteries, often results in hypertension. Fibromuscular hyperplasia, also called fibrous dysplasia, is more commonly encountered in white women under 50 years of age. A variety of pathologic lesions have been described but with little clinical relevance. Renal ischemia leading to excessive renin secretion and activation of the renin-angiotensin-aldosterone system causes elevated blood pressure. A continuous (systolic/diastolic) upper abdominal bruit that radiates to the side of the lesion is often present. Radionuclide renogram after 50 mg of oral captopril or 2.5 mg of IV enalapril shows a slower uptake and excretion of the radionuclide on the side of the lesion. The diagnosis is confirmed by renal angiography. The ACE inhibitors are particularly useful in controlling blood pressure in many patients. These drugs should be avoided in the presence of bilateral renal arterial stenosis or in patients with one kidney and renal arterial stenosis. The reason for this is that these patients need a high tone in the efferent glomerular arterioles to maintain glomerular filtration and the ACE inhibitors, by reducing the intrarenal synthesis of angiotensin II, lead to dilatation of the efferent arterioles, causing the glomerular filtration rate to drop and serum creatinine to rise. If blood pressure is not readily controllable with medical therapy, angioplasty or surgical treatment should be considered.

Angioplasty or dilatation of the narrowed segment by an inflatable balloon catheter and stent placement is the treatment of choice. Surgical treatment may be necessary to salvage the kidney, if medical therapy and angioplasty have failed or if angioplasty is deemed inappropriate. The surgery consists of resection of the stenotic lesion, bypass of the lesions using either a Dacron graft or a saphenous vein graft, or an endarterectomy with or without patch plasty. Nephrectomy is considered only as a last resort if a revascularization procedure is technically impossible or

has failed. Surgical treatment can cure hypertension in many of these patients. However, in some cases, fibromuscular hyperplasia is progressive and can recur after surgery.

Renal artery stenosis due to atherosclerosis usually occurs in patients over the age of 50. The atherosclerotic narrowing is most frequently present at the origin of the renal artery. In almost all cases, there is evidence of extensive atherosclerosis elsewhere. Most of these patients have a history of long-standing, untreated, essential hypertension. In most patients, blood pressure can be controlled on medical therapy with an ACE inhibitor. Selected patients can be treated with angioplasty. Surgical therapy should be undertaken only in patients with severe, uncontrolled hypertension or in those with inevitable risk of losing kidneys due to ischemia. Unilateral nephrectomy of an unsalvageable kidney, combined with contralateral revascularization, is sometimes lifesaving in properly selected patients. In those treated medically, serum creatinine and renal size using ultrasonography should be monitored every 3–6 months.

Adrenal Disorders

Adrenal cortical and medullary disorders can cause hypertension and are discussed in chapter 61 (Adrenal Disorders).

Coarctation of the Aorta

Coarctation of the aorta is a narrowing of the aortic lumen due to a localized deformity of the vascular media and a curtain-like infolding. While characteristically located distal to the origin of the left subclavian artery, it can, occasionally, occur proximal to it as well. Headache, spontaneous epistaxis and leg fatigue are the usual symptoms. Bicuspid aortic valve and an aneurysm of the circle of Willis may be associated. The hallmark of the condition is hypertension in the upper extremities. The femoral pulses are feeble and delayed. Collateral arteries may be seen and felt on the patient's back. Chest x-ray films may show rib notching due to enlarged intercostal-internal mammary collateral arteries and "3 sign" from

dilation of the aorta above and below the constriction (see also chapter 133). The diagnosis is confirmed by echocardiography and by color Doppler flow mapping. Reduced blood supply to the kidney can stimulate renin secretion, thereby activating the renin-angiotensin-aldosterone system which then leads to exacerbation of hypertension. Section of the narrowed segment with end-to-end anastomosis or bypass with a Dacron graft are the surgical procedures of choice. Postoperative hypertension requiring medical therapy is not uncommon. Angioplasty is being increasingly used and may become the treatment of choice.

CNS Disorders

Disorders causing increased intracranial pressure, such as may occur in respiratory acidosis, encephalitis, brain tumor and hemorrhagic stroke, can cause increased sympathetic outflow from the brain and hypertension

that can be very severe and often labile. Reduction of intracranial pressure by reversal of the underlying cause usually leads to normalization of blood pressure.

Sleep-Disordered Breathing

The majority of patients with sleep-disordered breathing are obese and snore habitually. It is associated with daytime and nocturnal hypertension. Activation of the sympathetic nervous system by hypoxia or acidosis appear to be the physiological cause of hypertensive episodes. Cardiovascular morbidity and mortality are increased in patients with sleep apnea. Further information on sleep-disordered breathing is provided in chapter 250.

CHAPTER 178 HYPERTENSIVE EMERGENCIES

A hypertensive emergency or hypertensive crisis is a clinical situation in which the blood pressure is so elevated as to constitute a threat to life or certain organ systems. The diastolic BP is usually above 120 mmHg. Such conditions as acute left ventricular failure and acute dissecting aneurysm of the aorta qualify as hypertensive emergencies, not so much because of the severity of hypertension but as a result of coexisting life-threatening complications. Some of the clinical situations which constitute hypertensive emergencies are listed in Table 178.1. Asymptomatic patients, despite a very high blood pressure are in no immediate danger and should not be treated as hypertensive emergencies.

The use of sublingual or oral nifedipine is no longer recommended in the treatment of hypertensive emergencies due to the serious adverse sequelae such as myocardial infarction and stroke. Intravenous administration of antihypertensive drugs is often necessary to sustain blood pressure control. The intravenous medications presently used include furosemide, sodium nitroprusside, diazoxide, labetalol, enalaprilat and nitroglycerine. The dose and side effects of these drugs are summarized in Table 178.2. During administration of these potent antihypertensive agents, close monitoring of arterial blood pressure, preferably using an intraarterial line, is essential; these patients are, therefore, best treated in an intensive care unit. Oral antihypertensive medications should be started as soon as possible to keep hypertension under control as evaluation of the patient proceeds.

TABLE 178.1. Examples of Hypertensive Emergencies

1. Hypertensive encephalopathy
2. Acute dissecting aneurysm of the aorta.
3. Acute pulmonary edema (hypertension with acute left ventricular failure).
4. Malignant or accelerated hypertension.
5. Intracerebral or subarachnoid hemorrhage.
6. Severe hypertension in a patient with acute coronary insufficiency or myocardial infarction.
7. Diastolic blood pressure >130 mm Hg without symptoms.
8. Hypertension associated with acute glomerulonephritis.
9. Curable conditions that may require prompt reduction in blood pressure: (A) pheochromocytoma; (B) toxemia of pregnancy; (C) oral contraceptive-induced severe hypertension; and (D) renovascular hypertension.

TABLE 178.2. Selected Intravenous Drugs for Hypertensive Emergencies

Drugs	Dose	Important side effects
Diazoxide (Hyperstat)	50–100 mg bolus or 15–30 mg/min infusion	Hypotension, tachycardia, angina, vomiting, hyperglycemia
Enalaprilat (Vasotec)	1.25–5 mg q 6 hrs	Hypotension, renal failure if bilateral renal artery stenosis is present.
Furosemide (Lasix)	40–160 mg q 4-6 hrs	Hypotension, hypokalemia, hyperglycemia on prolonged use.
Labetalol (Normodyne, Trandate)	20–80 mg by bolus q 10–15 min or 0.5–2 mg/min infusion	Hypotension, bronchoconstriction, heart block, bradycardia
Sodium nitroprusside (Nipride)	0.25–10 µg/kg/min. (Maximum dose for 10 min only)	Vomiting, twitching, thiocyanate intoxication, methemoglobinemia, cyanide poisoning
Nitroglycerine (Nitrobid IV)	5–100 µg/min.	Headache, vomiting, methemoglobinemia, tolerance.

■ Questions

Instructions: For each question below, select only **one** lettered answer that is the **best** for that question.

1. A 42-year-old woman has new onset hypertension. Her review of systems is unremarkable. Urinalysis is normal except for microscopic hematuria. Serum chemistries and blood counts are also normal. An ultrasound of the kidneys demonstrates multiple fluid collections. The most likely diagnosis in this patient is which of the following?
   A. Medullary sponge kidney
   B. Bilateral renal carcinomas
   C. Polycystic kidney disease
   D. Toxoplasmosis
   E. Echinococcus cysts

2. A 24-year-old man has malaise, bilateral leg edema above the knees and hypertension. His review of systems is otherwise unremarkable. Three of his six siblings were placed on dialysis, but he does not know the etiology of their renal disease. Examination is otherwise normal. Serum creatinine is 2.4 mg/dl; BUN, 28 mg/dl and 24hr. urine protein, 10 gms with a creatinine clearance of 60 ml/min. Urinalysis demonstrates 4+ protein and 5 to10 RBCs. Three different antihypertensive medications in sufficient doses only lowers blood pressure to 160/90 mmHg. The most likely diagnosis on a renal biopsy would be which of the following?
   A. Acute glomerulonephritis
   B. Chronic interstitial nephritis
   C. Focal segmental glomerulosclerosis
   D. Membranous nephropathy
   E. Goodpasture's syndrome

3. A 27-year-old woman reports left flank pain and hematuria. There is a history of frequent urinary tract infections with *Proteus mirabilis*. She is currently taking suppressive antibiotic therapy to prevent recurrence. A renal ultrasound shows a large left kidney stone. Her renal function is normal and urinalysis shows hematuria and crystals. Urine shows: pH, 7.5, trace blood and protein. Which of the following types of kidney stones is most likely in this patient?
   A. Calcium oxalate stones
   B. Calcium phosphate stones
   C. Cystine stones
   D. Struvite stones
   E. Uric acid stones

4. A 32-year-old man has recurrent attacks of gross hematuria, occurring after flu-like symptoms or colds. These bouts have been present only over the past year. His review of systems is otherwise normal.

His laboratory studies are normal; urinalysis reveals only microscopic hematuria. The most likely diagnosis is which of the following?
   A. Alport's syndrome
   B. Anti-glomerular basement membrane disease
   C. IgA nephropathy
   D. Acute glomerulonephritis
   E. Crescentic glomerulonephritis

5. A 58-year-old woman with oat cell carcinoma of the lung is admitted for obtundation. Her weight is 60 kg; BP, 130/80 mmHg with no orthostatic hypotension, and focal signs are absent. Serum sodium: 115 mEq/l, plasma osmolality: 240 mOsm/kg H2O; urine osmolality: 680 mOsm/kg H2O, normal renal function and other laboratory tests were normal. The most likely diagnosis is which of the following?
   A. Hyponatremia due to decreased effective circulating volume
   B. Inappropriate ADH release
   C. Pseudohyponatremia
   D. Nephrogenic diabetes insipidus
   E. Central diabetes insipidus

6. A 31-year-old epileptic suffers a grand-mal seizure. Laboratory tests taken immediately after the seizure reveal a pH, 7.14 PaCO$_2$, 45 mmHg, serum sodium, 140 mEq/l; potassium, 4 mEq/l; chloride, 98 mEq/l and bicarbonate, 17 mEq/l. Which of the following best explains this acid-base disorder?
   A. Metabolic alkalosis
   B. Combined metabolic alkalosis and respiratory alkalosis
   C. Respiratory acidosis with normal anion gap metabolic acidosis
   D. Combined respiratory and high anion gap metabolic acidosis
   E. Metabolic acidosis alone

7. A 29-year-old woman with end-stage renal disease has become dyspneic in the previous 24 hours, with orthopnea. During the past 2–3 months, she has missed at least one dialysis treatment every week. Bibasilar rates and bilateral leg edema to hips are noted. Arterial pH is 7.45 and PaO$_2$ is 90mm Hg. After being dialyzed for 5 minutes, she becomes severely hypotensive. Which of the following best explains her clinical picture?
   A. Myocardial infarction
   B. Pulmonary embolus
   C. Pericardial effusion
   D. Volume overload
   E. Dialyzer reaction

8. A 62-year-old man with chronic renal failure is started on a low-sodium diet for hypertension. Two

weeks later he reports being unable to lift himself out of a chair. His skin turgor is slightly decreased and there is marked proximal muscle weakness. The serum creatinine is 2.1 mg/dl, sodium, 130 mEq/L, potassium, 9.8 mEq/L, chloride, 98 mEq/L, bicarbonate, 17 mEq/L, and arterial pH, 7.32. Widened QRS complexes and peaked T waves are noted on ECG. Which of the following factors significantly contribute to the genesis of hyperkalemia in this patient?

A. Renal insufficiency
B. Superimposed volume depletion
C. Metabolic acidosis
D. Dietary potassium intake
E. All of the above

9. A 64-year-old man undergoes a routine physical examination. Pedal edema and heme positive stools are found. His laboratory chemistries and CBC are within normal limits, but 3+ proteinuria is found. A renal biopsy demonstrates membranous nephropathy. Given this clinical picture, what additional evaluation should be performed?

A. Immunologic workup to rule out collagen vascular disease
B. Hematologic workup to rule out a hemolytic process
C. Gastrointestinal workup to rule out malignancy
D. Bronchoscopy to evaluate for pulmonary renal syndromes
E. None of the above

10. A 65-year old man, a nursing home resident, is hospitalized for dehydration and a gram negative urinary tract infection. He was given ibuprofen three times daily over the past four days for his fever. Except for WBCs, his urinalysis is normal. In the hospital, he is started on gentamicin. Ten days later, at the time of discharge, his serum creatinine had doubled from his baseline value of 1.0 mg/dl. What is the most likely etiology for his acute renal insufficiency?

A. NSAID-induced nephropathy
B. Urinary Tract Obstruction
C. Aminoglycoside nephropathy
D. Volume depletion
E. Dehydration and aminoglycoside nephropathy

11. A 42-year-old man with 4 months of progressive azotemia is now hospitalized for increasing low back pain, lethargy and anorexia. Vital signs are normal, and pallor of mucous membranes and costovertebral angle tenderness are noted. Hemoglobin is 7g/dl, BUN, 45 mg/dl, creatinine, 5 mg/dl, calcium, 12mg/dl, K^+, 3.0 mEq/L, HCO_3,

18 mEq/L, and PO_4^-, 2.0 mg/dl; the blood sugar is normal. Urinalysis shows a pH of 6, no protein, glucose 2+ and occasional hyaline and granular casts. What is the most likely cause of this man's renal failure?

A. Urinary tract obstruction
B. Primary hyperparathyroidism
C. Multiple myeloma with nephropathy
D. Distal renal tubular acidosis
E. Metastatic oat cell carcinoma

12. A 37-year-old woman complains of polyuria. Her physical examination is normal. Urinalysis, including microscopy, is normal. Urine osmolality is 80 mOsm/kg H_2O, rsing to 120 after 12 hours of dehydration. Serum Na is133 mEq/L, K, 3.9 mEq/L, HCO_3, 25 mEq/L, Creatinine, 0.7 mg/dl, serum osmolality—268 mOsm/kg H_2O. What is the most likely diagnosis?

A. Central diabetes insipidus
B. Nephrogenic diabetes insipidus
C. Diuretic abuse
D. Psychogenic polydipsia
E. Essential hyponatremia

13. Which of the following statements concerning the incidence and severity of hypertensive disease in the United Stages is false?

A. The incidence of hypertension increases with age regardless of race.
B. The incidence of hypertension is higher in men than women.
C. The incidence of systolic hypertension is higher in young blacks than whites.
D. The incidence of diastolic hypertension is twice as high in blacks than whites.
E. Blacks suffer more severe complications of hypertension.

14. Laboratory investigation that need not be routinely performed in the evaluation of hypertension includes which of the following?

A. Urinalysis.
B. Blood glucose.
C. Serum potassium.
D. Plasma renin.

15. If lifestyle modifications prove inadequate and there is no contraindication or coexisting diseases, the antihypertensive of choice is a:

A. Calcium blocker.
B. Converting enzyme inhibitor.
C. Sympathetic inhibitor.
D. Diuretic.
E. Vasodilator.

16. Which of the following statements regarding diuretics is/are correct?
    A. Long-acting diuretics produce hypokalemia less often than short-acting diuretics.
    B. Loop diuretics are better antihypertensives than thiazides.
    C. Diuretic-induced hyperuricemia causes renal damage.
    D. Diuretics can cause hyperglycemia, hypercalcemia and hyperlipidemia.

17. Contraindication to β-blocker therapy includes:
    A. Hepatic insufficiency.
    B. Asthma.
    C. First-degree heart block.
    D. Diastolic heart failure.
    E. Renal insufficiency.

18. When hypertension remains uncontrolled despite the combination of a diuretic and a sympathetic inhibitor, which of the following drugs should be tried in place of the previous therapy?
    A. An ACE inhibitor
    B. Minoxidil
    C. Hydralazine
    D. Diazoxide

19. Which of the following are appropriate in the follow-up examination of a well-controlled hypertensive patient?
    A. Monthly serum potassium
    B. Annual general examination and laboratory tests of blood sugar, serum potassium, creatinine, uric acid, and lipids
    C. Annual rapid sequence IVP
    D. Annual plasma renin
    E. Annual chest x-ray

20. Drugs known to elevate arterial blood pressure include which of the following?
    A. Oral contraceptives
    B. Corticosteroids
    C. Appetite suppressants
    D. Phenylephrine nose drops
    E. Indomethacin
    F. All of the above

■ **Answers**

1. C	2. C	3. D	4. C	5. B
6. D	7. C	8. E	9. C	10. E
11. C	12. D	13. C	14. D	15. D
16. D	17. B	18. A	19. B	20. F

SUGGESTED READING
Textbooks
Brenner BM. The Kidney. 5th ed. Philadelphia, PA: W. B. Saunders Company, 1996.
Greenberg A. Primer on Kidney Diseases. San Diego, CA: Academic Press, 1994.
Heptinstall RH. Pathology of the Kidney. 4th ed. Boston, MA: Little, Brown & Company, 1992.
Izzo JL, Black HR, Taubert KA. Hypertension Primer. Dallas, Texas: American Heart Association, 1993.
Kaplan NM, Lieberman E. Clinical Hypertension. 7th ed. Baltimore, Williams & Wilkins, 1998.
Narins RG. Maxwell and Kleeman's Clinical Disorders of Fluid and Electrolyte Metabolism. 6th ed. New York, NY: McGraw Hill, Inc., 1994.

Initial Evaluation of Kidney Disease
Ahmed Z, Lee J. Asymptomatic urinary abnormalities. Hematuria and proteinuria. Med Clin North Am. 1997;81:641–652.
Cockcroft DW, Gault MH. Prediction of creatinine clearance from serum creatinine. Nephron. 1976;16:31–41.
Fogo A, Horn RG. A 51-year-old woman with nephrotic syndrome, hematuria, and renal insufficiency. Am J Kidney Dis. 1997;29:806–810.
Levine E. Acute renal and urinary tract disease. Radiol Clin North Am. 1994;32:989–1004.
McCarthy JJ. Outpatient evaluation of hematuria: locating the source of bleeding. Postgrad Med. 1997;101:125–128.

Nephrotic Syndrome
Cameron JS. Nephrotic syndrome in the elderly. Semin Nephrol. 1996;16:319–329.
Glassock RJ. Management of intractable edema in nephrotic syndrome. Kidney Int (suppl) 1997;58:875–879.
Ponticelli C, Passerini P. Treatment of the nephrotic syndrome associated with primary glomerulonephritis. Kidney International. 1994;46:595–604.

Renal Failure
Browne BJ, Kahan BD. Renal transplantation. Surg Clin North Am. 1994;74:1097–1116.
Buckalew VM Jr. Pathophysiology of progressive renal failure. South Med J. 1994;87:1028–1033.
Hood VL, Gennari FJ. End-stage renal disease. Measures to prevent it or slow its progression. Postgrad Med. 1996;100:163–166.
Malhotra D, Tzamaloukas AH. Nondialysis management of chronic renal failure. Med Clin North Am. 1997;81:749–766.
Thadhani R, Pascual M, Bonventre JV. Acute renal failure. N Engl J Med 1996; 334:1448–1460.

Nephrolithiasis
Resnick MI. Urolithiasis. Urol Clin North Am 1997;24:1–245.

Glomerular- and Tubulointerstitial Diseases
Appel GB, Valeri A: The course and treatment of lupus nephritis. Annu Rev Med 1994;45:525–537.
Austin HA, Antonovych TT, Mackay K, Boumpas DT, Balow JE. NIH conference: Membranous nephropathy. Ann Int Med. 1992;116:672–682.
Bolton WK. Rapidly progressive glomerulonephritis. Semin Nephrol. 1996;16:517–526.
Choudhury D, Ahmed Z. Drug-induced nephrotoxicity. Med Clin North Am. 1997;81:705–717.
Dhillon S, Higgins RM. Interstitial nephritis. Postgrad Med 1997;73:151–155.

Glassock RJ, Cohen AH. The primary glomerulopathies. Dis Mon. 1996;42:329–383.

Johnson RJ. The mystery of the antineutrophil cytoplasmic antibodies Am J Kidney Dis. 1995;26:57–61.

Lapuz MH. Diabetic nephropathy. Med Clin North Am. 1997;81:679–688.

Vascular Diseases of the Kidney

Harris RC, Ismail N. Extrarenal complications of the nephrotic syndrome. Am J Kidney Dis. 1994;23:477–497.

Ram CV, Clagett GP, Radford LR. Renovascular hypertension. Semin Nephrol. 1995;15:152–174.

Saleem S, Lakkis FG, Martinez-Maldonado M. Atheroembolic renal disease. Semin Nephrol. 1996;16:309–318.

Vidt DG. Cholesterol emboli: a common cause of renal failure. Annu Rev Med. 1997;48:375–385.

Cystic Disorders

Fick GM, Gabow PA. Hereditary and acquired cystic disease of the kidney. *Kidney Int* 1994;46:951–964.

HIV Nephropathy

Rao TK. Renal complications of HIV disease. Med Clin North Am 1996; 80:1437–1451.

Disorders of Water Balance

Ayus JC, Arieff AI. Abnormalities of water metabolism in the elderly. Semin Nephrol. 1996;16:277–288.

Fried LF, Palevsky PM. Hyponatremia and hypernatremia. Med Clin North Am. 1997;81:585–609.

Disorders of Potassium Balance

Kamel KS, Quaggin S, Scheich A, Halperin ML. Disorders of potassium homeostasis: an approach based on pathophysiology. Am J Kidney Dis. 1994;24:597–613.

Mandal AK. Hypokalemia and hyperkalemia. Med Clin North Am. 1997;81:611–639.

Acid-base Disorders

Laski ME, Kurtzman MA. Acid-base disorders in medicine. Dis Mon 1996; 42:51–125.

Smulders YM, Frissen PH, Slaats EH, Silberbusch J. Renal tubular acidosis: pathophysiology and diagnosis. Arch Intern Med 1996; 156:1629–1636.

Hypertension

Joint National Committee. The report of the Joint National Committee on detection, evaluation and treatment of high blood pressure (JNCVI). Arch Intern Med 1997;157:2413–2446.

Murphy C. Hypertensive emergencies. Emerg Med Clin North Am. 1995:13:973–1007.

SHEP Cooperative Research Group. Prevention of stroke by antihypertensive drug treatment in older persons with isolated systolic hypertension in the elderly program (SHEP). JAMA. 1991;265:3255–3264.

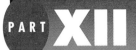

PART **XII**

Safwan Jaradeh
Theresa M. Braun
Eric F. Maas
Lorri J. Lobeck
Jeffrey R. Binder
L. Cass Terry

NEUROLOGIC DISORDERS

CHAPTER 179 · APPROACH TO THE PATIENT WITH A NEUROLOGIC DISORDER

■ History

After a detailed history is elicited, the physician should develop an initial working hypothesis that describes the location(s) and pathologic process that would explain the patient's symptoms. A neurological examination should follow, which is meant to prove one's hypothesis or suggest another if the findings refute the first. As the site/level of lesion is felt to be certain, one should outline the most likely (top three) pathologic processes. Then, one should select the most appropriate laboratory test(s) to confirm one's diagnosis. In most patients, the diagnosis is derived from the history, from an unexpected physical finding in some, and, occasionally, from a laboratory finding. The most important historical information concerns the onset and course of symptoms and signs (Figure 179.1). In diagnosing selected neurologic disorders (i.e., degenerative diseases), the family history may help significantly.

■ Neurologic Examination

Mental status examination

Level of consciousness and orientation to person, place, and time should be noted. Language function, attention, concentration, behavior, knowledge of current events, judgment, and mood can be assessed while taking the history. A mini-mental status examination is outlined in Table 114.1.

Evaluation of speech and language

Dysarthrias

Dysarthrias are the product of neurologic disorders affecting the mechanisms that control and coordinate speech. This is reflected by changes in the acoustic quality of speech without alteration of language per se. Written language is always spared.

Aphasias

Aphasia is a disturbance of language expression, comprehension or both. The dysfunction involves both spoken and written language, albeit to a variable extent. The examination assesses fluency of language production, language comprehension, ability to repeat, and presence of word substitutions known as **"paraphasias."** Fluency is impaired if the patient produces speech slowly or laboriously, utters unusually brief sentences, pauses frequently to find a word, or uses only the most essential words ("telegraphic speech"). Comprehension is tested by requiring the patient to answer

questions or carry out commands of varying complexity. Repetition of words and sentences measures the integrity of cortical regions surrounding the Sylvian fissure. Paraphasias usually indicate injury posterior to the peri-sylvian region. Patterns of aphasia are summarized in Table 179.1.

Cranial nerves

Assessment of **cranial nerve function** is summarized in Table 179.2.

Evaluation of sensory function

The main sensory modalities are primary (light touch, pinprick, temperature, vibration and joint position sensation) and complex (2-point discrimination, graphesthesia and stereognosis). **Impairment of sensory function** usually presents with **numbness.** One should ask for a description of the feeling in the patient's own words. Paresthesia (tingling or prickling) or dysesthesia (disagreeable sensory symptoms) may be associated. The isolated feeling of heaviness or deadness may be due to either sensory or motor impairment. If the history suggests sensory impairment, the sensory functions should be tested first. The **Romberg procedure** tests the posterior column and vestibular (not cerebellar) function because it eliminates **visual-spatial orientation.** Cerebellar pathology is manifest with or without the eyes closed. Patterns of sensory loss in various disorders are shown in Table 179.3

Motor system

Besides gait, the motor system is most efficiently assessed by checking **fine and gross coordination** (i.e., **finger and toe tapping**), observation for wasting or fasciculations (lower motor neuron), muscle tone, and individual muscle strength. Neuromuscular junction defects (e.g., myasthenia gravis) more often present with fatigue on exertion, rather than primary weakness (Table 179.4).

Striated muscles are composed of multiple motor units; each unit is a single motor neuron, its axon and the muscle fibers it innervates, together called the **lower motor neuron.** Various descending cerebral pathways (corticospinal tract being the most important) that control these units form the **upper motor neurons.** Diseases of either the upper or the lower motor neuron cause weakness, which may be partial **(paresis),** or complete **(paralysis).** Paralysis of one limb is **monoplegia,** and of both legs, **paraplegia;** paralysis of one side

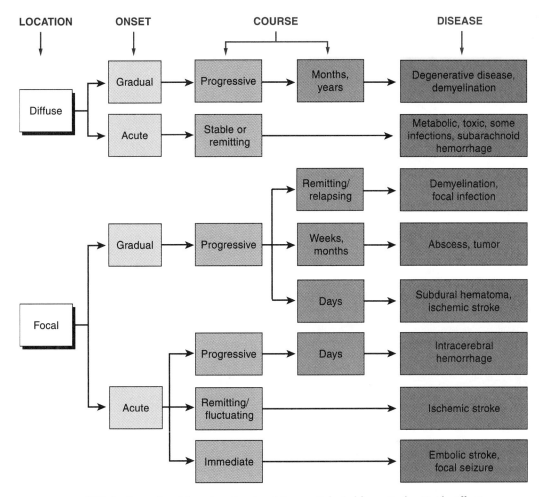

LOCATION	ONSET	COURSE		DISEASE

FIGURE 179.1. Examples of Symptom Onset and Course. (Adapted from: Caplan LR. The Effective Clinical Neurologist. Cambridge: Blackwell Scientific Publishers, 1990; 45-52.)

TABLE 179.1. Clinical Differentiation of Major Aphasias

Type	Fluency	Comprehension	Repetition	Lesion site
Broca	Impaired	Usually intact	Impaired	Usually left frontal, infero-posterior
Wernicke	Intact, paraphasic	Impaired	Impaired	Left temporal, supero-posterior
Global	Impaired	Impaired	Impaired	Left frontal and temporal
Conduction	Intact, paraphasic	Intact	Impaired	Left arcuate fasciculus, or left supramarginal gyrus
Transcortical motor	Impaired	Usually intact	Intact	Antero-superior to Broca's
Transcortical-sensory	Intact, paraphasic	Impaired	Intact	Infero-posterior to Wernicke's
Anomic	Intact, naming difficulty	Intact	Intact	Left angular gyrus, or left posterior temporal

(Adapted from: Damasio AR. N Engl J Med 1992;326:531-539. Used with permission.)

TABLE 179.2. Cranial Nerve Examination

Site to Examine	What to Look for:	Which Cranial Nerve Will This Examine?
Fundus	Optic disk, venous pulsations[a], visual fields	II
Pupils	Size, shape, symmetry, light reaction	III, cervical sympathetic[b]
Eye movements	Nystagmus, paralysis, dissociation, diplopia	III, IV, VI, VIII
Corneal reflex	Sensation[c], blink	V, VII
Facial symmetry	Upper versus lower motor weakness	VII
Gag reflex	Sensation (IX), motor	IX, X
Neck/shoulder	Turn neck from one side to the other; shrugging of shoulders; sternocleidomastoid/trapezius	XI
Tongue	Protrusion in midline	XII

[a]The ability to detect venous pulsations is very important; when present bilaterally, the probability (approx. 95%) is that intracranial pressure is not elevated.
[b]The cervical sympathetic is not a cranial nerve.
[c]Tests only cranial nerve V.

TABLE 179.3. Patterns of Sensory Loss in Various Disorders

Site/Disease	Pattern/Distribution of Sensory Loss
Thalamus or sensory cortex	Impaired complex sensory functions
Spinal cord lesion	Involves trunk plus upper and/or lower extremity
Root or peripheral nerve	Dermatome/peripheral nerve territory
Mononeuropathy	Territory of the involved nerve
Polyneuropathy	Symmetric, gradual transition from distal to proximal; stocking and glove distribution
Hysteria	None, sharp transition from anesthetic to normal areas

TABLE 179.4. Motor System in Various Disorders

Location	Tone	Bulk	Strength	Reflexes
Upper motor neuron	Spastic	+/−	Decreased	Increased, Babinski sign
Basal ganglia	Rigidity	No change	No change	No change
Cerebellar	Hypotonic	No change	No change	Pendular
Anterior horn cell	Decreased	Atrophy, fasciculations	Decreased	Decreased
Radiculopathy	+/−	+/−	Decreased	Decreased
Peripheral nerve (motor)	+/−	Decreased distally	Decreased distally	Decreased
Muscle	Decreased	Decreased	Decreased	Decreased
Neuromuscular junction	Variable	Variable	Fatigue	Variable

+/− = may or may not be abnormal.

is **hemiplegia,** and of all limbs, **quadriplegia.** Weakness of muscles innervated by the brain stem, such as face, tongue and pharynx is **bulbar palsy.** Differentiation between upper and lower motor neuron disorders is outlined in Table 179.4.

Gait

One useful screening test is to observe a patient's **gait,** including standing, walking, stopping, turning, and associated arm swing movements. These maneuvers require integration of sensory, motor, basal ganglia, cerebellar, vestibular, and visual processing, and are, therefore, sensitive indicators of abnormal function of one or more systems. In a unilateral **upper motor neuron lesion,** the patient walks by circumducting the affected leg while keeping the affected arm close to the body in a mildly flexed position. In extrapyramidal disorders, particularly Parkinsonism, there is mild stooping of the body, with difficulty initiating gait or performing rapid turns. Initial shuffling is seen once walking begins, with a mild increase in the speed (**"festinating" gait**). In mild disease, only reduced swinging of the arms may be noted. A **wide-based gait,** often with instability on turning, frequently follows cerebellar disorders. The patient is unable to perform a **heel-to-toe** tandem gait. The unsteady gait in vestibular or proprioceptive sensory deficits dramatically worsens when visual input is removed, such as walking in the dark. When joint position sense is severely impaired, patients lift their legs significantly before landing on the ground in a **"step-page"** manner (**"tabetic gait"**). A unilateral vestibular lesion, particularly when associated with a cerebellar lesion, results in veering to the side of the lesion. Finally, proximal weakness, as in myopathies or spinal muscular atrophies, cause **"waddling"** due to pelvic tilting. However, foot and leg weakness from a neuropathy results in a gait with foot drop.

Cerebellum

This system is most efficiently tested by observation of heel-to-toe tandem walking and **finger-to-nose** and **heel-to-shin** movements. Slurred, dysarthric speech, clumsiness or **ataxia, hypotonia, nystagmus,** dysarthria, and **gait dysfunction** usually result from cerebellar dysfunction. Patients also usually have an abnormal finger-to-nose and/or heel-to-shin testing (dysmetria). With severe cerebellar disease, an intention tremor is commonly observed.

Reflexes

Deep tendon reflexes (DTRs) test both sensory and motor limbs of the spinal reflex arc, besides the degree of upper motor neuron input. Amplitude, symmetry, proximal versus distal pattern, and an isolated diminution or absence of a single response are looked for. Most commonly tested reflexes are listed in Table 179.5, despite the anatomic variation in spinal segments. The plantar response, normally flexor, should be assessed in every patient. Extension of the great toe, with/without fanning of the other toes, is the **Babinski sign** and indicates upper motor neuron involvement.

Formulation

When assessing a neurologic problem, besides the probability of a neurologic disease, one should also consider its "treatability." Even though a diagnosis may not be the most likely, one should pursue it, if it is possible and reversible (i.e., hypothyroidism, vitamin B_{12} deficiency, subdural hematoma).

■ Localization

The following principles are very useful in neurologic diagnosis: 1) one lesion or process can often explain the neurologic symptoms and signs; 2) abnormal neurologic function can usually be localized to regions, and 3) it is often helpful if one neurologic sign is longitudinal (corticospinal, spinothalamic, posterior column) and another is segmental (sensory level, reflexes, cranial nerves, cerebellum). For example, in paraplegia with a sensory level, one can localize the lesion within one to three spinal segments.

■ Laboratory Studies

Lumbar puncture (LP)

LP is useful in diagnosing meningitis, encephalitis, encephalopathies, subarachnoid hemorrhage, inflammatory disorders, and multiple sclerosis. It is contraindicated if bleeding disorders are suspected, or with increased intracranial pressure, intracranial mass, and spinal cord mass. Often, it should be preceded by CT to exclude an intracranial mass. In the lateral decubitus position, normal cerebrospinal fluid (CSF) opening pressure is less than 200 mm water.

The CSF should be collected in 4 tubes. Tube 1 is usually for cell count if the fluid is bloody; cell counts should be done on tubes 1 and 4. Tube 2 is usually for

TABLE 179.5.	**Clinical Manifestations of Common Radiculopathies**		
Root	**Pain/Sensory Loss**	**Reflex Arc**	**Motor Deficit**
C5	Shoulder	Biceps	Shoulder abduction
C6	Lateral arm, forearm, thumb	Biceps, brachio-radialis	Elbow flexion
C7	Dorsal arm and fore-arm, middle finger	Triceps	Elbow extension
C8	Medial arm & forearm, little finger	Finger flexion	Finger flexion
L3	Anterior and medial thigh	Adductor, patellar	Thigh adduction
L4	Medial leg	Patellar	Leg extension
L5	Lateral calf and leg, posterior thigh, dor-sum of foot	Hamstring	Ankle dorsiflexion
S1	Posterior calf and leg, plantar surface	Achilles	Ankle plantar flexion

TABLE 179.6. CSF Findings in Main Neurologic Conditions				
Condition	Cell Type and Count	Protein	Glucose	IgG Index/Bands[a]
Acute meningitis: bacterial	PMN, elevated	Elevated	Decreased	Increased/none
viral	Lymph, elevated	Elevated	Normal	Increased/none
Chronic meningitis	Lymph, elevated	Elevated	Decreased	Increased/rare
Viral encephalitis	Lymph, elevated	Elevated	Normal	Increased/none
HIV				
Aseptic meningitis	Lymph, elevated	Elevated	Normal	Increased/rare
AIDS-related dementia	Lymph, elevated	Elevated	Normal	Increased/often present[b]
Multiple sclerosis	Rarely elevated	Slightly elevated	Normal	Increased/present
Subarachnoid hemorrhage	RBC, abundant	Slightly elevated	Normal	Normal/none
Leptomeningeal tumor	Malignant cells	Slightly elevated	Decreased	Normal/none

[a]Refers to oligoclonal bands.
[b]Depends on the stage of the disease; myelin basic protein is normal; β2 microglobulin in CSF is high.

TABLE 179.7. Laboratory Testing and Imaging Studies in Neurological Diagnosis	
Test	Indication/Comments
Electrophysiologic studies	
EEG	Suspected seizures, encephalopathies, changes in consciousness, and brain death
EP	Suspected multiple sclerosis, assess and prognosticate after brain trauma or hypoxia, evaluate spinal cord integrity after trauma or during spine surgery
EMG/NCV	Suspected motor neuron disease, radiculopathy, peripheral neuropathy, myasthenia gravis, and myopathy
Imaging studies	
Cranial	
Plain x-rays	Very limited
CT	Differentiate infarction from intracranial hemorrhage; evaluation of suspected subarachnoid hemorrhage, trauma, and tumor; good visualization of bony changes
MRI	Early (<48 hours) suspected non-hemorrhagic stroke, posterior fossa tumors, demyelination syndromes, and white matter edema associated with infections
Angiography	Intracranial aneurysms, AVMs, fistulae, TIA in surgical candidates, venous sinus thrombosis, meningiomas, dissecting aneurysms, and vasculitis
Spinal	
Plain x-rays	A good screening test for neck/low back pain since it shows congenital, traumatic, degenerative, and neoplastic bony abnormalities, as well as spinal stenosis
Myelography	Suspected spinal cord or nerve root compression; being supplanted considerably by MRI
CT	Lateral disk herniations (when combined with myelography); also helpful in evaluation of bony abnormalities
MRI	Visualize spinal cord, nerve roots, herniated disks, and spinal cord compression
Ultrasonography	
B-mode	Evaluation of extracranial carotid disease; screen for suspected ICA stenosis
Doppler	Measure velocity of carotid blood flow as a screening test
Biopsies	
Temporal artery	Suspected giant cell arteritis
Muscle/nerve	Suspected myopathies, polymyositis, vasculitides, and infectious and inflammatory disorders; not necessary for diagnosing peripheral neuropathy

a-v m = arteriovenous malformations; CT = computed tomography; EEG = electroencephalography; EMG/NCV = electromyography and nerve conduction studies; EP = evoked potentials; ICA = internal carotid artery; MRI = magnetic resonance imaging; TIA = transient ischemic attack.

glucose and protein; tube 3 for microbial stains, and tube 4 for cultures. Other tests include IgG and **oligoclonal bands** in suspected demyelination, and cytology for malignant cells. With a traumatic tap, the supernatant is usually colorless, the cell count is significantly less in tube 4 and, the WBC:RBC ratio is 1:1000, similar to peripheral blood. Following subarachnoid hemorrhage, CSF is usually pink. **Xanthochromia** (from conversion to bilirubin) appears within 8–12 hours and lasts up to 3 weeks. CSF findings in major neurologic diseases are shown in Table 179.6.

The role of additional laboratory, imaging and electrophysiological testing in neurological diagnosis is summarized in Table 179.7.

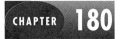 **180** COMA

■ Definition and Etiology

Coma is a medical emergency requiring simultaneous attention to treatment of life-threatening problems (e.g., ventilation, cardiovascular status, trauma, hypoglycemia) and evaluation to determine the cause, which may be apparent or elusive.

Defining coma and normal consciousness is not difficult. Disruptions of consciousness between these two extremes are variously described with confusing and often misapplied terminology. Consciousness has two facets—**arousal** and **content.** These are obviously codependent for normalcy but can be disrupted independently at variable intervals. For instance, a sedative overdose will acutely depress arousal with conscious content initially maintained. Conversely, **dementia of the Alzheimer type** disrupts memory and cognition with general sparing of arousal. *Coma is a state of unarousable unresponsiveness.* In practice, a statement recording the responses elicited with various stimuli should be used to define arousal states. Confusing terms may pose an impediment to the accurate portrayal of the clinical course. Nonetheless, certain terms deserve mention. **Lethargy** is simply a tendency toward sleepiness—**drowsiness.** The obvious presence of excessive amounts of sleep and inattention to the environment with the maintenance of spontaneous arousal may be described as **obtundation. Stupor** is a state where arousal is only maintained with constant vigorous stimulation.

Depression of arousal has an important neurologic localization, indicating impairment of the rostral brainstem (rostral pons and midbrain) or both cerebral hemispheres. If a comatose patient has a lesion that does not conform to this localization, then further investigation is necessary. A single, large, acute unilateral hemispheric lesion can depress arousal transiently. If the altered consciousness persists, then other pathology must be present. Diffuse processes such as metabolic encephalopathies or infection will, of course, disrupt both hemispheres and brainstem. The causes of coma are listed in Table 180.1.

■ Initial Management of the Comatose Patient

Coma is a medical emergency and assessment of the airway, respiration (breathing), and circulation (ABCs) take precedence over all other issues. Head and neck trauma must always be considered and excluded using radiographic studies of skull and cervical spine before proceeding with manipulation during the examination. Periorbital ecchymosis, hemotympani or CSF rhinorrhea and otorrhea indicate skull fracture. Early funduscopy will detect papilledema or hemorrhage as evidence for increased intracranial pressure. Intravenous access should be established and blood collected for laboratory studies, including CBC with differential and platelet count, basic chemistries with immediate glucose determination, liver tests, TSH, blood culture and toxicology screen. Urine should be sent for the additional toxicology tests as well as routine analysis and culture. Arterial blood gas analysis, chest x-ray and ECG should be done as soon as possible (comatose patients will not report chest pain). Oxygen, thiamine, and 50 ml of 50% dextrose are given. **Naloxone** is administered if narcotic overdose is suspected, and **flumazenil,** if benzodiazepine overdose is suspected.

TABLE 180.1. Causes of Coma
Supratentorial lesions
Mass effect from edema, hemorrhage, infection or tumor
Posterior fossa lesions
Vertebrobasilar occlusion
Pontine or cerebellar hemorrhage
Other mass lesions (abscess or hemorrhage into a tumor)
Diffuse and multifocal causes
Hypoxic ischemic insult following cardiac arrest
Meningoencephalitis, carcinomatous meningitis
Drug intoxication
Renal or hepatic failure
Hypothyroidism, Addisonian crisis, hyperglycemia, hypoglycemia, acid-base disturbances
Nutritional deficiencies
Acute demyelination (disseminated encephalomyelitis, central pontine myelinolysis)
Seizures, especially nonconvulsive status epilepticus

■ Bedside Examination of the Comatose Patient

As the initial urgent management measures are deployed, a history is obtained from the patient's family, friends and the medical record. Particular attention should be paid to the patient's recent health and behavior, medication changes, and the possibility of any recent trauma. The past medical history is of increased importance since little else may be known about the patient. Frequently, telephone calls to pertinent individuals may provide key information in diagnosing the cause of coma.

The five principal elements of the coma examination are assessment of arousal, respiratory pattern, pupils, ocular motility and motor responses (Table 180.2). Observation for any spontaneous movement or elements of arousal from internal or environmental stimuli is a useful, but often forgotten step. Next, the response to progressively increasing stimuli should be recorded. This begins with gentle verbal cues and progresses to more noxious stimuli by first calling the patient's name, then shouting or clapping, followed by perioral stimulation with a tongue blade and progressing to pressure in the supraorbital notch, over the sternum or to the nail beds. The patient should be uncovered so that any reactive movement can be observed. A one or two line statement describing the spontaneous and reflex responses is an accurate and useful way to record the state of arousal.

Spontaneous respiratory pattern is important. **Cheyne-Stokes respiration** is a pattern of periods of hyperpnea alternating with apnea. Bihemispheric lesions,

congestive heart failure with cerebrovascular disease and metabolic derangements (hepatic and renal failure and sedative intoxication) are causes. **Central neurogenic hyperventilation,** ascribed to lesions of the midbrain, is exceedingly rare, and a systemic cause for hyperventilation is invariably present. Cheyne-Stokes respiratory pattern may deteriorate into an irregular periodic pattern indicating progressive dysfunction, such as with rostral caudal deterioration due to an expanding supratentorial lesion.

Pupillary size, symmetry and reflexes are an essential part of the coma examination. Metabolic and toxic disturbances generally do not cause abnormalities of pupillary size and reactivity. Asymmetry in size and reactivity are most pronounced with midbrain and third cranial nerve lesions. *Probably the most important pupillary abnormality to recognize is the presence or development of a unilateral dilated and unreactive pupil suggesting compression of the midbrain from the medial aspect of the temporal lobe due to expansion of a laterally placed supratentorial lesion.* The pupillary change alone may herald this uncal herniation syndrome. On occasion, a pontine lesion will cause very small and weakly reactive pupils, sometimes referred to as **"pinpoint pupils."** One should suspect narcotic overdose when this is seen with no other brainstem abnormalities.

Ocular movements provide important information about brainstem function. Spontaneous full eye movements, while commonly roving and slow in coma, nevertheless indicate integrity of the third, fourth, and sixth cranial nerves. Horizontal dysconjugate gaze is relatively common in coma, while vertical separation more often indicates brainstem or cerebellar pathology. Any persistent gaze deviation suggests a destructive lesion, either in the ipsilateral cerebral hemisphere or contralateral pons. Ocular oscillations may be present. When the eyes seem driven downward and medially, insult to the diencephalon should be suspected, particularly as part of increasing pressure from a more rostral supratentorial lesion.

Assessment of oculocephalic and **vestibulo-ocular** reflexes should follow next. The term **oculocephalic responses** should be used instead of "dolls eyes," since the latter term is ambiguous. Any cervical spine trauma must be excluded prior to this test. The head is turned rapidly from one side to the other and the eyes are observed for any slow phase movement in the opposite direction. If the oculocephalic response is inadequate, then caloric stimulation of the vestibular labyrinth should follow, but only *after* careful examination of the external auditory canal and tympanic membrane for impacted cerumen or other pathology that might contraindicate the test. The absence of any response to oculocephalic maneuver and properly performed caloric stimulation

TABLE 180.2.	**Principal Elements of Examination of the Comatose Patient**

Assessment of arousal
  Spontaneous movement
  Response to exogenous stimuli
Respiratory pattern
  Cheyne-Stokes respiration
  Irregular respirations
Pupil size, symmetry and reflexes
Ocular motility
  Spontaneous eye movements
  Oculocephalic reflex
  Oculovestibular reflex
Motor responses
  Spontaneous movement
  Abnormal posturing
  Response to pain
  Tone

strongly suggests disruption of the vestibulo-ocular pathways between the rostral medulla up to the mid pons and midbrain.

The *motor examination* also begins with observation for any spontaneous movement. Any asymmetry in spontaneous movement is particularly important. Motor responses to noxious stimuli may be either purposeful and localizing or abnormal posturing movements. It can be difficult to determine which, although if the movement is toward the noxious stimulus, then this might indicate posturing. Abnormal upper extremity posturing can be either in flexion or extension. The latter indicates injury progressing below the diencephalon and into the brainstem, whereas flexion response occurs with hemispheric lesions above this level. Lower extremity posturing is extensor with both hemispheric and brainstem lesions, although becomes weakly flexor or flaccid with lower brainstem injury. Muscle stretch reflexes and plantar responses are tested, particularly looking for asymmetry and pathologic responses.

■ Laboratory Evaluation of Coma

A noncontrast CT scan of the head is needed in the acute stage to detect hemorrhage, mass lesion or edema. Imaging should always be obtained prior to lumbar puncture. A CSF examination is required for suspected subarachnoid hemorrhage, acute demyelination, vasculitis, infection or if the etiology is elusive despite initial studies. Electroencephalography (EEG) is important for the diagnosis of nonconvulsive status epilepticus, metabolic encephalopathies, encephalitis and psychogenic coma. EEG should also be performed whenever the cause of coma is elusive.

■ Continued Management of the Comatose Patient

Continued management of the comatose patient depends upon careful recording of serial examinations as treatment of the underlying cause is initiated. Nutrition management and usual precautions against complications of chronic immobility must also be remembered. Patients do not remain in a coma for longer than days or weeks and either begin to show recovery or progress to death or a persistent vegetative state. The latter is a condition where arousal patterns normalize with development of a sleep-wake cycle and yet are without evidence of conscious content. Studies using serial examination protocols to predict prognosis for comatose patients who have suffered hypoxic injury have been published.

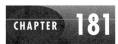

HEADACHES

■ Epidemiology and Pathophysiology

Headache is an extremely common symptom, with an estimated 40% of Americans having suffered from severe headaches at some point in their lives. Headaches may signal the presence of life-threatening illness, or be a chronic, recurrent, life-long condition. **Migraine** and **cluster headache** cause significant disability and days lost from work for some patients.

Pain-sensitive structures of the head and neck include the scalp, head and neck muscles, cerebral venous sinuses, dura, dural arteries, intracerebral arteries; the third, fifth, sixth, and seventh cranial nerves; and cervical nerves. Irritation of any of these structures will produce pain referred to the head, felt as headache. The neurotransmitter, serotonin, appears to play a role in at least the recurrent headache syndromes, since drugs which alter serotonin levels in the central nervous system affect headache frequency. Since such response is not universal, it indicates a role for other transmitters also.

Sudden, Severe Headache

Sudden, severe headache in a patient not otherwise prone to headache should not be attributed to migraine without careful evaluation. **Subarachnoid hemorrhage** (SAH) from ruptured **intracerebral aneurysm** or **arteriovenous malformation** (AVM) must be considered, particularly if there is neck stiffness. Headache, neck stiffness and fever suggests meningitis. **Intracerebral hemorrhage** usually produces focal neurological deficits. Seizures may accompany any of the foregoing. With chiefly retro-orbital pain, **acute glaucoma** should be considered. **Acute sinusitis** presents with sinus tenderness and fever. **Acute hydrocephalus** from tumor, hemorrhage or meningitis (cancerous or infectious) may present with altered consciousness, nausea, vomiting and headache.

■ Emergency Approach to Headache

Neuro-imaging should be performed on any patient presenting with a first, sudden, severe headache. A non-contrasted CT suffices to demonstrate an acute bleed in a subarachnoid, intraparenchymal, epidural or subdural locus. If tumor is suggested, a follow-up CT with con-trast or MRI can follow. If suspicion of SAH lingers despite a negative CT, a lumbar puncture (LP) should be done. Fever, headaches and nuchal rigidity strongly suggest acute bacterial or viral meningitis. This mandates LP and antibiotic therapy within one hour to cover for possible bacterial meningitis until CSF results become available. Proper use of CT in this setting is discussed in Chapter 153. Evaluation for pseudotumor involves a similar workup, imaging and LP; sedimentation rate (ESR) is necessary in persons older than 50 years to exclude temporal arteritis.

New, Progressive Headache

Conditions with prominent, new, progressive headache and subacute presentation include brain tumor, pseudotumor cerebri and temporal arteritis. Progressive neurological signs evolving over days to weeks suggest a **brain tumor;** a history of a known primary malignancy is helpful, but a malignant tumor may present initially with cerebral metastasis. Papilledema implies raised intracranial pressure and may be seen in brain tumor or hydrocephalus. It should prompt urgent neuro-imaging. If these processes are excluded, **pseudotumor cerebri** (papilledema, normal neural imaging and elevated CSF pressure on LP) should be considered. **Temporal arteritis** should be excluded in anyone over 50 years of age with new onset of headaches; jaw claudication, muscle aches (polymyalgia rheumatica), fever, anemia and weight loss may be associated. ESR is typically markedly elevated. Left untreated, this entity can cause blindness. **Subdural hematomas** can cause progressive headache and confusion, with or without focal signs; the preceding trauma need not be severe, especially if there is concurrent anticoagulant therapy. Non-neurologic systemic febrile illness also commonly cause headaches.

Recurrent Headache Syndromes

Migraine

■ Etiology

Migraine headaches, recognized since ancient times, more commonly affect women. They typically begin in young adulthood and have a familial tendency. Dietary migraine triggers include ingestion of caffeine, alcohol and food such as chocolate or aged cheeses. Disordered regulation of serotonin systems in the CNS has been implicated.

■ Clinical Features

Migraine has 2 broad categories, classic and common. **Classic migraine** begins with an aura, which is typically visual and often described as flashing lights in one visual field, with a jagged configuration, leading to the term "fortification spectrum." This spectrum may move slowly across the visual field, leaving in its wake, a hemianopia. This visual disturbance may last 20–60 minutes. Tingling or numbness may be reported in the hand or side of the face, which spreads slowly over minutes in contrast to the spread of a sensory seizure. As the aura subsides, the headache begins. Described as pounding or throbbing, it is often accompanied by photophobia, nausea, and vomiting. It typically peaks within minutes to an hour and lasts one to several hours. The patient usually seeks a dark, quiet place to lie down. Sleep may end the pain. In some, the pain may last a day or two. **Common migraine** lacks aura or neurological symptoms; the pounding headache may be associated with nausea and vomiting.

The term **complicated migraine** is used when objective neurological deficits accompany the headache. Aphasia, hemiparesis, or third nerve palsies may transiently follow migraine. However, other causes of headaches *and* focal deficits such as stroke, AVM, aneurysm or tumor must first be excluded.

■ Diagnosis

Migraine headaches should be differentiated from other causes of recurring headaches, such as cluster or muscular headaches, as well as AVM. AVM may present with a long history of recurring pounding headache with pain that is usually unilateral. **Cluster headaches** are primarily nocturnal and brief, associated with conjunctival injection and tearing. Features of cluster and migraine may overlap in some patients, and others may share features of migraine and **muscle contraction headache.** Diagnosing migraine requires an accurate headache history. With typical features, confusion seldom arises. Neurological examination should be normal. Atypical features in history, complicated migraine and abnormal examination call for neuroimaging. Even in the migraine patient, a change in headache character or lack of response to therapy may necessitate imaging. Migraine with a third nerve palsy may require cerebral angiography to exclude a cerebral aneurysm.

■ Management

Acute migraine

Although rest, combined with acetaminophen or nonsteroidal anti-inflammatory agents (NSAIDs) suffice in some patients to abort a headache, for many others, these are inadequate. Analgesic combinations that contain codeine or barbiturates can help occasional headaches; however, for those patients with frequent migraines, these agents may entail both drug dependence and withdrawal headaches. Limitation of weekly and monthly use is important in the successful use of these agents. Ergotamine given by tablet or aerosol can effectively abort migraine with aura. A dose taken at the onset of the aura can prevent the headache. Dihydroergotamine (DHE), given IM, can also help abort a refractory attack. Because it causes pronounced nausea, an antiemetic should be given simultaneously. Sumatriptan, a 5-hydroxytryptamine antagonist, is a very effective abortive therapy. It acts rapidly, usually within a matter of minutes, and is nonsedating. Its use must be limited to 2 injections per day.

Prophylaxis

When the number of migraine episodes exceeds 3–4 per month, prophylactic therapy, combined with abortive therapy, is reasonable. With any prophylactic agent, a few weeks of therapy must elapse before changing the dose or ascertaining effectiveness. Amitriptyline, usually begun with 25 mg at bedtime and increased gradually, is effective for prophylaxis. Side effects include dry mouth, constipation, blurry vision and sedation. Its sleep-promoting effect can be a boon when there is sleep disturbance. Calcium channel blockers, such as verapamil, or the beta-blocker, propranolol, in doses similar to that used for hypertension, can also be extremely effective for prophylaxis. Beta blockers may cause fatigue, dizziness, and exercise intolerance. Use of both these agents have been simplified by sustained release formulations.

Muscle Contraction Headaches

Muscle contraction headache is sometimes used as a nonspecific term for headaches that "do not fit the mold." Often referred to as tension headaches, the pain is reportedly steady, nonthrobbing, "band like" or "vise like," with no associated nausea, vomiting or visual changes. Onset is typically gradual. They generally do not interfere with work. Their pathophysiology is unknown. Physical examination is normal. Neuro-imaging is often not required, although cervical spine films may be necessary to evaluate for degenerative disease. Treatment depends upon the frequency and severity of these headaches. Acetaminophen and NSAIDs, taken on a daily basis, may be helpful. A tricyclic agent (amitriptyline) can be beneficial in refractory cases. Biofeedback may similarly be successful in motivated patients. Some consider this headache to be a manifestation of depression, and an assessment for depression is reasonable.

Cluster Headaches

Cluster headache is relatively uncommon but six times more prevalent in men. "Cluster" describes a tendency for recurrence over a period of a few to several weeks. These tend to occur at the same time of day and are particularly nocturnal, often waking the patient from sleep. Onset is usually between ages 20–50. The headache begins rapidly, without aura, peaks within minutes, and is intense and brief (30–120 min). It most often affects an eye and/or temple; face, neck, ear or head may or may not be involved. During an attack, tearing of the eye, conjunctival injection or transient **Horner's syndrome** may occur. A pain-free interval lasting months to years commonly follows a cluster. Family history of recurrent headaches is usually absent. Neurological examination and imaging studies are usually normal. Attacks may be aborted by inhaling 100% O_2 for 10–15 minutes, or aerosolized ergotamine or sumatriptan injection. Effective preventive agents include prednisone, lithium, cyproheptadine, methysergide (risk of retroperitoneal fibrosis), indomethacin and calcium channel blockers.

CHAPTER **182** DIZZINESS

■ Evaluation of the Dizzy Patient

Dizziness is a common complaint, and a variety of disorders produce symptoms evoking this description. A reasonable diagnosis can be determined in the majority of cases through a careful clinical assessment and selected ancillary tests. The four principal symptom categories that present with the complaint of dizziness are vertigo, syncope, disequilibrium, and lightheadedness. Syncope is discussed in Chapter 29.

The patient should describe the problem without using the word "dizziness"; the history is then refined with specific inquiries. An illusion of self motion or environmental motion—vertigo—or a sense of impending faint should be explicitly determined. Often, syncope is initially accompanied by a sense of floating, drifting or moving and, likewise, vertigo may evoke a fear of fainting. One of the two sensations will generally predominate. Precipitating, palliative and temporal fea-

tures must be detailed. Particular attention is given to the effect of physical activity and postural changes, as well as accompanying cardiac and neurologic symptoms.

The "dizzy" patient should receive a general physical examination, a standard neurologic examination and special or provocative tests. A careful cardiovascular examination should be done, searching for dysrhythmias, murmurs, cervical and supraclavicular bruits and evidence of peripheral vascular disease, and recording postural changes in blood pressure and pulse. Coordination should be tested and special attention paid to vision, eye movements, hearing and lower extremity sensory function. Natural and tandem gait should be observed for a good distance while ensuring the patient's safety. Romberg sign, and finger-to-nose, heel-to-shin, and rapid alternating movements should be examined, and nystagmus (spontaneous or position-induced) elicited.

Vertigo

Vertigo is an illusion of self motion or environmental motion. Most often rotational, this may also be a sensation of tilt or linear motion. Dysfunction of the vestibular system, either centrally (brainstem vestibular nuclei and vestibulocerebellar pathways) or peripherally (labyrinth and vestibular nerve) is responsible; the initial challenge is to determine which one of these is operative. Determination of the underlying cause should follow next.

Generally, peripheral vertigo is more severe; nausea and vomiting are prominent. Patients fall toward the side of the vestibular lesion and have a jerk nystagmus (direction of nystagmus is denoted by the direction of the fast phase movement) away from the lesion. Direction of peripheral nystagmus will not reverse with eye position, and the magnitude is more likely to dampen with fixation. Facial weakness might occur in both central and peripheral vertigo, but is most pronounced in conjunction with lesions of the eighth nerve, since the facial nerve runs directly proximate to it. Other features are shown in Table 182.1.

■ Peripheral Disorders

Peripheral vestibular disorders cause vertigo in the majority of patients with dizziness. Patients with labyrinthine or vestibular nerve lesions usually

report true rotational vertigo, often with a positional character. Common forms have distinguishing clinical features.

Benign paroxysmal positional vertigo (BPPV) is, perhaps, the most common form of peripheral vertigo; its incidence rises with age. The symptoms begin with a change in head position. Frequently, the patient notes the first attack when rolling over in bed. Hearing is usually not disturbed. A latency is present between the head rotation and the vertigo. Barany's maneuver (Figure 182.1) is important in eliciting the typical nystagmus of BPPV. In BPPV, there is a latency to the onset of nystagmus from 2–20 seconds. The nystagmus fatigues over a few seconds to a few minutes and may recur in the opposite direction on return to the sitting position. After repeating the maneuver a few times, there is habituation of the response. The nystagmus has a specific upward-rotatory character. Trauma and forms of labyrinthine inflammation or ischemia also manifest as BPPV. Most patients recover over days or weeks. A special exercise can hasten improvement. (Figure 182.2). A few repetitions of this cycle are completed two or three times a day. Vestibular suppressants (meclizine, promethazine, diphenhydramine, astemizole, diazepam) may help in the acute phase. Any deviation from the typical character of symptoms, signs, positional nystagmus or clinical course

TABLE 182.1. Differentiating Between Peripheral and Central Vertigo		
Criterion	Peripheral	Central
Direction of nystagmus	Unidirectional, fast phase away from lesion	Bi- or unidirectional; may change with direction of gaze
Pure vertical or rotary	Never	Possible
Pure horizontal without rotary	Uncommon; usually horizontal or vertical with rotary component	Common
Visual fixation	Inhibits nystagmus and vertigo	No inhibition
Intensity of vertigo and constitutional symptoms	Severe	Often mild to moderate; may be severe
Environmental movement	Toward fast phase of nystagmus	Variable
Romberg fall and past pointing	Toward slow phase of nystagmus	Variable
Tinnitus or deafness	Often present, unilateral; important clue	Usually absent
Latency to vertigo and nystagmus after position change, and habituation of response	Often present	Usually absent

(From: Danoff RB. In Harrison's Principles of Internal Medicine. Isselbacher KJ et al. (ed.). 13th ed. New York: McGraw Hill, 1994. Used with permission.)

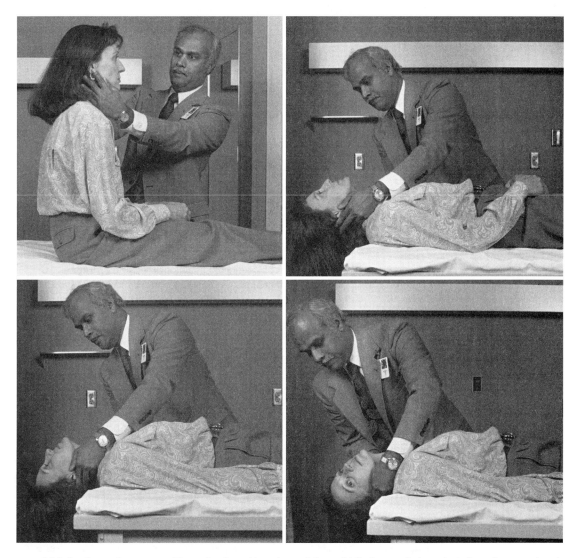

FIGURE 182.1. Barany's maneuver. The patient is positioned with the head hanging 30–45° over the table edge first in the midline, which is repeated with the head rotation to the right and left. Frames 1 through 4 show the procedure in sequence.

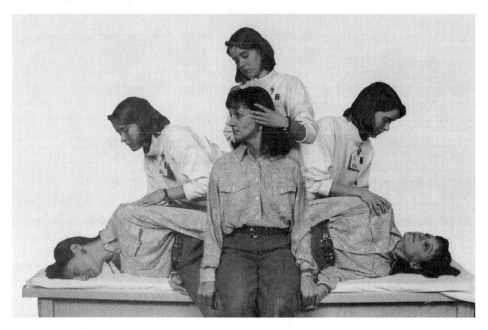

FIGURE 182.2. Special exercise to hasten improvement in BPPV, performed by sitting on the edge of a bed, turning head to one side by 45° and moving sequentially to the right or left and back to the sitting position, each time allowing the vertigo to nearly extinguish prior to making the next move. The entire sequence is shown with the motions superimposed.

should raise concern for another etiology or central disturbance.

In **Ménière's disease,** sudden, severe attacks of disabling rotational vertigo of variable durations (minutes to 24 hours) occur, heralded by tinnitus and aural fullness or pain. Symptoms are worse with head motion but a definite postural precipitation is absent. The vertigo recurs at variable intervals from weeks to months. Documentation of sensorineural hearing loss is important to the diagnosis. Tinnitus varies in conjunction with the attacks and becomes more persistent as the disease progresses. Treatment consists of a sodium- and caffeine–restricted diet, diuretics and vestibular suppressants. The most disabling, refractory forms may require surgical intervention. Serial audiograms (it may progress to bilateral disease) and neuro-otologic consultation are essential.

Labyrinthitis and **vestibular neuronitis** may be due to viral infection or a postinfectious, immune-mediated inflammation. The pattern is one of nonrecurrent, acute or subacute peripheral type vertigo occurring within a few weeks of a viral illness. Symptoms usually last days to weeks, although milder symptoms may persist longer. The vertigo gradually resolves as the inflammation subsides and central compensatory mechanisms evolve. Treatment is supportive in the acute phase, with hospitalization being required for disabling nausea, vomiting and ataxia. Short-term use of vestibular suppressants and a course of physical vestibular therapy help the recovery.

■ Central Disorders

A central lesion is suggested when the vertigo and constitutional symptoms are less intense, despite significant ataxia and nystagmus. The presence of brainstem symptoms (diplopia, dysarthria, dysphagia, vision loss) and signs (facial or appendicular motor and sensory changes) clearly point to a central localization. Abnormalities of eye movement or pupil function (e.g., Horner's syndrome) often betray a brainstem lesion. Limitation of eye movement, especially internuclear ophthalmoplegia, skew deviation (vertical dysconjugate eye position), gaze paresis or specific palsies of cranial nerves III, IV, or VI, implicates brainstem pathology. Cerebellar tremor and appendicular ataxia point to a direct lesion of the cerebellum or its pathways. Corticospinal tract dysfunction or hemisensory loss, which should be contralateral to brainstem findings strongly support a central lesion. Neuro-otologic consultation and electronystagmography (ENG) may help distinguish between peripheral and central lesions.

Central lesions causing vertigo involve the vestibular

nuclei, their projections to the ocular motor nuclei and cerebellum or the cerebellum itself. Contrasting features of central vs. peripheral vertigo and nystagmus are mentioned above and summarized in Table 182.1. A few causes of central vertigo deserve specific mention.

Brainstem ischemia due to thromboembolic disease of the vertebrobasilar circulation may cause acute and recurrent central vertigo. Generally, there are cranial nerve, cerebellar, visual field or long tract symptoms and signs. Transient ischemia, causing deficits lasting minutes, commonly precedes brainstem infarction and are often reported as "dizzy spells." Suspicion for such a vascular cause of vertigo increases when patients have risk factors for cardiac and cerebrovascular disease. These patients require a swift evaluation and initiation of stroke prevention therapy including antiplatelet aggregation agents or possible anticoagulation. Urgent hospitalization is necessary for presumed acute ischemia or if there is a history of increasing frequency and severity of transient vertigo with concern for progressive vertebrobasilar insufficiency.

In **multiple sclerosis** (MS) and other demyelinating disorders, vertigo is usually more subacute, worsening over hours to days, but can be rather rapid. Distinction from labyrinthitis and vestibular neuronitis rests on the central features and cranial nerve or long tract findings. Certainly, vertigo occurring in a patient with known MS is presumed to be from an acute demyelinating lesion, unless proof for a peripheral vestibular etiology is overwhelming. Patients with probable central vertigo having clinical features consistent with a demyelinating disorder should be referred to a neurologist for a more detailed examination. An MRI and CSF examination are often necessary.

Acoustic neuromas usually originate from Schwann cells in the vestibular portion of the eighth nerve at or near the internal auditory meatus. Their slow growth allows ample time for central compensation of the disordered vestibular input, making acute vertigo infrequent. However, when it occurs, it typically has more of a peripheral character. Progressive hearing loss with poor speech discrimination and tinnitus are typically the most prominent early symptoms. Enlargement of these tumors in the cerebellopontine angle causes compression of adjacent cranial nerves and brainstem, e.g., facial anesthesia and weakness. Ataxia and disequilibrium worsen and long tract signs begin to emerge. Early detection is paramount; surgical resection is the treatment. Brainstem auditory evoked responses are sensitive to changes early in the course.

Disequilibrium

Another important category of dizziness, best termed **disequilibrium,** is really a sense of imbalance and unsteadiness, worsened by walking, turning and in certain provocative situations. Postural stability depends on reliable sensory input from vision, vestibular function, joint position, skin pressure and light touch sensation. A disturbance of any one of these systems will cause some element of instability, with compensation through undue dependence on the other sensory inputs. Dysfunction in multiple systems destroy this compensatory agility. For instance, an elderly diabetic patient with peripheral neuropathy and mild labyrinthine disease who develops a retinal artery occlusion may become severely impaired, since maintaining posture was critically dependent on normal vision and stereopsis. More commonly, the alterations are slow to develop and less dramatic, resulting in a complaint of increasing "dizziness." Abnormal muscle strength and tone, skeletal/joint deformity and cervical spondylosis and myelopathy could compound the patient's difficulty.

Primary diseases of the cerebellum also lead to disequilibrium. Appendicular and gait ataxia, hypotonia, diminished reflexes, central nystagmus and ocular dysmetria may be found. Alcoholic cerebellar degeneration affects the anterior vermis preferentially and, therefore, the disturbance of axial stability and gait is much more pronounced than that of appendicular metrics.

Lightheadedness

This category represents a wide variety of causes. These patients find it difficult to characterize the sensation any further than dizzy or lightheaded, and yet may affirm any other symptom description suggested. They are more likely to report the experience as being constant and daily. The largest subset in this group is psychogenic dizziness, with depression and anxiety disorders most commonly encountered. Panic attacks, phobic disorders—especially agoraphobia, and somatization often feature dizziness as one of the presenting complaints. It is also important to remember that patients with episodic vertigo develop varying degrees of anxiety regarding recurrent attacks, especially toward the possibility of incapacitation in public. They may report features that closely resemble a primary neurosis or phobic disorder. Additionally, the cardiovascular and extrapyramidal side effects of many psychiatric medications easily cause syncope and postural instability. Finally, patients with early dementia and confusional states may report their advancing cognitive disability as dizziness.

CHAPTER **183** STROKE

S troke is the third leading cause of death and the leading cause of adult disability in the United States. It is increasingly considered a serious neurological emergency warranting expedient evaluation, acute treatment, and carefully considered preventive measures. Just as effective medical and surgical interventions for coronary artery disease have evolved over the past several decades, so has management of cerebrovascular disease evolved away from a nihilistic "watch and wait" attitude toward an increasingly interventional and analytical approach, bolstered by the results of several, recent, successful clinical trials.

Stroke is a sudden neurologic deficit or symptom attributable to vascular disease of the central nervous system, encompassing many diverse entities, including transient brain ischemia, brain infarction, brain hemorrhage, subarachnoid hemorrhage, and vascular disease of the spinal cord. The most common of these by far is brain infarction. Brain infarction may follow embolism, large artery atheroma, and small vessel occlusion. The term "transient ischemic attack" (TIA) has been applied to clinical syndromes lasting less than 24 hours. Many, if not most, "TIAs" lasting more than a few hours are associated with some degree of brain infarction.

Ischemic Stroke

■ Pathophysiology

Ischemic stroke is caused by embolic occlusion in one-third or more of cases. Potential sources of emboli include the heart (atrial fibrillation, sick sinus syndrome, myocardial infarction with mural thrombus, dysfunctional or artificial valves, congestive cardiomyopathy, and infective endocarditis), the proximal internal carotid and vertebral arteries, the aortic arch, and the deep venous system. Patent foramen ovale (PFO) is increasingly recognized as a conduit for paradoxical embolism. Emboli from the aortic arch and cervical vessels may arise from the irregular surface of atherosclerotic lesions. Hypercoagulable states, including pregnancy, oral contraceptive therapy and antiphospholipid syndrome may increase the likelihood of embolization by promoting thrombus formation at any of these sites. Emboli most typically cause large (>1 cm) infarcts involving the cortical surface, basal ganglia, or cerebellum.

The small vessel or **"lacunar"** stroke, seen in roughly 20% of ischemic strokes, arises from gradual occlusion of a small arteriole following hypertension-induced necrosis, atherosclerosis, and lipid deposition. Since the area supplied by the affected vessel is small, occlusion causes a small (<1 cm) infarct, located typically in the basal ganglia, internal capsule, thalamus, or pons. Ischemia may result, albeit less commonly, from occlusion or tight stenosis of a large artery (e.g., the carotid, vertebral, or basilar). In that case, infarction may be visible in the surface or deep white matter **"watershed"** areas (boundaries between main vascular territories). Uncommon causes of ischemic stroke include arterial dissection, vasospasm due to migraine, and cerebral vasculitis.

■ Clinical Features

Neurologic symptoms of ischemic stroke begin suddenly, although patients may be unaware or only gradually aware of their own deficits. This unawareness (anosognosia) is particularly likely with right hemispheric lesions. Common features of brain ischemia include unilateral weakness (**hemiparesis** or **hemiplegia),** unilateral visual field deficit in both eyes (**hemianopia),** impaired speech production or comprehension (**aphasia),** and unilateral sensory deficit. Brainstem ischemia (vertebro-basilar system) may cause nausea and vomiting, vertigo, gait imbalance, diplopia, dysphagia, dysarthria, or ptosis. Ischemic stroke may impair alertness, or cause sudden disorientation, inability to remember new information, deviation of the eyes or head to one side, and inability to read. These features may be isolated or combined with other impairments. While not a stroke by definition, retinal ischemia (brief monocular blindness, or **amaurosis fugax**) may be associated. Lightheadedness is not a symptom of stroke, and is possibly due to anemia, hypovolemia, autonomic dysfunction, vasovagal phenomena or cardiac arrhythmia.

Management

Despite the highly promoted distinction between "completed stroke" and TIA, there is no reason to treat these syndromes differently from a management point of view. Patients with TIA might be considered more urgently in need of attention, given the potentially greater opportunity to prevent permanent deficits. Acute management of ischemic stroke includes airway protection as needed, ECG to exclude arrhythmia and myocardial infarction, correction of anemia, dehydration, and glucose abnormalities, neurology consultation and urgent CT to exclude hemorrhage. Most patients with acute stroke are hypertensive at presentation, which may in part be a normal physiological pressor response to ischemia. Antihypertensive medications should be avoided or used with great caution in these cases, and only if the systolic pressure persists above 220 mm Hg. A recent multicenter trial found that systemic tissue plasminogen activator (tPA) administered within three hours of a stroke improved patient outcomes significantly. Careful evaluation is necessary before this drug is administered, given the significant risk of cerebral hemorrhage. Other thrombolytic and neuroprotective agents are currently being evaluated for their ability to minimize brain injury.

Intravenous heparinization is recommended for patients with cardiogenic embolism devoid of very large brain lesions (i.e., half of a hemisphere or more). However, stroke complicating bacterial endocarditis should be treated with antibiotics without any heparin, given the inherent risk of mycotic aneurysmal rupture. Heparin is given to reduce the risk of early recurrence of embolism, which probably exceeds 10% during the first 2 weeks after cardiogenic stroke. The risk of fatal hemorrhage is higher with a very large infarct, which outweighs the benefit of heparin in such patients. Heparin is usually given as a constant infusion, beginning with 800–1000 units per hour depending on age and body mass. The authors do not recommend an initial loading bolus. Heparin may also be used in patients with an unknown or uncertain mechanism of infarction, pending diagnostic tests to exclude a cardiac source. Heparin is often given to patients with TIAs in an attempt to prevent subsequent infarction and to help predict the response to oral anticoagulation. Heparin is indicated for cranial arterial dissection, as the usual mechanism of stroke in such patients is embolism from the dissection site.

An expedient evaluation should follow, to clarify the mechanism of ischemia. This determination is relatively straightforward using lesion size and location information from a brain image. At present, brain imaging between 2–7 days after onset with either CT or MRI perhaps most reliably distinguishes embolic, lacunar, and watershed infarctions (Figure 183.1 and Figure 183.2). Carotid and vertebral duplex Doppler studies can adequately detect severe extracranial stenosis. Large stenoses in the distal internal carotid or basilar arteries, if suspected, can be detected noninvasively by transcranial Doppler or MR angiography. Echocardiography is necessary in those with a suspected cardiac embolic source. Transesophageal echocardiography is superior for detecting PFO and for visualizing the left atrium, atrial appendage and aortic arch, and should be performed in patients with suspected embolism in whom the transthoracic echocardiogram is not revealing. Cardiac Holter monitoring or loop recording may occasionally detect paroxysmal atrial fibrillation. Catheter angiography is reserved for cases with suspected intracranial stenosis, dissection, or arteritis, in whom other tests have been not revealing. In young patients (<50 years) and older patients with no clear cause for stroke, a workup for occult hematologic abnormalities is recommended, including prothrombin time (PT), partial thromboplastin time (PTT), anti-nuclear antibodies (ANA), serum protein electro phoresis (SPEP), serological tests for syphilis (STS), sedimentation rate, lupus anticoagulant, anticardiolipin antibody, protein C, protein S, and antithrombin III.

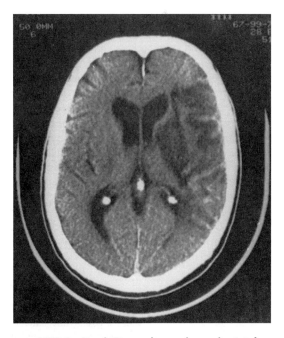

FIGURE 183.1. Head CT scan shows a hemorrhagic infarction of embolic origin involving the distribution of the left middle cerebral artery.

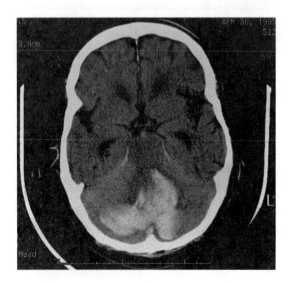

FIGURE 183.2. Head CT scan of a patient with cerebellar hemorrhage. This hypertensive woman developed dizziness and sudden inability to walk.

Long-term warfarin therapy is generally recommended to prevent recurrence in patients with emboli of cardiac source. Aspirin has been suggested as a treatment for patients with noncardiogenic causes of ischemic stroke, although the risk reduction associated with aspirin, regardless of the dose, is only 20–25%. Another alternative in this group is ticlopidine, an antiplatelet agent which, in one study, was slightly superior to aspirin for secondary prevention. Ticlopidine has some intolerable side effects; complete blood counts (CBC) must be monitored every 2 weeks during the first 3 months of therapy, given the risk of neutropenia during this interval.

Patients who are good surgical risk with significant carotid disease demonstrated by duplex imaging should undergo carotid angiography. With high-grade (>70%) carotid stenosis, surgery is superior to aspirin in preventing stroke recurrence. In such cases, carotid endarterectomy should be performed by an experienced surgeon, whose documented perioperative stroke and mortality rates are low (i.e., total <5%). The benefit of surgery in moderate (40–69%) stenosis is possibly below that in severe stenosis, but studies are ongoing to assess this; the skill of the surgeon would perhaps be crucial in this setting.

Intracerebral Hemorrhage

■ Etiology and Pathophysiology

The most common type of intracerebral hemorrhage is the "hypertensive" bleed, which occurs when a small, deep vessel weakened by chronic hypertension (**Bouchard's aneurysm**) ruptures. A large bleed may raise intracranial pressure sufficiently to impair consciousness, or cause brain herniation and death. Cerebellar hemorrhage is particularly ominous, given its proximity to the brainstem. Patients who survive the acute bleed, even a fairly large one, often recover remarkably well, because permanent damage is usually limited to the ischemic zone immediately surrounding the bleed. A bleed in the hemispheric white matter is not usually due to hypertension. Possible causes include vascular malformation, brain tumor, amyloid angiopathy, mycotic aneurysm, cerebral venous thrombosis, coagulopathy, anticoagulants, thrombolytic agents, vasculitis, and sympathomimetic drugs, including cocaine.

■ Clinical Features

Clinical signs of intracerebral hemorrhage are the same as those listed for ischemic stroke. While patients with intracerebral hemorrhage tend to be somewhat younger, more hypertensive, more stuporous, and report headaches more than patients with ischemic stroke, hemorrhage should be differentiated from infarction by CT scan rather than by the clinical presentation.

■ Management

Emergency evaluation includes airway management if needed, ECG, coagulation tests including PT, PTT, CBC, and platelet count, and emergent CT. Toxicology screen is useful in young patients. Blood pressure, if elevated, is reversed gently to maintain the systolic below 180 mmHg. Urgent neurology or neurosurgery consultation should be obtained. Alert patients with small hemorrhages may be observed on a general inpatient ward with frequent monitoring of vital signs and mental status. Patients with impaired alertness or large hemorrhages, being at high risk for deterioration, brain herniation, and death from increased intracranial pressure, should be admitted to an intensive care unit experienced in cerebral hemorrhage management.

Surgical evacuation of intracerebral hemorrhage/ hematoma, while controversial, is sometimes undertaken in patients who deteriorate despite intensive medical treatment for elevated intracranial pressure. However, surgical evacuation to prevent brainstem compression is usually recommended in cerebellar hemorrhage, if the hematoma exceeds 3 cm in diameter. For those with unexplained bleed and without hypertension, a search is made for the cause of bleeding. MR scan with gadolinium contrast will detect most vascular malformations and brain tumors. Catheter angiography is often necessary to detect or exclude aneurysm, vasculitis, venous thrombosis, and very small vascular malformations. Pressure effects during the acute period may obscure small aneurysms, tumors, and malformations. Definitive exclusion of these causes requires follow-up MRI and angiogram after resorption of the hematoma.

Subarachnoid Hemorrhage

■ Definition and Pathophysiology

Subarachnoid hemorrhage (SAH) results from rupture of an intracranial saccular aneurysm, most of which are located at the base of the brain near branch points of the major arteries. Bleeding into the subarachnoid space causes pain through elevation of intracranial pressure and meningeal irritation. Focal signs may occur from local pressure or ischemic effects on nearby brain tissue and exiting nerves. Recurrence of bleeding in the first few weeks after initial rupture is common (25%) and catastrophic. Vasospasm produces secondary infarction and is the most common cause of morbidity associated with SAH. It frequently occurs between 4–14 days after SAH and is due to irritation of blood vessels by subarachnoid blood. Other common complications of SAH are hydrocephalus, problems of antidiuretic hormone secretion (both inappropriate and deficiency), seizures, and brain injury from increased intracranial pressure.

■ Clinical Features

The cardinal symptom is sudden, symmetric or asymmetric, severe pain in the head or neck. In nearly one-half of cases, consciousness is lost briefly or for days. Many patients present with drowsiness, while some experience primarily neck pain and stiffness due to meningeal irritation, as the blood settles in the cervical subarachnoid space. Nausea and vomiting are common; photophobia may occur. Focal neurologic signs, most commonly, hemiparesis, aphasia, and paralysis of 3rd and/or 6th cranial nerves, may be present.

The diagnosis of SAH is missed in roughly 25% of cases. Misdiagnosis is particularly common when symptoms are less severe. The combination of neck stiffness and nausea may resemble a viral syndrome, while that of headache, nausea, and photophobia may simulate migraine. One should consider SAH when there is abrupt neck pain or headache, particularly if the patient perceives the pain symptoms to be in any way different from past experience(s).

■ Management

Urgent CT must be done when SAH is suspected. It is positive in nearly 90% of cases, the subarachnoid blood appearing as a bright area surrounding the brain or settling within the ventricular system on noncontrast images (Figure 183.3). Because CT may miss a small bleed, the diagnosis should be pursued using lumbar puncture (LP) when CT is negative and the suspicion is strong. The cerebrospinal fluid (CSF) is sent for cell count and other tests; a centrifuged sample is examined for xanthochromia. **Xanthochromia** in the CSF may take 3–4 hours to appear after symptom onset, as it entails breakdown of red blood cells. Xanthochromia may persist for more than a week; thus, patients presenting many days after the onset of symptoms may still be reliably diagnosed by LP. Once SAH is diagnosed, patients should be transferred urgently to an intensive care unit (or one where expert SAH management is available). Bed rest, stool softeners, analgesia, and treatment of high blood pressure are undertaken to minimize the risk of recurrence of bleeding. Nimodipine, a lipophilic calcium channel blocker, is effective in reducing brain injury from vasospasm after SAH, in a dose of 60 mg q 4h, given for 14–21 days after onset.

Definitive treatment for SAH consists of surgical clipping of the aneurysm responsible. Catheter angiography is required to locate the aneurysm and for planning a surgical approach. Timing of angiography depends on the planned timing of surgery. With improvements in surgical technique and a growing recognition of the dangers of early recurrence of bleeding, the trend is for surgery to be performed at the earliest possible opportunity. Many experienced centers now recommend urgent angiography and surgery on the first day after bleeding. Besides protecting against recurrence of bleeding, early clipping also makes possible the use of intravascular volume expansion therapy, which may lower the risk of vasospasm-induced ischemia.

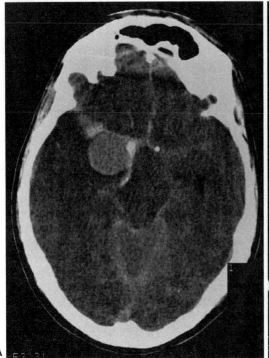

FIGURE 183.3. **A.** Head CT scan shows subarachnoid hemorrhage secondary to aneurysmal rupture. Midline shift is evident. The scan also shows a large aneurysm which was the source of the bleed. Aneurysms of this size are unusual. **B.** Same case as 183.3A, showing midline shift.

Primary Prevention of Stroke

The physician has a key role in the primary prevention of strokes by identifying patients at high risk and deploying suitable risk reduction strategies.

Hypertension is most strongly associated with stroke. Modern therapy of hypertension has probably brought forth the modest decline in strokes observed over the last several decades. Hypertension is the major cause in lacunar stroke and deep intracerebral hemorrhage, and contributes to accelerated atherosclerosis in larger cerebral arteries. Early diagnosis and therapy of hypertension, particularly in younger persons, remains the simplest and most effective means of stroke prevention. Diabetes mellitus and cigarette smoking are also strongly associated with stroke. Uncontrolled diabetes greatly accelerates cerebral atherosclerosis, particularly in small and medium-sized arteries. Cigarette smoking is most closely linked to large vessel disease, particularly, carotid bifurcation stenosis. Other modifiable stroke risk factors include elevated cholesterol and/or triglycerides, alcohol abuse, and obesity.

Nonvalvular atrial fibrillation (AF) increases stroke risk nearly fivefold, and accounts for about 75,000 strokes per year in North America alone. Nearly 1 in 3 persons with AF will experience a stroke. Warfarin reduces stroke risk in AF by roughly 70% (reductions range from 55–86% in different trials), with a risk of serious bleeding below 1% per year. The benefit of aspirin is less clear, with risk reductions ranging from 0–42%. It is now generally recommended that patients with AF be treated chronically with warfarin, maintaining the international normalized ratio (INR) between 2.0 to 3.0. This must be weighed against the perceived risks of anticoagulation in individual patients, and against the inconvenience and cost of monitoring and maintaining anticoagulation. The risk of major bleeding in the elderly (>75 yrs) treated with warfarin was 4.2% per year compared to 1.6% per year for aspirin in one study, although this finding requires further confirmation. There may also be subgroups of patients—e.g., younger patients with "lone" atrial fibrillation—in whom the risk of stroke is low enough that treatment costs and risks of warfarin outweigh any real benefits.

■ Asymptomatic carotid artery stenosis

In the Asymptomatic Carotid Atherosclerosis Study (ACAS; random assignment of patients with carotid stenosis exceeding 60% to either aspirin or aspirin plus surgery), the combined incidence of stroke or death from angiography and surgery was 3.5%. Despite this surgical/angiographic risk, the total stroke incidence in the surgical group was 4.8% compared to 10.6% in the nonsurgical group, a relative risk reduction of 55%. Therefore, it appears reasonable to recommend carotid endarterectomy in asymptomatic patients with angiographically defined stenosis exceeding 60% to reduce the risk of subsequent stroke. Patients must be appropriate surgical candidates and must undergo aggressive risk factor management and aspirin therapy before and after surgery. The success of the operation depends on an experienced surgical team with documented perioperative stroke and mortality rates of ≤3%, and on a low rate of angiographic complications.

CHAPTER 184 SEIZURES

Seizure is a sudden, excessive, electrical discharge in the brain leading to abnormal movement or alteration of consciousness. The causes of seizures are numerous, some benign, and some life-threatening. A seizure is a symptom, not a diagnosis. It is not synonymous with epilepsy, which refers to an underlying tendency toward having seizures, and may be an inherited tendency or due to trauma, malformation, tumor, surgery, cerebrovascular anomalies or idiopathic. Epilepsy can also be called seizure disorder, a term many patients prefer.

Generalized Motor Seizures

A generalized motor seizure may begin with sudden, tonic posturing which usually leads to a fall. Tonic contraction of the diaphragm causes apnea. Tonic-clonic activity follows with flexion and extension of the limbs, as apnea continues. The pupils dilate; incontinence and tongue biting may occur. The clonic movements then subside and respiration resumes. The pupils begin to react to light. The patient is now typically limp and poorly responsive. Postictal confusion and depression of consciousness follow, as the patient awakens tired and disoriented. Typically, there is amnesia for the seizure, part of the events preceding the seizure and part of the postictal state.

■ Focal Seizures

A focal seizure, depending on its brain locus, may lead to motor activity (motor cortex, focal motor seizure), sensory phenomenon (sensory cortex, sensory seizure; medial temporal lobe, olfactory hallucination), or alteration of consciousness (temporal lobe, partial complex seizure). Focal phenomena typically spread quickly, affecting contiguous areas of brain rapidly. Movement may spread from mouth to arm to leg because of contiguous representation of these areas in the motor cortex. Sensory phenomenon such as tingling or other paresthesias may quickly spread in a similar distribution. Mesial temporal lobe discharges may lead to olfactory hallucinations where a smell, which is frequently unpleasant, is perceived, or a rising abdominal feeling is noted. Temporal lobe discharges may also alter consciousness; the patient may become out of touch with the environment or stare or fumble with the hands. Posture is typically maintained. While there is typically amnesia for these events, consciousness is not lost.

Auras

Auras are phenomena the patient experiences from a focal electrical discharge and are actually focal seizures. Because amnesia from a partial complex or generalized seizure may involve the events immediately preceding the seizure, the memory for the aura or onset may be lost. If there is a history of an aura, the seizure is most likely focal in onset. If none, the seizure may be focal or generalized in onset. EEG can distinguish between these possibilities and help in the choice of anticonvulsant.

Considerations in Emergent Care of Seizures

Emergency considerations in seizures are numerous. Upon initial evaluation, besides the ABCs (airway, breathing and circulation), one must determine if the seizure is ongoing or has stopped. Status epilepticus is defined as ongoing seizure activity without return to normal consciousness. This includes continuous convulsions, as well as intermittent seizures which are interspersed with postictal confusion not proceeding to normal consciousness. Status epilepticus is a life-threatening condition requiring aggressive treatment. Glucose and thiamine should be administered at the onset, and blood obtained for anticonvulsant levels (if the patient was previously receiving them), general chemistry and toxicology screen. Benzodiazepines such as lorazepam control convulsions but may produce respiratory depression. A long-acting anticonvulsant, usually phenytoin, should be administered concurrently in a typical loading dose of 20 mg/kg. If seizures persist, phenobarbital 20 mg/kg may be added; however, significant respiratory depression necessitates intubation. If seizures continue, general anesthesia is next pursued to produce a burst suppression pattern on EEG.

The emergency approach to a self-limited seizure depends upon the history and examination. Is this an unprecedented or a breakthrough seizure in a patient already on anticonvulsant therapy? An unprecedented seizure merits careful analysis with a long differential diagnosis (Table 184.1). Seizures occur in 10–26% of cases of subarachnoid hemorrhage; blood is demonstrated by CT or lumbar puncture (LP). In meningitis and encephalitis, besides fever, headache and seizures; neck rigidity may be present. LP will demonstrate pleocytosis and other abnormalities, depending on etiology (viral versus bacterial). Drug intoxication should be considered and patient's medications reviewed; drug screen (both licit and illicit) is performed. Cocaine use and alcohol withdrawal are common causes of seizures at some medical centers. Brain tumors, both primary and secondary, are characterized by progressive neurological dysfunction over a period of days to months. Papilledema from increased intracranial pressure, or focal motor signs may be noted.

Emergency evaluation of a first-time seizure should include evaluation for metabolic disturbance, a drug

TABLE 184.1.	Differential Diagnosis of New Onset Seizures

Subarachnoid hemorrhage
Arteriovenous malformation
Subdural/epidural hematoma
Stroke
Meningitis/encephalitis
Abscess
Tumor
  Primary brain tumor
  Metastatic
Metabolic derangement
  Calcium, magnesium, sodium, glucose, others
Drug intoxication
  Theophylline
  Cocaine
Drug withdrawal
  Alcohol
  Benzodiazepines
  Barbiturates
  Anticonvulsants
  Non-compliance
Associated with degenerative disease
Cerebral malformation
Post-traumatic
  Birth injury
  Impact seizure
Idiopathic

screen and a neuroimaging study, either CT or MRI. CT is the initial procedure of choice in trauma, status epilepticus, and suspected subarachnoid hemorrhage. MRI is otherwise preferable because it demonstrates certain tumors and reveals smaller lesions than CT. EEG is generally not required urgently.

The differential diagnosis of chronic seizure disorder includes numerous entities. Symptoms suggestive of a seizure disorder include episodic impairment or loss of consciousness. Witnessed generalized seizures usually leave little doubt. Complex partial seizures may present with memory lapses which may initially be confused with other medical or psychiatric conditions. Witnessed staring spells or automatisms (e.g., lip smacking or fumbling with the hands) suggest partial complex seizures. Olfactory hallucinations just prior to events are highly suggestive of complex partial seizures.

Syncope and episodic metabolic disturbances are other causes of episodic alteration of consciousness. Syncope due to cardiac arrhythmias may be accompanied by a few clonic jerks which may mimic a seizure. Episodes of hyperglycemia or hypoglycemia may alter consciousness or cause actual convulsions. Cardiac evaluation including 24-hour cardiac monitoring and/or blood screening for glucose abnormalities may be needed, depending on the history. Further workup for seizures will usually include a neuroimaging study (CT or MRI). MRI may reveal subtle abnormalities such as mesial temporal lobe sclerosis, or evidence of tumor, stroke, trauma or vascular anomalies and is the test of choice, a contrast-enhanced CT being the next best. Commonly, the scan may be entirely normal. Further studies such as angiography usually depend on the CT or MR findings. Unless the seizures are extremely frequent, EEG usually does not capture an event itself. Thus, a normal EEG does not exclude seizure.

■ Pseudoseizures

Pseudoseizures mimic seizures, but are psychologically based. Many patients with pseudoseizures also have electrical (real) seizures. Diagnosis can be very difficult, and may be suggested by witnessing events with phenomena atypical for seizures. These include out-of-phase (asynchronous) clonic jerks, lateral head movements and pelvic thrusting. Pseudoseizures are not influenced by anticonvulsant medications. Video EEG monitoring may be confirmatory. Treatment is difficult; patients accept neither a psychological basis for the events, nor counseling.

■ Medication Management

The initial choice of an anticonvulsant depends upon the seizure type (Table 184.2). In general, it is best to maximize one medication before adding a second. When seizures escape their previous control, the most common cause is medication noncompliance. Others include lowered blood medication level due to drug interaction, alcohol withdrawal, sleep deprivation, or progressive neurologic lesion, particularly when new symptoms and signs appear.

The management should also include patient education to avoid precipitating events, e.g., alcohol use or sleep deprivation, and to be informed of their obligation to notify the Department of Motor Vehicles in their state regarding temporary suspension of driving privileges. Similarly, occupational adjustments need to be made. Tapering anticonvulsant therapy over a few months can be discussed with individuals who were seizure-free for 2 or more years, provided their examination, contrast imaging (CT or MRI) and EEG studies are all normal.

TABLE 184.2.	Medications for Seizures	
Petit Mal	**Primary Generalized**	**Focal; Generalization (±)**
Valproic acid	Phenytoin	Phenytoin
Ethosuximide	Valproic acid	Carbamazepine
	Carbamazepine	Valproic acid
	Phenobarbital	Primidone
	Clonazepam	

CHAPTER 185 NEUROLOGIC ASPECTS OF LOW BACK PAIN AND NECK PAIN

The rheumatologic aspects of low back and neck pain are reviewed in Chapter 252. Spinal pain can be classified into the following major categories: local, referred, and radicular.

■ Etiology

The pain of **acute disk rupture** is acute and radiating, with muscle spasm and stiffness, and exacerbated by coughing and Valsalva. Neurologic examination is abnormal. Because the first cervical root exits above C1, herniated intervertebral cervical disk affects the root corresponding to the lower vertebrae. The process reverses in the thoracic spine because the C8 root exits above T1, and therefore, a herniated thoracic intervertebral disk will affect the root corresponding to the higher vertebrae. This continues into the T12-L1 space. In the lumbosacral spine, the cauda equina roots angle in such a way that they exit above their corresponding vertebrae, and a herniated intervertebral disk at any level usually results in compression of the root one level below, unless the disk is extruded or far lateral in which case it compresses the root at that level (Table 179.5). Most herniations occur at the C5-C6, C6-C7, L4-L5, and L5-S1 levels.

Other causes of neck or low back pain can be compressive or noncompressive. The first category includes all spinal neoplasms, which can be intramedullary, extramedullary-intradural, or epidural. Early and severe spine pain, followed later by weakness, typifies an epidural spinal process (e.g., Schwannomas, meningiomas, and metastatic tumors) while early weakness and sensory symptoms in association with a mild and rather vague pain exemplifies an intramedullary spinal process (e.g., ependymomas, gliomas, and syringomyelic conditions). Vascular malformations may present in either form. Noncompressive etiologies are mainly comprised of infectious or inflammatory disorders of the spine. They are discussed in Chapter 252.

■ Approach to the Patient

History should focus on the location of the pain, its radiation, exacerbating/alleviating factors, associated neurologic symptoms, history of trauma or work injury, litigation, drugs and malignancy. The general examination should search for signs of systemic infection, occult malignancy, tenderness, muscle spasm, spine and hip range of motion and straight leg raising. The neurologic part of the examination should focus on the patient's affect and mood, presence or absence of muscle weakness, muscle atrophy, sensory loss, changes in the reflexes, and rectal examination, if there are sphincter complaints.

■ Management

If spinal bony pathology appears likely and further imaging is desired, CT scan of the cervical or lumbosa-cral spine would be helpful. However, the soft tissue images have a lower resolution than that obtained from MRI. Disk protrusions or herniations may be radiologically present in some healthy asymptomatic adults, and their importance should be weighed clinically. Patients with persistent neck or low back pain or abnormal neurologic findings should undergo electrodiagnostic testing. This helps differentiate between radiculopathies and neuropathies, confirms the presence of radicular involvement, evaluates its activity and allows its accurate localization.

The management of neck and low back pain depends chiefly on the underlying etiology. Conservative treatment, as outlined in Chapter 252, is the main therapy. Definite indications for surgical treatment include severe or progressive neurologic deficits, sphincter changes or the failure of conservative management with emphasis on spine rehabilitation for 6 weeks. Following surgery for spine pain, at least one-third of the patients will be left with persistent pain and one-fourth would not be able to return to their previous work.

CHAPTER 186 DISORDERS OF SPINAL CORD, NERVES, AND MUSCLES

Spinal Cord Diseases

The level of a spinal cord lesion is determined by the pattern of sensory and motor abnormalities. Because the spinothalamic fibers cross the midline over one to two segments, the location of a lesion may be one to two levels higher than found by dermatomal sensory examination. Acute cord lesions cause areflexia and hypotonia at, and below, the level of the lesion. With time, upper motor neuron signs (spasticity, hyperreflexia, extensor plantar responses) are present below the level of the lesion while lower motor neuron signs (atrophy, hyporeflexia) persist at the level of the lesion. Bowel and bladder dysfunction are hallmarks of spinal cord lesions. Lesions of the conus medullaris and cauda equina may be difficult to distinguish but should be suspected with early sphincter dysfunction, saddle anesthesia or radicular pain of the lower extremities. Compressive myelopathies require urgent evaluation. MRI is the procedure of choice as it is noninvasive and the entire cord can be viewed, if necessary, to exclude multiple lesions. Myelography should be used if MRI cannot be obtained, to prevent any delay in diagnosis. High-dose corticosteroids are indicated while definitive treatment is determined.

Compressive lesions may be extramedullary or intramedullary. **Extramedullary lesions,** which may be intradural or extradural, often begin as a radicular process with unilateral weakness and/or pain radiating into a limb. Upper motor neuron signs are present early with hyperreflexia, spasticity and Babinski sign. Sphincter abnormalities occur later. **Metastatic tumors** are classic examples of extradural extramedullary compressive lesions that cause cord compression, either by bony destruction or as epidural masses. Most frequent primary cancer sites are breast, lung or prostate; others include lymphoma, multiple myeloma, melanoma, renal cell carcinoma or sarcoma. **Primary bone tumors** may also cause bony destruction, as can osteomyelitis or tuberculosis (Pott's disease), leading to cord compression. **Epidural abscesses** occur more often in the immunocompromised, IV drug abusers or diabetics. Fever and leukocytosis may be present. **Cervical spondylitic myelopathy** from narrowing of the spinal canal, usually occurs in older persons. **Meningiomas** or **neurofibromata** are examples of intradural extramedullary lesions; their slow growth allows the cord time to accommodate; even large masses may thus produce sparse signs.

Spinal cord infarction may follow dissection, surgery or trauma of the descending aorta. Occlusion or narrowing of the anterior spinal artery, which supplies all areas of the cord except the posterior columns, leads to dysfunction of all modalities below the level of the lesion, except vibration and joint position sense. Infectious processes causing intrinsic cord damage include HIV vacuolar myelopathy or HTLV-1-associated myelopathy. HIV vacuolar myelopathy

generally involves the posterior and lateral cords and occurs with other neurologic symptoms of AIDS. HTLV-1-associated myelopathy occurs in only a small subset of infected patients, suggesting the myelopathy may be immune-mediated. Vitamin B_{12} deficiency, with or without megaloblastic anemia, causes posterior column and lateral corticospinal tract damage. Patients display hyperreflexia and Babinski signs; the associated peripheral neuropathy causes decreased ankle reflexes. Some intrinsic lesions (e.g., demyelinating disease) are well-visualized by MRI, whereas others (e.g., B_{12} deficiency) require further laboratory testing.

Neuromuscular Diseases

The disorders of the neuromuscular system may involve the motor neuron, the peripheral nerve, the neuromuscular junction, or the muscle, and all manifest weakness as their hallmark. Patterns of weakness and associated clinical features for each of these major components are shown in Table 186.1.

■ Motor Neuron Disease

The most common motor neuron disease is **amyotrophic lateral sclerosis** (ALS, Lou Gehrig's disease). This rarely familial, idiopathic disorder, usually begins after the fourth decade with often asymmetric weakness and wasting of the hands. Less frequently, the onset is with weakness and wasting in either one lower extremity or in the bulbar innervated muscles. Cramps and fatigue are other symptoms. In most patients, its relentless

progression is usually fatal in less than 5 years. The neurologic findings include scattered fasciculations, wasting of the affected muscles, and hyperreflexia with or without Babinski sign(s). Even when the onset is in one extremity, patients frequently develop progressive spastic dysarthria, dysphagia and dysphonia. The sparing of the extraocular muscles, sphincters, sensory perception, and cognitive functions is striking, and so is the unique and characteristic combination of upper and lower motor neuron dysfunction. The latter is due to degeneration of both motor neurons and corticospinal tracts. Electromyographic examination shows diffuse denervation and confirms the diagnosis. Symptomatic treatment, rehabilitation and support to the patient and family are important; there is no cure. Death is usually due to respiratory failure and/or aspiration pneumonia.

TABLE 186.1.   Differential Diagnosis of Weakness

Sign	Motor Neuron	Peripheral Nerve	Neuro-Muscular Junction	Muscle
Wasting	Yes	Yes	Absent	Late
Distribution	Distal	Distal	Cranial	Proximal
	Bulbar		Proximal	
Reduced reflexes	Late	Early	Late	Late
Brisk reflexes	Yes	No	No	No
Fasciculations	Common	Rare	Absent	Absent
Sensory loss	Absent	Present	Absent	Absent
Elevated CK	Rare	Absent	Absent	Frequent
Elevated CSF Protein	No	Yes	No	No
Nerve conduction	Normal	Abnormal	Normal	Normal
Motor decrement	Rare	Absent	Present	Absent
Electromyography	Neurogenic	Neurogenic	Normal	Myopathic
Muscle biopsy	Neurogenic	Neurogenic	Endplate	Myopathic

CK = creatinine kinase.

Peripheral Nerve Disease

Nerve dysfunction involving the sensory fibers, motor fibers, autonomic fibers, or a combination of these may afflict the cranial nerves, spinal nerve roots, brachial and lumbosacral plexus, and peripheral nerves. Sensory fiber dysfunction results in sensory loss, paresthesias and pain. Motor nerve involvement causes weakness, wasting and hypo- or areflexia. The involvement of the autonomic systems leads to trophic changes involving the bone and skin, in addition to sweating and cardiovascular abnormalities.

The most important step in approaching peripheral nerve disease is to characterize the pattern of deficit. **Mononeuropathy** refers to dysfunction in the territory of a single nerve, and is most often due to an acute compression or chronic entrapment of that nerve, e.g., carpal tunnel syndrome, peroneal neuropathy at the fibular head or ulnar neuropathy at the elbow. Asymmetric involvement of multiple nerves is usually termed **mononeuritis multiplex** and indicates an ischemic condition such as seen in diabetes or connective tissue disease. Proximal and distal weakness with hyporeflexia or areflexia indicates **polyradiculoneuropathy** or a polyradiculopathy, most of which are inflammatory in origin. Finally, bilateral symmetric involvement of the peripheral nerves, usually greater distally, indicates a polyneuropathy and is the most common but least specific presentation of the peripheral nerve diseases.

Polyneuropathy can be hereditary or acquired. Hereditary types include 1) motor and sensory (Charcot-Marie-Tooth, Dejerine-Sottas, Refsum, metachromatic leukodystrophy, and Krabbe disease); 2) sensory and autonomic; 3) porphyria; and 4) amyloidosis. Acquired causes can be remembered by the mnemonic "INDICATE" outlined in Table 186.2.

The approach to peripheral neuropathy begins by confirming the diagnosis, usually through nerve conduction studies (NCV) and electromyographic (EMG) examination. In addition, EMG-NCV may elucidate a certain pattern of neuropathy that was not apparent clinically, such as an asymmetry among limbs, or over various nerve trunks in one limb that could provide clues to the etiology. Once the diagnosis is confirmed, preliminary studies should include CBC with differential, sedimentation rate, fasting chemistry, serum B_{12} and folate, thyroid function tests and chest x-ray. If these tests are unrevealing, additional tests (antinuclear antibody, serum protein electrophoresis, urine protein electrophoresis, 24-hour urine for porphyrins and heavy metals) should follow. If the etiology is still elusive, it is important to again review the patient's family history, drug and occupational exposures. Further di-

TABLE 186.2.	Etiologic Diagnosis of Acquired Polyneuropathy
I	Immune: acute inflammatory demyelinating polyneuropathy or Guillain-Barré syndrome, chronic inflammatory demyelinating polyneuropathy, sarcoidosis, connective tissue disorders
N	Nutritional deficiencies and malabsorption: vitamins B_1, B_6, B_{12}, folate, and vitamin E
D	Diabetes mellitus
I	Infections: leprosy, Lyme disease, HIV, herpes zoster, diphtheria
C	Cancer and dysproteinemia
A	Alcoholism
T	Toxic-metabolic: pharmaceutical or environmental, renal- or hepatic failure
E	Endocrine causes: hypothyroidism, acromegaly

agnostic studies include CSF analysis before proceeding with a nerve biopsy.

■ Carpal Tunnel Syndrome

Carpal tunnel syndrome (CTS) is the most common entrapment neuropathy. Besides its occurrence in a variety of occupations involving frequent use of wrists and hands, as well as many medical conditions, CTS may occur for the first time during pregnancy, most probably because of volume expansion and fluid shifts. The symptoms reflect dysfunction of the median nerve underneath the flexor retinaculum, characterized by dysesthesias, which are more severe at night and involve primarily the first three digits. Pain at rest that may radiate more proximally up to the shoulder is another symptom. As the condition worsens, hypesthesia develops over the first three digits, sparing the palm, along with weakness in several of the thumb muscles and partial atrophy of the thenar eminence. Tinel's sign (paresthesia radiating into the fingers provoked by gentle tapping over the median nerve at the wrist) is helpful if found. The diagnosis is confirmed by NCV. Symptomatic relief may be obtained by using wrist splints during repetitive manual activities. Underlying causes such as diabetes mellitus, acromegaly, hypothyroidism, gout, or rheumatoid arthritis should be sought and corrected, if possible. However, the definitive treatment consists of surgical section of the transverse carpal ligament.

■ Guillain-Barré Syndrome

Also known as acute inflammatory demyelinating polyneuropathy (AIDP), Guillain-Barré syndrome (GBS) is the most dramatic of polyneuropathies, featuring acute onset of peripheral and cranial nerve dysfunction. No age or gender predilection is seen. Triggered by a viral illness, immunization or surgery within 1–3 weeks preceding symptoms, it usually presents with distal paresthesias that show proximal extension, along with rapidly evolving distal and proximal muscle weakness and symmetric areflexia. The deficit usually peaks 3 weeks after the onset. Unilateral or bilateral facial nerve paralysis occurs in approximately one-half of cases. Autonomic instability may occur, particularly in more severe cases. GBS can cause respiratory failure requiring mechanical ventilation. CSF examination is characteristic and shows significant elevation of the protein without pleocytosis, the so called albumino-cytologic dissociation. NCV-EMG reveal demyelinating polyneuropathy and confirm the diagnosis. Management includes close observation, supportive care, physical therapy, mechanical ventilation once the vital capacity falls below 15 ml/kg (see Chapter 247) and treatment of the autonomic instability syndrome when present. Plasmapheresis for 2 weeks lessens the duration and severity of the neurological deficit, and is indicated whenever ambulation becomes difficult. IV gamma globulin administered over 5 days can be substituted in children or in hemodynamically unstable patients. The prognosis is relatively good, particularly when NCV show well-preserved distal responses.

Neuromuscular Junction Diseases

■ Myasthenia Gravis

Myasthenia gravis (MG) is a common autoimmune disorder in which a cell-mediated immune response leads to the formation of various antibodies directed against the acetylcholine receptors. The initial rapid turnover of these receptors is followed by their later, complete destruction. The hallmark of MG is fatigability of the involved muscles, with predilection for the extraocular, other cranial and proximal limb muscle groups. The pupils are spared. Intermittent initially, the symptoms tend to follow exertion or occur at the end of the day. As the disease progresses, they become constant with superimposed fluctuations. The presence of acetylcholine receptor antibodies in the serum establishes the diagnosis. However, being highly sensitive for only generalized MG, these antibodies are not detectable in a significant number of patients with more focal forms of myasthenia. Such cases are diagnosed on EMG. Repetitive nerve stimulation produces a decrement of the motor evoked potential, at least in the weak muscles. When the disease is confined to the extraocular- or bulbar muscles, the

EMG is negative. The diagnosis can then be made by single fiber EMG. In the Edrophonium (Tensilon) test, the patient is given 2 mg of the drug, and if tolerated, an additional 8 mg; the test is positive if it reverses the patient's deficit within 1 minute, and if such reversal lasts 10 minutes. However, both false-positives and false-negatives occur. Atropine (0.4 mg) should be available to correct any muscarinic effects.

Definitive diagnosis of MG should be followed by thyroid function tests to detect any thyroid dysfunction, antistriated muscle antibodies (association with thymomas) and chest CT scan or MRI (to rule out an enlarged thymus). Patients should be made aware of drugs that could worsen their condition, such as aminoglycoside antibiotics, certain antiarrhythmics and sedatives.

Symptomatic management of MG is with anticholinesterase drugs. The prototype drug is pyridostigmine (Mestinon), in doses of 60–90 mg every 4–6 hours, depending upon the disease severity. Side effects include diarrhea, abdominal cramps and muscle twitching or fasciculations. Pyridostigmine overdose may result in paradoxical weakness of the muscles known as **"cholinergic crisis."**

Immunosuppressive treatment is also necessary, primarily with prednisone, with a low dose of 10 mg daily for several days begun in the outpatient setting. If no response occurs, the dose is gradually increased up to 1mg/ kg body weight; the dose is maintained for a few weeks, after which it can be tapered gradually, and an alternate day schedule adopted. An initial high dose may paradoxically worsen muscle weakness in a small subset of patients. Serum glucose, electrolytes, and blood pressure are monitored carefully. A tuberculin test is also done before instituting prednisone. Other immunosuppressive agents include Azathioprine (Imuran) and Cyclosporin. Thymectomy is indicated whenever chest imaging studies show thymic enlargement or a thymoma. Thymectomy is also indicated even when imaging is negative, in generalized MG, and in localized myasthenia that has failed to respond to anticholinesterase agents and prednisone.

Occasionally, MG may present with a rapidly progressive weakness of all extremities along with respiratory difficulties and bulbar weakness. This condition, known as **myasthenic crisis,** constitutes a neuromuscular emergency. Hospitalization and temporarily withholding anticholinesterase agents are necessary to rule out a cholinergic crisis. If the patient's vital capacity is poor, endotracheal intubation and mechanical ventilation are required. Once myasthenic crisis is confirmed, anticholinesterase therapy must be resumed, and a trial of plasmapheresis begun, at the rate of 3 sessions for the first week, after which the frequency may be reduced.

Pulmonary and supportive care are of prime importance. When recovered from the myasthenic crisis, the patient should undergo thymectomy.

■ Eaton-Lambert Myasthenic Syndrome

This is an autoimmune disorder in which various antibodies bind to the calcium channels located on the presynaptic axonal end. This reduces the amount of acetylcholine released from the axonal end and thus, the activation of the muscle membrane. The disease has a strong association with malignancy, particularly small cell lung cancer, but an association with autoimmune disorders seems to be emerging. The usual clinical features are fatigability and weakness that improve with exercise. A greater involvement of the limb and respiratory muscles is noted, with less frequent involvement of the extraocular muscles. Distal paresthesias, dryness of the mouth and orthostatic hypotension may be noted.

The diagnosis is confirmed by neurophysiologic testing. A single stimulus to a motor nerve evokes a low muscle action potential amplitude. A train of stimuli at low rate (2–3 Hz) results in a small decrement. Following brief exercise for 10 seconds, the motor evoked amplitude increases massively, usually by several fold; the decrement also improves. When the diagnosis is confirmed, work up for malignancy and connective tissue disease should follow.

Pharmacologic treatment with anticholinesterase agents may modestly benefit some patients. Presynaptic activating agents such as Guanidine and 4-aminopyridine do cause symptomatic relief, but with toxic side effects. A recent investigational drug, 3, 4-diaminopyridine, has proven useful in the symptomatic management of the disorder. The underlying condition should be treated, if possible. Immunosuppression with prednisone alone, or together with Azathioprine, can result in improvement. Plasmapheresis is indicated in moderately severe cases or when there is rapid deterioration.

Muscle Diseases

■ Myotonic Dystrophy

The most common adulthood dystrophy is myotonic dystrophy, an autosomal dominant disorder, where a gene defect is located on chromosome 19, and with an anticipation phenomenon, i.e., an earlier phenotypic expression in subsequent generations. Quite uniquely the myopathy is predominantly distal. Besides weakness of hands and feet, there are thin facies, ptosis, wasting of temporalis and masseter muscles, and thinning of the sternomastoids. Other features are percussion myotonia, high arched palate, frontal baldness, cataracts, intellectual deficit, endocrine changes and cardiac conduction abnormalities.

The clinical presentation, characteristic retrocapsular cataracts, and myotonic discharges on EMG form the basis for diagnosis. Confirmation is by DNA blood testing, which would also be useful in genetic testing and prenatal diagnosis. Serial electrocardiograms are necessary for early detection of conduction abnormalities. The treatment of muscular weakness is primarily supportive. Although myotonia responds to anticonvulsants (e.g., phenytoin) and Class Ia antiarrhythmics, the latter are generally contraindicated in this disease, because of the underlying cardiac conduction system involvement.

CHAPTER 187 MULTIPLE SCLEROSIS

■ Epidemiology

Multiple sclerosis (MS) is a relapsing-remitting, and sometimes progressive disease that affects roughly 350,000 persons in the United States. It is twice as common in women as in men. While it is most common in 20–40 year olds, no age is exempt. The disease may occur through genetic predisposition and subsequent environmental exposure to an as yet unknown, possible viral agent. Abnormal immune function is likely the underlying theme. In general, the prevalence of the disease increases at higher latitude. This risk is possibly acquired before age fifteen, as moving away from a higher prevalence area after this age does not seem to lower the risk of developing the disease. The high prevalence of disease in Italy and Sicily, but not in Spain, is an exception to this pattern. Multiple sclerosis is less common in African Americans than Caucasians, which raises the question of genetic influence. Further, the risk of developing the disease is increased in children or first degree relatives of a patient afflicted by multiple sclerosis. The risk is even higher for dizygotic twins.

■ Clinical Features

Patients most often present with sensory symptoms, which are varied, but a common symptom is an ascending abnormal sensation progressing from one foot to both lower extremities over several days. **Lhermitte's sign** is a brief but unpleasant electrical sensation passing down the back to the legs or arms when the patient flexes the neck. It is a common, but not exclusive symptom of MS. Frequent involvement of the posterior columns lead to balance or gait abnormalities. Weakness is characterized by upper motor neuron signs of spasticity and hyperreflexia. While spasticity may inhibit walking and be more disabling than actual weakness, it may also allow one to remain ambulatory if the spastic limb helps maintain an upright posture. Lesions of the pyramidal tract or cerebellum cause coordination difficulties. **Intention tremor** is unusual in early stages of the disease, but with progression, may prohibit use of the upper extremities.

Optic neuritis, manifest as loss of central vision or decreased visual acuity in one eye (rarely bilateral), poor color vision, and orbital pain may occur at anytime during the disease. An afferent pupillary defect (decreased pupillary response to light) may persist indefinitely as a residuum of previous optic neuritis. Blurring of vision on exercise may be the only symptom, possibly disabling, of an optic nerve lesion. While most notable for visual symptoms, many patients with multiple sclerosis also report worsening of their other symptoms when their body temperature rises even a few tenths of a degree. This is an effect of increased temperature on synaptic transmission and not a true exacerbation of the disease. Various ocular movement abnormalities may lead to diplopia, the most common of which is **internuclear ophthalmoplegia** (INO). In INO, difficulty with adduction of the eye is noted on the affected side with nystagmus in the abducting eye. The patient reports double vision when looking horizontally.

Vertigo, as an initial symptom in multiple sclerosis, may not be distinguishable from vestibular neuronitis unless other central nervous systems signs are evident. **Bladder dysfunction,** while rarely the sole presenting complaint, is very common. Most common is bladder dyssynergia where the detrusor contracts at the same time the sphincter closes, preventing expulsion of urine. Patients may also have incontinence, urgency, frequency, or nocturia. Fatigue is also very common. Depression occurs and the suicide rate for patients with multiple sclerosis is higher than the general population.

■ Diagnosis

There is no clinical sign that is unique to multiple sclerosis. Nor is any one test diagnostic. MRI is a sensitive tool, positive in most cases of clinically definite multiple sclerosis. It is, however, not specific for MS. Demyelinating plaques appear in the white matter as hypointense lesions on T1 and hyperintense on T2 weighted images (Figure 187.1). Lesions may be confined to either the spinal cord or brain; thus, clinical

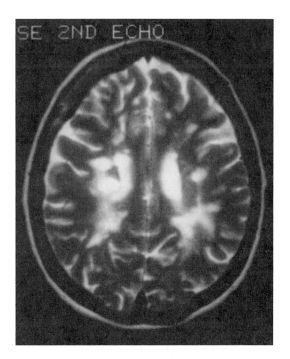

FIGURE 187.1. T2-weighted image of head MRI from a patient with multiple sclerosis, showing the presence of foci of hyperintense signal in the peri-ventricular white matter bilaterally ("Dawson fingers").

localization is important. A lumbar puncture may help exclude other abnormalities. While CSF total protein is normal in 60% of cases, it rarely exceeds 70 mg/dl. The leukocyte count is normal in two-thirds of patients. When high, it is usually below 20 cells/mm^3. Oligoclonal bands, elevated IgG synthesis rate and IgG index also help diagnostically, although they are not specific. Evoked potentials can document subclinical involvement of various areas of the central nervous system (e.g., abnormal visual evoked potentials in subclinical optic neuritis; somatosensory evoked potentials in subclinical spinal cord involvement).

■ Management

Symptomatic therapy is of utmost importance. Spasticity may respond to baclofen, diazepam, tizanidine, dantrolene or intrathecal baclofen. Tremor is very resistant to therapy although propranolol, primidone, or benzodiazepines may provide partial relief. Urinary incontinence may respond to anticholinergic agents such as oxybutynin. Cholinergic agents such as bethanechol are used to stimulate bladder emptying although usually patients require intermittent self-catheterization. Erectile dysfunction is treated in several ways, including penile intracorporeal papaverine injections. Paroxysmal sensory and motor symptoms often respond to carbamazepine, other anticonvulsants or baclofen. Treatment of chronic dysesthetic pain includes tricyclic antidepressants, carbamazepine and clonazepam, to name a few. Fatigue may require adjustment of the patient's daily schedule. Amantadine, pemoline, fluoxetine or selegiline may provide some relief, but their mechanism of action is not well established. Finally, depression should be treated aggressively, along with monitoring for suicidal tendency.

Acute exacerbations of multiple sclerosis may be treated with ACTH or methylprednisolone, but these agents do not affect the long term prognosis, and are not indicated for chronic use. In a recent study of optic neuritis, patients receiving IV methylprednisolone followed by oral steroids had more rapid recovery of vision than those on oral steroids alone. Those on oral steroids alone had higher risk of recurrence of optic neuritis. During the 2-year follow-up, fewer patients given methylprednisolone developed clinically definite multiple sclerosis. Thus, exacerbations of multiple sclerosis are not generally treated with oral steroids alone. Interferon β-1 b and β-1 a have been approved for the treatment of patients with relapsing-remitting multiple sclerosis who remain ambulatory. Studies have shown fewer exacerbations and less progression of white matter disease on MRI in patients receiving these therapies. However, long term disability seems unaffected. Glatirimar acetate is also effective in decreasing relapse rate. The future seems optimistic for treatment and possibly, prevention of this disease.

CHAPTER 188   MOVEMENT DISORDERS

Movement disorders may be **hypokinetic,** i.e., those lacking spontaneous movements, and hyperkinetic, i.e., those with excessive involuntary movements. **Hypokinetic disorders** feature slowness, muscular stiffness, postural instability, tremors and a tendency for the handwriting to become small (micrographia). Muscular rigidity on passive manipulation of the limbs, or decreased associated movements in walking such as poor arm swing, retropulsion (the tendency to tip backwards, demonstrated by a backward pull on the shoulders), or shuffling gait may all be seen on examination. Such generalized hypokinesia may occur in Parkinson's disease, drug-induced Parkinsonism, progressive supranuclear palsy and multiple systems atrophy. **Hyperkinetic disorders** are mainly chorea, dystonia, or dyskinesia, tremor and tic. Bedside differentiation of these movement disorders is shown in Table 188.1.

The extrapyramidal function is arranged in a series of closed loops. Cortical projections reach neostriatal small neurons, while neostriatal large neurons send efferents to the cortex via connections with the globus pallidus and thalamic nuclei. Acetylcholine and glutamate are important excitatory substances. The nigro-neostriatal system (dopaminergic) has inhibitory projections on neostriatal (cholinergic) neurons. The striatum and pallidum influence nigral dopaminergic neurons via GABA and substance P pathways. Reciprocal connections exist between

TABLE 188.1.	Differentiating Movement Disorders at the Bedside
Disorder	**Features**
Athetosis	Slow, writhing, flowing appearance
Ballismus	Rapid, flinging-like, non-repetitive
Chorea	Rapid, random, flowing, non-repetitive
Dystonia	Twisting, repetitive
Myoclonus	Rapid, non-twisting, stimulus-sensitive
Tic	Random, patterned, coordinated, "urge"
Tremor	Rhythmic, oscillatory, continuous

striatum and subthalamus, and between red nucleus and mesencephalon (partly serotoninergic).

Essential Tremor

Essential tremor is probably the most common movement disorder. A postural and kinetic tremor may affect the hands most commonly but also can affect the head and the voice. Essential tremor is not associated with any other neurologic abnormalities. Its relationship to Parkinson's disease has been debated. No brain pathology has been found. Treatment depends upon symptoms; ß-blockers (propranolol) or use of primidone, can be effective.

Parkinson's Disease

Parkinson's disease is characterized by four cardinal features: **resting tremor, muscular rigidity, bradykinesia,** and **postural instability.** Its onset is gradual and progression insidious over many years. The loss of the pigmented, normally dopaminergic neurons in the substantia nigra leads to declining dopamine levels in the striatum. Over many years, 70–80% of the neurons are lost in the substantia nigra, when symptoms appear. No clear etiology for Parkinson's disease has yet been identified. Associated features may include depression and/or dementia. The diagnosis of Parkinson's disease is clinical. Some consider the resting tremor to be nearly pathognomonic.

The treatment of Parkinson's disease depends on the severity of symptoms. Several factors should be taken into account including quality of life, and function in both employment and daily activity as well as social embarrassment. Several medications are currently in use. Deprenyl (Eldepryl) has been studied extensively and has been felt to slow disease progression. Some patients note minimal improvement in symptoms with this agent. Anticholinergic agents may be helpful when tremor is the dominant symptom, but, cognitive side effects, especially decreased memory, may limit their use. Amantadine, which acts as an anticholinergic agent and promotes dopamine release from CNS stores, may improve all aspects of disease. When there is a threat to employability, activities of daily life, or balance, carbidopa/levodopa (Sinemet) is indicated. Initial improvements and smooth response to this drug tend to be followed in several years by the development of a fluctuating response, and drug-induced dyskinesias. The addition of a dopamine agonist may improve Parkinsonian features as well as dyskinesias. Surgical procedures such as thalamotomy or pallidotomy improve the tremor significantly on the contralateral side of the procedure. However, bilateral thalamotomy leads to significant speech abnormalities. Pallidotomy appears promising for the control of motor symptoms. These procedures were popular before the advent of effective drug therapy of Parkinson's disease, but their use is now infrequent. Transplantation surgery continues to be evaluated, but its current role is only experimental.

Dopamine antagonists may produce secondary parkinsonism by blocking dopamine receptors in the striatum. Antipsychotic agents are most commonly associated with this syndrome; however, antiemetics such as prochlorperazine (Compazine) and metoclopramide (Reglan), also dopamine antagonists, may produce this syndrome. Withdrawal of the offending agent should alleviate the movement disorder. Debate continues as to whether those who develop drug-induced Parkinsonism are at a higher risk of ultimately developing Parkinson's disease.

Neuroleptic Malignant Syndrome

Neuroleptic malignant syndrome (NMS) is a life-threatening condition which can present as an akinetic rigid state. This occurs typically in a patient on dopamine antagonists, usually after a dose increase. The patient develops fever, confusion, and muscular rigidity. Serum creatinine kinase is elevated. Treatment of NMS involves withdrawing the dopamine antagonist. For mild cases, this may suffice as treatment. In more severely affected patients, dantrolene and bromocriptine can improve rigidity, reduce fever, and improve mental status.

CHAPTER 189 BRAIN DEATH

The advent of life saving and sustaining technologies lead to a re-appraisal of the concept of death. Respiratory and/or cardiac standstill leads to so-called somatic death. With severe brain injury including the brain stem, respiration and blood pressure control are lost. Such events also lead to somatic death, but artificial respiration and blood pressure support can maintain the vital signs in such a brain-injured patient for prolonged periods of time. When the severity of brain injury is such that there is irreversible loss of function of the brain and the brain stem, the patient is said to be brain dead.

Strict diagnostic criteria should be adhered to in confirming this diagnosis. The American Academy of

Neurology has recently published a statement with recommended guidelines (*Neurology* 1995; 45:1012–1014). The coma must be of an established and irreversible cause. Drug intoxication and hypothermia both may mimic brain death, but are reversible and must be excluded. Most patients with brain death from a primary neurological cause have suffered a head injury or subarachnoid hemorrhage; however, other etiologies occur, including large stroke with herniation and hypoxic ischemic injury.

On examination, the patient is comatose and unresponsive to any and all stimuli. Temperature must be greater than 32°C. All brain stem reflexes are abolished. Pupils show no light reaction. Oculocephalic maneuvers or caloric testing produce no eye movements. Corneal responses are absent. Gag and cough are absent. Spontaneous respiration is absent (testing methods vary; apneic oxygenation is best performed by delivery of 100% oxygen at the carina, removing ventilatory support until blood gases document $PaCO_2$ of ≥ 60 mm Hg). Posturing is not present. Muscle stretch reflexes may vary; diagnosis of brain death does not require their loss, as they reflect spinal cord function. CT is usually done to document the extent of cerebral injury, particularly with trauma.

Examination may be beset with some difficulties. Trauma with an unstable cervical spine makes oculocephalic maneuvers inadvisable. Preexisting pupillary abnormalities may be confounding. Chronic CO_2 retention may cloud interpretation of apnea testing. Spinal reflexes may produce movements difficult to distinguish from cortically based movement. With unambiguous features, two clinical evaluations performed 6–12 hours apart are widely accepted as conferring the diagnosis as brain death. Confirmatory testing may be desirable in difficult situations. EEG for 30 minutes should show no cerebral activity, or, a cerebral angiogram should show no cerebral perfusion at the level of the carotid bifurcation or circle of Willis. Technetium[99] brain scan should show no parenchymal tracer uptake.

It must be emphasized that these guidelines are for adults. The diagnosis of pediatric and in particular, infant brain death, is best made in consultation with a pediatric neurologist.

■ Questions

Instructions: For each question below, select only **one** lettered answer that is the **best** for that question.

1. A 36-year-old woman was found unconscious behind the steering wheel following a motor vehicle accident. Her neurologic examination in the ED showed mild drowsiness, normal oculocephalic reflexes and pupillary responses and a supple neck. She was moving all her extremities spontaneously and symmetrically. Her plantar response was extensor bilaterally. The most likely diagnosis is which of the following?
   A. Bilateral intracerebral hemorrhage
   B. Bilateral epidural hematoma
   C. Pontine stroke
   D. Post-ictal state
   E. Central cord syndrome

2. A 70-year-old man has progressive memory difficulties. The most important part of his neurologic examination would be which of the following?
   A. The mental status
   B. The cranial nerves
   C. The muscle strength
   D. The sensory examination
   E. The gait testing

3. A 65-year-old hypertensive man has intermittent cramping pain in the back of his thighs and legs after climbing steps or walking a variable distance. The lower extremity pulses are symmetrically reduced. The ankle jerks are absent on the left and slight on the right, while the right knee jerk is moderately decreased. Muscle strength is normal, and the sensory examination shows reduced pinprick over the dorsal aspect of both feet. The most likely diagnosis is which of the following?
   A. Arterial insufficiency with claudication
   B. Herniated L5-S1 disc
   C. Lumbar stenosis
   D. Buerger's disease
   E. Peripheral neuropathy

4. A 21-year-old woman complains of intermittent horizontal diplopia for the past 3 months. Her examination revealed mild bilateral weakness of her lateral rectus and her facial muscles. Her neck flexors were mildly weak. The rest of her neurologic examination was normal. The most likely diagnosis is which of the following?
   A. Lyme disease
   B. Pontine stroke
   C. Multiple sclerosis
   D. Myasthenia gravis
   E. Motor neuron disease

5. A 35-year-old man has intermittent horizontal diplopia and intermittent numbness of the right cheek for the past 2 months. During right lateral gaze, there is limited adduction of the left eye with nystagmus in the right. The right corneal reflex is mildly decreased. Rapid alternating movements are mildly decreased

on the left. The rest of his neurologic examination was normal. The most likely diagnosis is which of the following?

A. Lyme disease
B. Pontine stroke
C. Multiple sclerosis
D. Myasthenia gravis
E. Motor neuron disease

6. A 65-year-old man notes gradual weakness and numbness of the right hand and leg for the past 18 months. Mild wasting of his right hand muscles is evident with reduced vibration over both feet but greater on the right, and bilateral Babinski signs. The neurologic examination is otherwise normal. Useful diagnostic tests would be which of the following?

A. Serum Folate and B_{12} levels
B. Syphilis serology
C. MRI of the cervical spine
D. Nerve conduction and electromyography
E. All of the above

7. A 31-year-old woman reports intermittent stiffness in her legs for the past 4 months, followed 2 months later by urinary urgency. There is mild bilateral horizontal nystagmus, bilateral Babinski, and decreased vibration sense over hands and feet. The neurologic examination is otherwise normal. Which of the following tests will be useful?

A. Visual evoked responses
B. MRI of the brain
C. MRI of the cervical spine
D. CSF analysis
E. All of the above

8. A 27-year-old asthmatic woman was found by her husband to have episodes of brief staring followed by lip smacking, lasting less than 1 minute. Her only medication is theophylline. She does not remember the episodes. Her neurologic examination is normal. Which of the following would you do now?

A. Serum chemistry
B. Theophylline level
C. MRI of the brain
D. EEG
E. All of the above

9. A 21-year-old man was found unconscious by his parents. The paramedics noticed intermittent jerking of his arms and legs and twitching of his face during transport to the ED. While unresponsive to verbal stimuli, he was moving all his extremities symmetrically in response to pain, and had preserved oculocephalic reflexes and pupillary responses. The neck was supple. His plantar responses were extensor

bilaterally. His vital signs are stable. Which of the following is/are indicated?

A. Serum chemistry and toxicology screen
B. One ampule of 50% dextrose and thiamine
C. Intravenous phenytoin 20 mg/kg
D. EEG
E. All of the above

10. A 60-year-old woman notes shaking in her hands, greater on the right side, whenever she carries weights. It disappears at rest. Her father had similar problems around the same age. Her symptom is likely to respond to which of the following?

A. Propranolol
B. Primidone
C. Methazolamide
D. Alcohol
E. All of the above

11. A 30-year-old man has had three episodes of loss of consciousness preceded by brief "metallic taste" in his mouth lasting less than 1 minute. The neurologic examination is normal. Which of the following is most appropriate for this patient?

A. Phenytoin
B. Carbamazepine
C. Valproic acid
D. All of the above
E. None of the above

12. A 39-year-old man came to the ED complaining of abrupt headache after lifting weights at the gymnasium. He noticed transient visual blurring at the peak of his headaches. In the ED, he vomited once. His examination is normal. A noncontrast head CT scan is negative. The next step is which of the following?

A. Send home with analgesics
B. Schedule a head MRI
C. Repeat the head CT with contrast
D. Perform a lumbar puncture
E. None of the above

13. A 60-year-old man reports progressive walking difficulties over 6 days, with "numb, tingly" feeling in his fingers and feet. Mild weakness of the face and hand intrinsics is noted, along with moderate weakness of the lower extremities, absent ankle jerks, and diminished vibration sense over fingers and feet. Which of the following best describes his condition?

A. Brainstem stroke
B. Brainstem abscess
C. Guillain-Barré syndrome
D. Myelitis, subacute
E. None of the above

14. A 46 year-old man presents with 6 months of unilateral rest tremor. Unilateral cog-wheeling of the upper limb is noted. The initial treatment of choice is which of the following?
    A. Trihexyphenidyl
    B. Amantadine
    C. Bromocriptine
    D. L-Dopa
    E. None of the above

15. A 67-year-old hypertensive man had transient loss of vision in the right eye for 30 minutes. Other than a high-pitched bruit over the right carotid artery, examination is normal. The next step is which of the following?
    A. Intravenous heparin
    B. Carotid angiography
    C. Surgical consultation
    D. All of the above
    E. None of the above

■ ANSWERS

1. D	2. A	3. C	4. D	5. C
6. E	7. E	8. E	9. E	10. E
11. D	12. D	13. C	14. A	15. D

SUGGESTED READING

Approach to the Patient with a Neurologic Disorder

Caplan LR. The effective clinical neurologist. Blackwell Scientific Publications, 1990.

Fishman RA. Cerebrospinal fluid in diseases of the nervous system. 2nd ed. Philadelphia: WB Saunders, 1992.

Mayo Clinic & Mayo Foundation Clinical Examinations in Neurology. 6th ed. St. Louis: Mosby Year Book, 1991.

Disorders of Consciousness and Cognition

Plum F, Posner JB. The diagnosis of stupor and coma. 3rd ed. Contemporary Neurology Series, Vol 19. Philadelphia: F.A. Davis Co., 1980.

Headaches

Dalessio DJ. Diagnosing the severe headache. Neurology 1994;44 (5 Suppl 3):S6–S12.

Goadsby PJ, Olesen J. Diagnosis and management of migraine. Br Med J 1996;312 (7041): 1279–1283.

Kumar KL, Cooney TG. Headaches. Med Clin North Am 1995;79(2):261–286.

Welch KM. Drug therapy of migraine. N Engl J Med 1993;329(20):1476–1483.

Dizziness and Syncope

Brandt T. Vertigo and dizziness. In Asbury AK, McKhann GM, McDonald WI (eds.). Diseases of the Nervous System: Clinical Neurobiology. 2nd ed. Philadelphia: WB Saunders, 199: 451–467.

Baloh RW. Approach to the dizzy patient. Baillieres Clinical Neurology 1994;3(3):453–465.

McGee SR. Dizzy patients. Diagnosis and treatment. West J Med 1995;162(1):37–42.

Sloane PD. Evaluation and management of dizziness in the older patient. Clin Geriatr Med 12(4):1996;785–801.

Stroke

Adams HP Jr. Use of anticoagulants or antiplatelet aggregating drugs in the prevention of ischemic stroke. Advances in Internal Medicine 1995;40:503–531.

Barnett HJ, Meldrum HE, Eliasziw M. The dilemma of surgical treatment for patients with asymptomatic carotid disease. Ann Intern Med 1995;123 (9):723–725.

Brickner ME. Cardioembolic stroke. Am J Med 1997;157(6): 605–617.

Broderick JP, Brott T, Tomsick T, et al. The risk of subarachnoid and intracerebral hemorrhage in blacks as compared with whites. N Engl J Med 1992;326 (11):733–736.

Brott T, Toole JF. Medical compared with surgical treatment of asymptomatic carotid artery stenosis. Ann Intern Med 1995; 123 (9):720–722.

Gorelick PB. Stroke prevention. Arch Neurol 1995;52(4):347–355.

The National Institute of Neurological Disorders and Stroke rt-PA stroke study group. Tissue plasminogen activator for acute ischemic stroke. N Engl J Med 1995;333(241):1581–1587.

Raps EC, Galetta SL. Stroke prevention therapies and management of patient subgroups. Neurology 1995;45(2 Suppl 1):S19–S24.

Sherman DG, Dyken ML, Gent M, et al. Antithrombotic therapy for cerebrovascular disorders. An update. Chest 1995; 108(4 Suppl):S444–S456.

Seizure Disorders

Engel J. Seizures and Epilepsy. Contemporary Neurology Series, Vol 31. Philadelphia: F.A. Davis Co., 1989.

So EL. Update on epilepsy. Med Clin North Am 1993;77(1): 203–214.

Thomas RJ. Seizures and epilepsy in the elderly. Arch Intern Med 1997;157(6):605–617.

Wyllie E. The Treatment of Epilepsy: Principles and Practice. Philadelphia: Lea & Febiger, 1993.

Disorders of Spinal Cord, Nerves, and Muscles

Byrne TN, Waxman SG. Spinal Cord Compression: Diagnosis and Principles of Management. Contemporary Neurology Series, Vol 33. Philadelphia: F.A. Davis Co., 1990.

Griggs R, Mendell J, Miller R. Evaluation and Treatment of Myopathies. Contemporary Neurology Series, Vol 44. Philadelphia: F.A. Davis Co., 1995.

Schaumburg HH, Berger AR, Thomas PK. Disorders of Peripheral Nerves. 2nd ed. Contemporary Neurology Series, Vol 36. Philadelphia: F.A. Davis Co., 1992.

Multiple Sclerosis

Brod SA, Lindsey JW, Wolinsky JS. Multiple sclerosis: clinical presentation, diagnosis, and treatment. Am Fam Phys 1996; 54(4):1301–1306.

Lublin FD, Whitaker JN, Eidelman BH, et al. Management of patients receiving interferon beta-1b for multiple sclerosis: report of a consensus conference. Neurology 1996;46(1): 12–18.

McDonald WI. Diagnosis of multiple sclerosis. Br Med J 1989;299(6700):635–637.

Tourtelotte WW, Pick PW. Current concepts about multiple sclerosis. Mayo Clin Proc 1989;64(5):592–596.

Movement Disorders and Parkinson's Disease

Ahlskog JE. Treatment of early Parkinson's disease: are complicated strategies justified? Mayo Clin Proc 1996;71(7):659–670.

Jankovic J, Brin MF. Therapeutic uses of botulinum toxin. N Engl J Med 1991;324(17):1186–1194.

Krauss JK, Jankovic J. Surgical treatment of Parkinson's disease. Am Fam Phys 1996;54(5):1621–1629.

Quinn N. Drug treatment of Parkinson's disease. Br Med J 1995;310(6979):575–579.

Quinn N. Parkinsonism—recognition and differential diagnosis. Br Med J 1995;310(6977):447–452.

Stacey M, Brownlee HJ. Treatment options for early Parkinson's disease. Am Fam Phys 1996;53(4):1281–1287.

Head Trauma

White RJ, Likavec MJ. The diagnosis and initial management of head injury. N Engl J Med 1992;327(21):1507–1511.

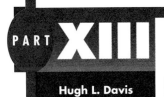

PART XIII

Hugh L. Davis
Tom Anderson

ONCOLOGY

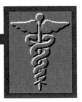

CHAPTER 190   CANCER AND CARCINOGENESIS

ancer ranks a close second to cardiovascular disease as the major cause of overall morbidity and mortality in the United States. With the continued aging of the population and recognition of the myriad genetic and environmental factors influencing carcinogenesis, cancer has profound implications for the twenty-first century. In 1997, an estimated 1,382,400 new cases of cancer and 580,000 cancer deaths will occur in the United States. These figures are based on data from the National Cancer Institute *S*urveillance, *E*pidemiology and *E*nd *R*esults (SEER) program as well as state cancer registries and the Bureau of Vital Statistics of the United States. The most common sites of cancer are listed in Table 190.1.

■ Etiology of Cancer

Age and heredity

Over 60% of all cancer deaths occur in persons over age 65 years. The increased incidence of common cancers with age may reflect the duration of exposure to environmental carcinogens. Certain cancers do cluster in the young, including brain tumors, Hodgkin's disease, bone sarcomas, testicular cancer, and some leukemias. Many common tumors have an increased genetic predisposition, including breast, colon, lung, ovary, and prostate cancers, which occur more commonly at an earlier age in those with first-degree relatives afflicted. Common neoplasms and conditions predisposing to malignancies that are inherited are shown in Table 190.2.

Carcinogens

Carcinogenesis is a multistep process with a period of variable latency between initiation and the development of premalignant and finally malignant changes. Chemical carcinogens, ubiquitous in our society, include dietary, industrial, and medicinal products. Most are metabolically activated derivatives of parent compounds in the environment. The activated carcinogen forms DNA adducts; these in turn lead to DNA strand breaks and/or interstrand cross-linking events which may cause muta-

TABLE 190.2.   Selected Inherited Cancers

Autosomal Dominant (neoplastic and preneoplastic)
  Retinoblastoma
  Neurofibromatosis
  Von Hippel-Lindau syndrome
  Li-Fraumeni syndrome
  Dysplastic nevus syndrome
Autosomal Recessive
  Xeroderma pigmentosa
  Ataxia-telangiectasia
X-Linked Recessive
X-Linked agammaglobulinemia
Wiskott-Aldrich syndrome

  Familial adenomatous
    polyposis
  Nonpolyposis colo-
    rectal cancer
  Hereditary breast
    cancer
  Hereditary breast/
    ovarian cancer

TABLE 190.1.   Major Cancers in the United States by Site and Gender—1997

Site	Total	Men	(%)	Women	(%)
Lung	178,100	98,300	(13)	79,800	(13)
Prostate	334,500*	334,500	(41)	0	
Breast	181,600	1,400	(–)	180,200	(31)
Colorectal	131,200	66,400	(9)	64,800	(11)
Melanoma	40,300	22,900	(3)	17,400	(3)
Oral-pharynx	30,750	20,900	(3)	9,850	(2)
Pancreas	27,600	13,400	(2)	14,200	(2)
Stomach	22,400	14,000	(2)	8,400	(1)
Urinary tract	85,400	58,000	(7)	27,400	(4)
Ovary	26,800	0		26,800	(4)
Uterus	49,400	0		49,400	(8)
Leukemia	28,300	15,900		12,400	
Lymphoma	61,000	34,200	(5)	23,900	(6)
All Other			(15)		(13)
Total	1,382,400	785,800	(100)	596,600	(100)

(Adapted from: Parker SL, et al. CA - A Cancer Journal for Clinicians 47:5–27, 1997.)
*The incidence of prostate cancer has been revised downward to 219,000 for 1997, and to 184,000 in 1998.

TABLE 190.3. Chemical, Physical and Biological Agents Linked to Cancer	
Agents	**Principal Tumors**
Tobacco	Lung, head/neck, esophagus, pancreas, bladder, kidney
Increased dietary fat	Colon, prostate, rectum, endometrium
Charred, smoked, salted, pickled foods	Esophagus, stomach
Low fiber diet	Colon
Alcohol	Oral cavity, esophagus (synergism with smoking)
Asbestos	Mesothelioma, lung (synergism with smoking), larynx
Benzene	Leukemia
Nickel, chloromethylether, arsenic, mustard gas	Lung
Aromatic amines	Bladder
Alkylating agents, nitrosoureas, etoposide	Leukemia
Estrogens	Breast, ovarian
Diethylstilbestrol	Vaginal adenocarcinoma; ingestion during pregnancy causes cancer in daughters
Androgens, oral contraceptives	Liver (?)
Immunosuppressives (azathioprine, cyclosporine)	Lymphoma, skin cancer
Sunlight (UV rays)	Basal and squamous cell cancers, melanoma
Radiation	Leukemia, lung
Epstein-Barr virus	Burkitt's lymphoma, nasopharyngeal cancer
Hepatitis B and C	Hepatocellular carcinoma
Human papilloma virus (HPV 16, 18)	Cervix, anus, penis, oral cavity
Herpesvirus	Kaposi's sarcoma
Clonorchis sinensis	Cholangiocarcinoma
Schistosoma hematobium	Urinary bladder cancer

tions and deletions in growth-regulating genes or tumor-suppresser genes. In addition to these chemicals, physical (e.g., sunlight, ionizing radiation) and biological (e.g., viruses, helminths) agents also may have carcinogenic potential (Table 190.3).

Promoting agents are noncarcinogenic compounds that induce cell-proliferation in tissues (e.g., estrogen in women). If a preexistent carcinogenic injury exists, promoting agents increase the frequency of progression from hyperplasia to neoplasia.

■ Molecular Genetics and Carcinogenesis

The discovery that certain viruses could induce neoplasia in infected animals by inserting a **viral oncogene** into the normal host cells unraveled many theories of the molecular events in carcinogenesis. Many oncogenes have been isolated and named for the tumors they cause in animals (e.g., c-*myc* for the avian myelo-cytomatosis virus, and *ras* group for rat sarcoma viruses) or after their discoverers (e.g., v-*abl* for the Abelson leukemia virus).

With the rapid development of molecular biology techniques, it became apparent that viral oncogenes were homologous to a wide array of genes in normal cells (called **cellular oncogenes** or **proto-oncogenes**) conserved through evolution in many classes and species of animals. Subsequent work showed the importance of these genes in normal growth and differentiation. Further laboratory studies uncovered a class of oncogenes called **tumor-suppresser genes** (anti-oncogenes or recessive oncogenes).

Some of the mechanisms of oncogene activation in cancer are shown in Figure 190.1. In dominant oncogenes, point mutations, translocations, amplification, and deletion of only one allele (gene copy) is sufficient to result in unregulated growth, which may result in malignant transformation. The tumor suppressor genes usually require a lesion in both alleles to alter the inherent growth-suppressive effect of the normal gene products. Dominant oncogenes and tumor-suppressor genes are listed in Tables 190.4 and 190.5, with the postulated function of their protein product. Whereas theoretically a single mutation creating a dominant gene should be capable of carcinogenesis, such single mutations rarely seem able to confer the malignant phenotype on a cell. At least two steps are required in the autosomal dominant cancers such as retinoblastoma, and it is believed that carcinogenesis is a multistep process involving mutations in *several* regulatory and growth-promoting genes. There are hereditary cancers characterized by the loss of one allele in the **germline** (loss of heterozygosity) wherein a second mutation, acquired due to some environmental insult, becomes

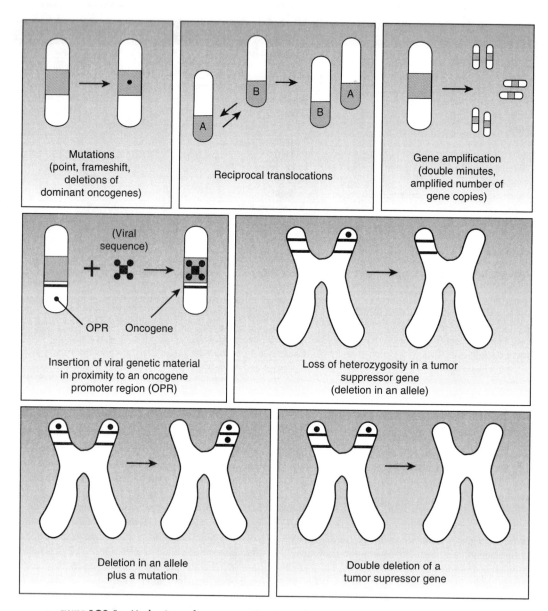

FIGURE 190.1. Mechanisms of oncogene activation and inactivation of tumor-suppressor genes.

the "triggering event" that causes cancer; hence, the propensity for increased risks of cancer within families. Examples would include retinoblastoma in children, familial polyposis coli and its resultant colon carcinoma, hereditary breast cancer, the Multiple Endocrine Neoplasia syndrome families. Such entities demonstrate that the neoplasia is genetically predisposed because of the transmission of the germ cell mutation, but is consistent with the "second hit" theory that requires another mutation, presumably induced by our environment, to cause the subsequent cancer. This explains why not everyone in a hereditary cancer family may suffer the disease; it requires both the genetic predisposition and the environmental insult. In contrast the concept of somatic mutations represents the observation of sporadic cancers, and implies that both mutations, on a random basis, were caused by separate environmental insults. Examples would include the cancers commonly associated with smoking, e.g.—lung, head and neck, esophagus, bladder.

TABLE 190.4.	Dominant Oncogenes in Human Cancer	
Oncogene	**Activation/Function**	**Tumors Associated**
ras family	Point mutation signal transduction	Multiple human solid tumors and leukemias
bcl-2 inner mitochondrial (membrane protein)	Translocation prevents apoptosis	B cell lymphomas (follicular)
abl tyrosine protein kinase	Translocation	Chronic myelogenous leukemia (Philadelphia chromosome) ALL
raf serine threonine kinases	Rearrangement	Gastric
Growth factor receptors and growth factors (erbB2 [Her2/Neu] int2, C-sis)	Amplification homology with growth factors and receptors	Many tumors, including breast
Cyclins	Translocation, regulate cell cycle	B cell lymphomas
MYC family (c-myc l-myc n-myc)	Translocation, amplification	Lymphomas, neuroblastoma, small cell lung carcinoma

TABLE 190.5.	Examples of Tumor Suppressor Genes	
Gene	**Chromosome**	**Tumors**
rb1	13q	Retinoblastoma, osteosarcoma, small cell lung cancer, sarcomas, breast, genitourinary
wt1	11p	Wilms tumor
nf1	17q	Neurofibromatosis, type 1
nf2	22q	Acoustic neuromas, neurofibromatosis type 2
men1	11q	Adenomas of multiple endocrine organs
men2	10q	Pheochromocytomas, medullary carcinomas of thyroid, parathyroid hyperplasia
p53	17p	Li-Fraumeni Syndrome, in many tumors as acquired mutations
BRCA1	17q	Hereditary breast, and breast-ovarian cancer as autosomal dominant
apc	5q	Familial adenomatous polyposis, sporadic colon cancer
dcc	18q	Sporadic and familial colon cancer
msh2	2p	Hereditary nonpolyposis colorectal cancer
Deletions	3p	Renal cell carcinoma, Von Hippel-Lindau disease, lung cancer (commonest in small cell)

■ Cancer Invasion and Metastasis

The fully developed malignant tumor represents a distinct pattern of cellular and subcellular processes referred to as its **phenotype,** due to the mutations that altered the cell's original genotype. Malignant cells often have decreased expression of cell surface adhesion molecules and loss of contact inhibition which otherwise restrain the growth of normal cell populations; receptors identify specific basement membrane proteins, and activation of proteolytic enzymes allow tissue invasion, with subsequent lymphatic and blood vessel invasion. The growth of cancer is clonal, but genetic instability leads to the development of subclones with minor genetic modifications. These subclones have variable affinity for metastasis to different tissues as well as autonomy in growth.

CHAPTER 191 PRINCIPLES OF CANCER THERAPY

■ Surgical Therapy

Surgical therapy for cancer has been employed since antiquity and remains the treatment of choice for most cancers, provided early diagnosis allows curative inter-vention and minimizes the extent of surgery. In the first half of the twentieth century, progressively more aggressive surgery was employed, based on the rationale that cancers grow in an orderly sequence of contiguous spread, from local tumor, to lymphatic extension, to distant metastasis. This belief fostered the routine use of radical surgery for many cancers (e.g., radical mastectomy, radical head and neck resections, limb amputation). In general, it was believed that *en bloc* resection involving wide excision of the primary tumor and its first or second echelon of regional nodal metastases offered the best chance of local regional cure. The subsequent realization that lymphatic involvement is in essence a metastasis, together with the recognition that hematogenous metastases occur coincident with lymphatic metastases, has led to the modern approach of using less-disfiguring surgical resection of the primary tumor (e.g., breast cancer).

Although surgery remains the major therapy option for most cancers, the current emphasis in clinical research is not how to perform more aggressive curative surgery for primary tumors, but rather how best to utilize additional therapeutic modalities, such as radiotherapy and chemotherapy, to augment the curative potential of currently available surgical techniques while producing less morbidity. Utilizing other modalities of treatment as adjuncts to surgery, the current trend is toward more-selective, less-radical surgery with better functional and cosmetic outcomes. However, the selective use of aggressive surgical resection of metastases has become highly effective as palliation for certain patients whose primary tumor is under control.

■ Radiation Therapy

Ionizing radiation has seen remarkable innovations in the twentieth century. Electromagnetic radiation and gamma rays exert their cytotoxic effects through free radical generation from interaction with intracellular water and molecular oxygen, leading to irreparable breaks in double-stranded DNA. Particulate radiation from subatomic particles also causes direct DNA damage (Table 191.1). Conventional radiation therapy utilizes a series of daily doses (fractions) given over several weeks to achieve the optimum cumulative dosage for tumor control while minimizing side effects in normal tissues. This external, fractionated form of radiotherapy is known by its historical term teletherapy, which utilizes electromagnetic radiation consisting of photons of varying energy delivered originally by Cobalt radiation sources, but now almost exclusively by modern linear accelerators. The latter provide a much greater range of energy levels, allowing for more diversity in dose fractionation, energy level (with its relationship to depth of penetration), and field design which allows much greater precision in treating the target tumor volume.

Brachytherapy, the implantation of radiation sources directly into the tumor bed, has the advantage of

TABLE 191.1. A Glossary of Terms in Radiation Oncology	
Term	Definition
Type of radiation	
Electromagnetic	External beam. Produced by machines
Gamma rays	Decay of isotopes, e.g., Cobalt[60]
Particulate	Decay producing subatomic particles
Dose Units	
Gray (Gy)	1 Joule/kg tissue absorbed dose.
Rad	Absorbed dose/gm tissue = 0.01 Gy
Beam energy	
Orthovoltage	100-400 KeV
Supervoltage	Usually 4–25 MeV; deeper penetration with higher energy units; less skin absorption
Administration	
Teletherapy	External beam therapy, e.g., linear accelerators, cobalt units.
Brachytherapy	Implanted in treatment area (interstitial, intracavitary)

limiting radiation exposure to a relatively precise body region. Successful applications include intracavitary implants for cervical and endometrial cancers and interstitial treatments for oral cancers. Radioactive isotopes of iodine have been the mainstay in treating well-differentiated thyroid cancers, both as an adjunct after surgical resection of the primary tumor and for effective long-term control of metastatic disease. Radioactive strontium, with its affinity for skeletal tissues, is useful in palliating pain from widespread bone metastases.

■ Systemic Chemotherapy

The use of cytotoxic drugs to treat cancer began in 1945 with the discovery of the effect of nitrogen mustard (mechlorethamine) on Hodgkin's disease and small cell lung cancer, followed in 1948 by the demonstration of the ability of the anti-folate compounds aminopterin and methotrexate to produce temporary remissions in childhood leukemia. Over the ensuing decades, combination chemotherapy programs have evolved, resulting in an increasing number of cures of childhood lymphoblastic leukemia, Hodgkin's disease, aggressive intermediate-grade non-Hodgkin's lymphoma, and germ cell tumors of the testes. Almost without exception the advances made in chemotherapy have resulted from the successful integration of multiple drugs into a comprehensive, concomitant treatment program. The principles of such combination chemotherapy relate to the design of regimens which have the following characteristics: (1) each drug utilized has demonstrably independent activity, or favorably affects the metabolism or binding of another drug in the program; (2) each drug can be given in therapeutic doses approximating that which can be used as a single agent when palliating the same disease; (3) each drug has an independent mechanism of action, making it more difficult for an individual tumor cell to express or acquire a resistance mechanism to that particular pharmacological challenge; (4) each drug's dose-limiting toxicity profile allows it to be combined with other drugs in the regimen, such that the use of one drug does not adversely affect the ability to utilize others. In general terms most successful regimens include alkylating agents, anti-metabolites, agents which interfere with tubulin required for mitosis, and agents which induce apoptosis.

Classes of chemotherapeutic agents and mechanisms

The major mechanisms of currently available antineoplastic drugs fall into several categories, with DNA damage being a common theme. These categories include alkylating agents, antimetabolites, antibiotics, plant alkaloids and miscellaneous agents (Table 191.2).

- **Alkylating agents,** such as cyclophosphamide, cisplatin, chlorambucil, melphalan, and mechlorethamine, produce cross-links between guanine nucleotide base pairs on opposite DNA strands, preventing subsequent DNA repair and replication.
- **Antibiotics,** such as daunorubicin, bleomycin, and doxorubicin (Adriamycin), interpose (intercalate) themselves between base pairs during DNA replication in such a way as to inhibit the interaction

TABLE 191.2. Major Cytotoxic Agents and Their Toxicity

Drug	Activity	Toxicity
Alkylating Agents		
Cyclophosphamide	Broad spectrum	N/V, My, cystitis, carcinogenic
Mechlorethamine	Hodgkin's disease	N/V, My, carcinogenic, vesicant
Chlorambucil	CLL, lymphoma	My, carcinogenic
Busulfan	CML	My, carcinogenic, pulmonary fibrosis
Melphalan	Myeloma	My, carcinogenic
Ifosfamide	Testicular, sarcomas	N/V, My, carcinogenic, cystitis, acidosis, confusion
Antimetabolites		
Methotrexate	Broad spectrum	N/V, M, My, renal failure, cirrhosis
5-Fluorouracil	Adenocarcinoma	N/V, My, M, cardiac ischemia, cerebellar ataxia
6-Mercaptopurine	Leukemia	My, hepatitis
Cytarabine	Leukemia	N/V, My, CNS, hepatic
Fludarabine, cladribine	CLL, low grade lymphoma	My, immunosuppression
Antibiotics		
Doxorubicin	Broad spectrum	My, M, N/V, alopecia, cardiotoxicity
Mitoxantrone	Lymphoma, breast	N/V, My, cardiomyopathy
Actinomycin D	Childhood tumors	N/V, M, My
Plicamycin	Hypercalcemia	N/V, My, hepatitis, coagulopathy
Bleomycin	Testicular, lymphomas	Dermatitis, fever, pulmonary fibrosis
Mitomycin C	Adenocarcinomas	My (delayed), hemolytic uremic syndrome
Plant Alkaloids		
Vincristine	Leukemia, lymphoma, breast cancer	Neurotoxicity
Vinblastine	Germ cell, bladder	My, neurotoxicity, myalgia
Etoposide	Germ cell, broad spectrum	N/V, My, leukemogenesis
Paclitaxel (Taxol)	Ovary, breast	My, myalgia, neuropathy, anaphylaxis
Miscellaneous		
Cisplatin	Broad spectrum	N/V, renal, otic, neuropathy, hypomagnesemia.
Carboplatin	Broad spectrum	My esp. thrombocytopenia
Carmustine, lomustine	Brain tumors	N/V, My (delayed), pulmonary fibrosis, leukemia
Hydroxyurea	CML	My, dermatitis
Streptozotocin	Endocrine tumors	N/V, renal failure, diabetes
L-Asparaginase	ALL	Anaphylaxis, pancreatitis, coagulopathy, thrombosis

ALL = acute lymphoblastic leukemia; CLL = chronic lymphocytic leukemia; CML = chronic myelocytic leukemia; M = mucositis; My = myelosuppression; N/V = nausea, vomiting.

TABLE 191.3.	Agents to Modify Chemotherapy-related Toxicity	
Agent	**Mechanism of Action**	**Clinical Use**
Interleukin-3 (IL-3)	Stimulates stem cells of WBC, RBC and Platelets	Investigational—shortens duration of neutropenia and thrombocytopenia after chemotherapy
Granulocyte-monocyte colony stimulating factor (GM-CSF)	Acts to stimulate granulocyte/monocyte precursors	Shortens duration of neutropenia after bone marrow transplantation
Granulocyte colony stimulating factor (G-CSF)	Stimulates proliferation of granulocyte precursors	Shortens neutropenia after chemotherapy; may reverse drug-induced neutropenia
Interleukin-6 (IL-6)	Stimulates platelet production	Investigational—reduces thrombocytopenia from chemotherapy
Erythropoietin	Stimulates red cell production	Reverses anemia of cancer and chemotherapy
MESNA	Binds toxic cyclophosphamide and ifosfamide metabolites in bladder urine	Prevents hemorrhagic cystitis
Amifostine	Scavenges free radicals	May prevent some radiation and alkylating agent toxicity
ICRF 187	Chelates free radicals	Reduces risk of cardiotoxicity from large doses of doxorubicin and other anthracyclines

of the enzyme topoisomerase II, leading to permanent DNA strand breaks.

- **Antimetabolites,** such as methotrexate, 6-mercaptopurine, and 5-fluorouracil, inhibit key enzymes in DNA synthesis, usually as competitive inhibitors.
- **Plant-derived agents** interrupt mitosis by altering the microtubules necessary to form mitotic spindles. The **vinca alkaloids** vinblastine and vincristine do so by disassembling microtubules, whereas the taxanes paclitaxel and docetaxel lead to polymerization of the microtubules, with excessive stabilization and functional incompetence. Epipodophylotoxins, another class of plant alkaloids, create DNA intercalation events similar to the anthracyclines and antibiotics noted above.
- **Topoisomerase inhibitors** are agents which disrupt the critical function of these agents. Topoisomerases I are enzymes which catalyze formation of single-strand DNA breaks; topoisomerases II catalyze both single, and double-strand breaks. These are critical for the faithful replication or transcription of DNA segments. Drugs which bind to these enzymes can lead to lethal damage by disruption of these critical replicative events. Camptothecin analogues are the only topoisomerase I inhibitors utilized as chemotherapy in human tumors; however, many of the drugs originally developed because of their anti-replicative effects are now known to also depend upon inhibition of topoisomerases II for their action—e.g., the an-

thracyclines (e.g., daunomycin and doxorubicin, the anthracenediones (e.g., mitoxantrone), and the epipodophylotoxins (e.g., VP-16).

It has been postulated that some cancer chemotherapeutic agents and radiation therapy act in part by promoting **apoptosis** (programmed cell death). Apoptosis, a natural process, provides a mechanism for removal of cells with DNA damage or mutations and eliminates the cells made defective or potentially neoplastic by toxic agents or radiation.

Drug resistance

Drug resistance may be intrinsic or acquired. Some tumors, such as renal cell carcinoma and pancreatic carcinoma, display a high degree of intrinsic resistance to virtually all chemotherapeutic agents. However, other cancers, such as malignant lymphomas and small cell lung cancer, are initially highly sensitive to many cytotoxic agents, but acquire resistance after exposure to them.

There are several well-defined mechanisms of resistance specific to particular drugs, including increased efficiency of DNA repair, gene overexpression (amplification) leading to increased production of the protein product, and production of enzyme with altered affinities. Of more clinical importance is the mechanism of resistance to a variety of naturally derived anticancer compounds mediated by the *MDR-1* **gene** (multidrug resistance), which codes for a cell membrane efflux pump that ejects chemotherapeutic compounds from the cell. Sublethal exposure to any one compound of several classes of natural products, (e.g., doxorubicin of other anthracyclines) often results in induction of *MDR-1-* mediated resistance to virtually all compounds in these classes. The protein product of the *MDR-1* gene is the p170 glycoprotein, a calcium channel-dependent pump.

Toxicity of chemotherapeutic agents

The available cancer chemotherapeutic agents act principally on cycling cells. (i.e., rapidly proliferating tissues) and therefore affect both tumors and normal tissues. The toxicity of chemotherapy is extremely pervasive and sometimes dose-limiting. Whereas some toxic effects are common to several agents, others are unique or especially severe with particular chemotherapeutic compounds (Table 191.2).

Nausea and vomiting depend on the agent, dose, and schedule. Although common with many drugs in the past, nausea and vomiting are now almost universally controllable with newer antiemetic agents which selectively block the 5-HT receptors in the brain responsible for most chemotherapy-induced nausea. **Myelosuppression,** affecting principally leukocytes but, to a lesser extent, platelets and erythrocytes, is common to alkylating agents, antimetabolites, and the antibiotics. In general, transient leukopenia appears early after exposure to antimetabolites and most alkylating agents, with a nadir at 10 to 14 days and subsequent rapid recovery. Its severity can be abrogated by judicious dose scheduling; the more recent advent of Granulocyte-Colony Stimulating Factors (G-CSF) or Granulocyte, Monocyte-Colony Stimulating Factor (GM-CSF) has made more aggressive chemotherapy regimens feasible because co-administration of such growth factors produces a more rapid recovery from the cytotoxic effects of chemotherapy. **Mucositis** and **enteritis** are also common, occurring principally with antimetabolites and antitumor antibiotics. The former can be ameliorated by mouth-rinsing formulations.

Treatment schedules usually involve the intermittent administration of drugs, with intervening rest periods to allow for recovery of normal tissue. Such schedules tend to maximize antitumor effects and minimize immunosuppression. Nevertheless, dose-limiting toxicity might disrupt the schedule. A variety of cloned growth factors and some chemical compounds may be used to alleviate chemotherapy-related toxicity and help maintain the dose and schedule (Table 191.3).

Supralethal doses of chemotherapy have been used in an effort to destroy widely metastatic cancers, with subsequent reconstitution of the bone marrow by **bone marrow** or **stem cell transplantation.** Allogeneic bone marrow transplantation (from haploidentical donors) has an established role in acute leukemia and chronic myelogenous leukemia. Autologous (self-donated) marrow reconstitution after high-dose therapy is under study in acute leukemias, Hodgkin's disease, non-Hodgkin's lymphomas, and breast cancer.

■ Hormonal Therapy

Because breast and prostate cancers proliferate on exposure to physiologic levels of hormones, initial hormonal therapies were ablative, (e.g., oophorectomy, orchiectomy). Pharmacologic doses of estrogens, androgens, and progestins, given in the appropriate settings (e.g., androgens in women with breast cancer, estrogens in men with prostate cancer), also produce responses, with subsequent down-regulation of the endogenous hormone production (Table 191.4). More recently, the antiestrogen tamoxifen has emerged as the primary hormonal therapy in breast cancer. Tamoxifen, actually a weak estrogen agonist rather than a true biochemical antagonist, binds to the estrogen receptor but, contrary to endogenous estrogen, fails to stimulate cancer cell growth.

■ Biologic Response Modifiers

The biotherapies comprise a heterogeneous group of compounds and natural agents that act by altering

TABLE 191.4.	Toxicity of Hormonal Therapy	
Agent	**Use in**	**Toxicity**
Prednisone	Lymphoma, breast	Iatrogenic Cushing's disease
Fluoxymesterone	Breast	Virilization, erythrocytosis, hepatic toxicity
Diethylstilbestrol	Prostate, breast	Nausea, gynecomastia, edema, cardiac failure
Megestrol	Breast, anorexia in AIDS	Weight gain, thromboembolism
Tamoxifen	Breast	Thrombosis, hot flashes, endometrial cancer
Leuprolide/Goserelin	Prostate	Hot flashes
Flutamide/Bicalutamide	Prostate	Diarrhea, hepatotoxicity
Aminoglutethimide	Breast, Cushing's disease	Drowsiness, rash, leukopenia

TABLE 191.5. Selected Biologic Response Modifiers in Clinical/Investigative Use		
Agent	**Mechanism of Action**	**Clinical Use**
Bacille Calmette Guérin (BCG)	Activation of macrophages, T and B cells	Intravesical therapy for superficial bladder cancer
Levamisole	Immunostimulatory	Modifies action of 5-Fluorouracil in colon cancer
Interferons	Antiproliferative, enhance immune responses	Chronic myelocytic leukemia, other hematologic malignancies, carcinoid tumors
Interleukin-2 (IL-2)	Enhances cytotoxicity of natural killer cells and T cells	Renal carcinoma, melanoma
Tumor necrosis factor	Mediator of sepsis, acute phase reactions	Investigational
Monoclonal antibodies	Antibodies to tumor antigens, carriers for radioactive isotopes and cytotoxic compounds	Investigational responses observed in lymphomas

immunity or suppressing proliferative activity (Table 191.5). **Alpha-interferons,** expressed by a wide variety of cells including leukocytes, have antiproliferative activity and are an established therapy for hairy cell leukemia, chronic myelogenous leukemia, multiple myeloma, and Kaposi's sarcoma (in AIDS). They result in toxicity at high doses, causing a flu-like syndromes, fever, myalgia, and malaise. **Interleukin-2** (IL-2) is a T-cell growth factor and is believed to stimulate the cytotoxic function of natural killer and cytotoxic T cells. High doses produce serious toxicity, including massive edema, hypotension, and respiratory failure. **Monoclonal antibodies** to lymphocyte determinants have been used to purge bone marrow of malignant B and T cells and to reduce graft rejection in transplant recipients.

■ Cancer Management

Cancer diagnosis

The diagnosis of cancer requires tissue confirmation, done by surgical biopsy. While traditional surgical methods are still widely used, fine needle aspiration and cutting core needle biopsy (which provides a larger tissue sample for histologic analysis) are increasingly being used. Many nonmalignant diseases mimic cancers, and a cytologic or histologic diagnosis is mandatory in virtually all suspected cancers.

Cancer staging

In general, stages range from I through IV, referring to early localized, regional, locally advanced, and metastatic cancers. The tumor-node-metastasis (TNM) classification is widely used to help determine the stage for prognostic and therapeutic decisions, particularly for solid tumors (Table 191.6).

Many additional variables are used to determine the prognosis of specific malignancies and supplement the

TABLE 191.6. TNM Staging—General Outline	
Primary tumor	
T_1	Tumor <2 cm confined to organ
T_2	Tumor 2–5 cm, may involve capsule or muscularis
T_3	Tumor >5 cm, involves adjacent structures
T_4	Massive tumor with extensive invasion of adjacent structures
Lymph nodes	
N_0	No clinically palpable adenopathy
N_1	Solitary ipsilateral mobile node <3 cm
N_2	Ipsilateral, contralateral, or bilateral >3 cm or multiple
N_3	Ipsilateral, contralateral, or bilateral >6 cm, multiple fixed
Metastases	
M_0	No evidence of metastases
M_1	Distant metastases present

prognostic determination from staging. **Performance status** (Table 191.7) is an assessment of the patients' degree of debility or overall functional level. The **histologic type** and **grade** of the tumor give an indication of its rate of growth and nuclear atypia. In addition, the presence of paraneoplastic syndromes, such as hypercalcemia, "B" symptoms, or weight loss, convey additional prognostic information.

Therapeutic approaches and goals

Following cancer diagnosis and staging, the clinician must design a therapeutic plan. Whenever possible, an initial strategy should be clearly defined: i.e., potentially curative; noncurative but prolonging life; or palliative.

Increasingly, tumors are treated with combined-modality therapy, either simultaneously or sequentially.

When used sequentially the primary curative modality of therapy is used first. Subsequent additional therapies are then used as an "adjunct" to reduce the risk of relapse. Traditionally post-operative radiotherapy has been the modality most commonly applied to such clinical situations. As the efficacy of chemotherapy has improved, the use of "adjuvant chemotherapy" has developed for those cancers responsive to chemotherapy in the relapsed setting. Use of such adjuvant chemotherapy has now been shown to significantly reduce the risk of relapse in colon, breast, esophageal, and head and neck cancers. Clinical trials are underway to determine such efficacy in cancers of the lung, stomach, pancreas, etc.

In some cancers (e.g., breast), adjuvant chemotherapy has replaced adjuvant radiotherapy for patients undergoing mastectomy; in patients undergoing breast lumpectomy and irradiation, the radiation becomes the primary modality of cure, and the chemotherapy assumes the adjuvant treatment role. For selected cancers such as the breast, such adjuvant therapy can be hormonal therapy. The term "neo-adjuvant therapy" alludes to the concept of using such treatment prior to the application of the curative modality. Rationale for such an approach includes the ability to test the efficacy of the adjuvant treatment in a setting where one can assess its efficacy to determine whether it is cost-effective to administer to the particular patient; it also can produce significant regressions of the primary tumor, perhaps leading to more successful primary treatment by shrinking tumor masses whose surgical removal is compromised by the tumor size, location, etc. Neoadjuvant chemotherapy is often used in Hodgkin's disease with large bulky mediastinal lymph nodes to avoid subsequent radiation injury to adjacent lung tissue.

Consultation and close cooperation among the practitioners of the different modalities—surgery, radiation oncology, and medical oncology—are vital for the optimum treatment of most cancers. Chemotherapy is curative in a few tumors when used alone and contributes significantly to curability in many cancers when used in conjunction with other modalities (Table 191.8). However, several tumor types are virtually unresponsive to chemotherapy, and in advanced-stage cancers, its use is principally palliative, or may not be indicated.

Several general factors are germane in the use of palliative chemotherapy: (1) the probability of therapeutic benefit, (2) the patient's general physical condition, and (3) the patient and family's preferences after a candid discussion of the benefits and risks of treatment. Patients with poor performance status (ECOG 3 or 4) rarely benefit from chemotherapy unless their particular tumor is known to be highly responsive to such treatment.

Outcome of treatment

In order to accurately define the disease status of a patient and the prognosis, physicians have developed definitions based on identifiable responses to therapy. With response to treatment, the survival and perhaps the quality of life are increased proportionately to the magnitude of response. The survival of patients whose treatment fails is analogous to the natural history of disease. Whenever the patient has one or more lesions, these allow reproducible measurements of the diameter of the lesion, usually in at least two dimensions over a period not less than 30 days. Patients with **stable disease** (or **no change**) are those whose tumors are unchanged. In patients with **progressive disease** the lesions(s) increase over 25% in product of bi-dimensional diameter, or new lesions develop.

TABLE 191.7. Performance Status Scales			
ECOG*		**Karnofsky**	
Score	Criteria	Score	Criteria
0	Asymptomatic	100	Asymptomatic
1	Symptomatic, fully ambulatory	90	Normal activity, minor signs and symptoms
2	Less than fully ambulatory but in bed <50% of the day	80	Normal activity with effort
3	In bed >50% of the day	70	Cares for self, unable to carry on normal activity or work
4	Bedridden	60	Requires occasional assistance but self-cares for most needs
		50	Requires considerable assistance
		40	Disabled; requires special care and assistance
		30	Severely disabled; hospitalization indicated
		20	Very sick; hospitalization needed
		10	Moribund
		0	Dead

*ECOG = Eastern Cooperative Oncology Group.

TABLE 191.8.	Response of Adult Tumors to Systemic Therapy

Frequent cures with Chemotherapy
ALL
    Gestational choriocarcinoma
    Hodgkin's disease
    Intermediate/high grade non-Hodgkin's lymphomas
    Germ cell tumors
Highly responsive—cure in a minority
    Adult AML
    Small cell lung cancer
    Ovarian cancer
Highly responsive and variably curable with combined
  modality therapy
    Sarcomas of bone
    Operable breast cancer
    Cancer of esophagus
    Bladder cancer
    Head and neck cancer
    Colon & rectal cancer
Responsive, essentially noncurable
    Metastatic breast cancer
    Metastatic prostate cancer
    Low grade non Hodgkin's lymphomas
    Chronic leukemias
    Multiple myeloma
    Endocrine tumors
Less responsive tumors
    Adult soft tissue sarcomas
    Gastrointestinal cancers (except operable colon and
      rectal cancer)
    Metastatic non small cell lung cancer, cancers of en-
      dometrial, cervical, head and neck origin, renal cell
      carcinoma and melanoma
    Hepatocellular carcinoma
    Primary brain tumors

Patients with **partial response** are those whose tumor diameter (as previously defined) decreases over 50%. Such patients survive longer than those with progressive disease. Those patients who have all evidence of their disease disappear after therapy are said to have **compete response.** Although clinical tools (physical examination, radiographic studies, etc.) are used for measuring such outcomes, occasionally it is necessary to re-examine the previous disease sites by repeat biopsy. Patients with a complete response survive the longest; a subset is potentially cured.

Other definitions used in outcome analysis of cancer include **overall survival (OS)** where all patients are followed from the time of diagnosis until death from any cause. **Disease-free survival (DFS)** denotes the time from initiation of treatment until relapse and/or death from disease. **Event-free survival (EFS)** is the time from diagnosis until either death from disease or from therapy.

In prostate cancer which affects an advanced age population, the deaths from co-morbid diseases are so frequent that an analysis of disease-free survival can establish treatment efficacy; but overall survival may not be improved if there are too many deaths from other diseases.

■ Supportive Care of the Cancer Patient

Good medical care of the cancer patient frequently requires more than treatment of the disease process. A general policy of honesty and open, compassionate communication with the patient and family will result in better cooperation and serve to lessen the anxiety derived from common misconceptions about the disease or the proposed therapy. Complications of the various treatment modalities result in multiple problems during therapy, which must be addressed. In the later stages of cancer, control of symptoms becomes paramount.

Nutrition

Nutritional concerns and weight loss may be addressed by dietary modifications, feeding through nasogastric or gastrostomy tubes, or, at times, parenteral support. Such supportive measures must be implemented in the context of the patient's disease and treatment options. Intensive, expensive, complicated, and inherently risky forms of nutritional support should be offered only if a potential exists for long-term survival. Megestrol acetate (800 mg/day for one month) has recently been recognized as an important adjunct for nutritional support. An appetite stimulant with minimal side effects, this agent allows many patients with advanced cancer (and AIDS) to regain their appetite, appreciate the enjoyment of eating again, and to gain weight which helps obviate inanition and cachexia. It is often so effective that more complex nutritional techniques can be avoided. If patients do not respond in 30–45 days it should be discontinued.

Pain management

Pain accompanies advanced or metastatic cancer in at least 60% of the cases. Cancer pain may result from the cancer itself, through direct pressure of the tumor on adjacent structures, infiltration of nerves and tissues, gastrointestinal tract infiltration or obstruction, or damage to bony structures. Pain may also arise as a treatment-related effect, such as with mucositis, edema, or nerve damage. Specific treatment, such as palliative radiation, chemotherapy, hormonal therapy, nerve blocks, or neurosurgical procedures may be designed to interrupt pain pathways.

Pain control needs to be individualized. A careful history and physical examination, a thorough evaluation of the pain intensity and its temporal relationships (preferably by using analog rating scales), and the development of a prospective management plan that seeks to minimize pain and cope with the frequent side effects of analgesic medications are necessary steps. In rating pain-control measures, the World Health Organization's "pain ladder" and similar schemata are useful. Each step is a response to increasing levels of pain and the need for increasing therapeutic intensity.

Step 1: Mild Pain

Often the patient has already utilized nonprescription analgesics. For control of mild pain, the use of acetaminophen, aspirin, or nonsteroidal anti-inflammatory agents (e.g., ibuprofen or naproxen) in effective, regularly scheduled doses is sufficient.

Step 2: Moderate Pain

Oral narcotic agents of moderate potency, usually in fixed dosages and combined with acetaminophen, are used for moderate pain. Examples include codeine, hydrocodone, or oxycodone, combined with acetaminophen. At higher doses, preparations such as oxycodone or codeine alone may better control pain without the potential for acetaminophen toxicity.

Step 3: More severe pain, uncontrolled by Step 2 agents

Strong oral narcotics are used after Step 2 agents fail and work best when used on a regular schedule, with additional doses for "breakthrough" episodes of increased pain. Unless there are problems with absorption or gastrointestinal intolerance, oral administration is desirable.

The prototypical agent is morphine, given at an initial oral dosage of about 30 mg every 3–4 hours. Sustained-release morphine preparations, administered every 8–12 hours, provide increasing flexibility since their dosage may be gradually increased to optimum levels, thus obviating interim dosing with immediate release morphine for breakthrough pain. Alternatives to morphine include hydromorphone, levorphanol, oxycodone, and methadone. Transdermal fentanyl patches, which are changed every 3 days, should be reserved for those patients who are less compliant or who have gastrointestinal problems, making oral administration unreliable.

Step 4: most severe pain

Severe pain often requires parenteral narcotics when consciousness is altered, the gastrointestinal tract is dysfunctional, or the pain intensity requires rapid relief. Examples include the immediate postoperative state, pathologic fracture, or intestinal obstruction.

Morphine can be administered every 3 hours around the clock, or by programmable pump which can deliver a constant or variable dose via IV or subcutaneous routes. **Patient-controlled analgesia** allows the patient to control the frequency of metered analgesic dosages, with additional boluses of drug for breakthrough pain, and provides an important physiologic and psychologic benefit to the patient and family. Continuous morphine infusion is frequently the preferred strategy for rapid control of severe pain and is especially appropriate in the moribund or disoriented patient.

Other adjuncts to pain management

Nonanalgesic adjuncts to enhance pain relief come under several classes: tricyclic antidepressants, phenytoin, and carbamazepine for neuropathic pain; antiemetics with anxiolytic effect for controlling nausea; and short courses of corticosteroids to enhance feelings of well-being. As cancer progresses and disability increases, the dose of pain medication required may escalate. It must be emphasized that there is no ceiling dose; an adequate dose is the amount of the analgesic that assures pain control, given regularly by whatever chosen route. The use of sedation at this time may be very important. Relatively short-acting benzodiazepines, barbiturates, or phenothiazines can be useful in this context.

Managing gastrointestinal alterations

Constipation is universal with opioid use and is compounded by patient inactivity and dehydration. Adequate fluid intake and stool softeners should be supplemented with oral peristaltic stimulants, suppositories, and enemas. Regularly scheduled use of stool softeners or mild laxatives is often preferable.

Another problem that plagues cancer patients is **nausea and vomiting.** If this is due to gastrointestinal obstruction, nasogastric suction may be the only effective measure for relief. Many chemotherapeutic agents and opiates are emetogenic, and for these, effective antiemetics are available. For minor degrees of nausea, a phenothiazine antiemetic, such as prochlorperazine, IV or orally, is usually effective and well-tolerated. If there is evidence of any dystonic complications, diphenhydramine or lorazepam may be coadministered. The prophylactic use of the new serotonin-blocking agents, ondansetron and granisetron, represents a major breakthrough in the control of nausea and vomiting.

Care of the terminal patient

As cancer progresses and life is shortened, close communication between the primary physician, specialist consultants, the patient, and family members is essential. A realistic plan for further care, discussion concerning limiting or terminating specific anticancer treatment, discussion of artificial life support and cardiopulmonary resuscitation ("code" status), and issues of home or hospice care become paramount. Hospice programs center around home care, with hospitalization for brief periods for crises and respite for the caregivers.

CHAPTER 192 HODGKIN'S DISEASE

Hodgkin's disease is a malignant lymphoma. The majority of the tumor mass is composed of nonmalignant lymphocytes, histiocytes, granulocytes, plasma cells, eosinophils, and fibrosis, all apparently reactive (unlike non-Hodgkin's lymphomas). The characteristic **Reed-Sternberg cells** and their variants form only a minority of the cellular component of the lymph node.

■ Incidence and Epidemiology

Hodgkin's disease is relatively uncommon, with 7500 cases expected in 1997. There is a striking bimodal age distribution, the first peak occurring in young adulthood and a second peak after age 50. Slightly more men than women are affected (1:1:1). Rare geographic clustering in neighborhoods have been observed.

■ Etiology and Pathogenesis

The disease is more common in upper socioeconomic groups and in persons with a prior history of infectious mononucleosis. Epstein-Barr viral DNA has been detected in the genome of Reed-Sternberg cells, suggesting an etiologic relationship to this agent. The origin of the Reed-Sternberg cell is unclear; it shows features of both B and T cells, varying with the histologic type of Hodgkin's disease.

■ Pathology

There are four main histologic types of Hodgkin's disease. These include, in order of decreasingly favorable prognosis, lymphocyte predominant, nodular sclerosis, mixed cellularity, and lymphocyte depletion subtypes. The first three subtypes tend to present with more limited disease, whereas lymphocyte-depleted Hodgkin's disease is often widespread at the time of diagnosis. Nodular sclerosing Hodgkin's disease has a predilection for the mediastinum, especially in young women.

■ Clinical Features

Most patients with Hodgkin's disease present with the complaint of a painless mass, usually in the neck but occasionally in the axilla or groin. On examination, rubbery, **lymphadenopathy** (usually painless) is noted. Occasionally, an **abdominal mass**, representing enlarged retroperitoneal nodes, or **splenomegaly** is the initial finding. Some patients are totally asymptomatic, and the physician may discover lymphadenopathy during the course of a routine physical examination or detect mediastinal adenopathy on a chest radiograph obtained for other indications (Figure 192.1). Gallium scans are helpful to confirm the biological activity of disease, but sometimes after apparently curative therapy the patient has a residual mass discernible by computed tomography (CT). A mediastinal mass which was "gallium positive" prior to therapy, and "gallium negative" after therapy is most likely a residual fibrotic mass. Most patients can be safely watched with no further therapy, and without invasive biopsy procedures.

Occasionally, extensive lymphadenopathy causes symptoms by **compression of adjacent organs**, (e.g., venous obstruction in an extremity, hydronephrosis [and renal failure if both ureters are compressed], superior vena cava syndrome, tracheal compression, dysphagia due to esophageal compression, and spinal cord compression). With early recognition and prompt treatment, compression of the adjacent organs are potentially reversible, but they may be medical emergencies.

A minority of patients (~25%) present with characteristic **systemic symptoms,** such as unexplained fever, weight loss, and night sweats. Designated by the suffix "B" to the clinical stage, these symptoms imply a less favorable prognosis in any given stage. Another, occasionally noted symptom is **pruritus**, which is typically intense and refractory to symptomatic treatment. An extremely rare, but almost pathognomonic symptom is localized pain in areas of lymphadenopathy following alcohol ingestion. Hodgkin's disease of unfavorable cell types (e.g., mixed cellularity and advanced stage) is frequently observed in HIV infected patients.

■ Diagnosis and Staging

The differential diagnosis of Hodgkin's disease consists primarily of infectious, inflammatory, autoimmune, or other neoplastic diseases. While Reed-Sternberg cells are the hallmark of Hodgkin's disease, their presence alone is insufficient for diagnosis, because similar cells may be seen in other conditions (lymphomas, carcinomas, infectious mononucleosis, toxoplasmosis, etc).

Even when Reed-Sternberg cells are observed in the appropriate cellular milieu, establishing this diagnosis is still arduous. Because careful tissue acquisition, preservation, fixation, and expert pathologic examination are key elements in the diagnosis, all lymph node biopsies should be presumed to be Hodgkin's disease until proven

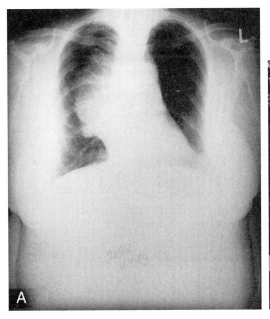

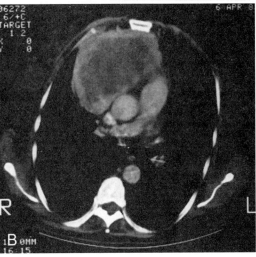

FIGURE 192.1. Hodgkin's disease presenting as a mediastinal mass. **A,** Posteroanterior chest radiograph shows a large mass to the right of the ascending aorta. **B,** CT scan showed it was an anterior mediastinal mass.

otherwise. The false presumption that a lymph node is "not lymphoma" often engenders inadequate tissue handling and thus a difficult diagnosis. Newer immunologic markers are making the diagnosis somewhat more accurate.

Staging of Hodgkin's disease is facilitated by the knowledge that it spreads most frequently by contiguous extension to adjacent nodal groups and structures. The clinical stage is established by a careful history, physical examination, laboratory studies (complete blood count with differential, platelet count, erythrocyte sedimentation rate, and liver and renal function tests), and imaging studies (CT of the neck, chest, abdomen, and pelvis; Figure 192.2). Besides determining the risk of extranodal disease in bone marrow and/or liver, laboratory studies help assess whether anemia of chronic disease, nephrotic syndrome, or other rare manifestations of Hodgkin's disease (or concomitant independent disease) are present. Bipedal lower-extremity lymphangiography (Figure 192.3) shows nodal architecture and size, but it is technically difficult and uncomfortable, and thus done only when critical to selecting between treatment modalities. A modified Ann Arbor staging system is shown in Table 192.1.

Bone marrow status is evaluated by bilateral iliac crest biopsies; such involvement is important to identify, but is rare without extensive, widespread adenopathy, "B" symptoms, a positive bone scan or an elevated

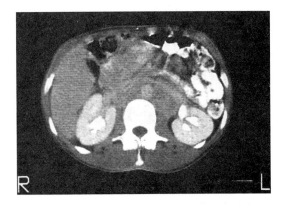

FIGURE 192.2. CT scan showing retroperitoneal lymphadenopathy.

alkaline phosphatase. Staging **laparotomy** or laparoscopy may help clarify an otherwise ambiguous assignment of stage category. As with lymphangiography, they are required only when precise staging would make a difference in selecting therapy. A staging laparotomy is a challenging procedure that requires multiple liver biopsies, splenectomy, biopsy of upper abdominal celiac nodes, and extensive sampling of periaortic and iliac nodes. A wedge liver biopsy and a wedge of the iliac crest are usually taken for larger marrow sample, and an intraoperative oophoropexy is performed in women with

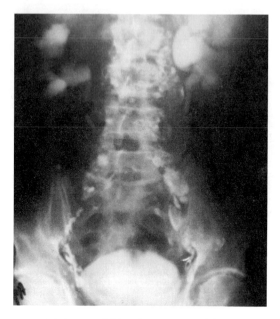

FIGURE 192.3. Bipedal lymphogram in Hodgkin's disease showing replaced lymph nodes and ureteral obstruction.

TABLE 192.1.	Modified Ann Arbor Staging of Hodgkin's Disease (and Non-Hodgkin's Lymphomas)

Stage*	Definition
I	Involvement of a single node group
IE	Stage I, accompanied by a single extranodal site
II	Two or more involved nodal groups on the same side of the diaphragm
IIE	Stage II accompanied by a single extranodal site
III	Involved nodes on both sides of the diaphragm
III_1	Upper abdominal nodes or spleen (S) involved
III_2	Periaortic, iliac, or mesenteric nodes involved
IV	Extranodal disease beyond that indicated by "E"

*The suffix A or B may be used with any stage, indicating:
A: No systemic symptoms
B: Documented fever, night sweats, or weight loss of >10% of body weight

the potential for childbearing. The postsplenectomy state is a risk factor for lethal pneumococcal sepsis, and whenever possible, patients should receive the pneumococcal vaccine preoperatively.

■ Management

The treatment options for Hodgkin's disease include radiation alone, radiation plus chemotherapy, and chemotherapy alone. Treatment decisions are based on stage more than histology. A simplified outline of treatment decisions by stage is shown in Table 192.2.

Definitive radiation therapy for early stage (stages I and IIA) Hodgkin's disease includes treatment of the upper mantle (cervical, mediastinal, and axillary nodes) and upper abdomen (celiac, portal, and splenic hilar nodes; the spleen if present; and periaortic nodes to the aortic bifurcation). Patients with stage III disease are sometimes divided into subcategories to allow for less extensive radiotherapy when possible, while still treating all known involved nodal sites plus the next contiguous uninvolved nodal area.

Combination chemotherapy has been used to treat Hodgkin's disease since 1970. MOPP (*m*echlorethamine, vincristine [*O*ncovin], *p*rednisone, *p*rocarbazine) was the standard regimen until recently, when ABVD (doxorubicin [*A*driamycin], *b*leomycin, *v*inblastine, *d*acarbazine) was introduced. Comparative trials favor ABVD because of its equal or superior efficacy and less toxicity, especially gonadal toxicity. In reality, there are a myriad of effective regimens.

Chemotherapy is used in patients who have advanced disease (most stage III and all stage IV) or who have relapsed after prior radiotherapy. A subset of stage II patients also may receive neo-adjuvant chemotherapy before definitive, curative radiotherapy, to reduce the size of large mediastinal masses, making subsequent radiotherapy more effective and less toxic (see below).

■ Prognosis

In contrast to the poor survivals seen in the 1960s, today the overall survival rate for patients with early-stage Hodgkin's disease is 75–90%, and for those with disseminated disease, 50% or greater. When Hodgkin's disease relapses following radiation therapy, full-course chemotherapy results in a high percentage of complete remissions (eradication of all evidence of disease) and a prolonged survival rate that approximates to that of previously untreated patients with advanced disease. With modern radiotherapy techniques and better staging and therapy, such occurrences are less frequent. Failure to obtain a complete remission with chemotherapy or relapse within 1–2 years after achieving a remission indicates survival less than 3 years, although bone marrow transplantation is promising in a small subset of such patients.

■ Complications

The complications of Hodgkin's disease are myriad (Table 192.3). **Infectious complications,** both acute and long-term, are probably more prevalent in Hodgkin's disease because of the inherent, and probably permanent, immunodeficiency in these patients, transiently worsened by the extensive radiotherapy and chemotherapy.

TABLE 192.2. Summary of Treatment Regimens for Hodgkin's Disease		
Stage	**Treatment Alternatives**	**5 Year Disease-Free Survival (%)**
IA, IIA (includes E)	Extended-field radiotherapy	80–90
IB, IIB	Chemotherapy alone, or extended field radiotherapy if pathologically staged	60–85
IIA with bulky mediastinal disease	Combination chemotherapy plus mantle radiotherapy	80
IIIA$_1$	Extended-field radiotherapy	60–85
IIIA$_2$	Combination chemotherapy ± total lymphoid radiotherapy	70–85
IIIB	Combination chemotherapy	60–80
IVA, IVB	Combination chemotherapy	50–70

TABLE 192.3. Complications of Hodgkin's Disease and/or Therapy Thereof	
Complications of splenectomy 　Infections with encapsulated bacteria (e.g., *S. pneumoniae*) Other infections 　Related to immunosuppressive therapy or corticosteroids 　Reactivation of varicella/zoster 　*Pneumocystis carinii* pneumonia (PCP) 　*Cryptococcus neoformans* meningitis Thyroid dysfunction 　Clinical hypothyroidism (6-25%) 　Progressive elevation in TSH (31–53%) Cardiovascular (mostly related to mantle irradiation) 　Accelerated coronary artery disease 　Acute and chronic pericarditis 　Pericardial effusion 　Acute and chronic myocarditis Pulmonary 　Acute radiation pneumonitis 　Airway obstruction 　Chronic pulmonary fibrosis 　Interstitial lung disease (related to chemotherapy) 　Opportunistic infection	Gonadal dysfunction 　Impaired spermatogenesis 　Decreased testosterone levels 　Transient amenorrhea 　Permanent ovarian failure 　Premature menopause 　Spontaneous abortion (if therapy given in first trimester) Second neoplasms 　Leukemia (acute non-lymphocytic leukemia) 　Non-Hodgkin's lymphoma 　Solid tumors (bone and soft tissue sarcoma, lung cancer, cancers of head and neck, melanoma, breast cancer) Hematologic 　Reduced circulating T-cells 　Secondary myelodysplasia Metabolic 　Hypercalcemia 　Lactic acidosis Neurologic 　Paraneoplastic cerebellar degeneration 　Neoplastic meningitis 　Epidural compression

Adapted from: Young RC et al. Monogr Nat Cancer Inst 1990; 10:55–60.

Radiation therapy causes immediate local (e.g., sore throat, dysphagia, nausea and diarrhea) and late complications (e.g., radiation pneumonitis or fibrosis, pericardial effusion, pericardial constriction, coronary artery disease, radiation spinal cord damage, hypothyroidism, and late-onset solid tumors of the skin, lung, esophagus, and breast). Acute leukemia, while an extremely rare complication of radiation therapy alone, occurs more frequently when both radiotherapy and chemotherapy are given together, especially salvage chemotherapy with MOPP after failure of radiation. Careful lifelong follow-up is necessary to detect such complications in patients.

CHAPTER 193

NON-HODGKIN'S LYMPHOMAS

The non-Hodgkin's lymphomas (NHL) are a heterogeneous group of malignant neoplasms of the immune system that, despite diverse origins, share a common link in the characteristic monoclonal proliferation of malignant B or T cells. In contrast to the predominantly reactive, polymorphic cells of Hodgkin's disease, those of the NHLs are monomorphic and monoclonal. Unlike Hodgkin's disease which tends to spread by contiguity, NHL often spreads hematogenously to involve diverse sites important in immune regulation and lymphocyte proliferation. The bone marrow is frequently involved, although NHLs can arise in diverse extranodal sites. Thus, the site of presentation and spread of NHL are more unpredictable and widespread than in Hodgkin's disease. Most patients present with stage III or IV disease, thus rendering NHL somewhat less curable.

Incidence and Epidemiology

Malignant lymphomas account for 6–7% of malignancies, with an estimated 53,600 new cases and 23,800 deaths in 1997. The incidence increases with age, although NHLs occur in all age groups. Burkitt's lymphoma and lymphoblastic lymphomas are common in youth, with the frequency of indolent (low-grade) lymphomas increasing with age. States of immunosuppression, rheumatoid arthritis, Sjögren's syndrome, phenytoin use, and a history of Hodgkin's disease are all associated with an increased incidence of NHL. NHL shows a slight preponderance among men.

Etiology and Pathogenesis

The precise etiology of NHL is elusive in most cases. African Burkitt's lymphoma, the post-transplant lymphomas, and those associated with AIDS are strongly associated with **Epstein-Barr virus** (EBV) infections. The human T-cell leukemia virus 1 (HTLV-1) is implicated in adult T-cell leukemia and the lymphomas endemic in southwestern Japan and the Caribbean basin.

Cytogenetic abnormalities accompany several types of NHL. The 8;14 translocation in Burkitt's and other high-grade lymphomas and the 14;18 translocation in most follicular small cleaved lymphocytic lymphomas are the most striking findings. In the 8;14 translocation, the c-*myc* oncogene on chromosome 8 is translocated to the region of the immunoglobulin heavy-chain gene locus on chromosome 14. In the 14;18 translocation, the *bcl*-2 gene on chromosome 18 is translocated to the immunoglobulin heavy-chain promoter region on chromosome 14. The 8;14 abnormality seems to cause unregulated transcription and rapid growth, and the 14;18 translocation leads to increased cellular longevity, probably by retarding apoptosis.

Pathology and Classification

The diagnosis of NHL is established by biopsy of an involved lymph node or other tissue, including bone marrow and the many extranodal sites where lymphomas arise. The lymph node histology must be distinguished from that of infection (cytomegalovirus, mononucleosis, toxoplasmosis, HIV, etc.), Hodgkin's disease, and various reactive lymphadenopathies. The hallmark, a clonal lymphocyte population, is established by immunohistochemical study, flow cytometry, or DNA analysis. Light microscopy can define the cell size and architecture.

Malignant lymphomas are classified according to either the Working Formulation or Rappaport histologic methods (Table 193.1). Indolent lymphomas almost invariably arise from B cells, whereas a sizable portion of the intermediate and high-grade lymphomas are of T-cell origin.

Clinical Features

The manifestations of NHL can best be described as protean. This group of diseases should always be included in the differential diagnosis of a patient with an unidentified organ disease process.

NHL commonly presents with lymphadenopathy similar to Hodgkin's disease, although hepatosplenomegaly and anatomically widespread, palpable adenopathy are more common. Conversely, clinically or radiographically significant mediastinal lymphadenopathy is less frequent. The adenopathy may be bulky, and large abdominal masses may be felt. Massively enlarged nodes may cause organ compression or obstruction. The nodes are usually described as discrete or rubbery, unlike the hard nodes of metastatic carcinoma. The bone marrow is commonly involved (20–40%), more frequently when hepatosplenomegaly or hematologic abnormalities are present and especially when the histology is low-grade.

Lymphomas with a large-cell component and a diffuse histologic growth pattern are known collectively as **high-grade,** or aggressive. They are most likely to be localized, limited-stage disease, but also likely to show locally aggressive, invasive characteristics; hence, the historical term reticulum cell sarcoma. High-grade NHLs may also involve the central nervous system (CNS),

TABLE 193.1. Basic Classification of Lymphocytic Lymphomas		
Working Formulation	**Rappaport**	**Cell of Origin**
Low-grade		
A. Small round lymphocytes, plasmacytic	Diffuse, well-differentiated lymphocytic	98% B-cell; 2% T-cell
B. Follicular predominantly small cleaved lymphocytes	Nodular poorly differentiated lymphocytic	B-cell
C. Follicular mixed, small cleaved and large cells	Nodular mixed lymphocytic-histiocytic	B-cell
	Nodular histiocytic	B-cell
Intermediate-grade	**Diffuse**	
D. Follicular, predominantly large cell	Well differentiated lymphocytic	B-cell
E. Diffuse small cleaved cell	Poorly differentiated lymphocytic	95% B-cell
F. Diffuse mixed small and large cell, including epithelioid component	Mixed lymphocytic histiocytic	85% B-cell
G. Diffuse large cell, cleaved and noncleaved	Histiocytic	85% B-cell
High-grade		
H. Large cell immunoblastic, including plasmacy-toid, clear cell, polymorphous, lymphoblastic	Histiocytic	85% B-cell
I. Lymphoblastic, convoluted and nonconvoluted cells	Lymphoblastic	85% T-cell
J. Small noncleaved cell, Burkitt's and non-Burkitt's	Diffuse undifferentiated	100% B-cell
Miscellaneous		
Cutaneous T-cell lymphoma		
Composite lymphomas		
Anaplastic large cell		
Unclassified		

manifesting as a lymphomatous infiltration of the meninges and cranial and/or spinal nerve roots, with resultant nerve dysfunction. Diplopia and facial weakness, myelopathy, or radiculopathy at any level may occur.

The presentations of **extranodal lymphomas** are legion, mimicking tumors of the brain, thyroid, gastrointestinal tract, lung, or genital tract of either gender. The B symptoms characteristic of Hodgkin's disease occur in NHL as well.

■ Evaluation and Staging

The evaluation of patients with NHL is similar to that of Hodgkin's disease. Physical examination and CT scanning of the abdomen and occasionally the chest are useful to show enlarged nodes. The mediastinum is infrequently involved, except in high-grade lymphoblastic lymphomas.

Bone marrow biopsy is required. The marrow is involved in most disseminated low-grade lymphomas but is not as prognostically important. In intermediate and high-grade lymphomas, marrow involvement is less frequent, but when present, it is more ominous. Additional investigation may be necessary, such as examination of the cerebrospinal fluid for malignant lymphocytes

and studies of the gastrointestinal tract in high-grade lymphomas.

The Ann Arbor staging system is shown in Table 192.2. The "E" category is frequently used in extranodal lymphomas. Indolent, low-grade lymphomas rarely present with localized disease (stages I or II), but intermediate and high-grade lymphomas are localized in up to 40% of cases.

■ Management

Treatment of lymphomas is complex, because the biology of disease varies with the subtype. Unlike Hodgkin's disease in which treatment decisions depend primarily on the stage of disease, in NHL, histologic features as well as stage frequently determine the treatment. An overview of the treatment options is shown in Table 193.2.

Low-grade lymphomas

Low-grade lymphomas, listed as subtypes A, B, or C in Table 193.1, are almost always stage III or IV disease. Initially, even patients with stage IV disease can often be observed without treatment. Palliative radiotherapy and/or oral-based chemotherapy may be utilized upon disease progression.

TABLE 193.2. Treatment Options in Non-Hodgkin's Lymphoma

Histology/Stage	Options	Results
Low grade	Observation, local radiation, chemotherapy	Median survival 7–10 yrs. Few cures
I-II		
III-IV	Observation, single or combination chemotherapy	Median survival 5–10 yrs.
Intermediate	Combination of radiotherapy + chemotherapy	80% 5 yr survival; 30-65% only with radiation alone
I-II including Extranodal		
III-IV	Combination chemotherapy; high dose therapy in some cases with marrow transplantation	Complete response 50–70% with 30–40% 5 yr survival
High-grade	Chemotherapy + radiation; intrathecal chemotherapy with or without radiation; maintenance therapy for 2 yrs	50–60% 5 yr survival
I-II including extranodal (E)		
III-IV	Combination chemotherapy; intrathecal chemotherapy with or without radiation; consider high dose therapy with marrow transplantation	20–30% 5 yr survival

Survival averages 7–10 years, with many patients living 10–20 years even if not treated to remission. This "watch and wait" approach has become the standard of care for such patients. However, such an approach requires regular, careful monitoring of disease status, and the more aggressive combination chemotherapy must be implemented if the indolent disease can no longer be managed conservatively. More aggressive intervention is generally used with younger patients, those with B symptoms, or symptoms due to bulky disease.

Complications and prognosis

About 5% of indolent lymphomas secrete a monoclonal immunoglobulin. Depending on the class of immunoglobulin secreted or the antigen it recognizes, patients may present with a syndrome of hyperviscosity (i.e., Waldenström's macroglobulinemia), renal failure, autoimmune hemolytic anemia, or autoimmune thrombocytopenia.

Complications of treatment include marrow failure from repetitive and prolonged radiotherapy or chemotherapy, increased susceptibility to infection, and occasional chemotherapy-induced leukemia.

Careful follow-up is necessary because of the propensity of low-grade diseases to transform into intermediate or high-grade, diffuse large-cell lymphomas. Such transformation markedly worsens the prognosis, and more-aggressive therapy must be offered.

Intermediate-grade lymphomas

Large-cell diffuse lymphoma is the most frequently diagnosed subgroup of intermediate-grade lymphomas.

Localized disease is managed with excisional biopsy, followed by combination chemotherapy and consolidative radiation, an approach particularly suitable for extranodal presentations (stage IE and, IIE). Initial excision is especially important in primary gastrointestinal lymphomas which may manifest rapid tumor lysis with combination chemotherapy, resulting in bleeding or perforation.

In stage III or IV disease, chemotherapy with CHOP (cyclophosphamide, doxorubicin, vincristine [Oncovin] and prednisone), given every 3 weeks for 6–8 cycles, results in a 50–60% rate of complete responses. Among these responses, 60–80% are durable, resulting in 30–45% long-term survival consistent with cure. Addition of methotrexate, cytarabine, and bleomycin has not consistently improved long-term results. High-dose consolidation therapy with autologous bone marrow or stem cell reconstitution is a promising approach for high-risk younger patients.

Complications and prognosis

Meninges and nerve roots are involved by lymphoma in 9–10% of patients with diffuse large-cell lymphomas, especially those with preexisting bone marrow infiltration. With suspected CNS involvement, cerebrospinal fluid should be analyzed.

Localized lymphomas and localized extranodal involvement can be cured with combined modality therapy in 50–80% of cases. Stage III and IV disease pose more of a problem, with only 20–40% of patients surviving disease-free for over 5 years. Failure to achieve a complete response to initial chemotherapy results in death in 1–2 years. Favorable prognostic factors include age less than 60 years, a normal lactate dehydrogenase level, stage III disease, stage IV without marrow or CNS involvement, and a rapid response to therapy (complete response in one to three cycles). One-fourth or fewer of older patients and those with adverse prognostic factors are cured.

High-grade Lymphomas, Including AIDS-associated Lymphomas

The high-grade lymphomas comprise three uncommon histologic types.

■ Large-Cell Immunoblastic Lymphomas

Large-cell immunoblastic lymphoma is so named because the cells resemble the normal immunoblasts of the follicular centers. Lymphomas of this histology are more aggressive than the intermediate-grades. They are frequently associated with the Epstein-Barr virus (EBV), organ transplantation, and HIV infection (where it is an AIDS-defining neoplasm).

These lymphomas are often extranodal in presentations, with a predilection for spread to the CNS when they present as widely disseminated disease. Combination chemotherapy is less successful than with the intermediate-grade, and opportunistic infections and associated HIV-induced myelosuppression in persons with AIDS make aggressive chemotherapy hazardous. Lymphomas arising in the setting of iatrogenic immunosuppression (e.g., after solid-organ transplantation) can represent polyclonal as well as monoclonal B-cell proliferations. Conventional therapies in this latter setting almost always fail.

■ Burkitt's Lymphoma

Burkitt's lymphoma, a diffuse B-cell lymphoma, has a distinctive histology, an aggressive course, and remarkable sensitivity to chemotherapy. In Africa, the EBV-associated form is endemic, but this lymphoma is rare in the United States. Here, it occurs generally in older children and young adults and presents with massive abdominal disease, with frequent bone marrow, peripheral blood, and meningeal involvement.

Whereas the African form of disease is often cured with single-agent chemotherapy, the American form requires more aggressive chemotherapy to achieve a respectable cure rate. With this intensive therapy, the prognosis for localized involvement is favorable (50–80% cure). With dissemination and organ or meningeal involvement, the prognosis is guarded (20% long-term survival).

This tumor is so responsive to chemotherapy that massive **tumor lysis** may ensue with the first cycle. Pretreatment with allopurinol, vigorous hydration, and diuresis with meticulous monitoring and intervention for hyperkalemia are imperative during the first few days of the first treatment cycle.

■ Adult Lymphoblastic Lymphomas

Adult lymphoblastic lymphomas are predominantly thymic T-cell lymphomas and are closely related to T-cell acute lymphoblastic leukemia. Their incidence clusters in the teens and young adulthood, predominantly in men. They are usually associated with prominent mediastinal masses, one of the few NHLs to present this way. Treatment is identical to that of acute lymphoblastic leukemia, with CNS prophylaxis and prolonged maintenance therapy, in contrast to the more limited duration of treatment for other high-grade lymphomas.

Angioimmunoblastic Lymphadenopathy

Angioimmunoblastic lymphadenopathy starts as a polyclonal, usually nonneoplastic proliferation of immune cells with similarities to, and frequent evolution into, a peripheral T-cell lymphoma. This disorder presents in older persons as generalized lymphadenopathy, hepatosplenomegaly, skin rash, fever, weight loss, anemia (frequently autoimmune hemolytic anemia), and polyclonal hypergammaglobulinemia. A polymorphous cell population and capillary proliferation are seen in affected lymph nodes. Treatment is with corticosteroids or cautious combination chemotherapy, but survival is usually only 1–2 years.

CHAPTER 194   MULTIPLE MYELOMA AND PLASMA CELL DYSCRASIAS

The plasma cell dyscrasias are a clonal proliferation of immunoglobulin-producing cells, including plasma cells and plasmacytoid lymphocytes. This proliferation leads to the production of a monoclonal immunoglobulin which may represent an intact antibody or just the light-chain component. The clinical manifestations depend on the proliferative and secretory characteristics of each patient's malignant clone of cells. The clonal proliferation and resultant diseases or syndromes can be classified into distinct syndromes, including the nonmalignant monoclonal gammopathy of unknown significance (MGUS), isolated plasmacytoma (essentially a malignant myeloma limited to a single osseous or extraosseous site), multiple myeloma, Waldenström's macroglobulinemia, or systemic amyloidosis.

■ Incidence and Epidemiology

The age distribution is similar for all the plasma cell disorders. MGUS is more common after the seventh decade of life, when approximately 2% of individuals over age 70 are thought to have this syndrome.

Multiple myeloma is an uncommon disease. Its incidence is 3–4/100,000 among Caucasians and 6.7–9.6/100,000 among African-Americans (for women and men, respectively) with 13,800 new cases in the US in 1997. Less than 2% of cases occur in persons under age 40; the median age is 68 years for men and 70 for women.

■ Etiology and Pathogenesis

The etiology of plasma cell tumors is elusive. Previous exposure to ionizing radiation may be a risk factor. The cell of origin is a precursor B cell. The clonal progeny (i.e., plasma cell or plasmacytoid lymphocytes) are terminally differentiated, usually functional cells, in that they can synthesize and secrete immunoglobulin molecules or fragments. This is in contrast to the malignant cells of non-Hodgkin's lymphomas which are arrested at intermediate stages of differentiation and do not routinely produce immunoglobulin.

Proliferation of myeloma cells is accompanied by secretion of β_2-microglobulin (the light chain of the major histocompatibility complex), which may be used as a marker of disease activity. The pathogenesis of amyloidosis involves the tissue deposition of light chains in a protein matrix secreted by a dysplastic clone of aberrant, albeit nonmalignant, plasma cells.

■ Pathology

Gross pathologic findings in the plasma cell disorders include osteolytic bone lesions, and in advanced cases, involvement of lymph nodes and other organs such as the kidneys. Light microscopy shows proliferation of plasma cells of variable phenotypic expression, with focal or diffuse infiltration of the bone marrow (Figure 194.1). The accompanying osteolysis seen on bone biopsies is caused by the proliferation of osteoclasts actively resorbing bone. Pathologic fractures may be seen.

The kidney may show amyloid deposition in the glomeruli. However, the most common lesion is **Bence-Jones kidney,** or light-chain nephropathy. Protein casts, degenerative changes, and inflammatory reactions in the renal tubules are characteristic and lead to renal failure.

■ Clinical Features

Persons with MGUS are asymptomatic. Multiple myeloma is sometimes found in patients in an asymptomatic stage, when routine blood tests or urinalysis reveals an increased sedimentation rate (ESR), mild anemia, or unexplained proteinuria. Such patients have a better prognosis and tolerate therapy better than debilitated patients in a more advanced stage.

Bone pain is the most frequent presenting symptom of overt myeloma. The pain is often sudden and severe, due to an incidental pathologic fracture. Radiographs usually reveal widespread, multiple osteolytic or "punched-out" lesions throughout the skeleton (Figure 194.2). On occasion, diffuse osteoporosis is seen, rather than lytic lesions. Skeletal surveys are preferred to

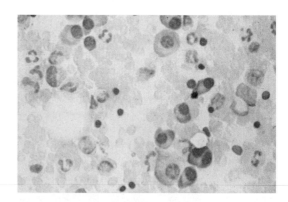

FIGURE 194.1.   Bone marrow in multiple myeloma showing a significant increase in plasma cells.
(Courtesy of Lawrence S. Hurwitz, MD, Milwaukee, Wisconsin.)

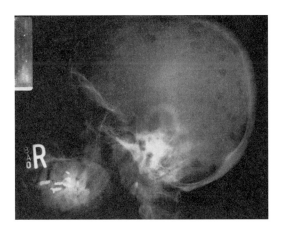

FIGURE 194.2. Lytic skull lesions with punched-out appearance in multiple myeloma.

radionuclide bone scans in myeloma, because the lytic bone lesions in myeloma do not evoke an osteoblastic response. As the disease progresses, the lytic lesions increase in size and number; vertebral compression fractures follow with resultant marked skeletal deformity and possible spinal cord compression. The patient may actually lose several inches in height.

Patients with myeloma have increased susceptibility to **bacterial infections,** particularly pneumococcal infections. Although 99% of patients with multiple myeloma secrete an aberrant antibody product, synthesis of functioning polyclonal antibody is routinely suppressed.

Impaired kidney function is found in up to 80% of patients and may be the presenting feature. Renal disease in myeloma most commonly results from tubular damage related to the reabsorption of large amounts of Bence-Jones proteins. Use of IV contrast media can exacerbate renal dysfunction and should be avoided if multiple myeloma is suspected or previously diagnosed. **Neurologic problems** develop in many myeloma patients and involve all levels of the nervous system, including peripheral neuropathies (from amyloid infiltration) and nerve root symptoms (from vertebral compression fractures). Spinal cord compression, due to vertebral involvement, is a medical emergency. Confusion and stupor may accompany azotemia, hypercalcemia, or hyperviscosity.

Certain patients present with solitary **plasmacytomas** of bone or soft tissue. Soft tissue plasmacytomas are most commonly located in the upper airway and progress less commonly to myeloma. However, myeloma develops within 5 years in many patients with a solitary plasmacytoma of bone.

Laboratory Features

In multiple myeloma, peripheral blood almost invariably demonstrates **rouleaux** formation and a markedly elevated ESR. Hypercalcemia, azotemia, and hyperuricemia are also frequent. Monoclonal immunoglobulin (Ig) composed of a single heavy-chain type and a single light-chain class (kappa or lambda) is characteristic of myeloma, MGUS, and Waldenström's macroglobulinemia, whereas secretion of light chains characterizes amyloidosis. The most frequent monoclonal myeloma protein type is IgG, followed by IgA or IgD. When associated with proven myeloma, these individual paraproteins are called myeloma proteins, or "M spikes," referring to the appearance on immunoglobulin electrophoresis. In about 25% of cases, Bence-Jones proteinuria (isolated light chains filtered so effectively by the glomeruli that they are absent in the serum) may be the sole evidence of a paraprotein secretion. Bone marrow examination in multiple myeloma generally reveals an excess of abnormal plasma cells, usually exceeding 30%, frequently in large coalescent masses that efface normal marrow architecture.

Diagnosis and Evaluation

Diagnostic criteria for **MGUS** include a 24-hour urine showing a monoclonal Ig (<3.5 g/dl for IgG, <2 g/dl for IgA, or <1 g of light chains), with less than 5% plasma cells in the bone marrow aspirate and no bone lesions or extraskeletal tumors. Reactive plasmacytosis, as seen in chronic diseases such as rheumatoid arthritis, is usually less than 15% and untenable with a diagnosis of myeloma unless other evidence is strong (e.g., lytic bone lesions). Monoclonal immunoglobulins are found in a few (<5%) patients with chronic lymphocytic leukemia, rarely in non-Hodgkin's lymphomas, and incidentally in some patients with a variety of chronic diseases.

Multiple myeloma is a fatal disease, and every effort must be made to avoid confusing MGUS and reactive states with myeloma. The diagnostic criteria of overt multiple myeloma (Table 194.1) include bone marrow plasmacytosis over 15%, presence of a serum or urine monoclonal Ig (0.5% of cases are nonsecretory), and lytic bone lesions or osteoporosis on skeletal survey. Those presenting with renal failure pose difficult diagnostic problems, especially if no serum paraprotein (M protein) is apparent; one must remember that renal failure due to secretion of only light chain (Bence-Jones nephropathy) and/or amyloid deposition might be present.

Once multiple myeloma is diagnosed, the tumor burden is determined, based on the number of bone lesions, the serum or urine levels of monoclonal Ig (M protein), and the presence or absence of hypercalcemia, anemia, or renal failure (Table 194.2).

TABLE 194.1. Diagnostic Criteria for Multiple Myeloma

Major	Minor
1. Biopsy-proven plasmacytoma	A. Lytic bone lesions
2. Marrow plasmacytosis (>30% plasma cells)	B. Marrow plasmacytosis (plasma cells 10–30%)
3. SPEP: M-spike with:	C. M-spike present, but less than that to fulfill major
IgG >3.5 g/dl, or	criteria
IgA >2.0 g/dl;	D. IgM normal, IgG <600 mg/dl, or IgA <100 mg/dl
UPEP: kappa or lambda light chains >1.0 g/24 h	

Diagnosis confirmed when:
- Any 2 major criteria are present, or
- One major (1) + minor A, C or D are present; or
- One major (2) + Minor A, C or D are present; or
- One major (3) + Minor B or A are present, or
- Minor criteria A, B and C are present; or
- Minor criteria B, C and D are present

Abbreviations: SPEP = serum protein electrophoresis. UPEP = urine protein electrophoresis.

TABLE 194.2. Staging of Multiple Myeloma

Stage*	Myeloma Cell Mass	Criteria
I	Low (0.6 × 10^{12} cells/m^2)	All of the following:
		Hemoglobin >10 g/dl
		Serum calcium† ≤12 mg/dl
		OR Normal bone survey or solitary lesion only
		M component production:
		IgG <5 g/dl
		IgA <3 g/dl
		Urine light chain <4 g/24 hr
II	Intermediate (0.6-1.2 × 10^{12} cells/m^2)	Values intermediate between those for Stages I and III
III	High (>1.2 × 10^{12} cells/m^2)	Any of the following:
		Hemoglobin <8.5 g/dl
		Serum calcium† >12 mg/dl
		OR Advanced lytic lesions on bone survey
		M component production:
		IgG >7 g/dl
		IgA >5 g/dl
		Urine light chain excretion >12 g/24 hr

*Stages subclassified according to serum creatinine (Scr) and blood urea nitrogen (BUN).
Subtype A = Scr <2 mg/dl or BUN <30 mg/dl; B = Scr ≥2 mg/dl or BUN ≥30 mg/dl.
†Should be corrected for serum albumin level.
(Reprinted with permission from: Durie BG, Salmon SE: Cancer 1975;36:842.)

Amyloidosis complicates multiple myeloma in about 15% of cases, or it may occur as a primary disorder with or without monoclonal immunoglobulin spikes on electrophoresis and significant marrow plasmacytosis. It is suggested by the presence of amyloid deposition in the tongue, peripheral nerves, kidney, heart, or gastrointestinal tract, leading to macroglossia, peripheral neuropathy, renal failure, cardiac failure, or intestinal malabsorption. The diagnosis is confirmed by amyloid staining of tissue sections of rectum, tongue, kidney, or aspirated abdominal fat.

■ Management

MGUS does not require therapy. About 10–25% of cases eventually evolve over years to decades into myeloma, macroglobulinemia, or systemic amyloidosis. This transformation can be detected through comprehensive follow-up. Most patients with this benign condition never develop a disease requiring therapy.

Occasionally a patient with myeloma will have an indolent course requiring little or no intervention for months or even years. These patients, classified as **smoldering myeloma,** should be followed closely with laboratory and radiological monitoring. Solitary plasmacytomas should be treated with irradiation and closely followed.

Chemotherapy

For overt, symptomatic **multiple myeloma,** chemotherapy is clearly indicated, with an alkylating agent (melphalan or cyclophosphamide) plus prednisone given intermittently every 3–6 weeks until maximum response, followed by observation until relapse. Subjective and objective responses occur in 50–70% of those treated, as manifested by a decline in the M protein levels and improvement in pain, anemia, and renal function. Combinations of multiple alkylating agents, nitrosoureas, vincristine, and doxorubicin usually lead to higher response rates, with some but not all studies showing an improvement in survival. Current research studies are focusing on the role of autologous or allogeneic bone marrow transplantation. Early analysis suggests that such therapies improve survival with acceptable degrees of toxicity. However, to date there is no evidence that this, or any other treatment, cures multiple myeloma.

Amyloidosis secondary to multiple myeloma may resolve with successful chemotherapy. However, primary amyloidosis treated with identical melphalan-prednisone regimens is more refractory, with the largest series reporting only an 18% response of limited duration.

Other measures

General supportive measures play an important role in the management of these patients. Careful attention to proper hydration, caloric intake, regular ambulation, and adequate analgesia will enhance patient comfort and avoid hypercalcemia and renal failure. Palliative radiotherapy to specific, painful bone lesions, while highly effective, cannot substitute for systemic chemotherapy. Prophylactic orthopedic stabilization may be necessary for impending pathologic fracture. Despite a suboptimal immune response in these patients, pneumococcal vaccine is recommended.

■ Complications

The complications of plasma cell disorders are listed in Table 194.3. Anemia may respond to erythro-

poietin or androgens. Hypercalcemia has been successfully treated with corticosteroids or the new bisphosphonates, such as pamidronate, and hydration. Infectious complications are more common in the first few months of treatment, when chemotherapy-induced granulocytopenia and disease-related antibody deficiency coexist. Late complications of chemotherapy include acute nonlymphocytic leukemia in 5–10 % of long-term survivors.

Late in the course of disease, myeloma may transform into an aggressive form that resembles large-cell immunoblastic lymphoma or leukemia and is especially fulminant.

■ Prognosis

Multiple myeloma is universally fatal. The prognosis varies with the stage of disease at presentation and the response to treatment. Median survival ranges from

---

TABLE 194.3. Complications of Multiple Myeloma

Mechanical
 Bone pain
 Pathologic fractures
 Epidural spinal cord compression
Infections
 By viruses and encapsulated bacteria (e.g., *S. pneumoniae*)
Hypercalcemia
 Due to osteolysis (IL-6, TNF-β, IL-1)
Marrow Failure
 Anemia, leukopenia
 Thrombocytopenia
 Plasma cell leukemia
Renal Insufficiency
 Light chain nephropathy
 Amyloid
 Hypercalcemia
 Hyperuricemia
 Renal failure due to IV contrast
 Plasma cell infiltration
Hyperviscosity
 With IgG$_3$ and IgM
Cryoglobulinemia
Amyloidosis
 Malabsorption
 Cardiomyopathy
 Renal failure, nephrotic syndrome
Second Malignancies
 Acute nonlymphocytic leukemia
 Myelodysplastic syndrome
 Undifferentiated, large cell or immunoblastic lymphoma

IL = interleukin; TNF = tumor necrosis factor.

2–3.5 years, with 20–30% survival at 5 years and less than 10% at 10 years. Progressive drug resistance, renal failure, infection, and second malignancies are the usual causes of death. Coexisting amyloidosis further worsens the prognosis.

Waldenström's Macroglobulinemia

Waldenström's macroglobulinemia is a low-grade malignant lymphoma of plasmacytoid lymphocytes, which secrete excessive amounts of a monoclonal IgM paraprotein. Bone marrow, lymph node, liver, and spleen infiltrations are typical.

Most patients with macroglobulinemia present with symptoms related to anemia or the presence of the macroglobulin, such as cryoglobulinemia (e.g., Raynaud's phenomenon), hyperviscosity (e.g., visual disturbances), and protein-protein interactions (e.g., platelet dysfunction with petechiae and ecchymoses). Unlike multiple myeloma, renal failure and lytic bone lesions are rare. The diagnosis requires the demonstration of a monoclonal IgM paraprotein in the serum and characteristic infiltration of plasmacytoid lymphocytes in the bone marrow and/or lymph nodes.

Because cell proliferation is low, this indolent lymphoma is usually treated with the same regimens as used in multiple myeloma, although patients usually respond to any typical treatment regimens used for lymphoma. Plasmapheresis is used to control hyperviscosity emergently or prophylactically when the serum viscosity rises above 4 units while waiting for response to chemotherapy (which may require weeks to be effective). Overall, the median survival in Waldenström's macroglobulinemia is 5 years.

CHAPTER 195 **BREAST CANCER**

Breast cancer is the most frequent cancer in women and the second leading cause (following lung cancer) of cancer-related death. Its incidence has been slowly increasing over the past 30 years, with a marked increase in the past decade due to wider screening.

■ Incidence and Epidemiology

In 1997, there were 181,600 new cases of breast cancer and 44,390 deaths from this cancer in the United States. Breast cancer shows striking international variations. It is most frequent in the northern latitudes and the western world and among Caucasians. Despite a low incidence in Asia and the tropics, Asian immigrants to western areas gradually assume the incidence patterns of their adopted new homes.

Various factors can be used to estimate an individual's risk for developing breast cancer (Table 195.1). In large populations of breast cancer patients studied for these risk factors, 20–40% had one or more of the "high-risk" characteristics. However, most women who develop breast cancer are not of unusually high risk. The current estimate of an overall lifetime incidence is 10–14%, with the greatest risk concentrated in the sixth decade and beyond.

■ Etiology and Pathogenesis

Hereditary susceptibility accounts for 5–20% of cases and is associated with recently discovered abnormalities on multiple chromosomes, including the BRCA-1, BRCA-2 the *BRCA-1* and *p53* genes. Amplification of the *HER2/NEU* gene, which codes for the epidermal growth factor receptor, is a later-occurring abnormality associated with cancer progression and a prognostic predictor of disease behavior, but not a risk factor for disease development.

Hormonal factors appear to play an important role in disease development and progression (Table 195.1). The effect of early menarche, delayed pregnancy, and late menopause is to prolong the cyclic stimulation. Diet and obesity may lead to a relative state of excess estrogens, and alcohol may alter estrogen metabolism. In these instances, prolonged estrogen stimulation probably acts as a promoter to more fundamental molecular perturbations. Prolonged estrogen therapy (hormonal replacement therapy) is likewise credible as a minor risk factor.

■ Pathology

Almost all breast cancers are **adenocarcinomas.** Cancer arising in the milk ducts, termed **infiltrating duc**

TABLE 195.1. Risk Factors for Breast Cancer	
Risk Factor	**Estimated Risk Magnitude**
Feminine gender	Overwhelming
Age over 30	Risk begins ~ age 30; escalates rapidly ~ age 50–60.
Obesity	Potentially a factor after menopause
Regular alcohol intake	A factor in case control studies
History of previous breast cancer	Risk is 1% annually in opposite breast
Previous premalignant breast disease	Relative risk:
Hyperplasia	1.6
Atypical hyperplasia	>4.0
LCIS	20-25% cancer risk in either breast over 2 decades
Heredity	
One affected first degree relative	1.5
Two affected first degree relatives	≥3.0
Premenopausal bilateral cancer in first-degree relatives	8.0
Hormonal Factors	
Age at menarche <12	1.5–1.7
Age at menopause >54	1.5–1.7
First pregnancy after age 30–35	1.5–2.0
Nulliparity	1.5
Early pregnancy, age <21	↓ risk by 60%
Early castration without hormone replacement	Marked reduction in risk
Prolonged hormone replacement	1.3
Prolonged oral contraceptives	Debatable effects; may be a risk factor when started at a very "young" age

LCIS = lobular carcinoma in-situ.

tal carcinoma, accounts for 60–80% of invasive breast cancer cases. Carcinoma arising from the lobules is termed **infiltrating lobular carcinoma** and comprises about 10–15% of cases. **In-situ carcinoma** is a tumor that has not broken through the basement membrane and invaded the surrounding stroma. It remains confined within the ducts or lobules. Whereas the lobular form is considered premalignant, with a 25% chance of progression into malignancy, the ductal form is considered a malignancy. Ductal carcinoma in-situ is six times more frequent than lobular carcinoma in-situ.

Other rare forms of breast cancer include **Paget's disease** of the nipple, which presents as an eczematoid dermatitis caused by infiltration of the nipple with an underlying carcinoma. **Inflammatory breast carcinoma** is a distinct clinical entity presenting as erythema and edema of the overlying skin due to extensive involvement of the dermal lymphatics from an underlying aggressive ductal carcinoma.

The current concept of breast cancer is that it may be systemic almost from inception. Involvement of the regional lymph nodes is a marker for likely metastasis to other sites.

■ Clinical Features

The usual clinical presentation is a painless "lump" or localized thickening (fibrosis) in the breast. The majority of breast lumps are discovered by the patient herself. However, most breast masses are not cancer. Breast masses in premenopausal women are usually due to fibrocystic disease or fibroadenoma. Additional causes for masses in the postmenopausal age group are sclerosing adenosis, fibrocystic disease, fibroadenomas or fat necrosis due to unappreciated trauma. However, the frequency of cancer increases with age.

With screening, early breast cancer may present as a mammographic abnormality, before it is detectable on breast examination. Typically, the physical examination reveals a localized, firm mass or thickening of the breast tissue. In more advanced cancer, there may be dimpling or puckering of the overlying skin, distortion of the breast or nipple, or palpable axillary or supraclavicular nodes. More locally advanced cancer is characterized by skin fixation, ulceration, adjacent skin nodules or inflammatory skin changes.

Pain or discomfort, while more common in nonmalignant breast conditions, is sometimes a presenting symptom in breast cancer. Rarely, the patient will report an axillary mass with or without an evident breast abnormality. Nipple discharge is most often due to benign intraductal papillomas, but cancer must always be excluded.

Metastases cause symptoms related to the area of involvement (e.g., bone pain). Less frequent symptoms are due to liver or CNS involvement.

■ Diagnosis, Clinical Evaluation, and Staging

When a breast mass is discovered clinically or on mammography, the diagnosis must be established pathologically. In premenopausal women, a painful, cystic mass may be observed for resolution through one menstrual cycle to exclude the possibility of fibrocystic disease, but any persistent or suspicious mass must be promptly biopsied. **Mammography** is always done before biopsy to evaluate the appearance of the mass and both breasts (Figure 195.1). **Ultrasonography** may also be valuable in distinguishing solid from cystic masses.

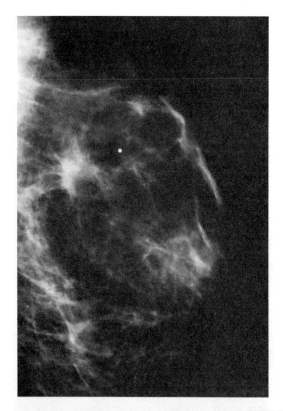

FIGURE 195.1. Mammographic findings in breast cancer. The characteristic findings associated with cancer are a spiculated irregular mass or clustered microcalcification. Only a biopsy procedure can establish whether a mammographically detectable lesion is benign or malignant.

TABLE 195.2.	TNM Staging of Breast Cancer
Tumor	
T_{1s}	Carcinoma in-situ
T_1	Tumor <2 cm in diameter
T_2	Tumor >2 cm but <5 cm
T_3	Tumor >5 cm
T_4	Extension to chest wall; skin edema, ulceration, satellite nodules on breast; inflammatory carcinoma
Nodes	
N_0	No clinically palpable nodes
N_1	Movable ipsilateral axillary nodes
N_2	Nodes (ipsilateral) fixed to one another or to axillary structure
N_3	Internal mammary nodes
Metastases	
M_0	No metastases
M_1	Metastases including ipsilateral supra-clavicular node

(American Joint Committee on Cancer. Manual for Staging of Cancer. 4th ed. Philadelphia, J.B. Lippincott Company, 1992. Used with permission.)

Palpable abnormalities may be biopsied by fine needle aspiration or direct excision. When mammography shows an abnormality but a mass is not palpable, radiologically guided fine-needle aspiration or excisional biopsy with needle or wire localization is necessary.

Fine-needle aspiration (FNA) of cystic lesions can accurately exclude cancer, but clinical and mammographic follow-up is necessary to ensure that the apparently benign disease process behaves as expected. FNA of tumors presenting as solid masses is about 90% sensitive. It is technically simple and, when positive for carcinoma, is reliable, the false-positive rate being 1–2%. Because virtually all solid masses will be subsequently excised for definitive diagnosis or therapy, the accuracy of FNA is acceptable and allows the patient and physician to plan subsequent treatment interventions. However, a negative or indeterminate cytologic result in a patient with a solid mass mandates subsequent excision and definitive histologic examination.

Further clinical evaluation after the diagnosis of cancer includes reevaluation of the physical examination, chest x-ray, and screening blood studies. Following primary surgery to remove the lump and the pathologic examination of the primary tumor and axillary lymph nodes, **TNM staging** can be completed (Table 195.2) and a decision made regarding further staging procedures and subsequent treatment. Additional tests may include CT scans of chest, abdomen, and pelvis, or a radionuclide bone scan to exclude metastases. These tests are not mandatory in low-stage disease (i.e., $T_1N_0M_0$), in the absence of signs or symptoms suggestive of metastases.

The size of the tumor and the presence of involved axillary nodes remain the principal **prognostic factors.** The presence of hormone receptors for estrogen (ER) or progesterone (PR) is important in deciding on the use of adjuvant hormone therapy. Flow cytometric analysis gives information on DNA content (ploidy) and proliferative activity (S phase). Table 195.3 lists the more important prognostic factors in the approximate hierarchy of relative importance.

■ Management

Management of noninvasive (in-situ) carcinoma

Lobular carcinoma in-situ does not present as a mass or mammographic findings but as an incidental histologic finding in biopsy specimens taken for other reasons. It signifies increased later cancer risk in either breast (20–30% incidence over 15–20 yrs). Careful annual screening for cancer is recommended. Prophylactic bilateral mastectomy is the only alternative for women unwilling to accept the risk of subsequent cancer.

Ductal carcinoma in-situ may present as a lump or mammographic abnormality. The size of the lesion and the histology influence the choice of treatment: tumor excision (lumpectomy) alone for very small lesions; or excision followed by radiotherapy for larger lesions to reduce the risk of local relapse. Alternatively, a mastectomy is usually curative, but for most patients it is cosmetically less desirable than a "breast-sparing" lumpectomy and radiotherapy.

Local therapy for invasive cancer

Surgery, radiation therapy, and systemic adjuvant therapy are all used in the treatment of localized invasive breast cancer. For local (primary) treatment, choices between lumpectomy plus radiotherapy, segmental resection plus radiotherapy, and total (modified radical) mastectomy depend on the disease stage and entail a thorough discussion between the patient and physician. Studies have established that **"breast-conserving" therapy** (lumpectomy plus radiation) is as effective as total mastectomy and axillary lymph node dissection for the treatment of most stage I and II cancers. Most women desire breast preservation for cosmetic reasons, but the slightly higher risk of local recurrence must be thoroughly explained.

In general the concept of breast-conserving therapy relates to the understanding that the control of local disease depends first upon the adequate surgical resection of the primary tumor. Cosmetic results depend upon the relative size of the tumor and breast. Thus unless there are unusual biological issues such as nipple involvement or multicentric disease (see below) patients have the options of either mastectomy or lumpectomy plus radiation. Even if technically feasible, removal of a large tumor from a small breast will result in an inferior cosmetic result. Such patients are better served with a mastectomy and reconstruction. As with all cancer operations there must be clear post-resection surgical margins. Thus some patients' tumors do not lend themselves to simple lumpectomy based upon the location of the tumor. Multiple tumors which are multifocal (more than one distinct tumor in the same quadrant of the breast) can be managed with such surgery, whereas patients with multiple tumors in different quadrants of the breast (multicentric tumors) should undergo mastectomy. This latter recommendation relates not only to cosmetic issues but also to the principle of conservative therapy.

Treatment of breast cancer mandates either removal of all breast tissue (mastectomy) or subsequent radiation to residual breast tissue after lumpectomy to eradicate not only any residual disease, but also to deal with possible occult additional microscopic primary tumors in other areas of remaining breast tissue. Experience has shown that patients with multicentric disease have an unacceptable risk of relapse after breast-conserving therapy. When mastectomy is selected, with rare exception, the classic "Halstead mastectomy" is almost never performed in the modern era. This surgical technique evolved a century ago when the concept of an "en bloc" cancer operation was invented. To accomplish this goal one had to remove not only the

TABLE 195.3. Prognostic Factors in Operable Breast Cancer		
Factor/Criterion	**Favorable**	**Unfavorable**
Nodal status	Histologically negative nodes	Increasing number of positive nodes
Tumor size	<1 cm	Increasing tumor size
Tumor grade	Well-differentiated	Poorly differentiated
Hormone receptors	ER+/PR+, ER−/PR+	ER+/PR− esp. ER−/PR−
DNA analysis	Diploid, low S phase (varies with laboratory)	Aneuploid, high S phase (usually >5)
Oncogene amplification	<5 copies HER2/NEU	>5 copies HER2/NEU

ER = estrogen receptor; PR = progesterone receptor.

breast, but the underlying pectoralis muscles and fascia. It included complete removal of all three levels of axillary nodes. While definitive, it had excessive morbidity, and most importantly did not dramatically change the risk of relapse. Rather, a modified or simple mastectomy is performed to accomplish the goal of removing the tumor, remaining breast tissue and to sample the ipsilateral axillary lymph nodes to assess potential spread of disease. By omitting resection of the chest wall musculature, and only "sampling" the axillary nodes, morbidity is significantly reduced, while disease control is unchanged. By doing a less morbid procedure, reconstructive surgery can more easily be performed, either simultaneously or at a later date, with excellent results. If lumpectomy is selected adjuvant radiotherapy is usually initiated within 3–6 weeks of lumpectomy and administered over 6–7 weeks, unless there was evidence of lymph node involvement [$TxN_{1-2}M_0$] disease, in which case adjuvant chemotherapy is usually interposed between the lumpectomy and radiation.

Systemic adjuvant therapy for operable breast cancer

Relapse after primary locoregional therapy usually occurs in distant sites and is primarily the result of prior occult micrometastases. Recurrent breast cancer is with rare exception incurable. Adjuvant (prophylactic) therapy can reduce the risk of relapse in all patients; studies are underway to determine the most optimal regimens and which patients benefit most of the various options noted in Table 195.4. Most patients with tumors exceeding 1 cm or with evidence of metastasis in the lymph nodes (node-positive) are routinely given **combination chemotherapy** following surgery and irradiation; in postmenopausal women, especially those with estrogen-receptor (ER) positive tumors, **hormonal treatment** with the antiestrogen drug tamoxifen is now standard, and it may be combined with chemotherapy. Combination chemotherapy for 4–6 cycles is most effective for patients below 50 years of age (premenopausal); hormonal therapy is more effective in older patients (postmenopausal). Both

TABLE 195.4.   Adjuvant Systemic Therapies for Breast Cancer

Regimen	Agents/Dosage	Duration/Adjuvant	Comments
Chemotherapy			
CMF	Cyclophosphamide, 100 mg/m² on days 1–14 Methotrexate, 40 mg/m² IV on days 1 and 8 5FU, 600 mg/m² IV on days 1 and 8	6–12 cycles q 28 days	40–50% response in metastatic disease
CMF(IV)	Cyclophosphamide, 600 mg/m² Methotrexate, 40 mg/m² 5FU, 600 mg/m²	6–12 cycles q 21 days	Less active in metastatic disease than CMF
CAF	Same as CMF, except Doxorubicin, 30 mg/m² IV instead of methotrexate on days 1 and 8	6 cycles q 28 days	50–70% response in metastatic disease
FAC	Cyclophosphamide, 500 mg/m²; Doxorubicin, 50 mg/m²; 5FU, 500 mg/m² IV on days 1 and 8	6 cycles q 22 days	Similar activity to CAF
AC	Doxorubicin, 60 mg/m² IV; Cyclophosphamide, 600 mg/m² IV	4 cycles q 21 days	Similar to CAF & FAC
Hormonal therapy			
Oophorectomy	Surgical, radiation or GnRH agonists	N/A	Used in premenopausal women; alternative to tamoxifen
Tamoxifen	10 mg BID	2–5 yrs	First-line endocrine therapy for postmenopausal patients
Megestrol	40 mg QID	N/A	Second line after tamoxifen
Androgens	Fluoxymesterone, 10 mg BID	N/A	Third line, rarely used
Aminoglutethimide	250 mg QID, plus Hydrocortisone, 30 mg qd	N/A	Third line

5FU = 5 Fluorouracil; GnRH = gonadotropin releasing hormone.

TABLE 195.5.	Recommendations for Adjuvant Therapy of Operable Breast Cancer		
Menopausal Status	**Nodal Status**	**Hormone Receptor (ER/PR)**	**Therapy Options***
Premenopausal	–	+	Chemotherapy + Tamoxifen†
Premenopausal or Postmenopausal	+	–	Chemotherapy
Postmenopausal	–	+	Tamoxifen ± chemotherapy††
Postmenopausal	+	+	Tamoxifen ± chemotherapy††
Elderly (>70–75 yrs)	Any	Any	Tamoxifen§
Tumor <1 cm (pre- and postmenopausal)	–	Any	Usually no adjuvant therapy

*Chemotherapy: 4–6 mo of standard combinations; tamoxifen for 2–5 years.
†Tamoxifen is an alternative in node-negative patients.
††Chemotherapy may add benefit.
§Fit patients of high risk may receive chemotherapy.

significantly lower the risk of relapse. Current recommendations are listed in Table 195.5.

In contrast to the excellent prognosis in patients with minimal disease (i.e., a small primary lesion and no nodal involvement), the prognosis worsens in patients with positive axillary nodes; over 85% with 10 or more positive nodes eventually relapse. A promising investigational regimen combines conventional therapy with combination chemotherapy followed by **high-dose chemotherapy with reconstitution** using previously harvested autologous bone marrow or peripheral blood stem cells.

Management of locally advanced breast cancer

Locally advanced disease is defined as tumors or axillary lymph nodes with fixation to the chest wall, extensive ulceration or satellite cutaneous nodules, or inflammatory cancer with diffuse dermal involvement. In all these presentations, mastectomy alone rarely effects local control. However, combining initial or **"neoadjuvant" chemotherapy** with subsequent radiotherapy and/or surgery leads to control of disease in 30–40% of patients.

Follow-up after primary treatment

Long term follow-up is essential after primary treatment. In asymptomatic patients, laboratory and radiological studies should only be performed if the patient is symptomatic, the physician concerned about persistent toxicities, or the patient is in an extremely high-risk group, and would be a candidate for unique follow-up therapy if there were relapse. Continued vigilance and prompt investigation of symptoms remain the best policy. New cancers occur in the contralateral breast at the rate of 1% annually. A relapse of the first cancer or a new cancer in the original breast will ultimately develop in 5–10% of patients. Thus, previously treated patients must be followed carefully and screened with annual breast examinations and mammog-

TABLE 195.6.	Decisions in Managing Recurrent/Metastatic Breast Cancer

- Confirm *first* apparent relapse by histology or cytology if feasible
- Re-stage using original spectrum of tests, including clinical, CT and bone scans, serum chemistries
- Select proper systemic therapy (Table 195.7)
- Hormone-receptor positive, long disease–free interval, few metastatic sites, soft tissue or bone → endocrine approach initially
  Hormone-receptor negative, multiple extensive metastases, symptomatic visceral metastases, failures of endocrine therapy → combination chemotherapy
  Radiation for palliation of locally refractory disease
  supportive care
- Identify, and pre-emptively treat impending emergent conditions
  Brain, epidural metastases → steroids, radiation
  Impending pathologic fracture → fixation, radiation

raphy. Historically, 5–30% of patients with negative axillary lymph nodes would relapse within 10 years, compared to 30–70% of those with positive nodes.

Being relapse-free for 5 years does not guarantee cure in breast cancer. Adjuvant therapy reduces the risk of recurrence by 5–20%, but the risk of metastasis is life-long. The most common sites of metastatic spread are bone (40–50%), soft tissue, regional lymph nodes, the contralateral breast (10–30%), and lung or pleura (25%).

Management of metastases

The approach to metastatic disease is summarized in Table 195.6. In general aggressive diagnostic evaluation is appropriate when relapse is suspected. In most instances circumstantial evidence is convincing that newly discovered lesions are relapsed breast cancer, but many older women are also at risk to develop other cancers (e.g., colon, lung). Therefore, if possible, biopsy documentation is desirable at the apparent first relapse. With the advent of fine needle aspirate (FNA) biopsies, most lesions can be successfully documented to be recurrent cancer. The diagnosis of metastatic disease has serious implications since it is rarely curable. The median survival of patients with relapsed breast cancer is 2–3 years; 15–25% will survive 5 years, and 5–10%, 10 years. Restaging is important once relapse has occurred. Patterns of involvement dictate specific interventions. Radiation with or without orthopedic stabilization of impending fractures can preserve mobility and prevent paraplegia; brain metastases which are relatively resistant to chemotherapy because of the blood-brain barrier can also be palliated by radiation.

Patterns of disease recurrence are important determinants of subsequent therapy. Hormonal therapy is often successful in patients who have had a long interval between initial therapy and relapse. This is especially true in post-menopausal women with exclusively or predominantly osseous metastases. A high proportion of such cancers in this age group are estrogen and/or progesterone receptor positive, which predicts successful hormonal therapy. Conversely women who are premenopausal often have receptor negative cancers. They are somewhat more likely to relapse earlier, and often have predominantly visceral disease such as liver or lung metastases. These patients rarely respond to hormonal therapies. Table 195.7 outlines treatment options in addition to emergent care. In general the selection of treatment modalities is based upon empiric knowledge, clinical trials, and hormonal status (positive estrogen and/or progesterone receptor analysis). The strategy in such patients is to maximize control of disease while minimizing morbidity of therapy. Thus, compared to initial adjuvant treatments, chemotherapy regimens are less intensive, utilize fewer drugs at any one time, and are given for more prolonged periods. In the case of hormonal treatments, response to one intervention often predicts the response to further hormonal treatment. Thus unless the pattern of disease changes, patients successfully treated with one hormonal program often benefit from further therapies (Table 195.7). Supportive care with pain management, nutritional support, and psychological counseling are all important aspects of good medical care.

■ Complications

Surgery with axillary dissection may result in postoperative lymphedema—swelling of the arm due to blockage of lymphatic vessels—which may develop months or even years later. **Radiation therapy** causes minor, transient, acute erythema and edema of the breast in most patients; later, scarring, shrinkage, and distortion

TABLE 195.7.	Treatment Options in Recurrent or Metastatic Breast Cancer
Hormonal Therapy	**Chemotherapy**
First line	First line
Oophorectomy–(surgical, radiation, or GnRH agonists)	CMF
Tamoxifen	CAF
Megestrol acetate	CNF
Second line	Second line
Androgens	Paclitaxel (Taxol)
Estrogens (DES)	Docetaxel (Taxotere)
Aromatase inhibitors (aminoglutethimide)	Vinorelbine (Navelbine)
	Vinblastine (Velban) + Mitomycin-C
Prednisone	Methotrexate + calcium leucovoran

CMF = cyclophosphamide, methotrexate, 5-fluorouracil; CAF = cyclophosphamide, adriamycin, 5-fluorouracil; CNF = cyclophosphamide, Novantrone (mitoxantrone), 5-fluorouracil.

of the breast, delayed lymphedema, radionecrosis of ribs or clavicle, and brachial plexus neuropathy may follow. **Chemotherapy** produces anorexia; alopecia, fatigability, and myelosuppression in most patients (see Tables 191.2 and 191.3). **Tamoxifen** therapy produces or worsens a hypoestrogenic state with menopausal-like symptoms and may induce the development of endometrial cancer (although the reduction in risk of breast cancer relapse far outweighs the possible risk of inducing endometrial cancer).

■ Prevention of Breast Cancer

Primary prevention by early pregnancy or dietary modification is neither feasible nor of proven value. A trial of secondary prevention using tamoxifen has recently demonstrated a 47% reduction in occurrence of breast cancer in high-risk patients. With the advent of genetic screening for high risk patients with the newly discovered BRCA-1 and BRCA-2 genes, the issue of prophylactic mastectomy has resurfaced. Of theoretical benefit in selected patients, such drastic interventions impact significantly upon the patient's body image; besides, the exact risk of breast cancer in such genetically prone families is still controversial.

■ Screening and Case-Finding in Asymptomatic Persons

Screening of women at risk for breast cancer is key to its early detection. **Breast examination** is not easy, and the skill of the examiner is pivotal to avoid missing or overdiagnosing cancers. Although breast examinations by physicians and other health professionals are important and cause a significant number of the cancers to be diagnosed, the physician must realize that patients can often feel masses which the physician can not. **Breast self-examination** has been recommended for years and is widely taught, but many older patients are reluctant to practice it. In addition, randomized trials have not yet confirmed its worth. The physician must always take the patient's report of a breast mass seriously; the report should either prompt immediate follow-up with mammography and consultation or initiate a careful follow-up at short intervals to determine whether it is related to cyclical hormonal changes as in premenopausal patients. The alleged failure of a physician to diagnose breast cancers earlier, especially if the patient's reported signs or symptoms are apparently ignored by her physician, constitutes a common cause for litigation.

Mammography has been used since the 1960s for screening asymptomatic women and evaluating palpable breast abnormalities. Screening asymptomatic women aged 50 years or more at intervals of 1–3 years has been widely accepted because of convincing data that breast cancer mortality can be lowered by 25–30%. Although similar data in younger women is less convincing, a recent consensus panel concluded that annual mammography should begin at age 40, or even earlier in high-risk cases based on family history and/or genetic predisposition. It remains uncertain whether women over 70 need yearly mammograms as opposed to every 2–3 years.

■ Breast Cancer in Men

Only 1400 cases of breast cancer occur annually in men in the United States. The disease biology and treatment are identical to those in women. Breast cancer typically is clinically advanced at diagnosis in men.

CHAPTER 196 CARCINOMA OF THE LUNG

■ Incidence and Epidemiology

Lung cancer was rare until cigarette smoking became endemic. The age-adjusted lung cancer mortality in men has risen from 11/100,000 in 1940 to 73/100,00 today. In women, whose endemic smoking patterns began a generation later, the rate rose from 5/100,000 in 1960 to 32/100,000 today. With nearly 178,100 new cases and 160,400 deaths yearly, lung cancer is by far the most important cancer in the United States. The incidence and mortality of these cancers has finally begun to decrease in men, although unfortunately they are still increasing in women.

■ Etiology

Cigarette smoking continues to be the major cause of lung cancer. Lung cancer is more prevalent in urban populations. Certain occupations predispose to lung cancer; these include asbestos exposure, uranium mining, exposure to arsenic and nickel. Known or suspected cofactors include exposure to radon, beryllium, mustard gas, and various hydrocarbons. Concurrent cigarette smoke exposure exerts a synergistic role in many of these. Passive smoke inhalation by the spouses of heavy smokers may account for as many as 8,000 cases annually.

Patients should be strongly encouraged and taught to stop smoking, because continued tobacco use results in an increased relative risk of 12 or greater. Smoking cessation lowers the risk after 5–10 years, but an increased relative risk, of about 1.5 compared to nonsmokers, remains indefinitely.

■ Pathogenesis

Tobacco smoke, ionizing radiation, and industrial carcinogens are believed to exert a multistep carcinogenic process in the bronchial epithelium, where areas of dysplasia and metaplasia progress to carcinoma in-situ and then to invasive cancer. Molecular genetic studies show frequent loss of alleles on chromosome 3, especially in small cell carcinoma; mutations and deletions in the p53 gene in all cell types; and reported mutations in the *RB, ras,* and c-*myc* genes.

■ Pathology

The four basic types of lung cancer are adenocarcinoma, small cell, epidermoid (squamous cell), and large cell (Figure 196.1). A simple, widely used classification divides lung cancers into **small cell** and **non-small cell** types, reflecting the generally systemic nature of small cell lung cancer, which entails a minor role for surgery. With the exception of adenocarcinomas, which frequently occur in peripheral lung zones, most lung cancers arise in proximal bronchi.

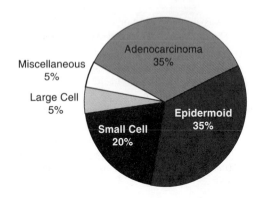

FIGURE 196.1. Lung cancer cell types. Epidermoid and adenocarcinoma are the two frequent histologic types. The miscellaneous group includes bronchoalveolar, giant cell, and mucoepidermoid types.

■ Clinical Features

The usual presentations in patients with lung cancer are outlined in Table 196.1. Asymptomatic **solitary nodules** are important because of their potential for cure. The frequency of lung cancer among solitary pulmonary nodules is variable and depends on age, characteristics of the nodule, and smoking history (see chapter 242).

Primary symptoms with all cell types include cough and wheezing from bronchial irritation or obstruction, variable degrees of sputum production, and bloody expectoration varying from blood-streaked sputum to frank hemoptysis. A bout of pneumonitis or a lung abscess may be the initial clue to underlying bronchial obstruction from tumor. A pleural effusion is another manifestation.

Chest wall invasion ultimately causes pain. Mediastinal invasion causes dyspnea and/or entrapment of the recurrent laryngeal nerve(s), producing a voice change due to vocal cord paralysis. If right-sided, it can cause the superior vena cava syndrome, featuring pain and swelling in the face and upper extremities. Cancers arising from the apex of the lung may invade the brachial plexus, leading to shoulder and arm pain or weakness ("Pancoast's tumor", or superior sulcus tumor, Figure 196.2).

Metastatic disease is seen at presentation in the majority of patients, justifying an extensive preoperative workup. Related paraneoplastic syndromes are listed in Table 196.1.

■ Diagnosis, Clinical Evaluation, and Staging

Additional information on diagnosing and evaluating lung cancer appears in Chapter 241. Physical examination may detect supraclavicular adenopathy, pleural effusion or atelectasis, the localized wheeze of bronchial obstruction, weight loss, clubbing of the fingers (Figure 196.3 A & B), or signs of gross metastatic disease. Laboratory tests are designed to uncover anemia (complete blood count), hepatic dysfunction (alkaline phosphatase, serum albumin, lactate dehydrogenase) hypercalcemia, hyponatremia, and metabolic alkalosis.

Cytologic examination of sputum may provide a definitive, noninvasive clue, especially in central lesions arising from the bronchi; it is less accurate with peripheral nodules ("coin" lesions). Cytologic and histologic specimens are obtained from peripheral lesions through transthoracic fine needle aspiration or core biopsy, and centrally located tumors are usually accessed via bronchoscopy. Fiberoptic bronchoscopy is an essential tool in the diagnosis and staging of bronchogenic carcinoma. Imaging studies used during preinvasive diagnostic studies and/or as staging studies after diagnosis include chest radiographs (Figure 196.4), CT scans of the chest, abdomen, and pelvis, radionuclide bone scans, and a CT or magnetic resonance scan (MRI) of the brain.

Small cell lung cancer is not treated surgically; it is "staged" as **limited** (confined to the ipsilateral thorax and supraclavicular nodes) or **extensive,** based on the same tests used for all lung cancer patients. Regardless of the clinical stage, this disease is virtually always widely disseminated. Thus, all patients undergoing treatment receive systemic chemotherapy. The cure rate for patients with disease limited to the chest is 15–30%; the disease is incurable for patients with extensive disease. In contrast, **non-small cell lung**

TABLE 196.1.	Clinical Features of Lung Cancer
Type/Extent	**Features**
Solitary pulmonary nodule	Asymptomatic
Primary symptoms	Cough, hemoptysis, dyspnea and wheezing, fever due to secondary infection
Regional effects	Hoarseness, superior vena cava syndrome, superior sulcus invasion, Horner's syndrome, pleural and pericardial effusions, esophageal compression, phrenic nerve paralysis
Metastasis	Brain, bone, liver, adrenal
Systemic	Paraneoplastic endocrinopathy: SIADH, Cushing's syndrome, hypertrophic pulmonary osteoarthropathy, gynecomastia, weight loss, Eaton-Lambert syndrome (Chapter 206)

SIADH = syndrome of inappropriate ADH secretion.

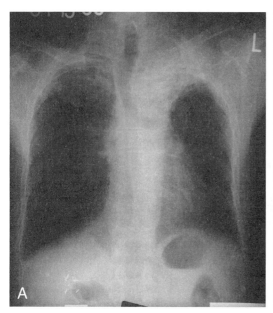
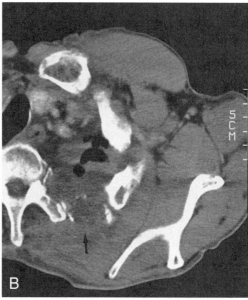

FIGURE 196.2. Pancoast's tumor (superior sulcus tumor) in lung cancer. A. Left shoulder pain and a new left apical lesion developed during long-term follow-up of this patient for previous tuberculosis. B. CT scan (magnified view) showed the lesion and associated destruction of the overlying rib (arrow).

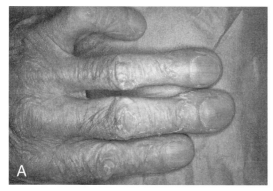
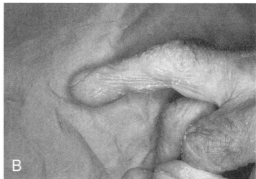

FIGURE 196.3. Finger clubbing in bronchogenic carcinoma. A. frontal view. B. profile.

cancer requires meticulous staging because of the potential for surgical cure (Table 196.2).

▪ Management

One cannot overemphasize the systemic nature of **small cell cancer** and the necessity of systemic chemo-

therapy, even in patients with **limited-stage** disease. Untreated patients with this cancer have a median survival of only months. However in most patients who undergo treatment the survival is meaningfully prolonged and the quality of life improved. Patients with disease limited to the ipsilateral thorax respond to chemotherapy with or without consolidation radiotherapy in almost

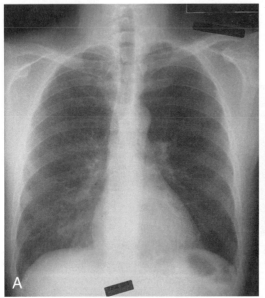

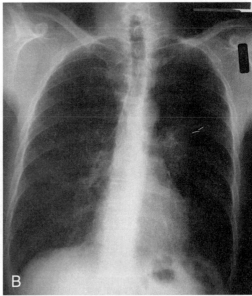

FIGURE 196.4. Chest radiographs in bronchogenic carcinoma. **A,** A prior chest radiograph was normal. **B,** Three years later, the chest film shows a left hilar mass *(arrow).* Adenocarcinoma was diagnosed by bronchoscopy.
(Courtesy of Jeffery Postles, MD, Wauwatosa, Wisconsin.)

TABLE 196.2.   Simplified Staging of Lung Cancer

Stage	Description
Small cell lung cancer	
Limited	Limited to one hemithorax
Extensive	Beyond one hemithorax
Non-small cell lung cancer	
TNM Stage	
I	T_1 (tumor <3 cm) or T_2 (tumor >3 cm); N_0
II	T_1 or T_2 tumors; N_1 (positive peribronchial or hilar nodes)
IIIA	T_3 (tumor invading chest wall, mediastinal pleura, or in main bronchus <2 cm from carina, or atelectasis of entire lung) N_0-N_1
	T_1-T_3 with N_2 (Ipsilateral mediastinal lymph nodes)
IIIB	Any T with N_3 nodes (contralateral or ipsilateral scalene, supraclavicular)
	T_4 (tumor invading deep mediastinal structures or malignant pleural effusion); any N
IV	M_1 (metastases)

(Manual for Staging of Cancer. 4th ed. See suggested reading list.)

90% of cases. Instead of a median survival of only 2-4 months in untreated cases, survival in treated patients exceed 1 year; most importantly a small subset (15–30%) of patients are alive and free of disease at two years, and are potentially cured. Patients with extensive disease also respond to therapy; about 80% of patients have a meaningful regression of disease, with improvement in their cancer symptoms. Their survival is also prolonged from 1–3 months to 8–12 months.

However, because virtually all such patients are doomed to relapse, experienced oncologists treat patients with advanced cancer with less toxic regimens than the potentially curable patient with limited stage disease. A large number of chemotherapy regimens exist, generally based on the use of a platinum-containing compound (cis-platin or carboplatin), combined with either VP-16 or Taxol. Treatment is given until best response is obtained, usually 4–6 cycles of treatment. Selected patients with limited stage disease are considered for thoracic radiation to areas of original involvement to maximize both local disease control and the chance of cure. In patients with advanced disease radiation is reserved for palliation of lesions not responsive to chemotherapy.

Non-small cell cancer is treated surgically, if possible, with the magnitude of resection being determined by the extent of involvement. Unfortunately the prognosis still remains dismal in most patients. About 60% of patients have unresectable disease prior to thoracotomy; another 25% are found to be unresectable during surgery. Thus, less than 20% of all patients undergo a potentially curative procedure. Furthermore, only about 50% of patients successfully undergoing such surgery are truly cured. Thus the overall survival of lung cancer patients is still dismal, and unlike in breast cancer, the survival rate is only minimally affected by adjuvant radiotherapy or chemotherapy.

Patients believed to have unresectable tumors, due to extensive locoregional disease, or having medical contraindications to surgery can be treated with radiation therapy. Long-term survival, and even a small chance of cure (<5–10%), can be obtained in selected patients. Chemotherapy has only modest palliative benefit in advanced stages of non-small cell lung cancer.

◼ Complications

Surgical procedures carry a 30-day overall mortality of 4%. Postoperative pulmonary compromise can be very limiting in patients with coexisting chronic obstructive lung disease. Radiation may cause transient esophagitis, bronchitis, and occasionally pneumonitis; delayed complications include constrictive pericarditis and small-vessel myocardial disease. Toxicity from chemotherapeutic agents include myelosuppression, renal dysfunction and possible neurotoxicity.

A second lung cancer or a cancer of the head and neck region may develop in survivors of an initial lung cancer of any type. Depending on risk factors (smoking being the most important), new cancers occur at a rate of 1–5% annually for at least 10 years after the successful treatment of the original cancer (rates even higher with continued smoking).

◼ Prognosis

As noted, only the small subsets of patients with limited stage disease are potentially curable. Thus, the overall 5-year survival of lung cancer patients is only 14% (Figure 196.5). Persons with lung cancer presenting as a **solitary nodule** (<3 cm) and no lymph node involvement ($T_1N_0M_0$) may have a 5-year survival rate of 80%. **Small cell lung cancer,** when limited in extent, has a median survival of 12–18 months, a 2-year survival of 15–30%, and a 5-year survival of 10–15%. Death occurring after 2 years following treatment is often due to a new cancer. Patients with extensive disease have a median survival of 7–12 months and survival of 2% or less at 2 or more years.

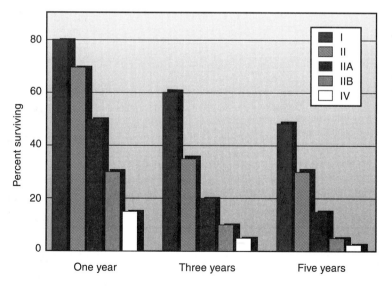

FIGURE 196.5. Survival in non-small cell lung cancer according to stage. Treatments for various stages included: stages I and II, surgery; stage IIIA, surgery and radiation; stage IIIB, radiation; stage IV, supportive care and chemotherapy.
(Adapted from: Mountain CF Semin Oncol 1988;15:2236–245.)

CHAPTER 197 GASTROINTESTINAL CANCERS

O f the 225,900 new cancers involving the gastrointestinal (GI) tract annually, roughly two-thirds (131,200) involve the colon and rectum. The other cancers are pancreatic (27,600), gastric (22,400), hepatobiliary (20,500), and esophageal (12,500). The incidence of gastric cancer continues to decline in the United States, and mortality from colorectal cancer, especially in women, has declined since 1940. Only colorectal cancers will be discussed in this chapter.

Colorectal Cancer

■ Epidemiology, Pathogenesis, and Pathology

The incidence and epidemiology of colorectal cancer (CRC) are reviewed in chapter 93; risk factors for CRC are shown in Table 197.1. The predominant histologic type in CRC is adenocarcinoma; sarcomas, lymphomas, and carcinoid tumors are very uncommon. Tumors are described as polypoid, flat, ulcerating, and constricting.

Regional lymph node **metastases** follow infiltration into the bowel wall, and the peritoneum may also be a major site of metastases, once transmural growth occurs. For colonic cancers, hematogenous spread occurs initially to the liver via the portal venous system. The rectal or anal areas drain via the inferior hemorrhoidal veins and thus bypass the hepatic capillary bed; cancers of these areas may present with pulmonary metastases.

Tumors in the cecum are frequently superficially ulcerated and bulky, but are less likely to infiltrate circumferentially within colonic musculature. These tumors are usually more advanced at the time of diagnosis. Conversely, most tumors of the descending colon or rectosigmoid tend to infiltrate the muscular layers, leading to luminal, concentric narrowing and thus, a "napkin ring" (or applecore) lesion on barium enema (Figure 197.1).

■ Clinical Features

The primary symptoms and signs of colorectal cancer depend on the location of the tumor (see chapter 93). More often, right-sided lesions produce subtle alterations in bowel habits and iron-deficiency anemia; **Rectal** cancer and **low sigmoid** cancers produce blood-streaked stools and obstructive symptoms. Obstruction may be the first feature and occur abruptly without antecedent symptoms. Weight loss, ascites, hepatomegaly, and multiple abdominal masses suggest metastases. More advanced lesions cause pain from nerve infiltration and invasion of neighboring structures. Urinary symptoms include bleeding and obstruction from invasion of the bladder or prostate. Lymphatic or venous obstruction may cause leg swelling.

■ Diagnosis, Clinical Evaluation, and Staging

Although many benign rectosigmoid lesions can bleed, any case of rectal bleeding should arouse a suspicion of cancer. The rectum extends to about 13–15 cm from the anal verge, and the digital rectal examination, while able to explore only 8–10 cm of the rectum, is still a useful first test, to be followed by proctoscopy if negative.

The prolonged preclinical phase (8–10 years) of colorectal cancer and its association with adenomatous

TABLE 197.1. Risk Factors for Colorectal Carcinoma	
Factor	**Association**
Age	>50 yrs
Diet	Increased incidence with high fat intake
Inflammatory bowel disease	Highest risk with ulcerative colitis of entire colon; less so with Crohn's disease
Previous adenomatous polyps	Believed to be precursor lesions; increasing risk with size >1 cm and villous or tubulovillous histology
Hereditary:	
Multiple polyposis/ Gardner's syndrome	Autosomal dominant
Hereditary non-polyposis colon cancer	Autosomal dominant
Family History	1.7–3.0× increase in first-degree relatives
Previous pelvic radiation	Rectal cancer
Ureterosigmoidostomy	Sigmoid cancer
History of breast, ovarian or endometrial cancer	Moderate risk factor

polyps have led to the recommendation of screening, case finding, and removal of any polyps encountered in asymptomatic persons. **Screening tools** include fecal occult blood testing (FOBT), digital rectal examination, proctoscopy, flexible sigmoidoscopy to 35–60 cm, and colonoscopy to examine the entire colon. Radiological

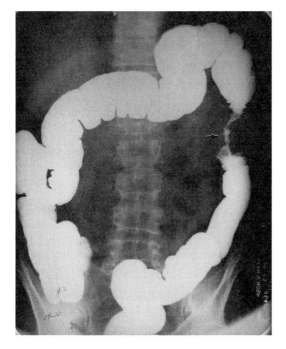

FIGURE 197.1. Barium enema showing an applecore lesion *(arrow)* in the sigmoid colon, indicative of a colorectal tumor circumferentially infiltrating the muscular layers.
(Courtesy of Radiology Museum, St. Joseph's Hospital, Milwaukee, Wisconsin.)

imaging consists of the **air-contrast barium enema.** The effectiveness of these screening tests in detecting colorectal neoplasms is shown in Figure 197.2.

Suggestions for screening and surveillance are provided in Table 93.2 (see chapter 93). Logically, screening in patients known to be at higher risk because of a family history or known predisposing conditions (Table 197.1) should begin at a younger age and be repeated frequently. All polyps should be removed if possible; polyposis patients must face the prospect of prophylactic colectomy. Because it takes years for transformation of a small precursor polyp into a malignant tumor, there are multiple opportunities to detect the disease before invasion occurs, as long as the patient and physician maintain a screening program.

Screening studies have shown that 1–4 % of FOBT will be positive. Most patients with a positive FOBT have hemorrhoids, anal fissures or diverticula and not cancer. The incidence of polyps in this group is 30%; only 5–10% of patients with a positive FOBT will have cancer. Initial endoscopy or radiological imaging will detect about 95% of cancers. If bleeding persists, tests should be repeated at least once, and then diseases of the stomach and upper GI tract excluded by appropriate studies. In performing fecal occult blood tests, one must remember that even advanced cancers may bleed only intermittently. Symptoms such as abdominal pain, change in bowel habits, and occult or visible bleeding introduce an extensive differential diagnosis, including diverticular disease, inflammatory bowel disease, and enteric infection by bacteria, viruses, or parasites. Abdominal and bowel complaints without apparent bleeding are extremely common symptoms and often due to irritable bowel syndrome.

When a lesion is identified, the diagnosis of cancer must be established by biopsy, usually obtained by

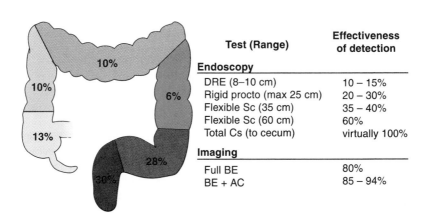

Test (Range)	Effectiveness of detection
Endoscopy	
DRE (8–10 cm)	10 – 15%
Rigid procto (max 25 cm)	20 – 30%
Flexible Sc (35 cm)	35 – 40%
Flexible Sc (60 cm)	60%
Total Cs (to cecum)	virtually 100%
Imaging	
Full BE	80%
BE + AC	85 – 94%

FIGURE 197.2. Distribution of large bowel cancers by anatomic site and their approximate rate of diagnosis by endoscopy and radiologic imaging. BE + AC = Air-contrast barium enema; Cs = colonoscopy; DRE = digital rectal examination; Procto = proctoscopy; Sc = sigmoidoscopy.

endoscopy. Subsequent **preoperative staging** is performed through abdominal and pelvic CT scans to evaluate the liver, kidneys, and ureters. The presence of iron-deficiency anemia confirms a prior significant and repeated blood loss; an elevated alkaline phosphatase or γ-glutamyl transpeptidase level may reflect liver metastases. The serum level of carcinoembryonic antigen (CEA), a tumor marker, is high in one-third of patients having small, early-stage tumors and in 90% of patients with metastases. Knowledge that the CEA level was high prior to surgical resection of a primary tumor allows subsequent rational decisions about the timing and frequency of repeat tests postoperatively. A chest radiograph and a general medical evaluation complete the preoperative workup. A chest CT scan is not indicated in patients with a negative abdominal CT scan if the IV contrast study confirms the liver is free of disease. The TNM and Dukes' staging systems are shown in Table 197.2.

■ Management of Colorectal Cancer

Surgical treatment

Early detection of CRC not only increases the rate of survival but also improves the quality of life for patients. The type and extent of surgery depend on the location of the tumor. In general, a curative surgical operation includes removal of the involved bowel segment, with disease-free surgical margins at each end, and en-bloc removal of the applicable blood vessels and lymphatics. Colostomy, if required, is only temporary. However, patients with extensive disease invading adjacent organs or with rectal tumors less than 5 cm from the anal verge are exceptions, and thus require permanent colostomy. When there is more than one primary tumor or associated multiple polyps, a subtotal or total colectomy may be required.

TABLE 197.2.	Stage Classification of Colon Cancer
AJCC Stage	**Dukes' Stage**
I $T_{1-2}N_0 M_0$	A, B_1
II T_3, $T_4 N_0 M_0$	B_2, B_3
III Any T, N_{1-3}, M_0	C_1, C_2
IV Any T any N M_1	D
T_1	Tumor spread into submucosa
T_2	Tumor spread into muscularis propria
T_3	Tumor spread through muscularis propria
T_4	Tumor spread through wall and visceral peritoneum or direct invasion of adjacent organs
N_1	1-3 involved regional nodes
N_2	4 or more involved nodes
N_3	Second-echelon nodes along a vascular trunk

(Modified from: Manual for Staging of Cancer. 4th ed. See suggested reading list.)

Palliative resections in the face of unresectable metastatic disease usually involve only resection of the colonic segment at risk of perforation or repeated hemorrhage. When the cancer cannot be resected because of adjacent organ infiltration, a "diverting" colostomy is constructed.

Adjuvant treatment of operable colorectal cancer

Postoperative radiotherapy is recommended for all Dukes' B2 or C patients having rectal cancers or colon cancers occurring below the peritoneal reflection (5–25 cm from the anal verge). Such therapy may contribute slightly to overall survival, but more importantly, reduces the risk of local recurrence. Lesions above 25 cm are usually not treated due to the risk of excessive bowel toxicity, and the lower risk of morbidity of recurrence in the tumor bed. Concomitant, or adjuvant chemotherapy decreases the risk of relapse, thus improving survival, especially when combined with radiotherapy.

All patients having colonic cancer with Dukes' C tumors (at high risk of relapse) and probably a subset of high-risk patients with Dukes' B tumors benefit from postoperative adjuvant chemotherapy. Regimens consist of 5-fluorouracil, combined with either calcium leucovorin or levamisole.

Follow-up after initial therapy

Surveillance of the remaining colon is carried out with yearly fecal occult blood tests. Colonoscopy is required at 1 year to exclude recurrence, and if normal, every 3 to 5 years, because these patients are at a higher risk for development of a second cancer as well as relapse of their first. Because of the nature of hematogenous spread via the portal circulation, metastases to the liver are important to identify. Resection of hepatic metastases can significantly prolong patients' lives, and indeed some may be cured by such "metastatectomies" if the number of lesions are limited.

Management of recurrent and metastatic disease

Surgical resection or ablation is offered in selected patients for anastomotic recurrences, new primary tumors, and isolated metastases to lung or liver. Radiation therapy can palliate local recurrence, pelvic masses, and bone metastases. Palliation with chemotherapy incorporates 5-fluorouracil (5-FU) and levamisole or leucovorin. In those patients with unresectable liver metastases without other sites of metastases, arterial perfusions with floxuridine, an analogue of 5-FU, can meaningfully palliate and control the disease over the short-term.

Complications

Diagnostic endoscopy is safe when done by experienced practitioners, and perforation or bleeding is rare. Surgical complications include wound disruption, anastomotic leak, and postoperative pulmonary complications common to older persons. Radiation therapy for rectal cancer can cause chronic cystitis or proctitis (5%). If the small bowel cannot be excluded from the field of radiation during the multiple treatments, late-onset adhesions or strictures may develop. Chemotherapy may cause mucositis, enteritis, and leukopenia. Levamisole may cause liver or CNS dysfunction.

Prognosis

Lesions confined to the mucosa or submucosa (stage I/ Dukes' A) carry an excellent prognosis with 90% or more cured by initial surgical resection. Most (60–85%)

tumors penetrating the bowel wall (stage II/Dukes' B) are still cured. In stage III/Dukes' C patients with 1–3 positive lymph nodes, the 5-year survival is 56%, and for those with 4 or more positive nodes, the survival is 30% or better. Adjuvant 5-FU-based chemotherapy reduces the relapse rate by about 40%, and thereby improves the survival in such patients by 15–20%; a lesser degree of improvement occurs in patients with high-risk stage II/Dukes' B tumors. The same statistics apply to rectal cancers; postoperative radiotherapy in these patients reduces local recurrence. Patients with advanced disease rarely survive beyond 2 years. Chemotherapy can improve the survival and quality of life for many patients; patients responding to chemotherapy live longer than untreated patients (6–12 months).

Cancer of the Esophagus, Stomach, Pancreas, and Liver

Esophageal cancer is discussed in Chapter 72, cancer of the stomach in Chapter 76, and pancreatic cancer, in

Chapter 97. Primary hepatocellular carcinoma is discussed in Chapter 106.

CHAPTER 198 CANCERS OF THE KIDNEY, URINARY BLADDER, AND PROSTATE

Renal Cell Carcinoma

Renal cell carcinoma (hypernephroma) accounted for 28,800 new cases, and 11,300 deaths annually in the United States 1997. It is more prevalent among men by a 2:1 margin. With the exception of familial syndromes, the only established risk factors are age and probably cigarette smoking.

Etiology, Pathogenesis and Pathology

Familial renal cell carcinoma occurs in 30–45% of patients with von Hippel-Lindau disease (syndrome of cerebellar hemangioblastoma and retinal angiomatosis with renal and pancreatic cysts) although clusters of disease occur in some families without this genetic disorder. A consistent deletion in chromosome 3p is seen in von Hippel-Lindau disease, and similar deletions are seen in sporadic renal cell carcinomas, indicating a probable tumor suppressor gene at that locus.

Ninety percent of renal cell carcinomas are adenocarcinomas of the tubular epithelium. The predominant

types are clear cell (most common), granular cell, sarcomatoid, or papillary. Renal tumors are highly vascular—both the primary and metastatic tumors bleed with minimal trauma—and often have a necrotic, cystic appearance.

Limited early by Gerota's fascia, the tumor spreads by direct extension through the kidney and adjacent structures. Regional lymph node metastases and a high incidence of renal vein invasion are common. The latter presents as a tumor thrombus, often extending into the inferior vena cava. Hematogenous metastases are frequent to the lung, liver, bone, and brain. Renal cell carcinomas (like melanomas) are notoriously unpredictable in their behavior.

Clinical Features

Renal cell carcinomas have a variable, often lengthy, preclinical period and may be detected when unrelated conditions lead to abdominal CT or intravenous pyelog-

TABLE 198.1. Manifestations of Renal Cell Carcinoma	
Manifestations	**Incidence %**
Local	
Hematuria	60
Flank pain	40
Mass	40
Surgical triad (hematuria, mass and flank pain)	10
Varicocele	2
Metastasis as the initial presentation	30
Unexplained weight loss	Variable
Systemic	
Fever	20
Anemia	20
Hypercalcemia	5
Erythrocytosis	3
Amyloidosis	1–2
Hypertension	20–30
Hepatic dysfunction without metastasis	10

raphy (IVP). Besides the surgical triad of **hematuria, flank pain,** and a **palpable mass,** there are a variety of associated symptoms related to chronic inflammation and tissue necrosis, such as fever, anemia, weight loss, and paraneoplastic syndromes (e.g., hypercalcemia, polycythemia) (Table 198.1). Because of the tumor's location and frequent lack of symptoms only 45% have disease within the renal capsule; many patients have locally invasive cancer, and 30% have metastatic disease on presentation.

■ Diagnosis, Clinical Evaluation, and Staging

IVP or ultrasound may show a mass. However, IVP is neither very sensitive nor specific, and further workup is indicated if the patient has persistent hematuria or other signs or symptoms. **Ultrasound** can reliably distinguish cysts from complex cystic and solid masses. **CT** is best suited for diagnosis and staging, because it provides information (including vascularity) on the primary tumor, lymph nodes, renal vein, and inferior vena cava. The differential diagnosis of a renal mass with or without

associated symptoms includes cysts, perinephric or renal abscess, renal lymphoma, renal tuberculosis, or benign tumor, as well as malignancy.

Patients are staged by the TNM classification or another simplified staging system. The latter system classifies stage I disease as tumor confined to the kidney; stage II, spread through the capsule; stage III, renal vein invasion or lymph node metastases; and stage IV, hematogenous metastases.

■ Management

Radical nephrectomy is the standard surgical procedure. Tumor thrombi in the renal veins and vena cava may require extensive vascular resection and reconstruction. **Postoperative radiotherapy** can reduce the risk of local recurrence but has not been shown to enhance survival.

Metastases occasionally may appear as a solitary focus in brain, lung, thyroid, or liver and should be evaluated and considered for resection the primary tumor has been resected. A 5-year survival of almost 35% has been reported after resection of solitary metastases. Nephrectomy in the presence of disseminated metastases is rarely (<1%) associated with temporary regression of metastatic disease and should not be performed for this purpose. However, it may reasonably palliate pain or hematuria. Radiation is useful in palliating bone metastases.

Renal cell carcinomas are drug-resistant, and chemotherapy is rarely useful. Objective, and occasionally durable responses occur in 15–20% of patients treated with **recombinant interleukin-2** and/or **alpha-interferon.**

■ Prognosis

Tumors confined within the kidney have a cure rate of 60–90%, depending on tumor size, although a minority of patients present with disease at this stage. Lymph node metastases, invasion of the inferior vena cava, and sarcomatoid histology are unfavorable prognostic factors. Survival in metastatic disease averages 8–10 months.

Carcinoma of the Urinary Bladder

Bladder cancer is the most common malignancy of the urinary tract, afflicting 39,500 men and 15,000 women annually in the United States. A disease of the urbanized, industrialized world, it is most prevalent in the fifth to seventh decades of life and is more common in Caucasians. In rural Egypt, chronic cystitis from bilhar-

ziasis (infection by *Schistosoma haematobium*) predisposes to bladder cancer.

■ Etiology and Pathogenesis

Cigarette smoking is the principal risk factor for bladder cancer, in addition to the well-documented occupational exposures to chemicals used in the rubber and aniline dye industries. Chronic cyclophosphamide use for cancer chemotherapy or immunosuppression and excessive phenacetin intake are causative in a few cases.

Pathology

Ninety-five percent of bladder cancers arise from the transitional epithelium, the urothelium. Carcinoma in-situ may be associated. Because the etiology involves carcinogenic chemicals excreted by the kidney, the entire urothelium is at risk for malignancy. Thus, patients with transitional cell carcinoma of the bladder have an increased risk of similar tumors involving the ureters and renal pelvis.

Bladder cancer spreads contiguously through the bladder wall into the adjacent structures; lymphatic spread is to pelvic and periaortic lymph nodes. Widespread hematogenous dissemination to lung, liver, and bone is common once the deep muscle and lymph nodes are involved. The grade of tumor directly relates to invasiveness. Patients with high-grade, low-stage disease have as poor a prognosis as some patients with lower-grade but higher-stage disease.

Clinical Features

Variable degrees of **hematuria** and **urinary frequency** are the most common presenting symptoms. Pain follows bladder wall invasion. Lymphatic obstruction can lead to lower extremity or genital swelling. Symptoms of distant metastases may coexist. Physical examination is rarely helpful unless the diagnosis is markedly delayed. The urinalysis reveals red blood cells, but hematuria may be intermittent and detected only through repeated urinalyses.

Diagnosis, Clinical Evaluation, and Staging

The key step in the diagnosis of bladder cancer is the careful evaluation of any unexplained episodes of hematuria. Hematuria can be caused by infection or cancer anywhere in the urinary tract, glomerular disease, urolithiasis, and prostatitis.

Cytologic analysis of voided urine, cystoscopy, and IVP are appropriate diagnostic steps. At cystoscopy, suspicious areas should be biopsied and bladder washings obtained for cytologic examination. The IVP may show obstruction at the ureterovesical junction. CT or MRI can assess bladder wall thickness and detect invasion of contiguous structures as well as pelvic or periaortic lymphadenopathy. Imaging can help rule out associated renal tumors as well. The Marshall-Jewett staging system is commonly used (Table 198.2).

Treatment

Carcinoma in-situ may be benign but is often extensive, involving the entire bladder surface and producing intractable symptoms of dysuria, frequency, and incontinence. Treatment with the immunotherapeutic preparation bacille Calmette-Guérin (BCG) may control some patients, but persistent disease, like frequent recurrence of invasive disease, mandates **cystourethrectomy.**

Low-stage, low-grade tumors are treated with limited **transurethral resection.** If the lesions recur or are high-grade, a chemotherapeutic agent or BCG, given intravesically, significantly reduces the risk of relapse. Up to 30% of patients so treated become permanently disease-free. About 30% develop multiple recurrences of low-grade, low-stage tumors requiring repeated therapy. The remainder ultimately develop invasive disease and require aggressive surgical intervention.

Most instances of invasive disease require **radical cystectomy** and urinary diversion. This procedure involves resection of the bladder, prostate, and seminal vesicles in men and the bladder, entire urethra, anterior wall of the vagina, uterus, and ovaries in women. This radical surgery allows for precise, pathologic staging.

Irradiation without cystectomy is usually reserved for patients whose comorbid conditions preclude radical surgery. Transurethral resection may be employed for invasive disease in patients who are not surgical candidates. In only highly individualized circumstances, partial cystectomy may be considered for small localized lesions. In metastatic disease, combination chemotherapy with a cisplatin-based regimen produces effective short-term palliation.

Prognosis

Recurrence after local treatment is frequent (40–80%), and patients must be followed for life. The 5-year disease-free survival for patients with localized, low-grade tumors (stage 0 or A) approaches 90%, but that for

TABLE 198.2.	Clinical Staging for Transitional Cell Bladder Cancer	
Stage	**Description**
0	Papillary noninvasive and carcinoma in-situ
A	Invades submucosa
B1	Invades superficial muscle
B2	Invades deep muscle
C	Invades perivesical fat
D	Extension to adjacent organs, lymph node, or distant metastases

high-grade lesions is less favorable (60–80%). Patients having invasive cancer (stages B1, B2, and C) have 5-year survivals of 20–50%, while those with stage D disease rarely have long-term survival.

Carcinoma of the Prostate

The recent introduction of serologic screening for prostate-specific antigen (PSA) has led to an artifactual explosive increase in the prevalence of prostate cancer. Earlier projections suggested that 340,000 new cases of prostate cancer will be diagnosed in 1997; however, revised estimates suggest 219,000 cases for 1997 and 184,000 cases for 1998. Even with these revisions, prostate cancer is the most frequently diagnosed cancer in the United States. By identifying previously occult and asymptomatic disease, PSA testing has ushered in a vigorous debate regarding how, and even whether, to treat patients with newly diagnosed disease, given the typical indolent nature of the disease and the older patient population it affects.

■ Incidence and Epidemiology

About 30% of men over age 50 have occult prostate cancer. Autopsy studies in men dying of cardiovascular or other disease, who have no history or evidence of prostate cancer clinically, show that almost all men in the tenth decade have one or more foci of prostate cancer upon careful pathologic examination. Clinically, less than 1% of prostate cancers occur in men under age 40. Most cases become clinically manifest over age 60, and death from prostate cancer is most common over age 75.

The estimated lifetime risk of developing clinically significant prostate cancer is about 20 %, with the lifetime risk of dying of the disease being 4 %. Racial factors are important: African-American men have a 1.5-fold higher incidence than Caucasians, and Asians have one-half the incidence.

■ Etiology, Pathogenesis, and Pathology

Prostate carcinoma is not seen in castrated men, and androgens are believed to play a permissive role. The international variation in incidence positively correlates with fat intake. There are inherent racial variations in the prostatic tissue level of 5-α reductase, the enzyme which converts testosterone into its more potent derivative dihydrotestosterone. The highest values are found in African-American and white men, and lower values in Asians. Age is the most important additional risk factor, with the others being prior vasectomy and a positive family history.

Virtually all prostate cancers are **acinar adenocarcinomas.** Rarely, there are small cell (neuroendocrine) carcinomas, squamous cell carcinomas, transitional cell carcinomas, or lymphomas. The **Gleason grading system,** which classifies prostate cancers into five grades, takes into account the two dominant histologic patterns, and sums them into a score; 2–4 are well differentiated, 5–7 moderately differentiated, and 8–10 are poorly differentiated. This system is universally used in assigning prognostic categories along with the anatomically staging information.

Unlike **benign prostatic hypertrophy** (BPH), which arises in the central periurethral zone, prostate cancers usually begin in the periphery of the gland, mainly the posterior lobe. Thus, obstructive urinary symptoms occur relatively late in the cancer's natural history; when manifest, the symptoms can mimic BPH, a disorder also common in this patient population.

As the disease progresses, local growth extends beyond the prostatic capsule to include the pelvic sidewalls and seminal vesicles. Regional pelvic lymph nodes are involved first, followed by the periaortic nodes. The pattern of hematogenous metastasis is unique, as almost all such patients have bone metastases. The axial skeleton is most commonly involved, typically with new bone formation causing increased radiographic density (osteoblastic metastases). Distant metastases (lungs, liver, elsewhere) usually occur late, signifying extensive metastatic disease.

■ Clinical Features

Low-grade, low-stage prostate cancer may remain asymptomatic for the patient's life. In asymptomatic men, the initial evidence may be a high level of PSA on screening or a prostatic nodule noted on rectal examination. Locally advanced disease may cause urinary obstruction, hematuria, or hematospermia. Bone pain or stiffness may occur from metastatic disease. The differential diagnosis of urinary complaints includes infection, prostatitis, and BPH, while skeletal complaints may simulate osteoarthritis, Paget's disease, or degenerative disc disease.

Leukoerythroblastic anemia is typical of bone marrow involvement. High blood urea nitrogen and creatinine levels may indicate ureteral obstruction. Alkaline phosphatase elevation suggests osteoblastic bone metastases.

PSA, a proteolytic enzyme from the prostatic acinar cells, serves to liquefy the seminal plasma coagulum. In healthy men, the PSA level is <4 ng/ml, and it may rise moderately in BPH and prostatitis (usually <10 ng/ml). Although prostate cancer may occur with normal PSA levels, higher PSA levels should raise the index of suspicion of prostate cancer.

■ Diagnosis, Clinical Evaluation, and Staging

Screening for the disease in asymptomatic patients can be done by **digital rectal examination (DRE)** and/or PSA. The DRE has been the historical test, and can be incorporated with a routine checkup, as well as to investigate the patient's symptoms of dysuria, frequency or hematuria. Its accuracy depends on physician experience, patient compliance, and co-existing benign prostatic hypertrophy. Even when thought to be suspicious, only 15–30% of patients have a positive biopsy. The availability of the PSA test has revolutionized the approach to prostate cancer screening. Its better acceptability by patients has led to a dramatic increase in cases diagnosed within the last few years. Cancer cells secrete PSA at about 3 times the rate of normal prostate cells. Thus, for a given volume of prostate tissue, the serum PSA value will be higher. The physician can then evaluate the PSA level, assess glandular size, and assess risk of early prostate cancer.

Because the level of the PSA is related to the volume of cancer present, it can not only suggest the presence of prostate cancer, but can also roughly predict the stage of the disease. In general, the higher the PSA level the higher the risk of disease outside the prostatic capsule, and the lower the chances of cure. Levels above 4 ng/ml are considered abnormal, although patients with significant BPH may sometimes exhibit values at this level or even higher. However, levels above 4 ng/ml should be presumed to be cancer until proven otherwise, and follow-up studies performed with directed biopsies. PSA levels of 4–10 ng/ml indicate a 20–25% risk of prostate cancer. Almost invariably these patients have early stage, highly treatable disease. When the PSA exceeds 10 ng/ml the risk of cancer increases to 40-60 %. With wider application of this test, a more comprehensive database of implications of PSA screening will emerge. **Transrectal ultrasound (TRUS)** helps distinguish known or suspected foci of prostate cancer from areas of BPH, infection, or calcification and can guide the urologist in selecting areas within the prostate for **needle biopsy.** Typically, multiple biopsies are done from both prostatic lobes to facilitate staging and grading analysis.

The staging of prostate cancer is shown in Table 198.3.

Stage A disease is clinically occult and discovered incidentally, by histologic evaluation of tissue resected to relieve urethral obstruction from BPH or obtained

TABLE 198.3. Clinical Staging of Prostate Cancer

Stage	Description
A	No palpable disease (T_1)
A_1	Well differentiated ≤3 chips
A_2	Poorly differentiated or disease in ≥4 chips
B	Clinically palpable, confined to prostate (T_2)
B_1	One lobe—single nodule
B_2	Diffuse disease in one lobe
B_3	Bilateral confined to prostate
C	Disease extending outside the prostate $(T_3\text{-}T_4)$
D	Metastases
D_1	Pelvic node metastases
D_2	Upper abdominal, osseous, or visceral metastases

by biopsy of all prostate quadrants to investigate an elevated PSA.

Stage B disease may be detected by DRE of the prostate. It is subdivided into unilateral, bilateral, or diffuse in its involvement. This has implications regarding curability and whether the "nerve-sparing" prostatectomy, designed to preserve sexual functioning, can be successfully performed.

Stage C disease, which signifies disease beyond the capsule, appears on DRE as an area of diffusely indurated enlargement, with loss of palpable landmarks of the prostate. This is not surgically curable; such patients are treated with radiotherapy.

In **Stage D,** besides local disease on DRE, distant metastases are apparent by bone scan, CT, and other imaging techniques (Figure 198.1).

Because of the crude stoichiometric relationship with the PSA level, a minimal PSA elevation (<10 ng/ml) is expected in localized disease; levels between 20–30 ng/ml usually suggest capsular invasion and/or hematogenous metastases. Since localized prostate cancer is curable and advanced disease is not, the PSA test is now integral in evaluating patients with prostate cancer.

■ Screening for Prostate Cancer in Asymptomatic Men

The asymptomatic period of prostate cancer is at least 10 years, thus making screening theoretically attractive with the goal of reducing the mortality through early intervention. The American Cancer Society recommends annual DRE for all men over age 40 and DRE and PSA for African-American men over age 45, for white men over 50, and for all men over 40 with an affected first-degree relative. However, other groups argue that the evidence for mortality reduction from screening is lacking and therefore do not endorse widespread screening for prostate cancer. Because of the long latency of the

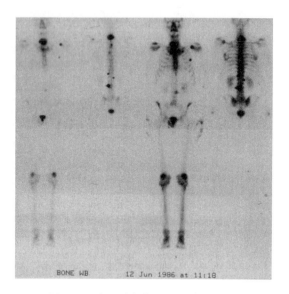

FIGURE 198.1. Radionuclide bone scan in prostate cancer showing scattered foci of uptake, which indicate metastases.

disease and the advanced age of this group, many patients will die of other diseases common to this age group, and thus no consensus may evolve that screening impacts survival in the overall patient population. At present, if the clinician feels that the patient's projected longevity exceeds 10 years, screening for prostate cancer is probably relevant.

■ Management

Treatment options for localized prostate cancer include **radical prostatectomy** or **radiation therapy** for relatively young and healthy patients. "Watchful waiting" is reasonable in asymptomatic men with comorbidities or those unwilling to undergo curative surgery or radiotherapy.

Specifically, patients with stage A1 disease are usually observed; except for especially young men or those with intermediate or high-grade disease. Over a 10-year period, the disease will progress in approximately 15%.

Patients with stages A2 and B1 to B3 disease, if medically fit, are normally treated for cure with radical prostatectomy or radiation therapy. Treatment selection depends on the patient and physician's preference and the complication rate. **Radical prostatectomy** entails 1% mortality, 1–5% incontinence, and 100% impotence. Recent "nerve-sparing" prostatectomy techniques for early-stage patients appear to reduce the postoperative impotence rate to below 50%. High-risk surgical patients usually receive **radiotherapy,** the late complications of which are significant chronic radiation cystitis and/or

proctitis in 2–5% of patients as well as impotence. All patients should be counseled extensively about the risks and benefits of both treatment options, and older patients (>75 yrs) should have the option of watchful waiting.

With rare exceptions, patients with nonmetastatic disease extending beyond the prostatic capsule, stage C (T3), are usually given radiation. Patients with stage D disease usually receive hormonal therapy, although a subset with positive pelvic nodes but no skeletal metastases (stage D1) are sometimes given radiotherapy as well. In patients with skeletal metastases, (stage D2), hormonal therapy is the mainstay of treatment, although temporary observation may be appropriate in asymptomatic persons.

In hormone-refractory disease, radiation to painful bone metastases or strontium-90 for systemic metastases may help. Corticosteroids may give short-term relief. Chemotherapy is generally ineffective.

Hormonal therapies

Options in **hormonal therapy** for prostate cancer are summarized in Table 198.4. Patient and clinician preferences dictate the choice of approach. **Orchiectomy** is the simplest, cheapest, and most rapid in onset of effect but also the least popular.

Monthly or quarterly injections of **luteinizing**

TABLE 198.4.	Options for Endocrine Therapy for Prostate Cancer
Orchiectomy	Achieves rapid androgen control
LHRH agonists (leuprolide; goserelin)	Control takes an average of 3 weeks; symptoms may flare dangerously (from increased androgens) in the first 2 wks
LHRH agonists or orchiectomy plus the antiandrogen flutamide	Produces total androgen blockade; flutamide blocks dihydrotestosterone receptors and prevents the flare from excess androgens; combined therapy modestly improves disease-free survival and is widely used.
Diethylstilbestrol	Decreases androgen secretion by feedback inhibition of hypothalamic-pituitary axis.

GnRH = Gonadotropin releasing hormone.

hormone-releasing hormone (LHRH) agonists have comparable effects and side effects but, in addition, have the theoretical advantage of reversibility, avoiding the patient's image of castration. Because a flare of the disease may occur from a transient rise of androgens soon after therapy starts, a short course of an antiandrogen must preferably accompany LHRH therapy, especially in those with impending spinal cord compression.

Exogenous **estrogen** therapy, although cost-effective and avoiding the hypoandrogenic syndrome ("male-menopause"), is rarely used because of its risks of gynecomastia and thromboembolic disease. It is contraindicated in patients with known hypertensive or atherosclerotic cardiac disease. **Flutamide** and **Casodex** are nonsteroidal antiandrogens which are of limited value when used alone, but when used in conjunction with either orchiectomy or LHRH therapy to produce "total androgen blockade", are thought to increase the duration of hormonal response.

Any of these hormonal interventions can generally produce responses in 60–80% of patients, typically lasting 18–36 months and occasionally over 5 years.

During this time, bone pain, obstructive urinary symptoms, and weight loss are under control. Failure is inevitable, and secondary hormone therapy (with progestational agents, adrenal suppression with ketoconazole, or the anticancer agent aminoglutethimide) is successful in inducing further remission in 20–30% of cases.

■ Prognosis

The prognosis depends on the stage and grade of tumor in localized disease. The 5-year survival is 88–95% for localized prostate cancer, 70–85% for locally advanced disease, and 20–30% for metastatic disease. Radical prostatectomy and radiation series achieve survival in the range of 70–75% at 10 years for stage A2 and B disease, but only 25–30% of patients with stage C disease survive 10 years (although a subset of patients with low-grade disease have prolonged survivals without active intervention). Fifty percent of patients with metastatic prostate cancer live 2–3 years, 20% survive 5 years, and only a few survive 10 years.

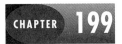

CHAPTER 199 CANCER OF THE TESTIS

Germ Cell Tumors

Nearly 7200 cases of germ cell testicular cancer occur annually in the United States. The peak age of incidence is 15–35 years. The only known risk factor is a history of cryptorchism. There is no convincing evidence that an orchiopexy, the surgical correction of this congenital problem, obviates the subsequent risk of testicular cancer.

■ Pathology

The basic classification divides these tumors into **seminomas** and **nonseminomas** (Table 199.1). All arise from the germinal epithelium of the testis. Grossly, the

tumors appear as firm nodules, often with areas of necrosis or hemorrhage. Because of their embryonic origin, lymphatic spread is via the spermatic cord to the perirenal and periaortic lymph nodes at the level of the renal vessels, not the anatomically adjacent pelvic or inguinal regions. Hematogenous metastases appear first in the lungs, with widespread dissemination following.

■ Clinical Features

A painless or minimally painful testicular mass is the usual presenting complaint in patients with testicular cancer. Spontaneous hemorrhage may cause rapid testicular enlargement and pain. Painful masses may erroneously be diagnosed as epididymitis or orchitis; painless masses are often erroneously considered to be hydroceles.

On examination, the testicular mass may be firm and irregular. Metastatic disease may cause abdominal and/or back pain from enlarged retroperitoneal nodes, cough, pleuritic chest pain, hemoptysis from lung metastases, and even gynecomastia if the tumor cells secrete an excess of β-human chorionic gonadotropin (β-HCG).

TABLE 199.1. Germ Cell Testicular Tumors	
Category	**Frequency (%)**
Seminoma	40
Embryonal carcinoma	25
Teratocarcinoma	25
Choriocarcinoma	<1
Yolk sac tumor	<1
Mixed histology	<10

Seminomas may be relatively indolent; often, the reported duration of symptoms is 1–2 years before diagnosis. Nonseminomas are often explosive in growth and dissemination and are diagnosed within months of onset of a testicular mass. Inguinal adenopathy is uncommon, unless antecedent scrotal surgery was performed, such as orchiopexy or a trans-scrotal biopsy.

■ Diagnosis, Evaluation, and Staging

Testicular **ultrasound** may be useful in diagnosing the tumor mass and making the distinction between a tumor and hydrocele. **Biopsy** should always be performed via a **high inguinal incision**, with immediate orchiectomy if cancer is diagnosed. **Serum marker** studies for β-HCG, alpha-fetoprotein (AFP), and lactate dehydrogenase (LDH) should be obtained before biopsy or orchiectomy.

Testicular neoplasms represent the ideal paradigm for utilizing blood tests to monitor the status of the patient's disease. β-HCG is modestly elevated in 7.5% of seminomas and markedly elevated in all choriocarcinomas and 50% of embryonal carcinomas. AFP is elevated in over 50% of embryonal and mixed histology tumors, but never in seminomas. Knowledge that such a marker was elevated prior to orchiectomy allows the physician to monitor for relapse effectively. Almost 80% of patients with advanced or recurrent nonseminomatous germ cell tumors will have a high β-HCG and/or AFP.

Staging should include CT of chest, abdomen, and pelvis, and if the primary tumor demonstrates a significant component of choriocarcinoma, the brain. Stage I disease is confined to the testis; Stage II disease includes the testis plus retroperitoneal nodes; Stage III includes lymphatic extension above the diaphragm or hematogenous metastasis to the lung, liver, or brain.

■ Management

Seminomas

Seminomas are highly sensitive to **radiotherapy.** Cure rates following orchiectomy and radiotherapy approach 100% for stage I disease and 75–85% for stage II. Patients with high-risk stage II disease with bulky (>10 cm) retroperitoneal masses are best treated with **chemotherapy** alone or with 2–3 cycles of neoadjuvant combination chemotherapy preceding radiotherapy. About 90% of patients with stage III are curable with combination chemotherapy.

Nonseminomas

In this group of patients, a baseline evaluation of β-HCG and AFP is crucial for following the disease. Stage I patients whose previously elevated tumor markers have returned to normal after **orchiectomy** can be observed without systemic therapy, unless relapse occurs. This careful surveillance approach demonstrates that nearly 75% of such patients are cured by orchiectomy alone. Because the potential for chemotherapy-induced cure is so high, patients should have monthly monitoring of tumor markers, with CT scanning every 3 months for 2–3 years.

For selected patients with stage II disease, **retroperitoneal lymph node dissection** is performed. **Chemotherapy** is also used and can achieve cure in 80–90% of patients, whether used as primary treatment for stage II disease or as salvage treatment in patients relapsing after surgical treatment for stage I or II disease.

Stage III disseminated disease

The treatment of nonseminomatous germ cell tumors represents one of the major successes in medical oncology. Over 80% of patients are now cured. Patients are classified as good- or poor-risk depending on the number, size, and site of metastases. β-HCG, AFP, and LDH levels help assess the "tumor burden" of the patient.

Chemotherapy is based on cisplatin with bleomycin and etoposide (VP-16); additional agents can be used but are probably unnecessary except in unusually poor-risk patients. Good-risk patients have an 80–95% cure rate after 3–4 cycles of chemotherapy, whereas the cure rate for poor-risk patients is only 40–70%.

A significant number of patients with stage II or III disease have persistent retroperitoneal adenopathy after definitive chemotherapy. Persistent elevation of the tumor markers β-HCG and AFP confirm the presence of residual disease, necessitating further chemotherapy or surgery. Conversely, if the tumor markers have returned to normal levels, patients may be followed carefully, although ideally such patients should undergo retroperitoneal dissection to rule out residual microscopic disease. Such surgical resection or restaging detects residual cancer in about 15% of patients; an additional two cycles of chemotherapy after successful surgical removal is occasionally curative in this subset of patients.

CHAPTER **200**   GYNECOLOGICAL NEOPLASMS

Carcinoma of the Ovary

In 1997, 26,800 new cases of ovarian cancer will occur, with 14,200 deaths. The incidence rises sharply after age 40, peaking at about 70 years. Hereditary ovarian cancer accounts for 5% of cases and may be associated with hereditary breast, ovarian, endometrial and/or colon cancers. This previously puzzling spectrum of cancers is now better understood as the use of the BRCA-1 and BRCA-2 gene probes are applied to such patients. The chief endocrine risk is believed to be related to an abnormal repair mechanism after ovulation, so that the number of ovulatory cycles is a risk factor. On the other hand, multiple births, lactation, and oral contraceptive use are partially protective.

■ Pathology

Eighty percent of malignant ovarian tumors arise from the surface epithelium (**epithelial tumors**). Half of these are papillary serous cystadenocarcinomas; mucinous papillary cystadenocarcinomas and endometrioid or undifferentiated tumors constitute 10–15% of cases each. **Stromal** and **germ cell** tumors are uncommon and include granulosa cell tumors and arrhenoblastomas. Germ cell tumors comprise only 1–2% and include dysgerminoma, malignant teratomas, embryonal carcinomas and the rare choriocarcinoma. A few primary epithelial ovarian tumors, termed **borderline,** are very low grade and may have a prolonged clinical course of years or even decades, regardless of whether they are localized or metastatic.

■ Clinical Features

Early ovarian cancer evokes few symptoms, and therefore, most patients present with more advanced stage II or III disease. Early symptoms of lower abdominal pain or cramping may be confused with the irritable bowel syndrome, diverticular disease, or other nonmalignant abdominal discomfort. Advancing disease causes single or multiple mass effects. With spread to peritoneal and diaphragmatic serosal surfaces, ascites and pleural effusion develop. Ascites may be the presenting complaint and may be confused to be due to liver disease. Three-fourths of patients have disease disseminated throughout the peritoneum at diagnosis. Death usually results from bowel obstruction, often at multiple sites. Additional complications include cachexia, refractory ascites, or renal failure from ureteral obstruction.

Of laboratory features, the tumor marker **CA-125** is elevated in proportion to the tumor bulk of ovarian cancer. However, CA-125 is not specific for ovarian cancer, being elevated in many other adenocarcinomas and benign diseases such as endometriosis, benign ovarian cysts, inflammatory peritonitis, and chronic liver disease. Nevertheless, it provides an index of disease activity in proven ovarian cancer and is often used to monitor the clinical course of therapy.

■ Diagnosis, Clinical Evaluation, and Staging

Unlike the case with breast cancer, there is no evidence that careful **screening** of asymptomatic women effectively detects early-stage disease. All tests, including pelvic examination, pelvic ultrasound, and CA-125 measurements, are limited by their lack of specificity or sensitivity for early ovarian cancer. Current screening methods are probably not cost-effective, given the relatively low prevalence of the disease.

However, patients with a history of breast or colon cancer or the familial ovarian cancer syndrome are at high risk. Evidence suggests that screening in this high-risk group may result in a survival benefit. Prophylactic **oophorectomy** is an option in this subset of patients.

Pelvic (ovarian) mass in a **postmenopausal** woman requires open or laparoscopic biopsy. In **premenopausal** women, masses exceeding 8 cm should be promptly diagnosed surgically; most often, masses under 8 cm are functional cysts and, if confirmed by ultrasound, should be observed for regression over 2–3 menstrual cycles. In more advanced abdominal presentations, cytologic evaluation of ascitic fluid, laparoscopy, or direct laparotomy are indicated.

Staging procedures including serum CA-125, pelvic ultrasound, and abdominal CT scans are useful. Precise staging is usually accomplished by laparotomy or laparoscopy. Staging is commonly done by the international system (Table 200.1).

■ Management

Surgical exploration is offered to most patients who have no contraindications to surgery. Localized disease is treated with total abdominal hysterectomy, bilateral salpingo-oophorectomy, and omentectomy. In more advanced disease, even when complete resection is not

TABLE 200.1.	FIGO Classification for Epithelial Ovarian Malignancy
Stage	**Description**
I	Growth limited to the ovaries
Ia	Single ovary involved
Ib	Both ovaries involved
Ic	Surface spread in one or both ovaries, rupture at surgery, ascites/peritoneal washing with positive cytology
II	Pelvic extension
IIa	Extensions/metastasis to uterus or fallopian tubes
IIb	Extension to other pelvic structures
III	Spread outside the pelvis
IIIa	Microscopically confirmed seeding of abdominal peritoneum (micrometastases)
IIIb	Grossly apparent spread to serosal surfaces outside of the pelvis (maximum diameter <2 cm); retroperitoneal nodes negative
IIIc	Implants >2 cm and/or positive retroperitoneal nodes
IV	Confirmed distant metastasis; cytologically positive pleural effusion; parenchymal liver metastases

FIGO = International Federation for Gynecology and Obstetrics. (From: Richardson et al. N Engl J Med 1985;312–417. Used with permission.)

possible, meticulous tumor reduction (debulking), with excision of all apparent abdominal disease, results in a more favorable prognosis with subsequent chemotherapy. The few patients with borderline malignancy or stage I disease without penetration of the ovarian capsule are usually cured by surgery. With adjuvant chemotherapy, a small group of stage II patients can also be cured.

Chemotherapy is the current principal treatment for advanced stages of ovarian carcinoma. Many chemotherapy regimens are moderately effective in this disease. Most recently, **Carboplatin** (or its parent compound cisplatin), combined with paclitaxel (Taxol) has become the treatment of choice with higher overall response rates, and occasional long-term survival.

■ **Prognosis**

The overall 5-year survival is 60–85% for patients with stage I ovarian cancer, 40–70% for stage II, 15–35% for stage III, and up to 5–15% for stage IV. At 10 years, only about 10% of stage III patients are alive and disease-free. Because most long-term survivors have been given chemotherapy with alkylating agents (cisplatin and/or cyclophosphamide), a small but finite risk of leukemia exists.

Endometrial Carcinoma

Annually, 34,900 cases of endometrial cancer occur in the United States, mostly in women aged 55–70 years. Adenocarcinomas, including those with squamous elements, constitute 90% of tumors. Clear cell papillary variants, endometrial stromal sarcomas, carcinosarcoma and leiomyosarcoma constitute the remainder.

Endogenous risk factors include obesity, diabetes mellitus, hypertension, polycystic ovaries, and prior granulosa cell tumors. Exogenous risk factors include hormone replacement therapy with unopposed estrogen, which increases the risk 4- to 10-fold. The concomitant administration of progestins markedly reduces this risk. Prolonged treatment with the weak estrogen agonist tamoxifen in breast cancer appears to increase the risk of endometrial cancer by 1.3–3-fold.

■ **Clinical Features**

Abnormal vaginal bleeding is the primary symptom, so that all women with postmenopausal bleeding require investigation. Advanced disease leads to pelvic and abdominal pain. Metastases may appear as supraclavicular adenopathy, hepatic metastases, or pulmonary nodules. Physical examination may reveal an enlarged uterus or pelvic masses.

■ **Diagnosis, Clinical Evaluation, and Staging**

Cytologic assessment of vaginal and cervical surface may be positive but are unreliable for screening. Although endometrial sampling is better, a thorough dilatation and curettage (D&C) is the most accurate test, and must be done if the disease is suspected.

Once cancer is diagnosed, preoperative sigmoidoscopy and cystoscopy help assess resectability, as do CT or magnetic resonance scans. Progesterone receptor determination and histologic grading provide additional prognostic data. Staging follows the anatomic spread of the disease: stage I, carcinoma confined to the uterus; stage II, affecting the uterus and cervix; stage III, spread to the pelvic structures; and stage IV, local invasion of bladder, rectum, and outside the true pelvis (stage IVa) or distant spread (Stage IVb).

Management

Surgical treatment is by total abdominal hysterectomy and bilateral salpingo-oophorectomy, with peritoneal washings and pelvic and periaortic node sampling. External beam and intracavitary radiation is an alternative to surgery in patients with poor surgical risks and as an adjunct to surgery in patients with high-risk stage I and II disease. Most patients with advanced stages III or IVA

Cervical Carcinoma

Incidence and Etiology

In 1997, 14,500 new cases of invasive cervical cancer and 55,000 cases of cervical in-situ cancer were diagnosed in the United States. The earliest precancerous manifestation, cervical dysplasia, begins to appear in women in their 20s, carcinoma in-situ is prevalent in women in their 30s, and invasive carcinoma is seen in women beyond their 40s. Because of screening and improved medical care, rates have decreased generally in the United States since the 1930s, but not among African-American and Hispanic women.

The chief epidemiological factors are age at first intercourse, socioeconomic status, and number of sexual partners. Cervical cancer is believed to result from a sexually transmitted infection: **human papilloma virus** (HPV) types 16 and 18 are strongly associated with premalignant lesions. Patients positive for HPV-16 or -18 at routine pelvic examination more often develop dysplasia or carcinoma in situ on follow-up. Cigarette smoking, HIV infection, and possibly herpes virus type 2 infection are cofactors.

Pathology

Ninety-five percent of cervical carcinomas are **squamous cell,** typically arising from the squamocolumnar junction of the cervical epithelium. The uncommon adenocarcinoma also has an in-situ counterpart. Unlike other disease sites, the influence of histologic grade in squamous cell carcinoma of the cervix is minimal; by far the most important prognostic factor is tumor stage.

Cervical cancer progressively invades the surface, then the base of the cervix, followed by extension to the parametrium and pelvic sidewalls. Involvement of the regional lymphatics, including the obturator and iliac nodes follow. Locally advanced disease invades the bladder and rectum.

cancer are given radiotherapy. Patients with metastatic disease can be given medroxyprogesterone or megestrol (progestational agents) for palliation if their tumor expresses progesterone receptors. Systemic chemotherapy is much less effective in endometrial than in ovarian cancer.

Prognosis

Localized stage I presentations are cured in 80–90% of patients, depending on the depth of myometrial invasion and tumor grade. The 5-year survival rate may reach 50–80% in stage II patients. Survival in stage III and IV is only 5–30%.

Clinical Features

Cervical dysplasia and carcinoma in-situ are usually asymptomatic and diagnosed incidentally during routine screening or during the evaluation of inflammatory or infectious diseases of the cervix. Until invasive tumors are well-established, there are no symptoms. Contact bleeding (postcoital) and discharge occur, which intensify with progression. Locally advanced disease causes pelvic pain, ureteral obstruction, and back pain. Edema of one or both lower extremities may occur. These symptoms of locally advanced disease portend a worse prognosis. Death results from infection, hemorrhage, or uremia due to ureteral obstruction. Distant metastases are relatively infrequent as a cause of death.

Diagnosis, Clinical Evaluation, and Staging

Because the premalignant phases of this disease normally span years, there is ample time for detection of premalignant changes, allowing successful treatment of dysplasia and carcinoma in-situ before invasive disease develops. **Annual pelvic examinations** with a **Papanicolaou (Pap) smear** from the cervix should begin at the onset of sexual activity or at age 18. After 2–3 negative annual examinations and if dysplasia and HPV infection are not present, the frequency of screening can be reduced to every 2–3 years. If premalignant changes have not developed on routine screening by age 65, invasive cancer is unlikely during remaining life.

Occasionally, a Pap smear may be nondiagnostic or even normal in the face of cancer. Therefore, a normal Pap smear does not negate a prior positive test or suspicious finding at pelvic examination. Once suspicion is aroused by an abnormal Pap smear or visualized cervical abnormalities, colposcopy and biopsy should

TABLE 200.2.	Staging and Prognosis in Cervical Carcinoma	
Stage	**Description**	**5 Year Survival (%)**
I	Confined to cervix	
IA	Microscopic	90
IB	Gross invasion	70–90
IIA	Upper ⅓ of vagina invaded	75–85
IIB	Parametrium invaded	60–65
III	To pelvic side walls or to lower ⅓ of vagina	30–50
IVA	Mucosa of bladder or rectum	<20
IVB	Distant metastases	<5

follow to obtain tissue from below the surface of the cervix. Staging and prognosis of cervical cancer are shown in Table 200.2.

▪ Management and Prognosis

For premalignant lesions, local treatments are used. Dysplasia is treated with cryosurgery or conization of the cervix. Carcinoma in-situ may be treated similarly or by hysterectomy. Microinvasive cancer is treated by radical hysterectomy. The treatment of higher stages of disease is frequently by external and intracavitary radiation. The prognosis depends exclusively on the stage of disease (Table 200.2).

CHAPTER 201   SELECTED ENDOCRINE GLAND TUMORS

Principal endocrine neoplasms represent a diverse group of malignancies (Table 201.1). Thyroid cancer is discussed in chapter 58; pheochromocytomas are discussed in chapter 61 (Adrenal Disorders) and chapter 177 (Secondary Hypertension).

Adrenal Neoplasms

Adrenal carcinoma is rare and occurs most frequently in children, with a second peak of incidence occurring in the fourth and fifth decades. Functional (secreting) adrenal tumors are more common in women, whereas the nonfunctioning variant is more common in men. Hormonally nonfunctional tumors are often quite large at diagnosis, given their anatomical location.

Clinical presentations of adrenal tumors include those due to tumor bulk or endocrine syndromes (preco-cious puberty in children, feminization, virilization, or Cushing's syndrome). Labeled iodocholesterol studies show uptake in benign adenoma, but only rarely in carcinoma. CT and magnetic resonance scans provide the best imaging of adrenal tumors. Adults usually present with more advanced disease, and only 20–25% are cured by surgery. Recurrent metastatic disease is treated with mitotane (o',p'-DDD), with partial responses in 60%. Nausea and CNS toxicity are dose-limiting effects.

Multiple Endocrine Neoplasia

The rare but fascinating multiple endocrine neoplasia (MEN) syndromes have been recognized for over 80 years. **Type I MEN** (Wermer's syndrome) involves the parathyroid and pituitary glands and pancreatic islet cells. Hyperparathyroidism is almost universal in these patients. The leading cause of death in MEN I is the Zollinger-Ellison syndrome, produced by a gastrin-secreting islet cell tumor causing intractable peptic ulcer disease. Less commonly, hyperparathyroidism-induced hypercalcemia or the complications of a space-occupying pituitary lesion result in death.

MEN type IIa consists of medullary carcinomas of the thyroid (MCT), pheochromocytomas, and hyperparathyroidism (Sipple's syndrome). Patients operated on for hyperparathyroidism or MCT may have unrecognized pheochromocytomas as part of MEN IIa and thus, are at risk for hypertensive crises. Blood relatives of patients with this syndrome should be screened for

TABLE 201.1. Endocrine/Neuroendocrine Tumors	

Thyroid
  Well–differentiated
    Papillary, mixed
    Follicular
    Hurthle cell variant
  Medullary
    Sporadic
    MEN IIa, IIb
  Undifferentiated (anaplastic) carcinoma
Parathyroid
  Adenoma
  Carcinoma
Adrenal cortex
  Adrenal cortical carcinoma
Adrenal medulla
  Malignant pheochromocytoma
	Islet cell tumors
	  Insulinoma
	  Gastrinoma
	  Glucagonoma
	  VIPoma
	  Somatostatinomas
	  MEN I
	Carcinoids
	  Foregut (bronchial)
	  Gastric
	  Intestinal (midgut)
	  Appendix, colon, rectum (hindgut)
	Extrapulmonary small cell carcinoma
	  Esophagus
	  Cervix
	  Prostate
	  Many other viscera

MCT using stimulated calcitonin assays. A test for the responsible gene, known as the *RET* proto-oncogene, is now available to facilitate identification of family members at risk.

MEN IIb consists of the same triad of conditions, plus mucosal neuromas, a body habitus resembling Marfan's syndrome, and a characteristic facies. With either MEN II syndromes, children and teenagers from these families must be screened for MCT. Total thyroidectomy is curative in either premalignant hyperplasia or early malignancy stage; however, cases of MCT that are diagnosed after the development of clinical symptoms are frequently metastatic and almost invariably fatal.

CHAPTER 202 CANCER OF THE HEAD AND NECK

Squamous cancer of the head and neck region accounts for approximately 41,650 cases and 12,670 deaths annually. These cancers have a predilection for men (3:1 for most sites and 5:1 for laryngeal tumors). The larynx is the most common site affected, followed by the oral cavity, pharynx, tongue, and lip. Nasopharyngeal cancer and carcinoma of the paranasal sinuses each account for less than 5% of cases.

■ Etiology and Pathology

Tobacco smoke (cigarette and, to a lesser extent, pipe and cigar) and smokeless tobacco are the prime etiologic factors, with alcohol being a potent cofactor. The Epstein-Barr virus is convincingly associated with nasopharyngeal carcinoma, particularly in the Orient. Industrial exposure to wood dust and oils is implicated in the etiology of nasal and paranasal tumors.

Most tumors are **squamous** and arise from the surface epithelium of the oral, pharyngeal, and laryngeal mucosa. In the nasopharynx, dense lymphocytic infiltration often occurs, and these tumors are termed **lymphoepitheliomas**. The rare adenocarcinoma arises from the major or minor salivary glands.

■ Clinical Features

Symptoms depend on the site of origin. Leukoplakia, a premalignant lesion, is usually asymptomatic, but often identified during routine dental examinations. Symptoms and signs of malignancy include an oral ulcer or plaque, sore throat, trismus, or dysphagia. A neck mass is a frequent presenting sign due to metastatic adenopathy, especially in tumors arising from tonsillar, nasopharyngeal, or pharyngeal sites. Persistent serous otitis media and unilateral deafness are clues to nasopharyngeal cancer. Hoarseness is a cardinal feature of laryngeal cancers.

Local invasion and regional node metastases are

more common than distant metastases, which occur late in the course of most of these cancers. Because of the underlying common risk factors, multiple primary tumors of the head, neck, lung, and esophagus are not unusual, either simultaneously or separated by months to years.

■ Diagnosis, Evaluation, and Staging

Screening in high-risk persons can be done by the dentist or primary physician. Those with any suspicious symptoms and signs should be seen by an otolaryngologist for a more detailed evaluation using specialized techniques, such as nasopharyngoscopy and fiberoptic laryngoscopy.

Careful biopsy of suspected lesions is necessary to distinguish leukoplakia, the premalignant lesion, from early cancer. CT and magnetic resonance scans of the head and neck are helpful in defining the anatomic extent of disease and enlargement of lymph nodes not palpable on examination. There are peculiarities of staging in several sites but the basic staging system illustrated in Table 202.1 provides a common basis for evaluation of treatment protocols.

■ Management

Because of the predominantly local nature of squamous cell cancers arising in head and neck, **surgery** and **radiation therapy** are the primary modes of treatment. The size and location of the primary lesion and the presence or absence of regional nodal metastases determine the choice of initial therapy. The functional and cosmetic sequelae of both radical surgery and radiation therapy are also major considerations.

In Stage I and II lesions of a number of sites, radiation and surgery yield similar long-term results, with 70–85% cure rates. Lymph node involvement adversely affects the overall survival rate. **Neoadjuvant chemotherapy** leads to rapid responses in Stage III and IV disease, but does not appear to increase resectability or

TABLE 202.1.	Basic TNM Staging of Head and Neck Cancer
Tumor	
T_1	Maximum diameter <2 cm
T_2	Maximum diameter 2–4 cm
T_3	Maximum diameter >4 cm or extension to adjacent structures
T_4	Massive lesion with deep invasion
Nodes	
N_0	No cervical adenopathy
N_1	Single homolateral node <3 cm
N_2	One node >3 cm or multiple homolateral nodes, none >6 cm or bilateral nodes <6 cm
N_3	Ipsilateral node/nodes >6 cm; bilateral nodes >6 cm
Metastases (M)	
M_0	No metastases
M_1	Metastases
Stage I	$T_1 N_0 M_0$
Stage II	$T_2 N_0 M_0$
Stage III	$T_3 N_0$ or $T_1\text{-}T_3, N_1$
Stage IV	$T_4 N_{0\text{-}2} M_0$; any T $N_3 M_0$; any T, any N, M_1

(AJCC Manual for Staging of Cancer. 4th ed. See suggested reading list.)

survival, except in nasopharyngeal cancer (in which chemotherapy and radiation lead to 50–60% cures). Metastatic disease can be treated palliatively with several chemotherapy agents given either singly or in combination, (e.g., methotrexate, cisplatin, 5-FU), but responses are usually incomplete and transient.

Smoking cessation is of paramount importance. Patients who continue to smoke respond less favorably to radiation. A second primary tumor of the head and neck region, esophagus and lung occurs at a rate of 3–4% annually after treatment of the first tumor at one of these sites. Secondary prevention with 13-*cis* retinoic acid is undergoing clinical study.

Malignant Melanoma

The epidemiology, clinical features, and treatment of melanoma and nonmelanoma skin cancer are presented fully in chapter 49.

■ Diagnosis, Evaluation, and Staging

Ideally all individuals should have a total skin inspection annually. Isolated dysplastic or suspicious lesions should be totally excised. Any excised lesion, no

matter how innocuous-looking, should be sent for pathologic examination.

When melanoma is diagnosed, a careful comprehensive physical examination together with radiological studies should be done to assess possible lymphatic spread or hematogenous dissemination. The most important assessment of melanoma is the careful evaluation of **depth of invasion,** using either Clark's or Breslow's system. Each is designed to allow for reproducible assessment of depth of invasion, which correlates with risk of relapse. The prognostic importance of depth of invasion is shown in Table 202.2. Survival is 60–70% for patients with localized disease, 15–40% with lymph node involvement, and <1% for distant disease. The prognosis is superior at all stages for women.

■ **Management**

Initial therapy for malignant melanoma is **local excision.** For thin lesions (<1 mm depth of invasion), 2-cm lateral margins give equivalent outcome but better cosmetic results than the older, traditional 5-cm margin of resection. Wider excisions with 2–3-cm margins are done for lesions that invade more deeply. Skin grafting may be required. Lesions on fingers and toes require amputation. Routine prophylactic regional node dissections are not indicated, but clinically suspicious nodes at the time of initial surgery or later should be dissected. Adjuvant alpha-interferon reduces the risk of relapse in high risk patients.

Metastatic melanoma shows an overall poor response to therapy; effective treatment regimens are lacking for this disease. **Radiation therapy** to the regional lymphatics may improve local control in head and neck melanomas. Isolated hyperthermic limb perfusion for extremity melanomas has led to a high rate of local control. **Combination chemotherapy** with cisplatin, carmustine, and dacarbazine, now usually given with tamoxifen, elicits a 40–50% response rate, although responses are usually short. For recurrent melanoma, intralesional BCG is locally effective, and systemic interferon therapy may be added to combination chemotherapy. Interferons produce a 10–15% response rate, and interleukin-2 (IL-2) produces a 15–20% response, however rarely are these durable beyond a matter of months. Many patients can benefit from resection of an isolated metastasis, or a regional lymphatic metastasis after prior therapy for the primary lesion.

TABLE 202.2.	Level of Invasion in Localized Melanoma and Prognosis		
Depth of Invasion		**Class**	**10 yr Survival (%)**
Clark classification			
Epidermis (in-situ)		I	100
Invades papillary dermis		II	>90
Invades junction of papillary dermis and reticular dermis		III	75
Invades reticular dermis		IV	60
Invades subcutaneous fat		V	20–40
Breslow's classification			
<0.76 mm			85–95
0.76–1.5 mm			75–95
1.51–2.5 mm			60
2.51–4.0 mm			45–55
4.1–8.0 mm			20–40
>8.0			20

(Adapted from: Balch and Milton Cutaneous Melanoma. J.B. Lippincott Company Philadelphia 1985, p. 329. Used with permission.)

CHAPTER **203** MALIGNANT TUMORS OF THE CENTRAL NERVOUS SYSTEM

Primary Brain Tumors

The incidence of brain tumors is bimodal, with an initial peak at age 4, a decline after age 15, a second rise after age 25–30, and then a plateau after age 65. Brain tumors in children differ from those of adults. The former are medulloblastomas, low-grade astrocytomas, and ependymomas, whereas the tumors affecting adults are predominantly high-grade astrocytomas, including grade III and IV lesions known as **glioblastoma multiforme**. In adults, benign meningioma is second to astrocytomas in inci-

dence. The other malignant tumors shown in Table 203.1 are less common.

■ **Etiology**

A number of hereditary disorders are associated with brain tumors. While uncommon, they include neurofibromatosis, tuberous sclerosis, the Li-Fraumeni syndrome (Table 190.2), and Turcot's syndrome, a

| TABLE 203.1. | Malignant Brain Tumors |

Astrocytomas
   Low grade (grade I-II)
   Anaplastic (grade III)
   Glioblastoma multiforme (grade IV)
Ependymoma
Oligodendroglioma
Medulloblastoma
Malignant meningioma
Primary CNS lymphoma
Pinealoma
Metastatic malignancies (breast, lung, colon, renal,
   melanoma)

rare entity in which patients with colonic polyposis and colonic cancer develop medulloblastomas or high-grade astrocytomas. Despite their obscure etiology, the incidence of astrocytomas have risen somewhat since 1973.

■ **Pathology**

The principal tumors in adults are gliomas, and over one-half of these are high grade, highly cellular, with new blood vessel formation, palisading of nuclei, and necrosis. Brain tumors rarely metastasize, but high-grade gliomas and medulloblastomas can seed the subarachnoid space along the spinal cord.

■ **Clinical Features**

The brain, being enclosed in the rigid cranium, is subject to compression by space-occupying lesions, with elevation of intracranial pressure and cerebral edema. Brain tumors often progress slowly, and so patients frequently do not seek medical attention until the disease is usually locally advanced. Progressive disease causes generalized headache, nausea, vomiting and lethargy.

Seizures occur in 20–50%. Investigation of new-onset of seizures in an adult rarely uncovers a latent brain tumor, but nevertheless, new-onset seizures should lead to appropriate diagnostic studies. Symptoms are often vague and include personality changes, depression, and fatigue. Primary or metastatic tumors may present with a hemispheric or cerebellar syndrome mimicking a vascular accident.

■ **Diagnosis and Evaluation**

CT and MRI are highly effective diagnostic tools, and can delineate the extent of disease, concomitant edema, and distortion and shifting of vital brain structures. Biopsy is performed at the time of resection. Lesions in unresectable locations or in patients with comorbidities may undergo a stereotactic needle biopsy.

■ **Management and Prognosis**

High-dose **dexamethasone,** to reduce edema and secondary symptoms, is often used to stabilize patients before and after initial surgery. Anatomy and limitations of surgery permitting, malignant brain tumors should be excised completely. Well-circumscribed, low-grade tumors (oligodendrogliomas, meningiomas, and low grade astrocytomas) may do well for long periods. High grade astrocytomas (anaplastic astrocytomas and glioblastoma multiforme) can usually be only subtotally resected. Prognosis improves in proportion to the extent of tumor resected.

Radiation is routinely given for anaplastic astrocytomas and glioblastoma multiforme following surgery. Nearly 50% of patients with the former will survive 2–3 years after this regimen, compared to less than 5% for glioblastoma. Chemotherapy adds only minimal benefit. Precisely targeted radiation (gamma knife or stereotactic radiosurgery) or brachytherapy with ^{125}I or iridium-^{192} may further benefit localized tumors. Reoperation is attempted in localized recurrence or in post-radiation brain necrosis.

Primary Central Nervous System Lymphomas

Primary CNS lymphomas are large-cell lymphomas formerly called **microgliomas** of the brain. They occur in near-epidemic proportions in immunosuppressed patients (e.g., AIDS patients, solid organ transplant recipients). The incidence also appears to be increasing in the normal population, predominantly in men in their sixth or seventh decade.

Multifocal presentations are common. CSF cytology may be positive. Patients respond dramatically and rapidly to steroid-based therapy with radiation, but control is usually only for a matter of months. Current studies are investigating the role of combined chemotherapy and radiotherapy.

Metastatic Brain Tumors

Cancers of the lung, breast, kidney, melanoma, and large bowel together cause most brain metastases. Usually, uncontrolled tumor is obvious elsewhere, but melanoma and renal cell carcinoma are notorious for isolated cerebral metastases, even after a long, disease-free interval. Solitary or multiple brain metastases may be the harbinger of lung cancer.

Intracranial metastases cause symptoms similar to those of a primary brain tumor, and the diagnostic workup and therapeutic interventions are similar, especially for patients with an isolated metastasis. About 60–80% respond to treatment, with an average survival of 6 months, depending on the volume of tumor in the brain and the degree of control elsewhere. A patient with solitary brain metastasis and minimal or no tumor burden elsewhere may survive months, or even years following surgery or radiotherapy. This is especially true in patients with a long, disease-free period from primary therapy.

Meningeal Carcinomatosis

Acute lymphocytic leukemia and intermediate and high-grade lymphomas may disseminate to the meninges, as can some solid tumors (e.g., breast and lung cancers, melanoma). A myriad of features result: confusion, headache, meningitis, back pain, and cranial or spinal neuropathies. Magnetic resonance imaging or CT may show paraventricular contrast enhancement.

The classic **cerebrospinal fluid** (CSF) findings include elevated pressure, elevated protein, and low glucose levels. Initially, the CSF may be nondiagnostic in 50% of patients, requiring multiple CSF examinations. Cytologic examination frequently (but not invariably) shows malignant cells.

Therapy may be considered in the appropriate clinical setting. Intrathecal methotrexate, cytarabine or thiotepa is given twice weekly until the CSF clears, and then weekly for 6–8 weeks. A reservoir (Ommaya) providing intraventricular therapy is more convenient and safer than multiple lumbar installations, and the distribution of drug (at least methotrexate) in the CSF is more uniform. Cranial irradiation is usually added. Intrathecal therapy can cause acute lethal demyelination, while chemotherapy plus radiation frequently elicits encephalopathy. Remissions are brief in carcinomatous and lymphomatous meningitis, but exceptions occur if the systemic disease is controlled.

CHAPTER 204 SARCOMAS

Sarcomas, malignant tumors arising from multiple types of connective tissue, are uncommon (6,600 soft tissue sarcoma and 2,500 bone sarcoma cases are diagnosed annually). Bone sarcomas occur predominantly in childhood. Soft tissue sarcomas occur at all ages.

■ Etiology and Pathology

Sarcomas may be inherited, as in the Li-Fraumeni syndrome. Previous radiation, neurofibromatosis, and Paget's disease of bone are predisposing conditions for the development of **osteosarcoma.** Industrial exposure to vinyl chloride has been associated with hepatic **angiosarcomas.** Post-transplant immunosuppression and HIV infection are associated with **Kaposi's sarcoma,** which is an AIDS-defining malignancy. Sarcomas are defined by the tissue of origin (Table 204.1). Histologic grade and cell type are the most important features in establishing a prognosis.

■ Management

Soft tissue masses should be biopsied by **core-needle** or careful **incisional** technique to enhance subsequent resectability. **Surgery** of all soft tissue and bone sarcomas is designed to ensure totally clear margins. Because these tumors tend to extend along tissue planes, wide excisions are necessary. Prior to modern reconstructive surgical techniques, this usually meant amputation for all patients whose tumor presented in an extremity. **Irradiation** is commonly employed postoperatively, thus producing "limb-sparing" approaches for patients with extremity lesions. **Adjuvant chemotherapy** is not routinely recommended for adult soft tissue sarcomas. Pediatric sarcomas, both soft tissue and bone, are frequently cured by combined modality therapy, including chemotherapy, surgery, and judiciously applied radiation therapy.

Kaposi's Sarcoma

Kaposi's sarcoma (KS) deserves special mention because of its association with HIV infection and immunosuppression. It has three forms:

Nonendemic KS occurs among the elderly, chiefly men of Mediterranean or Ashkenazi Jewish extraction. It presents as nodules and plaques on the extremities, with an indolent course averaging 10 years.

Endemic KS in young men in central Africa comprises the second group, manifested by frequent lymphadenopathy and spread to the lungs and gastrointestinal tract.

TABLE 204.1.	Sarcomas of Bone and Connective Tissue
Bone	Osteosarcoma
	Periosteal osteogenic sarcoma
	Malignant giant cell tumor
	Ewing's sarcoma
	Primary lymphoma
	Fibrosarcoma
	Fibrous histiocytoma
Cartilage	Chondrosarcoma
Fat	Liposarcoma
Fibrous tissue	Fibrosarcoma
Smooth muscle	Leiomyosarcoma
Striated muscle	Rhabdomyosarcoma
Mesenchyme	Mesenchymoma
Synovia	Synovial cell sarcoma
Vascular/lymphatic	Hemangiosarcoma
	Lymphangiosarcoma
	Hemangiopericytoma
	Kaposi's sarcoma
Nerve	Malignant schwannoma
	Malignant neurilemoma
Miscellaneous	Alveolar soft parts sarcoma
	Malignant fibrous histiocytoma
	Extraskeletal Ewing's sarcoma
	Primitive primary neuroectodermal tumors
	Clear cell sarcoma

Epidemic KS especially affects homosexual men with HIV infection; 1% of cases afflict recipients of solid-organ transplants. Because persons acquiring HIV through blood products or IV drug abuse rarely develop KS (unless sexual risk factors are also present), KS has long been suspected to have an infectious etiology. Recently, evidence of viral DNA in the tumor genome has pointed to a new virus of the herpesvirus family.

Pathologically, the tumor nodules show spindle cells and endothelial cell proliferation with a marked proliferation of small blood vessels. The lesions are distributed in the skin, mucous membranes, lungs, trachea and bronchi, and GI tract.

The **endemic form** of KS in elderly men usually starts as purplish nodules on the lower extremities. The course is indolent: years may pass before progressive lymph node involvement and, ultimately, spread to the lungs and GI tract supervene. **KS in HIV-infected persons** more frequently involves the skin of the trunk, head and neck, or mucous membranes of the oral cavity. Lymph node involvement is universal, and dysphagia, GI hemorrhage, or hemoptysis are common, as are cough and dyspnea from pulmonary metastases. In HIV-infected patients, KS may be relatively indolent if the patient has a reasonably intact immune system, but with progressive immunosuppression, KS may progress parallel to the increasing risk of opportunistic infections.

■ Management and Prognosis

Radiation is useful for local palliation. Alfa-interferon, in patients who are relatively immunocompetent, produces a 25–40% response, especially when combined with zidovudine. Single-agent chemotherapy with vinca alkaloids, etoposide, bleomycin or anthracyclines achieve responses in at least 40% of patients, but combination chemotherapy is only marginally more beneficial.

The prognosis depends on the degree of immunosuppression. With associated opportunistic infections, survival beyond 2 years is unusual.

CHAPTER **205** METASTATIC CANCER OF UNKNOWN PRIMARY SITE

Approximately 5% of cancer patients present initially with a metastasis, the primary tumor of which remains elusive. When a careful history and physical examination fail to uncover a primary, a targeted workup is undertaken, directed by symptoms, histologic type of malignancy, and possible sites of presentation.

About 60% of patients with metastatic malignancies of unknown primary site have easily recognizable adenocarcinomas, and 30% have a poorly differentiated

TABLE 205.1.	Clinical Features Useful in Determining the Source of a Malignancy of Unknown Primary Site
Feature	**Primary Tumors to be Suspected**
Cervical lymphadenopathy	Lymphoma
	Hodgkin's disease
	Head and neck squamous carcinoma
	Thyroid
Right supraclavicular node	Lung, mediastinum, lymphomas
Left supraclavicular node	Carcinoma originating below the diaphragm
Inguinal nodes	Cancer of the penis, vulva, anus, melanoma
Axillary nodes	Breast, melanoma
Brain tumor	Lung cancer
Pulmonary nodules	Many sites (Kidney, melanoma, germ cell tumors)
Abdominal carcinomatosis	Ovary, pancreas, other GI tract
Undifferentiated cancer in young man	Germ cell tumor
Undifferentiated cancer following pregnancy, abortion, or molar pregnancy	Choriocarcinoma

TABLE 205.2.	Special Pathologic Stains and Markers in Carcinoma of Unknown Primary Site
Tumors	**Immunostains and Serum Markers**
Lymphoma	Leukocyte common antigen (LCA)
Carcinoma	Cytokeratin (epithelial membrane antigen)
Sarcoma	Vimentin, desmin, factor VIII antigen
Ovary	CA125 (tumor and serum)
Breast	Hormone receptors
Prostate	Prostate-specific antigen (PSA)
Follicular thyroid	Thyroglobulin
Medullary thyroid	Calcitonin (tumor and serum)
Germ cell tumors	Human chorionic gonadotropin (β-HCG), alpha fetoprotein (AFP)
Neuroendocrine tumors	Chromogranin A, neuron-specific enolase
Melanoma	S100, HMB-45

neoplasm or poorly differentiated carcinoma. About 5% have squamous cancers, and a lesser proportion represent metastatic melanoma or malignant lymphoma.

■ Clinical Features

The features of malignancies with unknown primary sites are legion, but some recurrent themes should lead to suspicion of particular sites of origin (Table 205.1). Combining these presentations with pathologic features and special examinations may disclose a treatable neoplasm. Consultation with a pathologist is especially helpful in the subset of patients with poorly differentiated neoplasms. In these patients, a battery of pathologic examinations, including immunohistochemical staining, may be employed (Table 205.2).

■ Management

Metastatic squamous carcinoma of unknown primary that occurs in the neck region may be treated with radical neck dissection and radiation. In a considerable proportion of cases, long-term survivals may follow. The same is true for cancer of unknown primary involving the inguinal lymph nodes.

Patients who have disease presenting in the lungs, liver, or peritoneal cavity represent difficult problems because these areas are frequent sites of metastases from many different tumors. In general, the emphasis is on the search for a primary tumor that is known to respond well to palliative therapy (e.g., breast or ovarian cancer in women). Serum tumor markers associated with these diseases can sometimes provide supportive evidence for a possible diagnosis or at least allow the treating physician to make reasonable treatment decisions.

Patterns of disease also may be helpful. In women with diffuse peritoneal carcinomatosis, ovarian cancer should be strongly considered. Malignant axillary adenopathy in women is considered to be breast cancer unless proven otherwise. In young men, the possibility of occult testicular tumor or extragonadal germ cell tumor must be considered; presentation with multiple pulmonary nodules or with mediastinal, retroperitoneal, or supraclavicular adenopathy mandate testing for serum AFP and β-HCG as well as careful testicular examination and ultrasonography. In men with bone metastases, prostate cancer should always be suspected. Thyroid cancers are usually histologically apparent, but stains for thyroglobulin and calcitonin may provide further confirmation. Abdominal CT may be cost-effective because pancreatic cancer is one of the most common primary sites for metastatic adenocarcinoma of unknown primary.

■ Prognosis

Most patients whose tumor is suspected to be of lung, pancreatic, or other gastrointestinal origin tend to have a poor prognosis. Survival is usually brief, and chemotherapy is of minimal palliative benefit. Palliative chemotherapy may be offered to patients with excellent performance status and minimal tumor burden, but its use should be discouraged in patients severely disabled by their disease. Judicious radiotherapy to symptomatic sites of disease is often better therapy.

CHAPTER 206 PARANEOPLASTIC SYNDROMES

The paraneoplastic syndromes comprise a diverse group of systemic disorders which represent the remote effects of cancer due to the action of ectopic hormones, antibodies, and various tumor products.

Endocrine Syndromes

The endocrine syndromes (Table 206.1) include **Cushing's syndrome,** seen in 6% of small cell lung cancers and various other neuroendocrine tumors. **Ectopic secretion of antidiuretic hormone** (ADH) is also frequent in small cell lung cancer.

Hypercalcemia of diverse etiology is encountered in lung, breast, other solid tumors, multiple myeloma, and lymphomas. Tumor production of parathormone-related polypeptide [PTH-rp], with its partial homology to native parathormone, is a major cause of hypercalcemia in squamous carcinomas of head and neck, esophagus, and lung and in adenocarcinoma of the kidney. Calcitonin production in medullary carcinoma of the thyroid and small cell lung cancer is usually asymptomatic and serves as a marker for recurrent disease in both sporadic and familial types.

In contrast to hypercalcemia, **hypocalcemia** is quite rare and occurs occasionally in patients with osteoblastic bone metastases of breast and prostate cancer or in the syndrome of oncogenic osteomalacia in large mesenchymal tumors. **Hypoglycemia** is also rare and results from the secretion of insulin-like growth factors in massive retroperitoneal sarcomas or hepatoma; malignant insulinomas secrete endogenous insulin. **Gynecomastia** is seen occasionally in germ cell tumors in men and rarely in patients with large cell or adenocarcinoma of the lung.

TABLE 206.1. Paraneoplastic Endocrine Syndromes

Syndrome	Hormone	Associated Tumors
Cushing's syndrome	ACTH	Small cell lung cancer, other lung cancer, carcinoids
Syndrome of inappropriate ADH secretion (SIADH)	Arginine vasopressin	Lung cancer, mainly small cell
Hypercalcemia	PTH-rp, cytokines, Vitamin D	Lung (squamous), renal, breast cancer, myeloma, lymphoma
Gynecomastia	Unknown and β-HCG	Germ cell—lung
Hyperthyroidism	β-HCG	Choriocarcinoma, germ cell tumors
Hypocalcemia	Unknown	Osteoblastic metastases
Hypoglycemia	Insulin-like growth factors	Sarcomas, esp. large fibrosarcomas

PTH-rp = parathyroid-related peptide.

Hematologic Manifestations

Hematologic manifestations of malignancy are legion. **Anemia** can result from many mechanisms (Table 206.2). Besides chronic inflammation and blood loss from gastrointestinal cancers, immune hemolysis (Hodgkin's and non-Hodgkin's lymphoma, chronic lymphocytic leukemia, and ovarian teratomas), pure red cell aplasia (thymomas and chronic lymphocytic leukemia), and fragmentation (microangiopathy) hemolysis (disseminated intravascular coagulation [DIC] as seen in adenocarcinomas of diverse sites) are other mechanisms.

Leukemoid reactions and **eosinophilia** may occur in disseminated sarcomas, Hodgkin's disease and some metastatic carcinomas. **Erythrocytosis** due to ectopic erythropoietin production is observed in about 3% of renal cell carcinoma patients, as well as in rare patients with hepatocellular carcinomas, cerebellar hemangioblastomas, and benign renal conditions. **Thrombocytopenia** is seen with marrow replacement or following the development of an autoimmune phenomenon or secondary to DIC.

The most common coagulation abnormality in cancer is activation of the coagulation system. Isolated **thrombophlebitis** of multifactorial origin is common in the cancer patient, as is **migratory thrombophlebitis**. In severe cases, there is life-threatening decompensated **disseminated intravascular coagulation** with hemorrhage and consumption of platelets, fibrinogen, and factors V and VIII. Nonbacterial thrombotic endocarditis is due to fibrin deposition on the mitral or aortic valve, with systemic embolization to the brain, kidneys, and spleen or to the microcirculation of the extremities leading to peripheral ischemia and gangrene.

TABLE 206.2.	Hematologic Manifestations of Cancer
Anemia	Chronic disease
	Blood loss
	Marrow replacement
	Microangiopathic (±DIC)
	Pure red cell aplasia
	Immune hemolysis
Leukocytosis	Leukopenia
	Neutrophilic leukemoid reaction
	Eosinophilia
Erythrocytosis	Due to ectopic erythropoietin production
Thrombocytopenia	Marrow replacement
	Immune
	DIC syndromes

DIC = disseminated intravascular coagulation.

Neurologic Syndromes

The remote effects of cancer on the nervous system are pervasive (Table 206.3) and include **cerebellar degeneration**, **dementia**, **limbic encephalitis**, and many other neurologic disorders. A syndrome of uncoordinated, spontaneous eye movements termed **opsoclonia** or opsoclonus has been reported in breast and lung cancer. **Necrotizing myelopathy** is seen in leukemia, and a variety of sensory, motor, and autonomic neuropathies

TABLE 206.3.	Paraneoplastic Neurologic Syndromes
Brain	Dementia
	Subacute cerebellar degeneration
	Limbic encephalitis
	Optic neuritis
	Opsoclonia
	Progressive multifocal leukoencephalopathy
Spinal cord	Necrotizing myelopathy
	Amyotrophic lateral sclerosis
Peripheral nerve	Sensory neuropathy
	Sensory motor neuropathy
	Autonomic neuropathy with orthostatic hypotension
Neuromuscular junction	Myasthenia gravis
	Myasthenic (Eaton-Lambert) syndrome
Muscle	Dermatomyositis
	Polymyositis

are frequent in lung cancer. **Myasthenia gravis** is noted in association with thymomas (usually benign), and a

myasthenic-like syndrome (**Eaton-Lambert syndrome**) is seen with small cell lung cancer.

Dermatologic Syndromes

A myriad of dermatologic syndromes exist and most are associated with adenocarcinomas, especially of the gastrointestinal tract (e.g., syndrome of Laser-Trelat, which is the sudden appearance of large numbers of seborrheic keratoses). **Bowen's disease** is associated with internal malignancies of the lung, gastrointestinal tract, and genitourinary tract. Palmar and plantar **tylosis** is associated with cancer of the esophagus. **Acanthosis nigricans** (pigmentation involving axillae and belt areas

with a velvety appearance of the skin) is rare, but striking in its appearance as well as relationship to (gastric) adeno-carcinoma. The historically interesting Sister Mary Joseph's nodule, unlike the above mentioned paraneoplastic syndromes, is the result of direct retrograde extension of cancer along the umbilical lymphatics, producing a periumbilical mass. Synopses of the myriad of such syndromes can be found in comprehensive oncology or dermatology textbooks.

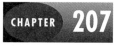

CHAPTER 207 ONCOLOGIC EMERGENCIES

A variety of cancer-related conditions may develop, typically as late complications, that require urgent or immediate treatment. The most common ones can be classified as mechanical, systemic, infectious, or iatrogenic complications (Table 207.1).

Mechanical Complications

■ Superior Vena Cava Syndrome

The superior vena cava (SVC) syndrome, though not always a medical emergency, occurs with primary tumors or adenopathy involving the right side of the mediastinum. Most cases are due to bronchogenic carcinoma, usually of the small cell type. The clinical syndrome results in edema of the upper extremity, thorax, neck, and face, neck vein distention, periorbital and conjunctival edema, and often headache, flushing, and cyanosis. Venous collaterals may be visible on the chest wall.

The clinical diagnosis is confirmed by a contrast-enhanced CT scanning or radionuclide flow study. Other diagnostic studies include biopsy of superficial nodes and/or bronchoscopy, bearing in mind that excessive bleeding may follow. Transthoracic fine-needle biopsies are probably safer, when possible. Blind therapy without an etiologic diagnosis should be avoided, if possible.

The underlying etiology of this syndrome is often a highly treatable, even curable neoplasm. Small cell lung cancer can be treated initially with radiotherapy or combination chemotherapy. Similar considerations may

apply in germ cell tumors, Hodgkin's disease, and non-Hodgkin's lymphoma. In contrast, non-small cell carcinoma and adenocarcinomas metastatic to the mediastinum are best managed with radiotherapy, at least initially. SVC obstruction due to thrombosis has been treated with fibrinolytic agents, anticoagulants, and stenting, but in general, the results are not satisfactory.

■ Upper Airway, Esophageal, and Bronchial Obstruction

Most airway obstruction syndromes are secondary to carcinoma of the lung and esophagus. Although chemotherapy and radiotherapy may be helpful in selected cases when a responsive tumor is known to be present, emergency management requires bronchoscopy and surgical creation of a lumen using a variety of techniques, including the neodymium-YAG laser. Esophageal obstruction may be treated by laser therapy, or placing a bypassing gastrostomy tube or an indwelling endoprosthesis. Tracheoesophageal fistula, likewise, may require an emergency endoprosthesis.

TABLE 207.1.	Cancer-related Emergencies

Mechanical Complications
  Superior vena cava syndrome
  Upper airway, esophageal and bronchial obstruction
  GI tract perforation and obstruction
  Cardiac tamponade due to pericardial effusion
  Increased intracranial pressure
  Spinal cord compression
  Pathologic fractures
Coagulopathies
  Thrombocytopenia
  Immune-mediated
  Cancer treatment-related
  Extensive marrow infiltration
  Disseminated intravascular coagulation (DIC)
  Life-threatening thrombosis/embolus
  Severe anemia may be a consequence
Renal Emergencies
  Obstruction of the urinary tract
  Urinary hemorrhage
  Tumors of bladder or prostate
  Treatment related:
  Radiation therapy
  Cyclophosphamide or ifosfamide therapy
Metabolic Emergencies
  Hypercalcemia
  Hyponatremia
    SIADH
      Small cell carcinoma of the lung
      Nausea from cancer chemotherapy
    Hypotonic fluid administration given with cancer
      chemotherapy
    Adrenal insufficiency
    Gastrointestinal fluid losses and dehydration
  Cushing's Syndrome
    Small cell lung cancer
    Carcinoids
    Benign neuroendocrine tumors
Emergencies Due to Cancer Treatment
  Neutropenia and sepsis
  Tumor lysis syndrome
    Initial treatment of acute lymphocytic leukemia, Burkitt's or other undifferentiated lymphomas

■ Perforation and Obstruction in the Gastrointestinal Tract

Gastrointestinal perforations and obstructions represent surgical emergencies. Before urgent surgical therapy or other maneuvers are undertaken (e.g., nasogastric suction, analgesia, and antibiotics), the patient's prognosis and fitness for surgery should be ascertained.

■ Cardiac Tamponade due to Pericardial Effusion

Neoplastic pericardial effusion and tamponade occur most frequently with carcinoma of the lung or breast, melanoma, and lymphomas. It may also follow thoracic irradiation therapy, and infections of the pericardium, and conditions such as uremia and hypothyroidism, which may or may not be related to cancer. The diagnosis may be suggested by an enlarged cardiac shadow on chest x-ray and by weakness, fatigue, dyspnea, distended neck veins, and pulsus paradoxus (>12 mm Hg). In florid cases, prompt drainage may prevent death. Echocardiography, which shows the effusion as well as the signs of tamponade, is diagnostic.

■ Increased Intracranial Pressure

Usually due to mass effects of primary or metastatic brain tumors, increased intracranial pressure is ushered in with headache, nausea, vomiting, visual blurring, and a variety of neurologic signs with subsequent lethargy, somnolence, and coma. The diagnosis of brain metastases is confirmed by CT scan of the head or MRI of the brain. Some cases, especially with cranial neuropathies and negative CT or MRI, may be due to meningeal carcinomatosis.

The emergency treatment of brain metastases includes high-dose corticosteroids, usually dexamethasone, to control edema (10–20 mg initially followed by 4–10 mg q6h until maximal neurological response is obtained). Emergent radiation therapy should follow unless surgical resection or decompression is possible. Meningeal disease is usually treated by intrathecal chemotherapy with methotrexate or cytarabine, accompanied in most cases by whole-brain radiotherapy.

■ Spinal Cord Compression

Most cases of spinal cord compression are due to tumor extension into the epidural space from the vertebral body. On occasion, pathologic fracture of the involved vertebra can add the additional mechanical hazard of compression by bone. The diagnostic approach first involves a high index of suspicion. Increasing back pain and findings suggestive of metastatic tumor should lead to prompt MRI of the spine (Figure 207.1). When spinal cord compression is manifested by sensory or motor defects—decreased sensation, voluntary motor weakness (paraparesis or paraplegia), or involuntary motor dysfunction (e.g., bowel or bladder incontinence)—it is a true emergency. If an MRI scanning facility is not available, myelography is the alternative procedure. When combined with CT scanning, myelography with contrast

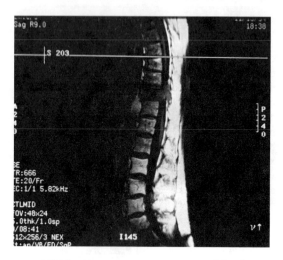

FIGURE 207.1. Magnetic resonance image of the thoracic spine showing metastatic prostate cancer invading the epidural space.

provides useful information as to encroachment on the dural sac.

Treatment options include emergent surgery or radiotherapy, if the underlying tumor is known, or highly suspected to be radioresponsive. High-dose corticosteroids, similar to those used in patients with intracranial neoplasms, should be given concurrently. If there is a pathologic fracture with spinal instability and compression of the cord by bone, the tumor is radioresistant and accompanied by neurologic deficit, or the cause of the spinal cord compression is unknown, one should proceed to surgery first. If the patient is ambulatory with minimal or no neurologic deficit, treatment by radiation or laminectomy followed by radiation will permit continued ambulation in 60–80% of patients, which drops to 40–45% or less if the patient has paraparesis and to 3–10% with paraplegia or quadriplegia. In few other conditions is an early diagnosis more vital.

■ Pathologic Fractures

Pathologic fractures of the femur and humerus, commonly from metastatic breast carcinoma, cause much disability. If a lesion is larger than 2.5×3 cm or causes thinning of the cortex, prophylactic orthopedic fixation should be performed, followed by radiation therapy.

Hematologic Emergencies

Many hematologic manifestations of cancer may present as emergencies. Severe anemia may require urgent transfusion. Thrombocytopenia and disseminated intravascular coagulation (DIC) may lead to bleeding, arterial emboli, and renal failure. Thrombocytopenia may be due to cancer treatment, extensive marrow infiltration, or immune-mediated mechanisms. After appropriate diagnostic studies, including bone marrow aspiration and biopsy, the etiology of the coagulopathy should be ascertained. The treatment of neoplastic DIC is difficult, as it involves the replacement of factors, cryoprecipitate, fresh frozen plasma, and platelets. Occasionally, heparin therapy may reverse DIC and nonbacterial thrombotic endocarditis. Warfarin therapy is almost universally unsuccessful. Thrombosis and/or embolus can be life-threatening emergencies. As in other consumptive coagulopathies, effective oral anticoagulation is difficult; recurrent, otherwise unexplained thrombosis/embolus should elicit a search for an occult malignancy.

Renal Emergencies

Obstruction of the urinary tract and urinary hemorrhage are the most common renal emergencies. Obstruction can occur in the pelvis or higher in a wide variety of malignant neoplasms and, if bilateral, can lead to rapidly progressive uremia. Ureteral stenting through the bladder with a double J-stent or by percutaneous nephrostomy allows palliation of this complication. Hemorrhage from the bladder may occur with tumors of the bladder or prostate, following radiation therapy or therapy with cyclophosphamide or ifosfamide. The emergency treatment is urethral catheterization with continuous bladder irrigation to flush out clots.

Metabolic Emergencies

■ Hypercalcemia

The most common hormonal syndrome causing a metabolic emergency is hypercalcemia. Its principal features (see Table 59.1 and chapter 59) are CNS depression, urinary frequency, polyuria and resultant polydipsia, nausea, vomiting, dehydration, and severe constipation from gastrointestinal tract atony. Dehydration is universal in symptomatic hypercalcemia; fluid replacement should be the initial therapy, followed by loop diuretics such as furosemide (thiazides must be avoided), which will maximize Na^+ coupled calcium excretion. This regimen will suffice for minimal elevations in serum calcium. In patients with compromised neurological states, bisphosphonates should be included, e.g., pamidronate. Medical therapy of hypercalcemic crisis is shown in Table 59.4.

Definitive treatment of malignancy-associated hypercalcemia consists of pamidronate infusion in doses of 60–90 mg every few days to control the serum calcium level. Hypercalcemia complicating multiple myeloma, some lymphomas, and breast cancer, commonly responds to corticosteroids. Mithramycin and gallium nitrate are two antitumor agents that are particularly useful in treating hypercalcemia. Specific antitumor treatment, appropriate to the type of neoplasm, may alleviate mild hypercalcemia and not require any specific calcium-lowering therapy.

A special case includes the hypercalcemic flare seen shortly after institution of **hormonal therapy in breast cancer** metastatic to bone. This effect had been encountered with estrogen and androgen therapy and now is seen with tamoxifen, and paradoxically, it was a marker for a subsequent good response to hormonal therapy. Frequently, tamoxifen can be continued while the hypercalcemia is being treated by specific measures.

■ Hyponatremia

Euvolemic hyponatremia, resulting from the syndrome of inappropriate secretion of antidiuretic hormone (SIADH), may be seen in a variety of malignancies and nonneoplastic disorders. The chief cause is small cell lung cancer. Mild cases can be treated with water restriction and demeclocycline. This antibiotic is phototoxic, and sun exposure should be avoided to prevent severe sunburn.

Management of severe hyponatremia is shown in Figure 57.4 in chapter 57. Emergencies can be managed by partial correction of the serum sodium with isotonic or hypertonic saline and administration of a loop diuretic to remove excess water. This must be done with care, correcting the serum sodium by no faster than 0.5 to 1 mEq/hr to avoid central pontine myelinolysis.

■ Cushing's Syndrome

Paraneoplastic Cushing's Syndrome can lead to hypokalemia, muscle weakness, and acute psychosis. It is most common in small cell lung cancer, with more indolent types seen with carcinoids and benign neuroendocrine tumors. That seen with small cell carcinoma of the lung is usually associated with muscle wasting, hypokalemia, hypertension, and severe weakness and progresses rapidly to death. Treatment with high-dose ketoconazole, 1200–1800 mg/day, or aminoglutethimide and hydrocortisone is indicated. Acute Cushing's syndrome in small cell carcinoma of the lung portends a poor prognosis.

Emergencies Associated with Cancer Treatment

■ Neutropenia and Sepsis

Neutropenia and subsequent fever commonly follow chemotherapy. Sepsis, which is rare when neutrophil counts exceed 1500/mm³, is increasingly common with falling counts, especially those below 500/mm³. Fever above 38.3°C (>101°F) with a neutrophil count below 500 mandates prompt examination, chest radiography, urinalysis, and cultures of blood, urine, and blood from venous access devices.

The most common organisms are gram-negative rods of the *Escherichia coli-Klebsiella* group, followed by *Pseudomonas*. Gram-positive infections are becoming much more common. Empiric broad-spectrum antibiotics should be started immediately to cover gram-negative organisms.

When fever persists, vancomycin and subsequent antifungal therapy with amphotericin-B should be instituted. Cultures may be negative in over one-half of cases, and therapy is largely empirical. With positive cultures or identification of a specific infection site, therapy can be individualized. Prolonged, severe neutropenia, systemic fungal infections, or uncontrolled bacterial sepsis are unfavorable signs. Antibiotics can be discontinued in the culture-negative, afebrile patient when the absolute neutrophil count exceeds 500/mm³. **Colony-stimulating factors** should be considered for prophylactic administration in subsequent courses of chemotherapy, but are not of proven benefit in patients presenting with neutropenic fever.

■ Questions

Instructions: For each question below, select **one** lettered answer that is the **best** for that question.

1. In the past two decades, which cancer has increased in incidence?
   A. Carcinoma of the cervix
   B. Carcinoma of the breast
   C. Carcinoma of the stomach
   D. Carcinoma of the rectum

2. Tobacco-associated malignancies include:
   A. Head and neck cancer
   B. Bladder cancer
   C. Esophageal cancer
   D. Pancreatic cancer
   E. All of the above

3. A 30-year-old man has had daily fever for two months and has lost 25 lbs. The only positive physical finding is an enlarged right axillary lymph node. CT scanning shows periaortic adenopathy. Bone marrow biopsies show a hypercellular marrow. The node shows lymphocyte-depleted Hodgkin's disease on biopsy. The patient's stage and management should be:
   A. The stage is undefined; he should have a staging laparotomy.
   B. He has Stage IIIB disease and should have a staging laparotomy to determine treatment options.
   C. Stage IIIB or higher. He should receive at least six cycles of ABVD or similar chemotherapy.
   D. Stage IIIB. He should receive total lymphoid irradiation.

4. Drugs used in chemotherapy have myriad toxicities. Those that may cause lung injury include:
   A. Methotrexate
   B. Busulfan
   C. Bleomycin
   D. Mitomycin C
   E. All of the above

5. A 36-year-old woman presents with a 2.5-cm non-tender breast mass that fails to disappear after her subsequent menstrual period. There are no palpable axillary nodes. Mammography shows bilateral dense breast tissue without a dominant mass. Correct management now is:
   A. Reassure the patient because the mammogram is negative.
   B. Discontinue the oral contraceptives she is taking; observe at 3-month intervals.
   C. Magnetic resonance imaging of the breast.
   D. Ultrasonography and fine needle aspiration; if no fluid is obtained, proceed directly to surgical excision.

6. A 25-year-old man complains of cough and wheezing. A lymph node is palpable in the right lower neck. A chest radiograph shows a large superior mediastinal mass with tracheal deviation. The next step would be:
   A. Biopsy the lymph node.
   B. Proceed with radiation without histologic diagnosis.
   C. Start combination chemotherapy with MOPP without histologic diagnosis.
   D. Initiate a comprehensive workup for infectious diseases, including TB, infectious mononucleosis, fungal infections, and HIV.

7. A 40-year-old woman with a 2.5-cm breast cancer with three positive axillary nodes is treated with six cycles of CMF. She asks you what is the estimated absolute benefit in terms of 10-year mortality reduction. You answer:
   A. 5%
   B. 3–6%
   C. 10–12%
   D. 50%

8. A 75-year-old man with coronary heart disease and chronic obstructive lung disease has palpable adenopathy in the neck and inguinal regions. He feels well and has normal blood counts. Lymph node biopsy shows follicular, small cleaved lymphocytic lymphoma. Bone marrow biopsy shows paratrabecular infiltrates of small cleaved lymphocytes. His lactate dehydrogenase is normal. The most reasonable management would be to:
   A. Initiate comprehensive combination chemotherapy with doxorubicin, cyclophosphamide, vincristine, and prednisone (CHOP). Tell the patient he has a 50% chance of cure.
   B. Discuss the potential indolent and incurable nature of this low-grade lymphoma; recommend close follow-up with palliative chemotherapy and/or radiotherapy only if/when progression is apparent.
   C. Institute palliative radiation therapy to all the enlarged lymph nodes.
   D. Institute non-toxic palliative chemotherapy using daily chlorambucil to be given indefinitely.

9. A 70-year-old man with known prostate cancer develops chronic back pain of 2 months' duration and is seen in the emergency department because of severe midthoracic pain with radiation to the left anterior chest. He reports difficulty in starting his

urinary stream. Appropriate steps in this situation include:

A. Tell the patient to use heat; prescribe an even stronger narcotic, encourage him to use stool softeners to prevent constipation since he may have this as well as urinary hesitancy due to narcotics.

B. Refer the patient to see his urologist expeditiously.

C. Obtain a CBC, ESR, and PSA.

D. Obtain spine films and an MRI of the thoracic spine immediately

10. A 68-year-old man has been diagnosed with pancreatic cancer. His wife reports he cannot sleep because of abdominal and back pain. He states his pain is mild, but he is visibly distressed and depressed. The best techniques for management are:

A. Sustained-release morphine every 8–12 hours with oral immediate-release morphine as needed for breakthrough pain.

B. Self-administration of meperidine (Demerol), 100 mg IM every 3 hours.

C. Administer PRN oxycodone with acetaminophen.

D. Prescribe ibuprofen, 800 mg orally every four hours.

11. A patient with known HIV infection develops a malignancy. Which of the following neoplasms are associated:

A. Squamous anal cancer

B. Cervical carcinoma

C. High-grade non-Hodgkin's lymphoma

D. Kaposi's sarcoma

E. All of the above

12. A 70-year-old woman with recently diagnosed metastatic breast cancer has generalized bone pain. She has widespread lytic bone metastases. Her original breast cancer was both estrogen- and progesterone-receptor-positive, but she has had no treatment since her original surgery 7 years ago. The best initial approach is:

A. Endocrine manipulation; radiation to weight-bearing bones with large lytic lesions.

B. Chemotherapy with cyclophosphamide and doxorubicin. Reserve radiation until pathologic fractures begin to develop.

C. Radiation treatment to sites of most severe pain followed by radioactive strontium if her pain is not immediately relieved.

D. Supportive care only

13. A patient presents with severe hyponatremia and vomiting. His serum sodium is 105 mEq/L; the blood urea nitrogen, 3 mg/ml; uric acid, 2.2 mg/ml. The most likely cause of a mediastinal mass in this setting is:

A. Hodgkin's disease

B. Teratoma of the mediastinum

C. Small cell lung cancer

D. Mesothelioma

14. Immediate and long-term management for the above patient includes:

A. Correct serum sodium to 140 mEq/L in 4 hours.

B. Correct serum sodium to 120 mEq/L in 10–15 hours with hypertonic saline and furosemide followed by fluid restriction and demeclocycline.

C. Allow unrestricted fluid intake.

D. Administer long-acting morphine sulfate.

15. In cancer of the colon, adjuvant chemotherapy using 5-fluorouracil and levamisole is beneficial in:

A. Duke's A

B. Dukes B1

C. Stage C

D. Stage D

16. A 45-year-old man has carcinoma of the larynx, stage II. He is treated with laryngectomy. Three years later, he develops a 2- cm nodule in the right upper lobe of his lung. The most likely etiology is:

A. Hamartoma

B. Metastasis of his laryngeal cancer

C. Granuloma

D. Primary lung cancer

17. Risk factors important in invasive cervical cancer include:

A. Early onset of sexual activity and multiple sex partners

B. Smoking

C. HIV infection

D. Absence of prior screening in an elderly woman

E. All of the above

■ Answers

1. B	2. E	3. C	4. E.	5. D
6. A	7. C	8. B	9. D	10. A
11. E	12. A	13. C	14. B	15. C
16. D	17. E			

SUGGESTED READING

General

Books and Monographs

DeVita VT Jr., Hellman S. Rosenberg SA. Cancer: Principles and Practice of Oncology. 5th ed. Philadelphia: Lippincott-Rowe, 1997.

Murphy GP, Lawrence W Jr., Lenhard RE. Jr American Cancer Society Textbook of Clinical Oncology. Atlanta: The American Cancer Society, 1995.

Holland JF, Frei E III, Bast RC et al. Cancer Medicine 4th ed. Philadelphia: Lea & Febiger, 1997.

Abeloff, MD, Armitage JO, Lichter AS, et al. Clinical Oncology. New York: Churchill Livingstone, 1995.

Casciato DA, Lowitz BB, Manual of Clinical oncology 3rd ed. Boston, Little, Brown and Company; 1995.

American Joint Committee on Cancer. Handbook for Staging of Cancer from Manual for Staging of Cancer 4th ed. Philadelphia: J.B. Lippincott Company, 1993.

Articles

Parker SL, Tong T, Bolden S, et al. Cancer statistics 1997. CA-A Journal for Clinicians. 1997;47:7–26.

Riparmonti C, Brucera E. Pain and symptom management in palliative care. Cancer Control 1996;3:204–213.

US Preventive Services Task Force. Guide to clinical preventive services. 2nd ed. Alexandria, VA: International Medical Publishing, 1996.

US Department of Health and Human Services Public Health Service. Clinical Practice Guidlines #9 Management of Cancer Pain Adults. Agency for Health Care policy and Research (AHCPR) 1994:592.

Lymphomas and Plasma Cell Dyscrasias

Urba WJ, Longo DH. Hodgkin's disease N Engl J Med 1992; 236:678–687.

Armitage JO. The treatment of Non-Hodgkin's lymphoma. N Engl J Med 1993;328:1023–1030.

Kyle RA. "Benign" Monoclonal Gammopathy—after 20 to 30 years of follow-up Mayo Clin Proc 1993;68:26–36.

Bataille R, Harousseau JL. Medical progress: multiple myeloma N Engl J Med 1997; 336:1657–1664.

Breast Cancer

Venta LA, Goodhartz LA. Age and interval for screening mammography: whom do you believe? Sem Surg Oncol 1996;12:281–289.

Donegan WL. Evaluation of a palpable breast mass. N Eng J Med 1992;327:937–942.

Hudis CA, Norton L. Adjuvant drug therapy for operable breast cancer. Semin Oncol 1996;3:475–493.

Goldhirsch A, Gelber RD Endocrine therapies for breast cancer Semin Oncol 1996;23:494–505.

Lung Cancer

Patel AM, Peters SG. Clinical manifestations of lung cancer. Mayo Clin Proc 1993;68:273–277.

Kunsell PR. Diagnostic Tests for lung cancer. Mayo Clin Proc 1993; 68:288–296.

Gastrointestinal Cancers

Ransohoff DF, Lang CA. Clinical guidlines part II: screening for colorectal cancer with the fecal occult blood test: a background paper. Ann Intern Med 1997;126:811–822.

Genitourinary Cancer

Coley CM, Barry MJ, Fleming C, et al. Clinical guidlines part I: early detection of prostate cancer: prior probability and effectiveness of tests. Ann Intren Med 1997;126:394–406.

Figlin RA, Belldegran A. Renal cell carcinoma. Semin Oncol 1995;22:1–91.

Frydenberg M, Stricker, PD, Kaye KW. Prostate cancer diagnosis and management. Lancet 1997;349:1681–1687.

Gurpeide DP. Endometrial cancer: biochemical and clinical correlates. JNCI 1991;83:405–416.

Kantoff PW, Scher HI. Bladder cancer. Hematol Oncol Clin North Am 1992;6:1–201.

McGuire WP, Hoskins WJ, Brady MF, et al. Cyclophosphamide and cisplatin compared with paclitaxel and cisplatin in patients with stage III and stage IV ovarian cancer N Engl J Med 1996;334:1–6.

Roth BJ, Nichols CR. Testicular cancer. Semin Oncoly 1992; 19:117–216.

Cancer of the Head and Neck

Balch CM, Houghton AN, Milton GW, et al (eds.). Cutaneous melanoma. Philadelphia: J.B. Lippincoll Company; 1991.

Vokes EE. Head and neck cancer. Semin Oncol 1994;21:279–399.

Cancer of Unknown Primary Site

Hainsworth JD, Greco FA. Drug Therapy: Treatment of patients with cancer of an unknown primary site. Semin Oncol 1993;20:205–294.

Paraneoplastic Syndromes and Oncologic Emergencies

American Society of Clinical Oncology recommendations for the use of hematopoetic colony stimulating factors: evidence-based clinical practice guidlines. J Clin Oncol 1994;12:2471–2508.

Cascino TL. Medical complications of systemic cancer. Med Clin North Am 1993;77:265.

Moore GP, Jorden RC. Hematologic/oncologic emergencies. Emerg Med Clin North Am 1993;11:273–555.

Patel AM, Davila DG, Peters SG. Paraneoplastic syndromes associated with lung cancer. Mayo Clin Proc 1993;68:278–287.

Pizzo, PA. Drug therapy: Management of fever in patients with cancer and treatment-related neutropenia N Engl J Med 1993;328:1323–1332.

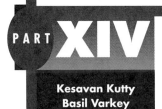
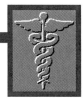

PART XIV

Kesavan Kutty
Basil Varkey

PULMONARY DISEASES

CLINICAL EVALUATION OF LUNG DISEASE

ippocrates believed that the purpose of breathing was to "cool the heart", whose function it was to generate heat and thereby maintain life. Through centuries of scientific progress has evolved the correct concept that the prime function of the lungs is sustenance of life through respiration, effecting oxygenation of blood and removal of carbon dioxide. The lungs also perform some metabolic functions. Despite the recent great strides in diagnostic procedures, (e.g., fiberoptic bronchoscopy, computed tomography), the initial diagnostic tools for a patient with lung disease remain traditional: history, physical examination, the roentgenogram, and differential diagnosis, in that order.

■ Presenting Complaints

Cough

Cough, a very common symptom, generally implies airway disease. Its onset (acute or chronic) and the presence or absence of sputum should be noted. Associated fever suggests an infection. An acute cough of a few days is commonly caused by acute bronchitis. A cough lasting longer than 4 weeks is **chronic persistent cough** (Table 208.1). Rhinosinusitis with postnasal drip, asthma, and gastroesophageal (g-e) reflux cause most instances of chronic persistent cough in nonsmokers; chronic bronchitis is the most common cause among smokers. Other causes in nonsmokers and smokers are left ventricular

---

TABLE 208.1. Common Causes of Chronic Persistent Cough: Features, Diagnosis, and Therapy

	Causes		
Rhinosinusitis with Postnasal Drip	**Asthma**	**GE Reflux**	**Chronic Bronchitis**
Features			
• "Tickle" in the throat • Frequent throat clearing • Nasal twang to voice • Nasal discharge (±purulence), nasal stuffiness or sneezing • Relation to supine posture • Recent viral infection with sinusitis	• Cough may be the only symptom • Cough may be productive • Wheezing • Relationship to cold air, exercise, or ingestion of cold liquids or ice cream • Other atopic symptoms • Relationship to supine posture • Dyspnea on exertion • Nocturnal periodicity	• Hoarseness • Heartburn • Chest pain • Relation to supine posture • Nocturnal periodicity	• Productive cough • Smoking history • Symptom diminishes or disappears after smoking cessation • Wheezing • Hemoptysis
Diagnosis			
Based on history and findings as above.	If spirometry is normal, perform methacholine bronchoprovocation test, which has a 100% sensitivity for asthma presenting as cough.	Causes 15–20% of chronic cough. Suspect if a basic evaluation reveals no cause. Ambulatory pH monitoring quite useful in diagnosis.	Essentially a clinical diagnosis. Pulmonary function tests commonly show airflow obstruction. High risk for lung cancer, which should be appropriately excluded.
Therapy			
Empiric therapy with antihistamines, decongestants. Others include intranasal corticosteroids; antibiotics for infection.	Inhaled corticosteroids and β2 agents (as needed).	H2-blocking agents.	Smoking cessation.

failure, interstitial lung disease, and viral infection (postviral cough). Combinations are not uncommon (e.g., postnasal drip in an asthmatic). While sinusitis and g-e reflux can also cause a persistent cough in smokers, lung cancer should be excluded in this group.

Management of chronic cough

A careful history and physical examination are key to an accurate diagnosis (Table 208.1). Pulmonary function tests and a methacholine bronchoprovocation study may also be necessary. Chest x-ray is generally not useful unless considerations include heart failure (history of heart disease, edema, dyspnea, orthopnea, paroxysmal nocturnal dyspnea, interstitial lung disease (dry cough, dyspnea, finger clubbing, "Velcro" rales) or bronchogenic carcinoma (hemoptysis, weight loss, chest pain). Once a definite cause is obvious, treatment should follow (Table 208.1). Among nonsmokers, a **stepwise management** is advocated (Figure 208.1), in which further treatment is recommended if the patient does not respond to the initial treatment and compliance by the patient is not in question. Cough may be due to multiple causes in the same patient, requiring multiple agents simultaneously. Medications (angiotensin-converting en-

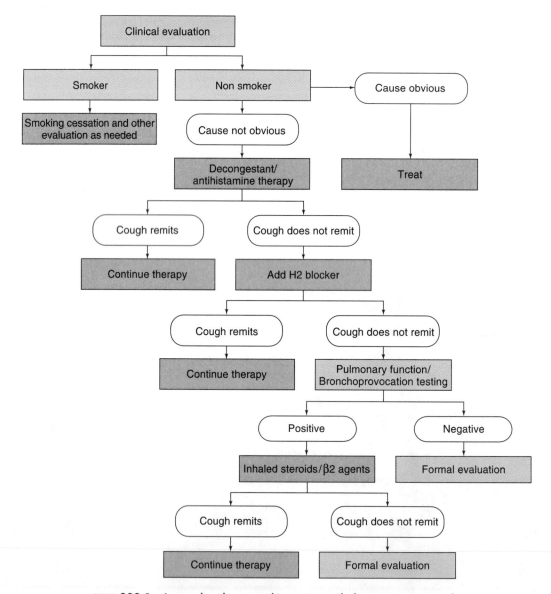

FIGURE 208.1. Approach to the nonsmoking patient with chronic persistent cough.

zyme inhibitors and/or β-blocking agents) may need to be withdrawn if it appears that they are causing the cough. Generally, **fiberoptic bronchoscopy** is not very useful in the nonsmoker unless the chest x-ray (if taken) is abnormal or a foreign body is suspected. In most smokers, the cough disappears after smoking cessation; if it does not, other causes must be pursued. If the patient does not stop smoking, some evaluation (at a minimum, a chest x-ray) is necessary, depending on the likelihood of lung cancer.

Sputum production

Sputum is mucus produced by mucin-secreting bronchial glands and cleared by the airway cilia. Expectoration of sputum is abnormal. Cough and sputum are integral features of **chronic bronchitis.** Yellow **sputum** is most commonly from bacterial bronchitis, stasis in the tracheobronchial tree, or asthma exacerbation when eosinophil-laden. **Abundant mucopurulent sputum** signifies bronchiectasis; **foul-smelling sputum** signifies anaerobic lung abscesses.

Dyspnea

Dyspnea is awareness of one's breathing. In clinical terms, **it means shortness of breath.** Dyspnea at rest is always abnormal, but during exercise it is contextual. If the patient previously tolerated similar levels of exertion well, then the dyspnea is significant. **Acute dyspnea** may be from acute airway obstruction, acute pulmonary edema, pneumothorax, or pulmonary embolism. Postoperative dyspnea is commonly from pulmonary embolism, massive atelectasis, or acute pulmonary edema from fluid overload. Associated cough, sputum production, or hemoptysis are useful clues in assessing **chronic dyspnea.** Orthopnea or paroxysmal nocturnal dyspnea suggests heart failure. With a normal chest x-ray, the causes are pulmonary embolism, interstitial lung disease, airway obstruction, chest wall or neuromuscular disorders, or anxiety. Abnormal chest x-rays accompany dyspnea due to heart failure, interstitial lung disease, large pleural effusion, or advanced emphysema. Worsening of pre-existent dyspnea in a smoker, whatever the chest x-ray results, should always alert the physician to possible bronchogenic carcinoma. In evaluating chronic dyspnea, an occupational history is also very important.

Chest pain

Chest pain has varying patterns, among them angina (chapter 23); pleural, muscular, and costochondral pain; and intercostal neuralgia. Pleuritic pain worsens upon inspiration, cough, or even movement of the chest wall. Commonly encountered in emergency departments, it is caused by pulmonary embolism in about one-fourth of the cases; other causes are pneumonia, or viral pleuritis.

TABLE 208.2. Common Causes of Hemoptysis	
General Category	**Specific Diseases/Causes**
Infectious/inflammatory	Chronic bronchitis[a]
	Mycobacterial diseases (tuberculosis and others)[b]
	Bronchiectasis[a,b]
	Lung abscess[b]
	Blastomycosis
Cardiovascular diseases	Pulmonary thromboembolism
	Mitral stenosis[a,b]
Neoplasms	Pulmonary
	Primary: bronchogenic carcinoma,[b] bronchial carcinoid[a]
	Metastatic
	Extrapulmonary
	Laryngeal carcinoma
	Nasopharyngeal carcinoma
Autoimmune	Pulmonary hemorrhage syndromes
	Wegener's granulomatosis
	Lupus pneumonitis
Miscellaneous	Inhaled foreign body
	Bleeding dyscrasias/anticoagulant ingestion[b]
	Expectoration of aspirated blood (from vomiting/epistaxis)

[a]May cause recurrent episodes.
[b]May cause massive hemoptysis.

Muscular pain is superficial and may follow strenuous movements of the chest wall muscles or trauma-induced muscle bruising. There may be rib fractures as well. Costochondral pain is typically along the costochondral articulations. **Tietze's syndrome** affects the upper costochondral joints. **Intercostal neuralgia** is a pain shooting from the back forward and characteristically worsened by movement but not generally by respiration. It is a pre-eruptive symptom of herpes zoster and occasionally persists after the eruptions have resolved.

Hemoptysis

Hemoptysis—expectoration of frank blood—signifies a serious underlying disease (Table 208.2). (Patients with acute respiratory infections, acute bronchitis, or bacterial pneumonia may have blood-streaked sputum, which is different.) The first step—distinguishing hemoptysis from hematemesis (vomiting of blood), is generally easy with a history. The historical data that should be collected in hemoptysis, and their implications, are shown in Table 208.3. Clinical assessment includes examination of the ears, nose, and throat (epistaxis, lesions

TABLE 208.3.	Hemoptysis: Clinical Implications of Historical Data
Data	**Implication**
Amount	Massive hemoptysis can be lethal by asphyxiation.
Prior cough and sputum	Chronic bronchitis.
Prior episodes	Episodes of blood-streaked sputum common in chronic bronchitis.
Provocating factors	Repetitive, severe cough can cause hemoptysis, but is a diagnosis of exclusion.
Associated symptoms	
Chest pain	Complicates pulmonary embolism, tuberculosis.
Fever	Suggestive of infectious, inflammatory, or neoplastic process.
Weight loss	Suggestive of neoplasm or tuberculosis.
Leg pain/swelling	Suggestive of venous thromboembolism/heart failure.
Loss of consciousness	May have predisposed to a lung abscess.
History of smoking	Bronchogenic carcinoma; chronic bronchitis.
Prior recurrent pneumonia	Endobronchial obstruction or residual bronchiectasis.

of Wegener's granulomatosis). Telangiectasia of the lips may suggest a pulmonary arteriovenous fistula. Stridor, wheezing, clubbing (intrathoracic neoplasm or bronchiectasis), and mediastinal or tracheal shift indicating atelectasis are important findings that offer clues to a cause for hemoptysis.

Helpful laboratory studies include a complete blood count, platelet count, coagulation studies, oximetry or arterial blood gases, and sputum examination for cytology and fungi. A chest x-ray is pivotal. With a normal chest x-ray, likely causes are pulmonary embolism, acute exacerbation of chronic bronchitis, and bronchiectasis. If the x-ray suggests tuberculosis, the sputum should be examined for mycobacteria. Otherwise, a fiberoptic bronchoscopic examination is undertaken within 48 hours to establish a site and cause of bleeding. Massive hemoptysis, defined as 600 ml of blood within 24 hours (prorated for smaller intervals of time), carries a 75% mortality—urgent rigid bronchoscopy is the first step; bronchial arteriography and embolization, and/or surgical resection are options.

Wheezing

A wheeze is a high-pitched, whistling or squeaking continuous sound with a frequency of ≥ 400 Hz, lasting over 250 msec, produced by the passage of air across a narrowed airway. Wheezing is best heard at the mouth, often without using a stethoscope. Upper airway obstruction below the thoracic inlet causes wheezing rather than stridor. Diffuse wheezing with a uniform pitch and intensity in both lungs suggests central obstruction; focal wheezing suggests localized bronchial obstruction. Since wheezing in itself is nondiagnostic, the integration of clinical history, physical findings, and laboratory studies is essential. Asthma may occasionally appear for the first time after the age of 60, but unprecedented wheezing in someone of this age group more typically signifies left heart failure ("cardiac asthma"). Other causes of wheezing are listed in Table 208.4.

■ Bedside Clinical Assessment

Besides a succinct history of present illness, a detailed history of all illnesses, particularly respiratory illnesses, should be obtained. It is important to inquire about past chest roentgenograms and their availability for review. All current and past use of drugs (legal and illicit), alcohol, and tobacco (quantitated in pack-years) should be reviewed. The patient's hobbies and the presence of household pets should also be recorded. Travel history is important, especially in endemic mycoses and some viral illnesses. One should ascertain all the jobs held, from the first one to the most recent. It is well known that some occupations may cause lung disease, but the long interval between exposure and manifest disease is not so readily appreciated.

Physical findings in some pulmonary processes are shown in Table 208.5.

TABLE 208.4.	Causes of Wheezing
Category	**Specific Diseases/Causes**
Upper airway obstruction (below the thoracic inlet)	Angioedema
	Epiglottitis
	Foreign body
	Goiter
	Tumor
	Vocal cord paralysis
Lower airway obstruction	Asthma
	Bronchiolitis
	Left heart failure
	Chronic obstructive pulmonary disease
	Cystic fibrosis
	Foreign body
	Tumor
	Tenacious secretions
Extrapulmonary disorders	Carcinoid syndrome

TABLE 208.5. Typical Physical Findings in the Chest in Common Pulmonary Disorders

Disorder	Mediastinal Shift	Percussion	Breath Sounds	Adventitious Sounds	Vocal Resonance	Other
Atelectasis	Present, toward side of lesion	Impaired over affected area	Reduced or absent	None	Reduced or absent	Diminished chest wall movement over affected side
Consolidation	None	Impaired over affected area	Bronchial	Mid to late inspiratory rales[a]	E to A changes, whispering pectoriloquy	Splinting from pain may reduce ipsilateral chest wall movement
Cavitation	May or may not occur, but if present, to side of lesion if there is fibrosis	Impaired	Bronchial	Rales	Increased E to A changes	
Asthma	None	Normal	Normal with prolonged exhalation	Wheeze, mostly expiratory	Normal	Accessory muscle use and pulsus paradoxus may be present
Emphysema	None	Increased	Reduced with prolonged expiration	Rhonchi ±	Reduced	Pursed-lip breathing; pink and cherubic
Chronic bronchitis	None	Normal	Normal with prolonged expiration	Expiratory rhonchi, rales throughout inspiration	Normal	Cyanosis ±, often obese
Pleural effusion	Present, to opposite side	Dull	Reduced or absent over the effusion	None	Reduced or absent	—
Pneumothorax	Present, to opposite side	Normal to hyperresonant	Normal to reduced	None	Reduced	Affected side may move less

[a]Râles (crackles) are best classified according to their timing. Rales occurring in early and mid-inspiration suggest airway disease. Those in late inspiration are mostly representative of alveolar disease.

CHAPTER **209** BASIC LABORATORY TESTS

■ Skin Tests

A **tuberculin skin test** is used to diagnose tuberculosis infection, and is done using an intradermal injection of 0.1 ml (= 5 tuberculin units [TU]) of Tween-stabilized purified protein derivative (PPD-S). Tests for skin reactivity are also given, using mumps and Trichophyton antigens (or tetanus toxoid if the patient has previously had vaccination against tetanus). The extent of induration is carefully noted after 48 hours. Negative reactions to antigens indicate anergy. Tuberculin reactivity wanes with time and therefore, the test is repeated one week later if the initial test is negative. The person is considered infected or noninfected based on the results of the second ("boosted") test. If Bacille Calmette Guérin (BCG) inoculation was not done within the preceding 6–7 years, a positive PPD test denotes infection with *Mycobacterium tuberculosis*. Atypical mycobacterial infections may cause false positive tests. Revised criteria for PPD tests are shown in Table 209.1.

■ Sputum Examination

The sputum should be collected in a clean, sterile container. If the patient does not expectorate, induction may be needed. Gross characteristics such as viscidity, color, odor, and the presence of blood should be noted. Reliable results depend on prompt delivery of the specimen to the laboratory. A reliable sputum specimen will reveal several alveolar macrophages (round, large cells with granular inclusions and an oval, eccentric nucleus). Abundant squamous cells (large, flat cells, with a central nucleus) signify contamination with oral/pharyngeal secretions, making the sample unreliable. Many neutrophils (≥25 at 10x power) signify infection, most often bacterial. More than 20% eosinophils means atopic disease.

Staining procedures

Bacteriology is evaluated by a Gram stain. Acid-fast (Ziehl-Nielsen) staining is done for *Mycobacterium tuberculosis,* and pretreatment with 10% potassium hydroxide for visualizing fungi. Gram-positive cocci may be pneumococci (pairs or chains) or staphylococci (groups). Gram-negative bacilli may be *Haemophilus influenzae* (small, pleomorphic) or *Klebsiella pneumoniae* (large, often encapsulated). These results should be integrated with the clinical history and culture results; in the setting of a pulmonary infection, they provide a guideline for initial antibiotic therapy.

While a reliable microbiologic diagnosis of a pulmonary infection helps in determining effective treatment, routine sputum microbiologic tests are probably of limited use in community-acquired pneumonias (especially in an otherwise healthy, immunocompetent adult); also, the availability of broad-spectrum antibiotics that are effective against the majority of pathogens causing community-acquired pneumonias might preclude the need for a microbiological diagnosis prior to therapy. However, in the hospitalized or immunocompromised adult, sputum should be examined if available, and if not, after induction. Cultures for fungi and mycobacteria are also useful.

Cytologic examination

The results of cytologic examination vary, depending on the number of sputum samples submitted and the proficiency of the cytopathologist. In bronchogenic carcinoma, sputum cytology has a high (69–80%) sensitivity, with a specificity of nearly 96%. Slightly over half of all metastatic lung cancers are diagnosable with three or more good samples.

■ Arterial Blood Gas Analysis

Arterial blood gas analysis provides significant information about the gas-exchanging function of the

TABLE 209.1.	Tuberculin Skin Test: New Centers for Disease Control Guidelines for Positive Reactions
Tuberculin Test is Considered Positive with an Induration of at Least:	**Affected Population**
5 mm	• In recent contacts • When fibrotic lesions in chest x-ray simulate old healed tuberculosis • With co-existent HIV infection

10 mm	• In medically underserved, economically disadvantaged minorities
	• In those with
	  – other medical risks for tuberculosis
	  – residence in endemic areas or long-term care facility
	  – IV drug abuse
	• All others with increased prevalence of tuberculosis

15 mm	• All others

lung. A sample of arterial blood is obtained in a heparinized syringe from the brachial or the radial artery. The syringe with the sample should be placed in ice immediately and the sample analyzed for the pH and the tensions of oxygen (PaO_2) and carbon dioxide ($PaCO_2$). The following stepwise approach is recommended for interpreting the data:

Step 1. Estimate the partial pressure of inhaled oxygen (PIO_2).

Principle: Atmospheric air, with water vapor removed, is essentially a mixture of oxygen (O_2) and nitrogen (N_2) in a ratio of 0.21:0.79. Their combined partial pressures make up the total pressure of the mixture—namely, barometric pressure (P_B)—with their individual partial pressures in this mixture bearing the same ratio (Dalton's law). At sea level, P_B is 760 mm Hg and water vapor pressure (PH_2O) at body temperature is 47 mm Hg.

Formula:

$$PIO_2 = (P_B - PH_2O) \times 0.21$$
$$= (760\text{-}47) \times 0.21$$
$$= 149.7 \ mm \ Hg$$

Note: If the person is breathing supplemental oxygen, the appropriate fraction for 0.21 should be substituted.

Step 2. Estimate the alveolar oxygen tension (PAO_2).

Principle: The ratio of gases is altered in the alveoli because of the entry of CO_2 from the pulmonary capillaries. The rate at which O_2 is exchanged for CO_2 is determined by the respiratory exchange ratio, or R, which is usually 0.8. For purposes of calculation, the alveolar PCO_2 ($PACO_2$) is assumed to be equal to arterial CO_2 ($PaCO_2$).

Formula:

$$PAO2 = PIO_2 - (PACO_2/R)$$
$$But \ PACO_2 = PaCO_2$$

Therefore,

$$PAO_2 = PIO_2 - (PaCO_2 / 0.8)$$

or

$$PAO_2 = PIO_2 - (PaCO_2 \times 1.25)$$
$$At \ sea \ level, \ with \ PaCO_2 \ of \ 40 \ mm \ Hg,$$
$$PAO_2 = 149.7 - (40 \times 1.25)$$
$$= 99.7 \ mm \ Hg$$

Step 3. Estimate the alveolar-arterial (A-a) oxygen gradient.

Principle: The normally small difference between the PAO_2 and the PaO_2 is called the A-a gradient for oxygen, or $P(A\text{-}a)O_2$. It is age-dependent, rising from 10 mm Hg in a young adult to around 27–30 mm Hg in a nonagenarian. An abnormally widened age-adjusted gradient indicates lung disease.

Formula:

$$P(A\text{-}a)O_2 = PAO_2 - PaO_2$$

Step 4. Define the adequacy of ventilation.

Principle: $PaCO_2$, which maintains an inverse relationship to alveolar ventilation, is the sole harbinger of the adequacy of ventilation. A low value indicates hyperventilation and a high value reflects hypoventilation.

Step 5. Assess the hypoxemia.

Principle: The hypoxemia (a low PaO_2) may be due to several mechanisms, the most common being a *mismatching of ventilation-perfusion (V/Q) relationships*. Hypoxemia due to V/Q mismatch readily improves with supplemental oxygen administration or induced hyperventilation. Another mechanism is *hypoventilation*, since PaO_2 and $PaCO_2$ maintain a reciprocal relationship. The sum of [PaO_2 + ($PaCO_2 \times 1.25$) + the applicable gradient for age] approximates the calculated PIO_2 when hypoxemia is due to pure alveolar hypoventilation. A *shunt* (anatomic, as in a right-to-left intracardiac shunt) or *shunt effect* (as in various intrapulmonary processes, such as widespread atelectasis or adult respiratory distress syndrome) also causes hypoxemia, where the PaO_2 responds poorly at best to supplemental oxygen. Finally, *diffusion defects*, by precluding equilibration of alveolar gas with the pulmonary end-capillary blood, can sometimes contribute, albeit trivially, to hypoxemia.

Step 6. Estimate the oxygen content.

Principle: Oxygen is transported in hemoglobin-bound and dissolved forms. Oxygen saturation (SaO_2), which represents the saturation of hemoglobin, may be determined by direct measurement as part of a blood gas analysis, or estimated from the oxyhemoglobin dissociation curves. Each gram of hemoglobin, upon full (100%) saturation, carries 1.34 ml of oxygen. Oxygen also dissolves in the plasma at a rate of 0.003 ml for every mm Hg of PaO_2.

Formula:

$$Hb\text{-}bound \ oxygen = 1.34 \times Gm \ of \ Hb \times SaO_2\%$$
$$Dissolved \ Oxygen = 0.003 \times PaO_2$$

The sum of the above (Hb-bound oxygen + dissolved oxygen) represents the total oxygen transported by every 100 ml of blood. Many blood gas laboratories automatically provide this information in the blood gas report.

Step 7. Assess the pH and acid-base status.

Principle: Normal pH varies from 7.35 to 7.45. A pH above 7.45 indicates **alkalosis,** and a pH below 7.35 indicates **acidosis.** (The range of acid-base disturbances is shown in Table 172.1.) Compensatory mechanisms that follow a primary disturbance bring the pH toward but not completely back to normal. The extent and effectiveness of such compensation varies with the primary disorder. Because renal HCO_3 retention takes several days, acute respiratory acidosis is least well compensated. Thus, the most effective therapy for acute respiratory acidosis is to increase alveolar ventilation, often through an endotracheal tube and mechanical ventilation, if indicated.

CHAPTER 210 IMAGING IN PULMONARY DIAGNOSIS

■ Conventional and Special Studies

For most practical purposes, a posteroanterior (PA) chest x-ray is adequate. But unless supplemented by a lateral view, processes in the retrosternal and retrocardiac areas as well as a very small pleural effusion in the posterior costophrenic sulcus may be missed. Additional examinations may be dictated by circumstances (e.g., rib films in suspected rib fractures).

A small pleural effusion is most commonly manifested by a blunted costophrenic angle. To distinguish a pleural effusion from pleural fibrosis or thickening, an ipsilateral decubitus view is very helpful. An effusion that does not layer out is loculated. Loculations often portend an underlying infection in the pleural fluid. **Inspiration-expiration films** are most valuable for detecting a small pneumothorax. A **barium esophagogram** may also be helpful in investigating unexplained, recurrent lower lobe pneumonia that may be secondary to a Zenker's diverticulum esophageal stricture and/or achalasia. **Pulmonary arteriography** is used mainly in investigating pulmonary thromboembolism (chapter 226). It is also useful in diagnosing vascular anomalies such as pulmonary arteriovenous fistulae.

■ Computed Tomography

With computed tomographic (CT) scanning, one can obtain an image of a transverse slice of the body. An x-ray beam, as it passes through organs of varying tissue density, gets variably attenuated. Computer analysis of such attenuations generates images of various organs, yielding valuable information about the density of a particular organ or tissue—for example, solid, cystic, and metallic (calcification). Using contrast media, vascular structures can be distinguished from nonvascular densities.

Chest CT offsets the blind spots of the conventional radiographs and is, therefore, invaluable in evaluating mediastinal structures and masses and pleural-based densities. It is essential in the preoperative staging of bronchogenic carcinoma, except perhaps those that present as a small (<2 cm), single nodule. **Spiral (helical) CT** shows promise for diagnosing pulmonary embolism in larger (proximal) vessels. The physician should consider both its cost and its usefulness before ordering it.

■ Magnetic Resonance Imaging

While very effective in detecting soft tissue contrast and visualizing in multiple planes, magnetic resonance imaging (MRI) requires no contrast media and has no ionizing radiation. Its disadvantages are its high cost, lack of general availability, the hazard to individuals with various prosthetic devices, and the problems caused by air-containing lungs and their physiologic motion. MRI can diagnose large but not small, peripheral pulmonary emboli. While it can image hilar and mediastinal areas very well (e.g., evaluating mediastinal or vascular invasion by neoplastic process) it is unable to distinguish between reactive lymphadenopathy and malignant infiltration of lymph nodes. Its ability to image in multiple—especially coronal and sagittal—planes makes it an invaluable tool in the management of **superior sulcus tumor,** a distinct advantage over CT.

■ Radionuclide Scans and Ultrasonography

Perfusion, ventilation, and **gallium scanning** are three categories of commonly performed radionuclide scans of the lung. Perfusion scans assess the vasculature of the lung. Intravenously administered Tc^{99}-labeled albumin microspheres enter the lung and become trapped in pulmonary capillaries. External imaging of the radioactivity of these trapped particles can assess the perfusion in each area. Areas devoid of perfusion are free of radioactivity. In pulmonary embolism, these defects usually have a lobar or segmental pattern. Ventilation scanning, performed by using a radioactive tracer gas (usually 133^{Xe}), helps detect abnormal ventilation patterns such as air trapping. The gas is inhaled and equilibrated within the lung; during exhalation the washout is detected by imaging. In normally ventilated areas, the radioactivity clears in approximately 3 minutes. Gallium (67^{Ga}) has an affinity for leukocytes and when given parenterally it accumulates in inflammatory foci and tumor tissue. It is quite useful in detecting opportunistic infections in immunosuppressed patients and potentially useful in detecting other types of inflammatory lung or pleural disease.

Ultrasonography is used mainly as guidance for thoracentesis of very small or loculated pleural effusions.

Segmental Anatomy

The lungs consist of two general components: **conducting airways** and the **terminal respiratory units.** Conducting airways (trachea, bronchi, and nonrespiratory bronchioles) transport air. Respiratory units (respiratory bronchioles, alveolar ducts, and alveoli) accomplish gas exchange. The trachea divides into right and left main bronchi at the carina. Because this angle of bifurcation is less acute on the right, gravitational (aspiration) processes occur more commonly in the right lung. Each lung has several bronchopulmonary segments, and each segment is supplied by a segmental bronchus and its corresponding segmental branch of the pulmonary artery. The right lung has 10 segments: three (apical, posterior, and anterior) in the right upper lobe, two (lateral and medial) in the middle lobe, and five (superior, medial basal, anterior basal, lateral basal, and posterior basal) in the right lower lobe. The left lung has 8 segments. The upper division bronchus of the left upper lobe has two segments, the apical-posterior and anterior. The lower division bronchus has two segments—namely, superior lingular and inferior lingular. The lower lobe has four segments: superior, anteromedial basal, lateral basal, and posterior basal (Figure 211.1).

Bronchopulmonary segmental anatomy is clinically relevant since certain disease processes tend to affect certain segments—for example, tuberculosis in apical and posterior segments of the upper lobes and gravitational pneumonia and lung abscess in posterior segments of the upper lobes and superior segments of the lower lobes.

Physiology

Ventilation is the intake and distribution of air from the external environment to the alveolus and its return to the exterior. The process of gas exchange in the alveolus is **diffusion,** which involves the passive movement of gases based on concentration gradients. Gas exchange is facilitated by the maintenance of a constant blood flow—**perfusion**—through the pulmonary parenchyma. Optimal performance of the system requires careful matching of the body's metabolic needs with pulmonary ventilation and perfusion.

Ventilation

Tissue oxygen demands increase substantially during exercise, febrile states, and other metabolic stresses. Impulses from the peripheral and central chemoreceptors as well as from the receptors in the lung are received in the medulla, where the information is assimilated and appropriate changes in ventilation initiated. These receptors are stimulated in pneumonia, asthma, various neurologic disorders, and following the ingestion of drugs (e.g., aspirin). Depression of these receptors leads to hypoventilation as seen in obesity, severe chronic bronchitis, severe metabolic alkalosis, and myxedema.

The various compartments of ventilation are represented in Figure 211.2. Even in healthy persons, the amount of inhaled air is distributed somewhat unevenly because of variations in intrapleural pressures. In an erect person, the intrapleural pressure tends to be maximally negative at the apices and less negative at the bases. This leads to more distention of the alveoli at the apex than at the bases and, thus, a slow breath from the functional residual capacity (FRC) level is distributed preferentially to the lower lobes. During rest, therefore, when the lower lobes get the maximal share of blood supply, ventilation is also preferentially distributed there. But with increasing breathing frequency and increasing rates of air flow, the distribution becomes more uniform. During exercise, a more equitable distribution of blood flow occurs; this is matched by a redistribution of ventilation.

Abnormal ventilation

The two abnormal patterns of ventilation are obstruction and restriction. **Obstructive impairment,** characterized by obstruction to air flow, occurs in asthma, chronic bronchitis, emphysema, bronchiectasis, and cystic fibrosis. **Restrictive impairment,** characterized by a limitation of the amount of air in the lungs, manifests with diminished lung volumes, especially the total lung capacity. Examples are pulmonary fibrosis, fibrothorax, and lung resection.

Diffusion

The quantity of a gas that diffuses across the alveolar-capillary membrane per unit time, based on gas-pressure gradients between the alveolus and the blood, is known as the **diffusing capacity of the lung** (DL) for that gas. The most common gas used for measuring DL is carbon monoxide (CO). The measurement (DL_{CO}) is expressed as ml/min/mmHg. It has a membrane (D_m) and capillary blood volume (V_c) components. The values correlate well with lung volume and body size. The single-breath (SB) determination is easy to perform, although it involves breath-holding for about 8–10 seconds.

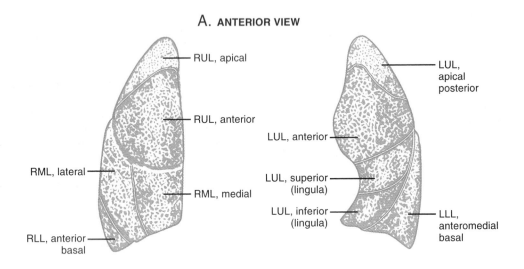

A. **ANTERIOR VIEW**

RUL, apical

LUL, apical posterior

RUL, anterior

LUL, anterior

RML, lateral

LUL, superior (lingula)

RML, medial

LUL, inferior (lingula)

LLL, anteromedial basal

RLL, anterior basal

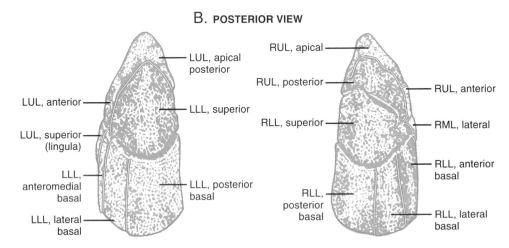

B. **POSTERIOR VIEW**

LUL, apical posterior

RUL, apical

RUL, posterior

RUL, anterior

LUL, anterior

LLL, superior

RLL, superior

RML, lateral

LUL, superior (lingula)

LLL, anteromedial basal

LLL, posterior basal

RLL, anterior basal

RLL, posterior basal

LLL, lateral basal

RLL, lateral basal

FIGURE 211.1. Bronchopulmonary segments.

Elevated values for DL_{CO} are often seen in asthmatics (presumably from the augmented intrathoracic blood volume, V_c, due to increased negative intrathoracic pressure) and in intrapulmonary hemorrhage. DL_{CO} often declines in anemia and in diseases that affect or destroy pulmonary vasculature, such as pulmonary vasculitis, thromboembolism, interstitial lung diseases, emphysema, and pulmonary resection.

Perfusion

The distribution of blood flow in the lungs is uneven since the low-pressure circulation is vulnerable to gravity. Consequently, blood flow is scarce at the apices and considerable at the bases. In a normal person, this probably leads to very slight ventilation-perfusion mismatching, but its effects can be considerable in patients with underlying lung disease.

■ Pulmonary Function Testing

Pulmonary function testing (PFT) evaluates the physiologic status of the lungs, which may be impaired to varying degrees and patterns by various diseases. Taken in conjunction with the clinical history and roentgenographic evaluation, PFT offers a strong clue to the underlying disease. Pulmonary function tests may be classified as (1) **commonly used tests**— e.g., forced expiratory spirometry (often performed using a flow-volume loop), lung-volume studies, DL_{CO}, and arterial blood gases, (2) **those with special applications**—e.g., bronchoprovocation testing and body plethysmography, and (3) **those yet to gain clinical usefulness**—e.g., closing volume and frequency dependence of compliance. Some laboratories use body plethysmography for measuring lung volumes. PFT has many clinical applications (Table 211.1).

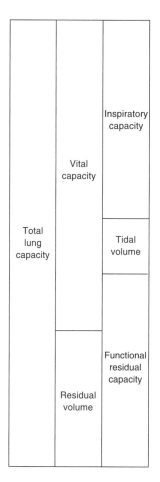
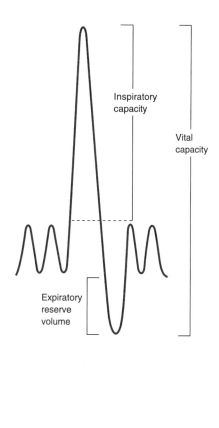

FIGURE 211.2. Compartments of ventilation.

TABLE 211.1.	Clinical Uses of Pulmonary Function Tests
Purpose	**Identified Outcome**
Detection	Lung disease early
Evaluation/	Respiratory status prior to surgery
diagnosis	Dyspneic states
	Severity and progression of lung disease, and response to specific therapy
	Extent of pulmonary disability
Screening	Patients being given medications with adverse pulmonary effects
	In epidemiologic surveys
	Persons working in environments hazardous to lung function

Forced expiratory spirometry

This is the recording of a forced, rapid, and complete exhalation from a position of maximal inspiration. (Figure 211.3 shows a normal test.) The entire volume constitutes the **forced vital capacity (FVC),** and the volume of the FVC exhaled in the first second constitutes the **1-second forced expiratory volume (FEV$_{1.0}$).** Normally, FEV$_{1.0}$ exceeds 87% of the FVC, and the ratio of FEV$_{1.0}$ to FVC must exceed 0.7 (or 70%). Airway obstruction is present when the ratio is below this level. FVC is reduced in restrictive disorders and often in obstructive disorders. FEV$_{1.0}$ is reduced primarily in airway obstruction (Figure 211.4) and secondarily (due to reduced FVC) in restrictive conditions; the FEV$_{1.0}$/FVC ratio helps differentiate these. If obstructive impairment is found, a bronchodilator aerosol is given and spirometry repeated to evaluate for reversibility.

The rate of flow of the exhaled air is computed from the forced expiratory spirogram. The standard measurements are the forced expiratory flow between the initial 200 and 1,200 ml of the FVC (FEF$_{200-1,200}$), also known as the **peak expiratory flow rate** (PEFR), and that between 25% and 75% of the FVC (FEF$_{25\%-75\%}$). Reduction of the latter is a sensitive guide to the presence

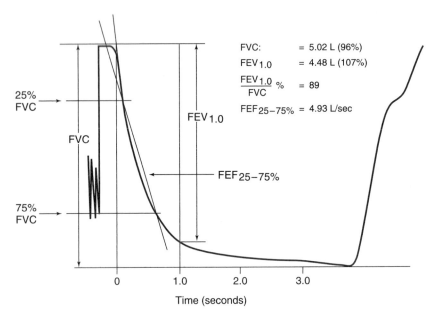

FVC:	= 5.02 L (96%)
$FEV_{1.0}$	= 4.48 L (107%)
$\dfrac{FEV_{1.0}}{FVC}$ %	= 89
$FEF_{25-75\%}$	= 4.93 L/sec

FIGURE 211.3. A normal forced expiratory spirometry. FVC = forced vital capacity; $FEV_{1.0}$ = 1-second forced expiratory volume; $FEF_{25-75\%}$ = forced expiratory flow between 25% and 75% of FVC.

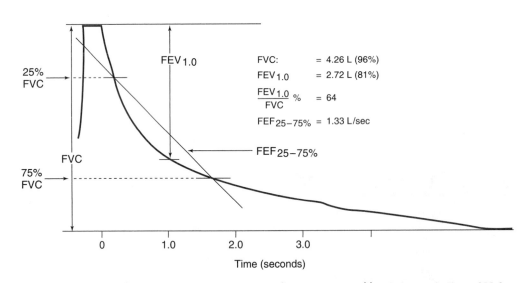

FVC:	= 4.26 L (96%)
$FEV_{1.0}$	= 2.72 L (81%)
$\dfrac{FEV_{1.0}}{FVC}$ %	= 64
$FEF_{25-75\%}$	= 1.33 L/sec

FIGURE 211.4. Forced expiratory spirometry in airway obstruction. Same abbreviations as in Figure 211.3.

of airway obstruction. However, flow rates also may be reduced in restrictive lung disease secondary to a low vital capacity. Review of the spirograms, use of the $FEV_{1.0}/FVC$ ratio, and clinical correlation are necessary under such circumstances. Most laboratories now perform spirometry using the **flow-volume loop**, in which a computer measures flow throughout inspiration and exhalation, and plots the flow against volume. Because instantaneous flows are measured throughout the vi-

tal capacity, they facilitate early diagnosis of upper-airway obstruction (chapter 224) and small airways dysfunction.

Lung volumes are determined using **helium dilution** or **nitrogen washout** or **body plethysmography.** Diffusion capacity is measured using a nontoxic concentration of carbon monoxide. Patterns of ventilatory impairments as seen on clinical pulmonary function testing are outlined in Table 211.2.

Bronchoprovocation testing

Bronchoprovocation testing (BPT) detects enhanced airway reactivity, most commonly using methacholine or histamine. The end point is attaining a 20% decline in $FEV_{1.0}$. BPT helps only to determine nonspecific bronchial hyperreactivity (BHR). BHR is an ingrained feature of asthma, correlating well with severity of symptoms, bronchodilator responsiveness, and medication requirements. However, BHR may also be seen in allergic rhinitis, cystic fibrosis, sarcoidosis, idiopathic pulmonary fibrosis, and even in the absence of apparent respiratory diseases. BPT is used principally to diagnose bronchial asthma, especially in atypical presentations (e.g., cough as the sole manifestation, with a normal spirometry) or when episodic symptoms accompany a normal spirometry without significant bronchodilator responsiveness. BPT is also quite useful in the diagnosis or exclusion of occupational asthma.

TABLE 211.2. Typical Pulmonary Function Abnormalities in Obstructive and Restrictive Ventilatory Impairments

Type of Impairment	VC	FVC	$FEV_{1.0}$	$FEV_{1.0}/FVC$	$FEF_{25-75\%}$	FRC and RV	TLC
Obstructive	May be normal	Usually reduced	Always reduced	<70	Reduced	High	Normal or high
Restrictive	Reduced	Reduced	May be normal or reduced	>70	Normal	Normal or reduced	Always reduced

VC = vital capicity; FVC = forced vital capacity; $FEV_{1.0}$ = 1-second forced expiratory volume; $FEF_{25-75\%}$ = forced expiratory flow between 25% and 75% of FVC; FRC = functional residual capacity; RV = residual volume; TLC = total lung capacity.

CHAPTER 212 BRONCHOSCOPY AND BIOPSY PROCEDURES

Bronchoscopy, performed using a fiberoptic or a rigid instrument, is indicated for the conditions shown in Table 212.1. **Rigid bronchoscopy** is the method of choice for foreign body retrieval, vascular tumors, massive hemoptysis, or upper airway obstruction. It requires general anesthesia, and the patient's neck must be extended, causing discomfort; only proximal (segmental) visualization is possible. **Fiberoptic bronchoscopy** (FOB) can be done transnasally or through an oral endotracheal tube and involves minimal discomfort; general anesthesia is generally not required and visualization to the sub-subsegmental level is easily accomplished. Bronchoalveolar lavage (BAL), brushings, and biopsies from abnormal areas can be performed during FOB. Brushings, biopsies, and needle aspirates can be fluoroscopically guided where appropriate. Postbronchoscopic sputa are collected when bronchogenic carcinoma is suspected.

■ Bronchoalveolar Lavage

Bronchoalveolar lavage, performed during fiberoptic bronchoscopy, consists of segmental lavage with isotonic saline, which is suctioned back and examined. BAL is particularly useful in evaluating diffuse lung infiltrates and/or opportunistic infections in the immunosuppressed. While it can diagnose 86–87% of cases of *Pneumocystis carinii* pneumonia complicating acquired immune deficiency syndrome (AIDS), the yield is appreciably lower for other infections and in immunosuppression from other causes. Normal cellular content is mostly macrophages (>90%) and lymphocytes (10%). A more lymphocytic response is seen in sarcoidosis and hypersensitivity pneumonitides and a more neutrophilic response in idiopathic pulmonary fibrosis. BAL can also be useful in the diagnosis of Histiocytosis X and alveolar proteinosis.

■ Biopsy Techniques

Tissue for diagnostic purposes may be obtained by biopsy of the pleura (chapter 243), lung, mediastinal lymph nodes, and scalene nodes.

Lung biopsy

Any persistent pulmonary lesion undiagnosed by conventional methods, when a specific tissue diagnosis would change the line of management, is an indication for lung biopsy. Available methods are the **transbronchoscopic (via bronchoscopy) approach, transthoracic needle biopsy, open (thoracotomy) incision,** or **video-assisted thoracoscopic technique.** The easiest and the least invasive approach should be tried first, unless circumstances dictate otherwise. The severity of the illness, urgency for treatment, x-ray appearance, exper-

TABLE 212.1.	Indications for Bronchoscopy
Purpose	**Indication**
Diagnostic	Hemoptysis, to determine cause and location of bleed
	Diagnosis of lung cancer
	Positive sputum cytology, with negative chest x-ray
	Paralysis of recurrent laryngeal nerve (hoarseness)
	Staging of known lung cancer
	Atelectasis from suspected endobronchial obstruction
	Cough of unclear etiology (see discussion in chapter 208)
	Acute inhalational injury
	Assessment of tracheal damage during mechanical ventilation with endotracheal tube
	Diagnosis of interstitial lung disease
	Diagnosis of pulmonary infections in both immunocompetent and immunosuppressed patients
Therapeutic	Foreign body in tracheobronchial tree
	Tracheobronchial toilet for excessive secretions
	Atelectasis (due to secretions)
	Aspiration
	Lavage
	Endobronchial brachytherapy

tise available, most likely diagnosis, and sample size the pathologist needs to provide a definite diagnosis should all be considered when selecting an approach. Transbronchoscopic lung biopsy is the preferred method to diagnose sarcoidosis. Open lung biopsy, performed through a 4″–6″ thoracotomy, always provides a definite pathologic diagnosis, but a definitive etiologic diagnosis may still be elusive in about 20–30% of the cases, especially in the immunosuppressed. Finally, needle biopsy of the lung is often employed in the diagnosis of lung nodules, particularly those located peripherally.

Mediastinal node biopsy

Mediastinal node enlargement is the prime indication for mediastinal node biopsy, which is generally accom-

plished by a mediastinoscopy. The latter, performed through a suprasternal or anterior approach, is often used in the staging of bronchogenic carcinoma. However, its role in this setting compared with that of CT varies widely. For right-sided lesions, a suprasternal approach is appropriate; however, for left-sided lesions, an anterior approach is performed (Chamberlain procedure). Its yield in lung cancer varies with the histological type, the location and size of the tumor, the location of abnormal nodes within the mediastinum, and the presence or absence of abnormality detected in the mediastinal area by chest radiographs or computed tomography.

CHAPTER **213** GENERAL ASPECTS OF ENDEMIC MYCOSES

Histoplasmosis, coccidioidomycosis, and **blastomycosis** are the most common endemic fungal infections in the United States, caused by *Histoplasma capsulatum*, *Coccidioides immitis*, and *Blastomyces dermatitidis*, respectively. *H. capsulatum* and *C. immitis* grow in the soil. Growth of *H. capsulatum* is favored by black bird, chicken, or bat droppings. When the soil or area of habitat is disturbed, the infecting conidia become airborne. The main endemic area for histoplasmosis in the United States is around the Mississippi and Ohio rivers; the disease is also common in

Missouri, Tennessee, Kentucky, and Ohio. Coccidioidomycosis is seen mostly in the Southwestern United States and the lower Sonoran Life Zone. The major endemic areas for blastomycosis are the southeastern United States and the Mississippi Valley area including the Midwestern states. However, within these **endemic areas,** scattered foci of hyperendemicity occur, which share common characteristics of **acidic soil** with a **high organic content, abundant moisture,** and **proximity to waterways.**

■ Pathogenesis and Pathology

Both *H. capsulatum* and *B. dermatitidis* occur in two forms—**a mold (mycelial) form** in the natural habitat and in artificial media, and as **yeast** in the human host (**dimorphic fungi**). *C. immitis* is also dimorphic (grows and reproduces as mold and yeast), but the arthroconidia of the mycelia evolve into spherules (sac-like structures) containing endospores. Rupturing mature spherules release endospores, each forming another spherule and thus completing the cycle.

Pathogenetic processes common to these fungi include, in sequence, initial entry into the lungs by inhalation, conversion into yeast forms and multiplication, a host response that is initially by neutrophils and, later, macrophage-mediated, systemic dissemination to many organs, and finally, containment of infection once specific, cell-mediated immunity is acquired through T-cell proliferation. While mild infections resolve without significant pathologic residuals, more intense infections lead to caseating granulomas, which heal by fibrosis and calcification. Minor variations in this theme occur with specific entities. While the **portal of entry** is the lungs, coccidioidomycosis can be acquired, though rarely, through cutaneous inoculation. In histoplasmosis, a granulomatous change predominates, whereas in blastomycosis, the polymorphonuclear neutrophils remain in the area of inflammation, causing a picture of a mixed pyogranulomatous exudate. Both neutrophilic and granulomatous responses occur in coccidioidomycosis, but the neutrophilic response almost approximates that in blastomycosis.

While these mycoses have been increasingly recognized in immunocompromised patients who live in or travel to endemic areas, more often they occur in healthy persons. The shared common clinical characteristics are **asymptomatic** and **pneumonic forms** of the disease, **common drug therapy** and **diagnostic clues** (clustering of cases in family members or groups engaged in a common activity—e.g., camping, hiking, hunting, canoeing, excavating), a history of travel to an endemic area, failure to respond to antimicrobial treatment of a suspected bacterial pneumonia, and the presence of extrapulmonary disease, particularly involving the skin.

Antifungal agents used for treating deep mycoses are **Amphotericin B** (AmB) and the **azoles.** AmB may be infused intravenously (IV) in 60–90 minutes, thus obviating the traditional, longer infusion time. Infusion may cause fever and chills, which can be reduced by premedicating with aspirin and diphenylhydramine, although occasionally codeine or meperidine may be needed. If infused through a peripheral vein, adding a small dose of corticosteroids to the infusion can reduce the incidence of phlebitis. Drug toxicity due to AmB primarily affects the kidney. Renal tubular toxicity results in potassium wasting and progressive decline in renal function, which necessitates weekly or twice-weekly monitoring of renal function. The dose should be reduced when the serum creatinine level reaches 2 mg/dl, and the treatment should be stopped temporarily if it reaches 3 mg/dl. Saline loading before the infusion of AmB would reduce nephrotoxicity. Hypokalemic patients would need potassium supplementation.

Ketoconazole and itraconazole are orally administered and have gastrointestinal toxicity. Ketoconazole, in particular, may cause nausea, vomiting, and liver-function abnormalities. Because of its interference with testosterone biosynthesis, loss of libido may result. Both agents require gastric acidity for absorption; therefore, concurrent H2 blockers and antacids should be avoided. Ketoconazole (as well as erythromycin) blocks the metabolism of terfenadine, and polymorphic ventricular tachycardia (torsade de pointes) has followed the concurrent use of terfenadine with these agents.

CHAPTER 214

HISTOPLASMOSIS

Histoplasmosis is caused by *Histoplasma capsulatum*. Its epidemiology and pathogenesis are discussed in chapter 213. When the soil dries out or is disturbed, the infectious microconidia (<5μ) of this fungus become airborne and may be inhaled.

■ Clinical Features

The incubation period is 1–3 weeks (mean of 2 weeks). Inoculum size, the host's immunocompetence, and previous chronic lung disease may all change the clinical picture. Initial infection is most often asymptomatic. In others, the diagnosis may be missed because of trivial symptoms. **Acute histoplasmosis** in symptomatic, normal persons resembles influenza with abrupt fever, chills, chest pain, a nonproductive "brassy" cough, headaches, arthralgias, and body aches. Physical examination may be normal or reveal transient râles, and skin lesions such as erythema nodosum and erythema multiforme. Hepatosplenomegaly is rare. Chest x-rays usually show single or multiple areas of infiltrates with lymph-adenopathy. A parenchymal infiltrate with ipsilateral hilar adenopathy is a strong clue. Symptoms usually clear in 1–3 weeks. Most often, the x-ray changes also fully resolve; however, residual lesions include punctate parenchymal or hilar lymph node calcifications ("buckshot" and "mulberry" calcifications, respectively) or calcified or uncalcified parenchymal nodules (chapter 242).

Complications include pericarditis (not direct infection) and obstruction of adjacent mediastinal structures by adenopathy. In patients with emphysema, histoplasmosis infection may mimic tuberculosis in two ways: either during initial infection (apical cavities) or during progressive disease (apical cavities, low-grade fever, and weight loss). With a large infecting dose, a rapidly progressive illness may evolve with diffuse pulmonary infiltrates and severe hypoxemia, progressing to adult respiratory distress syndrome (ARDS), which may be lethal.

Progressive disseminated histoplasmosis

Progressive disseminated histoplasmosis (PDH) is a progressive and often fatal systemic form of histoplasmosis in a host **immunocompromised** by medications (especially glucocorticoids), hematologic malignancies, or HIV infection. PDH may follow reactivation of a previously healed primary focus or an initial infection

that the host cannot contain. High fever, weight loss, hepatosplenomegaly, and mucocutaneous ulcers are characteristic, with or without respiratory symptoms. Involvement and destruction of the adrenals may cause

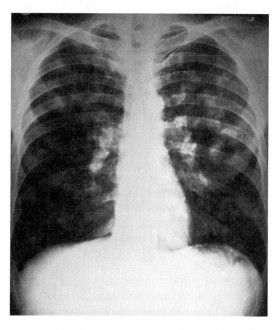

FIGURE 214.1. Primary histoplasmosis; multiple nodular infiltrates and hilar adenopathy.

TABLE 214.1. Histoplasmosis: Usefulness and Limitations of Diagnostic Studies		
Test	**Result/Usefulness**	**Comment**
Bone marrow biopsy	Good method in severely ill patients with PDH.	—
Blood cultures with lysis centrifugation	High diagnostic yield in immunocompromised patients with PDH.	Blood concentration of the organism is high in this population.
Sputum cultures for fungus	Should be performed in patients with cavitary disease.	If negative, bronchoscopy, lavage, brushings, and biopsies should follow.
Histoplasmin skin tests	Epidemiologic tool without clinical usefulness.	Avoid using this test.
Complement fixation (CF) test	Titer of 1:32 to the yeast phase antigen or a four-fold rise in the presence of consistent clinical disease strongly suggests diagnosis.	Becomes (+) 3–6 weeks after infection; remains (+) for a long time. Low sensitivity, especially in those with chronic cavitary disease and those with PDH.
Precipitating antibodies to H and M antigens of *Histoplasma capsulatum*		—
Immunodiffusion	Low sensitivity.	—
RIA	High sensitivity but less specific than immunodiffusion or CF.	—
Urinary histoplasma antigen	Discoverable in most patients with PDH-complicating HIV infection.	HIV-infected patients have an increased density of organisms.

PDH = progressive disseminated histoplasmosis; RIA = radioimmunoassay.

TABLE 214.2.	Histoplasmosis: Summary of Treatment Options		
Indication	**Agent**	**Dose/Duration**	**Comments**
Severe illness (diffuse infiltrates, hypoxemia)	IV AmB (see chapter 213)	35 mg/kg (some use 0.5–1.0 g as total dose)	AmB is the drug of choice
Massive adenopathy/ symptoms >1 week	IV AmB	Same as above	
PDH	IV AmB	Accelerate dose rapidly	Relapses uncommon after full AmB dose
PDH + HIV-infection	AmB full dose IV, plus weekly AmB or daily Itra	1.0 g AmB + AmB (50 mg) weekly or Itra 200 mg/ daily	Long-term treatment necessary
Mild cases of PDH	Itra	200–400 mg/daily for many months	May suffice as primary treatment
PCH	Itra	200–400 mg/d × 6 mo.	Excellent results

AmB = Amphotericin B; Itra = Itraconazole, PCH = progressive cavitary histoplasmosis; PDH = progressive disseminated histoplasmosis.

adrenal insufficiency. Rarely, other sites may be involved (e.g., the central nervous system, with mass lesions or meningitis). Abnormal liver function tests, pancytopenia, and, in some cases, disseminated intravascular coagulation may occur. Chest x-rays may be normal, or may show localized findings or a classic miliary pattern.

■ Diagnosis and Management

In most cases, the diagnosis depends mainly on the clinical and x-ray findings. Other diagnostic tests in histoplasmosis are reviewed in Table 214.1. Diagnosis is confirmed by isolation of the organism from biologic material or tissue. All biopsied material should be examined with specific stains such as Giemsa, periodic acid Schiff (PAS stain), or Gomori methenamine silver stain. If characteristic yeast morphology is seen on microscopy, treatment should be started since the culture results may be delayed by weeks. Most cases of acute histoplasmosis do not require treatment. Indications for treatment and appropriate agents are shown in Table 214.2.

CHAPTER 215 COCCIDIOIDOMYCOSIS

■ Clinical Features

Acute coccidioidomycosis, caused by *Coccidioides immitis,* is a **mild respiratory illness** in most persons, but may become progressively worse. Fever, cough, headache, and pleuritic chest pain are the most common symptoms. Erythematous rash, erythema nodosum, and, less commonly, erythema multiforme are nonspecific features. Chest x-rays are abnormal in most cases, usually showing a pneumonitis with or without ipsilateral hilar lymphadenopathy. Isolated hilar adenopathy may also be seen. Spontaneous resolution occurs within 3 weeks.

In some patients, the symptoms and x-ray abnormalities persist beyond 6–8 weeks (**persistent pulmonary infection),** with the original pneumonia evolving radiographically into nodules and thin-walled cavities (Figure 215.1). Generally asymptomatic, these cavities can also cause hemoptysis or they can enlarge and rupture into the pleural space, causing a bronchopleural fistula. **Progressive primary coccidioidomycosis** (persistent symptoms of fever and cough with progressive radiographic worsening) is more likely among those with underlying immune defects and perhaps dark-skinned races. Rarely, pulmonary coccidioidomycosis may progress slowly with symptoms and x-rays that mimic pulmonary tuberculosis.

In a few patients, **systemic dissemination** follows. Patients at risk are the immunocompromised (patients receiving glucocorticoid or cytotoxic treatment patients, organ transplant recipients, and HIV-infected patients) and probably African Americans and Native Americans. Those at extremes of age and perhaps the pregnant are also at risk. Skin (draining pustules, ulcers, sinus tracts, and multiple abscesses), bones (vertebrae, skull and long bones, with osteomyelitis, large paraspinous abscesses), joints, and the genitourinary system may be involved. Meningitis occurs in about one-third of patients with disseminated disease; it may be present with no other evidence of the disease.

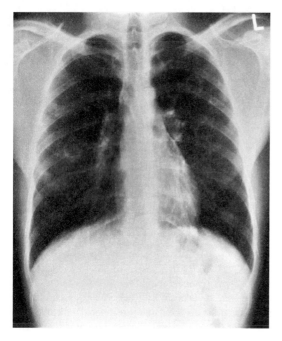

FIGURE 215.1. Coccidioidomycosis; multiple thin-walled cavities and nodules.

■ Diagnosis

Given the nonspecific nature of the symptoms and x-ray findings, the diagnosis is confirmed by recovering the fungus from a **culture** of tissue or biologic fluids. However, with traditional methods for culture, accidental infection of laboratory personnel is a definite risk. **Serologic tests,** in the appropriate setting, are very helpful. Various available tests and their usefulness are summarized in Table 215.1.

■ Management

Drug therapy is not required in most cases of acute coccidioidomycosis. Treatment with Amphotericin B (0.5–2.0 g) or oral fluconazole is indicated for immunosuppressed patients or those at risk for dissemination; symptomatic, persistent disease; progressive lung disease simulating tuberculosis; or persistent (>2 years), enlarging, or symptomatic cavities. Thin-walled cavities do not need treatment; small ones usually resolve. Disseminated disease or dissemination with AIDS requires aggressive therapy with Amphotericin B (2.0–3.0 g), given over several months, followed by suppressive fluconazole therapy. Disseminated disease with AIDS has a poor prognosis. Coccidioidal meningitis requires prolonged intrathecal or intracisternal Amphotericin B or oral fluconazole, because of relapses. Complications (subcutaneous abscesses, excision of cutaneous lesions, osteomyelitis, rapidly enlarging or hemorrhaging cavity) require surgery.

TABLE 215.1. Diagnostic Tests in Coccidioidomycosis	
Test	**Comment**
Skin tests with coccidioidin or spherulin	Not diagnostic by themselves, but conversion from (–) to (+) in the setting of clinical infection strongly supports the diagnosis. False-negatives occur.
Tube precipitant test; latex particle agglutination (LPA) or immunodiffusion (ID)	LPA and ID are recent innovations. Detects IgM antibodies, which rise early; LPA is sensitive but not very specific.
Complement fixation (CF) or immunodiffusion (ID)	Detects IgG antibodies, which rise later. Rising CF titers may imply dissemination; serial titers can help assess treatment efficacy. Sensitivity and specificity of ID is similar to the CF test.
Microscopy of sputum, BAL, aspirated pus, or other body fluids	Best diagnostic method to detect spherules. Sputum and BAL Papanicolaou stains more sensitive than KOH digestion.
Tissue biopsy	H & E and special stains (i.e., silver stain or PAS) can detect both spherules and endospores.

BAL = bronchoalveolar lavage; H & E = hematoxylin-eosin; KOH = potassium hydroxide; (–) = negative; (+) = positive; PAS = periodic acid Schiff stain.

CHAPTER 216 BLASTOMYCOSIS

Blastomycosis is caused by *Blastomyces dermatitidis,* which has a characteristic appearance (Figure 216.1): spherical, multinucleated, double-contoured, and refractile, displaying a single, broad-based bud of 5–15μ. In the largest point source outbreak, reported in 1984 in Eagle River, Wisconsin, the organism was isolated from the soil. Its pathogenesis and pathology are discussed in Chapter 213.

▪ Clinical Features

Epidemiologic studies clearly identify a subclinical form of blastomycosis. In symptomatic patients, **acute blastomycosis** may be mild, simulating an upper respiratory viral infection, or severe, simulating a bacterial pneumonia, with productive cough, pleuritic pain, and fever. Extrapulmonary involvement is uncommon and skin lesions are very rare. Physical findings in mild, acute cases are unremarkable but if the disease mimics a bacterial pneumonia, signs of consolidation (shown in Table 208.5) may be noted. Other than leukocytosis and left shift in the pneumonic presentation, laboratory features are nonspecific. X-rays commonly show alveolar infiltrates, some with a typical consolidation pattern, solitary nodules, and nodules combined with infiltrates and cavitation. Lymphadenopathy and pleural effusions are uncommon. Acute blastomycosis may cause a rapidly progressive diffuse lung involvement, leading to adult respiratory distress syndrome. Radiographically, this picture of ARDS is indistinguishable from ARDS due to other causes.

Most cases of blastomycosis are sporadic in nature, with a **chronic** presentation. With low-grade fever, cough productive of mucopurulent sputum, weight loss, and hemoptysis in one-fifth of the cases, the resemblance to tuberculosis or bronchogenic carcinoma may be striking. With more chronicity, skin lesions are common, usually involving the face, hands, and legs. The lesions are characterized by an ulcerated center with heaped-up edges that contain microabscesses. With time, the ulcer enlarges and its edges become more verrucous. Chest x-rays show mass-like lesions, miliary and reticular nodular patterns, and/or cavitary disease.

Blastomycosis also occurs in patients who are immunocompromised from HIV disease, hematologic malignancy, long-term glucocorticoid use, and so forth. **Extrapulmonary dissemination** is common and the disease is rapidly progressive. The risk of mortality is high.

▪ Diagnosis

Skin tests are not useful. Blastomycosis is diagnosed by the isolation of the organism from **cultures** of biologic fluids or tissue. However, given the distinctive morphology of the fungus and the time lost in culture, all biologic material should be examined microscopically. This is best done by mixing a smear of the material (e.g., sputum) with an equal amount of 10% potassium hydroxide, and examining it as a wet mount. **Morphologic identification** is sufficient to institute treatment in symptomatic cases. Generally speaking, acute blastomycosis presenting as pneumonia can be diagnosed in this manner in over 75% of the cases.

Secretions and/or biologic materials may also be obtained by fiberoptic bronchoscopy, bronchial brushings, transbronchoscopic lung biopsy, and thoracentesis if a pleural effusion is present. Cytological preparations from these are a potentially reliable method to identify the organism. Involved extrapulmonary sites (e.g., skin lesions) should be biopsied. Microscopic examination of pus from the microabscesses around the edges of the lesion or biopsy of the lesion itself may be diagnostic. **Serological tests** have limitations in clinical practice. Complement fixation tests and immunodiffusion for antibody detection are not sensitive enough for diagnosis. Enzyme immunoassay to detect antibody against A antigen is more sensitive and the antibody is detected about 2 weeks after the onset of illness. Titers 1:32 or greater by this test strongly support the diagnosis. However, the time-delay factor limits its usefulness.

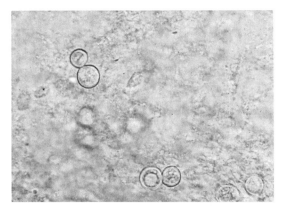

FIGURE 216.1. Yeast forms of *Blastomyces dermatitidis.*
(From: Chest 1980;77:789. Reprinted with permission.)

■ Management

Symptomatic blastomycosis should be treated. Blastomycosis in the immunocompromised host, severe, life-threatening, or fast progressive disease and blastomycosis of the central nervous system should be aggressively and promptly treated with Amphotericin B, with a total dose of 2.0 g in adults. Another reasonable approach, though not rigorously studied, is to control the disease initially with Amphotericin B with a dose of 1.0 g,

followed by itraconazole for several months. In persons with mild to moderate nonmeningeal disease, itraconazole is the preferred drug, as it is taken orally and does not have the renal complications of Amphotericin B. The usual dose is 200 mg daily (400 mg daily, maximum), continued for about 6 months. Good results have also been reported with ketoconazole. The use of Amphotericin B is preferred for any extrapulmonary involvement besides skin.

CHAPTER 217 ASPERGILLOSIS

A spergilli (*Aspergillus fumigatus* and many other species) are ubiquitous (soil, decaying organic matter, etc.) fungi responsible for a variety of human ailments. Infection is acquired through inhalation of Aspergillus spores (conidia). The development and form of the clinical disease depend on the intensity and frequency of exposure and on host factors (atopy, pre-existing cavitary disease, im-

munosuppressed state). Despite an extensive knowledge base on Aspergillus lung disease, the nosology still lags. The distinct clinical forms of the disease caused by Aspergilli are summarized in Table 217.1. The three most commonly recognized forms of Aspergillus lung disease are **allergic bronchopulmonary aspergillosis** (ABPA), **aspergilloma**, and **invasive aspergillosis**.

TABLE 217.1. Aspergillus-related Pulmonary Disorders	
Syndrome/Disorder	**Comment**
Allergic bronchopulmonary aspergillosis, aspergilloma, and invasive aspergillosis	The three most commonly recognized forms of Aspergillus lung disease. See discussion in text, pages [TK]–[TK].
Extrinsic asthma	Aspergillus may act as a specific allergen; inhalation of spores cause mediator release from mast cells and bronchospasm.
Hypersensitivity pneumonitis (chapter 234)	Result from inhalation of Aspergillus organisms present in moldy barley or moldy oats, corn, or hay. Occurs primarily in nonatopic individuals.
Chronic necrotizing pulmonary aspergillosis	Indolent, invasive infection affecting and limited to the lung, occurring in immunocompetent persons.
Aspergillus tracheobronchitis	Seen in immunocompromised patients; some have ulcers and pseudomembranes

Allergic Bronchopulmonary Aspergillosis

■ Pathogenesis and Pathology

In atopic individuals, the inhaled Aspergillus may continue to reside in the bronchi; the host responds with IgE and IgG antibodies against the fungus. The immune reaction (type I and type III) of these antibodies against the fungal antigens causes **bronchospasm** and, probably, **immune complex injury** to the bronchi. **Proximal**

saccular bronchiectasis is a serious complication of allergic bronchopulmonary aspergillosis ABPA.

■ Clinical Features

Wheezing, recurrent fever, cough productive of thick, brownish sputum, and sputum and blood eosinophilia are the common manifestations of ABPA. Roentgenographic findings are varied: transient pulmonary infiltrates, band-like densities, and atelectasis secondary to mucus plugging of bronchi. Contraction of lobes, pulmonary fibrosis, and extensive bronchiectasis may follow. Pulmonary function varies with the stage of the disease. Obstructive ventilatory impairment is common. In later stages, restrictive impairment and diminished diffusing capacity may result.

■ Diagnosis and Management

The major criteria for the diagnosis of ABPA are asthma, blood and sputum eosinophilia, recurrent pulmonary infiltrates, and skin-test allergy to *Aspergillus* antigens (immediate wheal and flare reaction and late reaction). Virtually all patients with ABPA react to the skin test; therefore, immediate skin test (test) reactivity is useful as a screening test. Others include markedly elevated IgE, Aspergillus in sputum, Aspergillus precipitins in serum, a history of recurrent fever or pneumonia, and a history of coughing up sputum plugs. Specific IgE antibody to *A. fumigatus* (greater than 2 times the levels seen in asthmatics with aspergillus skin reactivity, but without other criteria for ABPA) is considered a specific diagnostic finding of ABPA. CT findings of central bronchiectasis are highly specific for the diagnosis of ABPA in an asthmatic.

Antifungal agents are not useful. Glucocorticoids effectively reduce the symptoms, along with a decline in the serum IgE level, which is a useful index for adjusting the steroid dose. Long-term treatment is usually necessary.

Pulmonary Aspergilloma

■ Pathogenesis and Pathology

Aspergilloma is a mycelial mass formed by colonization and growth of Aspergilli within an area of destroyed lung. Thus, diseases that cause parenchymal necrosis or bronchiectasis—namely, tuberculosis, sarcoidosis, pulmonary infarct, lung abscess, neoplasm, ankylosing spondylitis, and various pulmonary mycoses—predispose to the development of aspergilloma. Nearly 11% of patients with healed tuberculosis and residual cavities will develop aspergilloma in 3–4 years, the likelihood being higher in patients with a positive precipitin test by immunodiffusion. The cavitary wall and adjacent area may be highly vascular.

■ Clinical Features

The most common symptom of a well-established aspergilloma is hemoptysis, which is usually minimal and recurrent and occurs in more than one-half of patients. However, severe, massive hemoptysis may occur, ostensibly from friction between the mycetoma and the cavitary wall, an endotoxin, and/or an anticoagulant liberated by Aspergillus and possible local vascular invasion. Other symptoms include chronic cough and shortness of breath. Aspergillomas have a very variable natural history, with stability, increase in size, and gradual or spontaneous lysis all possible.

■ Diagnosis

Aspergilloma is mainly an x-ray diagnosis. It typically appears as an intracavitary oval, round or irregular density surrounded by a crescent of air (Figure 217.1). It is usually solitary and located in the upper lobe. This typical x-ray appearance is not pathognomonic, since other processes (intracavitary hematoma, lung necrosis, neoplasm, and other mycoses) can mimic it. The absence of Aspergillus in the sputum does not exclude the diagnosis; however, a negative precipitin test virtually excludes it. A positive precipitin test with a typical x-ray appearance makes its diagnosis certain.

■ Management

The prognosis and eventual outcome of aspergilloma depends on the severity of the underlying diseases rather

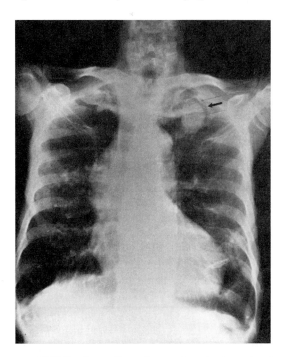

FIGURE 217.1. Aspergilloma; intracavitary density and typical crescent (arrow).

than on the aspergilloma itself. Systemic antifungal therapy has not been shown to be effective. Routine surgical resection of an aspergilloma is not indicated. Patients with mild or intermittent hemoptysis should be carefully observed; usually these episodes are self-limiting. Massive or life-threatening hemoptysis calls for localization of the bleeding site followed by surgical resection or bronchial artery embolization.

Invasive Aspergillosis

■ Pathogenesis and Pathology

Invasive aspergillosis is an acute, severe, rapidly progressive infection of the lung with Aspergillus, with a tendency for systemic dissemination. The degree of immune suppression rather than the dose of the infecting agent determines the severity of infection. Prolonged and intense neutropenia is the most important predisposing factor. Invasive aspergillosis occurs in the immunosuppressed or myelosuppressed; the typical patient is **neutropenic,** with a **hematogenous malignancy** and undergoing **cytotoxic chemotherapy,** or an **organ transplant recipient.** Corticosteroids and immunosuppressive drugs are also predisposing factors.

Although invasion of the lung can occur through the walls of the trachea or main bronchi, more often the first infection is a distal pneumonia. Hyphae have a propensity to grow into blood vessels causing hemorrhagic infarction and cavitation of the lung. Aspergillomas may form within these cavities.

■ Clinical Features

Abrupt fever, dyspnea, and cough are the most common symptoms. **Pleuritic chest pain** may be present, usually associated with a **pleural friction rub.** Hemoptysis, at times severe, may be a symptom. The x-ray features are usually those of a bronchopneumonia and the infiltrates may be miliary, patchy, or dense. Follow-up x-rays are likely to reveal progressive infiltrates and cavitation. Since Aspergillus has a **propensity for vascular invasion and thrombosis,** the clinical and x-ray features may mimic pulmonary embolism and infarction. Increasing size of a pneumonic consolidation toward the periphery, cavitation, and intracavitary density are roentgenographic clues to invasive Aspergillosis. CT of the chest and MRI can identify target-like lesions due to cavitation. MRI after gadolinium enhances the intensity of the rim of the cavity. The progressive worsening that follows is usually lethal within 1–2 weeks. Early therapy (medical and surgical) has been successful in some cases.

■ Diagnosis

Correct diagnosis depends on a high index of suspicion. If an immunocompromised patient (especially one with a hematogenous malignancy) with bacterial pneumonia fails to respond to antibacterial therapy, the possibility of aspergillosis should be considered. However, proving this diagnosis is often difficult. Absence of Aspergilli in the sputum does not exclude invasive aspergillosis. Lung tissue should be obtained promptly, preferably through an **open biopsy.** The finding of septate, acutely branching hyphae of Aspergilli in tissue is diagnostic (Figure 217.2). If the patient's condition does not permit lung biopsy, presumptive treatment is justified when clinical and roentgenographic findings are consistent. In this context, the discovery of Aspergilli in the sputum is sufficient reason to start Amphotericin B. Serologic tests for antibody detection are not very reliable for diagnosis and antigen detection is still not applicable for clinical use.

■ Management

Untreated, invasive aspergillosis is lethal; even with treatment, only a minority survive. The drug of choice is Amphotericin B. Because the disease is life-threatening, rapid increments of dose and larger doses are both necessary. In markedly neutropenic patients, 1.0–1.5 mg/kg of AmB is given daily until clinical improvement is noted. The latter is correlated with an increase in neutrophil count. Liposomal AmB is promising, as large doses can be delivered without the risk of significant nephrotoxicity. Itraconazole has also been used successfully, either as a sequel to AmB, or alone in less severe cases (300 mg twice daily, followed

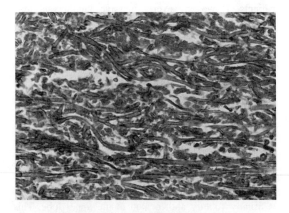

FIGURE 217.2. Aspergillus hyphae in tissue.

by 200 mg twice daily). Besides medical treatment, single localized pulmonary lesions may be excised to prevent complications of hemoptysis, pneumothorax, or relapse of aspergillosis.

Multiple prophylactic regimens are being studied in susceptible populations. Oral Itraconazole, alone or together with intranasal AmB, appears to be a reasonable prophylaxis.

CHAPTER 218 TUBERCULOSIS

The term "tuberculosis" arises from "tubercle," which is its histopathological hallmark. A worldwide disease, it is caused by *Mycobacterium tuberculosis, Mycobacterium bovis,* or *Mycobacterium africanum.* Virtually all cases of tuberculosis in the United States are caused by *M. tuberculosis.*

Epidemiology

Tuberculosis incidence in the U.S. has been declining since 1948. An intercurrent rise in the 1980s in the U.S. was attributed to human immunodeficiency virus (HIV) infection and weakened tuberculosis control efforts owing to health care funding cuts. In the United States (as of 1996), non-Hispanic blacks, Hispanics, immigrants from Asia, and inmates of correctional institutions appear most vulnerable to tuberculosis. The 25–44-year age group is strikingly vulnerable, a group also most affected by HIV.

Pathogenesis and Pathology

Tuberculosis is transmitted by infectious droplets from an active case of pulmonary tuberculosis. Normal respiratory aerodynamics generally carry inhaled droplets into the lower or middle lung zones. Phagocytosis by alveolar macrophages follows, but in the previously uninfected, the organism replicates within and outside the cell. The macrophage processes and presents mycobacterial antigens to the CD-4 lymphocytes, which generate lymphokines, thereby sensitizing the macrophage. Through cell-mediated immunity (CMI), granulomatous inflammation, and caseation, the infection is contained. Mycobacteria encased in the caseation fail to replicate and remain dormant. However, they may later replicate; their contact with the sensitized lymphocytes triggers immunologic memory. Tissue damage (necrosis, inflammation, and cavitation) follows through delayed type hypersensitivity. With mycobacterial replication, the host hypersensitivity to the tuberculoprotein generates a vicious cycle of tissue liquefaction and cavitation, bacterial replication, and dissemination.

A pneumonitis follows infection. Multiplying bacilli spread into the lymphatics, causing hilar lymph node enlargement. The initial pneumonitis together with the

TABLE 218.1. Tuberculosis: Selected Factors that Favor Development of Disease Following Infection

Age (infancy, childhood, old age)
Race
Impaired integrity of the cellular immune mechanisms
    Acquired immune deficiency syndrome (AIDS)
    Corticosteroid, cytotoxic, or other immunosuppressive therapy
    End-stage renal disease
    Malnutrition
    Hematological and reticuloendothelial malignancies
Associated diseases
    Diabetes mellitus
    Silicosis
    Prior gastrectomy
    Infection with measles virus
    Alcoholism

lymphadenopathy characterize the **primary (Ghon) focus.** Hematogenous bacillary dissemination occurs next, causing formation of the **secondary (Simon) foci.** Generally, both Ghon and Simon foci resolve and heal; the organisms in most of these foci are killed. Residual organisms remain in these foci, contained by caseation. In some cases, Simon foci involving upper lobes of the lung, growing ends of bones, and renal cortices either progress immediately or, more commonly, reactivate after a period of latency. Bacterial replication, once begun, is perpetuated by a conducive local environment; a high local availability of oxygen is the alleged mechanism.

The formation of Ghon foci and Simon foci is generally a subclinical event. Clinical tuberculosis occurs mostly from endogenous reactivation of the dormant bacilli in the Simon foci; in areas for endemic tuberculosis, exogenous reinfection may also be responsible. Among all those infected, roughly 10% will develop subsequent disease—5% within 2 years of infection and another 5% in the years following. Many conditions and factors enhance this propensity, as shown in Table 218.1.

Pleural tuberculosis occurs from contiguous extension of a subpleural Ghon focus or when tuberculosis bacillemia spreads to the pleura. In either case, hypersensitivity to tuberculoprotein plays a role. Such effusions usually resolve spontaneously, only to be followed by frank pulmonary tuberculosis in over two-thirds of the cases within 2 years. A liquefying, cavitating caseous focus may erode a blood vessel, resulting in massive hematogenous dissemination and causing miliary tuberculosis, characterized by tiny lesions that resemble a spill of millet seeds.

Tuberculosis and HIV co-infection

Tuberculosis complicating HIV generally occurs early in the course of HIV, but its effect on the course of HIV is unknown. However, HIV co-infection profoundly affects clinical tuberculosis. It clearly impairs the host's ability to contain new tuberculosis infection. Immunity against tuberculosis is thwarted; thus, a previously infected and immune individual is no longer protected against reinfection. HIV infection is the strongest known risk factor for endogenous reactivation of tuberculosis, with a risk of 7.9% per year in tuberculin-positive HIV-infected individuals (compared with 10% per lifetime for tuberculin-positive, HIV-negative persons). In a significant proportion of HIV-positive patients with proven tuberculosis infection, a tuberculin skin test evokes little or no response. Granulomas are poorly formed and cavitation seldom occurs. Thus, the chest x-rays may be deceptively normal or reveal minor abnormalities. However, the unfettered bacterial replication leads to a large bacillary load, and the infectious threat from these persons becomes formidable.

■ Clinical Features

Primary tuberculosis, which often goes unnoticed or is mistaken for a viral illness, occurs most commonly in childhood and youth; however, 15% of primary tuberculosis in the United States occurs in the elderly. In all forms of tuberculosis, symptoms lag until the disease is moderately advanced. Weight loss, night sweats, and fever are general symptoms. **Pulmonary tuberculosis** is manifested by chest pain, cough, sputum, and hemoptysis, which is occasionally massive and life-threatening. A chronic unresolving or slowly resolving pneumonia is an infrequent but deceptive presentation in the elderly. It can mimic an acute bacterial pneumonia or present with catastrophic respiratory failure. Physical findings include signs of inanition and fever, and in pulmonary tuberculosis, signs of cavitation, consolidation, and/or pleural effusion. **Extrapulmonary tuberculosis** begins insidiously, often involving the kidneys, bones, and meninges. Fever, weight loss, progressive respiratory insufficiency, and prostration characterize **miliary tuberculosis;** men-

ingitis is frequent. While miliary tuberculosis is sometimes the cause of a **fever of unknown origin (FUO),** this recognition is often delayed. The insidious presentation can delay the diagnosis.

■ Ancillary Studies

Anemia and **hyponatremia** are common. **Abnormal liver function tests** may signify hepatic involvement. Acid-fast stains of sputum may show the organism, depending on the bacillary load and the extent of cavitation. The cerebrospinal fluid (CSF) in **tuberculous meningitis** is characteristically clear, with a high cell count that is neutrophilic initially and lymphocytic later. The protein is high; glucose is decreased to around 45 mg/dl. While the organism may be detected in the CSF, especially through polymerase chain reaction (PCR), the key feature that should arouse suspicion of tuberculous meningitis in most cases is the associated pulmonary or other extracranial disease. Tuberculous pleural effusion is discussed in chapter 243.

The slow growth of *M. tuberculosis* delays its identification. The **BACTEC-TB** system can detect mycobacterial growth in culture, reliably ascertain drug susceptibility, distinguish tubercle bacilli from atypical mycobacteria, and, in the febrile AIDS patient, help recover mycobacteria from the blood. **DNA probes** (single-stranded DNA sequences that hybridize with the counterparts of the mycobacterial DNA or RNA) hasten species identification. The combination of DNA probes with PCR can further hasten this process. PCR amplifies the *M. tuberculosis* DNA, making adequate nucleotide sequences available for testing with a DNA probe. This sophisticated technique is highly sensitive and specific, but cross-contamination may cause false positive results.

Roentgenographic features

Primary infection generally manifests with a hazy, unilateral, peripheral, middle, or lower lung **infiltration, with hilar lymphadenopathy** and without cavitation. **Reactivation tuberculosis** manifests with generally bilateral, but not necessarily symmetrical **upper-lobe infiltrates,** involving the apical and/or posterior segments. Cavitation and fibrosis are common but hilar adenopathy is not (Figure 218.1). With HIV co-infection, atypical x-ray patterns occur often. In general, the greater the immunosuppression, the closer the x-ray findings simulate primary tuberculosis. Furthermore, pulmonary tuberculosis with HIV co-infection can present with no significant pulmonary infiltration.

■ Diagnosis

A tuberculin skin test (PPD), chest x-ray, and sputum acid-fast smears should be done when pulmonary

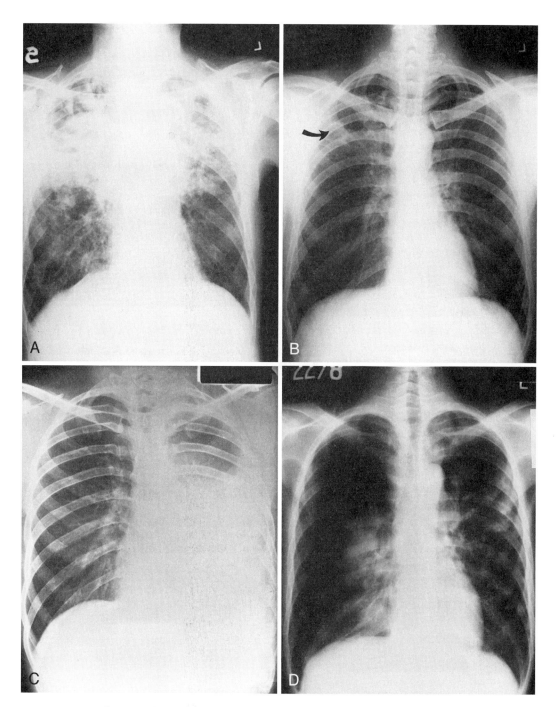

FIGURE 218.1. X-ray features of pulmonary tuberculosis. **A.** Extensive bilateral upper lobe cavitary disease, most pronounced on the right side. **B.** Right upper lobe cavity (arrow). **C.** Pleural effusion. **D.** Right pneumothorax from rupture of one of the subpleural lesions into the pleural space; nodular infiltrates on the left side.

tuberculosis is suspected. PPD is positive in most cases (>85%) of active tuberculosis. A positive sputum smear does not necessarily mean tuberculosis, but is enough to initiate isolation precautions and drug therapy if the clinical picture is compatible. When smears are negative, transbronchoscopic biopsy of the lung infiltrates rapidly and reliably provides a diagnosis, if caseating granuloma is seen. Bronchial brushing of pulmonary infiltrates or

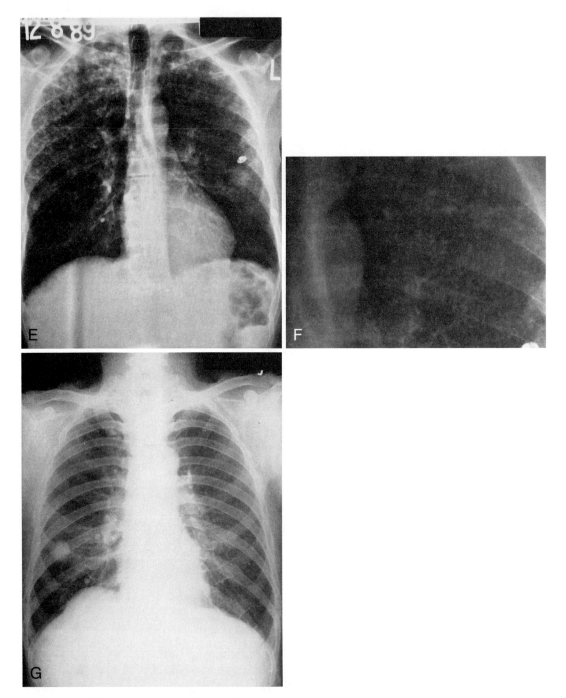

FIGURE 218.1—*continued.* **E. Extensive miliary tuberculosis. F. Magnified view of miliary nodules. G. Tuberculoma of the right lower lobe. Nodular lesions such as this may be** confused for a bronchogenic carcinoma. **A, B,** and **C** are more common and **D, E, F,** and **G** are unusual.

(Adapted from: Emergency Med 1983;15:133. Used with permission.)

transthoracic needle aspiration biopsy of pulmonary nodules may also provide material for microbiologic studies. Antimicrobial sensitivity testing should follow the identification of any positive cultures. There are no reliable, rapid diagnostic tests that could supplant culture identification. However, culture is possible in most (75%) cases, making a presumptive diagnosis of tuberculosis inevitable in some. To diagnose extrapulmonary tuberculosis, pathologic material obtained from infected sites should be processed as described above. Presumptive treatment is not recommended in extrapulmonary tuberculosis.

■ Management

Three groups of mycobacteria exist in tuberculous lesions: actively growing intracavitary (10^8), slow-growing intracellular ($<10^5$), and a very slowly or intermittently multiplying group inside caseous foci ($<10^5$). Mutants with primary resistance to one standard antituberculosis drug commonly occur in the larger groups ($>10^6$). With single drug therapy, mutants will selectively grow and replicate ("selection"). Their slow replication causes inadequate bacillary eradication and "relapse" on cessation of therapy. In the smaller ($<10^6$) groups, drug resistance and selection are not a problem. Thus, the treatment objectives are (1) to rapidly eliminate the first group, obviate selection, and make the patient rapidly noninfectious, and (2) to sterilize the tissues and prevent relapse. The first step involves simultaneous use of multiple drugs and the second one involves the extended use of agents to kill intracellular organisms.

Isoniazid (INH), rifampin (RFN), streptomycin (SM), and pyrazinamide (PZA) are mycobactericidal. Others, including ethambutol (EMB), are mycobacteriostatic (see also Table 145.4). Recent outbreaks of multidrug-resistant tuberculosis have necessitated several initial drug regimens (Table 218.2). Droplet spread is prevented by various isolation methods (mask, negative flow ventilation, etc.). antituberculosis agents should be given in a single daily dose, since mycobacteria replicate only once per day. Baseline liver function studies are obtained before treatment. Treatment rapidly renders patients noninfectious, probably in about 2 weeks. Alcohol is best avoided during treatment. Directly observed therapy is the only proven way to ensure compliance. Common side effects of antituberculous drugs are abnormal liver tests and hepatitis (INH, rifampin, pyrazinamide), peripheral neuropathy (INH), orange discoloration of secretions and urine (rifampin), hyperuricemia (pyrazinamide), vestibular toxicity, nephrotoxicity (streptomycin), and optic neuritis (ethambutol). INH is given with pyridoxine (50 mg daily) to prevent neurotoxicity. One-fifth of patients taking INH will show abnormal liver function tests (LFTs), which should be taken into account in the case of routine monitoring of LFTs. The exact LFT correlates of early hepatotoxicity are open to debate. When there is HIV co-infection, the treatment incorporates the same principles but for a longer duration.

Immediate contacts of the patient should be identified and given PPD testing and, if positive at least 5 mm induration, (see Table 209.1), a chest x-ray examination. All immediate contacts are given chemoprophylaxis with INH and pyridoxine; those with positive PPD are given this combination for 6 months; those who are negative are retested 3 months later, and prophylaxis is stopped if the results remain negative. Indications for tuberculin skin testing and chemoprophylaxis appear in Table 218.3.

TABLE 218.2.	Current Recommendations from the Centers for Disease Control for Initial Therapy of Tuberculosis				
Option	Agents and Frequency	Duration	Follow with	Add	Total
1	Daily INH, RFN, PZA	8 weeks	INH, RNF daily or 2–3 x/week	EMB, SM until sensitivity is reported to INH and RFN	At least 6 months; 3 months beyond negative culture
2	Daily INH, RFN, PZA, SM, or EMB	2 weeks	Same agents 2x/week for 6 weeks by DOT; INH, RFN 2x/week for 16 weeks by DOT	—	6 months
3	INH, RFN, PZA, EMB/SM 3x/week by DOT	6 months	—	—	6 months
TB + HIV	Use options 1, 2, or 3	9 months	—	—	9 months and at least 6 months beyond culture conversion

Note: Consult a TB expert if symptoms persist or smear/culture remains positive after 3 months.
Source: *MMWR* 1995; 42:RR-7: 1–8.
DOT = directly observed therapy; EMB = ethambutol; INH = isoniazid; PZA = pyrazinamide; RFN = rifampin; SM = streptomycin.

TABLE 218.3. Indications for Tuberculin Skin Testing and Chemoprophylaxis

Indications for tuberculin skin testing
  Suspected active tuberculosis
  Recent contacts of persons with or suspected to have active tuberculosis
  HIV infection
  Abnormal chest x-rays compatible with, but not definitely diagnostic pf past tuberculosis
  Medical conditions that increase the risk of tuberculosis (Table 218.1)
  Medically underserved populations
  Long-term institutional residence (nursing home, prisons, psychiatric institutions)
  Prior residence in areas of the world endemic for tuberculosis
  Health care workers
Indications for tuberculosis preventive therapy (chemoprophylaxis)[†]
Conditions irrespective of age
  HIV infection
    Definite
    Risk factors for and suspicion of HIV infection, but HIV status unknown
  Close contacts of recently diagnosed tuberculosis
  Recent infection (PPD test conversion)
  Associated medical conditions that increase risk of tuberculosis
Preventive therapy acceptable if age less than 35
  Persons born in countries with high prevalence of TB
  Medically underserved low-income populations
  Residence in long-term care facilities (prisons, nursing homes, psychiatric institutions)
  Health care workers in whom development of tuberculosis would pose a risk to many patients

†Requirement: positive tuberculin skin test; see criteria in Table 209.1.

CHAPTER 219 ATYPICAL MYCOBACTERIOSES

The term "atypical mycobacteria" (AM) rests on the premise that *M. tuberculosis* produces a typical form of the disease and the others do not—a premise on which there is no universal agreement. These ubiquitous organisms cause colonization through clinically silent infection to frank disease.

■ Clinical Features

Among the AM that cause lung disease, the most frequent etiologic agents are *M. avium-intracellulare* complex (MAC) and *M. kansasii*. Compared to tuberculosis, pulmonary disease caused by these agents occurs more often in older, immunocompetent individuals. They frequently are asymptomatic and the disease is detected because of an abnormal chest x-ray (indolent or slowly progressive bilateral or unilateral upper lobe infiltrates) or because the organism is cultured from a resected, granulomatous pulmonary nodule. Symptoms, when present, and the chest x-ray appearances closely mimic those of *M. tuberculosis*. Mediastinal disease and pleural involvement are unusual. Generally, systemic dissemination is uncommon in the immunocompetent host.

Disseminated disease due to AM is emerging as a common problem among patients with AIDS, and as a general rule is occurring in those with more advanced immunosuppression. Although symptoms are numerous and nonspecific, intermittent fever, weight loss exceeding 20 pounds, anorexia, abdominal pain, and diarrhea are the most notable. Fever, hepatosplenomegaly, and generalized lymphadenopathy are the usual findings. Disseminated disease associated with AIDS is diagnosed by isolation of the organism from blood, stool, and/or bone marrow. In rare cases, biopsy and culture of other sites, such as the lymph nodes, liver, and small bowel, may be needed. Granulomas are usually absent, and abundant organisms are seen within foamy macrophages.

■ Diagnosis

Initially, when only the sputum acid-fast stain is positive, the patient must be presumed to have *M. tuberculosis*. However, when the sputum culture finally yields AM, disease must be distinguished from colonization. This consideration arises from the general need to employ multiple, potentially toxic agents to attain a cure that is otherwise unattainable. Recently, clarithromycin and azithromycin have been found to be effective in the therapy of this disease and its prophylaxis in AIDS.

Practitioners should consult up-to-date journal articles that discuss the criteria for diagnosing AM-related diseases and their therapy.

CHAPTER 220 OBSTRUCTIVE DISORDERS OF THE AIRWAYS

Airway obstruction, which limits airflow, occurs in many pulmonary disorders. In **chronic obstructive pulmonary disease** (COPD), the single, common feature is airway obstruction. The American Thoracic Society defines COPD as a "disorder characterized by abnormal tests of expiratory flow that do not change markedly over periods of several months of observation." In this restrictive definition of COPD, only chronic bronchitis, emphysema, and peripheral airways disease are included; diseases characterized by reversible airflow obstruction—that is, asthma and other specific disorders—are not.

The American Thoracic society considers **chronic bronchitis** to be "associated with prolonged exposure to non-specific bronchial irritants and accompanied by mucus hypersecretion and certain structural alterations in the bronchi." Some consider chronic bronchitis to be present when cough and sputum (productive cough) occur on most days for at least 3 months in a year for 2 successive years, after other causes of productive cough (e.g., tuberculosis and bronchiectasis) are excluded. Mucus hypersecretion without airflow obstruction is

simple chronic bronchitis, whereas mucus hypersecretion, significant airway obstruction, hypoxemia, and (sometimes) hypercarbia represent **chronic obstructive bronchitis.** In emphysema, according to the American Thoracic Society, there is "abnormal, permanent enlargement of airspaces distal to the terminal bronchiole, accompanied by destruction of their walls, and without obvious fibrosis." In **peripheral airways disease,** which primarily involves the small conducting airways, epithelial damage causes inflammation with resultant luminal narrowing and/or obliteration of the airway.

Thus, COPD represents a spectrum of diseases that have histopathological definitions but are diagnosed clinically. Since they are most commonly due to tobacco smoke, the component disorders do not generally occur as pure entities. Although COPD, asthma, and even bronchiectasis and/or cystic fibrosis are not component disorders, they tend to be associated with each other. For example, in **asthmatic bronchitis,** asthmatic symptoms (wheezing) co-exist with chronic bronchitis (cough and sputum). Bronchitis and bronchiectasis also share similar associations.

CHAPTER 221 CHRONIC BRONCHITIS AND EMPHYSEMA

Chronic Bronchitis

■ Etiology, Pathology, and Pathogenesis

Inhalation of tobacco smoke is the principal cause of chronic bronchitis, but exposure to environmental pollutants and irritants may also be causative. Chronic bronchitis is characterized by the hypersecretion of mucus. The subepithelial mucus glands and their acini hypertrophy and airway smooth muscles become hyperplastic. Goblet cell hyperplasia, intrabronchial mucus plugging, and distension of respiratory bronchioles with destruction of the wall (centrilobular emphysema) are other findings.

Tobacco smoke stimulates bronchial mucus secretion, impairs mucociliary clearance, and disrupts alveolar

macrophage function. A vicious cycle of respiratory infections, bronchial damage, and further impairment of ciliary function follows. However, airflow obstruction develops in only a minority (20–25%) of smokers, suggesting that host susceptibility is an important prerequisite for this complication. In this context, both smoking-related airway irritation and bronchial hyperreactivity (BHR) have been implicated in the genesis of airflow obstruction. Nonetheless, current evidence suggests that COPD evolves through smoking-induced BHR. Finally, cholinergic innervation is abundant (and sympathetic innervation sparse) in the large and medium airways. Vagal stimulation causes bronchospasm and bronchial gland secretion. Cholinergic airway tone increases significantly following airway damage. In susceptible persons, various provocative stimuli could thus produce bronchoconstriction through vagal reflex.

Airway obstruction produces unventilated or under-ventilated alveoli; continued perfusion of these alveoli leads to hypoxemia (low PaO_2) from mismatching of ventilation and blood flow (V/Q mismatch). Hypoxemia occurs early in chronic obstructive bronchitis, and when sustained leads to pulmonary hypertension. Ventilation of unperfused or poorly perfused alveoli increases dead space (V_d), causing inefficient CO_2 removal. Hyperventilation normally compensates for this, thus producing a normal $PaCO_2$. However, hyperventilation, which further increases the work required to overcome the already increased airway resistance, ultimately fails, resulting in CO_2 retention (hypercapnia).

■ Clinical Features

The cardinal symptoms of established chronic bronchitis are cough and expectoration, which tend to be maximal in the morning and reflect pooling of secretions overnight. A productive cough, intermittent at first, becomes almost a daily occurrence with time. Sputum is clear and mucoid, but may become thick, tenacious, and yellow, and even blood-streaked during intercurrent bacterial respiratory infections. Blood-streaking may also be from repetitive coughing or intercurrent lung malignancy. Chronic bronchitis is the most frequent cause of frank hemoptysis. However, the amount of bleeding is generally modest and only infrequently life-threatening. Wheezing is generally present, especially during respiratory infections.

Dyspnea, usually absent in **chronic simple bronchitis,** is a feature of **chronic obstructive bronchitis,** which develops over many years. In addition to dyspnea, chronic obstructive bronchitis is characterized by cyanosis and marked wheezing, and is often complicated by heart failure. Physical examination is generally normal in simple chronic bronchitis, but reveals expiratory prolongation, rhonchi, and, less often, basilar râles in obstructive bronchitis. **Digital clubbing is not a feature of chronic bronchitis or COPD** and, when present, should arouse suspicion of another disorder, especially bronchogenic carcinoma.

■ Ancillary Studies

Sputum examination may show a mixed bacterial population. Erythrocytosis occurs, characteristically without leukocytosis or thrombocytosis, triggered by chronic arterial hypoxemia. Roentgenograms may be normal or show increased lung markings, with or without cardiomegaly. Pulmonary function studies, while normal in chronic bronchitis, show airway obstruction in chronic obstructive bronchitis. Hypoxemia occurs early; hypercapnia complicates advancing disease, usually when the $FEV_{1.0}$ falls below 1.0 L.

■ Course, Complications, and Prognosis

Symptoms of chronic bronchitis persist with continued exposure to irritants, and generally improve with cessation of such exposure. Long-term decline in pulmonary function appears to be less severe in those who stop smoking. Expiratory flow rates may improve more rapidly following smoking cessation.

The main complications of chronic obstructive bronchitis are bacterial colonization of the lower respiratory tract, respiratory infections, respiratory failure, erythrocytosis, and cor pulmonale. Most respiratory infections are initially viral, but soon evolve into bacterial bronchitis and sometimes into pneumonia. Increased cough with thick, tenacious, yellow sputum laden with numerous bacteria and neutrophils, along with a worsened respiratory status, characterize these bacterial infections. Respiratory failure is usually caused by a respiratory infection; heart failure, uncontrolled oxygen therapy, sedation, chest trauma, pneumothorax, surgery under general anesthesia, and pulmonary thromboembolism are others. Hypoxemia, hypercarbia, increased blood viscosity from erythrocytosis, and the destruction of pulmonary vessels all contribute to cor pulmonale (chapter 227).

Pulmonary function generally declines progressively, and while less accurately predictable in a given patient, the average yearly loss in $FEV_{1.0}$ is 50–100 ml. Activity is markedly limited when the $FEV_{1.0}$ is about 1.0 liter. With lower values, dyspnea may even limit conversation. COPD definitely shortens the life span, especially in persons younger than 65 years, but various investigators report highly variable survival statistics (Figure 221.1). Among the many variables that apparently influence survival (Table 221.1), the most important are age and the postbronchodilator $FEV_{1.0}$. Survival also improves with ambulatory, long-term oxygen therapy (LTOT) in appropriately selected patients.

■ Diagnosis and Differential Diagnosis

Chronic bronchitis is a clinical diagnosis, based on history; lung examination is generally abnormal. Chronic obstructive bronchitis involves airflow obstruction but no decrease in the diffusion capacity (DL_{CO}) unless significant emphysema is present. Wheezing and dyspnea are symptoms common to chronic bronchitis, asthma and emphysema; helpful distinguishing features are listed in Table 221.2).

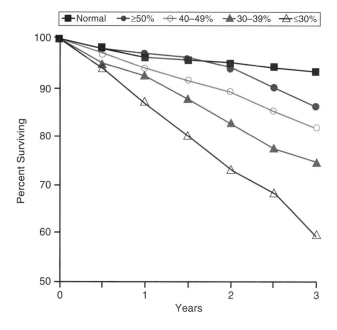

FIGURE 221.1. Survival curves from the National Institutes of Health-Intermittent Positive Pressure Breathing trial, based on baseline postbronchodilator $FEV_{1.0}$.

(From: Anthonisen NR, et al. Am Rev Resp Dis 1986;133:14–20. Reprinted with permission.)

TABLE 221.1. Factors of Prognostic Significance in Chronic Obstructive Pulmonary Disease (COPD)	
Factors Correlating with Survival	
Positively[a]	**Negatively[b]**
Predominant chronic bronchitis	Age
$FEV^{1.0}$	Progressive decrease in $FEV_{1.0}$
PaO_2	High resting heart rate
Reversibility of airflow obstruction	Increased $PaCO_2$
Exercise capacity	Pulmonary hypertension/cor pulmonale
Diffusing capacity	Total lung capacity
Vital capacity	Continued smoking
Atopy	Malnutrition/weight loss
	α-1-antitrypsin deficiency

[a]Presence of one of these or a higher value indicates a better prognosis.
[b]If present or high, the prognosis is worse.
(Adapted from: Hodgkin JE. Clin Chest Med 1990;11(3):556. Used with permission.)

■ Management

Bronchodilators

All patients with the diagnosis of chronic obstructive pulmonary disease should be given a trial of bronchodilators (Table 221.3), whether or not the spirometry shows bronchodilator responsiveness. Repeat spirometry and review of symptoms after several weeks of treatment may help in determining the continued course of therapy.

Anticholinergic agents

Anticholinergics are the most logical bronchodilators to use in COPD (see previous discussion). **Ipratropium bromide,** a quaternary ammonium compound, is most widely used. When given as an aerosol, ipratropium is poorly absorbed from the airways, relatively nontoxic, and has little effect on mucociliary clearance. In contrast to other bronchodilators, ipratropium perturbs V/Q mismatch only minimally; thus, it only slightly worsens arterial hypoxemia, if at all.

Theophylline

Theophylline has a narrow therapeutic window. Its bronchodilatory action is serum level–dependent. It improves mucociliary clearance, reduces pulmonary hypertension, improves right ventricular performance in COPD, and augments diaphragmatic contractility by

TABLE 221.2.	Differentiating Between Asthma, Bronchitis, and Emphysema		
Criterion	**Asthma**	**Chronic bronchitis†**	**Emphysema**
Principal symptom	Wheezing, paroxysmal dyspnea	Productive cough for many years	Progressive dyspnea for many years
Pattern of wheezing	Paroxysmal	Perennial	Perennial
Relationship of attacks to allergens	Temporal	None	None
Seasonal nature of symptoms	Seasonal; symptom-free intervals	None	None
Worsening/improvement over time with or without treatment	Characteristic	Not seen	Not seen
History of smoking	Variable	Integral part of history	Integral part of history
Personal/family history of asthma or atopy	Supports diagnosis	Incidental, not helpful in diagnosis	Incidental, not helpful in diagnosis
Exacerbations of the disease	Usually no purulent sputum; recovery from exacerbations generally rapid and nearly complete	Sputum ± purulent. Exacerbations from infection and/or heart failure. Recovery often prolonged.	Exacerbations from infection and/or heart failure. Recovery often prolonged.
Physical examination	Normal between paroxysms	Rhonchi, râles, wheezing, cyanosis ±, ↑ FET.	Barrel-shaped chest, breath sounds ↓, wheeze, ↑ FET.
Laboratory	Blood and sputum eosinophilia. Atopy and high IgE levels helpful.ᵃ Reversibility of airflow obstruction >25%. DLCO nl, often ↑. CXR nl when stable.	Erythrocytosis. Atopy not a feature. PaO$_2$↓↓, PaCO$_2$ may rise. Reversibility of airflow obstruction minimal. DLCO nl or ↓. CXR: "dirty lungs."	Atopy not a feature. PaO$_2$ slightly ↓; PaCO$_2$ ↓. Reversibility of airflow obstruction minimal. DLCO ↓. Emphysematous changes in CXR.

†Refers to chronic obstructive bronchitis.
Note: Disorders are described here when they occur as "pure" entities. However, in clinical practice, these diseases often co-exist.
ᵃAtopy and high IgE levels are seen only in allergic asthma. Thus, the absence of these features does not exclude asthma.
↑ = increased; ↓ = decreased; ± = may be; CXR = chest x-ray; DLCO = diffusion capacity; nl = normal; FET = forced expiratory time (normal <6 sec).

enhancing diaphragmatic blood flow. This beneficial effect on diaphragmatic function may help minimize or prevent diaphragm fatigue or respiratory failure in advanced COPD.

Theophylline metabolism, influenced by many factors, is 90% hepatic. For rapid dosing, IV loading is infused at 5–6 mg/Kg in 20–30 minutes, if the drug has not been recently used. Because maintenance dose regimens are not highly reliable, drug-level monitoring is critical. In nonsmoking adults, an acceptable dose is 0.5 mg/kg/hr, and in smokers it is 0.7 mg/kg/hr; the aim is a serum level between 10 and 13 mg/ml. The oral starting dose of anhydrous theophylline for adults is 400–600 mg daily in divided doses. Drug-level monitoring and dosage changes should follow until therapeutic levels are reached. Toxic side effects, uncommon with a therapeutic drug level (<20 mg/ml), include irritability, nausea, vomiting, diarrhea, palpitations, tachycardia, cardiac arrhythmias, confusion, agitation, and seizures. Follow-up drug-level monitoring is needed only for

suspected toxicity, suboptimal response, or intercurrent factors that affect clearance of the drug.

β-Adrenergic Agonists

These agents mimic the effects of β-adrenergic receptor stimulation (see Table 221.3). Because the β receptors have both cardiovascular (β-1) and bronchodilatory (β-2) effects, β agonists with selective β-2 effects are highly desirable; such exclusive selectivity is unavailable at present. β agonists presumably stimulate adenyl cyclase, increasing intracellular cyclic adenosine monophosphate (c-AMP), thus causing bronchodilation.

Sequential therapy of COPD is shown in Figure 221.2. It is best to administer all bronchodilators except theophylline via metered dose inhalers (MDIs), providing fixed-dose, targeted delivery into the airway and thus minimizing systemic effects. In one-third of all patients, lack of dexterity may preclude activation of MDI during inspiration ("hand-lung incoordination"), thus making MDIs less effective. Solutions include

TABLE 221.3.	Commonly Used Bronchodilators		
Agent	**Action**	**Dosage**	**Route**
Ipratropium bromide	Anti cholinergic	2 puffs qid	MDI
(Atrovent)®		0.5 ml qid, diluted in 3 ml saline	Via nebulizer
Albuterol	β-2 adrenergic	2 puffs q 4–6h;	MDI,
(Proventil®; Ventolin®)		2–4 mg[b] qid	Tablets and syrup
Metaproterenol	β-2 adrenergic	1–2 puffs q 4–6 h;	MDI,[a]
Alupent®, Metaprel®		0.3 ml in 3 ml saline	Via nebulizer
		q 4–6h 20 mg tid/qid.	Tablets and syrup
Salmeterol	β-2 adrenergic	1–2 puffs q 12 h.	MDI[a]
Serevent®			
Terbutaline	β-2 adrenergic	1–2 puffs q 4–6 h.	MDI[a]
		2.5 to 5.0 mg tid/qid	Tablets
		0.25 ml q 4–6h.	Parenteral solution
		subcutaneous injection	
Theophylline	See text.	See text.	Oral and intravenous

[a]Preferably administered as two separate puffs with an interval of a minute between each.
[b]Sustained release (long-acting) preparation available with b.i.d. (twice daily) dosing.
MDI = Metered dose inhaler.

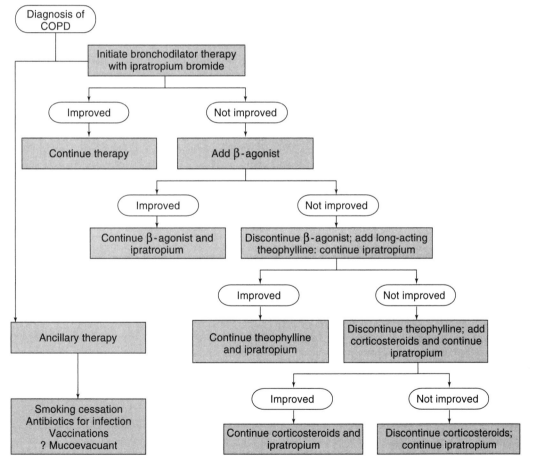

FIGURE **221.2.** Sequential application of drug therapy in COPD. Ancillary therapy should also include oxygen, where appropriate.

(Adapted from: Ferguson JF, Cherniack RM. N Engl J Med 1993;328:1017. Used with permission.)

careful patient education, use of spacers or use of hand-held, compressor-driven nebulizers. Nebulizers deliver a larger dose, involve bulky equipment, and require skills in equipment care and medication dispensing.

Control of secretions

It is critical that the patient stop smoking and avoid irritants. Avoiding passive smoke or pollutants may require a change in occupation, the use of filter masks, or modifications in the workplace and/or home. Increasing water intake is beneficial only when dehydration is present. Physical therapy with chest clapping and postural drainage is helpful for coexistent bronchiectasis or excess secretions. Expectorants have no proven benefit, but mucolytics (e.g., acetylcysteine by aerosol, 1–4 ml, q 4–6 h) may help liquefy tenacious secretions by breaking the sulfhydryl bonds in the mucus. Because it causes bronchospasm, a concurrent bronchodilator aerosol should be given.

Long-term oxygen therapy

In properly selected patients with COPD, ambulatory LTOT significantly improves the quality of life and survival. The criteria for LTOT are target organ dysfunction from hypoxemia (e.g., erythrocytosis or cor pulmonale) and/or PaO_2 50mm Hg or less ($\leq$55 mm Hg according to some) on room air and with optimal treatment of the underlying disease and its complications. LTOT effectively treats erythrocytosis in the bronchitic; concurrent smoking, besides being risky, counteracts this benefit. Equipment involves oxygen tanks with gaseous or liquid systems, or oxygen concentrators, which, by removing most of the nitrogen from the atmospheric air, deliver 93–94% pure oxygen. Proper patient selection is crucial because LTOT is expensive and may be cumbersome.

Corticosteroids

Corticosteroids, despite their frequent adjunct use, are controversial in COPD. They might benefit a subset of COPD patients with wheeze, atopy, labile or reversible airflow obstruction, or a progressive decline in $FEV_{1.0}$ exceeding 80 ml/year. Prednisone, initiated at 30–40 mg daily for 10–14 days, is continued at the minimum necessary dose to maintain objective improvement. If none is apparent, prednisone is tapered rapidly.

Other ancillary measures

Prophylactic vaccinations against influenza should be given yearly, generally in early autumn. Pneumococcal vaccine is recommended, but the immunity wanes after about 5 years. While most patients with COPD are managed on an ambulatory basis, hospitalization may be required for exacerbations unresponsive to the usual care, for occurrence of serious complications, and for operations or procedures that entail serious risk to the patient, significant analgesia, or anesthesia.

Treatment of exacerbations

Generally, 1-2 exacerbations occur yearly, precipitated by either respiratory infection or heart failure. It is critical to recognize and treat exacerbations, as they are notorious for precipitating respiratory failure. Usual features are increasing dyspnea, cough and sputum, and, when caused by infection, purulent sputum. Most infections are viral, generally caused by bacterial secondary infection resulting from *Hemophilus influenzae*, pneumococci, and *Moraxella catarrhalis*, in that order of frequency. When respiratory infection is suggested or when sputum becomes yellow, antibiotics should be started. Ampicillin (2.0 gm/d), Doxycycline (200 mg/d), or sulfamethoxazole/trimethoprim (400/160 mg, respectively, twice daily), for 7–10 days, are all acceptable. Given the increase in β-lactamase–producing bacteria, the newer macrolides (e.g., clarithromycin) may have a role in these cases. The use of corticosteroids remains controversial even in COPD exacerbations with worsening respiratory distress; however, their use in this situation is appropriate (methylprednisolone, 2.0 mg/kg initially, followed by 0.5 mg/kg q 6 h for 3 days). Exacerbations caused by heart failure call for the determination of etiology/mechanism for heart failure and appropriate therapy. Exacerbations that do not respond to the usual measures often require hospitalization.

Pulmonary rehabilitation

When customized for the patient with COPD (or other debilitating respiratory disorders), a comprehensive program using bronchodilators, oxygen, exercise reconditioning, and psychosocial rehabilitation will be beneficial. These programs do not improve longevity or pulmonary function, but they enrich the quality of life and reduce hospitalizations.

Pulmonary Emphysema

■ Etiology and Pathogenesis

Cigarette smoke is strongly implicated in the genesis of human emphysema. It is thought to result from an imbalance in the elastase-antielastase system. On exposure to tobacco smoke, alveolar macrophages secrete elastases and chemotactic factors for neutrophils, which

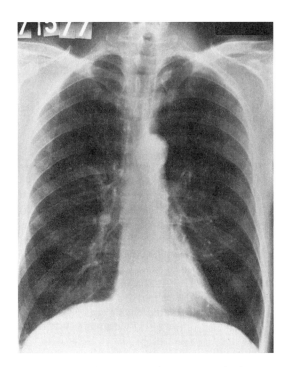

FIGURE 221.3. Pulmonary emphysema: note the hyperinflated lungs and flattened diaphragms.

in turn also release elastases. An anti-elastase system (e.g., α-1 antitrypsin) protects against elastase-induced lung injury. When anti-elastases are naturally defective or rendered ineffective by components of the smoke, lung injury follows. Collagen synthesis and repair are also impaired by the tobacco smoke.

■ Pathology and Pathophysiology

The acinus distal to the terminal bronchiole enlarges and the alveolar septa are destroyed. Early ruptures in airway walls later become confluent, finally destroying the walls. Ultimately, the orderly appearance of the acinus and its components is disturbed and lost. Loss of elastic recoil and the resultant compressibility of large airways upon exhaling, as well as the loss of radial traction on the airways, all lead to expiratory obstruction and decreased expiratory airflow. As a result, α-1 antitrypsin, a normal element in the airway lining fluid, is damaged or destroyed; both emphysema and airway damage follow. Expiratory airflow obstruction compromises bronchial hygiene and lung defenses, causing chronic bronchitis to be associated.

■ Clinical Features

The patient, generally a man in his fifties, reports dyspnea and, if chronic bronchitis is associated, a

productive cough. Findings include use of accessory muscles during inspiration, pursed lips on exhaling (which prevents premature airway collapse), barrel-shaped chest, hyperresonance to percussion, and obliteration of cardiac and hepatic dullnesses. Breath sounds are markedly diminished and exhalation prolonged, often with a wheeze. The precordial heart sounds are distant, but generally well heard in the epigastrium.

■ Ancillary Studies

Because chest x-rays are normal in early emphysema, they are unsuitable for screening. However, they are a good adjunct to the clinical evaluation of emphysema. The most accepted radiographic criteria for emphysema are overinflation of the lungs, low, flat diaphragms, and a large (>3.0 cm) retrosternal airspace. The heart is vertical and narrow. Lung vasculature is attenuated peripherally with prominent central pulmonary arteries (Figures 221.3 and 221.4). Spirometry shows airflow obstruction; DLCO is decreased.

■ Management

Respiratory function declines in most patients with time. (See the discussion of chronic bronchitis, above). Hypercapnia, resting tachycardia, and the presence of cor

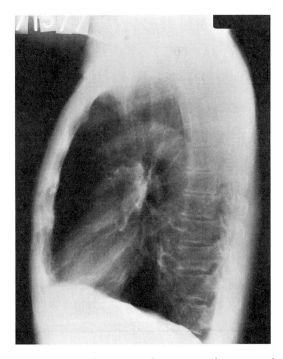

FIGURE 221.4. Pulmonary emphysema: note the attenuated vasculature, flattened diaphragms and increased retrosternal airspace.

pulmonale indicate a poor prognosis. There is no specific therapy for emphysema, other than the management of associated chronic bronchitis—that is, relief of any reversible bronchospasm, oxygen therapy when appropriate, and prevention and treatment of bacterial pulmonary infections. In selected patients, the elimination of some bullous lesions by lung volume reduction surgery ameliorates symptoms, although it is not known who might best benefit from this procedure and whether it can alter the long-term prognosis.

CHAPTER 222 SMALL AIRWAYS DISEASE

First described in the 1960s, small (peripheral) airways disease—also known as **bronchiolitis**—consists of dyspnea, airflow obstruction, reticular changes in the chest x-rays, and pathological findings confined to the small (<2 mm diameter) airways. The disease is heterogeneous and involves the small conducting airways, with several forms having since been described. **Diffuse panbronchiolitis,** primarily seen in Japan and predominantly involving middle-aged men, manifests with dyspnea, cough, purulent sputum airflow obstruction, and sinusitis. Untreated, the 5-year mortality rate is about 40%. Long-term erythromycin, unrelated to its antibacterial properties, is beneficial. The epidemiology of **adult bronchiolitis** is not well known. Airflow obstruction develops over many years and without associated features of asthma, chronic bronchitis, or emphysema. Corticosteroid therapy has been found to be useful.

Bronchiolitis obliterans (BO) may be idiopathic or may have disparate causes, including viral infections, noxious dust and fume exposure, heart and/or lung transplants, bone marrow transplants, and connective tissue disorders (particularly rheumatoid arthritis being treated with penicillamine). BO following heart/lung transplant occurs 3 or more months after the transplant, and represents chronic rejection. BO following bone marrow transplant develops within 6–12 months of the transplant and is associated with graft versus host disease. The features are relentlessly progressive dyspnea, dry or minimally productive cough, and evidence of airflow obstruction. Treatment options are augmentation of immunosuppression and/or retransplantation. Corticosteroid therapy produces equivocal results. **BO with Organizing Pneumonia (BOOP)** has features of interstitial lung disease and produces a restrictive impairment (see chapter 232).

CHAPTER 223 CYSTIC FIBROSIS AND BRONCHIECTASIS

Cystic Fibrosis

Cystic fibrosis (CF) is a common, fatal genetic (autosomal recessive) disorder characterized by chronic bronchopulmonary suppuration, exocrine pancreatic insufficiency, and elevated sweat electrolytes. A heterozygous state for CF is said to be present among 2–5% of Caucasians. Pulmonary problems in CF account for most of the morbidity and almost all the premature deaths. (Malabsorption and exocrine pancreatic deficiency are discussed in chapter 96.)

■ Pathology and Pathogenesis

Approximately 70% of CF arises from a genetic mutation—deletion of three base pairs causing a phenylalanine deletion at F508 locus (ΔF508) on the CF gene, located in the long arm of chromosome 7. This gene encodes for a protein, **cystic fibrosis transmembrane conductance regulator** (CFTR). The defective gene produces a defective protein, which interferes with normal chloride ion permeability, causing intracellular entrapment of chloride ions. The chloride and sodium ions osmotically draw water from the airway mucus, causing its dehydration, inspissation, viscidity, and tenaciousness; glandular ducts are obstructed, bacteria are trapped, and infection results. Bacterial proteases and leukocyte elastases cause tissue injury, leading to bronchitis, bronchiolitis, and bronchiectasis, which perpetuate the infection; then the vicious cycle repeats itself. Pulmonary infection, especially by Pseudomonas strains, causes most of the morbidity and mortality in

CF. The same genetic defect causes elevated sodium and chloride levels in the sweat and saliva. Pancreatic fibrosis is common.

Clinical Features

The onset is usually in infancy or childhood—for example, intestinal obstruction from **meconium ileus** in infancy, and **pancreatic insufficiency** (chapter 96) by 2 years of age, with bulky, greasy, foul-smelling stools and failure to thrive. In others, **cough, sputum production**, repeated **respiratory infections**, and **asthmatic symptoms** develop and, as the severity of bronchiectasis increases, bloody sputum and frank hemoptyses become frequent. Finger clubbing and nasal polyps are common. Recurrent pneumothoraces and/or repeated respiratory infections with mucoid *Pseudomonas aeruginosa, Pseudomonas cepacia,* or *Staphylococcus aureus* are clues to underlying CF. Cor pulmonale eventually develops and cardiac or respiratory failure is the usual cause of death. A list of complications of CF is provided in Table 223.1.

TABLE 223.1. Complications of Cystic Fibrosis and Their Frequency	
Complication	**Incidence (%)**
Pneumothorax (adults)	17–20
Massive hemoptysis	8
Intestinal obstruction	17
Circulating immune complexes	28–100
Pancreatic insufficiency	85–90
Gallbladder disorders (stones, cholecystitis)	50
Biliary cirrhosis	25
Nasal polyps	41
Sinusitis	90
Azoospermia (men)	>95
Systemic amyloidosis	Unknown

Ancillary Studies

A sweat chloride level exceeding 80 mEq/L in adults (>60 mEq/L in infants) after **pilocarpine iontophoresis** is diagnostic. False positive results occur in hereditary nephrogenic diabetes insipidus, glucose-6-phosphate dehydrogenase deficiency, and untreated adrenal insufficiency. Genetic testing can help confirm diagnosis or screen for carriers in first-degree relatives when CF is diagnosed. Pulmonary function testing shows airway obstruction in most cases. Sputum cultures may help antibiotic selection. Chest x-rays show peribronchial thickening, cystic and bullous lesions, and branching linear densities indicative of fluid-filled bronchi. Unresolved pneumonitis, atelectasis, and apical lesions mimicking tuberculosis are frequent.

Prognosis and Management

The individual prognosis varies, but appears to be better for boys/men, and with lack of respiratory symptoms on presentation, and residence in a temperate climate. Survival has been related to the abnormalities in the chest roentgenograms: the worse they are, the poorer the survival rate.

Pulmonary infection, airflow obstruction, nutritional failure, pancreatic insufficiency, and psychological issues need to be addressed. Segmental postural drainage with chest clapping should be performed about four times per day. Bronchodilators are indicated when airway obstruction is demonstrated by pulmonary function tests. Antibiotics must be given for respiratory infections in full therapeutic doses for 3–4 weeks. Antibiotics and bronchial hygiene may help eradicate staphylococci, but Pseudomonas generally persists. Prophylactic antibiotics are not recommended. The use aerosolized, recombinant dornase alpha (DNAse) has been shown to reduce the number of infectious respiratory exacerbations requiring parenteral antibiotics, and decrease the rate of hospitalizations, the number of days missed from work or school, and the frequency of CF-related symptoms.

Bronchiectasis

Bronchiectasis is a permanent, abnormal dilatation of bronchi with destruction of elastic and muscular layers of their walls. Three varieties have been described: **saccular, tubular,** and **fusiform.** With the availability of antibiotics, its incidence has declined.

Pathology and Pathogenesis

Purulent secretions usually occupy the abnormal bronchial lumen. Dilated bronchial mucus glands, squamous metaplasia of the bronchial epithelium with ulcerations and fibrosis, and destruction of the elastic and muscular layers of the bronchus are the chief pathologic findings. The involved areas may contain extensive bronchial-pulmonary artery anastomoses.

Bronchiectasis may be acquired or congenital. Acquired bronchiectasis may follow an inflammatory process (postinflammatory) or mechanical bronchial obstruction (obstructive). Viral respiratory infections (respiratory syncytial virus or adenovirus), allergic bronchopulmonary aspergillosis, cystic fibrosis, and chronic bronchitis account for most acquired cases.

Ciliary dysfunction causes bronchiectasis. All cilia have the same architecture, whether they are in the respiratory epithelium or the flagella of the spermatozoa. Generalized ciliary dysfunction in immotile cilia syndrome (ICS) impairs airway mucus clearance and sperm motility, and bronchiectasis and male infertility follow. Bronchiectasis, infertility, sinusitis, and situs inversus constitute **Kartagener's syndrome.** Situs inversus presumably occurs when embryonic clockwise visceral rotation fails, as a result of the absence of ciliary activity within the archenteron. Bronchiectasis and male infertility also complicate **Young's syndrome** (the epididymal head becomes enlarged, palpable, and obstructed due to inspissated secretions) and cystic fibrosis. **IgG subclass deficiencies** have also been recently found to cause bronchiectasis.

■ Clinical Features

Cough and abundant mucopurulent or purulent sputum are principal symptoms. In severe cases, a collection of expectorated mucus may settle into three layers: a top mucoid, middle salivary, and bottom layer of purulent debris (Figure 223.1). Other symptoms are recurrent pneumonias involving localized areas and hemoptysis. Finger clubbing, wheezing, and rales that occur throughout inspiration are frequent findings. Lung abscess and empyema may arise as complications, although amyloidosis and brain abscesses are unusual. Sinusitis and otitis are important clues to ciliary disorders.

■ Diagnosis

Clinical history and physical examination often suggest the diagnosis. Serum immunoglobulin levels may be low when immunodeficiencies are the underlying etiology. Arterial hypoxemia is common, from ventilation-perfusion mismatch. Chest x-rays are rarely normal; typical findings are increased bronchial markings, "tramline" shadows (parallel lines that resemble tracks of a tram), and cystic areas. Computed tomography has an acceptable degree of sensitivity and extremely high specificity; "signet rings" are diagnostic (the hollow, dilated, thick-walled bronchus is the ring, and accompanying pulmonary artery is the signet). Pulmonary function ranges from normal to obstructive and/or restrictive patterns.

■ Course and Complications

Repeated episodes of pneumonia lead to further worsening of bronchiectasis, creating a vicious cycle. Necrotizing infection may lead to a lung abscess. In the pre-antibiotic era, bronchiectasis often caused brain abscesses; although rare, they still represent a dreaded complication. Bronchial-pulmonary artery anastomoses, which line the bronchiectatic cavities, are liable to rupture, causing frequent (and occasionally massive, life-threatening) hemoptysis.

■ Management

Dependent postural drainage and chest physiotherapy should be practiced daily, about three to four times if possible, preceding meals. Antibiotics are indicated for respiratory infection. The usual pathogens are *S. pneumoniae* or *Haemophilus influenzae*. Even though cultures may not yield these pathogens, empiric therapy is indicated, similar to that of bacterial infections in COPD (see Treatment of Exacerbations, chapter 221). Prompt therapy and good bronchial hygiene together prevent further bronchial damage. Smoking is forbidden; so is exposure to irritating fumes. Yearly influenza vaccine and pneumococcal vaccine every 5 years are indicated. Severe, localized, disabling disease or severe recurrent hemoptysis may require surgery, although its role has dwindled owing to the generalized nature of the disease and the effectiveness of medical management.

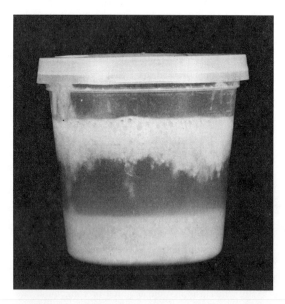

FIGURE 223.1. Sputum from a patient with bronchiectasis showing the characteristic three layers.

BRONCHIAL OBSTRUCTION, ATELECTASIS, AND UPPER AIRWAY OBSTRUCTION

Bronchial Obstruction

Besides obstructive airway disease, bronchial obstruction may result from intraluminal lesions (e.g., a mucus plug, inhaled foreign body), mural lesions (e.g., benign and malignant neoplasms), and extrinsic compression (e.g., hilar or mediastinal lymph node enlargement, mediastinal tumors, and aortic aneurysms). In these, the manifestations arise from both the primary disease *and* the effects of the obstruction.

Bronchial obstruction most commonly results from a neoplasm. Obstruction of a large bronchus may cause dyspnea, cough, and focal wheezing. With sig-

nificant atelectasis, there is mediastinal shift. Obstruction, regardless of cause, may produce localized hyperinflation from air trapping, distal atelectasis, bronchiectasis, and, with distal infection, pneumonia and/or lung abscess. Bronchial obstruction should be suspected when pneumonias resolve slowly or lung abscesses present without apparent risk factors. In suspected endobronchial obstruction, bronchoscopy is the most important diagnostic test. Computed tomography alone is not reliable. Treatment should be directed toward the etiology.

Atelectasis

With complete endobronchial obstruction, absorption of air in the lobe or segment distal to it causes a process known as **absorption atelectasis** (mediastinum shifts ipsilaterally); a similar result from pneumothorax or large

pleural effusion is called **compression atelectasis** (contralateral mediastinal shift). Absorption atelectasis signifies bronchial obstruction and should be managed appropriately.

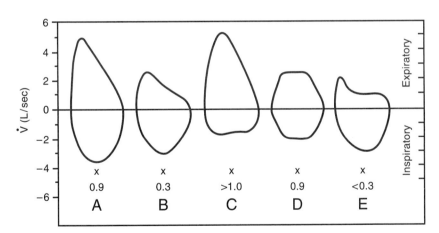

FIGURE 224.1. Flow volume loops in airway obstruction. $\dot{V}$ = flow rate. Numbers below each graph represent ratios of expiratory to inspiratory flow at the mid-vital capacity point (x). A = normal (ratio = 0.9); B = asthma or COPD; C = variable extrathoracic obstruction; D = fixed intrathoracic obstruction; E = variable intrathoracic obstruction. (Note the plateau in the expiratory phase.)

Upper Airway Obstruction

■ Tracheal Obstruction

Local extension of esophageal or bronchogenic carcinoma into the trachea, impaction of food in the esophagus with compression of the posterior tracheal wall ("cafe coronary"), and tracheal stricture following endotracheal intubation are the common causes of tracheal obstruction. Primary tracheal tumors are rare. Intrathoracic tracheal obstruction causes wheezing; extrathoracic obstruction leads to stridor. More chronic cases can be diagnosed by computed tomography and flow volume loop. Representative flow volume loops in various types of airway obstruction are shown in Figure 224.1. Management of tracheal obstruction is dictated by the acuteness of onset. Emergency intubation, rigid bronchoscopy, tracheostomy, and tracheal stents are options. In suspected upper airway obstruction, fiberoptic bronchoscopy is best avoided. In selected cases, obstruction may be relieved by laser therapy.

■ Laryngeal Obstruction

Laryngeal obstruction, distinguished by stridor, characteristically occurs when a foreign body, usually food, is inhaled. Other causes are angioneurotic edema, croup, bilateral vocal cord paralysis, laryngeal tumors, laryngospasm, and "rebound" edema following removal of an indwelling endotracheal tube. The victim with impaction of a foreign body in the larynx is unable to cough, speak, or breathe. Heimlich's maneuver (sudden, firm pressure with the fist in the area between the xiphoid and umbilicus) may dislodge the obstruction. Digital extraction of the foreign body may also be attempted. Emergency tracheostomy will be life-saving if other measures fail. In acute laryngeal obstruction due to hereditary angioedema, parenteral epinephrine is the treatment of choice.

CHAPTER 225 PULMONARY EDEMA

■ Definition and Pathogenesis

Pulmonary edema is a pathological state in which the extravascular lung water is increased. The normally small, constant egress of fluid from the microvasculature of the lung into the lung interstitium is removed by the lymphatics of the lung. Pulmonary edema is a dynamic extension of this process, where excessive filtration or excessive permeability of the microvasculature overwhelms the clearance capacity of the lymphatics.

Four major forces (also called **Starling's forces**) govern the transvascular fluid flow: a pair of hydrostatic forces (microvascular and perimicrovascular) and a pair of osmotic forces (microvascular and perimicrovascular). The components of each pair operate in opposite directions (Figure 225.1). Another determinant is the filtration coefficient of the capillary endothelium. The normal orientation of Starling's forces produces a net efflux of fluid from the capillary lumen into the pericapillary interstitial space, estimated to be about 10–20 ml/h, which is then cleared by the lymphatics. The pulmonary capillary endothelium is restrictive in its permeability for various molecules depending on their molecular weights. Its conductivity for fluid itself is low. The permeability of the alveolar epithelium is perhaps even more limited, mainly because of its intricate structure with tight intercellular junctions.

Thus, pulmonary edema may follow excessive fluid filtration (from increased hydrostatic pressure) or increased permeability of the capillary endothelium. Excessive fluid filtration, characterized by elevated left atrial pressures—pulmonary capillary wedge pressure (PCW)—and low protein levels in the edema fluid, is generally due to cardiogenic causes (left ventricular failure, arteriosclerotic heart disease, mitral stenosis, and fluid overload, discussed in chapter 30). Adult respiratory distress syndrome (chapter 249), drug-induced pulmonary edema, neurogenic pulmonary edema, and perhaps high altitude pulmonary edema all result from increased capillary permeability. Not only is the left atrial pressure normal or even low, but the edema fluid protein is high.

In early pulmonary edema, the excess fluid accumulates around the pulmonary capillaries accompanying the bronchiole, forming a perivascular and peribronchial fluid cuff. As the fluid accumulates, it raises the pressure in this cuff, and begins to leak into the alveoli at the bronchoalveolar junction. Lung compliance decreases and, with the flooding of the alveoli, the work of breathing (i.e., the oxygen cost of breathing) rises profoundly; gas exchange is severely disturbed and respiratory distress becomes manifest.

Drug-induced Pulmonary Edema

Opiates (most classically heroin) are the best-known drugs that cause pulmonary edema. Pulmonary edema

Pulmonary capillary

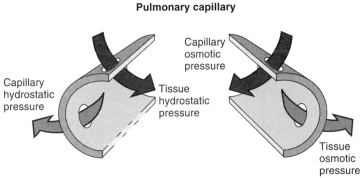

FIGURE 225.1. Starling's forces govern the transvascular fluid flow: the pair of hydrostatic forces (microvascular and perimicrovascular), operate against a pair of osmotic forces (microvascular and perimicrovascular). The hydrostatic and osmotic forces within the same compartment are also oriented in opposite directions.

with miotic pupils is typical, especially when the patient has a background of drug abuse. Enhanced capillary permeability from hypoxia, contaminants (in the heroin), or histamine released by opiates is the alleged mechanism. Naloxone (0.4 mg IV q 3–5 min) is the specific antidote for opiate intoxication. Respiratory failure and pulmonary edema may require endotracheal intubation.

Drug screens of urine and blood are useful since multiple drug poisonings are quite common. Other less well-known drugs and chemicals that may cause pulmonary edema are salicylates, ethchlorvynol (refer to Figure 249.2), nitrofurantoin, propranolol, radiographic contrast media, paraquat, cyanide, and blood transfusions.

CHAPTER 226 PULMONARY THROMBOEMBOLISM

Pulmonary embolism (PE) is not a disease in itself, but a complication of a thrombotic process elsewhere, often a deep vein thrombosis (DVT). Since PE and DVT are but two sides of the same coin, the process is frequently referred to as **venous thromboembolism** (VTE). More than 90% of all PE occurs in the hospitalized population.

■ Pathogenesis

The factors that predispose to VTE are summarized in Table 226.1. In deficiencies of anti-thrombin III, protein S, and protein C, the thrombotic process is recurrent. VTE without predisposing factors is considered idiopathic. In VTE complicating malignancy, the VTE might precede, accompany, or follow a malignancy. The risk of a subsequent neoplasm seems highest in those with idiopathic and recurrent VTE. Cancer-related VTE is highly complex and may be due to a hypercoagulable state (from products of cell-tumor cell interaction), from inadequate fibrinolysis (release of tumor-derived clotting factors), or from venous stasis (e.g., venous obstruction from a tumor).

■ Pathophysiology

The sequelae of pulmonary embolism depend upon the extent of obstruction and the previous state of the

TABLE 226.1. Predisposing Factors for Pulmonary Embolism

Specific predisposing factors for lower-extremity DVT
  Previous history of DVT
  Postoperative states (hip, prostate, abdominal/thoracic surgery)
  Trauma (pelvis, spine, or legs, all requiring a cast or immobilization)
  Prolonged bed rest (stroke, respiratory failure, paraplegia)
  Myocardial infarction where anticoagulation is not employed
Factors enhancing thrombotic risk
  Obesity
  Peripheral vascular disease (sluggish blood flow)
  Active cancers
    highest risk: pancreatic
    intermediate risk: lung, genitourinary, colon, and breast
    lowest risk: lymphoma and leukemia
  Oral contraceptives, risk relative to the estrogen content (high correlation with activated protein C resistance)
  Congenital disorders
    Anti-thrombin III deficiency
    Protein S deficiency
    Protein C deficiency
    Activated protein C resistance (see chapter 129)

cardiopulmonary system. Obstruction of the main pulmonary artery, generally at its bifurcation, may be lethal whether or not it is preceded by shock. In massive embolism the right ventricle must maintain a mean pressure above 40 mm Hg to sustain forward blood flow. A previously normal right ventricle (i.e., no cardiopulmonary disease) is unaccustomed to this, and thus fails. Acute cor pulmonale and shock follow (Table 226.2).

The physiologic disturbances in pulmonary embolism are shown in Figure 226.1. Pulmonary vascular resistance rises, with the extent of the increase depending on the magnitude of vascular obstruction, vaso-active agents released from the clot itself, prior cardiopulmonary disease, and perhaps reflex events. Hypoxemia has many causes (atelectasis, shunting, perfusion of unventilated alveoli, the severe desaturation of mixed venous blood from decreased cardiac output, etc.). Fragmentation and mechanical reshaping of an embolized clot, which together with endogenous fibrinolysis helps restore pulmonary blood flow, causes the initial improvement seen in some cases of massive pulmonary embolism. Clot resolution is highly variable and fails altogether in 0.5–12% of all cases. Large emboli (occlusion >35% on a perfusion lung scan), coexistent cardiac disease, and simultaneous, clinically apparent DVT all not only predispose to recurrent PE but also to poor clot resolution.

Pulmonary infarction (necrosis of lung tissue) is an uncommon sequel of PE (5–10% of cases) and results from peripheral, rather than central embolism. Because necrosis requires total cessation of oxygen supply, pulmonary infarction generally indicates diseased bronchial circulation and/or cardiopulmonary disease. Congestive atelectasis mimics pulmonary infarction clinically and radiographically, except for the quick and complete resolution and the lack of tissue necrosis.

■ **Clinical Features**

In many cases of PE, a predisposing factor to DVT is identifiable in the history. Despite the many symptoms

and signs (Table 226.3), three broad patterns of presentation of PE can be recognized: acute cor pulmonale, unexplained dyspnea, and acute pulmonary infarction. In acute cor pulmonale, which implies massive pulmonary embolism, acute dyspnea occurs with or without accompanying chest pain, and the patient's clinical status suddenly deteriorates, and may even result in a collapse. Findings include hypotension, shock, pulmonary hypertension (increased intensity of pulmonary valve closure [P_2], right ventricular heave, right-sided third or fourth heart sound), and significant elevations in right-sided pressures on cardiac catheterization. The second pattern (unexplained dyspnea) may be confused with worsening of pre-existent heart failure or lung disease in persons with these processes. In contrast, hemoptysis and pleuritic chest pain herald the (more dramatic) presentation of pulmonary infarction. Physical examination generally discloses fever and splinting of the chest wall. Ipsilateral consolidation and pleural effusion occur. Pleural friction rub is generally audible, at least early in the illness.

■ **Ancillary Studies**

Leukocytosis is common, but it seldom exceeds 15,000/mm³. In most cases, besides sinus tachycardia, an electrocardiogram (ECG) reveals no unique features and primarily helps exclude a myocardial infarction. Arrhythmias such as atrial flutter and fibrillation, and varying degrees of A-V block, may be demonstrated. Massive embolism may be associated with P pulmonale, S in lead I, and a Q with T wave inversion in lead III (the so-called S_1-Q_3-T_3 pattern). Changes from the previous ECG (e.g., a change in axis) are more important. Hypoxemia and hyperventilation-induced hypocapnia are common, but neither one is specific for pulmonary embolism. In patients without prior cardiopulmonary disease, the extent of hypoxemia correlates well with the severity of embolism. PaO_2 exceeding 85 mmHg with the patient breathing room air makes pulmonary embolism less likely, but does not exclude it.

TABLE 226.2. Pulmonary Embolism with Previously Normal Cardiopulmonary System: Classification of Severity				
Extent of Occlusion	**P̄A**	**RAP**	**CO**	**Clinical Correlates**
<50%	<20	<10	Maintained	Usually not lethal if no other disease.
50–75%	25–40	<10	Usually maintained	Submassive embolism; clot fragments and migrates distally, reducing cross-sectional obstruction. Survival depends on this.
>75%	≯40	>10	Decreased	Massive embolism; acute right ventricular failure. Lethal unless treated; shock may or may not precede death.

P̄A = PA mean pressure; RAP = right atrial pressure; CO = cardiac output.

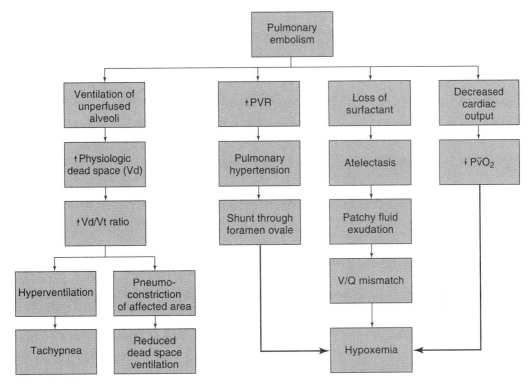

FIGURE 226.1. Physiologic disturbances in pulmonary embolism. PVR = pulmonary vascular resistance; Vd = dead space; Vt = tidal volume; $P\bar{v}O_2$ = mixed venous oxygen tension.

TABLE 226.3.	Symptoms and Signs of Pulmonary Embolism

Symptom	Incidence (%)
Pleuritic pain	74
Dyspnea	85
Apprehension	59
Cough	53
Hemoptysis	30
Chest pain	14
Syncope	13
Sign	
Tachypnea	92
Râles	58
Increased P_2	53
Tachycardia	44
Fever	43
Diaphoresis	33
Gallop	34
Phlebitis	32
Edema	24
Cyanosis	19

(From: Bell WR, et al. Am J Med 1977;62:355–360. Used with permission)

Owing to the varying pathogenetic mechanisms, pleural effusions in association with pulmonary embolism display a wide spectrum of features. In pulmonary infarction, the fluid is almost always an exudate and tends to be bloody or blood-stained, resolving with time. Lack of resolution or an intercurrent increase in size denotes coincident complications such as infection and/or reinfarction, or heart failure if other factors support that diagnosis.

Imaging studies

Chest roentgenograms, which are generally normal, primarily help exclude other conditions that can produce a similar picture (heart failure or pneumothorax). In pulmonary infarction, the classic finding is a wedge-shaped opacity with ipsilateral pleural effusion. Effusions may be seen without apparent infiltrate and are generally unilateral.

Perfusion (Q) scanning using technetium (^{99}mTc) macroaggregated albumin is a very sensitive test and, therefore, the mainstay of pulmonary embolism diagnosis. A normal six-view lung scan ("negative" scan) excludes clinically significant pulmonary embolism.

However, not all positive scans indicate pulmonary emboli. In obstructive airway disease, atelectasis, bullae, heart failure, lung cancer, and respiratory failure, perfusion defects are usual. A ventilation (V) scanning can then augment the accuracy of perfusion scans. Perfusion defects with normal ventilation are **mismatched defects** and are the hallmark of pulmonary embolism (Figure 226.2). Perfusion defects with ventilation anomalies in the same area are **matched defects,** which usually portend a non-embolic disorder (e.g., heart failure, obstructive airway disease, etc). Large (segmental or larger), mismatched defects correlate well, and subsegmental defects, matched or mismatched, correlate poorly, with pulmonary embolism. The criteria for probability estimates of pulmonary embolism based on V/Q scanning vary, but a generally accepted set is shown in Table 226.4.

Pulmonary angiography

Pulmonary angiography is invasive and may not be readily available in all institutions; even when available, its application may be precluded by several patient factors, or technical factors may severely limit the information it can provide. Nevertheless, it is the "gold standard" for the diagnosis of pulmonary embolism. The indications for pulmonary angiography (arteriography) in the setting of pulmonary embolism are summarized in Table 226.5.

The diagnostic findings are intraluminal filling defects and vessel cut-offs (Figure 226.3). Other findings such as localized avascularity or sluggish blood flow are not diagnostic. In experienced hands, pulmonary angiography is safe, with a mortality and morbidity less than 0.5% and 1%, respectively.

Diagnosis of deep vein thrombosis as a surrogate marker for pulmonary embolism

PE is a consequence of DVT, and treatments for isolated DVT and for PE without shock are generally the same. Thus, documented DVT in a patient with a compatible picture for PE supports the diagnosis of pulmonary embolism. Contrast venogram is the "gold standard," but other noninvasive tests such as impedance plethysmography (IPG) and B-mode ultrasonography are excellent for diagnosing DVT (Table 226.6). In most centers B-mode ultrasonography has superseded IPG. The acoustic Doppler test is commonly combined with B-mode ultrasonography (duplex imaging). The vein's lack of compressibility and, to a lesser extent, internal echoes from within are diagnostic. The less-than-ideal ability of duplex imaging to detect small calf thrombi is clinically insignificant because, without extension above the knee, pulmonary embolism from isolated calf thrombi is unusual.

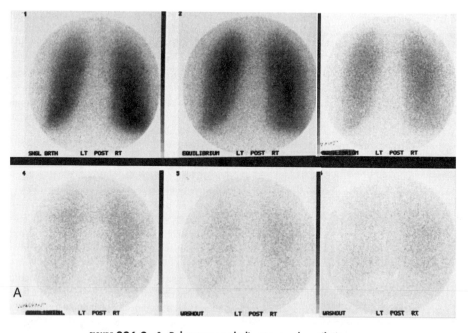

FIGURE **226.2** **A.** Pulmonary embolism: normal ventilation scan.

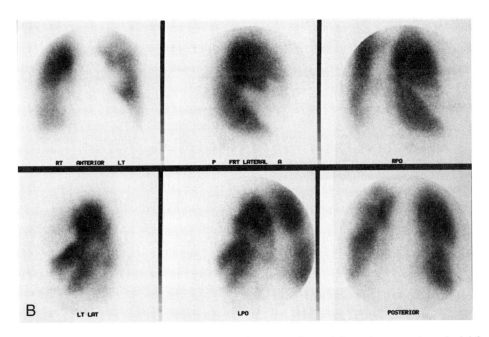

FIGURE **226.2. B.** Pulmonary embolism: perfusion scan showing perfusion defects. These are mismatched defects, which together with **A** constitute a high-probability lung scan.

TABLE 226.4.	Probability of Pulmonary Embolism Based on Ventilation-Perfusion Scan Patterns			
Probability	Perfusion Scan Abnormality	Mismatch	Match	Frequency of Pulmonary Embolism (%)
High	One or more segmental or greater defects	+		86
Intermediate	One or more segmental or greater defects		+	36
	One or more subsegmental defects	+		40
Low	One or more subsegmental defects		+	25
Indeterminate	Perfusion defect with chest x-ray abnormality corresponding to the perfusion defect			21

(Adapted from: Hull RD, et al. Chest 1985;88:819–828. Used with permission.)

■ Diagnosis

The strength of clinical suspicion together with the patient's condition dictate the extent of the workup for pulmonary embolism (Figure 226.4). Diagnosis of pulmonary embolism in hypotensive patients is by pulmonary angiography; in all others, V/Q scan is the initial study. A normal perfusion scan excludes clinically and/or hemodynamically significant pulmonary embolism. Abnormal V/Q scans are either **high probability** (Table 226.4, Figure 226.3) or **non-high probability** types; in the latter, perfusion defects are smaller than segmental, with or without abnormalities in corresponding areas of the chest x-ray. With a high probability scan and a strong clinical suspicion, pulmonary embolism is definite and treatment should proceed. If the lung scan is of a non-

high probability type, and suspicion of pulmonary embolism moderate, additional diagnostic tests should follow.

Venous thromboembolism leads to high levels of **D-dimer** in the peripheral blood. A specific degradation product of cross-linked fibrin, it may be detected through latex agglutination, enzyme-linked immunosorbent assay (ELISA), or whole blood agglutination assay. Elevated D-dimer in assays using ELISA have a high sensitivity, but low specificity for VTE but the latex test is much less sensitive. The whole blood agglutination method is easy, very rapid and reliable, can be performed at the bedside using a drop of whole blood, and depends on the use of a specific antibody that has epitopes that are portions of D-dimer and red blood cells (RBC). With high D-dimer, the antibody agglutinates the patient's RBC. False

TABLE 226.5.	Indications for Pulmonary Angiography in Pulmonary Embolism

Any of the following, where:
V/Q scans are unreliable for definitive diagnosis:
    Co-existent lung disease
    Heart failure
    Respiratory failure
Diagnosis is emergent or where pulmonary embolectomy or fibrinolytic therapy or pulmonary endarterectomy are active considerations:
    Shock with suspected massive pulmonary embolization
    Chronic pulmonary embolism, prior to thromboendarterectomy
Substantial risk from anticoagulation obligates a positive diagnosis:
    Bleeding diathesis
    Recent stroke
    Active/potential for active internal bleeding
One needs to differentiate PE from other conditions that cause a similar picture:
    Distinction between pneumonia and pulmonary infarction
Inferior vena caval interruption is being considered for recurrent PE.

contraindications, a bolus dose of 10,000 units of heparin is given IV, followed by continuous IV infusion (15–20 units/kg/h) until and after the diagnosis is confirmed. Activated partial thromboplastin time (aPTT) is measured once before and repeated every 4–6 hours for the first 24 hours, the goal being its prolongation by two to two-and-a-half times above baseline (Table 226.7). Platelet count is measured initially and daily thereafter to detect any thrombocytopenia from heparin (see chapter 132). Warfarin, 10 mg, is begun on the second day, and the dose adjusted to produce an international normalized ratio (INR) of 2.0–3.0. Heparin is discontinued on the fifth day or when satisfactory INR is reached; warfarin alone is then continued. Anticoagulant therapy merely inhibits further thrombosis; established clots or emboli are lysed by endogenous mechanisms. The exact duration of warfarin treatment, while subject to debate, generally is about 6 months following the initial episode of VTE.

Use of the international normalized ratio

The prothrombin test (PT) reflects the level of factors II, VII, and X. PT depends on the intensity with which factor X activates factor VII, and the responsiveness of

positive tests may occur with recent surgery, trauma, stroke, acute myocardial infarction, disseminated intravascular coagulation, pregnancy or recent (10 days) delivery, metastatic cancer or collagen vascular disease. These common predisposing factors for VTE limit the potential usefulness of the test.

Several useful clinical patterns emerge from limited studies using both IPG and D-dimer together: a normal IPG with negative D-dimer reliably excludes DVT, especially proximal DVT, and a positive IPG and a positive D-dimer reliably diagnoses DVT. A negative IPG with a positive D-dimer mandates serial testing, whereas an abnormal IPG with a positive D-dimer necessitates venography or duplex imaging. Combined use of D-dimer and V/Q scans require further elucidation. **Helical CT** has a high sensitivity for diagnosing proximal PE, but its sensitivity for distal, small PE is not satisfactory. Also, a dyspneic patient may not be able to breath-hold long enought for a reliable study. Finally, **MR angiography** appears very sensitive and specific, but its role requires additional large-scale studies.

■ Management

Heparin and oral anticoagulants

Heparin is the mainstay of treatment of VTE. For suspected massive or submassive embolization without

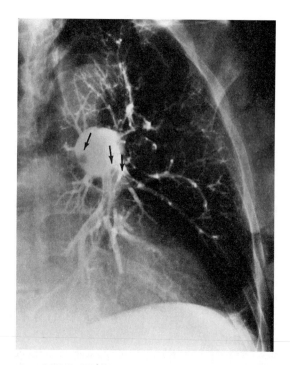

FIGURE 226.3. Pulmonary angiogram in a patient showing intraluminal filling defects (arrows).

TABLE 226.6.	Studies to Detect Deep Vein Thrombosis: Sensitivity, Specificity, Advantages, and Disadvantages			
Method	**Sensitivity (%)**	**Specificity (%)**	**Advantages**	**Disadvantages**
Contrast venogram	90	100	Visualizes the entire deep vein system and the pelvic and iliac veins and, possibly, inferior vena cava. Generally easily available; "gold standard."	Not well suited for repetitive use in the same patient. Dye allergy is a contraindication. Expensive.
IPG	95 (range, 87–100)	95 (range, 92–100)	Noninvasive; highly reliable.	Conditions with reduced arterial inflow or reduced venous outflow of blood cause false-positive tests. Facilities may not be available everywhere. Technical factors may cause false-positive and false-negative results.
Venous (acoustic) Doppler	77	50–60 for proximal DVT	More reliable than IPG in patients with peripheral vascular disease, congestive heart failure or limbs in plaster casts.	Very operator-dependent. Reliable graphic reproduction is not possible.
Real time ultrasound + acoustic Doppler (duplex imaging)	100 for proximal DVT	99 for proximal DVT	Effective and accurate. Results most reliable for veins above the thigh. Can diagnose other conditions causing symptoms such as Baker's cyst.	Results not reliable for isolated DVT in pelvic veins, or femoral vein in the adductor canal. Much less reliable for calf veins.

DVT = deep vein thrombosis; IPG = impedance plethysmography.

the thromboplastin. A sensitive thromboplastin causes less stimulation of factor X, and thus a lower PT; an unresponsive thromboplastin does the opposite. Because commercial thromboplastins vary in sensitivity, the same plasma sample may yield many PT values. INR represents normalization of these values using an international reference. INR values may be calculated from a nomogram. The effective INR varies for different clinical conditions.

Thrombolytic therapy

Emboli resolve faster and hemodynamic instability reverses quicker with thrombolytic agents in massive and submassive pulmonary embolism. It is uncertain whether they improve mortality. Early restoration of venous patency, early alleviation of the discomfort and pain, and, theoretically, less damage to the venous valves follow the use of thrombolytic agents in DVT. However, long-term benefits or a reduction in the incidence of post-phlebitic syndrome (an indicator of venous valve damage) have not been shown.

Thrombolytic agents are mainly indicated in patients who have no bleeding disturbance and have an established diagnosis of either a proximal DVT or pulmonary embolism accompanied by hemodynamic disturbances. Active internal or intracranial bleeding, stroke within the preceding 2 months, or any other active intracranial process are absolute contraindications. Others include recent major surgery, recent gastrointestinal bleeding, and severe arterial hypertension. Careful dose monitoring and meticulous avoidance of any but absolutely essential invasive procedures are essential. If such procedures are performed, proper hemostasis should be secured. Available agents are streptokinase, urokinase, and recombinant tissue plasminogen activator.

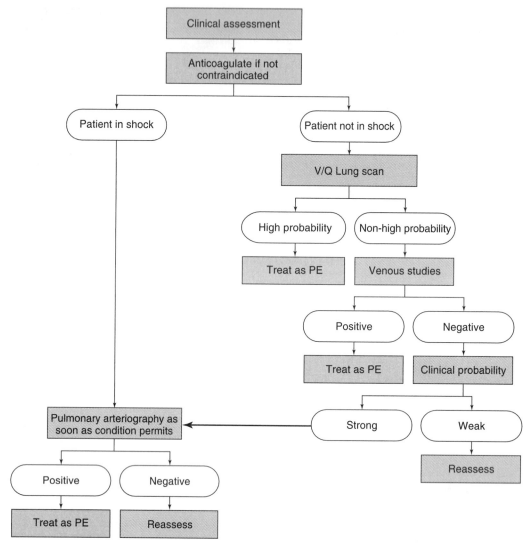

FIGURE 226.4. Suggested approach to the patient with suspected pulmonary embolism (PE). Rectangular boxes represent interventions/actions; boxes with rounded corners represent conditions.

TABLE 226.7.	Weight-Based Nomogram for Heparin Therapy				
	APTT Sec/(x C*)	Bolus (U/Kg)	Basic Infusion Rate (U/Kg/h)	↑ Basic by (U/Kg/h)	↓ Basic by (U/Kg/h)
Initial	—	80	18	—	—
	<35/<1.2	80	Same	4	—
	35–45/1.2–1.5	40	Same	2	—
Subsequent	46–70/1.5–2.3	—	Same	—	—
	71–90/2.3–3.0	—	Same	—	2
	>90	—	Hold 1 h	—	3[†]

*C = control APTT rate †: when resumed.
(Adapted from: Hirsh J et al. Chest 1995;108:262S. Used with permission.)

Embolectomy and inferior vena caval interruption

If there is refractory shock, if massive or submassive emboli are angiographically demonstrable, and if proper facilities are available, emergency pulmonary embolectomy is an option. The procedure itself carries a high mortality. Clots may be successfully removed using a specially devised suction catheter advanced into the pulmonary circulation. A variety of devices are available (Greenfield stainless steel vena caval filter, titanium Greenfield filter, and the bird's nest filter) to interrupt clots in the inferior vena cava (IVC), without affecting the blood flow. The indications for IVC interruption are listed in Table 226.8.

■ Venous Thromboembolism and Pregnancy

VTE commonly complicates pregnancy, particularly in the second trimester. The risk to the mother continues postpartum. Pregnancy is characterized by both venous stasis and hypercoagulability. DVT during pregnancy should be unequivocally confirmed before treatment. The initial study may be IPG or duplex imaging. Anticoagulation can follow a positive study if the pregnancy is within the first or second trimester. A positive study during the third trimester should be confirmed by a limited venogram; if it is not confirmatory, then a complete study should follow. If IPG or real-time ultrasound is unavailable, a limited venogram will suffice; if it fails to confirm DVT, then a complete venogram should be performed.

For suspected PE during pregnancy, a chest x-ray and a V/Q scan are appropriate initial tests. Normal results exclude PE. When clinical suspicion is strong, a high probability scan is sufficient indication for anticoagula-

tion. A non-high probability scan requires additional studies, such as IPG or duplex imaging. When DVT is thus confirmed, anticoagulation can follow. With strong clinical suspicion, negative IPG/duplex imaging, and a non-high probability scan, a pulmonary angiogram with appropriate shielding of pelvis and abdomen is the next step.

Heparin is the drug of choice because it does not cross the placenta. An IV bolus of 5,000 units is followed by continuous IV infusion, at 2,000–3,000 U/h. Following initial therapy, subcutaneous heparin is continued through the rest of the pregnancy and for 4–6 weeks after delivery. Complications are osteoporosis and thrombocytopenia. Labor is induced electively, and subcutaneous heparin is stopped 24 hours before. Low molecular-weight heparin is ideal for use during pregnancy; its longer half-life is conducive to once-daily use. Warfarin crosses the placenta, is teratogenic, and is contraindicated in pregnancy. Warfarin embryopathy—stippled epiphyses and nasal hypoplasia—is related to its use between 6 and 12 weeks of gestation.

■ Prognosis and Prevention

Appropriate and timely therapy reduces the high mortality from pulmonary embolism. Effective anticoagulation during the acute episode significantly decreases VTE recurrence. If the precipitating factor for the initial event is evanescent, the prognosis is good. Pre-existing left ventricular failure and coronary artery disease adversely affect long-term survival in pulmonary embolism. In a small minority (0.15–2%), a syndrome of postembolic pulmonary hypertension evolves insidiously, with progressive dyspnea and eventual severe disability. Pulmonary hypertension is detected clinically and confirmed on right heart catheterization. Perfusion lung scans show large, lobar, or segmental defects. Untreated, the mortality depends on the severity of pulmonary hypertension (90% 5-year mortality with mean pulmonary artery pressure exceeding 50 mmHg). Gratifying results follow early diagnosis and timely surgery.

Early ambulation following surgery, trauma, and other illnesses is key to reducing the incidence of VTE. The risk of VTE and the appropriate methods of prophylaxis are shown in Table 226.9. Low-dose heparin is not appropriate following surgery of the eye or central nervous system and in those with bleeding diathesis. Low-molecular weight heparin can effectively prevent VTE in susceptible populations; its efficacy is comparable to conventional heparin, but with a much lower incidence of thrombocytopenia and bleeding.

TABLE 226.8.	Indications for Inferior Vena Caval Interruption

Recurrent pulmonary embolism despite adequate anticoagulation
Documented VTE with any of the following:
  Contraindication to anticoagulation
  Necessity for premature discontinuation of anticoagulation
Chronic, recurrent pulmonary embolism in the setting of pulmonary hypertension and cor pulmonale
  During pulmonary embolectomy
  Septic pelvic thrombophlebitis
  Paradoxical embolism
  Residual, large, free-flowing iliofemoral thrombus in the setting of massive pulmonary embolism

TABLE 226.9.	Risk of Thromboembolism in Various Disease Categories and Guidelines for Prophylaxis		
Condition	**Risk (%) DVT**	**Type of Prophylaxis (either/or)***	**Risk reduction**
General surgery >40 years	16–30	1 LDH 2 EPC	67% DVT 50% PE

Orthopedic surgery
Hip surgery
	27–75	1 Moderate dose warfarin (PT to
		  16–18 sec.)
		2 LMWH
		  5,000 U/d or std heparin
		  5,000 U tid
			50% DVT

Urologic surgery	10–40	1 LDH 2 EPC	75%

Gynecology
<40 years
>40 years
>40 year & added risk
	3
	10–40
	40–70
		Early ambulation and graduated
		  stockings
		1 LDH
		2 EPC
		1 LDH plus external pneumatic
		  compression
		2 Dextran
		3 Moderate dose warfarin	

Pregnancy	5× control (Cesarean section, postpartum previous PE)	1 LDH 2 EPC	Not proven
Neurosurgery	9–50	1 EPC 2 For extracranial: LDH	
Stroke	75	1 EPC 2 If not hemorhagic, LDH	
Trauma	20–40	1 LDH 2 Dextran 3 EPC (if possible)	64% DVT
Congestive heart failure	70	LDH	31–84% DVT
Myocardial infarction	40	LDH	81–85% DVT

LDH = low dose heparin; EPC = external pneumatic compression; LMWH = low molecular weight heparin; std heparin = standard heparin; tid = 3 times a day. * = numbers represent desirability of option; 1 = primary, 2 = secondary, 3 = tertiary.
(From Briggs DD (ed.). Medical Knowledge Self-Assessment Program in the Subspecialty of Pulmonary and Critical Care. Philadelphia: American College of Physicians, 1994, p. 208. Reprinted with permission.)

CHAPTER **227** **PULMONARY HYPERTENSION**

■ **Physiologic Background**

The pulmonary circulation is a low-pressure system, with a normal resting pulmonary artery (PA) pressure of 25/10 mm Hg and a (resting) mean of about 15 mm Hg. The end-diastolic pulmonary artery pressure reflects the left ventricular end-diastolic pressure in persons without underlying lung disease. The pressure recorded after a catheter has been "wedged" into a small pulmonary artery to occlude its lumen is the pulmonary capillary wedge pressure (PCW), which is the left atrial pressure (normally 5–12 mm Hg). Exercise evokes little change in the systolic, whereas the diastolic may rise to 15 mm Hg and the mean to 20 mm Hg. A mean PA pressure exceeding 20 mmHg or a systolic PA pressure higher than 30 mmHg indicates definite pulmonary hypertension. In early pulmonary hypertension, resting pressures are often normal and only exercise, by increasing flow, may unmask it.

■ Pathogenesis

Although the entire cardiac output passes through the pulmonary circulation, it remains a low-pressure circuit, owing to the balance between various pressor influences (hypoxia, excessive blood flow) and the homeostatic dilatory mechanisms (ability to recruit blood vessels, distensibility of capillaries, the maintenance of vascular tone and patency by the endothelial cell, etc). The endothelial cell can modulate the pulmonary vascular tone, ward off in-situ thrombosis, and influence the migration and replication of vascular smooth muscle.

The pathogenesis of pulmonary hypertension is shown in Figure 227.1. Abnormal pressor influences (hypoxia, shear stress, excessive blood flow) cause pulmonary vascular tone to rise. The endothelial cell

normally responds to these influences through the release of endothelium-derived relaxing factor (EDRF), prostacyclin, and various agents that oppose platelet activation/adhesion and thrombin generation. EDRF appears to be nitric oxide (NO). NO stimulates guanylate cyclase, which increases cyclic guanosine monophosphate in vascular smooth muscle; vasodilatation follows. However, the endothelial cell can be damaged and become dysfunctional; these homeostatic mechanisms then fail. Consequently, the pressor response evolves into sustained pulmonary hypertension. The damaged cell also releases various cytokines and growth factors, which cause cell proliferation and intimal thickening in the small precapillary pulmonary arterioles. In-situ thrombosis and proliferation and extension of smooth muscle in the vessel walls soon follow. These changes are

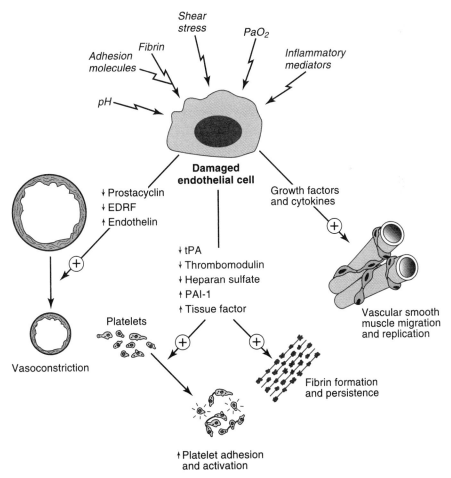

FIGURE 227.1. Pathogenesis of pulmonary hypertension following damage and/or dysfunction of the pulmonary vascular endothelial cell. Abbreviations: EDRF= endothelium dependent relaxing factor; PAI-1 = plasminogen activator inhibitor 1; tPA =tissue plasminogen activator; + = stimulation or permissive action.

collectively called vascular remodeling. Pulmonary hypertension is most often seen as secondary to another disease process. Primary or idiopathic pulmonary hypertension is uncommon. Regardless, it evolves from sustained pulmonary hypertension and structural remodeling.

Secondary Pulmonary Hypertension

Common causes of secondary pulmonary hypertension are left-sided heart disease, pulmonary vasoconstriction (high altitude, COPD, massive obesity), excessive blood flow (congenital heart disease), sleep-disordered breathing, and obliteration of the pulmonary vasculature (pulmonary embolism). It has no unique symptoms. Physical signs include large "a" waves in the jugular venous pulse, a left parasternal heave due to a prominent right ventricular impulse, loud pulmonary valve closure (P_2), a right ventricular gallop, ankle edema, and pulsatile and often tender hepatomegaly if right ventricular dilatation has caused frank tricuspid insufficiency. The most reliable way to diagnose pulmonary hypertension is right heart catheterization. Useful measurements include PA pressures (PAP), PCW, cardiac output during rest, oxygen, and exercise. Doppler echocardiography can noninvasively estimate pulmonary artery pressures. With the integration of clinical evidence, it is usually possible to ascertain the cause of secondary pulmonary hypertension. For example, since the mean PAP seldom exceeds 40 mm Hg even in massive, acute pulmonary embolism, a mean PAP of 50 mm Hg during acute pulmonary embolism indicates prior pulmonary vascular disease, either primary or secondary to prior thromboembolism with incomplete resolution or other causes.

Hypoxia-mediated pulmonary hypertension responds well to oxygen therapy. Pulmonary hypertension due to left-sided valvular heart disease often abates after replacement of the diseased valve. Some pulmonary hypertension will persist if the vasculature has undergone secondary changes. The course of postembolic pulmonary hypertension is improved by early diagnosis and pulmonary endarterectomy (chapter 26). Pulmonary hypertension due to sleep-disordered breathing responds well to therapy of sleep apnea.

Primary Pulmonary Hypertension

Primary pulmonary hypertension (PPH) occurs predominantly in women in their thirties or forties. Pathological findings include organized microemboli, intimal fibrosis, and medial hypertrophy with well-developed and hypertrophied longitudinal muscles. Intraluminal angiomatoid changes, adventitial vascularization, and perivascular lymphocytic collections are other changes. Whether recurrent thromboembolism causes or effects these changes is uncertain.

Exertional dyspnea, lasting months to years, effort syncope (from diminished left ventricular output because the right ventricle is unable to increase pulmonary blood flow against a fixed, high pulmonary vascular resistance), and chest pain (which often mimics angina) are common symptoms. Raynaud's phenomenon (a triphasic color reaction on exposure to cold, consisting of *pallor*, followed by *cyanosis*, and further followed by a *red color*) may occur. (Inquiries about Raynaud's phenomenon should be discrete, since leading questions generally produce positive answers, indicating the susceptibility of the complaint to suggestion.) Signs of pulmonary hypertension may be evident. A tender, pulsatile liver, ascites, and edema (signs of right-sided heart failure) represent advanced disease. Chest x-rays may show right ventricular enlargement, a prominent central pulmonary artery, and even a dilated main pulmonary artery. Pulmonary angiography and, to a lesser extent, perfusion lung scans could be lethal in these patients.

■ Management and Prognosis

Despite occasional cases of prolonged survival and spontaneous remissions, the prognosis is poor. The response of pulmonary vascular resistance to Prostacyclin (epoprostenol, PGI_2) during right-heart catheterization is used to select patients for high-dose nifedipine or diltiazem therapy. Intravenous infusions of Iloprost, a prostacyclin analog, have also produced more sustained reductions in pulmonary artery pressures. For those with more advanced disease, heart-lung transplantation and single-lung transplantation offer additional avenues of therapy.

CHAPTER 228

COR PULMONALE

Cor pulmonale is any structural or functional change in the right ventricle imposed by pulmonary hypertension which, in turn, results from a disease process (or processes) primarily involving the lungs, pulmonary vasculature, chest wall, or respiratory gas exchange; congenital or left-sided heart disease is excluded. Cor pulmonale may be acute, (e.g., massive pulmonary embolism) or chronic (e.g., COPD).

■ Etiology and Pathogenesis

Pulmonary vasoconstriction is the initial event, usually brought about by hypoxemia, hypercarbia, and/or obliteration of the pulmonary vascular bed. Hypoxemia is the mechanism in early COPD and in residents of high altitudes, whereas hypoxemia and hypercarbia are responsible in patients with **alveolar hypoventilation** (chest wall abnormalities, neuromuscular respiratory failure, or sleep-disordered breathing). **Obliteration of the pulmonary vasculature** (recurrent pulmonary thromboembolism, advanced pulmonary emphysema, interstitial lung disease, schistosomiasis, and sickle cell disease) and hypoxemia may operate together in some cases.

The pathogenesis of cor pulmonale in COPD, from which it most commonly results, is shown in Figure 228.1. Obliteration of the vascular bed, increased blood flow brought about by exercise, hypoxemia, compression of resistance vessels from increased alveolar pressure, vasoconstriction from hypoventilation in advanced COPD, hypercapnia, and acidemia are the major con-

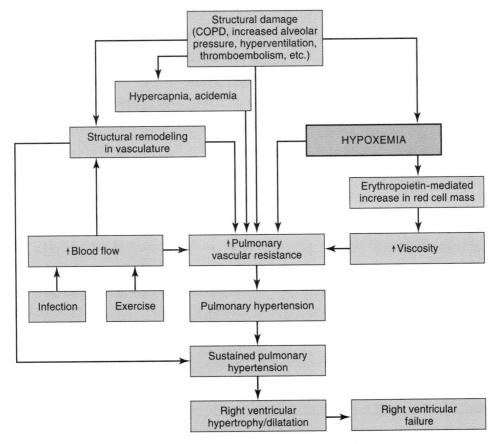

FIGURE 228.1. The pathogenesis of cor pulmonale.

tributors to pulmonary hypertension. Acidemia enhances the pulmonary vasoconstriction for any given level of arterial hypoxemia.

Arterial hypoxemia is compensated by an excess peripheral extraction of oxygen and, over time, **erythrocytosis**. Arterial hypoxemia lowers mixed venous oxygen saturation, and erythrocytosis raises blood viscosity; both exacerbate pulmonary hypertension. Heart failure as traditionally defined is absent; however, the cardiac output is inadequate for the extent of hypoxemia. This inadequate rise in cardiac output shortens survival. Oxygen therapy, by correcting hypoxemia, might be expected to improve the cardiac output but not completely. Finally, coronary artery disease, hypoxemia, and erythrocytosis with increasing blood viscosity may all evoke left ventricular dysfunction, which may follow as a secondary event.

■ Clinical Features and Diagnosis

Cor pulmonale has no unique symptoms. Dyspnea, weakness, and changes in cerebral function, despite being frequently reported, most likely are due to the underlying disease and the attendant hypoxemia. Pulmonary hypertension may cause chest pain. Symptoms of the underlying lung disease also may be evident. Physical findings are the same as those of pulmonary hypertension (chapter 227). The diagnosis of cor pulmonale depends on determining the presence of a disease that can cause cor pulmonale and the clinical features described above. ECG and x-ray criteria of cor pulmonale are listed in Table 228.1. Erythrocytosis may be evident. Distinguishing cor pulmonale from pulmonary hypertension due to left heart failure caused by disease is important, but could be difficult. Unless the patient has pulmonary edema or congestion, significant arterial hypoxemia (PaO_2 <60 mmHg) and hypercapnia favor the diagnosis of cor pulmonale. Pulmonary function tests (PFTs) generally reflect the underlying lung disease, but if PFTs are normal in the presence of cor pulmonale, **sleep-related hypoxemia** should be suspected. However, even in those with underlying lung disease, sleep-related hypoxemia contributes on its own to cor pulmonale.

■ Management and Prognosis

Besides appropriate treatment of the underlying disease, the following agents are important in cor pulmonale: oxygen, phlebotomy, digitalis, diuretics, and theophylline.

Long-term controlled oxygen therapy (LTOT) in hypoxemic patients with cor pulmonale lowers pulmonary artery pressures and improves survival. Concurrent smoking offsets the benefits of oxygen for

TABLE 228.1.	Electrocardiographic and Radiographic Manifestations of Cor Pulmonale
Measure	**Manifestations**
Electrocardiographic[a]	Right axis deviation of QRS complex, +110 or greater
	R wave to S wave ratio >1 in V_1[b]
	R wave to S wave ratio <1 in V_6
	P pulmonale
	$S_1 S_2 S_3$ or S_1, Q3 pattern
	Clockwise rotation of electrical axis[b]
	Incomplete right bundle branch block pattern[b]
Radiographic	Cardiomegaly with right ventricular and often right atrial enlargement
	Prominent central pulmonary artery with attenuated peripheral branches
	Features of the associated lung disease that leads to cor pulmonale[b]

[a]Any two of first six would confirm presence of cor pulmonale.
[b]Most characteristic when associated airway obstruction is present.

pulmonary hypertension. The lowest dose of oxygen that will keep the PaO_2 at or slightly above 60 mm Hg should be used; no attempt should be made to normalize the PaO_2. Hematocrit >55% raises blood viscosity, impairs myocardial performance seriously, and aggravates pulmonary hypertension. Exercise tolerance and maximal oxygen consumption improve after phlebotomy when the initial hematocrit exceeds 55%. Following phlebotomy the volume removed should be restored, since right ventricular performance depends on optimal filling pressures. LTOT is the prime therapy for erythrocytosis.

Digitalis might improve right ventricular ejection fraction in only those who have a concomitant decline in the left ventricular ejection fraction. Digoxin may increase the risk of arrhythmias in the presence of hypoxemia. Fluid overload often complicates cor pulmonale, especially with frank right ventricular failure. However, the line between excessive volume and that needed to maintain adequate right ventricular filling is a thin one. Bed rest and oxygen therapy in most cases cause prompt diuresis. Diuretics, if needed, should be used judiciously, and electrolytes and volume should be closely monitored. Theophylline, specifically in cor pulmonale due to COPD, reduces pulmonary artery pressure, improves right ventricular performance and pulmonary vascular resistance, and prevents diaphragm fatigue. A serum level of 10–13 µg/ml should be the goal.

The prognosis in cor pulmonale is essentially dependent on the underlying lung disease and how effectively it is being managed.

CHAPTER **229** INTERSTITIAL LUNG DISEASE

Definition, Etiology, and Classification

The **lung interstitium** is a layer of connective tissue between the epithelial layers of the alveoli and the endothelial layer of the capillaries. This layer contains connective tissue, macrophages, and fibroblasts. The lung interstitium may be infiltrated by many disorders that primarily affect the lungs or by a myriad of systemic diseases. Regardless, the resultant pulmonary process is called interstitial lung disease (ILD). If there is no identifiable primary process, the condition is termed **idiopathic pulmonary fibrosis,** which is the prototype of ILD. The more common entities are shown in Table 229.1.

Pathogenesis and Pathology

Regardless of etiology, interstitial lung diseases share a common pathway and some common clinical features. An initial **alveolar epithelial injury** leads to an **alveolitis;** changes in the lung interstitium and collagen along with infiltration by inflammatory and immune effector cells follow. Fibrosis and disordered architecture culminate in **"end-stage lung."** In any tissue injury, a balance ordinarily prevails between inflammation and repair. This balance is disturbed in ILD, and the inflammation is perpetuated. The type, route, and duration of the injury, the genetic predisposition of the host, and co-morbid factors all determine the breadth and severity of the resultant lung disease.

Following an alveolar epithelial injury, leukocytes transmigrate into the alveoli, duly influenced by chemoattractants (leukotriene B [LTB] 4 and interleukin [IL]-8) released by activated alveolar and interstitial macrophages. During phagocytosis, the neutrophils release an array of oxygen radicals, peptides, cationic proteins, and proteases, all of which can cause lung injury. Monocytes ultimately evolve into macrophages, thus controlling the inflammation and repair. The tissue repair is influenced by cytokines and growth factors released by macrophages such as platelet-derived growth factor (PDGF) and insulin-like growth factor (IGF). Neutrophils, lymphocytes, and other mononuclear phagocytic cells infiltrate the alveolar wall. Type I pneumocytes are damaged and type II cells show hypertrophy. Alveolar wall damage, proliferation of mesenchymal cells (fibroblasts), and collagen and matrix protein deposition can also occur. Depending on the disorder and the inciting event, other changes might be evident (e.g., granulomas in sarcoidosis or interstitial inorganic dust deposition in the pneumoconioses).

Clinical Features

Because ILD often follows a primary systemic disorder, the manifestations of the primary disease may overshadow the pulmonary symptoms. Symptoms of ILD are often chronic, but an acute onset with rapid progression is well known. The usual symptoms are

TABLE 229.1.	Classification of Interstitial Lung Diseases (ILD)

I. Collagen vascular disorders/connective tissue diseases/pulmonary-renal syndromes
II. Granulomatous disorders
    Cause unknown
        Sarcoidosis
        Histiocytosis X
    Cause known
        Hypersensitivity pneumonitis
        Drug-induced
III. Hereditary disorders
    Tuberous sclerosis
    Neurofibromatosis
    Metabolic storage disorders
IV. ILD from inhalational agents
    Occupational (pneumoconioses)
        Silicosis
        Asbestosis
    Environmental
V. Idiopathic pulmonary fibrosis (IPF)
VI. Miscellaneous entities
    Bronchiolitis obliterans (±organizing pneumonia)
    Eosinophilic pneumonia
    Lymphangitis carcinomatosa
    Irradiation
    Lymphangioleiomyomatosis
VII. Infectious/inflammatory disorders in the immunocompromised host

(Adapted from: Raghu G. Am J Resp Crit Care Med 1995, 151:909–914.)

gradually progressive dyspnea, dry cough, and chest pain, which may be pleuritic. Hemoptysis may follow severe cough or signify pulmonary hemorrhage syndromes that manifest as ILD. Histiocytosis X and lymphangioleiomyomatosis may present with recurrent pneumothoraces. In diagnosing occupational pneumoconioses, hypersensitivity pneumonitis (HP), and drug-induced ILD, it is critical to obtain a history of exposure to possible offending agents (e.g., silica, moldy hay or cytotoxic drugs). While smokers do not seem to develop HP, they are virtually singled out for ILD in histiocytosis X and Goodpasture's syndrome. Tachypnea is an early and constant feature of ILD. Finger clubbing and/or end-inspiratory râles vary, depending on the disease entity. Because the rales simulate the tearing apart of Velcro®, they are called **"Velcro râles."** A distinct feature of idiopathic pulmonary fibrosis, they are less commonly heard in granulomatous ILD (sarcoidosis, HP, silicosis, and histiocytosis X).

■ Ancillary Studies

Chest x-rays are abnormal in roughly 90% of ILD cases. Besides the features of the primary disease, other findings may include small lungs and/or diffuse interstitial (nodular, reticular, or reticulo-nodular) infiltration. High resolution computed tomography (HRCT) has a higher sensitivity than specificity in diagnosing ILD and in determining the underlying process. The debate continues as to its ability to help select appropriate areas for biopsy by differentiating inflammatory from fibrotic areas.

Pulmonary infection in the immunocompromised patient often presents with interstitial infiltrates. Thus, human immunodeficiency virus (HIV) infection should be excluded if risk factors for it exist. Because of the autoimmune basis of many of these disorders, laboratory studies addressing them are quite useful. Some disorders have characteristic laboratory abnormalities that foster their diagnosis—for example, elevated creatinine kinase in polymyositis, specific antinuclear antibody patterns in scleroderma and lupus erythematosus, or anti-glomerular basement membrane (anti-GBM) antibody in Goodpasture's syndrome. ILD occurring in these settings may be attributed to these specific disorders without resorting to lung biopsy.

Pulmonary function studies show a restrictive impairment in ILD (as was shown in Table 211.2). The DL_{co} is typically reduced, but may be spuriously normal or even increased in alveolar hemorrhage syndromes. (Hemoglobin binds the CO.) The PaO_2 and $PaCO_2$ are low. The PaO_2 declines further and the alveolar-arterial oxygen gradient ($P[A\text{-}a\ O_2]$) widens during exercise. In the absence of such signs, clinically significant interstitial lung disease can be considered unlikely.

■ Diagnosis

Diagnosis involves two steps: the first confirms an interstitial disease, and the second determines its etiology (Figure 229.1). A clinical assessment (focused history and examination) is the first step. Specific inquiries should be made about the following:

– symptoms, their progression, and how they alter work and daily activities,

– the presence or absence of underlying heart disease,

– the presence of immunosuppression,

– exposure to tobacco smoke, various noxious agents, or organic matter in the workplace and/or through hobbies, and the temporal relationship of such exposure to symptoms (especially important in diagnosing hypersensitivity pneumonitis),

– medication use,

– radiation exposure during the treatment of prior neoplasia, and

– family history of pulmonary disease (familial pulmonary fibrosis and sarcoidosis).

Pulmonary function tests, chest x-ray, and review of old x-rays to determine progression should follow. Heart disease should be excluded, since chronic left ventricular failure may mimic ILD. If a potentially removable or remediable cause is found, it should be eliminated/avoided/treated, as appropriate; if clinical recovery follows, no further work-up may be needed.

If no avoidable/removable process is identified, an attempt should be made to exclude a connective tissue disease or vasculitis by appropriately directed biopsies, if necessary (muscle for polymyositis, skin for vasculitis, etc.). If none is identified—and sarcoidosis, alveolar proteinosis, eosinophilic pneumonia, or lymphangitis carcinomatosa merit serious consideration—a transbronchoscopic lung biopsy is undertaken. Bronchoalveolar lavage (BAL) might help in obtaining samples for microbiological studies (mycobacteria and fungi). If no specific diagnosis is established by this time, a "large specimen" of lung is obtained through the video-assisted thoracoscopic method or through open chest incision (open biopsy). Most disorders that cause ILD, including idiopathic pulmonary fibrosis, will ultimately require this step to establish a specific diagnosis and determine the prognosis. Cellular processes (alveolitis) respond better to therapy, and fibrotic lesions respond poorly.

Management

There is no uniformly successful or satisfactory therapy for ILD. If an offending agent (especially medication or inhaled organic antigens) is identified, its removal might stop further progression and even result in

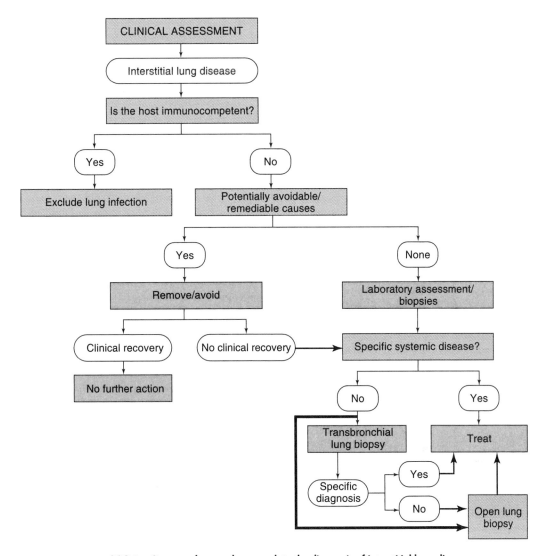

FIGURE 229.1. Suggested general approach to the diagnosis of interstitial lung disease.
(Adapted from: Raghu G. Am J Resp Crit Care Med 1995;151:909–914. Used with permission.)

some improvement. Treatment also depends on the type of ILD diagnosed. In general, corticosteroids produce short-term improvements in one-half and a sustained response in one-fourth of the cases. The generally recommended doses of prednisone (1–2 mg/kg) produce distressing side effects, especially in the elderly. A dose of 50–60 mg, which is more acceptable, is gradually tapered over several months, using clinical and physiological data as markers of effectiveness. However, there are no *reliable* markers. Azathioprine may be combined with prednisone in the treatment of IPF. Supportive care using long-term oxygen therapy and—while not proven—pulmonary exercise reconditioning may be beneficial. The age and the medical condition of the patient permitting, and depending upon the diagnosis,

single- or double-lung transplantation offers the best hope for some.

■ Prognosis

The prognosis varies depending on the underlying condition or process. Spirometric values, DL_{CO}, and gas exchange progressively decline, and eventually pulmonary hypertension and cor pulmonale supervene. Survival is shortest in lymphangitis carcinomatosa and in some very acute and relentlessly progressive forms of ILD. Long-term survivals, however, do occur in idiopathic pulmonary fibrosis. Many instances of drug-induced interstitial lung disease, sarcoidosis, and hypersensitivity pneumonitis have a favorable prognosis.

CHAPTER 230 SARCOIDOSIS

Definition and Epidemiology

Sarcoidosis is a systemic disease of unknown etiology. Its essential features are a compatible clinical picture along with noncaseating epithelioid cell granulomas in several affected organs and tissues that either resolve or become featureless hyaline connective tissue. Ninety percent of the patients with sarcoidosis are between 20 and 40 years of age with a higher prevalence in the United States among African Americans. The predilection for race, certain HLA types, and family clustering indicates a genetic basis.

Etiology, Pathogenesis, and Immunology

The noncaseating granuloma, which is a reaction against an as-yet elusive antigenic stimulus, contains epithelioid cells, giant cells, lymphocytes, and plasma cells with variable fibrosis and hyalinization. The CD_4 T-cells are increased in all affected tissues and decreased in the peripheral blood, which indicates their redistribution. Mononuclear phagocytes, epithelioid cells, and giant cells are transformed monocytes, which are attracted into the lung by monocyte chemotaxis, initiated by sarcoid lung T-lymphocytes. Proliferation of all these cells perpetuates the granuloma. The products of the accumulated cells (i.e., proteases, elastase, myeloperoxidase cationic proteins and oxidants from neutrophils and type IV collagenase, tumor necrosis factor [TNFα], and oxidants from macrophages) cause lung injury (alveolitis). Macrophages and epithelioid cells promote in-situ proliferation of fibroblasts, and fibrosis follows.

Clinical Features

Sarcoidosis is often detected initially by an **abnormal chest x-ray,** obtained generally while evaluating another illness or, less commonly, during a preemployment physical examination. Symptoms of sarcoidosis (Table 230.1) arise from the granulomatous involvement of various organs. The lungs are often involved; thus, pulmonary symptoms predominate. **Cough** is generally dry, and sputum and hemoptysis are infrequent. The reported extent of **extrapulmonary involvement** (Figure 230.1 and Table 230.2) varies depending on the histologic versus clinical criteria and the specialty of the investigator (pathologist, dermatologist, etc). Hepatic granuloma are prolific in sarcoidosis but clinical liver dysfunction is infrequent. Sarcoidosis may rarely present with **chronic renal failure;** prompt diag-

nosis and therapy may be rewarding. Such extrapulmonary involvement is suggested by signs and symptoms of respective organ dysfunction, especially with an established diagnosis.

Laboratory Features

Cutaneous anergy and leukopenia reflect T-cell kinetics, and serum immunoglobulins rise due to the B-cell overactivity. Hypercalcemia is from calcitriol (1,25 dihydroxycholecalciferol), one of the many biologically active agents secreted by activated macrophages. Other important anomalies are hypercalciuria, hyperuricemia, elevated serum angiotensin converting enzyme (SACE), and lysozyme. SACE is elevated in nearly 80% of sarcoidosis patients. While SACE rises also in Gaucher's disease, leprosy, and coccidioidomycosis, these conditions are clinically distinguishable from sarcoidosis. Thus, while the diagnosis must not be based on a SACE level, a high SACE level makes the clinical diagnosis of sarcoidosis credible.

Roentgenographic Features

Sarcoidosis most characteristically features bilateral hilar adenopathy (BHL) along with paratracheal adenopathy. Parenchymal infiltrates may or may not accom-

TABLE 230.1. Presenting Symptoms in Sarcoidosis	
Symptom	**Frequency (%, Range)**
None	12–34
Constitutional	
Weight loss	20–28
Fatigue	20–27
Fever	17–22
Malaise	0–15
Night sweats	0–14
Chills	0–13
Pulmonary	
Cough	30–32
Dyspnea	28
Chest pain	15–24
Sputum	11–12
Miscellaneous	
Skin lesions	14–32
Visual complaints	10–21
Lymph node enlargement	8–73
Joint symptoms	5–12

(Adapted from: Thrasher DR, Briggs DD Jr. Clin Chest Med 1982; 3:546. Used with permission.)

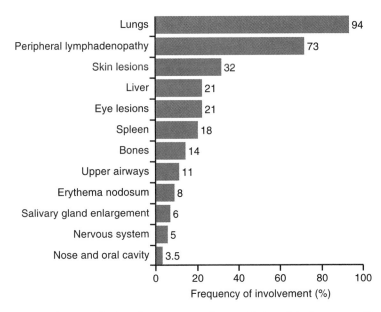

FIGURE 230.1. Involvement of selected organ systems in sarcoidosis and the frequency of involvement.
(Data from: Mayock RL et al. Am J Med 1963;35:67–89.)

TABLE 230.2.	**Extrapulmonary Involvement in Sarcoidosis: Frequency and Patterns of Cutaneous, Ocular, and Neurologic Lesions in Sarcoidosis**					
Cutaneous Lesions (32%)		**Ocular Lesions (21%)**		**Neurologic Lesions (5%)**	
Maculopapular lesions	46%	Uveitis	37%	Extremity paresis	16%
Subcutaneous nodules	14%	Blindness	8%	Facial paralysis	12%
Hypopigmentation or depigmentation	12%	Blurred vision	3%	Paresthesias	12%
Alopecia	7%	Scotoma	3%		
E. nodosum	6%	Conjunctivitis	3%		
Lupus pernio	≤1%				

(Adapted from: Mayock RL et al. Am J Med 1963;35:67–89. Used with permission.)

pany the adenopathy. This variable picture enables a clinical classification of sarcoidosis into three groups (we prefer the term "group" to "stage," since the latter suggests that a patient necessarily progresses from one stage to the next): group 1 with BHL alone (Figure 230.2), group 2, BHL with parenchymal infiltration (Figure 230.3), and group 3, parenchymal infiltrates alone (Figure 230.4).

■ Diagnosis

Differentiation is mainly from lymphomas (Hodgkin's disease; see Table 230.3) and other causes of mediastinal adenopathy. Tissue confirmation is recommended in all cases; transbronchoscopic lung biopsy is the recommended initial procedure. It is a simple, safe, uniformly applicable, low-morbidity procedure with a

yield of 95–100% in group 1, and virtually 100% in groups 2 and 3. The high yield on lung biopsy in group 1 reflects the widespread microscopic lung involvement despite the normal lung fields in chest x-ray. If sarcoidosis is strongly suspected, other, albeit less desirable biopsy sites are skin or conjunctival lesions, palpable scalene lymph nodes, or enlarged mediastinal or paratracheal nodes. Mediastinoscopy for diagnosis of sarcoidosis is seldom necessary or indicated at present.

■ Management

Our suggested management approach to sarcoidosis is shown in Figure 230.5. Spontaneous resolution is so frequent in group 1 that all that is needed is observation until resolution or classification into another group. Erythema nodosum and/or arthritis may require nonste-

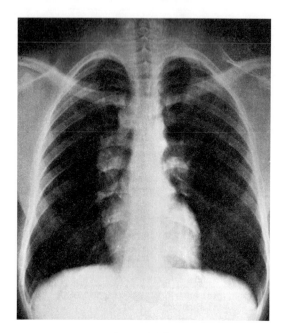

FIGURE 230.2. Sarcoidosis with bilateral hilar and paratracheal adenopathy (group 1).

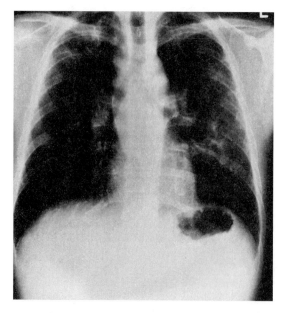

FIGURE 230.3. Sarcoidosis with BHL and parenchymal infiltration (group 2).

hypercalcemia and disfiguring skin lesions, and progressive pulmonary disease (best indicated by worsening pulmonary function tests) are indications. Prednisone, 40–60 mg, is given every other day (q.o.d) for 8–12 weeks. If improvement follows or if worsening has been halted, then the dose is tapered by 10 mg every 8–12 weeks with clinical, physiologic, and x-ray monitoring. The minimum steroid dose needed to maintain the improvement is then given q.o.d. Therapy is discontinued after two years; observation is continued for possible relapse. Shorter therapy with smaller doses has been used. Serial SACE determinations may be helpful in monitoring progression of the disease and/or its response to therapy. The initial enthusiasm for using bronchoalveolar lavage findings to guide therapy has not been realized.

■ Prognosis

Spontaneous resolution occurs in 80% of group 1 and almost 100% of patients with Lofgren's syndrome (acute onset, arthralgia, erythema nodosum, and BHL). In group 2 and group 3, spontaneous resolution occurs in only 30–50% of the cases; it is less frequent in older persons and in those with bone and skin lesions. Pulmonary fibrosis occurs in some cases, which predisposes to cor

roidal anti-inflammatory agents. Despite a lack of consensus regarding their overall role, corticosteroids are the major drugs available for treatment of sarcoidosis. Vital organ involvement (e.g., eye, heart, kidney),

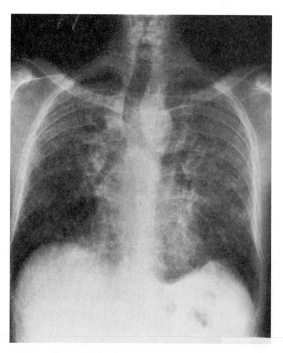

FIGURE 230.4. Sarcoidosis with parenchymal infiltrates alone (group 3). Upward displacement of minor fissure and buckling of the trachea indicate volume loss.

TABLE 230.3.	Differentiating Sarcoidosis from Hodgkin's Disease	
Criterion	**Sarcoidosis**	**Hodgkin's Disease**
Symptoms		
Fever	May occur	Common
Pruritus	Not seen	Common
Weight loss	Uncommon	Common
Findings		
Erythema nodosum	Frequent	Exceptional
Pleural effusion	Rare	Frequent
Enlarged spleen	Uncommon	Frequent
Skin lesions	Common, show NCG	±, characteristic histopathology
Intrathoracic-lymphadenopathy	Bilateral hilar and paratracheal	Bilateral or unilateral; isolated paratracheal adenopathy
Eosinophilia	Not a feature	May occur

NCG = noncaseating granuloma; ± = may or may not occur.

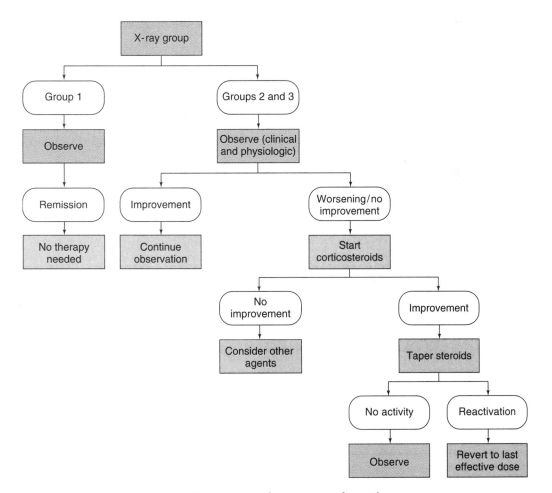

FIGURE 230.5. Suggested management of sarcoidosis.
(Adapted from: DeRemee RA. Mayo Clin Proc 1995;70:177–181. Used with permission.)

pulmonale. Cystic areas within the fibrotic lungs may harbor aspergillomas. Progressive respiratory insuffi-

ciency and massive hemoptysis from aspergillomas together account for the 5–10% mortality in this disease.

CHAPTER 231 PLEURO-PULMONARY MANIFESTATIONS OF COLLAGEN-VASCULAR DISORDERS AND VASCULITIDES

The abundance of vasculature and connective tissue in the lungs makes them vulnerable for involvement in many collagen-vascular disorders and vasculitides. The patterns and predominant sites of involvement may vary depending on the primary disease and the criteria employed (clinical, roentgenographic, or histopathologic). Since connective tissue and blood

vessels may be diffusely affected in these disorders, dysfunction of other organ systems might precede lung dysfunction and dominate the clinical picture. Depending on the type of disease, pleural involvement may also occur (Table 231.1). Despite the representation of various disorders here as pure entities, overlaps in their clinical picture are common.

TABLE 231.1. Patterns of Pleuropulmonary Involvement in Connective Tissue Disorders

Disorders	Involvement
Rheumatoid arthritis and systemic lupus erythematosus	See text
Polymyositis-dermatomyositis	Interstitial fibrosis, aspiration pneumonia from pharyngeal muscle weakness
Progressive systemic sclerosis	Interstitial fibrosis, pneumothorax, basilar pleural thickening, aspiration pneumonia, increased risk of broncho-alveolar cell carcinoma
Sjögren's syndrome	Interstitial fibrosis, pleural effusions, pseudolymphomas
Ankylosing spondylitis	Apical fibrobullous disease, diffuse pleural thickening, aspergilloma formation in apical bullae
Goodpasture's syndrome	Hemoptysis
Necrotizing vasculitis of the polyarteritis nodosa type	Allergic angiitis with granulomatosis
Wegener's granulomatosis	Sinusitis and upper airway involvement, nodular infiltrates, cavitation, airway obstruction
Lymphomatoid granulomatosis	Bilateral, multiple pulmonary densities, pleural effusion

Rheumatoid Disease

More common patterns of pleuropulmonary involvement in rheumatoid disease (RA) include diffuse interstitial fibrosis, pleurisy, and lung nodules. **Diffuse interstitial fibrosis** is characterized by a nonspecific interstitial pneumonitis with lymphocytes, plasma cells, macrophages, polymorphs, and eosinophils. Manifestations are

exertional dyspnea, cough, pleuritic pain, clubbing, end-inspiratory râles, and, in advanced stages, cor pulmonale. It is more frequent with subcutaneous nodules or when RA is more advanced. Restrictive ventilatory impairment and resting or exercise-induced hypoxemia may be present. The chest x-ray shows small nodular or punctate lesions in the early stages and medium to coarse reticulation and progressive loss of lung volume in the later stages. Pleural effusion or pleural thickening may coexist. Mild disease needs only observation. Corticosteroids may be needed for progressive disease.

Pleuritis *with/without effusion* is remarkably more common in men and may antedate RA. Often an asymptomatic and incidental finding, the effusion is exudative, generally unilateral with low glucose and high neutrophils, and may remain stable for months to years. There is no specific treatment. Repeated thoracentesis, corticosteroids, and decortication have all been tried. Pleuritis without effusion may cause a restrictive ventilatory impairment.

Rheumatoid nodules may be *nonpneumoconiotic* or *pneumoconiotic.* Nonpneumoconiotic rheumatoid nodules show a central zone of fibrinoid necrosis surrounded by a palisading layer of fibroblasts arranged perpendicular to the area of necrosis, and a layer of cellular or sclerotic granulation tissue surrounding the palisading layer. They are relatively uncommon and asymptomatic unless they enlarge or cavitate or become infected. Rheumatoid nodules may be present elsewhere and eosinophilia may be noted. X-rays show the nodules to be well-circumscribed, multiple, 2–7 cm in diameter, and generally peripheral. They often cavitate, leaving thick walls. Nodules may resolve or progress. Pleural effusion and **spontaneous pneumothorax** may coexist. Restrictive ventilatory impairment may be found. Unless complications occur, no treatment is necessary.

Caplan's syndrome refers to a (pneumoconiotic) rheumatoid nodule occurring in coal miners or those who have been exposed to silica or asbestos. The syndrome involves a central necrosis with peripheral fibroblasts arranged perpendicular to the necrotic zone containing the inorganic dust, with mononuclear, polymorphonuclear, or giant cell infiltration. A dark, concentric ring surrounds the central core. Other clinical features are the same as those in a nonpneumoconiotic rheumatoid nodule. On x-ray, the nodules are well circumscribed, round, 0.5–5.0 cm peripheral densities; they may cavitate, calcify, and become fibrotic. They may appear rapidly in "crops." No definite treatment is necessary.

Other patterns of respiratory affliction include bronchiolitis and bronchiolitis obliterans, apical fibrobullous disease mimicking tuberculosis, upper airway obstruction from vocal cord dysfunction caused by arthritis of the crico-arytenoid joints, and respiratory paralysis from atlanto-axial dislocation.

Systemic Lupus Erythematosus

The extent of lung and pleural involvement may vary from 50–70% in systemic lupus erythematosus (SLE). The kidneys and central nervous system may also be involved.

Pleurisy with or without effusion is the most common manifestation of SLE. Pleuritic pain may be an early symptom. Effusions are frequently small and bilateral or may be massive. They are exudative and may have a low glucose level. LE cells may be seen in effusion. Pericardial effusion and cardiomegaly may coexist. Treatment is corticosteroid therapy. **Acute lupus pneumonitis** presents with dyspnea, fever, cough, and sputum. The patients are severely ill. **Pulmonary infection** should be excluded first, since infectious complications are far more frequent than lung involvement by lupus. On x-ray, infiltrates are non homogenous and may be localized or diffuse. Cardiomegaly may be seen. Diagnosis is one of exclusion. Biopsy may show alveolar wall thickening and mononuclear cell infiltration. Evidence of vasculitis may be seen. Immunologic studies show granular IgG and C3 immunofluorescence. Treatment is corticosteroids with or without azathioprine. **Acute pulmonary hemorrhage** is a rare but serious manifestation of SLE.

Diaphragmatic dysfunction presents with dyspnea, striking orthopnea, and, characteristically, restrictive ventilatory impairment. Chest x-ray shows elevated diaphragms, which show very little movement on fluoroscopy. Lungs appear small as a consequence. There is no specific therapy.

Vasculitis

In vasculitis, the lung may be the major site of involvement in Wegener's granulomatosis, allergic angiitis (Churg-Strauss syndrome), and lymphocytic angiitis. In many other vasculitic disorders, the lung may be involved either as part of a systemic process or in a minor way. Only Wegener's granulomatosis will be considered here.

Wegener's Granulomatosis

This disorder, characterized by necrotizing granulomatous vasculitis of the respiratory tract, glomerulonephritis, and small vessel vasculitis, involves the upper and/or lower respiratory tract and/or kidneys. (See chapter 259.)

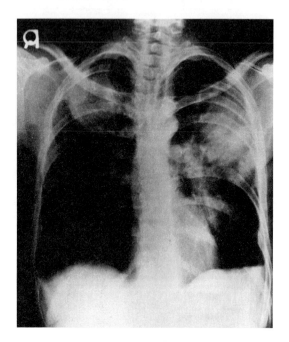

FIGURE 231.1. Wegener's granulomatosis. Bilateral opacities are present. Right upper-zone density is cavitated.

The extent of lung involvement approaches 95%, followed by paranasal sinuses (90%), kidneys (85%), nasopharynx (70%), and eyes (60%). A limited form involving only the lungs is well known. Symptoms include nasal discharge, sinusitis, otitis media, and nasal ulcerative lesions. Cough, hemoptysis, and chest pain signify lung involvement. Wegener's granulomatosis may present as a pulmonary-renal syndrome with alveolar hemorrhage and nephritis or, less commonly, as diffuse capillaritis. Chest x-ray shows bilateral nodular infiltrative lesions that cavitate (Figure 231.1). Mass densities, airway obstruction from endobronchial lesions, and pleural thickening or effusions are uncommon.

In those without renal failure, cyclophosphamide is started at 1–2 mg/kg and continued for two weeks. If needed, the dose may be raised by 25 mg increments, keeping the WBC count over 3,000/mm^3. The duration of treatment is generally 12-18 months after a complete remission. When renal failure is associated, cyclophosphamide is started IV in 4 mg/kg for three days with a reduction in the dose thereafter to 1–2 mg/kg per day. Associated corticosteroid therapy is needed in both instances.

CHAPTER 232   INTERSTITIAL LUNG DISEASE ASSOCIATED WITH BRONCHIOLITIS

■ **Definition**

Bronchiolitis is inflammation of the bronchioles, which are small airways 1–2 mm in diameter. The terminal bronchioles are conducting airways; the respiratory bronchioles exchange gases, since alveoli open into them through fenestrations in their walls. There are five histological subtypes of bronchiolitis: cellular bronchiolitis, diffuse panbronchiolitis, constrictive bronchiolitis obliterans, respiratory bronchiolitis-associated interstitial lung disease (RB-ILD), and bronchiolitis obliterans organizing pneumonia (BOOP). The first three produce pure airway disease; the latter two, which are discussed in this chapter, present as interstitial lung disease.

Respiratory Bronchiolitis Associated-Interstitial Lung Disease

RB-ILD may follow inhalation of cigarette smoke and mineral dusts (asbestos, silica, etc.), viral infections, connective tissue disease, and exposure to drugs. The disease is characterized by submucosal mononuclear cell infiltration of the respiratory bronchioles, goblet cell hyperplasia, and airway epithelial metaplasia. Also, fibrosis and bronchiolar metaplasia may extend into immediately adjacent alveolar walls.

Tan-brown-pigmented macrophages accumulate within and around the respiratory bronchioles, alveolar ducts, and alveoli.

■ **Clinical Features and Diagnosis**

Cough and dyspnea are the most common symptoms of RB-ILD, followed by chest pain, weight loss, and fever. A history of current or past cigarette smoking is almost invariably present. Pan-inspiratory (lasting over the entire inspiration) râles are present at the lung bases. Finger clubbing is not a feature. Pulmonary function studies generally show a restrictive ventilatory impairment; airflow obstruction may co-exist. The DL_{CO} is often reduced, and resting or exercise-induced arterial hypoxemia may be noted. The chest x-ray shows a fine, diffuse, reticulonodular infiltrate; peripheral ring-like shadows and bronchial wall thickening may be associated. Diffuse, patchy, "ground-glass" opacities or fine nodules may be seen on computed tomography.

■ Management

The generally quite favorable prognosis in RB-ILD contrasts sharply with other forms of ILD, which bespeaks the need for accurate diagnosis (Figure 232.1). Given the significant relationship to smoking, smoking cessation is the most logical first step. Corticosteroids have reportedly been quite beneficial.

Bronchiolitis Obliterans Organizing Pneumonia

Alveolar edema and inflammatory cellular infiltration follow a lung injury with necrosis of alveolar epithelia, alveolar ducts, and bronchioles. Fibroblasts and myofibroblasts then migrate into the alveoli, proliferate, and secrete type II collagen and fibronectin. Intraluminal fibroblastic plugs ("Masson bodies") form and foamy macrophages collect in the airspaces. Ultimately, proliferating bronchiolar cells and type 2 pneumocytes return these fibroblastic plugs to the lung interstitium, where they resolve by unknown mechanisms. While this proliferative bronchiolitis occurs in a variety of conditions (hypersensitivity pneumonitis, collagen-vascular disorders, vasculitis, infections, and drug exposure), the **essential aspects** of BOOP diagnosis are **histology** (proliferative bronchiolitis), **exclusivity** (no other primary entity), and **intensity** (involvement of a majority of alveoli and bronchioles).

■ Clinical Features

The disease commonly occurs in the sixth or the seventh decade, with no apparent relationship to smoking. Symptoms often last longer than 2–3 months. An antecedent flu-like illness occurs in nearly one-third of the cases; the onset is subacute, with a dry, persistent cough and progressive dyspnea. Fever, malaise, and weight loss may each be noted in one-half of cases. Tachypnea and râles may be noted. Wheezing is rare and clubbing is absent.

■ Ancillary Studies

While nonspecific, the erythrocyte sedimentation rate is high (often >100 mm), with leukocytosis and elevated C-reactive protein. Biochemical cholestasis may be noted. Pulmonary function tests

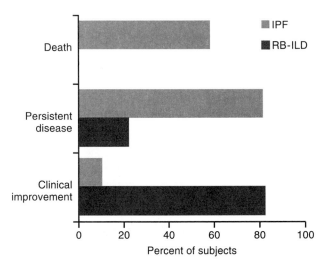

FIGURE 232.1. Treatment outcome and prognosis of patients with respiratory bronchiolitis–associated ILD and those with idiopathic pulmonary fibrosis. (Adapted from: King TE Jr. Clin Chest Med 1993;14:693–698. Used with permission.)

commonly show a restrictive impairment. Hypoxemia is common. Chest x-rays are seldom normal and show diffuse, bilateral, peripheral alveolar opacities. CT shows patchy, peripheral, lower-zone airspace shadows, small nodular densities, and bronchial wall thickening.

■ **Diagnosis and Management**

Given its favorable prognosis, BOOP should be considered a possibility in any patient who presents with an undiagnosed, subacute respiratory illness, compatible physiologic abnormalities, and an interstitial pneumonitis. An open lung biopsy is generally needed, in order to confidently exclude an alternative diagnosis. Corticosteroids confer a 65–80% response. Prednisone (1–1.5 mg/kg) is started and continued for 2–3 months; whether smaller doses might suffice is not known. If the response is satisfactory, the dose is reduced over the next several months to 0.5–1 mg/kg and gradually tapered over a year. If the response is inadequate, cyclophosphamide may be added.

CHAPTER **233** INTERSTITIAL LUNG DISEASE IN HISTIOCYTOSIS X

Langerhans cells are dendritic histiocytes and descendants of marrow stem cells that present antigen to lymphocytes. Their proliferation is a shared feature of eosinophilic granuloma, Letterer-Siwe disease, and Hand-Schuller-Christian disease, collectively called histiocytosis X.

The pathogenesis of histiocytosis X is elusive. Smokers and patients with histiocytosis X share an excess of Langerhans cells in their BAL fluid and an increased number of pulmonary neuroendocrine cells. The preponderance (>90%) of histiocytosis X among smokers suggests a role for smoking in its pathogenesis. Pulmonary histiocytosis X may occur as isolated lung disease or as part of a systemic disease. Pathologically, there is severe interstitial fibrosis with collections of histiocytes, lymphocytes, and eosinophils.

■ **Clinical Features and Diagnosis**

Histiocytosis X occurs mostly among young adults. Cough, sputum, dyspnea, chest pain, recurrent pneumothorax, hemoptysis, weight loss, and fever herald lung involvement. If it is part of a systemic disease, splenomegaly, lymphadenopathy, and diabetes insipidus may occur. Peripheral eosinophilia is absent. X-rays most commonly show miliary nodules with a reticular pattern; cystic lesions and "honeycombing" are less frequent. There is generally a restrictive ventilatory impairment, but airway obstruction is not uncommon. Diagnosis is generally made by thoracotomy and open lung biopsy.

■ **Management**

Spontaneous improvement may occur, but with extremes of age or with diffuse extrapulmonary or pulmonary disease, a poor outcome is likely. Thoracotomy and pleurodesis may be needed for recurrent pneumothoraces. No treatment regimen, including corticosteroids and vinblastine, has been found to be consistently effective, but several promising agents remain— for example, thalidomide, 2-chlorodeoxyadenosine, allogenic bone marrow transplantation, and cyclosporin.

CHAPTER **234** HYPERSENSITIVITY PNEUMONITIDES

■ **Definition**

Hypersensitivity pneumonitis (HP), an immunologically mediated lung inflammation, follows inhalation of a variety of organic antigens, many of them fungal. Selected causative agents and the occupations that predispose to them are shown in Table 234.1. The immunologic reactivity and atopic status of the host are key factors, since HP develops only in a minority of those who are exposed. Atopic persons show airway obstruction immediately, followed later by a parenchymal reaction, whereas nonatopic persons generally show only the late reaction.

■ **Pathogenesis and Pathology**

The basic mechanism of HP is an Arthus (type III) reaction in the lung. Cell-mediated immune mechanisms

TABLE 234.1.	The Hypersensitivity Pneumonitides: Selected Sources of Exposure and Causative Agents	
Disease	**Source of Exposure**	**Specific Agent**
Cheesewasher's lung	Moldy cheese	*Penicillium casei*
Malt worker's lung	Moldy barley	*Aspergillus clavatus* and *Aspergillus fumigatus*
Maple bark stripper's lung	Moldy maple bark	*Cryptostroma corticale*
Pigeon breeder's lung	Avian protein	None known
Ventilation pneumonitis	Humidifier water	*Acanthamoeba castellani* and *Acanthamoeba polyphaga*
Wheat weevil disease	Wheat flour	*Sitophilus granarius*
Wood pulp worker's disease	Moldy wood pulp	Alternaria
Isocyanate HP†	Resins	Toluene diisocyanate, diphenylmethane diisocyanate
Trimellitic anhydride (TMA)†	Paints, resins, plastics	Trimellitic anhydride

† = More often produces occupational asthma; HP is less frequent.

may also be involved. Lymphocytes and plasma cells infiltrate the lung interstitium and alveolar walls in a bronchocentric distribution. Granuloma formation, necrosis, Langhan's giant cells, epithelioid cells, and foreign body giant cells are also noted. The alveoli may contain foamy histiocytes and plasma cells. In chronic HP, there is interstitial and focal peribronchial fibrosis with alveolar septal thickening and lymphocytic infiltration.

■ Clinical Features

In acute HP, myalgia, fever, chills, chest tightness, cough, and dyspnea occur 4–6 hours following exposure to the offending organic dust. The patient is acutely ill with tachypnea, tachycardia, and late inspiratory, basilar râles. Symptoms subside in 12–18 hours, with spontaneous recovery, but recur on re-exposure. Wheezing is conspicuously absent. Leukocytosis and elevated serum IgG, IgM, and IgA are generally present. IgE is elevated only with concomitant atopy (asthma or rhinitis). Serum precipitins to the offending organic material, while frequent, only indicate exposure. Chest x-rays may be normal or may show a patchy, diffuse infiltrate or a fine, symmetrical, nodular pattern. Pulmonary function studies show a restrictive impairment with diminished DL_{CO}.

Cough and insidious dyspnea characterize the subacute form. Prolonged organic dust exposure may cause chronic HP, manifested by progressive dyspnea and diffuse interstitial fibrosis, often with "honeycombing." A progressive restrictive ventilatory impairment, hypoxemia, and low DL_{CO} are notable.

■ Diagnosis and Management

HP should be suspected when recurrent, stereotyped, self-limited respiratory and constitutional symptoms develop on exposure to specific environments. A thorough history and pulmonary function test following careful challenge (controlled exposure) can be diagnostic. Precipitins and chest x-rays are only supportive. A search of the patient's work environment or home may help identify the antigenic material from dusts or molds. Lung biopsy is especially useful in chronic HP.

Identification and avoidance of the offending antigen are key factors in management, these alone being sufficient in the acute phase. In selected cases, corticosteroids may hasten the recovery. In chronic HP, corticosteroids may be useful, but once irreversible fibrosis has occurred they may confer only minimal benefit.

CHAPTER **235** SILICOSIS

S ilicosis, caused by inhalation and retention of silicon dioxide (silica), is associated with many occupations (e.g., mining or tunneling, quarrying, chipping, grinding, sandblasting, grinding or polishing in pottery and in foundry work, and cutting or manufacturing heat-resistant bricks). Based on the x-ray picture,

silicosis may be **simple** (small nodules throughout the lungs) or **complicated** (large, confluent masses). **Acute silicosis** follows a relatively brief exposure (several months to 3 years). A subset of acute silicosis is **silicoproteinosis**, which appears in an x-ray as homogenous alveolar infiltrates simulating pulmonary alveolar proteinosis.

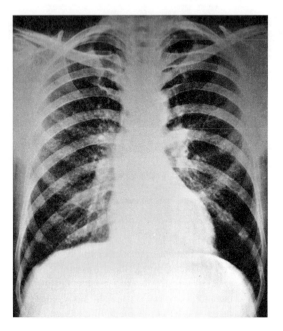

FIGURE 235.1. Simple silicosis; diffuse calcified nodules and prominent calcified (eggshell) hilar nodes.

■ Pathogenesis and Pathology

Inhaled silica particles of 1–5 μ in size reach the respiratory units of the lung. They are ingested by the alveolar macrophages, some of which succumb to the cytotoxic effects of silica and some of which are activated. Activated macrophages release interleukin (IL)-1, which activates T-lymphocytes, which, by releasing cytokines (e.g., macrophage activating factor), further increase the number of activated macrophages. Chemoattractants released by macrophages attract blood monocytes, which are macrophage precursors. These amplification loops maintain an increased number of macrophages. The products of activated macrophages, IL-1, macrophage-derived growth factor for fibroblasts, and fibronectin are key players in causing fibrosis.

Silicotic nodules, the characteristic histopathologic finding, are mostly seen close to the respiratory bronchiole. Each nodule comprises refractile particles of silica, surrounded by whorled collagen centrally and in concentric layers, surrounded by macrophages, fibroblasts, and lymphocytes. Emphysematous blebs (large flaccid vesicles) surround the silicotic nodules, especially in the subpleural areas. Infection, a pathogenetic factor in complicated silicosis, may be due to *Mycobacterium tuberculosis*, atypical mycobacteria, fungi, or bacteria. The morbidity of complicated silicosis is also increased by associated collagen vascular disease (rheumatoid arthritis, scleroderma, and lupus erythematosus). Finer

particle size and intense exposure are critical to the pathogenesis of silicoproteinosis.

■ Clinical Features

Simple silicosis may be asymptomatic. It is recognized by its roentgenographic manifestations which usually follow about 20 years after initial exposure. Exertional dyspnea, cough, and sputum production are frequent but concomitant cigarette smoking often makes their evaluation difficult. In complicated silicosis, besides dyspnea and cough, constitutional symptoms (malaise, weight loss) are also usually present. Physical findings vary with the extent of the disease. Expiratory prolongation, râles, and rhonchi may be present. Clubbing is unusual. Features of complicating infection or collagen vascular disease may be noted if complicated silicosis is present. Pulmonary function tests may reveal airflow obstruction; restriction or a combined impairment is less frequent. Lung compliance and diffusing capacity may be decreased and hypoxemia may be noted at rest or on exercise.

■ Roentgenographic Features

Clinically significant disease does not arise without roentgenographic abnormalities. Simple silicosis manifests as multiple nodules of several millimeters each, scattered throughout but more noticeable in the upper

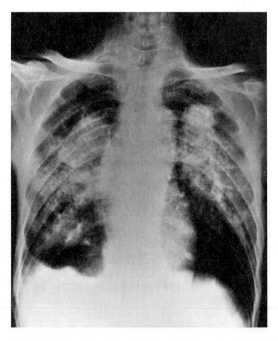

FIGURE 235.2. Complicated silicosis. Note the bilateral upper- and middle-zone confluent masses.

lung fields. The nodules may calcify infrequently; associated hilar node enlargement and **"egg shell" calcification** may occur (Figure 235.1). Complicated silicosis manifests as bilateral, confluent, upper-lobe masses that may be necrotic in the center. As these masses retract toward the hilum because of the fibrosis, the nodules present in the lower lung fields become less obvious because of overinflation (Figure 235.2). Caplan's syndrome represents rheumatoid pulmonary nodules (0.5–5.0 cm) complicating pneumoconioses (silicosis, coal workers' pneumoconiosis).

■ Diagnosis and Management

Diagnosis of silicosis depends on history of exposure and the chest x-ray findings. With discordant clinical or x-ray features, an open lung biopsy may be necessary for diagnosis. The excised lung tissue is examined for silica through microscopy with polarized light, scanning electron microscopy, or energy-dispersive x-ray analysis.

There is no specific treatment for silicosis. The main **complications** are infections (particularly mycobacterial), progressive respiratory insufficiency, cor pulmonale, and respiratory failure. Efforts should be aimed at preventing the disease (use of respiratory protection in susceptible occupations) and preventing and treating the complications. Evidence for mycobacterial infection should be sought by tuberculin testing; if found, antituberculosis chemoprophylaxis is recommended.

CHAPTER 236 ASBESTOSIS

Pulmonary fibrosis caused by asbestos inhalation is called asbestosis. Asbestos describes a group of heat-resistant fibrous minerals. Chrysotile, crocidolite, amosite, and anthophyllite are four of the more important forms. Because asbestos has thousands of industrial uses, occupational asbestos exposure is common (among, e.g., boiler makers, brake lining makers or workers, construction workers, dock workers, filter workers, insulation workers, gasket makers, pipe coverers or cutters, plumbers, rock miners, ship builders, and steam fitters).

A latent period of 20 years or more usually follows exposure before clinical or x-ray manifestations appear. Because the development of asbestosis is dose-dependent, this latent period may be shorter with more intense exposure.

■ Pathogenesis and Pathology

Chemoattractants are released when the inhaled asbestos activates both macrophages and dual complement pathways. Chemoattractants recruit neutrophils (PMN), which interact with asbestos to produce oxygen radicals (superoxide anion, hydrogen peroxide, and hydroxy radicals) that damage proteins and lipid membranes. Lipid peroxides may autocatalyze and perpetuate damage even without further asbestos exposure. Pathologic findings include both diffuse interstitial fibrosis and asbestos bodies (asbestos fibers coated with protein and iron). The respiratory bronchioles are thickened with connective tissue and fibrosis proceeds centrifugally. Macrophages accumulate, but granuloma or nodules (similar to silicosis) are absent. In advanced asbestosis, extensive fibrosis causes airspace distortion and a honeycomb pattern with cyst-like spaces.

■ Clinical Features

Dyspnea on exertion is the most common symptom, usually manifesting after 20 or more years of asbestos exposure. **Cough,** usually dry, may also be present. Tightness or pain in the chest may be reported, especially in advanced cases. Basilar "cellophane" (or **"Velcro"**) **râles** and **finger clubbing** are the most important findings.

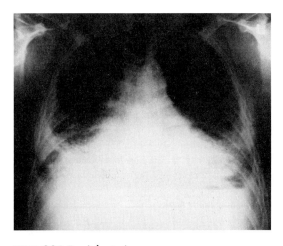

FIGURE 236.1. Asbestosis.
(From: Varkey B. Postgrad Med 1978;64:48. Reprinted with permission.)

■ Ancillary Studies

Pulmonary function shows a restrictive impairment, with reduced DL_{CO}; hypoxemia is present at rest or on exercise. Chest x-rays show interstitial, predominantly lower-zone infiltrates. Pleural thickening and hyaline pleural plaques are typically seen in the axillary areas and calcified pleural plaques are typically seen over the diaphragm (Figure 236.1). Hilar node enlargement or calcification is rare.

■ Diagnosis and Management

Diagnosis depends on obtaining a history of exposure, clinical features, typical x-ray findings, and the restrictive impairment. The more discordant the features, the more the burden of proof for diagnosis; thus, a lung biopsy is occasionally needed. Both asbestos bodies (Figure 236.2) and interstitial fibrosis, the hallmarks of asbestosis, are essential for a pathologic diagnosis. Electron microscopy aids in the detection of smaller uncoated fibers.

No specific treatment exists for asbestosis. Besides efforts directed at prevention (i.e., avoiding exposure to asbestos), prompt treatment of respiratory infections is necessary because infections may accelerate the fibrosis.

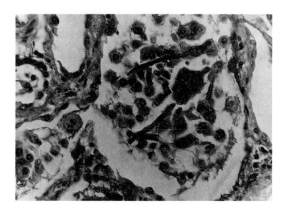

FIGURE 236.2. Asbestos bodies: asbestos fibers with an acid mucopolysaccharide and iron coating seen as elongated beaded bodies with clubbed ends.
(From: Varkey B. Postgrad Med 1978;64:48. Reprinted with permission.)

Complications of asbestosis are progressive fibrosis leading to cor pulmonale and respiratory failure. The risk of bronchogenic carcinoma is high in persons exposed to asbestos. Smokers are at an even higher risk, as smoking and asbestos are synergistic co-carcinogens.

CHAPTER 237 **IDIOPATHIC PULMONARY FIBROSIS**

Idiopathic pulmonary fibrosis (IPF), a disease of unknown etiology, is the prototypic interstitial lung disease (ILD). It is also known as **cryptogenic fibrosing alveolitis** (CFA). Its symptoms include inflammation and fibrosis of the pulmonary interstitium; it has been described under several other synonyms. Despite its distinct clinical, histologic, and roentgenographic aspects (described below), it is largely diagnosed after excluding other entities (a disease of exclusion).

■ Pathogenesis

In IPF, an elusive **alveolar epithelial injury** (a viral infection in some cases) initiates a cascade of events that culminate in **chronic alveolitis.** The initial injury causes immune complexes to develop locally; neutrophils and macrophages are brought in by chemotaxis. Activated macrophages release cytokines, which attract lymphocytes and more neutrophils. Neutrophil collagenase destroys lung collagen, which is replenished preferentially with type I collagen by fibroblasts. This process alters the normal (2 : 1) ratio of type I to type III lung collagen, but the total collagen remains the same. Thus,

the lung collagen undergoes **sustained lysis and disordered resynthesis;** the process, with abundant scar tissue, has been compared to "excessive" wound healing.

■ Pathology

In early IPF, alveolar walls and alveolar ducts show hyaline membrane formation and fibrin deposition. Alveolar walls, thickened with inflammatory cell infiltration, collapse from adhesions. Desquamated cells occupy the alveoli. Granulomas, arteritis, and mineral deposits are absent. As the disease progresses, peribronchiolar fibrosis, lymphoid hyperplasia, and hypertrophy of the media become noticeable, with intimal proliferation of the muscular pulmonary arteries. The lung architecture is grossly disturbed, with injury and repair seen simultaneously in different areas of the lung. In later stages, little inflammatory activity is evident and extensive widespread fibrosis supervenes.

■ Clinical Features

The incidence of IPF peaks in the fifth and sixth decades of life, without apparent gender preference. It is known to run in families. The onset is often with a flu-like illness. Exertional dyspnea and nonproductive cough are common; weight loss, fever, myalgias, and arthralgias are other symptoms. With significant hypoxemia, central cyanosis may appear. Clubbing occurs in the majority and in virtually all of the familial cases. Tachypnea occurs early. "Velcro râles" may be audible. Cardiac examination is normal, but pulmonic valve closure (P_2) may be loud, indicating pulmonary hypertension.

■ Ancillary Studies

The erythrocyte sedimentation rate may be high. Immunologic abnormalities—including cryoglobulins, rheumatoid factor, antinuclear antibodies, and elevated serum immunoglobulins—are frequent. Circulating immune complexes correlate well with cellular infiltration in the biopsied lung specimen. Arterial hypoxemia is present at rest or on exercise, and is mostly due to ventilation-perfusion mismatching. Pulmonary function studies show a restrictive ventilatory impairment. The DL_{CO} is reduced. Chest roentgenograms may be normal in about 10–15% of the cases. In the remainder, the roentgenogram may reveal (1) small lungs, (2) a ground glass appearance, or (3) reticular, reticulonodular, or nodular infiltrates. Honeycombing signifies advanced disease (Figure 237.1).

■ Diagnosis

A general approach to the diagnosis of ILD is presented in chapter 229. A definitive diagnosis of IPF depends on a lung biopsy. However, a constellation of findings including "Velcro rales," finger clubbing, and altered immune activity may suggest IPF, sometimes so strikingly that a biopsy is not essential (e.g., in an elderly person with no noxious dust exposure, "Velcro râles," clubbing, and honeycombing in the x-ray). Biopsy, however, makes it possible to reliably differentiate IPF from vasculitis and pneumoconioses, and to predict the severity and responsiveness to therapy and, thus, the prognosis. Because the minuscule tissue obtained by transbronchoscopic biopsy is inadequate for diagnosis, an open lung biopsy is the recommended method to procure tissue.

■ Management

Treatment of IPF is similar to that of ILD (chapter 229) and aims to prevent its progression by suppressing the alveolitis. In general, the shorter the duration of illness and the more cellular and less fibrotic the findings on lung biopsy, the greater is the likelihood of corticosteroid-responsiveness. The duration of steroid therapy is indeterminate. Azathioprine has also been found to be beneficial and may be combined with corticosteroids. Oxygen therapy is indicated for resting- or exercise-induced hypoxemia (PaO_2 <55 mm Hg). Consideration for lung transplant is appropriate in patients younger than 60 years with no other serious ailments. The average survival in IPF is 47 months from the onset of the symptoms.

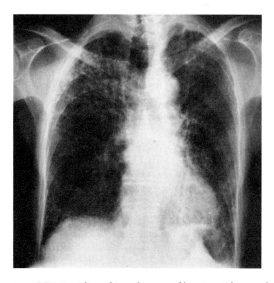

FIGURE 237.1. Idiopathic pulmonary fibrosis: widespread interstitial infiltration with honeycombing.

CHAPTER 238 # RADIATION PNEUMONITIS AND RADIATION FIBROSIS

Radiation-induced lung damage manifests in two syndromes, radiation pneumonitis and radiation fibrosis. Radiation toxicity is potentiated by some chemotherapeutic agents (e.g., dactinomycin [actinomycin-D], cyclophosphamide, bleomycin, and vincristine), previous radiation therapy, withdrawal of corticosteroid therapy, and infection.

■ Pathogenesis and Pathology

An early dose-related effect of radiation is the formation of free radical -OH, which damages structural macromolecules, resulting in leaky cell membranes. The free radicals also directly damage DNA, and the broken DNA strands are incorrectly repaired or form cross-links. In severe cases, the cell dies. The surviving cells may divide abnormally, resulting in asymmetric mitosis or anaphase arrest. Inflammation, initiated and continued by unknown mechanisms, and mediated by neutrophils, lymphocytes, and alveolar macrophages through mediator release, causes tissue damage.

How radiation pneumonitis progresses to fibrosis is unknown. Irradiation alters the normal balance between synthesis and lysis of collagen. The connective tissue matrix may be damaged by the radiation or inflammatory mediators, and cytokines may alter the repair process.

In animal models, vascular permeability increases within 24 hours. Swelling of endothelial cells, alveolar capillary congestion, neutrophil accumulation, and focal alveolar hemorrhage occur in 2 months. In animals surviving a lethal radiation dose, leukocytes infiltrate gas-exchanging units and blood vessels. Vascular inflammatory infiltration, intimal thickening, and thrombi may cause obliteration of the vessel lumen. Animals surviving for 6 months after exposure develop a focal or diffuse interstitial pulmonary fibrosis. The exact onset of fibrosis following radiation is unknown.

■ Clinical Features

Clinical **radiation pneumonitis** (RP) usually develops **2–6 months after** and occasionally as early as 2 weeks after the completion of radiation therapy. **Progressive exertional dyspnea** and a **dry cough** are the cardinal symptoms. **Fever** is common and usually low-grade; occasionally, it is high and intermittent. **Pleuritic chest pain** may be reported. **Tachypnea** is common. Auscultation is normal; occasionally, basilar rales and friction rub are present. RP may spontaneously resolve or may progress to acute hypoxemic respiratory failure and cor pulmonale. There are no characteristic laboratory findings, besides an increased sedimentation rate and neutrophilic leukocytosis. Restrictive ventilatory impairment and a decreased DL_{CO} are typical; hypoxemia and widened $P(A\text{-}a\ O_2)$ are common.

Early x-rays show a **ground-glass appearance** in the area of irradiation. Patchy alveolar infiltrates with air bronchograms may follow. One important diagnostic clue is a **"straight-edge effect"**—that is, an infiltrate with sharp boundaries that correspond to the radiation field

(port) but not to anatomic lung boundaries. However, in RP, infiltrates do occur outside the radiation field and even in the contralateral lung. Possible mechanisms for the latter include obstruction to the pulmonary lymphatic flow, absorption of radiation by lungs outside of the field, and inflammatory mediator release.

Radiation fibrosis (interstitial infiltrates radiating from the area of previous RP and often extending beyond the radiation field) becomes noticeable in x-rays about 1 year after the completion of treatment. Exertional dyspnea is common, but some persons may be asymptomatic. Progressive radiation fibrosis causes worsening dyspnea and orthopnea. Cyanosis and cor pulmonale may develop.

■ Diagnosis

RP is diagnosed when its characteristic clinical picture occurs at least 2 weeks after the completion of radiation therapy. Differential diagnosis includes an infectious pneumonia and lymphangitis carcinomatosa. It is useful to compare previous x-rays with current ones and to compare the areas of x-ray abnormalities with the radiation port. Nonpurulent sputum and negative microbiologic studies are also helpful. Lymphangitis carcinomatosa involves the lung bases more with prominent septal lines and pleural effusions. Mediastinal or hilar adenopathy may be present. When differentiating these entities is difficult, bronchoscopy with bronchoalveolar lavage, quantitative bacterial cultures, and transbronchoscopic lung biopsy are helpful.

■ Management

In symptomatic RP, **prednisone** therapy (60 mg/day) is recommended. However, there are no controlled human clinical trials of corticosteroids in RP, nor have the available studies shown uniform results. The steroids should be tapered slowly after a complete response, as pneumonitis may worsen markedly upon steroid withdrawal. Whether corticosteroids given before and during irradiation will prevent RP remains unknown. Supportive therapy includes supplemental oxygen, analgesics, antipyretics, and cough suppressants.

CHAPTER 239 PULMONARY ASPIRATION SYNDROMES

The clinical syndromes caused by aspiration are variable and depend on the quantity and nature of the aspirated material, the frequency of aspiration, and the host response. The major aspiration syndromes are described in Table 239.1. The term

"aspiration pneumonia" used in an all-inclusive sense has been confusing and, therefore, is better reserved to describe a chemical pneumonitis caused by the aspiration of gastric contents.

TABLE 239.1.	Pulmonary Aspiration Syndromes
Aspirated Material	**Manifestation**
Irritant liquids	Acute aspiration of gastric contents (acute aspiration pneumonia)
Bacterial pathogens	Gastric contents contaminated with pharyngeal organisms
	Gravitation of gingival secretions and saliva
Inert substances	Airway obstruction ("cafe coronary")

Acute Aspiration Pneumonia

In 1946 Mendelson described the clinical syndrome caused by the aspiration of gastric contents. Risk factors for aspirating gastric contents are shown in Table 239.2. Radionuclide studies have shown occult aspiration occurring even in normal sleeping subjects. However, in normal persons, significant parenchymal lung disease does not follow these episodes.

■ Pathogenesis

Animal studies show that lung injury due to aspiration depends on several characteristics of the aspirate, including the pH, volume, presence of food, particulate antacid, inert foreign body, bile, tube feeding formula, fecal contamination, and bacterial concentrations. Host factors such as alveolar macrophage function, nutritional status, functional status, structural lung disease, and the ability to cough are also important. Gastric juice with a pH of 2.4 in rabbits produces chemical injury; the severity correlates inversely with the pH. Increasing the aspirate volume from 0.5 to 4 ml/kg causes injury independent of pH. Both pH and volume are important; a **25 ml of aspirate with a pH <2.5 is critical** to produce a chemical pneumonitis in humans. Infection plays no role in the early chemical pneumonitis of acute aspiration pneumonia.

■ Clinical Features and Diagnosis

Cough, dyspnea, and **acute respiratory distress** immediately follow a witnessed aspiration. Tachypnea, tachycardia, râles hypotension, and shock are other features. Apnea may be noted, and wheezing occurs in about one-third of the cases. Low-grade fever and râles are almost always present. Sputum initially may be scant and the initial gram stain may show neutrophils without predominant bacteria. Chest x-ray findings are variable and may follow the clinical syndrome, without specific diagnostic patterns. Alveolar infiltrates, unilateral or bilateral, may occupy any lung zone, but the right lower lobe is commonly affected. In the early phases, pleural effusion or cavitation is very uncommon. An isolated area of atelectasis is rare, but when present suggests solid

particle aspiration. Hypoxemia, often quite severe, starts early, caused by ventilation-perfusion mismatching and **intrapulmonary shunting.** Inflammation leads to capillary **endothelial damage;** as edema fluid leaks into the alveoli, the shunt increases and hypoxemia worsens further. In severe cases, the fluid shift leads to **hemoconcentration,** low pulmonary artery wedge pressure, and decreased cardiac output. Pulmonary artery pressures may increase.

The clinical course depends on the nature and volume of the aspirate, and the severity of underlying diseases. In one-third of high-risk patients who aspirate, adult respiratory distress syndrome (ARDS) follows. Some of these patients rapidly deteriorate and die within days. Others stabilize or improve initially, only to develop a bacterial superinfection or ARDS. A third group that ostensibly aspirate a small volume or less acidic material rapidly improve within a week, even radiographically and physiologically. Given the variability in its clinical features and its severity, acute aspiration pneumonia has a **wide range of mortality risk.** Aspiration of highly acidic material, multilobar involvement, initial shock or apnea, and development of ARDS or bacterial pneumonia indicate a poor prognosis.

Bacterial infection that develops in a significant proportion of patients after days of stability or improvement is usually accompanied by a new fever or worsening radiographic infiltrates, leukocytosis, and purulent sputum. In the hospitalized patient, the likely pathogens are gram-negative bacilli, but others include *Staphylococcus aureus* as well as mixed aerobic and anaerobic bacteria, especially in those who have gingivitis.

■ Management

The initial step is to provide **adequate airway;** a bronchoscopy should be performed, if needed, to remove any solid material, but large-volume bronchial lavage is unnecessary. Intravascular volume needs to be maintained with a crystalloid. Hypoxemia should be corrected by supplemental oxygen. Ventilation should be ensured, if necessary, by mechanical ventilation and positive

TABLE 239.2. Aspiration of Gastric Contents: Predisposing Factors

Involved Organ	Problem	Predisposing Factors
Larynx and pharynx	Impaired function	Decreased level of consciousness (sleep, anesthesia, shock, drug overdose, ethanol, seizures, stroke)
		Extremes of age
		Postextubation, endotracheal or nasoenteric tube
		Tracheostomy
		Structural lesions (tumor, polyp)
		Neuromuscular disease (myasthenia gravis, poliomyelitis, amyotrophic lateral sclerosis, Guillain-Barré syndrome, myopathies)
Esophagus	Decreased antegrade propulsion	Esophageal dysmotility (scleroderma, achalasia, presbyesophagus, gastroesophageal reflux disease)
		Structural lesions (tumor, stricture, web, fistula)
	Decreased lower sphincter pressure	Increased gastric acidity (stress, anesthesia, peptic ulcer)
		Ethanol, caffeine, tobacco, fatty foods, drugs, nasoenteric tube
Stomach	Increased volume	Gastric tube
		Delayed gastric emptying (diabetes, outlet obstruction, ileus, drugs, pregnancy, trauma)
		Food ingestion, tube feedings
	Increased pressure	Nausea and vomiting
		Upper abdominal surgery
		Pregnancy, labor
		Obesity, ascites

TABLE 239.3. Prevention of Aspiration Pneumonia in High-Risk Patients

1. Use nonparticulate antacids and H2 blockers to reduce acidity and the residual gastric volume.
2. Use antiemetics selectively to increase lower esophageal sphincter pressure.
3. Confirm tube tip location radiographically prior to initiation of enteral tube feeding.
4. Elevate the head of the bed to 30 degrees.
5. Check residual gastric volume regularly. Residual should be <150 ml before the next feeding for those on bolus tube feeding.

end-expiratory pressure (PEEP). Corticosteroids have no therapeutic role in acute aspiration pneumonia. Given the lack of controlled studies on empiric antibiotic therapy in this disorder, they are best withheld unless clinical, microbiologic, or radiographic features suggest a need.

Unwitnessed aspiration may mimic an atypical pneumonia. Clues to diagnosis include the clinical presentation (wheezing, sudden onset of respiratory distress that is disproportionate to the level of fever or radiographic infiltrates, etc.), predisposing factors, and sputum gram-stain (more neutrophils and few organisms). In mechanically ventilated patients, a low-grade fever, shifting rales or rhonchi, diffuse and/or migratory infiltrates, and increasing amounts of (purulent) tracheobronchial secretions are potential clues.

■ Prevention

Preventive measures (Table 239.3) should be considered in patients predisposed to aspiration (those undergoing general anesthesia or enteral alimentation with feeding formula, and those with impaired pharyngeal and laryngeal function). Neither a gastrostomy tube nor a jejunostomy tube is totally protective; those with g-e reflux may still aspirate.

Aspiration of Pathogenic Bacteria

Pathogenic bacteria aspirated along with gastric contents may cause a bacterial pneumonia. A different mechanism is pneumonia caused by a gravitational process that transports bacteria—predominantly anaerobes—from the mouth into the dependent segments of the lung (most classically the superior segments of the lower lobe and posterior segments of the upper lobe). The predisposing factors are gingivitis and states of altered consciousness brought on by alcoholism, central nervous system diseases, drug overdoses, and seizures, among others.

Pathogenesis

The aspirated material is largely oropharyngeal secretions, containing bacteria that are pooled on the tongue, gingiva, buccal mucosa, and pharynx. Oral anaerobes predominate, outnumbering aerobes by 5:1. In persons with poor oral hygiene and gingivitis, anaerobe concentrations may rise to 10^{11}/ml. The most important pathogens are anaerobic streptococci, *Fusobacterium*, and *Bacteroides*. The lesion, initially a pneumonitis, evolves into an abscess.

Clinical Features and Diagnosis

Typically, symptoms occur 1–2 weeks following the gravitational event. An indolent presentation with symptoms lasting several weeks or even months is not uncommon. The initial symptom is a productive cough with purulent sputum; the sputum infrequently has a putrid odor. Dyspnea and chest pain may be present, especially if an abscess or empyema has formed. Most patients are febrile, with low-grade fever. Auscultatory findings (bronchial breath sounds occasionally and râles) are localized, predominantly in the involved areas. Finger clubbing occurs in chronic cases.

The gram-stain of sputum shows multiple organisms; a culture is not helpful, as the predominant causative organisms are anaerobes (which the laboratory reports as "oral flora"). Cavitation often complicates the pneumonia, which involves the dependent segments (see Figure 211.1). Parapneumonic effusions are common and most evolve into an empyema. Diagnosis is by clinical, roentgenographic, and laboratory features, taken together with the circumstances. Complications are lung abscess (single or dominant cavity with an air-fluid level in a dependent lung segment, as shown in Figure 239.1) and empyema.

Management

Antibiotics effective against anaerobic organisms are used to treat aspiration of pathogenic bacteria. Clinda-

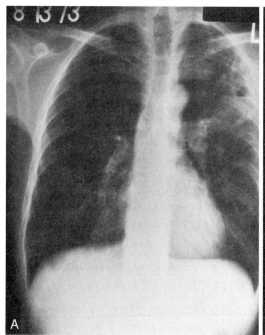
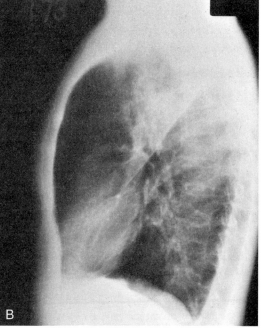

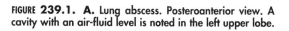

FIGURE 239.1. A. Lung abscess. Posteroanterior view. A cavity with an air-fluid level is noted in the left upper lobe. **B.** Lung abscess. Lateral view showing lesion in the apical-posterior segment of the left upper lobe.

mycin (600 mg t.i.d.) is the antibiotic of choice. Treatment duration depends on the resolution of symptoms as well as the radiographic findings. Patients with a lung abscess will require many weeks of treatment, until the symptoms resolve x-rays resolve or stabilize. A concomitant pleural effusion calls for a diagnostic thoracentesis and, if an empyema is found, intercostal closed chest tube drainage.

Aspiration of Inert Substances

Aspiration of foreign bodies into the tracheobronchial tree is the leading cause of accidental death at home for children under 1 year of age. Most of the patients with aspirated foreign bodies are below 12 years of age. In adults, sudden, unexpected obstruction of the upper airway (**cafe coronary**) is not uncommon and could be lethal. Meat is the most commonly aspirated solid that causes a cafe coronary. Older age, poor dentition, alcohol consumption, and use of sedative drugs are all predisposing factors.

■ Clinical Features and Diagnosis

The initial symptoms depend on the degree of obstruction, which depends on the size of the particle. Larger objects, such as poorly chewed meat, usually lodge in the larynx or trachea and cause **abrupt respiratory distress, inability to speak,** and **cyanosis.** Unrelieved, the obstruction is lethal. With significant, but incomplete tracheal obstruction by a foreign body, **stridor** and **intercostal retractions** may be noted. Obstruction in the distal trachea or in a mainstem bronchus may cause coughing and wheezing. Asymmetric breath sounds, unilateral wheeze, and unilateral decrease in air entry are clues. In general, the right lower lobe is more commonly affected than the left. Expiratory x-rays are useful to reveal air trapping on the affected side, manifested by a shift of the mediastinum to the opposite side. In difficult cases, endoscopy is the final arbiter. Smaller particles cause partial or distal obstruction in the tracheobronchial tree. Cough is the usual initial symptom, followed by shortness of breath, wheezing, chest pain, fever, nausea, and vomiting.

■ Management

In foreign body–related upper airway obstruction, immediate **Heimlich maneuver** is indicated, with the rescuer performing abdominal thrusts between the xiphoid process and the umbilicus. This elevates the diaphragm and expels enough air from the lungs to expel the foreign body. For **nonemergent foreign body removal,** a **rigid bronchoscope** is preferable to a fiberoptic bronchoscope. Fiberoptic bronchoscopy is suitable for a peripheral foreign body or when rigid bronchoscopy is inadvisable because of neck or face injury. Occasionally, bronchoscopy may fail, necessitating a **thoracotomy.** Long-term sequelae of chronic foreign body impaction are **bronchial stenosis** and **bronchiectasis.**

CHAPTER **240** **DRUG-INDUCED PULMONARY DISEASE**

D rug-induced pulmonary disease has a very wide spectrum (e.g., the life-threatening anaphylaxis due to penicillin, heroin-induced acute pulmonary edema, and pulmonary fibrosis from bleomycin). Table 240.1 will be helpful in approaching this important clinical problem. A number of drugs not listed in the table cause pleural or mediastinal disorders. For example, **nitrofurantoin** causes a **pleural effusion; procainamide, hydralazine, diphenylhydantoin,** and **isoniazid** cause **pleural effusions** through **drug-induced lupus erythematosus** mechanism; and corticosteroids or phenytoin cause mediastinal and hilar prominences on x-rays (mediastinal lipomatosis and lymphadenopathy, respectively).

Because there are **no specific diagnostic** tests, a comprehensive history, supplemented by an assessment of the time from exposure to the development of symptoms and roentgenographic findings, is critical to diagnosis. The physical findings and x-ray findings vary, depending on the types of pulmonary reactions and sites of injury. In selected situations and under physician supervision, a **challenge with the suspected drug** may prove the diagnosis. An open lung biopsy is helpful in selected situations (e.g., newly developing infiltrates in a leukemic patient receiving cytotoxic therapy). A biopsy in these situations helps exclude infections or other causes and might possibly find a characteristic histologic picture to confirm the diagnosis of drug-induced pulmonary disease. The general principle of treatment is **further avoidance of the drug;** specific treatments vary with the type and severity of the disease.

TABLE 240.1. Drug-Induced Pulmonary Disease*		
Type/Location of Reaction	**Class of Drug**	**Specific Drugs (Partial List)**
Pulmonary edema (noncardiac)	Narcotics	Heroin, methadone, morphine
	Analgesics	Aspirin, D-propoxyphene
	Others	Ethchlorvynol, hydrochlorothiazide
Pulmonary infiltrate with eosinophilia	Antibiotics and chemotherapeutic agents	Nitrofurantoin, penicillin, sulfonamides, methotrexate, procarbazine
	Others	Imipramine, cromolyn sodium
Diffuse alveolar/interstitial infiltrates	Chemotherapeutic agents	Bleomycin, busulfan, nitrofurantoin, cyclophosphamide, methotrexate, chlorambucil, azathioprine, gold, chloroquine
	Miscellaneous agents	Methysergide, oxygen, marijuana smoke, mineral oil, amiodarone, talc, tocainide
Pulmonary thromboembolism	Estrogens	Diethylstilbestrol, progesterone
Bronchospasm	Antibiotics	Penicillin, ampicillin
	Cholinergic agents	Mecholyl, neostigmine
	β-adrenergic blocker	Propranolol
	Analgesics	Ethyl ether
	Others	Piperazine, tartrazine
Respiratory muscle weakness	Antibiotics	Aminoglycosides, Polymyxin B
	Neuromuscular blockers	Tubocurarine, succinylcholine
Respiratory depression/acute respiratory failure	Narcotics	Heroin, methadone, morphine, cocaine
	Sedatives	Barbiturates
	Tranquilizers	Diazepam, chlordiazepoxide

*Not a complete list.

CHAPTER 241

BRONCHOGENIC CARCINOMA

Lung cancer, the most important malignant neoplasm in the United States, may be symptomatic on presentation, with cough, wheezing, new onset or worsening of sputum production, and bloody expectoration varying from blood-streaking of sputum to frank hemoptysis. Other well-known patterns of presentation of symptomatic lung cancer include postobstructive pneumonia, lung abscess, pleural effusion or an extrathoracic metastasis. Asymptomatic lung cancer classically presents as a solitary pulmonary nodule.

■ Diagnosis

Given the high rate of metastases (80%) even at initial presentation, the goal of diagnostic evaluation is to establish an unequivocal diagnosis of lung cancer, including identification of the cell type and to stage the disease. The staging determined by all studies up to the time of surgery and lymph node dissection represents the **clinical staging;** clinical staging duly modified by operative and histological findings constitutes **pathological staging.** Tumor-node metastasis (TNM) staging for lung cancer is shown in Table 196.2.

The yield from cytological examination of sputum varies from 50% in peripheral lesions to almost 90% for central lesions; the yield is higher with repeated samples. If small cell carcinoma is thus unequivocally diagnosed and the chest x-ray shows a central lesion, further surgical therapy or staging mediastinoscopy are not indicated. However, staging procedures should follow for peripheral lesions; mediastinal nodal involvement (N_2) will obviate surgery.

Flexible fiberoptic bronchoscopy (FFB) is used in the following instances: (1) when lung cancer is suspected with normal or equivocal sputum cytological examination and (2) to assess resectability when sputum examination discloses malignant cells other than the small cell type. With visible endobronchial lesions, FFB diagnoses over 99% of cases. However, this drops to between 30% and 60% in cases with no visible endobronchial lesions; the yield may be augmented by post-bronchoscopy sputum cytology. If paratracheal and subcarinal nodes are enlarged on CT scan, FFB may facilitate their transbronchoscopic aspiration for cytology.

If the foregoing methods are unrevealing, the clinical settings should dictate the diagnostic approach. Palpable lymph nodes should be biopsied. If the chest CT scan shows no significant mediastinal pathology, direct thoracotomy is the next step, cardiovascular/pulmonary function permitting. In general, mediastinal pathology on CT needs confirmation with mediastinoscopy or mediastinotomy before a nonoperative management is elected. Metastatic involvement of scalene nodes, contralateral

TABLE 241.1.	**Contraindications to Thoracotomy and Resection in Bronchogenic Carcinoma**
Operability	Poor cardiac reserve (uncontrolled heart failure, uncontrollable arrhythmias, recent myocardial infarction, etc.)[a]
	Poor pulmonary reserve[a]
	Resting PaO_2 <50 mm
	Resting $PaCO_2$ >45 mm Hg
	Age over 70[b]
	Small cell carcinoma, unless it is a localized pulmonary nodule[a]
Resectability	Any disease beyond Stage IIIA
	Distant metastases[a]
	Malignant pleural effusion[a]
	Contralateral mediastinal lymph node involvement[a]
	Superior vena caval obstruction[a]
	Esophageal/phrenic nerve involvement[a]
	Recurrent laryngeal nerve involvement[a]
	Involvement of trachea, carina or lesion within 2.0 cm of carina[a]

[a] = absolute.
[b] = relative.

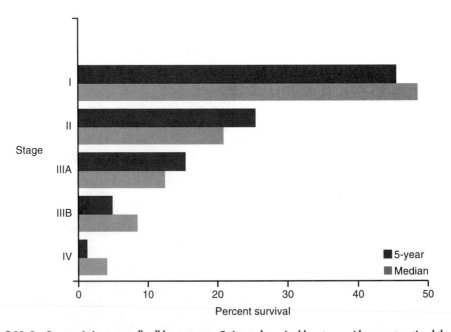

FIGURE 241.1. Prognosis in nonsmall cell lung cancer. Estimated survival by stage with current optimal therapy.
(Data from: Briggs DD et al. MKSAP in the Subspecialty of Pulmonary and Critical Care. Philadelphia: American College of Physicians, 1994, p. 136. Used with permission.)

TABLE 241.2.	Prognostic Factors in No Small-Cell Lung Cancer	
Factor	Favorable	Unfavorable
Age (operative cases)	Younger	Older
Gender	Women	Men
Histology (operative cases)	Squamous	Nonsquamous
LDH (inoperable cases)	Elevated	Normal
Liver/bone/brain metastases	None	Present
Mediastinal nodes (surgically resected)	Negative	Positive
Performance status	Fully ambulatory	Not fully ambulatory
TNM stage	See Figure 241.1	See Figure 241.1
Tumor-related symptoms	None	From metastases

(Adapted from: Ihde DC, Minna JD. Curr Prob Cancer 1991; 15:91. Used with permission.)

mediastinal nodes (Stage IIIB), or ipsilateral mediastinal node involvement (Stage IIIA) with nonsmall cell lung cancer (NSCLC) and/or poor pulmonary reserve would obviate resectional surgery. If cardiovascular/pulmonary function prohibits resection, further attempts to obtain tissue should be made only if necessary to carry out a treatment plan. In accessible lesions, CT-guided transthoracic needle aspiration (TNA) may be attempted. Pneumothorax from this procedure occurs in 20–30% of the cases, and bleeding occurs in about 20%. A definitive diagnosis may be obtained in over 90% of the cases, depending on the operator's expertise. TNA is superfluous if the patient is otherwise a candidate for surgery, and it is inadvisable if the lesion is close to the major vessels.

■ Management and Prognosis

Unless contraindicated (see Table 241.1), surgical resection offers the best cure rate for bronchogenic carcinoma. The best index of pulmonary function is the $FEV_{1.0}$. The entire neoplasm should be removed, preserving as much lung function as possible. Wedge resection, another potential choice in limited situations, has been associated with an increased risk of local recurrence. Surgical procedures carry a 30-day overall mortality of 3.7% (pneumonectomy, 6.2%; lobectomy, 2.9%). The age-related mortality in the eighth decade and beyond exceeds 7.1%. Prognosis depends on the staging (Figure 241.1) and other factors (Table 241.2).

(Additional information on bronchogenic carcinoma appears in chapter 196.)

CHAPTER **242** THE SOLITARY PULMONARY NODULE

■ Definition and Etiology

Solitary pulmonary nodule (SPN), a roentgenographic diagnosis, is a single, well-circumscribed (surrounded by aerated lung tissue), nodular pulmonary density. It is less than 3.0 cm in diameter (densities exceeding 3.0 cm in diameter are usually designated as mass lesions), calcified or uncalcified, and, if cavitated, the cavitation does not involve most of the lesion. Generally, the patient is asymptomatic.

A significant proportion of SPNs is malignant. Bronchogenic carcinoma tops the list and metastatic neoplasms constitute most of the remainder. The incidence of bronchogenic cancer varies with advancing age and smoking status of the study cohort. However, most SPNs are benign, comprising granulomas (predominantly mycotic and mycobacterial), hamartomas, and miscella-

neous entities including intrapulmonary lymph nodes, pulmonary infarction, and localized pulmonary scars.

■ Management

The high incidence of lung cancer and the highly favorable prognosis (5-year survival rate in 50–80% of all cases) for lung cancer that presents as an SPN necessitate an organized approach to the management of SPN. CT, high-resolution CT (HRCT), and the application of probabilistic reasoning (a high pre-test probability of a lesion being benign or malignant) have made the decision process somewhat more complex than it was at one time. The essentials in decision-making include a thorough clinical history, physical examination, and review of current and old roentgenograms if available. Age, history of smoking, presence of coexistent lung

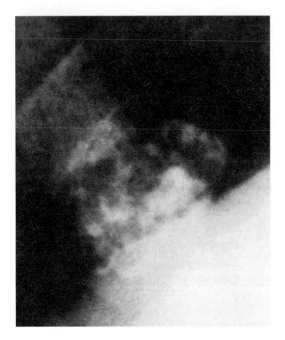

FIGURE 242.1. Solitary pulmonary nodule. "Popcorn" calcification in a benign lung nodule.

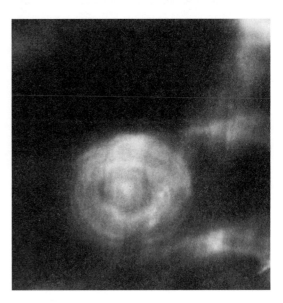

FIGURE 242.2. Solitary pulmonary nodule: benign concentric calcification in a histoplasmoma.

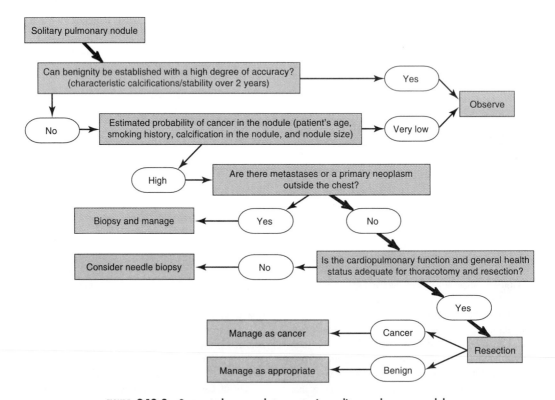

FIGURE 242.3. Suggested approach to managing solitary pulmonary nodule.

disease, and roentgenographic (and, if available, tomographic) appearances of the nodule are important considerations. While CT has widely replaced conventional tomograms, fluoroscopy and conventional tomography are still used to manage SPN in several medical centers, thus obviating the routine use of expensive studies such as CT and HRCT.

The **emphasis** in managing SPN continues to be **on resection,** unless benignity can be established with a high degree of accuracy. The two generally accepted criteria of benignity are **stability of the lesion** as seen from old x-rays and **characteristic patterns of calcification,** which include "popcorn" (Figure 242.1) or concentric (Figure 242.2) or central, "bull's eye" patterns. Younger age (<35 years) and an absence of smoking history also support a benign etiology. The management of SPN is outlined in Figure 242.3.

The **search for an extrapulmonary neoplasm** producing a metastatic SPN is indicated only when a previous history of neoplastic disease exists or when a review of systems or clinical examination suggests that possibility (e.g., a change in bowel habits or the presence of occult blood in the stools). Similarly, a search for metastases from a malignant SPN is indicated only if clinical features (pain and tenderness in long bones, enlarged nodular liver, localizing neurological findings, etc.) or basic laboratory studies (complete blood counts, urinalysis, liver function tests, and serum calcium) suggest that possibility. Bronchoscopy and brushing have no routine use. Mediastinoscopy is utilized for mass lesions (≥3 cm in diameter) and CT scans show significant mediastinal pathology. When the resected nodule demonstrates bronchogenic carcinoma, postoperative, life-long follow-up is necessary. Postoperative irradiation may be necessary, if residual disease is possible or suspected.

Fine needle aspiration biopsy (FNAB) of SPN yields a positive result for malignancy in over 90% of the cases when the nodule is malignant. However, these results vary widely and thus cannot be embraced universally. Benign disease, however, is definitively diagnosed by FNAB much less frequently (30–40%). It is indicated when resection is not feasible and a diagnosis is essential. Other possible indications include a patient with borderline pulmonary function, in whom a definitive diagnosis of malignancy could lead to surgical resection.

CHAPTER 243 PLEURAL EFFUSION

Pleural disease most commonly presents as a pleural effusion. It is an abnormal accumulation of fluid in the pleural space, caused by an imbalance in oncotic or hydrostatic pressures (transudate) or by an intrinsic abnormality of the pleura (exudate). Causes of pleural effusion are listed in Table 243.1.

■ Pathogenesis

The pleural space, the vacuum between the parietal and the visceral pleura, contains a small amount (approximately 10 ml) of clear fluid with a low-protein content. Fluid enters and exits the space through capillaries or the lymphatics in the parietal or visceral pleura. Because an equilibrium prevails between the physiologic formation and removal of pleural fluid, a pleural effusion results from an increase in the formation or a decrease in the lymphatic removal of fluid or a combination of the two.

■ Clinical Features

The symptoms of pleural effusion include dyspnea, pleuritic or nonpleuritic chest pain, and nonproductive cough. Sometimes it may be asymptomatic. Both a mechanical disadvantage of the diaphragm and restrictive ventilatory impairment resulting from the effusion cause the dyspnea. In addition, the underlying disease that caused the effusion may also cause symptoms and signs. Some of the historical clues to the etiology of the pleural effusion are listed in Table 243.2. Physical findings of pleural effusion are decreased tactile fremitus, dullness to percussion, and decreased breath sounds on auscultation. Large effusions (>1,000 ml) may cause contralateral mediastinal shift.

■ Roentgenographic Features

Free pleural fluid has a characteristic x-ray appearance: a meniscus in the costophrenic angle in the posteroanterior (PA) view (Figure 218.1c) and blunting of the posterior gutter in the lateral view (Figure 243.1). The former requires at least 500 ml fluid. Free fluid layers out on a lateral decubitus view. Pleural fluid may assume other appearances, including that of a pseudotumor or tumors (Figure 243.2). Absence of contralateral mediastinal shift with a massive effusion suggests prior mediastinal fixation due to malignancy. Loculated pleural effusions may be detected using ultrasonography.

TABLE 243.1.   Causes of Pleural Effusions

Frequency	Transudates	Exudates
Common	Congestive heart failure Cirrhosis of liver	Parapneumonic Malignant neoplasm Pulmonary embolism
Less common	Nephrotic syndrome Pulmonary embolism	Tuberculosis Nonbacterial infections Collagen vascular diseases Dressler's syndrome Drugs Pancreatitis Iatrogenic trauma endoscopic sclerotherapy, subclavian vein catheters
Rare	Peritoneal dialysis Urinothorax Atelectasis Superior vena caval obstruction	Subphrenic/liver abscess Esophageal rupture Chylothorax Benign asbestos effusion Uremia Sarcoidosis Meig's syndrome Yellow nail syndrome

TABLE 243.2.   Diagnosing Etiology of Pleural Fluid: Clues from History

History/Feature	Diagnosis Suggested by History/Feature
Asbestos exposure	Benign asbestos pleural effusion, malignant mesothelioma
Smoking with or without asbestos exposure	Malignant effusion due to bronchogenic carcinoma
Drugs (see text)	Drug-induced pleural effusion
Exposure to tuberculosis; positive tuberculin skin test	Tuberculous pleural effusion
Cough with purulent sputum, chills, fever	Parapneumonic effusion
Immobilization, postoperative states, obesity, cardiac failure, past or present deep venous thrombosis	Pulmonary embolism
Joint pains, swelling, stiffness	Rheumatoid effusion
Chest trauma	Hemothorax
Recent subclavian venous line insertion	Hemothorax or infusion into pleural space
Urinary obstruction	Urinothorax
Abdominal pain, alcoholism	Pancreatic effusion
Vomiting, upper G.I. endoscopy, sclerotherapy	Esophageal rupture/post-sclerotherapy
Parturition, upper abdominal surgery	Self-limited pleural effusion
Cirrhosis, ascites	Transudative effusion due to cirrhosis
Orthopnea, paroxysmal nocturnal dyspnea, pedal edema	Congestive heart failure

■ Differential Diagnosis and Diagnosis

Sometimes, the cause is evident (e.g., bilateral effusions in clinically obvious congestive heart failure or asymptomatic, small effusions within 48 hours of abdominal surgery or parturition). A repeat chest roentgenogram in a few days after appropriate treatment or observation will suffice. When the cause of the effusion is unknown, an evaluation is necessary to ascertain it. The physician must formulate a clinical diagnosis first, then obtain a pleural fluid sample by thoracentesis and determine whether it is a transudate or an exudate, and finally determine the exact cause by additional tests or invasive procedures.

To safely perform a thoracentesis, a lateral decubitus roentgenogram is helpful, but not essential. If the fluid layers along the inner chest wall and the "layer" is at

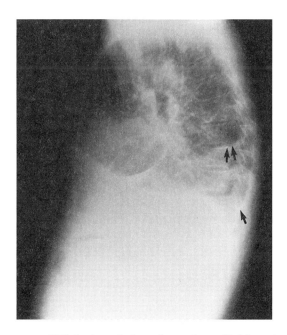

FIGURE **243.1.** Lateral view of a patient with bilateral effusions showing blunting of the posterior costophrenic sulcus (single arrow) representing one side and a posteriorly located meniscus (double arrows) representing the other.

least 10 mm thick, then one may proceed with thoracentesis. If the pleural effusion does not layer, it may be loculated and must be differentiated from pleural thickening or a pleural neoplasm, perhaps through an ultrasound. While computed tomography (CT) is not generally necessary, in select cases it gives useful information about the underlying lung and mediastinum and defines pleural loculations. An expiration chest x-ray is advisable after thoracentesis to detect a pneumothorax. Other complications are bleeding and infection.

The gross characteristics of the fluid should be noted. Yellow-green thick fluid is pus—that is, bacterial empyema. Foul-smelling fluid implies anaerobic empyema. Milky white fluid is either a chylous or a chyliform effusion; a grossly bloody fluid is likely a hemothorax. Protein and lactate dehydrogenase (LDH) of the pleural fluid along with simultaneous serum values can differentiate exudate from a transudate (Table 243.3). Exudates fulfill at least one of the following criteria: (1) pleural fluid: serum protein ratio ≥0.5; (2) pleural fluid: serum LDH ratio ≥0.6, or (3) an absolute LDH exceeding two-thirds of the upper limits of "normal" for the serum LDH. Transudative effusions meet none of these criteria.

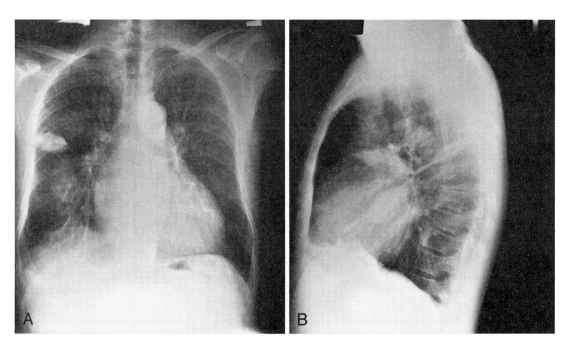

FIGURE **243.2. A.** Interlobar effusion (pseudotumor). Posteroanterior view. **B.** Interlobar effusion, lateral view. Figures **A** and **B** show accumulation of fluid in the major and minor fissures.
(Courtesy of Lawrence R. Goodman, MD, Medical College of Wisconsin, Milwaukee.)

TABLE 243.3. Pleural Fluid Tests and Their Usefulness		
Tests	**Usefulness**	**Comments**
LDH	Separates transudates and exudates.	Useful in all.
Protein	Separates transudates and exudates.	Simultaneously obtain serum LDH and protein.
Gram stain, cultures	If positive, diagnostic of empyema.	Useful in all exudates.
Glucose	↓ compared to a serum value in complicated parapneumonic effusions and empyema, rheumatoid pleural effusion, some malignancies, and TB.	Generally useful in all exudates.
Cytology	If positive, diagnostic of malignant effusion.	
Stains, cultures for mycobacteria, fungi	If positive, diagnostic.	
Antinuclear antibody (ANA)	ANA titer ≥1:160 and pleural fluid to serum ANA ratio ≥1 are indicative of SLE pleuritis.	Only selective use (rarity of the diagnoses). However, diagnostic if clinical suspicion is high.
LE cells	Diagnostic of SLE pleuritis.	Same as ANA.
Amylase	↑ and exceeds serum level in pancreatic effusion. Increased amylase of salivary origin in esophageal rupture, malignancies.	
Triglycerides	>110 mg/ml indicates chylothorax.	Selective use only.
Chylomicrons	Presence diagnostic of chylothorax.	
Hematocrit	↑, approaching that of blood diagnostic of hemothorax. ≥1%, but not hemothorax, suggests malignancy, trauma or tuberculosis.	Useful only if combined with a strong pre-thoracentesis clinical diagnosis.
Red cell count	>100,000/mm^3 suggest same diagnoses as hematocrit >1%.	Same as hematocrit.
White cell count	>10,000/mm^3 in parapneumonic effusion, pulmonary embolism, malignancy, tuberculosis, Dressler's syndrome, lupus pleural effusion.	
Differential count	↑ Neutrophils: indicates acute inflammation. ↑ Lymphocytic: malignancy or tuberculosis.	
pH	<6.0 accompanied by elevated amylase strongly suggests esophageal rupture. <7.20 due to a variety of causes. <7.00 in a parapneumonic effusion is a strong indication for chest tube drainage.	Useful in suspected esophageal rupture and parapneumonic effusions only.

↑ = elevated; ↓ = decreased; cytology = for malignancy; LDH = lactate dehydrogenase; LE = lupus erythematosus; SLE = systemic lupus erythematosus; TB = tuberculosis.

Transudative Pleural Effusions

Congestive heart failure is the most common cause of a transudate. Effusions are typically bilateral, but if unilateral, they are generally right-sided. The notion that diuresis converts a transudate into an exudate is unproven. Associated pleuritic pain or unilateral left-sided effusion should arouse the suspicion of pulmonary embolism. Liver cirrhosis is another cause of transudates, due to the egress of ascites from the peritoneal cavity into the pleural space through the diaphragmatic lymphatics. Ascites and stigmata of chronic liver disease are found in such cases. Typically, the effusion is right-sided; less commonly, it is bilateral. Other causes are listed in Table 243.1.

Exudative Pleural Effusions

The most common cause of an exudative pleural effusion is parapneumonic—that is, an ipsilateral effusion associated with a bacterial pneumonia. Such effusions complicate 40% of bacterial pneumonias and typically contain >10,000/μl of WBCs with a predominance of neutrophils. Some are uncomplicated and resolve with appropriate antibiotics alone. Others are an empyema (gross pus or bacteria seen on microscopy or culture) or a "complicated" effusion (a transitional fluid between uncomplicated parapneumonic effusion and an empyema), which requires chest tube drainage to avoid persistent infection, bronchopleural fistula, or adhesions. Parapneumonic effusions with a pH below 7.0 or a glucose below 40 mg/dl should be treated as an empyema. Those with a pH above 7.2 usually resolve on treatment of pneumonia. In the remainder, the pH and glucose trends should be determined by repeat thoracentesis in 12–24 hours to help formulate treatment decisions.

Malignant effusion, a common cause of exudative effusion, results from pleural invasion by the malignancy. Cancers of the lung and breast are the leading causes and, along with lymphomas, constitute 75% of the cases of malignant effusions. Pleural fluid cytology is diagnostic in 60–80% of malignant effusions. Pleural effusions may occur in malignancy without actual malignant pleural involvement. These cytology-negative effusions, best designated as **paramalignant effusions,** result from tumor invasion of mediastinal lymph nodes, atelectasis, or pneumonia.

A pleural effusion occurs in approximately one-half of patients with pulmonary embolism; about 80% of these effusions are exudative. It is usually unilateral and may be bloody and associated with a pulmonary infiltrate. Bloody pleural fluid in pulmonary embolism does not contraindicate anticoagulation. Pleural tuberculosis often causes a unilateral, exudative pleural effusion (see chapter 218 for pathogenesis). Parenchymal abnormalities are generally absent in the chest x-ray. A tuberculin skin test is positive only infrequently. The fluid is lymphocyte-preponderant with sparse (<5%) mesothelial cells. Fluid culture alone has a low diagnostic yield (<25%) but percutaneous pleural biopsy showing granulomas markedly increases the diagnostic yield. Although the effusion resolves spontaneously, if untreated, most of these patients develop active tuberculosis within 5 years.

Acute and chronic pancreatitis can cause a high-amylase, generally left-sided, exudative effusion. A pleural effusion that follows vomiting and is associated with chest pain and dyspnea, might signal spontaneous esophageal rupture; fluid analysis characteristically shows high (salivary) amylase, a low pH, and, on gram stain, a polymicrobial flora; ingested food particles are often seen. Finally, some medications cause exudative pleural effusions—for example, agents used in chemotherapy (methotrexate, procarbazine) and esophageal sclerotherapy, tocolytics (used in premature labor), bromocriptine, dantrolene, methysergide, L-tryptophan, nitrofurantoin, and amiodarone. Hydralazine, phenytoin, isoniazid, and procainamide can induce a lupus syndrome, an integral feature of which is a pleural effusion. Exudative pleural effusions may also occur in rheumatoid arthritis (RA), systemic lupus erythematosus (SLE), and Dressler's syndrome, also known as **postcardiac injury syndrome** (PCIS). The glucose in RA pleural effusions is typically low.

■ Indications and Utility of Procedures

To fully and cost-effectively utilize the diagnostic potential of pleural fluid tests (Table 243.3), all clinical information should be integrated and a pretest clinical diagnosis formed. Appropriate tests can then follow. Tuberculosis can be diagnosed in about 90% of the cases by combining percutaneous pleural biopsy (PPB) and pleural fluid smears and cultures. Pleural fluid cytology is superior to PPB in diagnosing malignancy. However, diagnostic yield improves by about 7% when PPB is added to a negative cytological study.

When a PPB is nondiagnostic, the options are clinical follow-up or thoracoscopy/fiberoptic bronchoscopy. Thoracoscopy with biopsy is particularly useful in the diagnosis of suspected tuberculous and malignant effusions and malignant mesothelioma. Fiberoptic bronchoscopy has a low yield in pleural effusion, unless there is hemoptysis, or a mass or complete or partial atelectasis is seen in the chest x-ray or CT scan. Even with an extensive work-up, a cause for pleural effusion may be elusive in 15–20% of the cases. However, the course and outcome of these patients are often favorable and the majority of such effusions resolve spontaneously.

■ Management

The management of pleural effusion depends on the cause of effusion. Pleural fluid drainage is necessary in some cases for therapy or palliation. Empyema and complicated parapneumonic effusions require closed chest tube drainage. Inadequate drainage calls for further surgical procedures. An undiagnosed lymphocytic effusion and a positive PPD skin test is tuberculosis unless proven otherwise. Pleural effusion and pleuritis due to PCIS respond to nonsteroidal anti-inflammatory agents or corticosteroids. Effusions due to esophageal rupture or pancreatic pseudocyst require prompt surgical consultation. Pleural fluid drainage followed by chemical pleur-odesis with talc or tetracycline frequently relieves dyspnea from a recurrent malignant effusion. A decision to do pleurodesis depends on the patient's overall condition and how the effusion is affecting the patient's well-being.

CHAPTER 244 PNEUMOTHORAX

Pneumothorax, or air in the pleural space, may be induced, traumatic, or spontaneous. **Induced pneumothorax** (deliberate introduction of air into the pleural cavity) was used to collapse tuberculous cavities. **Traumatic pneumothorax** results from penetrating or blunt injury or from surgical procedures (e.g., thoracentesis, subclavian vein catheterization, needle biopsy of lung). **Spontaneous pneumothorax** may be either primary or secondary. Primary spontaneous pneumothorax occurs more commonly in men (young, tall, asthenic) than in women. Its pathogenesis is elusive, but rupture of subpleurally located blebs is one reasonable theory. The configuration of the thoracic cage and traction pressures exerted onto the alveolar walls are presumed predisposing factors. Secondary spontaneous pneumothorax is usually due to underlying lung disease (Table 244.1).

TABLE 244.1.	Causes of Secondary Spontaneous Pneumothorax
Common	Obstructive disorders
	Emphysema
	Bronchial asthma
	Cystic Fibrosis
	Infections
	Tuberculosis
	Necrotizing pneumonia
	Lung abscess
	Diffuse Infiltrative diseases
	Histiocytosis X
	Sarcoidosis
	Complicating ventilator management
	Associated with PEEP
	High airway pressures
	Airway obstruction
Rare	Malignant neoplasm of lung or pleura
	Pulmonary infarction
	Marfan's syndrome
	Ehlers-Danlos syndrome
	Tuberous sclerosis
	Catamenial (associated with menstrual periods)

Pathogenesis

The pressure in the normal pleural space is negative with reference to atmospheric and alveolar pressures. A communication between pleura and the atmosphere (as in penetrating trauma), or between the pleura and the lung (as in a ruptured bulla), causes air to enter the pleural space until the pleural and atmospheric pressures equalize. This increased pleural pressure causes the lung to collapse. In some instances, air that enters pleural space cannot leave it because of a "ball valve" mechanism. Intrapleural pressure then exceeds atmospheric pressure throughout expiration and often during inspiration also. The resulting "tension pneumothorax" is life-threatening because it compromises ventilation via mediastinal shift and diminishes cardiac output by impairing venous return. Tension pneumothorax is more likely with mechanical ventilation or other secondary pneumothoraces than with primary spontaneous pneumothorax.

Clinical Features and Diagnosis

The clinical features depend on the volume of air in the pleural cavity and the nature and degree of the underlying lung disease. Most patients have some dyspnea; a few may be asymptomatic. The degree of dyspnea depends on the severity of the pneumothorax and the underlying disease. Chest pain is usually sudden. Physical findings include hyperresonance on percussion and diminished to absent tactile fremitus and breath sounds on the affected side. Underlying severe emphysema, particularly bullous emphysema, could make the diagnosis of pneumothorax by physical examination very difficult.

Tension pneumothorax is a respiratory emergency, manifested by respiratory distress, tachypnea, and tachycardia often accompanied by distended veins, thready pulse, and hypotension. Bulging of the ipsilateral intercostal spaces and mediastinal shift to the contralateral side may be detected.

The chest x-ray is diagnostic. The air separates the margin of the collapsed lung from the parietal pleura (Figure 244.1); mediastinal shift is present in tension

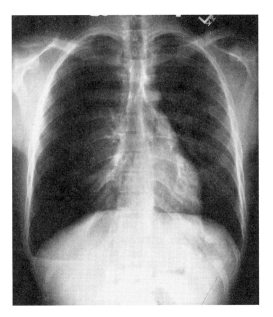

FIGURE 244.1. Spontaneous pneumothorax: entire right lung is collapsed.
(Courtesy of Lawrence R. Goodman, MD, Medical College of Wisconsin, Milwaukee.)

pneumothorax. Occasionally, there is an air-fluid level in the pleural cavity. An expiratory chest roentgenogram is helpful in delineating a pneumothorax after procedures (e.g., following thoracentesis, transbronchial lung biopsy) that can cause this complication.

Management

A variety of treatment options are available and the choice clearly depends on the severity of the pneumothorax, predisposing state, and underlying disease. Most cases of asymptomatic unilateral and small (approximately 10–20% of lung volume) primary spontaneous pneumothorax resolve within a week, and can be observed. A chest x-ray should be repeated in 6–12 hours to detect any progression. Supplemental oxygen may speed the resorption of air. Progressive increases in spontaneous pneumothorax and symptomatic pneumothorax require evacuation of pleural air, done by a small catheter thoracostomy, using a Heimlich valve attachment. If needed, suction could be added. Chest tube drainage is the preferred method in tension pneumothorax, hydropneumothorax, and pneumothorax with underlying pulmonary disease. Tension pneumothorax is a medical emergency and, if the diagnosis is suspected, a large-bore needle should be immediately inserted into the second anterior intercostal space of the affected side to evacuate the air. Large amounts of air coming through the needle with relief of symptoms confirms the diagnosis. The needle should be left in place until a chest tube is inserted and the air drained under water seal. Primary spontaneous pneumothorax recurs in about one-half of all cases in 2 years. Chest tube drainage and chemical pleurodesis are recommended for ipsilateral recurrence. Any further occurrence is best treated by thoracotomy or thoracoscopy and pleural abrasion.

CHAPTER 245 ASBESTOS PLEURAL DISEASE, FIBROTHORAX, AND PLEURAL TUMORS

Asbestos Pleural Disease

Owing to their size and shape, asbestos fibers that enter the lungs are only minimally cleared. The retained fibers generate a chronic inflammatory response that causes both parenchymal and pleural injury. Five pleural disorders are associated with asbestos exposure: benign asbestos pleural effusion, pleural plaque, pleural fibrosis, rounded atelectasis, and malignant mesothelioma.

Pleural Effusion and Pleural Plaques

Benign asbestos pleural effusion (BAPE) is the most common asbestos-related disorder that occurs within 10 years of asbestos exposure. It may be incidentally discovered on chest x-ray or may simulate a pneumonia with pleuritic pain and fever. The effusion is often unilateral and generally self-limited, but tends to recur. The fluid usually is blood-tinged and may be eosinophilic. The diagnosis depends on a history of asbestos exposure, a consistent clinical presentation, and an otherwise unexplained exudative effusion.

Pleural plaques commonly occur in the lateral areas and in the diaphragmatic pleura, and may be calcified. They occur at least 20 years after asbestos exposure and are the most common sequel thereof. Bilateral diaphragmatic pleural calcification is nearly pathognomonic of asbestos-induced pleural disease (Figure 245.1). Pleural plaques alone cause neither symptoms nor pulmonary function abnormalities; nor do they undergo malignant transformation. No therapy is needed. However, diffuse pleural fibrosis, which involves both the visceral and parietal pleura, commonly causes restrictive ventilatory impairment.

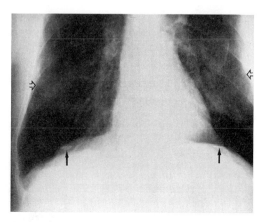

FIGURE 245.1. Chest x-ray of a patient showing several features of asbestos-related pleuropulmonary disease, including calcified pleural plaques (open arrows) and diaphragmatic calcification (solid arrows).

Fibrothorax

Fibrothorax results from the deposition of fibrous tissue, causing a thick fibrotic visceral pleura, which limits the expansion of the underlying lung. It is a late complication of empyema, hemothorax, or pleural tuberculosis. Conditions causing chronic pleuritis (uremia, collagen vascular disease, pancreatitis, and asbestos pleural disease) may cause fibrothorax. Patients present with exertional dyspnea. Findings include decreased expansion and narrowed intercostal spaces on the affected side with ipsilateral mediastinal shift. Chest x-rays show the ipsilateral mediastinal shift and dense pleural fibrosis, often calcified, surrounding the lung. Pulmonary function tests show restrictive ventilatory impairment. Decortication—removal of the fibrous pleural peel—is the only effective treatment.

Pleural Tumors

Primary tumors of the pleura are usually mesotheliomas that arise from mesothelial lining cells. They may be local or diffuse, benign or malignant. In histology, they may appear as epithelial, fibrous, or mixed types. However, the vast majority of pleural malignancies are metastatic, the most common sources being cancers of the breast and lung. Hodgkin's and non-Hodgkin's lymphoma, and carcinomas of the ovary, stomach, and colon may also metastasize to the pleura. However, a pleural effusion in conjunction with a past history of one of these neoplasms need not necessarily mean that the effusion is malignant; it may well be due to other causes. (See "Exudative Pleural Effusions" in chapter 243.)

CHAPTER 246 DISORDERS OF THE MEDIASTINUM

Pneumomediastinum

Pneumomediastinum means the presence of air in the mediastinum. This may be of no clinical consequence or could indicate a serious disease (e.g., rupture of the esophagus or bronchus). The causes are many: coughing, straining, traumatic compression of the chest, asthma, pneumonia, miliary tuberculosis, diabetic ketoacidosis, abuse of inhaled illicit drugs such as marijuana and crack cocaine, and mechanical ventilation, particularly with positive end-expiratory pressure. All these share an abrupt change in the pressure gradient between alveoli and interstitium, resulting in shearing of alveolar walls. The free air moves along the perivascular sheaths into the mediastinum and then along the great vessels and vascular sheaths into the subcutaneous tissues of the neck.

■ Clinical Features, Diagnosis, and Management

Typically, sudden substernal chest pain, radiating to the neck or arm, follows an episode of coughing or straining. Dyspnea is often present and may be aggravated by swallowing. Diagnosis is made by the feel of crepitus in the subcutaneous tissues of the neck. Roentgenographic demonstration of air in the mediastinal tissues is characteristic. The mediastinal structures, particularly the heart border and the aortic knob, are often outlined with unusual clarity. The lateral view shows free air anterior to the cardiac shadow.

No treatment is necessary in most cases since decompression occurs by the dissection of air in the subcutaneous tissues and the air is absorbed eventually. However, if large amounts of air progressively accumulate, venous return to the heart may be diminished. Treatment then would be a subcutaneous incision in the neck or a tracheostomy. If the pneumomediastinum follows a rupture of the esophagus or bronchus, the rupture should be surgically corrected.

Mediastinal Masses

Primary neoplasms and cysts of the mediastinum may occur at any age. Their manifestations vary from no symptoms to nonspecific symptoms to chronic symptoms and even to acute, life-threatening cardiorespiratory emergencies.

The mediastinum may be divided into anterior, middle, and posterior compartments. This division, based on anatomic landmarks, is useful in the roentgenographic localization of mediastinal masses. Besides, certain masses have a predilection to be localized in certain compartments. The anterior mediastinum, which lies between the sternum anteriorly and the pericardium and brachiocephalic vessels posteriorly shows a predilection for thymomas (see below). Other important tumors in this compartment are germ cell neoplasms, thyroid, parathyroid adenoma, malignant lymphoma (see Figure 192.1), primary carcinoma, and mesenchymal tumors. The middle mediastinum, which is between the anterior compartment and the anterior spinal ligament, has a predilection for congenital cystic lesions (pericardial, bronchogenic, enteric, thymic, etc.). The posterior mediastinum extends from the anterior spinal ligament to the posterior chest wall, medial to the pulmonary sulci. Neurogenic tumors are the most common (>90%) masses arising in this compartment.

Approximately 75% of all mediastinal masses are benign. The most common tumor in adults is **thymoma,** which represents 21% of all lesions. The frequency of other tumors is shown in Figure 246.1.

■ Clinical Features

In adults, most mediastinal masses and cysts are asymptomatic and are unexpectedly discovered on chest x-ray. The presence of symptoms increases the probability of malignancy from 50% to approximately 95%. Symptoms (chest pain, cough, dyspnea, dysphagia, hoarseness, stridor, respiratory infections, and hemoptysis) result from direct invasion or compression of adjacent mediastinal structures by the mass. Other manifestations include obstruction to pulmonary outflow tract, pericardial effusion, cardiac tamponade, superior vena caval syndrome, vocal cord paralysis, Horner's syndrome, chylothorax, and chylopericardium. Prominent systemic manifestations may occur from hormonal products of the mediastinal tumors (e.g., hypercalcemia from a parathyroid adenoma, thyrotoxicosis from an intrathoracic goiter, and hypertension due to a pheochromocytoma). Other notable associations are thymoma and myasthenia gravis, neurogenic tumors and osteoarthropathy, and Hodgkin's disease and Pel-Ebstein fever.

■ Diagnosis and Management

Rarely does a clinical assessment provide a definitive diagnosis in a mediastinal mass. However, it provides a framework for an orderly diagnostic evaluation. The major steps in the correct diagnosis of a mediastinal mass are localization, excluding a mass of vascular origin, and obtaining a definitive histologic diagnosis. Chest x-rays, particularly a lateral view, help in localization. Comparison with previous roentgenograms, if available, is very helpful. Increasing size of the mass is more indicative of a neoplasm. Computed tomography with contrast injection can localize and define the mass, its vascular origin, density (cystic, solid, or calcified), relationship to adjacent structures, and any local invasion. Myelography or MRI can detect invasion of the intervertebral foramina

FIGURE 246.1. The etiology of mediastinal masses and their relative frequencies.

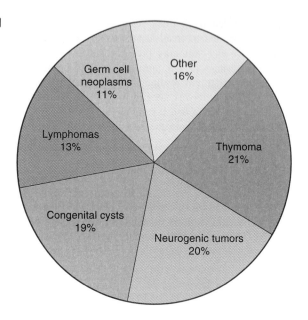

by a posterior mediastinal lesion. Other tests include serum parathyroid hormone level in suspected parathyroid adenoma and measurement of α-fetoprotein and carcino-embryonic antigen in suspected germ cell neoplasms and primary carcinomas.

While many procedures are available, they should be used selectively, depending on the localization, presentation, and, most importantly, the probable diagnosis in a given patient. Anterior mediastinoscopy and mediastinotomy are the most useful procedures for a histologic diagnosis, followed by exploratory thoracotomy in some cases.

Specific treatment depends on the nature of the mediastinal neoplasm or cyst. Surgical treatment—that is, excision of the mass—is recommended in many; the operative mortality for all mediastinal tumors ranges from 0% to 4%. Complications such as infections, hemorrhage, and injury to the phrenic or recurrent laryngeal nerve may occur in 4–11% of patients. The extent of the disease plays a large role in determining the type of treatment. Radiation therapy is useful in certain situations. Chemotherapy, either alone or combined with other modalities, is used in the treatment of some neoplasms.

CHAPTER **247** ACUTE RESPIRATORY FAILURE

■ **Definition**

The components of normal respiration include arterial oxygenation (represented by PaO_2, hemoglobin, and hemoglobin binding of oxygen), alveolar ventilation (represented by $PaCO_2$), and tissue oxygenation (represented by arterial oxygen content [CaO_2] and cardiac output). In broad terms, acute respiratory failure (ARF) indicates a failure of one or more of these components. (A comprehensive definition characterizes ARF as "a state in which the arterial oxygen tension [PaO_2] is below the predicted normal range for the patient's age at the prevalent barometric pressure [in the absence of intra-cardiac right-to-left shunting], or the arterial carbon dioxide tension [$PaCO_2$] is above 50 mm Hg [not due to respiratory compensation for metabolic alkalemia]." Narrowly defined, respiratory failure is the inability of the lungs and heart to maintain adequate arterial oxygenation and/or adequate CO_2 elimination. A more practical and simple definition is the sudden development of PaO_2 below 50 mm Hg with or without CO_2 retention.) Depending on its evolution, respiratory failure may be acute or chronic. Causes of ARF are listed in Table 247.1.

Clinical methods and oximetry are resolutely inadequate for diagnosing ARF, although they are

TABLE 247.1.	Respiratory Failure: Classification and Some Causes
Classification/General Cause	**Specific Causes**
Ventilatory failure	
Thoracic diseases	• Lung and airway diseases: chronic obstructive pulmonary disease, asthma, bronchiolitis, epiglottitis, laryngeal edema, foreign body, • Pleural diseases: pleural effusion, pneumothorax, fibrothorax • Chest wall disorders: kyphoscoliosis, thoracoplasty, flail chest
Neuromuscular diseases	• Brain disorders: infections, cerebrovascular disease, drugs (sedatives, tranquilizers, analgesics, anesthetic agents), myxedema, primary alveolar hypoventilation • Muscular and myoneural junction disorders: muscular dystrophy, myotonia, drugs (curariform drugs, aminoglycosides), myasthenia gravis, tetanus • Neural and spinal cord disorders: Guillain-Barré syndrome, poliomyelitis, amyotrophic lateral sclerosis, peripheral neuritis, cervical cord transection
Oxygenation failure	
Diffuse interstitial diseases	• Interstitial pneumonitis, fibrosis, sarcoidosis, pneumoconioses, lymphangitis carcinomatosa, interstitial pulmonary edema
Alveolar diseases	• Pneumonias, pulmonary edema, diseases with increased alveolar capillary permeability (see ARDS)
Vascular diseases	• Pulmonary embolism, fat embolism, vasculitis
Adult respiratory distress syndrome	• (see Table 249.1)

commonly used for that purpose. The diagnosis of ARF rests on arterial blood gas analysis, which measures both the adequacy of oxygenation and CO_2 elimination. An acute rise in $PaCO_2$ (hypercapnia) to above 50 mm Hg is called **acute ventilatory failure;** an acute decline in PaO_2 below 50 mm Hg without CO_2 retention is termed **acute oxygenation failure.** This distinction has important pathogenetic and therapeutic implications.

■ Clinical Features

While symptoms of hypoxemia have been likened to those of alcohol intoxication (restlessness, combativeness, agitation, and loss of judgment), and symptoms of hypercapnia to those of an anesthetic administration (headache, vasodilation, gradual onset of drowsiness, and coma), this correlation mainly emphasizes the nonspecific nature of the symptoms of respiratory failure and the circumstances in which one needs to be vigilant for its appearance. Besides these manifestations caused by gas exchange abnormalities, features of the causative disorders would also be present.

■ Diagnosis and Management

At one extreme, the onset of ARF may be dramatic (e.g., respiratory arrest or cyanosis) and at the other, quite subtle (e.g., acute ventilatory failure superimposed on chronic respiratory failure due to COPD). A lack of pathognomonic clinical features often makes the clinical diagnosis of ARF difficult. Thus, the first prerequisite for diagnosis is an awareness of the conditions that may lead to respiratory failure. Blood gas results, which follow, should be interpreted in the light of clinical circumstances and in comparison to previous results, if available. Finally, the clinician should also assess the underlying disease and precipitating cause(s) of the acute respiratory failure.

Conceptually, the treatment of acute respiratory failure differs little from that of acute failure of other systems—that is, to support the failed system while maintaining the functioning of all other systems until the failure is corrected or repaired to functional stability. The treatment can be considered in two phases: (1) support of respiration and circulation, and (2) treatment of precipitating factors and complications.

CHAPTER 248   ACUTE VENTILATORY FAILURE IN CHRONIC OBSTRUCTIVE PULMONARY DISEASE AND NEUROMUSCULAR DISEASES

Ventilatory Failure in Chronic Obstructive Pulmonary Disease

Patients with COPD generally live precariously balanced between deteriorated muscle function and an altered mechanical load. Muscle dysfunction results from alterations in the chest configuration and shortening and flattening of the diaphragm. A shortened diaphragm cannot generate a good contractile force, a problem only worsened by its loss of curvature. The mechanical load comprises the airway characteristics (resistance) and characteristics of the lung parenchyma and the chest wall (elastance).

Airway and parenchymal alterations in COPD lead to ventilation-perfusion (V/Q) mismatching. Perfusion of unventilated alveoli leads to hypoxemia. Ventilation of unperfused or underperfused alveoli increases dead space (V_d). As disease worsens, V_d increases and a higher proportion of the tidal volume (V_t) ventilates the V_d; alveolar ventilation (V_A) falls (since $V_A = V_t - V_d$). A rise in total ventilation (V_E) can compensate for a declining V_A, provided the mechanical load can be overcome by increased respiratory muscle work. Normal resting humans devote roughly 1% of the cardiac output to supply working respiratory muscles; the energy equivalent of this is called **"work of breathing."** Work of breathing rises several-fold to overcome the increased mechanical load. Increased work of breathing diverts a disproportionate amount of cardiac output to the respiratory muscles. In the patient with COPD, increased muscle work often causes respiratory muscle fatigue or worsens it if it is already present. If, however, the V_E cannot increase, the abnormal V_d/V_t ratio causes hypercapnia.

The hypercapnia triggers (renal) retention of bicarbonate, which offsets the acidosis of hypercapnia, and hypoxemia triggers tissue as well as other adaptive mechanisms to improve the oxygen delivery. When hypoxemia and hypercapnia evolve insidiously and fulfill the criteria for respiratory failure, a state of chronic respiratory failure prevails. While acute ventilatory failure in COPD often represents a further escalation of this entity, prior chronic respiratory failure may not have prevailed in others. Although the mechanical load and the muscle function are liable to many influences, the most important precipitating condition is airway infection, followed by congestive cardiac failure, bronchospasm (often from medication noncompliance), pulmonary embolism, and pneumothorax. The typical manifestations are increasing dyspnea, worsening exercise intolerance, and, as the gas exchange worsens, changes in mental status. Besides tachypnea, cyanosis, respiratory distress, and depressed sensorium, signs of right-sided heart failure may also be present.

■ Management

Oxygen therapy

The priorities are to assure adequate oxygenation and ventilation. **Controlled oxygen therapy** is the cornerstone of managing ventilatory failure in COPD. Oxygen should be used as a drug in the appropriate dose. The correct dose of oxygen is the dose that satisfies the oxygen needs of the tissues. Too little oxygen places the patient at risk for vital organ dysfunction, damage, and death while too much oxygen may cause progressive hypercapnia, CO_2 narcosis, and acidosis. Because tissue oxygenation is not directly measurable, the PaO_2 remains the most useful measure.

Because of the shape of the **oxyhemoglobin dissociation curve**—that is, the oxygen tension/saturation relationship—relatively small rises in PaO_2 lead to a substantial increase in oxygen saturation and, thus, CaO_2. An acceptable PaO_2 to aim for in this context is one between 50 and 60 mm Hg, achieved by using a Venturi mask or a nasal cannula. Venturi masks can deliver oxygen at inspired concentrations of 24–35% (fiO_2 0.24–0.35). Oxygen can also be given using nasal cannula at a low flow of 1–2 L/minute, each liter of supplemental oxygen raising the fiO_2 by nearly 0.04 points (4%). Compared with the mask, a nasal cannula delivers oxygen uninterruptedly even when the patient is eating or talking; however, the fiO_2 cannot be adjusted as precisely with cannula as it can with a Venturi mask. A modest hypercapnia (10–12 mm Hg) often follows oxygen treatment, which in itself is neither a cause for discontinuing oxygen nor a cause for initiating mechanical ventilation.

If possible, endotracheal intubation and mechanical ventilation should be avoided in COPD patients because of the associated complications and because of the difficulty in liberating the patient from the ventilator. However, with uncontrolled oxygen therapy, or in some cases even with controlled oxygen therapy, hypercapnia and acidosis may escalate. Controlled oxygen therapy may also fail in initially severely hypoxemic and acidotic patients or when ventilatory drive is depressed (e.g., central nervous system (CNS) depressants). Although many criteria have been proposed for intubation and mechanical ventilation (see Table 248.1), evaluation over a period of time of changes in mental status (confusion, restlessness), effectiveness of cough mechanism, and changes in arterial blood gases is more helpful than any particular criterion in making a decision.

For mechanical ventilatory assistance, a volume-cycled ventilator is used to deliver a tidal volume of 8–10 ml/kg and an inspiratory/expiratory (I/E) time ratio of 1:3 or greater. The respiratory rate (RR) should be adjusted to maintain an appropriate I/E ratio. In making any adjustment in the ventilator setting (fiO_2, V_t, RR), the goal of mechanical ventilation is to maintain arterial blood gas tensions that existed at a previous stable state, if known, but not necessarily to normalize them. With the availability of low-pressure cuffed tubes, strict deadlines need not be followed for performing a tracheostomy. However, it is appropriate to evaluate the need for it if prolonged (>1–2 weeks) mechanical ventilation is anticipated. A list of monitoring aids in respiratory failure is shown in Table 248.2.

Any precipitating factors should be treated and all reversible elements corrected. The role of bronchodilators, corticosteroids, and antibiotics is discussed in the treatment of exacerbations of COPD in chapter 221. Optimal tracheobronchial secretion clearance should be

TABLE 248.2.	Monitoring Aids in Respiratory Failure

- Arterial blood gases: PaO_2, $PaCO_2$, $P(A-a)O_2$
- Mixed venous oxygen tension ($P\bar{v}O_2$)
- Hematocrit and hemoglobin
- Electrolyte status, intake and output, daily weight
- Tidal volume, minute ventilation
- Endotracheal tube cuff pressure
- Vital capacity
- Maximum static inspiratory pressure (P_iMax)[a]
- Chest x-rays
- Bedside pulmonary artery catheterization
- Electrocardiogram
- Lung compliance
- Shunt fraction (Qs/Qt)

[a]Synonymous with inspiratory force, negative inspiratory force, or maximum inspiratory force, etc.

achieved with inhaled bronchodilators; the patient should then assume a sitting posture, and coughing should be encouraged. This approach could be supplemented by nasotracheal suctioning. Adequate nutritional support, progressively increasing sitting periods, and early ambulation are important but generally are not stressed enough.

Bedside assessment is necessary to determine when to initiate weaning. In general, a period of 24 to 48 hours of ventilatory assistance is necessary to "rest" the fatigued respiratory muscles. Premature discontinuation could easily lead to a recurrence of muscle fatigue. Many criteria for weaning are suggested (Table 248.1), but none is appropriate for all instances. The patient should be alert and responsive, with an improved and stabilized clinical condition, and oxygenation should be adequate at an fiO_2 of <0.4 (40%). A trial of spontaneous breathing or intermittent mandatory ventilation or pressure support may be used for weaning. Several hours of this trial should precede the extubation. In the immediate postextubation period, the patient should avoid eating and drinking because of the danger of aspiration. Intensive respiratory care, including attention to secretion clearance by cough and postural drainage, are of paramount importance in the first 24–48 hours after extubation.

TABLE 248.1.	Criteria for Mechanical Ventilatory Assistance	
Respiratory rate		>35
Vital capacity (ml/kg)		<10
Inspiratory force (cm H_2O)		−25 or less
PaO_2 (mm Hg)		<50 on room air
		<70 on mask oxygen
$P(A-a)O_2$ (mm Hg)		>450 on 100% oxygen
$PaCO_2$ (mm Hg)		>55 (with acidosis)
V_d/V_t		>0.60

Note: Reverse of these criteria may be used for eligibility for weaning.

Acute Ventilatory Failure in Neuromuscular Diseases

The common causes of neuromuscular respiratory failure are Guillain-Barre syndrome, myasthenia gravis, and demyelinating, degenerative, or infectious neuromuscular diseases. Ventilatory failure may occur even despite normal lungs and airways in these disorders. Often, weakness of inspiratory muscles and a poor cough mechanism are responsible. Chronic hypoxemia and cor pulmonale are generally not seen in neuromuscular respiratory failure. Acute, chronic, or periodic bouts of ventilatory failure may be seen in spinal cord and myoneural junction diseases.

Management

Respiratory muscle paralysis may be very subtle, yet has the potential to progress rapidly and culminate in a respiratory arrest. For that reason, clinical assessment and blood gases alone are not reliable; measurements that can assess respiratory muscle function—for example, vital capacity (VC) and maximum inspiratory pressure (P_i max)—should be regularly monitored. Intubation and mechanical ventilation are indicated when the VC falls to twice the predicted tidal volume or $P_i$max falls below -20 cm H_2O (measured by an aneroid pressure manometer). Dysphagia, maximum expiratory pressure ($P_e$max) of <40 cm H_2O, and hypercapnia are also indications for mechanical ventilatory support. Ventilator management approximates that used for a COPD patient in ventilatory failure, except that ventilation is more easily achieved, complications are less common, and tracheostomy is more often necessary. Physical therapy also plays an important role in the management of these patients.

CHAPTER **249** ADULT RESPIRATORY DISTRESS SYNDROME

Definition

Adult respiratory distress syndrome (ARDS) includes an array of features, namely, progressive respiratory distress, severe hypoxemia refractory to oxygen supplementation, diffuse pulmonary infiltrates, lack of another credible mechanism for these findings, and an antecedent major medical or surgical illness or trauma. The pulmonary infiltrates are due to edema, which is noncardiogenic, as evidenced by normal left ventricular filling pressures. The term **acute lung injury** has recently become synonymous with ARDS. Acute lung injury incorporates noncardiogenic pulmonary edema of *all degrees of severity,* but ARDS describes a subset with severe, acute lung injury. In contrast to respiratory failure in COPD, oxygenation failure generally requiring mechanical ventilation is the key issue in ARDS.

Pathogenesis and Pathology

Many clinical states lead to ARDS (Table 249.1), albeit with different relative risk levels (Figure 249.1). Following a systemic or pulmonary injury, leukocytes and macrophages are activated. Endothelial cells are injured from their mediators (tumor necrosis factor, proteases, prostaglandins, oxygen radicals, leukotrienes, platelet activating factor, and interleukin [IL]-1). Capillary integrity is damaged and its permeability enhanced. This excessive capillary permeability is widespread—thus the notion of ARDS as a "pan-endothelial" disease. Interstitial and alveolar pulmonary edema follow, with inactivation of surfactant. Lung compliance and volume decline. Edema, congestion, hemorrhage, microatelectasis, and microvascular thromboses are pulmonary pathologic findings. In later stages, alveoli fill with granulation tissue. Capillaries and myofibroblasts migrate into the alveoli, causing intra-alveolar fibrosis.

Clinical Features

Sepsis syndrome has emerged as the most frequent predisposing illness to ARDS (Figure 249.1). If trauma is the predisposing illness, the initial shock and resuscitation is often followed by a latent period of stability before acute lung injury sets in rather dramatically. This stability is deceptive, because fever, tachypnea, respiratory alkalosis, a widened alveolar-arterial oxygen gradient P(A-aO_2), and often hypoxemia, are usually present during this period, although the chest x-rays are generally normal. As ARDS develops, progressive dyspnea, intercostal retractions, rhonchi, and râles develop, along with progressive, diffuse pulmonary infiltration on x-rays

TABLE 249.1.	Clinical States Predisposing to ARDS
General	**Specific**
Infections	Pneumonias from viral, bacterial or fungal agents
	Miliary tuberculosis
Inhalation injury	Smoke inhalation
	Oxygen toxicity
	Hydrocarbon ingestion
	Aspiration of gastric acid
	Near drowning
Trauma	
Shock	Hemorrhagic or septic
Fat embolism	
Narcotic and illicit drug overdose	
Pancreatitis	
Neurogenic pulmonary edema	
Postcardiopulmonary bypass	

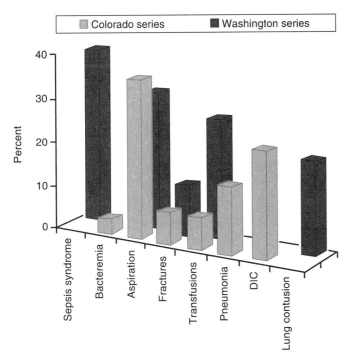

FIGURE **249.1.** The risk of adult respiratory distress syndrome (ARDS) in various predisposing conditions from two large series. Aspiration: aspiration of gastric acid. Pneumonia: pneumonia developing in the intensive care unit. Transfusions: defined as multiple (hyper) transfusions ≥10 units in 24 hours in Colorado series and ≥10 units in 6 hours in Washington series.
(Modified from: Fowler AA et al. Ann Intern Med 1983;99:593–598, Colorado series; Pepe PE et al. Am J Surg 1982;144:124-130, Washington series. Used with permission.)

(Figure 249.2). Hypocapnia and refractory hypoxemia are evident at this time. As illness advances, CO_2 retention and a combined metabolic and respiratory acidosis evolve, which are ominous.

Diagnosis

Suspicion is critical to the diagnosis of ARDS. The presence of a disease with the potential for ARDS (see Table 249.1) should arouse suspicion about the likelihood of its development. Frank hypoxemia and/ or widening of the $P(A-aO_2)$ during an acute severe medical or surgical illness often herald early ARDS, and should be pursued with serial blood gas analysis, chest x-rays, and oxygen therapy. ARDS cannot be differentiated clinically or on the basis of an x-ray from cardiogenic pulmonary edema. Bedside pulmonary artery catheterization is the only reliable means to making this distinction, but it may not always be necessary. Uniform criteria have been proposed for grading the severity of ARDS.

Management

The major objectives are to stabilize the patient, ensure adequate tissue oxygenation, adequately treat the underlying process, and recognize and manage complication(s). Hypoxemia is refractory and a progressive increase in inhaled oxygen concentrations (fiO_2) is necessary to achieve acceptable oxygenation. For alert

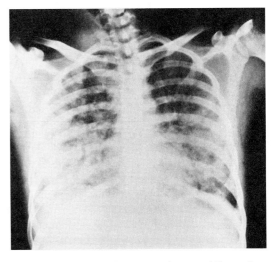

FIGURE **249.2.** ARDS: chest x-ray showing diffuse pulmonary opacification. ARDS followed IV abuse of ethchlorvynol (Placidyl).

and cooperative patients, at least initially, noninvasive pressure-mask ventilation is appropriate. These tight-fitting face masks often cause aerophagia and vomiting; the vomit can suffocate the obtunded. General indications for mechanical ventilation are shown in Table 248.1; however, most cases will ultimately require it. Thus, early anticipation and "elective" endotracheal intubation are appropriate when mental status and/or gas exchange progressively decline. Mechanical ventilation is only supportive; no specific type or mode (the usual modes are shown in Table 249.2) is superior.

Being very tachypneic, patients with ARDS usually require sedation and/or muscle relaxants when mechanically ventilated. One should aim for a satisfactory oxygenation—that is, a PaO_2 of 60–65 mm Hg (or PO_2, if monitored, of 35–40 mm Hg), using the lowest possible fiO_2. Varying criteria exist for the application of positive end-expiratory pressure. We use the "least PEEP," defined as just enough PEEP, generally below 10 cm H_2O but not exceeding 15, to maintain a PaO_2 at a previously specified level. These levels of PEEP call for less fluid administration to offset the hypotensive effect of PEEP and, consequently, less need for invasive monitoring. PEEP, started at an initial level of 5 cm H_2O, is increased in increments of 3–5 cm until a desired response is obtained. Finally, in order to avoid barotrauma, clinicians increasingly favor ventilation modes with lower peak and plateau airway pressures, lower tidal volumes, and consequently, a somewhat elevated $PaCO_2$ ("permissive hypercapnia"). With improving lung function—that is,

steady PaO_2, decreasing fiO_2, $P(A\text{-}a\ O_2)$, and shunt fraction— weaning may be initiated.

Other important objectives in ARDS management are meticulous control of fluid and electrolytes, skilled nursing care, control of infection, and treatment of underlying conditions. Careful diuresis to reduce extravascular lung water should be balanced against the need for fluid to counteract the hypotension from PEEP. The lung injury in ARDS is a pan-endothelial disease, encompassing other organ failure(s), the extent and severity of which vary. Such failing organs should be properly supported. When the gut fails, its compromised mucosal integrity causes bacteremias. Preventing further episodes of sepsis, drainage of any localized abscesses, and, in the case of the trauma patient, definitive treatment of long bone fractures are all important goals.

■ Prognosis

The outcomes of ARDS range from complete recovery to severe disability to death (Table 249.3). ARDS from various causes also carries varying prognoses (e.g., ARDS from fat embolism carries a relatively good prognosis compared with the one from sepsis syndrome), which underscores the importance of identifying and treating the underlying cause. Among those who recover, 50–75% suffer residual pulmonary dysfunction. Pulmonary function improves more rapidly during the first 3–6 months after recovery and more gradually in the next 6 months; the outlook for recovery is, therefore, better in the first year than thereafter. Residual impairments, in the order of frequency, are a reduced DL_{CO}, airflow obstruction, and a restrictive ventilatory impairment. Tracheal stenosis related to endotracheal intubation may also cause symptoms. Patients who recover from ARDS should have ongoing, regular follow-up.

TABLE 249.2.	Commonly Applied Ventilator Settings in ARDS
Tidal volume (V_t)	7–10 ml/kg
Setting	Assist-Control
Resp. rate	12–20 (highly variable)
fiO_2	1.0 initially, titrated along with PEEP to keep PaO_2 between 60 and 65 mm Hg
I:E ratio	1:2 to 1:4
PEEP	5–15 cm H_2O

PEEP = positive end-expiratory pressure; fiO_2 = fraction of inspired oxygen; I:E ratio = inspiratory:expiratory ratio.

TABLE 249.3.	Prognostic Factors in ARDS	
Criterion	**Favorable**	**Unfavorable**
Age	<40	>40
Nonpulmonary organ failure	None	One or more
Etiology	Postoperative state	Sepsis syndrome
	Transfusion-related	Trauma
	Fat embolism	
$C\text{-}_{stat}$ on day 3[a]	>50	<25
PaO_2/fiO_2 on day 3	>250	<150
Secondary bacteremia/sepsis	None	Present

[a]C_{stat} = static compliance.

SLEEP-DISORDERED BREATHING

Sleep-disordered breathing includes a variety of breathing disturbances that occur during sleep, exemplified by snoring, hypoventilation, apnea, increased upper airway resistance, Cheyne-Stokes' breathing, and nocturnal asthma.

This chapter is devoted to a discussion of obstructive sleep apnea and central sleep apnea as well as their pathophysiology and management.

Sleep Apnea

■ Definition

Sleep apnea (SA), defined as cessation of airflow (apnea) for 10 or more seconds during sleep, may arise from an obstruction to airflow at the upper airway (**obstructive sleep apnea**), from decreased respiratory muscle action (**central apnea**), or a combination of the two (**mixed or combined sleep apnea**). Mixed apneas are most common, followed by the obstructive and then central types. The term "hypopnea" (also similarly classified as mixed, obstructive, and central types) describes a significant reduction in ventilation during sleep rather than a total cessation of it. Detection and categorization of these disorders require polygraphic studies obtained during sleep. Arterial hypoxemia often follows apnea and hypopnea; however, its severity depends on the type (obstructive versus central) and duration of apnea, on the state of sleep—rapid eye movement (REM) versus non-REM phase—in which apnea or hypopnea occurs, and, finally, on the extent of associated lung disease and/or prior gas exchange abnormalities.

Obstructive Sleep Apnea

■ Pathogenesis

The upper airway walls have many muscles, which dilate or constrict its lumen. The tonic activity of dilator muscles maintains the lumen's potency during wakefulness, while their hypotonicity during sleep causes it to narrow. In obstructive sleep apnea (OSA), this physiologic collapse of the upper airway is magnified. It worsens when the patient is in a supine position, and it is prevented by mechanical activity of the upper airway muscles. Anatomic abnormalities, such as fat deposition, enlarged tonsils, or enlarged and hypertrophied uvula may further exacerbate the airway narrowing.

Upper airway size is determined by a balance of forces: pharyngeal muscles dilate the upper airway, whereas forces generated by the chest wall muscles constrict it. When ventilatory stimulation is low, chest wall inspiratory muscle activity predominates over that of inspiratory muscles of the upper airway, causing a diminution in upper airway lumen. However, when the ventilation is stimulated, the situation is reversed and the inspiratory muscles of the upper airway prevail; consequently, the upper airway caliber increases. The result, as shown in Figure 250.1, is similar to what occurs in OSA. During sleep, high and low ventilatory drives alternate and periods of normal ventilation, hypopnea, and apnea result—leading to periods of arousal and sleep in the OSA patient, which fragment sleep architecture.

Apneic spells lead to hypoxemia, desaturation of hemoglobin, and elevations in pulmonary and systemic arterial pressures. In some cases, there is left ventricular dysfunction, causing elevation of pulmonary capillary wedge pressures and pulmonary congestion, thus aggravating the hypoxemia. Cardiac arrhythmias are quite common during these sleep-wake cycles, with bradycardia during apnea and tachycardia on resumption of ventilation.

■ Clinical Features and Diagnosis

OSA is very common. Despite its distinct clinical features (see Table 250.1), it may merely be an expression of many other clinical disorders including nasal obstruction, tongue enlargement (macroglossia), jaw and pharyngeal abnormalities, laryngeal obstruction, acromegaly, Cushing's disease or syndrome, goiter, hypothyroidism, and obesity. Both obstruction and the sleep fragmentation cause OSA symptoms. Interview of the spouse or bed partner is crucial to elicit a history of obstructive events. **Loud snoring** of many, many years often underlies marital discord or other social problems. **Sleep fragmentation** causes excessive sleepiness (**daytime hypersomnolence**), the severity of which may vary. While the "fat boy" from Charles Dickens' *Pickwick Papers* represents a flagrant form of OSA, less severe forms may present with accidents at work or while operating an automobile. They may also be deceptively benign—for example, falling off to sleep

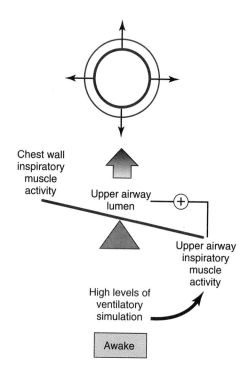

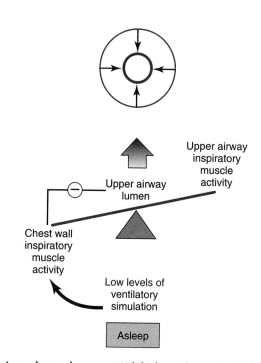

FIGURE 250.1. The balance of forces in sleep apnea. With low ventilatory stimulation (right side of diagram), the pump action generated by the chest wall inspiratory muscles [shown by (−) sign] collapses the upper airway. The upper airway lumen decreases. With high ventilatory stimulation (left side), the airway lumen dilates.
(Modified from: Hudgel DW. Chest 1992;101:541-549. Used with permission.)

TABLE 250.1.	**Clinical Features of Obstructive Sleep Apnea**

Excessive daytime sleepiness
Obesity
Loud snoring or apnea (usually reported by spouse/bed partner)
Hypertension
Nocturnal or morning headaches
Impotence
Nocturnal enuresis
Violent movements, mistaken for seizures
Personality changes
Changes in mental status
Dementia
Postanesthetic respiratory failure
Inability to wean from a mechanical ventilator
Laboratory abnormalities
  Polycythemia
  Proteinuria rarely in the nephrotic range

Patients occasionally perceive arousals as gasping or choking. The intellectual decline, personality changes, and the morning headache may simulate an intracranial tumor and/or space-occupying lesion. Impotence is another symptom, albeit with an unclear pathogenesis.

In many cases, physical examination is normal, and consequently, a normal physical examination does not exclude OSA. Other patients may present with obesity, a short, fat neck, congestion, edema and swelling of the uvula, or jowls around the jaw and upper neck. The clinician should look carefully for anatomic abnormalities mentioned previously, since their correction may be followed by clinical improvement or cure. Systemic hypertension, drowsiness, pulmonary hypertension, and/or cor pulmonale are other possible findings.

Laboratory studies may show elevated $PaCO_2$ and, in some cases, erythrocytosis. While OSA from acromegaly is self-evident at presentation, it is important to remember that OSA from hypothyroidism may remain clinically inapparent; thyroid function should, therefore, be evaluated in all cases of OSA.

Central Sleep Apnea

True, isolated central sleep apnea (CSA) is uncommon. It may especially follow encephalitis, poliomyelitis, and

while watching a (favorite) television show. Sometimes, patients misinterpret sleep fragmentation as insomnia. The consequent self-administration of ethanol or prescription of a hypnotic merely worsens the obstruction.

head trauma. The classification of CSA is based on $PaCO_2$ while awake, into hypercapnic and nonhypercapnic subsets. In contrast to OSA patients, those with CSA usually perceive awakenings from sleep. They may complain of an inability to fall off to sleep. Fatigue, depression, and sexual dysfunction have been reported. Apneic events may be reported by the spouse or the bed partner. Physical examination generally is normal. Episodes of hypoxemia during apneic spells in CSA are less severe than those in OSA.

■ Diagnosis

Although the clinical history may strongly suggest SA, confirmation and classification of its type require polysomnograms. The extent of desaturation can be determined and the apnea index (AI, the number of apneic spells per hour, also called RDI, respiratory disturbance index) calculated, which has been shown to influence prognosis. Besides, the severity of the abnormalities noted may affect the immediate management. Finally, these studies also offer the opportunity to apply therapy as well as to titrate its dose and directly observe the effects. Both types of SA characteristically involve cessation of airflow at the mouth and nostrils. However, diaphragmatic and intercostal muscle activity, which are absent during apnea in CSA, are noted in OSA.

■ Management and Prognosis

Untreated OSA, especially with a high AI (RDI), carries a high mortality. The general management of OSA is shown in Figure 250.2. The patient should stop using alcohol and/or hypnosedatives. In obese patients, weight

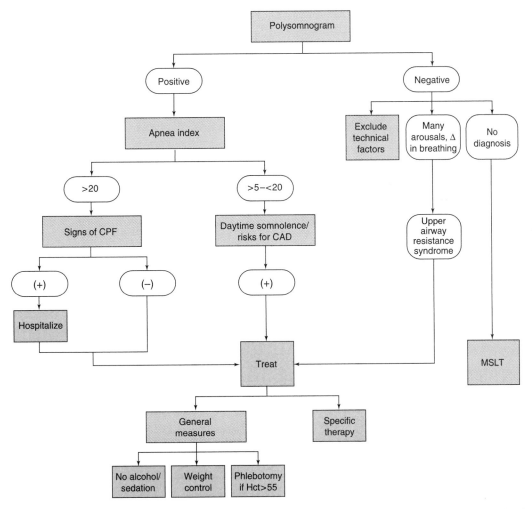

FIGURE 250.2. General management of obstructive sleep apnea. See text for discussion. Abbreviations: (+) = present; (−) = absent; CPF = cardiopulmonary failure; CAD = coronary artery disease; Δ = change; MSLT = multiple sleep latency test.

reduction is a useful general measure, but it is difficult to accomplish and arduous to sustain. Certain tasks, such as driving, may be impaired when OSA is left untreated. Statutes regarding the reporting requirements for driver impairments vary from state to state; physicians should contact the motor vehicle department in their state to find out which impairments must be reported.

Application of continuous positive pressure to the airway (CPAP) through the nose (NCPAP) or via a tight-fitting face mask is effective. Being easy to apply and titrate, it is the initial therapy for all patients with OSA with an AI of 20 or greater and for those with an AI between 5 and 20 when accompanied by daytime hypersomnolence. CPAP presumably stabilizes the upper airway, but its mechanism of action is speculative. Ideally, during the initial sleep study, the level of pressure needed to eliminate apneic episodes should be determined, which is usually between 7.5 and 12.5 cm H_2O. Some patients may not tolerate CPAP and such patients should undergo evaluation by a physician with expertise in the management of sleep disorders.

Other approaches are removal of redundant palatal and pharyngeal tissue (uvulopalatopharyngoplasty [UPPP]), progesterone, tricyclic antidepressants, and tracheostomy. UPPP uniformly relieves snoring and in many cases resolves the OSA. However, very skilled postoperative care is required, so the procedure should be performed only in institutions with proven experience. OSA in hypothyroidism responds quite well to thyroxine. Tracheostomy, the most definitive treatment, is socially and psychologically unacceptable for OSA.

Treatment of CSA is less than satisfactory, although variable successes have been reported with progestational agents and tricyclic antidepressants. For those with hypercapnia while awake, intermittent positive pressure ventilation administered through a tight-fitting nasal mask may be useful during sleep. In those with nonhypercapnic CSA, a trial of CPAP is worthwhile, since it can be effective if tolerated.

■ Questions

Instructions: For each question below, select only **one** lettered answer that is the **best** for that question.

1. A 60-year-old man has recently worsening dyspnea and a long history of productive cough, sputum production, frequent wheezing, and a 55-pack-year smoking history. He is on no medications. He is alert and in moderate respiratory distress. The pulse is 100/min; respirations, 29/min; and BP 190/95 mm Hg. Diffuse wheezing and mild lower-extremity edema are noted. Hemoglobin is 18.0g and hematocrit is 53%. The initial PaO_2 is 35 mm Hg; $PaCO_2$,

85 mm Hg; and pH, 7.28. One hour after oxygen and bronchodilator, he is alert and responsive. Pulse is 95/min; BP, 170/92 mm Hg; and respiration, 26/min. The pH is 7.26; $PaCO_2$, 90 mm Hg; and PaO_2, 54 mm Hg. Which of the following will you do now?
   A. Increase the oxygen dose and repeat blood gases in 1 hour.
   B. Administer aerosolized albuterol now; repeat blood gases in 1 hour.
   C. Arrange for endotracheal intubation, because of the rise in $PaCO_2$.
   D. Continue present management.

2. On the night of an elective cholecystectomy and common bile duct exploration, a 68-year-old woman develops sudden respiratory distress. She had quit chronic, heavy smoking 2 weeks previously. Her pulse is 120/min; BP, 160/90 mm Hg, respirations, 34/min, and temperature, 99° F. Breath sounds are normal and symmetrical, with diffuse end-inspiratory rales. Heart sounds are distant but otherwise normal. Her pH is 7.32; $PaCO_2$, 32 mm Hg; and PaO_2, 46 mm Hg. No preoperative blood gas results are available. Which of the following entities is MOST likely now?
   A. Acute exacerbation of chronic obstructive pulmonary disease.
   B. Atelectasis due to pain and secretions.
   C. Acute pulmonary edema.
   D. Acute respiratory failure from massive pleural effusion.
   E. Acute, submassive pulmonary embolism.

3. Besides administering oxygen, which of the following will you do now?
   A. Give analgesia to control pain and take measures to effect lung expansion.
   B. Perform an immediate ventilation-perfusion lung scan.
   C. Get consent for and proceed to thoracentesis.
   D. Give morphine sulfate and furosemide; perform 12-lead ECG.
   E. Give ipratropium bromide by hand-held nebulizer and IV corticosteroids.

4. A 25-year-old man is found comatose. His pulse rate is 130/min; respiratory rate, 28/min; BP 100/50 mm Hg; and temperature, 103° F. Trachea is deviated to the left. Movement and percussion note are diminished and breath sounds are absent in the left lower chest posteriorly. The entire lower half of the left chest is opacified on chest x-ray. His arterial blood gases initially are as follows: pH, 7.35; PaO_2, 48; $PaCO_2$, 50. After oxygen (15L/min by non-

rebreathing mask) his arterial blood gases are: pH, 7.36; PaO_2, 56; $PaCO_2$, 50. Which ONE of the following best represents your assessment?

A. Acute ventilatory and oxygenation failure related to ARDS.

B. He has acute, predominantly oxygenation failure due to left lower lobe atelectasis.

C. Acute, predominantly oxygenation failure due to a large left pleural effusion, which is very likely an empyema.

D. Acute, predominantly oxygenation failure due to pneumonia.

5. Which one of the following best explains the hypoxemia in the patient described in question 4?

A. It is caused by ventilation-perfusion abnormalities.

B. It is entirely explained by the hypoventilation.

C. It is caused by left-to-right shunting.

D. It is related to a severe diffusion abnormality.

E. It is caused by right-to-left shunting.

6. A 58-year-old man has had productive cough, almost daily wheezing, and progressive exertional dyspnea for the last 5 years. He is a smoker. Which ONE of the following sets of tests best fits his condition?

	FVC (L)	$FEV_{1.0}$ (L)	DL_{CO} (observed/ predicted)	PaO_2	$PaCO_2$
A.	3.5	2.95	12/24	55	35
B.	3.75	3.50	14/24	65	28
C.	3.1	1.01	15/24	58	49
D.	3.8	3.5	22/24	79	44

7. Which of the following will you now recommend for management of the patient described in question 6?

A. Long-term, low-flow oxygen; ipratropium bromide (2 puffs every 4-6 hours); smoking cessation.

B. Long-term, low-flow oxygen; sustained release theophylline (300 mg b.i.d.), and albuterol by metered dose inhaler (2 puffs q.i.d.).

C. All items in (B) above plus cessation of smoking and avoidance of atmospheric irritants.

D. All items in (C) above plus antibiotics when sputum changes in color or when symptoms indicate respiratory infection.

8. A businessman has a hematocrit of 61% and hemoglobin of 20.0 g. He has noted morning headaches, but no cough, sputum, or wheezing. He is a nonsmoker. Obesity, swelling, and redness of the uvula and mild lower-extremity edema are noted. Which of the following data would match his clinical situation?

	PA pressure	PCW	PaO_2	$PaCO_2$	pH
A.	48/30	20	76	38	7.48
B.	58/30	12	70	35	7.39
C.	52/28	22	55	44	7.34
D.	50/28	8	50	48	7.34

(PA = pulmonary artery; PCW = pulmonary capillary wedge pressure).

9. What would you recommend now for managing the patient described in question 8?

A. Furosemide, 40 mg; digoxin, 0.25 mg; theophylline, 600 mg; all daily.

B. Furosemide, 40 mg, and digoxin, 0.25 mg daily; albuterol metered dose inhaler, 2 puffs q.i.d.

C. Evaluation through a polysomnogram.

D. Captopril, 12.5 mg q 6 h; and oxygen, 2 L/min.

10. A 20-year-old student has had episodic wheezing, productive cough, and febrile episodes for the last several years, with further worsening in the last 18 months. He does not smoke. A family history of atopic disease is noted. His symptoms improved briefly after a course of tetracycline. Chest x-ray shows a left upper-lobe infiltrate with cystic lucencies and a non homogeneous right lower-zone infiltrate. Which ONE of the following studies would be most helpful?

A. Tuberculin skin test.

B. A histoplasmin skin test.

C. Sweat chloride level.

D. Serum α-1 antitrypsin level.

11. In which of the following situations will you prescribe mini (low-dose) heparin therapy to prevent development of deep venous thrombosis?

A. Elderly man with a prior history of DVT having a cataract surgery.

B. Elderly woman undergoing a colectomy for cancer.

C. Middle-aged woman having a craniotomy for meningioma excision.

D. All of the above.

E. None of the above.

12. A 55-year-old asymptomatic steam fitter has a new, uncalcified 2-cm left upper lobe solitary nodule. He has a 50 pack-year history of smoking. Review of systems is normal. A PPD skin test shows 13 mm induration at 48 hours. Urinalysis, liver function tests, and complete blood counts are normal. The MOST appropriate management for this patient is:

A. Abdominal CT, barium enema, and upper GI series, in that order.

B. Careful follow-up every 3 months with chest x-rays.

C. Six months of isoniazid with pyridoxine.

D. Thoracotomy and resection of nodule.

13. A 25-year-old African American man has redness and swelling involving the shins bilaterally, fever, dry cough, and arthralgias. A chest x-ray shows bilateral hilar and paratracheal lymphadenopathy. Which of the following abnormalities is most compatible with his diagnosis?

A. Increased sedimentation rate and increased peripheral T-lymphocytes.

B. Increased B-lymphocytes and decreased T-lymphocytes (both in the lung).

C. Serum calcium of 12.5 mg/dl.

D. Positive tuberculin skin test.

14. What is the most appropriate management for the patient in question 13?

A. Bronchoscopy, transbronchial lung biopsy; no corticosteroids.

B. Bronchoscopy, transbronchial lung biopsy, and corticosteroids.

C. Lymph node biopsy through mediastinoscopy.

D. Open lung biopsy.

15. A reduced pleural fluid glucose of 30 mg/100 ml (simultaneous plasma glucose 105 mg/100 ml) is consistent with a diagnosis of effusion caused by:

A. pancreatitis.

B. rheumatoid arthritis.

C. nephrotic syndrome.

D. hepatic cirrhosis.

16. In a patient with myasthenia gravis, which of the following can help the physician decide whether to use mechanical ventilatory assistance?

A. Forced vital capacity and maximum inspiratory pressure.

B. Arterial blood gases.

C. $FEV_{1.0.}$

D. Lung compliance.

■ **Answers**

1. D	2. C	3. D	4. B	5. E
6. C	7. A	8. B	9. C	10. C
11. B	12. D	13. C	14. A	15. B
16. A				

SUGGESTED READING

Books and Monographs

Briggs DD et al. Medical Knowledge Self-Assessment Program in the Subspecialty of Pulmonary and Critical Care. Philadelphia: American College of Physicians, 1994.

Centers for Disease Control. Guidelines for Preventing the Transmission of Mycobacterium tuberculosis in Health-Care Facilities, 1994. MMWR. 1994;43:RR13:1–132.

King TE, Jr. Idiopathic Pulmonary Fibrosis. In: Schwarz MI, King TE, Jr. (eds.). Interstitial Lung Disease. 2nd ed. St. Louis: Mosby–Year Book, Inc., 1993, p. 367–403.

Reichman LB, Hershfield ES. Tuberculosis. A Comprehensive International Approach. New York: Marcel Dekker, Inc., 1993.

Sarosi GA, Davies SF. Fungal Diseases of the Lung. 2nd ed. New York: Raven Press, 1993.

Schwarz MI. Clinical Overview of Interstitial Lung Disease. In: Schwarz MI, King TE, Jr., eds. Interstitial Lung Disease. 2nd ed. St. Louis: Mosby–Year Book, Inc., 1993 p. 1–22.

Articles
Clinical Evaluation of Lung Disease

Bartlett JG. Diagnosis of bacterial Infections of the lung. Clin Chest Med 1987;8:119–134.

Braman SS. Pulmonary signs and symptoms. Clin Chest Med 1987;8:177–337.

Braman SS, Corrao WM. Cough: differential diagnosis and treatment. Clin Chest Med 1987;8:177–188.

Braman SS, Corrao WM. Bronchoprovocation testing. Clin Chest Med 1989;10:165–176.

Ettinger NA. Invasive diagnostic approaches to pulmonary infiltrates. Semin Resp Infect 1993;8:168–176.

McPherson D, Buchalter SE. The role of bronchoalveolar lavage in patients considered for open lung biopsy. Clin Chest Med 1992;13:23–31.

Pratter MR, Bartter T, Akers S, et al. An algorithmic approach to chronic cough. Ann Intern Med 1993;119:977–983.

Shure D. Fiberoptic bronchoscopy. Clin Chest Med 1987;8:1–13.

Pulmonary Mycoses and Mycobacterial Diseases

Centers for Disease Control. Initial therapy for tuberculosis in the era of multidrug resistance. Recommendations of the Advisory Council for the Elimination of Tuberculosis. MMWR 1995;42:RR–7:1–8.

Davidson PT. M. avium Complex, M. kansasii, M. fortuitum, and other mycobacteria causing human disease. In: Reichman LB, Hershfield ES (eds.). Tuberculosis. A Comprehensive International Approach. New York: Marcel Dekker, Inc, 1993, pp. 505–530.

Davies SF, Sarosi GA. Epidemiological and clinical features of pulmonary blastomycosis. Semin Resp Infect 1997;12:206–218.

Salfinger M, Morris AJ. The role of the microbiology laboratory in diagnosing mycobacterial diseases. Am J Clin Path 1994;101:S6–13.

Van Scoy RE, Wilkowske CJ. Antituberculous agents. Mayo Clin Proc 1992;67:179–187.

Chronic Obstructive Pulmonary Disease, Cystic Fibrosis, and Bronchiectasis

Aitken ML, Fiel SB. Cystic fibrosis. Dis Mon 1993;39:1–52.

Celli BR. Current thoughts regarding treatment of chronic obstructive pulmonary disease. Med Clin North Am 1996;80:589–609.

Crystal RG. Gene therapy strategies for pulmonary disease. Am J Med 1992;92:44S–52S.

Hagedorn SD. Acute exacerbations of COPD. How to evaluate severity and treat the underlying cause. Postgrad Med 1992;91:105–7.

Marwah OS, Sharma OP. Bronchiectasis. How to identify, treat, and prevent. Postgrad Med 1995;97:149–50.

Meduri GU. Noninvasive positive pressure ventilation in chronic obstructive pulmonary disease patients with acute exacerbation. Crit Care Med 1997;25:1631–1633.

O'Donohue WJ, Jr. Home oxygen therapy. Med Clin North Am 1996; 80:611–22.

Rogers RM, Sciurba FC, Keenan RJ. Lung reduction surgery in chronic obstructive lung disease. Med Clin North Am 1996;80:623–644.

Pulmonary Thromboembolism

Anonymous. Opinions regarding the diagnosis and management of venous thromboembolic disease. ACCP Consensus Committee on Pulmonary Embolism. American College of Chest Physicians. Chest 1998;113:499–504.

Hillarp A, Zoller B, Dahlback B. Activated protein C resistance as a basis for venous thrombosis. Am J Med 1996;101: 534–540.

Hirsh J: Oral anticoagulant drugs. N Engl J Med 1991; 324:1865. Heparin. N Engl J Med 1991;324:1565.

Moser KM: Venous thromboembolism: State of the art. Ann Rev Respir Dis 1990;141:235.

Tapson VF, Hull RD. Management of venous thromboembolic disease. The impact of low-molecular weight heparin. Clin Chest Med. 1995;16:281–294.

Wells PS, Brill-Edwards P, Stevens P, et al. A novel and rapid whole-blood assay for D-dimer in patients with clinically suspected deep vein thrombosis. Circulation 1995;91: 2184–2187.

Interstitial Lung Disease

DeRemee RA. Sarcoidosis. Mayo Clin Proc 1995;70:177–181.

Fink JN. Hypersensitivity pneumonitis. Clin Chest Med 1992; 13:303–309.

King TE, Jr. Respiratory bronchiolitis-associated interstitial lung disease. Clin Chest Med 1993;14:693–698.

Raghu G. Interstitial lung disease: a diagnostic approach: are CT scan and lung biopsy indicated in every patient? Am J Resp Crit Care Med 1995;151:909–914.

Rosiello RA, Merrill WW. Radiation-induced lung injury. Clin Chest Med 1990;11:65–71.

Wiedemann HP, Matthay RA. Pulmonary manifestations of the collagen vascular diseases. Clin Chest Med 1989;10:677–722.

Pulmonary Aspiration Syndromes

Bartlett JG. Anaerobic bacterial infections of the lung and pleural space. Clinical Infectious Diseases 1993;16 Suppl 4:S248–55.

Tietjen PA. Kaner RJ. Quinn CE. Aspiration emergencies. Clin Chest Med 1994;15:117–35.

Drug-induced Lung Disease

Rosenow, ECIII. Drug-induced pulmonary disease. Dis Mon 1994;40:253–310.

Pleural Disease

Light RW. A new classification of parapneumonic effusions and empyema. Chest 1995;108:299–301.

Light RW. Pleural diseases. Dis Mon 1992;38:261–331.

Pistolesi M, Miniati M, Giuntini C. Pleural liquid and solute exchange. Am Rev Resp Dis 1989;140:825–847.

Lung Cancer

Matthay RA. Lung Cancer. Clin Chest Med. 1993;14:1–200.

Viggiano RW, Swensen SJ, Rosenow EC III. Evaluation and management of solitary and multiple pulmonary nodules. Clin Chest Med 1992;13:83–95.

Pulmonary Disease Due to Inorganic Agents

Banks DE, Cheng YH, Weber SL, Ma JK. Strategies for the treatment of pneumoconiosis. Occupational Medicine. 1993; 8:205–32.

Lapp NL, Parker JE. Coal workers' pneumoconiosis. Clin Chest Med. 1992;13:243–52.

Lordi GM, Reichman LB. Pulmonary complications of asbestos exposure. Am Fam Phys. 1993;48:1471–7.

Respiratory Failure

Bone RC. Treatment of respiratory failure due to advanced chronic obstructive lung disease. Arch Int Med 1980;140: 1018–1021.

Curtis JR, Hudson LD. Emergent assessment and management of acute respiratory failure in COPD. Clin Chest Med 1994;15:481–500.

Jasmer RM, Luce JM, Matthay MA. Noninvasive positive pressure ventilation for acute respiratory failure: underutilized or overrated? Chest 1997;111:1672–1678.

Sleep-Disordered Breathing

Hudgel DW. Mechanisms of obstructive sleep apnea. Chest 1992;101:541–549.

Strollo PJ Jr., Rogers RM. Obstructive sleep apnea. N Engl J Med 1996;334:99–104.

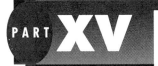

PART XV

Paul B. Halverson

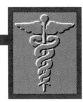

RHEUMATIC DISEASES

■ History

Rheumatic diseases are usually managed in the outpatient setting. Pain is the most common complaint that brings the patient to the doctor, but others include joint swelling or enlargement, stiffness, loss of joint mobility, weakness, and, occasionally, numbness or tingling.

Pain may vary from mild and aching to severe and disabling. Its pattern (intermittent, chronic low-grade, progressive worsening), location, and evolution over time should be determined. Some patients may report episodes of arthritis, but none may be seen on examination. A history of intermittent pain, swelling, and erythema in the great toe may suggest gout.

Sometimes, the main concern is **joint enlargement,** often noticed in the proximal interphalangeal (PIP) and distal interphalangeal (DIP) joints of the hands when osteoarthritis is developing. Joint symptoms and the physical abnormalities of the joints may be discordant, and thus, some joints with advanced joint damage manifest surprisingly little pain. Patients may also report **joint swelling,** which women may perceive as difficulty in removing rings. Sometimes, patients confuse fluid retention or edema with actual joint swelling. Thus, joint swelling must be confirmed by physical examination.

Stiffness, defined as discomfort in attempting to move joints after a period of inactivity, is common to most forms of arthritis. It may still provide some clues about the type and severity of arthritis. Morning stiffness lasting for over 30 minutes (What time do you get up? When are you as good or as loose as you're going to be?) suggests an inflammatory process. While morning stiffness lasting at least 1 hour (but often much longer) is one of the diagnostic criteria for rheumatoid arthritis, it also occurs in most other forms of "inflammatory" arthritis. However, in "noninflammatory" conditions such as osteoarthritis, morning stiffness usually is brief (30 min). Persons with osteoarthritis also report recurrent stiffness throughout the day following periods of inactivity (**gelling**). New-onset, severe morning stiffness in an older individual, even to the point of causing difficulty in getting out of bed, may suggest polymyalgia rheumatica.

Loss of joint motion is likely to be noticed in the shoulders or hands. Impaired glenohumeral motion often results in reduced shoulder abduction and rotation, thus making combing one's hair or dressing difficult. Similarly, making a fist or fully extending the fingers may not be possible.

Although **numbness** and **tingling** suggest a neurologic disorder, they may also reflect musculoskeletal disease. Hand numbness and tingling are common and are most often related to compression of either the median nerve at the wrist or ulnar nerve at the elbow or cervical spine disease. Sciatic pain and tingling or numbness may reflect a **radiculopathy** (disease of the spinal nerve roots), such as may occur with a herniated disc. Buttock pain with radiation down the leg or sensory symptoms associated with walking or standing may suggest neurogenic claudication from spinal stenosis (usually in the elderly). Sometimes, the cause of numbness and tingling in the extremities may be elusive if nerve conduction testing and imaging studies do not correlate.

A feeling of **weakness** is another common complaint that may be difficult to relate to physical findings. Proximal muscle weakness greater than distal weakness is usually due to a myopathic process (e.g., myositis), whereas the reverse is usually true in neurologic diseases.

Although nonspecific, **fatigue** is a frequent component of systemic rheumatic diseases. This fatigue follows activity and does not resolve after rest; the time for its onset after arising correlates inversely with the extent of inflammation. Fatigue on arising is more compatible with fibromyalgia or many nonrheumatic disorders (anemia, cancer, metabolic disorders, sleep apnea, insomnia, or a psychogenic problem).

The physician should assess the patient's reaction to a symptom by exploring its impact on his or her ability to perform activities of daily living, on sleep, employment, mental status, and family relationships. A family history of "arthritis" or "rheumatism" should be clarified to determine the type, disability or deformity, and treatment. A review of systems may provide clues to specific rheumatic syndromes (Table 251.1).

■ Physical Examination

Because rheumatic diseases can affect multiple organs, the physical examination must be thorough. The skin should be examined for rashes (e.g., purpura seen in vasculitis; psoriatic plaques which may be hidden in the hair, umbilicus, or gluteal folds), thickening or tightness, erythema, ulceration or scarring in the fingertips or on the forearms and lower extremities, nail pitting, subcutaneous nodules, or calcifications. The nail folds should be examined, preferably with an ophthalmoscope for magnification, for capillary abnormalities (e.g., giant

TABLE 251.1.	Review of Systems for Clues to Specific Rheumatic Diseases
Systemic	Fever, weight loss
Mucocutaneous	Rash, ulcers, nodules, sun sensitivity, alopecia, oral or genital sores
Head and neck area	Red painful eyes, dry eyes or mouth, jaw claudication
Cardiopulmonary	Pleurisy, cough, dyspnea, Raynaud's phenomenon, edema, claudication
Gastrointestinal	Dysphagia, abdominal pain, diarrhea, bloody stools
Genitourinary	Dysuria, bloody or cloudy urine, urethral discharge
Musculoskeletal	Weakness, myalgias, arthralgias; joint swelling, pain, warmth, redness, or decreased motion
Neurologic	Numbness, paraesthesias, urinary or fecal incontinence, radicular pain, weakness, exercise-induced pain or weakness, seizures, cranial or peripheral nerve abnormalities, visual disturbance, headache, vertigo

loops and reduced numbers of nail fold vessels in scleroderma).

A red eye or ciliary flush suggests conjunctivitis or iritis, respectively. Ulcerations of the nose or mouth and lymphadenopathy should be sought. Pericardial or pleural friction rubs suggest serositis. Dullness to percussion (pleural effusion) and crackles on auscultation (interstitial fibrosis) are important findings in the chest.

All joints and surrounding structures should be examined for tenderness (joints should be squeezed just enough to blanch the examiner's fingernail), swelling, warmth, erythema, limitation of motion, and flexion contractures. Moving the joints actively and passively through a range of motion can detect pain and crepitus (audible or palpable grating or crunching occurring during joint movement). Loss of joint integrity is suggested by instability and deformity. Swelling may follow several processes: joint effusion (most easily assessed in the knee), synovial thickening, periarticular soft tissue inflammation (e.g., bursitis), bony enlargement, or extra-articular fat pads.

Muscle strength and atrophy should be noted, as well as motor and sensory deficits and reflexes. Tapping over a nerve at the site of compression may elicit tingling (e.g., Tinel's sign at the wrist in carpal tunnel syndrome).

Laboratory Tests

Definitive diagnostic tests exist for few rheumatic disorders. In most cases, diagnosis depends on a combination of test results and clinical findings. The history and physical examination remain more essential tools for diagnosis than in most other specialties of medicine. In broad terms, rheumatologic testing includes synovianalysis, serologic tests, imaging and miscellaneous tests (Table 251.2).

Synovianalysis

Arthrocentesis is the process of aspirating synovial fluid from suspicious joints for analysis (**synovianalysis**). Synovial fluid analysis should be performed whenever synovial fluid is obtainable (Table 251.3). The **gross appearance** of synovial fluid can provide important clues about etiology. Clear fluid is noninflammatory and is typical of osteoarthritis, whereas slightly cloudy or translucent fluid with increased cellularity suggests an inflammatory condition (gout or rheumatoid arthritis). Bloody fluid (hemarthrosis) suggests traumatic arthritis, whereas purulent (opaque) fluid suggests septic arthritis.

TABLE 251.2.	Common Laboratory Tests in Rheumatic Diseases
Synovianalysis	**Result**
Appearance	Clear, cloudy
Mucin clot	Intactness of hyaluronic acid
Leukocyte count	>2000 suggests inflammatory arthritis
Polarized light	Monosodium urate, calcium pyrophosphate
Gram stain, culture, glucose	Suspected infection
Serum tests	**Result**
Rheumatoid factor	Present in 80% of patients with RA; 5% false positives
Anti-nuclear antibody	Screening test for autoimmune disease Present in: >95% of patients with SLE >95% of patients with scleroderma 15–50% of patients with RA 15–50% of patients with inflammatory myositis
Complements C_3, C_4	Reduced levels in some patients with SLE, cryoglobulinemia, and some cases of vasculitis
CH_{50}	As above. Also reduced in inherited complement deficiency states

SLE = systemic lupus erythematosus; RA = rheumatoid arthritis.

TABLE 251.3. Synovial Fluid Analysis

	Group 1 (Non-inflammatory)	Group 2 (Inflammatory)	Group 3 (Purulent)
Gross examination			
Color	Yellow	Pink to yellow to white (red if traumatic)	Purulent
Clarity	Transparent	Translucent to opaque	Purulent
Viscosity	High	Medium to low	Low
Mucin clot	Good	Fair	Poor
Microscopic examination			
WBC/mm^3	<2,000	5,000–20,000	>20,000
Neutrophils	<25%	<25-90%	>50%

The synovial fluid **leukocyte count** reflects the degree of inflammation (Table 251.2). Whereas counts exceeding 2,000/mm^3 are considered inflammatory, there are no "diagnostic" cell counts. As the leukocyte count increases, so does the proportion of polymorphonuclear leukocytes (PMN). Synovial fluid from patients with active rheumatoid arthritis, Reiter's syndrome, or gout often contain 30,000 or more cells/mm^3, whereas only 5,000–10,000 cells/mm^3 may be seen in gonococcal arthritis. Very high cell counts are more likely to occur with infection.

The **mucin clot** and **viscosity** tests reflect the intactness of polymeric hyaluronic acid, which gives "noninflammatory" synovial fluid its syrupy consistency. Low viscosity leading to a watery consistency and a poor mucin clot result when hyaluronic acid has been digested by inflammatory enzymes, as in rheumatoid arthritis.

In cases of suspected joint sepsis, useful tests include glucose levels, Gram stain, and culture. Synovianalysis is definitive when compensated **polarized light microscopy** shows crystals or a Gram stain shows microorganisms. Negatively birefringent crystals of **monosodium urate** indicate gout (see Color Plate 32). In acute gout, these needle-shaped crystals are often found inside PMNs. When aligned with the direction of the red compensator, the crystals will appear yellow, and when rotated 90°, they appear blue. Although highly sensitive and specific for gout, gout crystals may rarely coexist with septic or other arthritides. **Calcium pyrophosphate** crystals, in contrast, are positively birefringent, rhomboidal crystals found in pseudogout; they appear blue when aligned with the compensator and yellow when rotated 90° (see Color Plate 33).

matoid factor and antinuclear antibody. These tests are usually ordered when symmetrical joint swelling is suggested by history or observed on examination.

Rheumatoid factor (RF), antibody to the Fc portion of immunoglobulin G, occurs in approximately 80% of rheumatoid arthritis patients (seropositive). Absence of RF, however, does not rule out rheumatoid arthritis, because nearly 20% of patients with the disease are seronegative. RF may also occur in some other types of arthritis and in some chronic inflammatory states (Table 251.4). Rheumatoid factors may consist of any immunoglobulin class, but the agglutination methods used in most diagnostic laboratories detect essentially only pentameric IgM-RF.

The **antinuclear antibody** (ANA) is a screening test for the so-called connective tissue diseases (Table 251.5). Few tests engender more confusion because of the notion that a positive ANA may signify systemic lupus erythematosus (SLE). A negative ANA essentially excludes SLE, because over 95% of SLE patients have a positive ANA; however, a positive ANA by itself does not strongly suggest SLE. With high sensitivity for SLE but only low specificity, ANAs are frequent in other autoimmune diseases (Table 251.5). In addition, 5–15% of normal individuals have ANA, or they may be induced by drugs (e.g., procainamide, hydralazine). A positive ANA test becomes significant only when other features of SLE or another autoimmune disease are found by history, physical examination, other routine laboratory testing or with more specific serologic testing (e.g., antibodies to native DNA or to Smith antigen, which are rare in other conditions). With a positive ANA, tests for other nuclear antigens may help either to confirm or refute diagnoses of other connective tissue diseases.

Serologic studies

The two most often ordered serologic tests in the investigation of rheumatic diseases are the serum rheu-

Other blood tests

The **erythrocyte sedimentation rate** (ESR) has limited diagnostic value, especially in a patient with nonspecific symptoms. However, a markedly high ESR may be the sole laboratory finding in polymyalgia rheumatica or temporal arteritis. As a test of inflammation, some use the ESR to monitor response to therapy in chronic inflammatory arthritides (e.g., rheumatoid arthritis).

The serum **creatine kinase** (CK) may rise in many congenital and acquired inflammatory muscle disorders and may aid in evaluating patients with muscle pain or weakness. Hypothyroidism may also manifest myalgias, arthralgias, weakness, and, in some, an elevated CK.

Serum **complement** may be consumed in immune complex diseases (e.g., lupus nephritis), bacterial endocarditis, mixed or monoclonal cryoglobulinemia, rheumatoid arthritis with vasculitis (rarely), or severe sepsis. Quantitative measurement of C3 and C4 proteins, while readily available, does not distinguish the activated from the unactivated components. Because levels of C3 in closed spaces, such as pleura or joints, and in some sera may represent already activated protein, the **hemolytic assay (CH50)** may be preferred, as it assesses the function of the entire complement cascade. Individual complement components may be congenitally low, the most common being the C2 heterozygous deficiency. Search for a complement component deficiency may be prompted by an absent CH50 with normal or near-normal C3 and C4 levels.

Cryoglobulins (serum proteins which precipitate at 4° C) may occur in many patients with rheumatoid arthritis or SLE. Occasionally, they may be the sole serologic anomaly, as in infective endocarditis or essential cryoglobulinemia.

TABLE 251.4. Rheumatoid Factor: Frequency of Occurrence in Various Conditions

Disease	% Positive
Rheumatoid arthritis	80
Systemic lupus erythematosus, scleroderma, polymyositis	30
Bacterial endocarditis	70
Sarcoidosis	10
Aging (>60 yrs old)	15–50
Syphilis	10
Tuberculosis	15
Leprosy	25
Chronic liver disease	25

■ Imaging in Joint Disease

Joint radiographs are rarely diagnostic in acute arthritis, the exception being acute pseudogout or calcific tendinitis, in which cartilage calcification (chondrocalcinosis, see Figure 253.2) or tendon calcification are seen on the films. Radiographs also may detect stress fractures or tumors. Early radiographs in septic arthritis, osteomyelitis, SLE, rheumatoid arthritis, and other inflammatory arthritides typically show only nonspecific soft tissue swelling. In more chronic arthritis, radiographs may document the extent (progression) and severity of the disease process.

TABLE 251.5. Antinuclear Antibodies: Frequency of Positive Finding in Various Rheumatic Diseases

Antibody	SLE	Scl	CREST	PM/DM	RA	DLE	MCTD	SS
ANA	>95	95	95	20–50	15–35	>95	>95	75
Anti-native DNA	50	—	—	—	—	—	—	—
Sm	40	—	—	—	—	—	—	—
RNP	40	15	10	15	—	—	>95	15
Centromere	—	—	50	—	—	—	—	—
Histones	30	—	—	—	20	>95	—	—
Scl-70	—	40	15	—	—	—	—	—
SS-A/Ro	25*	—	—	10	10†	—	—	50
SS-B/La	15	—	—	—	—	—	—	25
PM-1	—	—	—	30–50	—	—	—	—

*Positive in subacute cutaneous lupus, in which ANA may be negative.
†SS-A/Ro positive patients usually have secondary Sjögren's syndrome.
ANA = antinuclear antibody; CREST = *c*alcinosis, *R*aynaud's, *e*sophageal dysmotility, *s*clerodactyly, *t*elangiectasia; DLE = drug-induced lupus; DM = dermatomyositis; MCTD = mixed connective tissue disease; PM = polymyositis; RA = rheumatoid arthritis; RNP = ribonucleoprotein; Scl = diffuse scleroderma; SLE = Systemic lupus erythematosus; SS = Sjögren's syndrome.

CHAPTER 252

CLINICAL PRESENTATIONS OF RHEUMATIC CONDITIONS AND PRINCIPLES OF THERAPY

■ Clinical Approach to Diagnosis

Diagnosis of rheumatic diseases may be facilitated by a stepwise approach, in which responses to a series of questions gradually limit the diagnostic possibilities (Figure 252.1).

- *What is the source of pain?* The examiner should determine, through clinical assessment, whether

the pain is based in joint-related or nonarticular tissues.
- *Is there evidence of a joint abnormality?* Tenderness, bony enlargement, intra-articular fluid, thickening of joint tissues (capsule and synovium), loss of joint motion, or joint instability are signs of an abnormal joint.

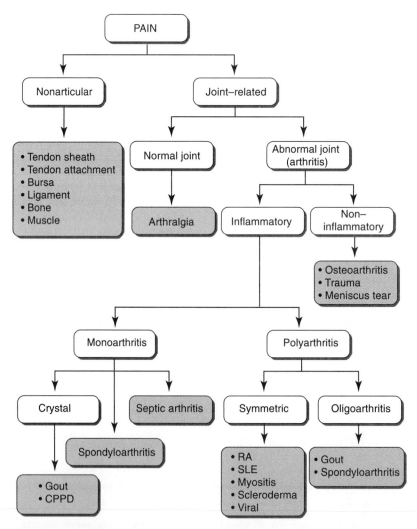

FIGURE 252.1. Classification and diagnostic algorithm of rheumatic diseases. CPPD, calcium pyrophosphate dihydrate crystal deposition disease; RA, rheumatoid arthritis; SLE, systemic lupus erythematosus. (Adapted from Lawrence M. Ryan MD, Medical College of Wisconsin, Milwaukee, Wisconsin.)

- *Is inflammation present?* The cardinal signs of inflammation are pain, warmth, swelling, erythema, and loss of function. Their complete presence is most likely in gout or septic arthritis, but even without erythema or warmth, inflammation is still possible. Many persons with rheumatoid arthritis may have joint thickening and tenderness without significant warmth or erythema.
- *Is the inflammatory arthritis monoarticular, oligoarticular, or polyarticular?* Monoarticular indicates that a *single* joint is affected; oligoarticular indicates *several* (≤4) joints; and polyarticular indicates 5 or more joints (Table 252.1). Descriptions of specific syndromes follow; a glossary of definitions is provided in Table 252.2.

TABLE 252.1.	Differential Diagnosis of Mono-/ Oligoarticular Arthritis

Non-inflammatory
  Trauma
  Osteoarthritis
  Meniscus/ligament tear
Inflammatory
  Gout
  Pseudogout
  Septic joint
  Spondyloarthritis
    Reactive arthritis
      Reiter's syndrome
    Psoriatic arthritis
  Rheumatoid arthritis, lupus (unusual)

■ Monoarthritis and Oligoarthritis

A **monoarthritis** in which the joint examination and synovial fluid show little or no signs of inflammation should suggest osteoarthritis, internal derangement of the knee (e.g., meniscal tear), or a traumatic arthritis.

In **inflammatory monoarthritis** (warm, red, swollen, painful *single* joint), the two primary considerations are **septic arthritis** and **crystal-induced synovitis.** Any inflammatory monoarthritis should be considered septic (i.e., infectious arthritis) until proven otherwise. The patient's age or immune status may suggest a responsible organism (e.g., gonococci in a young, sexually active patient, or gram-negative rods in a nursing home resident with an indwelling catheter). Crystal-induced synovitides include gout and pseudogout.

Synovianalysis is critical to the initial evaluation and management of a monoarthritis. If only a single drop of fluid is obtained, it should be cultured and examined for crystals; any remaining fluid should be sent for Gram stain and full synovianalysis. If crystals are found, therapy with a nonsteroidal anti-inflammatory drug (NSAID) or colchicine should be initiated unless contraindicated. With suspected infection, antibiotics should be started and the clinical response monitored for the first 24–72 hours; anti-inflammatory or antipyretic drugs should be avoided. Lack of a response requires re-evaluation of the suspected diagnosis.

If, after 72 hours, a crystal arthritis has been ruled out and cultures (including blood and genital cultures for gonococci) are negative, one may start therapy with an NSAID or, possibly, an intra-articular corticosteroid injection. When the monoarthritis is proven nonbacterial and a diagnosis or response to treatment is lacking for more than 2 months, alternative diagnoses should be

TABLE 252.2.	A Glossary of Rheumatic Disorders	
Osteoarthritis	Arthritis featuring cartilage degeneration in weight bearing joints and small joints of the hands	
Gout	Inflammatory arthritis, usually mono- but may be oligo- or polyarticular, mediated by mono-sodium urate crystals	
Pseudogout	Similar to gout but mediated by calcium pyrophosphate crystals	
Spondyloarthropathy	A group of diseases with frequent back inflammation, peripheral joint arthritis, common extra-articular features, and increased frequency of HLA-B27	
Ankylosing spondylitis	A spondyloarthropathy with prominent back pain, stiffness and progressive fusion of spinal joints	
Reactive arthritis	A spondyloarthropathy associated with infection by enteric pathogens	
Reiter's syndrome	A form of reactive arthritis, usually associated with genitourinary infection, and characterized by lower extremity arthritis, uveitis, skin and mucous membrane lesions	
Rheumatoid arthritis	Inflammatory arthritis in which the synovial lining becomes thickened and causes damage to joints	
Systemic lupus erythematosus	Multisystem inflammatory disorder mediated by autoantibodies	

considered, such as **spondyloarthropathies** (Table 252.2), atypical presentations of polyarthritis, osteonecrosis, articular neoplasm, or mycobacterial or fungal arthritis. A **synovial biopsy** may be helpful, particularly if cultures for these organisms are negative.

Oligoarthritis involves four or fewer joints, but may present initially as a monoarthritis. One or several joints, usually in the lower extremity, may be involved in spondyloarthropathies (e.g., Reiter's disease or psoriatic arthritis); skin and nail lesions may be a clue. Polyarticular gout usually follows gout that has been monoarticular. Systemic lupus erythematosus or rheumatoid arthritis may present atypically in up to 20% of patients with mono- or oligoarthritis.

■ **Polyarthritis**

The etiology of **inflammatory polyarthritis** is broader (Figure 252.2). The presence or absence of inflammation and the pattern of joint involvement are useful clues. For instance, the small joints tend to be involved in a symmetric pattern in rheumatoid arthritis or systemic lupus erythematosus, whereas the weight-bearing joints, distal interphalangeal (DIP), proximal interphalangeal (PIP), and first carpometacarpal joints are affected, but not inflamed, in osteoarthritis. Associated clinical features, synovianalysis, and serum tests are often diagnostic. Sometimes, the initial diagnosis is only presumptive until the evolving course verifies or alters the original diagnosis.

Inflammatory spondyloarthropathies include ankylosing spondylitis and the arthritis associated with Reiter's, inflammatory bowel disease, and psoriasis. Reiter's disease is more likely to involve large, lower extremity joints. Both Reiter's and psoriatic arthritis may

present with one or more "sausage digits" **(dactylitis).** Psoriatic arthritis may also present with predominant involvement of DIP joints and nail lesions (5%), arthritis mutilans (osteolysis of the phalanges and metacarpal joints, 5%), or symmetric polyarthritis with a distribution similar to that of rheumatoid arthritis (15%); the remainder present as oligoarthritis (70%) or ankylosing spondylitis (5%). Inflammatory bowel disease may also present or be associated with an inflammatory peripheral oligoarthritis, primarily in the lower extremities.

Infectious arthritis may occasionally present as acute polyarthritis. Lyme disease and viral infections (polyarthritis of rubella, either primary infection or vaccine-related; pre-icteric phase of hepatitis B and C; and human parvovirus) are examples. Gonococcal arthritis, acute rheumatic fever, and bacterial endocarditis may be associated with a migratory polyarthritis (arthritis which moves from joint to joint).

■ **Muscle Weakness or Pain**

To assess a patient's complaint of muscle weakness, one should grade muscle strength with a scale, albeit an arbitrary one. Early, primary myopathies present almost entirely as **proximal weakness.** Altered functional capacity may be a clue, as difficulty in combing hair suggests a proximal upper-extremity myopathy and trouble climbing stairs or getting out of a chair or tub suggests proximal lower-extremity myopathy. Muscle pain may or may not accompany weakness. A variety of conditions must be considered in a patient with true muscle weakness (Table 252.3). Polymyositis, dermatomyositis, and inclusion body myositis are the predominant rheumatic diseases that present with proximal weakness (Table 252.4). While patients with polymyalgia

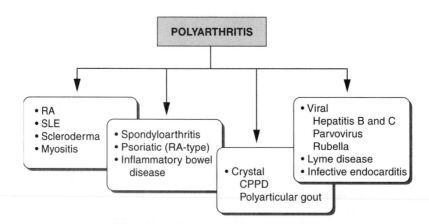

FIGURE 252.2. Possible causes of polyarthritis. CPPD, calcium pyrophosphate dihydrate crystal deposition disease; RA, rheumatoid arthritis; SLE, systemic lupus erythematosus.

TABLE 252.3.	Differential Diagnosis of Weakness

Inflammatory myositis
  Polymyositis
  Dermatomyositis
  Inclusion body myositis
Drugs
  Alcohol
  Corticosteroids
  Cocaine
Endocrinopathies
  Glucocorticoid excess
  Glucocorticoid deficiency
  Hyperthyroidism
  Hypothyroidism
Electrolyte abnormalities
  Hypokalemia
Neurologic disorders
  Upper motor neuron (e.g., amyotrophic lateral
    sclerosis)
  Lower motor neuron (e.g., Guillain-Barré syndrome)
  Myasthenia gravis, Eaton-Lambert syndrome
Muscular dystrophy
Congenital myopathies
  Glycogen storage disease and others
Viral infection

TABLE 252.4.	Myositis: A Glossary

Polymyositis	Inflammation of muscle resulting in progressive muscle weakness and muscle enzyme elevation
Dermatomyositis	Similar to polymyositis with characteristic facial (heliotrope) rash and rash on knuckles (Gottron's sign)
Inclusion body myositis	Similar to polymyositis but more insidious in onset; biopsy shows inclusion bodies in muscle fibers by light microscopy

rheumatica may report weakness because of trouble getting out of a bed, this is due to pain and stiffness mostly in the neck, shoulder, and pelvic girdle.

The physician must also consider **neurologic causes** of muscle pain and weakness. Upper or lower motor neuron diseases, nerve root, or peripheral nerve disease usually display altered reflexes and sensation. Myoneural junction disease may be confused with a primary myopathy, because muscle weakness in these disorders may be proximal. Myasthenia gravis is associated with muscle

weakness that increases with exertion and decreases with rest. Eaton-Lambert syndrome is readily differentiated from myasthenia gravis by electromyography.

Drugs (e.g., corticosteroids, potassium-depleting agents such as diuretics or cathartics), toxins (e.g., alcohol), and rhabdomyolysis (e.g., from heroin or cocaine use, exertion, or crush injury) may cause muscle weakness and/or pain. Although any endocrinopathy (hyper- or hypofunction) may cause a proximal myopathy, the commonest is hypothyroidism.

The **muscular dystrophies** represent a group of primary muscle diseases with onset usually before the third decade; however, both limb-girdle and myotonic dystrophy present in early adult life. In limb-girdle dystrophy, shoulder or pelvic girdle muscles are involved initially, and serum muscle enzymes are slightly increased. In myotonic dystrophy, weakness is distal and serum muscle enzymes are usually normal. Diagnosis of these dystrophies and the rare congenital myopathies rests on associated symptoms and signs, family history, and muscle biopsy (including special stains for carbohydrates and lipids). Less common causes of myopathy include disorders of glycogen, purine, and lipid metabolism and infectious myositis.

■ General Principles of Therapy

The principles of management of rheumatic diseases are largely similar to those employed in other illnesses, but they differ in that response is often measured over weeks or months instead of days and is based more often on clinical response than changes in laboratory measurements. Response time, quantification of response, and the decision to continue the current regimen as a more advanced drug is started all need assessment.

Rheumatic diseases are predominantly chronic, outpatient problems, with only a minority requiring hospitalization. Conditions requiring hospitalization include septic arthritis or bacteremia, visceral involvement (e.g., pericardial tamponade, neural vasculitis, or nephritis), or severe inflammation that renders the patient unable to care for self.

A variety of medications are employed in the treatment of musculoskeletal diseases (Table 252.5). Patients with joint inflammation commonly receive initial treatment with nonsteroidal anti-inflammatory drugs (NSAIDs) or aspirin, the exception being a suspected septic joint because NSAIDs may mask fever. In such instances, it is preferable to use analgesics such as codeine or propoxyphene until the diagnosis is clearer. Some cases of osteoarthritis may require only analgesics. Control of rheumatoid arthritis often requires additional medications (hydroxychloroquine, immunomodulating agents, gold, penicillamine). Acute gout is treated with

TABLE 252.5.	Medications Used in the Treatment of Musculoskeletal Diseases
Class	**Example**
Non-steroidal anti-inflammatory drugs	Indomethacin, ibuprofen, naproxen, etc.
Analgesics	Acetaminophen, tramadol, narcotics
Corticosteroids	
Oral	Prednisone, methylprednisolone
Injectable	Methylprednisolone acetate, triamcinolone hexacetonide
Anti-malarial	Hydroxychloroquine
Gold	
Oral	Auranofin
Injectable	Aurothioglucose (IM)
Immunomodulators	Azathioprine, methotrexate, cyclophosphamide
Tricyclic antidepressants	Amitriptyline

NSAIDs or colchicine. Recurrent attacks of gout are prevented by probenecid or allopurinol. Patients with arthritis may require several medications to control their disease but polypharmacy does expose patients, particularly the elderly, to increased risks of drug side effects, greater likelihood of drug interactions, and also high costs from multiple medications.

Aspirin and other nonsteroidal anti-inflammatory drugs

While **aspirin,** given in doses to attain a serum salicylate level of 20–25 mg/dl, is the traditional first-line NSAID, other NSAIDs hold distinct advantages over it. Other NSAIDs, unlike aspirin, do not irreversibly inhibit platelet prostaglandin function. Most of the newer NSAIDs produce less gastric damage than aspirin, although gastrointestinal bleeding remains a serious, potentially lethal complication of all NSAIDs (except for the nonacetylated salicylates). NSAIDs may further impair renal function in patients with underlying renal disease. In addition, the indole-pyrrole derivatives (e.g., indomethacin, sulindac, tolmetin) are more effective in acute gout and most spondyloarthropathies. Long-acting preparations requiring only once- or twice-daily dosing offer the advantage of better patient compliance; however, compounds having a longer duration of action typically take longer to achieve steady-state therapeutic levels.

Physical and occupational therapy

In musculoskeletal diseases, the goals of physical and occupational therapy are to maintain proper joint alignment, preserve range of motion, maintain muscle strength, minimize joint trauma, and to maximize the ability to carry out activities of daily living. In general, extremely inflamed joints should be rested, preferably in the anatomic position, using resting splints frequently. As inflammation abates, gentle assisted range-of-motion exercises may be started to help prevent loss of motion. At a later stage, muscle strengthening exercises may be begun, initially as isometric exercises to minimize joint trauma. Later, when the inflammation has been sufficiently suppressed, active resistive muscle strengthening may be started. Stiff joints and painful muscles may respond to heat (hydrocollator packs), massage, or ultrasound treatments. Neck or back pain may respond to cervical or lumbar traction respectively.

A complete discussion of the surgical management of arthritis is beyond the scope of this discussion. Severe arthritis of hips and knees is generally managed with total joint arthroplasty. Total joint arthroplasty is available but less commonly employed for other joints because of less favorable outcomes. Arthroscopic surgical procedures are being increasingly used for soft tissue repairs in the knee, shoulder, and ankle.

CHAPTER 253 CRYSTAL-INDUCED SYNOVITIS

Crystals associated with synovial inflammation include monosodium urate, calcium pyrophosphate dihydrate (CPPD), and, less often, hydroxyapatite, oxalate, and adrenocorticosteroid esters. Cholesterol crystals that are occasionally found in chronic joint effusions are probably inert.

The pathophysiology of crystal-induced synovitis is incompletely understood. The presence of a crystal in synovial fluid is insufficient to implicate it in acute synovitis because the crystal may occasionally be seen in quiescent joints as well. The precise inciting event in vivo is unknown but may involve crystal shedding from preformed cartilaginous or synovial deposits. Crystal phagocytosis by neutrophils in vitro induces release of lysosomal enzymes, humoral mediators, and chemotactic factors associated with acute inflammation.

Monosodium urate and CPPD crystals commonly

cause acute synovitis and chronic joint damage. Acute crystal-induced arthritis is rapid in onset and self-limited.

Differences in crystal morphology and clinical features are helpful in diagnosis.

Gout

Gout is a metabolic disease in which hyperuricemia and arthritis are variably expressed. Three possible stages exist: acute gouty arthritis, intercritical gout, and tophaceous gout. Urolithiasis (renal calculi) or other renal disease may also be associated with hyperuricemia.

Hyperuricemia

Hyperuricemia, a biochemical abnormality defined solely by the serum urate concentration, results from increased production of urate, decreased excretion, or both (Table 253.1). Decreased renal clearance is responsible for most cases of hyperuricemia. By the uricase method, the upper limit of normal for serum urate is 7.0 mg/dl in men and 6.0 mg/dl in premenopausal women. Plasma is saturated with urate at 6.4–6.8 mg/dl at 37˚C. Most clinical laboratories, however, use a colorimetric method and may report higher normal levels than the uricase method.

Normal urinary uric acid excretion is <600 mg/24 hr on a purine-free diet and <800 mg/24 hr on a regular diet. Approximately 150 mg of urate is secreted into the normal intestinal tract every 24 hours, but this rate is increased in hyperuricemia.

Acute Gout

Acute gout features acute inflammatory arthritis, which is usually **monoarticular** and most often involves **lower extremity joints.** Acute gout is precipitated by trauma, alcohol ingestion, acute medical illness, surgical procedures, and certain drugs (Table 253.1). Not all factors responsible for the precipitation of urate crystals are known, however, because hyperuricemia does occur without urolithiasis or gout. Gout occurs primarily in men, with onset in the fourth through sixth decades; in women, it is more likely to follow menopause.

An acute gouty attack is very painful. In 60% of cases, the first attack involves the first metatarsophalangeal (MTP) joint (**"podagra"**) or other joints in the foot. Acute gout may also occur in other joints of the foot or ankle, the prepatellar or olecranon bursae, and midfoot (gouty cellulitis). Within a few hours, the affected joint becomes red, swollen, warm, and tender, but usually the attack resolves on its own within a few days to a few weeks without leaving apparent sequelae. Fever may be present. In a minority, the initial episode may be polyarticular. **Tophi** (see below) usually follow years of gout and are rare in conjunction with the first attack.

Although hyperuricemia is characteristic of gout, normal serum urate values may be seen during the acute attack. Synovial effusions in acute gout are typically inflammatory (5,000–50,000 leukocytes/mm³, mostly neutrophils). Characteristic **needle-shaped, strongly negatively birefringent** crystals of monosodium urate crystals are seen either intra- or extracellularly on synovial fluid examination with a compensated polarizing microscope (See Color Plate 32).

Intercritical Gout and Polyarticular Gout

As the acute gouty attack subsides, the patient becomes asymptomatic (*intercritical gout*). A second attack occurs in most patients within 6 months to 2 years. Ensuing attacks may become polyarticular, more severe, and of longer duration, yielding a different clinical picture from early gout. During this period, gout is suggested by prior hyperuricemia, and acute arthritis, with clinical response to **colchicine;** but definitive diagnosis requires identification of monosodium urate crystals from a tophus or even from an asymptomatic (e.g., first MTP) joint.

TABLE 253.1. Conditions Associated with Hyperuricemia

Urate Overproduction	Urate Renal Underexcretion
Idiopathic (primary) gout	Idiopathic (primary) gout
Inherited enzymatic defects	Clinical disorders
Purine overproduction	Hypertension
Paget's disease	Dehydration
Hemolytic diseases	Obesity
Psoriasis	Sarcoidosis
Obesity	Renal insufficiency
Myelo- and lymphoprolif-	Lead toxicity
erative diseases	Starvation
Drugs	Acidosis
Cytotoxic agents	Toxemia of pregnancy
High-dose salicylates	Salt restriction
Ethanol	Drugs
Uricosurics	Ethanol
	Diuretics
	Low-dose salicylates
	Cyclosporine
	Levodopa

Chronic Tophaceous Gout

If recurrent gout is untreated, tophi can develop on the extensor surfaces of the elbows, in joints, and in surrounding tissues, especially the interphalangeal joints of the hands or feet and the helix of the ear. **Tophi** are usually firm, and when aspirated, yield a chalky white material containing monosodium urate crystals.

Chronic tophaceous gout may mimic rheumatoid arthritis, with arthralgias, progressive stiffness, nodules, joint swelling, and deformity (Figure 253.1), and even a high erythrocyte sedimentation rate and positive rheumatoid factor. While acute attacks manifest only soft tissue swelling on radiographs, chronic gout manifests punched-out erosions at the ends of phalanges, most commonly at the medial aspects of the head of the first MTP joint. These are highly typical of tophaceous gout. Tophi may be first detected on radiographs, before their clinical recognition.

Renal Disease Associated with Hyperuricemia

Hyperuricemia is associated with several renal diseases: renal stones (chapter 164), urate nephropathy, and uric acid nephropathy. The risk of renal failure from hyperuricemia alone is low. **Uric acid renal stones** occur in 10–25% of patients with gout but actually occur more often without gout or hyperuricemia. **Urate nephropathy** is due to deposition of sodium urate crystals in the renal tubular epithelium and adjacent interstitium. It is rare in the absence of gout and is a late event in the natural history of gout with very high serum urate levels. Aging and coexistent diseases, especially hypertension (rather than hyperuricemia), correlate with decreased renal function. **Uric acid nephropathy** is a rare, reversible form of acute renal failure due to uric acid crystal precipitation in collecting ducts and ureters. It most often occurs in patients with leukemia or lymphoma who are receiving chemotherapy.

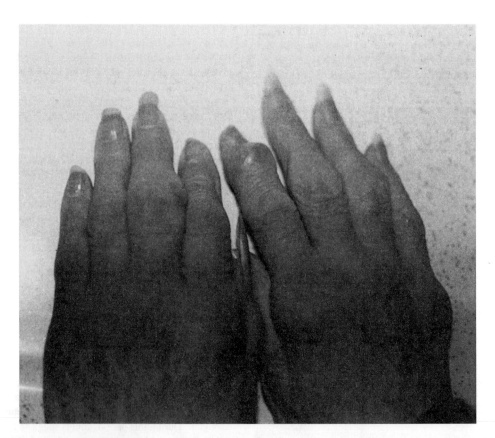

FIGURE 253.1. Hands of an elderly woman with *chronic tophaceous gout*. Some of the tophi appear to have formed in joints having previous osteoarthritic changes.

Management

Symptomatic hyperuricemia

NSAIDs or colchicine are the usual first line of treatment for acute gout. Oral **colchicine** is given in doses of 0.5–0.6 mg every 1–2 hours until either gout improves, gastrointestinal side effects (nausea, vomiting, or diarrhea) occur, or a total of 3.0–4.0 mg have been given. Colchicine should be used in lesser doses in the elderly or those with impaired renal function to avoid bone marrow suppression. It is not specific for gout because other crystal arthropathies, such as acute pseudogout or calcific tendinitis, may also respond.

Indomethacin, up to 200 mg/day in divided doses for usually 4–5 days, is effective and more convenient than colchicine, but the maximal dosage often produces CNS and gastrointestinal side effects. Other NSAIDs may be similarly effective but have been used less commonly in acute gout. In the unusual instances when oral therapy is not possible, alternatives include local intra-articular corticosteroid injection, IV methylprednisolone (20–50 mg/day), ACTH (40–80 U/day), or IV colchicine.

As **prophylaxis** against recurrent attacks, small doses of colchicine (0.5 g once or twice daily), indomethacin, or another NSAID may be prescribed, but this prophylaxis does not prevent crystal deposition and possible joint destruction. Instead, after acute gout resolves, chronic hypouricemic therapy is begun using **probenecid** or **allopurinol** (see below). Such therapy is indicated in patients with frequent recurrent attacks, tophi (clinically or radiographically manifest), or nephrolithiasis. A dosage achieving a serum urate concentration below 6.4 mg/dl prevents further monosodium urate crystal deposition (although some patients may require even further lowering of the serum urate).

Noncompliance is the usual reason for ineffective control of hyperuricemia.

Decreased uric acid excretion accounts for hyperuricemia in at least 90% of cases. A 24-hour urinary uric acid estimation should differentiate the overproducer from the underexcretor. The uricosuric drug **probenecid** may be used if the daily uric acid excretion is <800 mg/24 hr on a regular diet or when allergy to allopurinol is present; it is contraindicated with creatinine clearance below 60 ml/min or nephrolithiasis. **Allopurinol** and its metabolite **oxypurinol** inhibit xanthine oxidase to decrease uric acid synthesis. It is used in patients who excrete in excess of 800 mg uric acid/24 hr on a regular diet and in those with severe tophaceous gout, chronic renal insufficiency, or allergy to uricosurics. Probenecid should be avoided in the overproducer because of the risk of nephrolithiasis.

Toxic reactions to probenecid occur in about 5% of patients and are usually related to skin rashes or gastrointestinal complaints; serious side effects such as vasculitis, granulomatous hepatitis, or agranulocytosis are rare. The dose should be reduced in patients with chronic renal failure or on azathioprine therapy.

Asymptomatic hyperuricemia

Asymptomatic hyperuricemia need not be treated since the incidence of gout is low and the first attack is easily managed. The only exception is the patient with very high levels of serum urate (>10.5 mg/dl) which may cause **urate nephropathy.** Patients with uric acid nephrolithiasis should increase their fluid intake to increase urine volume, maintain alkaline urine to decrease urate precipitation, and reduce total uric acid excretion, usually by using allopurinol.

Calcium Pyrophosphate Dihydrate Crystal Deposition Disease

CPPD crystal deposition in hyaline cartilage and fibrocartilage is associated with several different patterns of arthritis. The incidence of CPPD deposition rises with age (5% at age 70; >40% at age 90). CPPD crystal deposition is idiopathic in most cases but may occur in hyperparathyroidism, hemochromatosis, hypomagnesemia, hypophosphatasia, and hypothyroidism. Younger patients should be screened for these disorders. Diagnosis is based on radiographic findings or the demonstration of characteristic **positive, birefringent rhomboid or rod-like crystals** by compensated polarized light microscopy in synovial fluid (See Color Plate 32).

Clinical and Laboratory Features

Probably, the most common form of CPPD deposition is asymptomatic radiographic **chondrocalcinosis,** consisting of punctate and linear radiodensities in cartilage (Figure 253.2) with minimal or no joint symptoms. Nearly 25% of patients will have *pseudogout,* which mimics gout with self-limited, often monoarticular attacks that may last from 1 day to 4 weeks without treatment. Severe medical illness, surgical procedures, and trauma may precipitate attacks, although the mechanism of release of crystals from cartilaginous deposits remains elusive. Pseudogout more commonly involves large

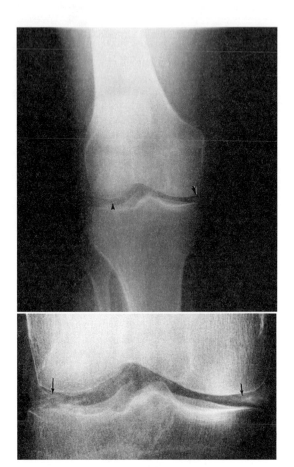

FIGURE 253.2. Radiograph of a knee and a magnified view of the joint space (inset) showing chondrocalcinosis in the hyaline articular cartilage and meniscus fibrocartilage (arrows), suggesting calcium pyrophosphate crystal deposition.

joints, especially the knees and wrists, and may coexist with gout (5%) and hyperuricemia (20%).

Synovial fluid during the acute attack is typically inflammatory (4,000–20,000 leukocytes/mm³, with mostly neutrophils). The leukocytes show ingested CPPD crystals during acute attacks (See Color Plate 32). The crystals may also persist in joint fluid even after the attack has resolved. Radiographs in most cases show chondrocalcinosis.

Nearly 50% of patients present with a picture simulating **symmetric osteoarthritis,** most commonly in the knees, followed by the wrist, metacarpophalangeal (MCP), hip, spine, shoulder, elbow, and ankle joints. Within this subgroup, one-half will have a history of episodic acute attacks. In patients with "osteoarthritis" affecting joints not usually involved in osteoarthritis, radiographs of the knees, hands, wrists and pelvis are useful to detect CPPD deposition.

Another 5% of patients present with polyarthritis resembling rheumatoid arthritis. In almost 10% of this subset, the rheumatoid factor is positive in low titers. The inflamed joints tend to be more asymmetric than those in rheumatoid arthritis and, radiographically, have CPPD deposition and osteophytes without typical erosive disease.

■ Management

Treatment may be with **colchicine** (IV or oral), NSAIDs, joint aspiration alone, or intra-articular corticosteroid injection (similar to that of symptomatic hyperuricemia).

Hydroxyapatite-associated Synovitis

Hydroxyapatite (HA) crystals refer to a group of crystals called basic calcium phosphates and include hydroxyapatite, octacalcium phosphate, and tricalcium phosphate. (For simplicity, they are referred to as HA here.) These crystals have been detected by electron microscopy in **acute calcific periarthritis** (most commonly of the shoulder), **tendinitis,** and **bursitis.** More recently, HA crystals have been found in synovial fluids of patients with several forms of arthritis, including osteoarthritis.

In one form of HA-induced disease, the **Milwaukee shoulder/knee syndrome,** elderly patients, usually women, present with glenohumeral joint stiffness, decreased motion, often a large effusion, and pain with use of the dominant shoulder. Bilateral disease is often noted clinically. One-half also have knee instability and pain

with ambulation, but other joints are rarely affected. Radiographs show severe glenohumeral joint degeneration with small osteophytes and bony destruction of the humeral head. Soft tissue calcifications occur in 40%. Rotator cuff lysis is evident by upward subluxation of the humeral head or by arthrogram.

Synovial fluids from affected joints have low leukocyte counts (<1000/mm³, usually mononuclear). HA crystals are not birefringent and thus, are not usually detectable by polarized light microscopy; scanning or transmission electron microscopy or x-ray diffraction are required for crystal identification. In some synovial fluids, both HA and CPPD coexist. **Treatment** is unsatisfactory but includes NSAIDs, reduced shoulder use, and joint aspiration.

■ **Steroid Crystal-Induced Synovitis**

In about 2% of patients receiving intra-articular crystalline corticosteroid injections, a brief (1–3 days) acute synovitis occurs several hours afterwards. Its early occurrence after injection helps distinguish it from the extremely rare infection caused by injection itself. On compensated polarized light microscopy, the crystals appear as positive and negative birefringent chunks, rods, or globular material.

CHAPTER **254** OSTEOARTHRITIS

Osteoarthritis (OA) is the commonest form of arthritis, with a prevalence that rises with age, and most people exhibit some roentgenographic evidence of OA after age 60. Its etiology is unknown. OA may best be viewed as the final common pathway for many pathologic articular processes (Table 254.1).

OA occurring in patients without known predisposing factors is termed **primary OA.** These are usually women with a history of similar disease in women kindreds, suggesting possible genetic and/or hormonal factors. Recent reports of inherited biochemical defects in Type II collagen account for some families with premature OA.

■ **Pathogenesis**

In the earliest stage of OA, chondrocytes, activated by unknown means, begin remodeling cartilage. Synthesis of proteoglycans is increased but so is also secretion of enzymes, including collagenase, stromelysin, and other metalloproteinases, which disrupt the cartilage matrix.

Osteoarthritis occurs in cartilage that has lost a significant portion of its glycosaminoglycan content. The surface cartilage initially shows microscopic fibrillation; deep fissuring follows, as shear forces disrupt the cartilage. Chondrocytes replicate within lacunae but eventually die. Underlying bone becomes sclerotic, and new bone growth occurs as a ridge around the margin of the joint (**osteophytes).** Ultimately, the cartilage fragments and disappears completely, leaving a bare surface of eburnated bone. Unlike rheumatoid arthritis, in which the cartilage thins diffusely as a result of more uniform damage, cartilage loss in the OA joint tends to be more asymmetric and confined to the area of greatest mechanical stress. Histologic examination of synovial tissues shows patchy hyperplasia.

■ **Clinical Features**

OA most commonly manifests with pain, usually made worse by activity and relieved by rest. Morning stiffness, if present, is usually short (<30–60 min). **Gelling** is stiffness that occurs after 1 or more hours of rest and is relieved by activity. Primary OA most often involves the PIP and DIP and first carpometacarpal (CMC) joints of the hand, the knees, first metatarsal joints, and apophyseal joints of the spine. It is useful to remember that knee pain can be referred from the hip and vice versa.

TABLE 254.2. Common Deformities in Osteoarthritis

Joint	Deformity
Distal interphalangeal	Heberden's node
Proximal interphalangeal	Bouchard's node
First carpometacarpal	Squaring (shelf sign)
First metatarsophalangeal	Hallux valgus (bunion)
Knee, medial femorotibial compartment	Genu varus (bow legs)
Knee, lateral femorotibial compartment	Genu valgus (knock knees)

TABLE 254.1. Conditions Predisposing to Osteoarthritis

Mechanical trauma
Weight bearing joints in obesity
Prior joint trauma
Excessive joint use (occupational)
Previous inflammatory arthritis
Congenital joint dysplasias
Avascular necrosis of bone
Metabolic diseases affecting cartilage
Hemochromatosis
Ochronosis
Calcium pyrophosphate crystal deposition
Neurologic disorders
Diminished pain perception

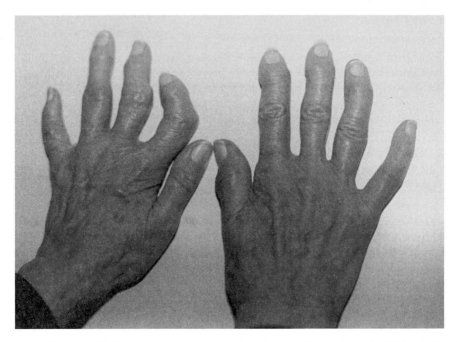

FIGURE 254.1. Hands of an elderly woman with *osteoarthritis* showing osteophytic enlargement of the PIP joint (Bouchard's nodes) and DIP joints (Heberden's nodes) as well as angulation deformity in some joints.

Patients may report bouts of acute pain, sometimes with swelling, which leave fibrous or bony enlargement in their wake. A few patients may have more persistent inflammation with synovial thickening and increased pain in one or a few of the small hand joints ("erosive osteoarthritis"). Some elderly women with underlying renal disease receiving thiazides may have gouty, tophaceous deposits with inflammation in osteoarthritic hand joints.

On examination, the involved joints exhibit variable pain and tenderness. Surprisingly, pain is often minimal, despite markedly abnormal finger joints. Enlargement in OA joints reflects underlying joint effusion or formation of osteophytes. Osteophyte formation of the DIP and PIP joints of the hands are called Heberden's nodes and Bouchard's nodes respectively. Wearing away of cartilage on one side of the joint leads to bony crepitus and malalignment (Table 254.2). Together, the bony enlargement and malalignment cause loss of motion (Figure 254.1).

OA of the spine occurs as the nucleus pulposus begins to liquefy in young adulthood, and the annulus fibrosus begins to desiccate and split. Disc collapse and extrusion follow, causing instability of the posterior (facet) joints, which later develop OA. The resultant vertebral and facet osteophytes and disc space narrowing can impinge on nerve roots and cause radiculopathy or spinal stenosis (see Low back pain, Chapter 252).

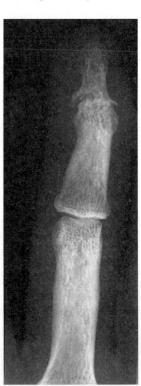

FIGURE 254.2. Radiograph of the third digit of a patient with osteoarthritis (erosive type) showing osteophyte formation, joint erosion, and mild sclerosis.

Ancillary Studies

Routine laboratory studies are normal in otherwise uncomplicated OA. Synovianalysis can help exclude crystal-induced and other inflammatory diseases. Joint fluid in OA has less than 1500 leukocytes/mm^3, predominantly mononuclear. Radiographs eventually show regional (asymmetric) thinning of the joint space, osteophytes, subchondral sclerosis, and cyst formation; however, symptoms only weakly correlate with radiographic severity (Figure 254.2). Such findings are very common in the elderly and may fortuitously be present along with other forms of arthritis.

Management

Therapy for OA is directed at relieving pain, minimizing further joint trauma, and preserving motion, alignment, and muscle strength. Treatment is started with mild analgesics (e.g., acetaminophen) and progressed to low-dose NSAIDs, and then high-dose NSAIDs if needed. In general, the response inversely correlates with severity of joint damage.

Physical and occupational therapy can provide instruction in joint protection to minimize additional joint trauma and exercises to preserve or increase range of motion and maintain muscle strength. The joint with severe destructive change can often be helped only by reconstructive surgery, which may include realignment of weight-bearing to a less involved area of the joint surface (e.g., tibial osteotomy), joint arthroplasty (e.g., first CMC joint), prosthetic joint replacement (e.g., total hip or knee replacement), or fusion to relieve pain in some joints where motion is not crucial to function (e.g., ankle, lumbar spine).

CHAPTER 255 RHEUMATOID ARTHRITIS

Etiology and Pathogenesis

Rheumatoid arthritis (RA), a systemic disorder of unknown etiology, afflicts almost 1% of the population. Eighty percent of patients with RA are seropositive for **rheumatoid factor** (RF), which consists of autoantibodies of the IgG, IgM, or IgA classes that react with antigenic determinants on the Fc portion of IgG. In the 80% of patients having RF, the disease is usually more sustained, more systemic, and more destructive. About 70% of seropositive Caucasian patients are positive for HLA type DR4, which occurs in only 16% of the normal population and a similar proportion of patients with seronegative RA.

In RA, the synovium is infiltrated with T lymphocytes, plasma cells, and macrophages, which may be attracted to the synovium by expression of **intercellular adhesion molecules (ICAM)** in synovial venules. Within the synovium, immunoglobulins including RF are actively synthesized. Formation of RF-IgG complexes and perhaps other immune complexes locally activate the complement, **kinin,** and other inflammatory cascades. Thus, complement levels may be low in synovial fluid.

Neutrophils predominate in RA joint fluid. As they phagocytize immune complexes, they locally release lysosomal enzymes and generate reactive oxygen species, both of which may cause cartilage destruction. Prostaglandins are elevated in such joint fluids. Cytokines, including interleukins 1 and 6, tumor necrosis factor, and probably other growth factors, activate synovial fibroblasts and possibly chondrocytes.

Proliferation of synovial fibroblasts causes expansion of the synovial membrane, demonstrating functional properties of a benign tumor, the so-called **pannus.** Upon contact with bone, cartilage, and ligaments, collagenase from dendritic cells in the pannus destroys their collagen framework. Large synovial effusions reduce synovial blood flow, causing ischemia of the joint tissues. Unchecked rheumatoid synovitis causes sustained inflammation with eventual thinning of cartilage, erosion of bone, and weakening of ligamentous structures, resulting in joint instability.

Clinical Features

RA has a variable natural history. Most patients experience recurrent and protracted exacerbations with a gradual, cumulative, and irreversible tissue destruction. Less commonly, a single episode may be followed by lasting remission. A rare patient will have progressive unremitting systemic disease, causing crippling disability and death.

The musculoskeletal system is the most commonly and the most visibly afflicted. Virtually any **diarthrodial (synovial) joint** may be involved, including the cricoarytenoid. The onset of systemic and musculoskeletal symptoms is insidious over weeks to months in most (55–70%) patients, but more rapid (and sometimes acute) in the remainder.

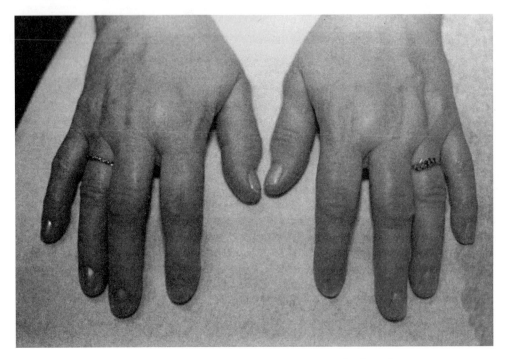

FIGURE **255.1.** Hands of a woman with *early rheumatoid arthritis* showing synovial thickening of the MCP and PIP joints.

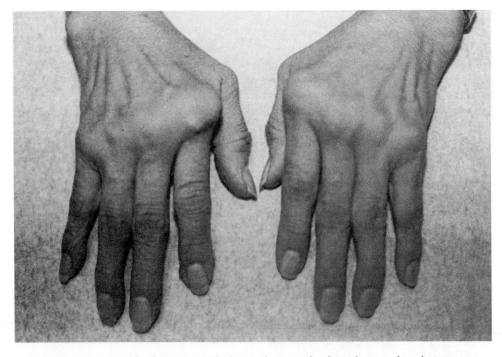

FIGURE **255.2.** Hands of a woman with *chronic rheumatoid arthritis* showing ulnar deviation, MCP subluxation, and swan neck deformities.

Symmetric involvement is more common, but even if the initial presentation is asymmetric, with time, symmetry usually prevails. **Morning stiffness** may last for 1 or more hours. Muscle atrophy may occur around involved joints, so that activities of daily living (e.g., household and self-care activities) become difficult. In some, there may be severe flares in one or a few joints or periarticular structures that last only a few days (palindromic rheumatism).

The most common **joints involved** are the proximal interphalangeal (PIP), metacarpophalangeal (MCP), and wrist, followed by the knee, ankle, metatarsophalangeal (MTP), shoulder, and elbow. Joint enlargement is due to soft tissue swelling (**synovitis**) and/or synovial fluid accumulation (Figure 255.1). With time, joint deformities may occur (see Figures 255.2 and 258.1, and Table 255.1).

Tenosynovitis at the wrist may produce carpal tunnel syndrome or cystic enlargement around the extensor tendons. Prolonged tenosynovitis may cause attrition and, eventually, rupture of extensor tendons, usually the fourth and fifth, resulting in inability to actively extend those digits. At the knee, expansion of the gastrocnemius-semimembranosus bursa by one-way flow of synovial fluid may produce a **Baker's cyst** in the popliteal space. This cyst is usually asymptomatic but may cause pain behind the knee or may rupture into the calf, simulating a deep vein thrombosis.

Neck pain in a patient with long-standing RA should prompt an evaluation of the cervical spine for C1-2 subluxation. Cervical spine radiographs in flexion and extension may reveal widening of the space between the odontoid process and anterior arch of C1, suggesting laxity of supporting ligaments. This type of cervical instability and also vertical subluxation of the odontoid

TABLE 255.2.	Extra-Articular Manifestations of Rheumatoid Arthritis

Skin
  Rheumatoid nodules
  Vasculitic lesions
Mucous membranes
  Sjögren's syndrome (20%)
Eyes
  Sjögren's syndrome
  Episcleritis
  Scleromalacia perforans
Heart
  Pericarditis (usually asymptomatic)
Lungs (see Chapter 231)
  Pleurisy
  Pulmonary rheumatoid nodules
  Interstitial pneumonitis
  Bronchiolitis obliterans
  Pneumoconiosis (Caplan's syndrome)
Nervous system
  Compression neuropathy
  Median nerve
  Posterior interosseous syndrome
  Peripheral neuropathy
  Mononeuritis multiplex (in vasculitis)
  Cervical cord compression (C1-2 subluxation)
Hematologic
  Anemia
  Leukopenia
  Felty's syndrome
  Leukocytosis
  Thrombocytosis
Vascular
  Rheumatoid vasculitis

into the foramen magnum may cause impingement on the spinal cord with paralysis and respiratory failure. (It is important for an anesthesiologist to be aware of any cervical spine abnormalities prior to any contemplated surgery and intubation.)

■ Extra-articular Manifestations and Associated Disorders

Although the joints are the most visibly afflicted, the systemic nature of RA produces prolific extra-articular manifestations (Table 255.2). About 60% of patients will have at some time either pleuritis or pericarditis (usually asymptomatic). With active disease, anemia of chronic disease is usually present. Serious forms of pulmonary disease include interstitial pneumonitis producing restrictive lung disease and bronchiolitis obliterans.

Granulomatous rheumatoid nodules occur in 20% of patients, virtually all seropositive for RF. These can occur in any organ, but the most common are, in

TABLE 255.1.	Common Joint Deformities in Rheumatoid Arthritis

Deformity	Joint Involvement
Swan-neck	Hyperextension of PIP and flexion of DIP
Boutonniere	Flexion of PIP and extension of DIP
Ulnar deviation of fingers	Radial deviation of carpal bones
Cock-up toes	Metatarsal head subluxation
Hammer toes	Metatarsal head subluxation leading to pressure necrosis of dorsal PIPs
Bunion (hallux valgus)	First MTP

diminishing order, subcutaneous, pulmonary (Figure 255.3), and myopericardial. Interestingly, the kidneys are virtually never affected in RA, and the appearance of significant proteinuria should prompt a search for other causes (e.g., amyloid, medication-induced).

Sjögren's syndrome (sicca complex) is found in RA, systemic lupus erythematosus, or other connective tissue diseases or by itself, without another associated disease. Lymphocytic infiltration of lacrimal and salivary glands produces dysfunction and damage, followed by reduced formation of tears and saliva. Prominent symptoms include eye dryness as well as burning, matter formation, and dryness of the mouth. Patients require frequent instillation of artificial tears or gels to prevent symptoms and corneal ulcers. In some, lymphocytic infiltration of lungs, kidneys, or other sites may evoke organ dysfunction. The risk of lymphoma is higher in patients with primary Sjögren's syndrome.

Felty's syndrome, affecting 5% of patients, is a triad of RA, splenomegaly, and cytopenia, usually leukopenia. Nearly all such patients are seropositive for RF in high titers, with more erosive, destructive arthritis than the average patient with RA. Such patients are at high risk for life-threatening pyogenic infections, although the actual peripheral blood leukocyte count and risk for infection are poorly correlated. Many RA patients have significant leukopenia without splenomegaly.

Signs of **vasculitis** occur in 8% of RA patients. In most, this includes minor digital infarcts (brown spots). In 1%, nearly all RF seropositive in high titers, a severe systemic vasculitic syndrome occurs, with fever, skin

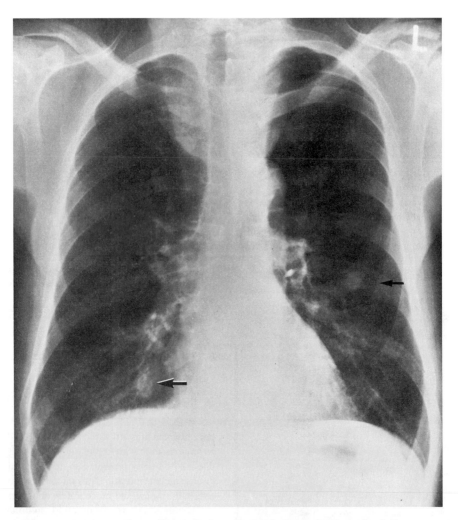

FIGURE **255.3.** Chest radiograph of a patient with chronic rheumatoid arthritis showing *rheumatoid lung nodules.*

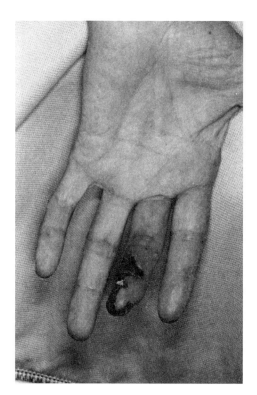

FIGURE 255.4. Digital infarction in a patient with *rheumatoid vasculitis.*

ulcers, digital gangrene (Figure 255.4), and organ infarction.

Whereas nodules, Felty's syndrome, and vasculitis occur predominantly in those with more severe joint disease, they frequently flare asynchronously with the joint disease. It is common to see patients whose joint disease seems quiescent, but in whom severe Felty's or vasculitis is occurring.

■ **Diagnosis**

A committee of the American College of Rheumatology developed a set of 7 clinical criteria for epidemiologic and demographic use. These criteria, being nonspecific, generally only indicate that an inflammatory arthritis is present (Table 255.3).

■ **Ancillary Studies**

Almost 80% of patients are seropositive for RF. The ESR may be high, but thrombocytosis and anemia of chronic disease also indicate active inflammation. Initially radiographs may show only soft tissue swelling. Classically, periarticular demineralization, symmetric joint space narrowing, and marginal articular erosions are

seen. In severe cases, marked bony destruction due to bony resorption, and malalignment due to weakened capsular, tendinous and ligamentous structures, may occur (Figure 255.5). Joint ankylosis is unusual in RA.

■ **Management**

Therapy for RA is directed at minimizing inflammatory signs and symptoms, halting progressive joint erosion, interrupting visceral involvement, and maintaining muscle strength, joint alignment, and joint mobility while awaiting remission. Because the disease course varies widely, medical therapy should be tailored to suppress synovitis or extra-articular manifestations of RA, if feasible, without exposing the patient to excessive risks of drug therapy. Considerable debate continues as to what represents optimal therapy. The consensus is that **early aggressive treatment** is warranted, given the serious disability and premature mortality due to RA.

Therapy is begun with a full dose of **NSAIDs** or high-dose **salicylates** (aspirin, 3.0 g/d usually) in order to attain a serum salicylate level of 20–25 mg/dl. Response is graded in terms of relief of pain, morning stiffness, and joint swelling and tenderness. Patients should also be questioned regarding potential side effects of NSAIDs including headache, rash, weight gain, dyspepsia, abdominal pain, or any other gastrointestinal symptoms. Many RA patients report some response to NSAIDs or aspirin but continue to have pain, morning stiffness, and joint swelling. If NSAIDs or aspirin fail to control pain and joint swelling adequately after 2 months, second-line drug therapy should be initiated.

The second-line agents, sometimes called **disease-modifying antirheumatic drugs (DMARDs)** or slow-

TABLE 255.3.	Revised American College of Rheumatology Criteria for Rheumatoid Arthritis (1987)*
1. Morning stiffness for at least one hour and present for at least six weeks
2. Swelling of three or more joints for at least six weeks
3. Swelling of wrist, metacarpophalangeal or proximal interphalangeal joints for six or more weeks
4. Symmetric joint swelling
5. Hand roentgenogram changes typical of rheumatoid arthritis that must include erosion or unequivocal bony decalcification
6. Rheumatoid nodules
7. Serum rheumatoid factor by a method that yields positive results in less than 5% of normals

*With exclusion of other joint disorders and fulfillment of 4 or more criteria, the diagnosis of RA is likely.
Reference: Arnett et al. Arthritis Rheum 1988; 31:315–324.

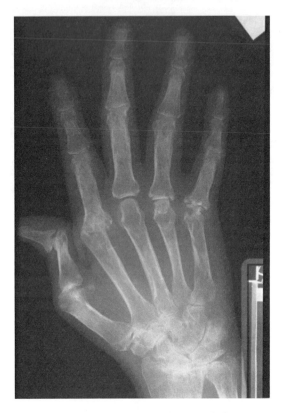

FIGURE 255.5. Radiograph of the right hand of a woman with chronic rheumatoid arthritis. Joint erosions are present in the carpal bones and second MCP joint. Joint space narrowing and subluxation are also present.

acting antirheumatic drugs (SAARDs) are listed in Table 255.4. Hydroxychloroquine, auranofin (oral gold), or sulfasalazine may be useful in milder cases. In more severe cases, intramuscular gold, methotrexate, azathioprine, or penicillamine are more likely to be beneficial. Each of these agents has its own unique, and in some cases potentially severe, toxicity which requires monitoring. Their delayed onset of action is a drawback of these drugs.

The last decade has witnessed a striking increase in the use of **immunosuppressive agents,** particularly methotrexate. Although cyclophosphamide and other alkylating agents clearly suppress RA, an increased risk

of malignancy is an important consideration, relegating their use for serious complications of RA, such as rheumatoid vasculitis.

Systemic corticosteroid therapy has a profound, immediate ameliorative effect on inflammation. However, the long- and short-term side effects of high, or even moderate, doses of steroids argue against their use except in a few limited situations, including life-threatening visceral disease (e.g., pericardial tamponade, systemic vasculitis). Low-dose steroids, usually prednisone (5 mg/ day), are sometimes used in patients with more severe RA who are beginning a remittive regimen in order to maintain function and employability while awaiting a therapeutic response. The long-term goal is always to discontinue steroids, although a few patients with the most severe RA may require low-dose treatment for years.

Intra-articular steroids are of value when the clinical picture is dominated by one or two joints, and this approach may control the local inflammatory response for months. It is inadvisable to inject a given joint any more than 3–4 times/year, since excess exposure to intra-articular steroids has been reported to result in a Charcot-like arthropathy.

TABLE 255.4.	Second-Line Drugs Used for Rheumatoid Disease
Agent	**Usual Dose**
Intramuscular gold	50 mg weekly during induction, less frequently later
Oral gold (Auranofin)	3 mg. bid.
Antimalarials-hydroxychloroquine	200 mg bid. initially, once daily later
Methotrexate	5.0–7.5 mg initially orally, subcutaneously or IM weekly, progressing to 15 mg weekly
Azathioprine	50 mg once daily, progressing slowly to 150–200 mg daily
D-Penicillamine	250 mg once daily, progressing slowly to 750–1500 mg daily
Sulfasalazine	2000–3000 mg daily

CHAPTER 256 INFECTIOUS ARTHRITIS

Infectious arthritis is curable if appropriate therapy is initiated promptly to prevent joint destruction. Synovial fluid culture, Gram stain, and synovianalysis are mandatory when infection is suspected.

Bacterial Arthritis (Septic Arthritis)

Among the 3 million cases of gonococcal (GC) infection that occur annually in the United States, nearly 1% will become bacteremic and develop arthritis, making GC infection the most common cause of joint sepsis. Additional information on septic arthritis is provided in chapter 156. The septic joint is usually inflamed, with marked redness, heat, swelling, tenderness, and limited motion. Usually monoarticular, the disease may be polyarticular in up to 10% of patients, generally in the immunosuppressed. Although any joint may become septic, large joints, especially the knees and hips, are the most vulnerable.

Most septic arthritides evolve hematogenously. Rarely, it originates by contiguous spread. Predisposing factors are extra-articular infection, a previously damaged joint, coexistent arthritis, chronic medical illness (malignancy, cirrhosis, diabetes mellitus, and IV drug use), and immunosuppression from any cause.

■ Clinical Assessment and Diagnosis

Clinical assessment and directed studies may reveal a nidus of infection. Patients, often febrile, may report rigors.

Disseminated gonococcal infection (chapter 150) may present uniquely as a polyarthritis. Most patients with gonococcal arthritis have no genitourinary symptoms, despite positive cultures at these sites. They may report migratory or additive polyarthralgias. Patients with gonococcal infection tend to have tenosynovitis at multiple sites and multiple skin lesions that are usually painless, hemorrhagic macules which may evolve into pustules or vesicles. Patients with monoarthritis have the dermatitis less often (40%).

Peripheral leukocytosis is common and acute phase reactants are elevated in septic arthritis. At least 2 blood cultures should be drawn, and cultures of any suspected portal of entry (skin lesion, urine, sputum) obtained.

When gonococcal arthritis is suspected, rectal, urethral, cervical, and possibly pharyngeal cultures are mandatory. Gram stains of the urethral swabs are a useful initial screen in men, but the finding of gram-negative diplococci in cervical smears is nonspecific in women. In gonococcal arthritis, genitourinary cultures provide the best yield (>70% cases), as cultures of skin lesion and joint fluid are usually unrevealing. In contrast, in over two-thirds of cases of nongonococcal bacterial arthritis, Gram stain and culture of joint fluid yield an organism. Radiographs show only soft tissue swelling initially, but may be of use in follow-up if osteomyelitis or joint damage is suspected.

Synovianalysis is mandatory when a septic joint is suspected. The fluid is usually cloudy, with decreased viscosity and poor mucin clot, and contains 5,000–250,000 leukocytes/mm^3 (mostly neutrophils). The fluid glucose is frequently 50% of a simultaneous serum level.

■ Management

Although Gram stain and culture are essential for a correct diagnosis and to guide appropriate therapy (Table 256.1), occasionally therapy must begin despite a negative Gram stain (Table 256.2). For gram-positive cocci, a penicillinase-resistant penicillin or vancomycin should be begun, and for gram-negative cocci, an extended spectrum cephalosporin is selected.

When no organisms are seen, treatment should be further individualized, keeping the clinical setting in mind (e.g., immunosuppression enhancing the risk for gram-negative rods or IV drug use increasing the risk of *Pseudomonas*). Cultures should be plated on blood agar routinely and on chocolate agar if *Neisseria gonorrhoeae* or *Haemophilus influenzae* is suspected. When indicated, fungal, mycobacterial, and anaerobic cultures must also be done. When the organism is identified, therapy

TABLE 256.1.	Intravenous Antibiotic Therapy Based on Culture Results	
Organism	**Antibiotic**	**Alternate**
Staphylococcus†	Nafcillin	Vancomycin
Streptococcus†	Penicillin G	Vancomycin, cefazolin, clindamycin
Neisseria gonorrhoeae†	Ceftriaxone	Spectinomycin
Haemophilus	3rd generation cephalosporin	Chloramphenicol
Enterobacteriaceae		
Escherichia coli, Salmonella, Klebsiella, Enterobacter, Proteus	Gentamicin	Tobramycin, amikacin
Pseudomonas	Antipseudomonal penicillin + gentamicin	

†Common organisms

TABLE 256.2. Initial Antibiotic Therapy for Suspected Septic Arthritis with a Negative Gram Stain Based on Patient's Age

Age (Yrs)	Suggested regimen	Alternate	Coverage
<½	Penicillinase-resistant penicillin + aminoglycoside		Gram positive cocci, Coliforms
½–6	Third generation cephalosporin		Haemophilus influenzae, Streptococci
6–15	Penicillinase-resistant penicillin	Vancomycin	Staphylococci, Streptococci
15–60	Third generation cephalosporin		Neisseria gonorrhoeae, Staphylococci
>60	Penicillinase-resistant penicillin	Vancomycin + third generation cephalosporin	Staphylococci, Coliforms

should be modified accordingly and continued for at least 7–10 days after the inflammation abates. For *Staphylococcus aureus* and gram-negative bacilli, 3–4 weeks of parenteral therapy is recommended, followed by 2–4 weeks of oral therapy.

Initially, the joint should be immobilized to relieve pain, but passive range of motion exercises should be gradually added to prevent joint contracture (reduced range of motion of the joint). Until a microbe is identified or a clinical response apparent, analgesics without antipyretic effect should be used. Joint effusions should be drained by simple aspiration, usually daily initially and then later, as often as necessary. Synovial fluid volume, cell count, and cultures should be monitored.

If needle aspiration cannot accomplish adequate drainage, early orthopedic consultation should be sought for open drainage. Prompt surgical drainage is required if the hip is infected, pus is loculated, or the arthritis does not respond to treatment after 3–4 days.

Tuberculous Arthritis

Diagnosis of tuberculous arthritis is often delayed because its symptoms are generally less severe and indolent. Furthermore, skeletal tuberculosis is uncommon, and tuberculosis itself is nonendemic in the United States. Mycobacteria enter the joint hematogenously or from an adjacent osseous focus. Active pulmonary tuberculosis is usually absent, and constitutional symptoms are generally lacking.

One-half of all skeletal tuberculosis occurs in the spine **(Pott's disease),** followed by weight-bearing joints (hip and knee, 15% each; ankle and wrist, 5–10%). Back pain and muscle spasm are usual symptoms of spinal tuberculosis, and findings include local tenderness, kyphosis, and referred pain from root compression. Radiographs show disc space narrowing and vertebral collapse; a paraspinous abscess may be seen.

Articular tuberculosis usually presents insidiously with chronic low-grade monoarthralgia; swelling and stiffness is less frequent. Most patients have both osseous and synovial infection. Initially, radiographs show soft tissue swelling and osteopenia. Later, subchondral marginal erosions appear and eventually, joint space narrowing and bony destruction occur without osteophyte formation.

Diagnosis depends on a high index of suspicion. Tuberculin skin test (PPD) is positive in 90% of cases, but older or very ill patients may be anergic. Synovial fluid shows leukocytosis (10,000–20,000 cells/mm^3, mostly neutrophils), elevated protein, and usually low glucose. Acid-fast smear is positive in 20%, and culture, in 80%. **Synovial biopsy** provides the quickest and most reliable diagnosis. Biopsy, culture, and DNA probe techniques (see chapter 218) can provide the diagnosis in over 90% of cases.

Treatment is similar to that of pulmonary tuberculosis, utilizing 3–4 mycobactericidal drugs for 6–9 months. Surgical drainage is reserved for cases with severe joint destruction or, in spinal tuberculosis, those with paraparesis.

Lyme Disease

Lyme disease, a systemic illness, is caused by the spirochete *Borrelia burgdorferi*. Initial infection produces flu-like symptoms, followed in 70% of cases by a characteristic rash, **erythema migrans** (EM), at the site

of an *Ixodid* (deer) tick bite. A secondary phase leading to cardiac conduction defects or neurologic abnormalities (e.g., Bell's palsy) develops weeks to months later in some patients. A tertiary phase accompanied by intermittent or chronic arthritis appears months to years later in untreated patients. Most cases of Lyme disease in the United States occur in the summer and in three locations (Northeast, upper Midwest, and the Pacific coast).

EM is a rapidly expanding annular erythematous rash that develops usually at the site of the tick bite. About 50% of patients develop multiple annular secondary lesions. Intermittent symptoms that often accompany the rash include malaise, fatigue, headache, fever, chills, stiff neck, myalgias, and arthralgias. Initially, **migratory arthralgias** occur; a large-joint **oligoarthritis** (60%) evolves later. Recurrences follow without sequelae for several years, but a chronic destructive oligoarthritis occurs in 10%.

Viral Arthritis

Viral arthritis is usually accompanied by nonspecific symptoms related to the systemic viral infection, such as lymphadenopathy and rash. Arthritis is often **symmetric** with varying signs of inflammation. Rubella, human parvovirus B19, and hepatitis B and C are the common viral pathogens. Hepatitis B may present with polyarthritis, low serum complement, and urticaria that clear as jaundice appears.

Laboratory abnormalities are nonspecific. Most commonly, the erythrocyte sedimentation rate is high, and synovial fluid is inflammatory. The patient's history (rubella immunization, exposure to en-

Special spirochetal culture techniques are not routinely available. Specific IgM antibody titers or rising titers suggest a recent infection. False-positive tests and background positivity in endemic areas render diagnosis and evaluation of level of activity difficult. Western blot testing provides more specific evidence of infection. Polymerase chain reaction (PCR) on synovial fluid and cerebrospinal fluid may be employed when other testing is inconclusive.

Oral doxycycline or penicillin shortens the early stages and can prevent later major multisystem disease, although 50% still have recurrent bouts of headache or musculoskeletal pain. High-dose IV penicillin or ceftriaxone for 2–3 weeks is used to treat the later neurologic, musculoskeletal, and cardiac involvement.

demic area and seasonal onset, IV drug use for hepatitis B) and serologic tests provide the diagnosis. The course is usually short and uneventful. Treatment is symptomatic.

Human immunodeficiency virus (HIV) infection has been associated with a severe form of Reiter's syndrome, manifested as widespread joint involvement and generalized rash resembling pustular psoriasis. Disease associations with HIV infection include polymyositis, dermatomyositis, vasculitis, and "diffuse infiltrative lymphocytosis syndrome," with some similarity to Sjögren's syndrome.

CHAPTER 257 SERONEGATIVE SPONDYLOARTHROPATHIES

The seronegative (rheumatoid factor negative) spondyloarthropathies comprise a group of disorders with frequent back involvement (sacroiliitis or spondylitis), enthesopathy (inflammation at ligamentous or tendon insertions onto bone), and peripheral arthritis. They include ankylosing spondylitis, reactive arthritis and Reiter's syndrome, psoriatic spondyloarthropathy, and the spondyloarthropathy of inflammatory bowel disease (see Table 257.1).

The peripheral arthritis is typically **oligoarticular** and **asymmetric.** Involvement of the MCP, PIP, and DIP joints on a single digit with sparing of adjacent digits leads to a **"sausage digit"** (dactylitis), which is typical of these diseases. On radiographs, juxta-articular osteoporosis is lacking, and entheses may show periostitis (new bone formation in the periosteum), erosions, and fluffy whiskering (small spicules of new bone

TABLE 257.1. Spondyloarthropathies: A Glossary of Conditions

Ankylosing spondylitis	Inflammation of spinal joints resulting in back pain, stiffness, and progressive fusion of the spine.
Reactive arthritis	Usually oligoarticular lower extremity large joint arthritis following bowel infection by enteric pathogens.
Reiter's syndrome	A form of reactive arthritis, usually associated with genitourinary infection (e.g., Chlamydia), and characterized by arthritis, uveitis, urethritis, and skin and mucous membrane lesions.
Psoriatic arthritis	Arthritis affecting peripheral joints or spinal joints in association with psoriasis.
Colitic arthritis	Arthritis affecting peripheral joints or spinal joints in association with ulcerative colitis or Crohn's disease.

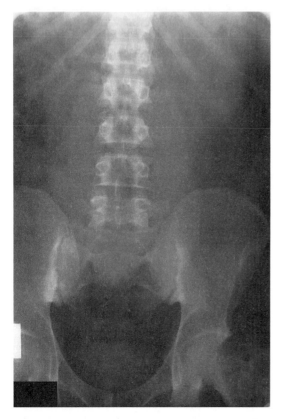

FIGURE 257.1. Roentgenogram of the pelvis showing *bilateral sacroiliitis* with sclerosis and irregularity of the joint margins in a young man with Reiter's syndrome. The sacroiliitis was asymptomatic.

formation). On presentation, radiographs in most patients show erosive **sacroiliitis**, which is often asymptomatic (Figure 257.1).

Patients with these diseases show an unusually high frequency of HLA-B27 (Table 257.2). HLA-B27 is noted in 8% of normal whites and even fewer blacks. Epidemiologic data suggest that the HLA-B27-positive person is susceptible to the development of a spondyloarthropathy following an infection or exposure to an antigen. For example, bacillary dysentery or nongonococcal urethritis often precedes reactive arthritis and Reiter's syndrome. A large proportion of patients with these diseases have incomplete or overlapping presentations of disease, which preclude formation of acceptable classification criteria.

TABLE 257.2. Frequency of HLA-B27 in Spondyloarthropathies	
Disease	**Frequency %**
Ankylosing spondylitis	85–90
Reiter's syndrome	
All patients	60–75
With sacroiliitis	90–100
Inflammatory Bowel Disease	
Peripheral arthritis	No increase
Spondylitis	30–50
Psoriasis	
Peripheral arthritis	No increase
Spondylitis	40–50
Normal Caucasian men	8–9

Ankylosing Spondylitis

The incidence of ankylosing spondylitis is about 0.1–0.2%. Symptomatic ankylosing spondylitis usually begins before age 40, with men predominating 9:1. The most common symptom is **low back pain,** which differs from the common discogenic or mechanical causes of back pain in that it is worse upon arising, associated with morning stiffness, improves with light exercise, interferes with sleep, and infrequently causes radicular or neurologic deficits. In late cases, the cauda equina syndrome may occur rarely.

Physical findings in early cases can be normal. About one-third of patients develop peripheral joint disease at some time (Table 257.3), with ankylosing (causing progressive fusion) arthritis of the hips and shoulders being the most common nonaxial involvement.

Although most cases are probably not progressive, a minority of patients develop **ascending spinal inflam-** **mation.** Roentgenograms may progress from normal initially to sacroiliitis, followed by squaring of the vertebral bodies, and later ligamentous ossification **(syndesmophytes)** and joint fusion **("bamboo spine").** Involvement of the costovertebral joints can cause pleuritic pain and immobility of the rib cage which limits chest expansion. Eventually, fusion of the entire spine may occur.

Iritis occurs in 20% and may be the presenting complaint. In 5% of patients inflammation of the aortic root causes aortic insufficiency or atrioventricular conduction disturbances.

Early diagnosis of ankylosing spondylitis can be difficult. Testing for HLA-B27 in those with back pain offers minimal diagnostic help, because back pain is a very common disorder. **Treatment** consists of physical therapy to maintain mobility and posture, combined with NSAIDs. Probably, indomethacin is the most

TABLE 257.3. Features of Spondyloarthropathies								
	Sacroiliitis	**Spine**	**Peripheral arthritis**	**Iritis**	**Aortitis**	**Cutaneous**	**Gastrointestinal**	**Genitourinary**
Ankylosing spondylitis	+++[1]	+++[2]	+	+	++	–	–	–
Reiter's syndrome	+++[3]	+++[4]	+++[5]	++[6]	+	+++	++	+++
Psoriatic arthritis	++[3]	++[3]	+	+	+	+++	–	–
Inflammatory bowel disease	+++[1]	+++[2]	+	+	+	–	++++	–

[1] Bilateral involvement
[2] Ascending pattern
[3] Can be asymmetric, i.e. unilateral syndesmophyte or one side larger than the other
[4] Tendency toward "skip pattern," i.e., skips vertebral segments
[5] Usually in lower extremity
[6] Conjunctivitis is the first manifestation in most patients.

effective NSAID; it may be used in divided doses up to 150–200 mg/day. Sulfasalazine or methotrexate may confer some benefit, but medications do not seem to halt progression of the disease.

Reiter's Syndrome and Reactive Arthritis

The classic triad of Reiter's syndrome consists of arthritis, conjunctivitis, and nongonococcal urethritis. The arthritis is usually oligoarticular, affecting joints in the lower extremity more than the upper extremity. The enthesitis is most often detected at the insertion sites of the plantar fascia and the Achilles tendon. Other features include spondylitis, shallow and usually asymptomatic ulcers on tongue and palate, circinate balanitis of the penis, and a characteristic desquamative rash on the soles or palms termed **keratoderma blennorrhagicum.** Spondylitis may involve the sacroiliac joints and vertebral column asymmetrically and may skip to the dorsal or cervical spine rather than ascending contiguously.

Acute attacks subside in several weeks to a few months in 95% of cases, with the remaining becoming chronic. Remissions carry a 10% annual risk of recurrence, with recurrences occurring in half the cases.

One-half of patients with Reiter's syndrome have evidence of *Chlamydia* infection, with antichlamydial antibodies, synovial biopsies showing chlamydial antigens and organism fragments, or by isolation of chlamydia from the urethra. Urethritis may also be due to *Ureaplasma urealyticum.* Epidemics of Reiter's-like illness, virtually all in HLA-B27-positive persons, have followed outbreaks of *Shigella flexneri* dysentery. Similar illnesses that have followed *Salmonella, Campylobacter, Yersinia enterocolitica,* and *Clostridium difficile* infection are termed **reactive arthritis** because the arthritis is in some way occurring as a reaction to the infection.

There is no specific laboratory test for Reiter's syndrome, and the diagnosis is made on the constellation of clinical features. Initial **treatment** is similar to that for ankylosing spondylitis. Sulfasalazine, methotrexate, and azathioprine have been successful in controlling persistent synovitis in many of these patients.

Psoriatic Arthritis

Arthropathy occurs in 6% of patients with psoriasis. In about 75%, the skin disease precedes the arthritis, and in 15%, the arthritis precedes the dermatitis, and in the remainder, the two manifestations begin concurrently. The severity of the skin disease and joint involvement correlate poorly, and in some patients, nail pitting (see Figure 44.2) may be the only clue to the diagnosis.

An asymmetric oligoarthritis occurs in 70% of patients. In 5–15%, the peripheral arthritis involves the DIP joints almost exclusively. In about 15%, the arthritis is symmetric and mimics rheumatoid arthritis, with some cases even being RF-seropositive. (These probably represent the incidental occurrence of both diseases.) Severe, osteolytic, disfiguring arthritis of the hands, termed **arthritis mutilans,** occurs in 5%. Inflammatory spondylitis that tends to spare the sacroiliac joints occurs in 40% of patients; men are predisposed 6:1 over women.

Treatment is similar to that for rheumatoid arthritis, although the role of gold therapy is less well established. Although antimalarials have led to improvement in the arthritis, they can cause a severe flare of the skin disease and should be used with caution. Methotrexate, azathioprine, and sulfasalazine have proven effectiveness. PUVA

Arthritis and Inflammatory Bowel Disease

Peripheral arthritis occurs in 12% of patients with ulcerative colitis and 20% of those with Crohn's disease, typically with symmetrical, large-joint arthritis in the lower extremities (colitic arthritis). The activity and severity of the arthritis usually parallels that of the bowel disease. About 7% of patients with inflammatory bowel disease have ankylosing spondylitis, the majority being

therapy given to control skin symptoms may improve the peripheral joint disease. Remission of spinal disease remains undocumented.

positive for HLA-B27 (Table 257.1); however, little correlation is seen between the spondylitis symptoms and activity of the bowel disease.

Therapy for the joint disease should be directed at the underlying bowel disease. The spine disease is treated similarly to ankylosing spondylitis.

CHAPTER **258** **SYSTEMIC LUPUS ERYTHEMATOSUS**

Systemic lupus erythematosus (SLE), first described in 1905 by Sir William Osler, predominantly affects women (95%) between 15 and 40 years. It afflicts about 0.1% of the general population but appears to be slightly more common and more severe in nonwhites.

■ Etiology And Pathogenesis

The cause of SLE is unknown. Its predilection for women suggests the influence of estrogen on the immunologic abnormalities. An increased frequency of HLA-B8, -DR2, and -DR3 and the occurrence of disease in monozygotic twins but not dizygotic twins strongly suggest a genetic predisposition. Environmental factors, such as UV light, may activate not only skin disease but also systemic disease. A panoply of antibodies against various tissue antigens may be found in such patients' sera.

Elevated immunoglobulin levels reflect B-cell stimulation. However, specific autoantibodies cause disease by direct reaction with a target tissue (e.g., immune thrombocytopenia) or by tissue deposition of the resulting immune complex (e.g., SLE nephritis, immune complex vasculitis). These immune complexes are poorly cleared by the reticuloendothelial system, perhaps due to inherited deficiencies of several complement components.

Some **drugs** can induce antinuclear antibody (ANA) and occasionally, overt clinical symptoms of SLE. Despite the long list, **procainamide, hydralazine, isoniazid, diphenylhydantoin,** and **penicillamine** are the most common offenders. Over 60% of patients taking procainamide develop ANAs with time, whereas only 5% of these develop symptoms of SLE. Most often, such

patients have only fever, serositis, and arthritis. Generally, cessation of the drug leads to alleviation of symptoms over several weeks to months (although the serologic changes may persist for years).

■ Clinical Features

SLE potentially involves every body system (Table 258.1). However, not all systems are affected in any given case, which may lead to insufficient criteria to make a definitive diagnosis of SLE at initial presentation. Over time, other features will appear that confirm the diagnosis.

The integument is commonly affected in SLE. A faint, relatively nonspecific **malar rash** is seen in 25% of patients, but the classic, **florid butterfly rash** is seen in only about 5%. Discoid lesions occur in about 10%. Other skin lesions include urticaria, macular or papular eruptions, bullae, and panniculitis. Livedo reticularis, Raynaud's phenomenon, nailbed telangiectasia, splinter hemorrhages, and Osler's nodes (tender, erythematous thickenings in the finger pads) reflect the underlying vasculitis. Oral mucosal or nasal septal ulcerations are often painless and, therefore, frequently missed. Patchy alopecia or brittle hair ("lupus hair") is seen in about 15% of cases and reflects involvement of the skin appendages.

Joint pain and **swelling** together represent the most frequent manifestation of SLE, being seen in 95% of patients. Typically, the arthritis is nondeforming and nonerosive, unlike that in rheumatoid arthritis. However, a minority can develop rheumatoid arthritis-like ulnar deviation and swan-neck deformities secondary to periarticular soft tissue changes (Figure 258.1). Aseptic

TABLE 258.1.	1982 Revised American College of Rheumatology Criteria for the Diagnosis of Systemic Lupus Erythematosus*

Criterion	Comment
Malar (butterfly) rash	Spares nasolabial folds
Discoid skin lesions	Atrophic scarring may occur in older lesions
Photosensitivity	Unusual reaction to sunlight
Oral ulcers	Usually painless; may be nasopharyngeal
Nonerosive arthritis	Involves >2 peripheral joints
Serositis	Pleuritis (pleurisy, pleural rub, or effusion) or pericarditis (abnormal ECG, rub, or pericardial effusion)
Renal disorder	Persistent proteinuria >0.5 g/24 hr, or >3+ proteinuria on dipstick, or cellular casts
Neurologic disorder	Seizures or psychosis in the absence of offending drugs or metabolic derangements
Hematologic disorder	Cytopenias on >2 occasions: hemolytic anemia with reticulocytosis, leukopenia <4000/mm^3, or lymphopenia <1500/mm^3, or thrombocytopenia <100,000/mm^3
Immunologic disorder	Anti-native DNA or anti-Smith (Sm) antibodies or positive LE cell prep, or false-positive VDRL
Antinuclear antibody	Abnormal ANA titer in the absence of drugs associated with drug-induced lupus

*For the purposes of case definition, diagnosis of SLE requires the presence of 4 of these 11 criteria, either serially or simultaneously. (Adapted from: Tan et al. Arthritis Rheum 1992, 1271-1277.)

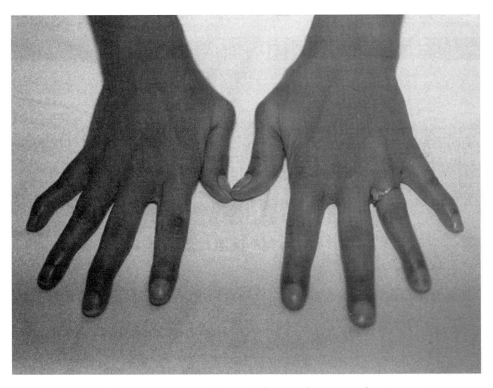

FIGURE 258.1. Hands of a woman with systemic lupus erythematosus, showing synovitis in several PIP joints and swan-neck deformities.

necrosis of bone, most often involving the femoral or humeral heads, can follow steroid therapy or vasculitis.

Serositis may occur as pericarditis, pleuritis, or peritoneal inflammation. Pericarditis occurs in 25% but rarely causes cardiac malfunction. Angina or myocardial infarction can result from vasculitis of the small coronary vessels or from coronary atherosclerosis as a result of corticosteroid therapy. Aortic or mitral insufficiency is seen in the rare patient with valvulitis. Libman-Sacks (verrucous) endocarditis is typically asymptomatic but may predispose to bacterial endocarditis.

Pleuritis, the most common pleuro-pulmonary manifestation, is seen in 30% of cases. Lupus pneumonitis is uncommon. Thus, a pulmonary infiltrate in SLE is more apt to be infectious than due to the underlying pulmonary disease (chapter 231).

Approximately 25% of patients exhibit some form of neurologic involvement. Virtually any central or peripheral neurologic structure can be affected, although seizures, cerebrovascular accidents, and organic mental syndromes predominate. CNS disease is the second leading cause of death. Lupus cerebritis leading to diffuse cortical atrophy, irreversible dementia, and organic brain syndrome is especially ominous.

Another pathogenetic mechanism for CNS lupus is that of vaso-occlusive stroke. These patients usually present with physical signs of one or more specific ablative neurologic defects, which may be detectable on computed tomography, magnetic resonance imaging, or arteriography. Vascular occlusion in these patients is due to vasculitis or thromboembolism, the latter being related to antiphospholipid antibodies (lupus anticoagulant).

Proximal muscle weakness may reflect myositis with elevation of muscle enzymes and other features of myositis (See Ch. 259).

About one-half of patients with SLE develop clinically apparent **renal disease** suggested by hematuria and/or proteinuria (see chapter 165). In general, the more diffuse the glomerulitis, the worse the prognosis. Patients with minimal or focal change on light microscopy have a generally benign prognosis, and those with pure membranous change, an intermediate prognosis. About one-third of patients with focal or membranous change, however, can progress in time to diffuse **lupus glomerulonephritis.** Thus, it is likely that every patient with clinically apparent renal involvement warrants treatment. Renal biopsy plays an important role in the management of lupus nephritis. Evidence suggests that the degree of chronic change on biopsy (e.g., scarring, crescents) identifies patients who do less well over several years.

Most patients with SLE have the anemia of chronic disease. In 5% or less, the anemia is an autoimmune hemolytic type. Granulocytopenia or lymphopenia can also occur. Although mild thrombocytopenia occurs in one-third, severe autoimmune thrombocytopenia develops in 5%.

■ Laboratory Features

Antinuclear, anti-DNA, and the variety of other autoantibodies possible in SLE are listed in Table 251.5.

A peripheral (rim) pattern of nuclear staining on the ANA strongly suggests SLE. Whereas the presence of anti-Smith or high titers of antinative DNA are virtually diagnostic, they are only 40–50% sensitive. Conversely, a negative ANA virtually excludes SLE-except in "subacute cutaneous lupus," in which ANA is negative but anti-Ro (SSA) antibodies are present. This subgroup of SLE patients features primarily photosensitivity, causing annular skin lesions and arthritis.

Depressions of serum hemolytic complement correlate with immune complex nephritis or, alternatively, may reflect congenital absence of one of the complement components (C2 deficiency is the most common). The latter patients are significantly more likely to develop SLE, polymyositis, or another autoimmune disease than the general population.

Twenty percent of SLE patients have a false-positive VDRL test, which may antedate full-fledged SLE by decades. Among these, 5% have a prolonged partial thromboplastin time, attributable to an antibody against the platelet factor III-factor X-factor V complex **(lupus anticoagulant).**

Radioimmunoassay results suggest that up to 50% of patients may have **anticardiolipin antibodies.** Hemorrhagic problems are rare in such patients. Instead, about one-third are at risk for thromboembolic disease, which may take the form of venous thromboembolism, stroke, or other vascular occlusive syndromes. Anticardiolipin antibody also identifies a group with recurrent spontaneous abortions, some of whom have no evidence of SLE.

The **antiphospholipid syndrome** should be considered in persons with a hypercoagulable state (younger persons without risk factors or those with recurrent thrombotic episodes) if other causes of hypercoagulability are excluded. A prolonged partial thromboplastin time or thrombocytopenia may be the tip-off.

Synovianalysis in active arthritis reveals 2000–5000 leukocytes/mm³. In patients with renal disease, a nephritic picture (microscopic hematuria or red cell casts), serum creatinine, blood pressure and serologic changes, and the degree of proteinuria can predict quite accurately the changes on biopsy. The closest correlate of lupus glomerulonephritis is a low serum complement, the second being a high level of anti-native DNA.

■ Diagnosis

The American College of Rheumatology criteria for diagnosis of SLE are useful in illustrating the protean clinical and serologic features of SLE (Table 258.1). For the purpose of clinical studies, the case definition requires that 4 or more criteria be met serially or simultaneously for an unequivocal diagnosis of SLE. Many patients with SLE acquire 4 criteria only after some years.

Management and Prognosis

Treatment of SLE is based on its severity. Rapid onset and the presence of both anti-DNA antibodies and low serum complement suggest more severe disease. Arthritis and, often, serositis respond to aspirin or other NSAIDs. Both arthritis and dermatologic manifestations can be treated with antimalarials, but ophthalmologic monitoring is required to detect early toxicity.

Indications for high-dose corticosteroid therapy (prednisone, 60–100 mg/day or equivalent, in divided doses) include severe multisystem disease, serositis unresponsive to NSAIDs, central or peripheral nervous system disease, vasculitis, hemolytic anemia, immune thrombocytopenia, and glomerulonephritis. Controlling blood pressure in hypertensive lupus patients is critical to prevent further renal deterioration. If corticosteroids fail to suppress disease activity, cytotoxic drugs (e.g., cyclophosphamide or azathioprine) are indicated, especially in active renal disease.

Drug-induced lupus is treated by withdrawal of the offending agent, which leads to the gradual disappearance of symptoms and eventually of the ANA.

The prognosis for SLE patients has improved. Since the introduction of corticosteroids, 5-year survival rates of 93–94% are reported. The use of cytotoxic agents delays the onset of renal failure requiring dialysis. Infection is the most common cause of death, and those with renal and CNS disease have the worst 5-year survival rate.

CHAPTER **259** OTHER CONNECTIVE TISSUE DISEASES

Myositis

Polymyositis (PM), dermatomyositis (DM), and inclusion body myositis are inflammatory disorders of the skeletal muscle, typically featuring symmetric proximal muscle weakness. These disorders are distinguished from each other by the presence of a rash in DM or by muscle biopsy findings. They may be associated with malignancy and may overlap with other connective tissue disorders, such as systemic sclerosis, systemic lupus erythematosus, mixed connective tissue disease, rheumatoid arthritis, and polyarteritis nodosa.

Clinical Features

The incidence of the muscle disorders is about 1:100,000. Most cases develop in the fifth or sixth decade, predominantly in women (2:1). Cases associated with neoplasia have no gender predilection and usually present in the seventh decade.

The presenting symptom in most patients (70–95%) is insidious **proximal muscle weakness** (e.g., difficulty in arising from a low chair, going up steps, combing hair, or placing dishes in upper cupboards); others develop a waddling gait with severe weakness. Muscle pain and tenderness, which are not always prominent, occur at some time in two-thirds.

Although proximal muscles are weaker than distal muscles, distal muscle weakness occurs in 20%. Profound muscle atrophy and joint contractures may develop as the disease progresses. More severe cases (15%) develop dysphagia due to skeletal muscle weakness in the posterior pharynx and proximal third of the esophagus; the consequences are regurgitation and aspiration pneumonia. While distal esophageal hypomotility may be seen in 50% on careful search, it is usually clinically insignificant. Interstitial lung disease is seen in 5–10%, but in a minority, dyspnea is due to intercostal muscle weakness. The ECG is abnormal, usually showing conduction defects in one-half, but without symptoms. Arthralgias without synovitis are common (25%), but these are more likely to have an associated connective tissue disease. Myocarditis is rare.

The classic rash of DM—a **dusky-red facial eruption** commonly affecting the malar and periorbital areas but also the neck, shoulders, and upper chest—occurs in 30% of adults and 7% of children with myositis. The eyelids may be lilac-colored (heliotrope rash), which is highly suggestive of DM, and these patients may also have periorbital edema and telangiectasia. A second rash is a deep-red papular plaque usually involving extensor surfaces, especially the knuckles, followed by elbows, knees, and medial malleoli (**Gottron's sign).** Whitish scaling may be noted. Nail-fold capillaries may be dilated, with hyperemia and telangiectasia in the periungual area. Cutaneous vasculitis, with tender nodules, periungual infarctions, and digital ulcerations, is seen more commonly in adults with neoplasia or in children.

Inclusion body myositis is a more recently described form of myositis with a more subtle presentation. Inclusion bodies are basophilic rimmed vacuoles seen on light microscopy and masses of filamentous material on electron microscopy. Inclusion body myositis tends to develop insidiously in older persons, affecting men more frequently and being less responsive to conventional agents. Thus, apparently ineffective therapy should be withdrawn so as to avoid needless risks from medications.

A **malignancy** is associated with myositis in about 5–20% of cases, with cancers of the lung, ovary, breast, and stomach being the most common. Myositis precedes the clinical appearance of cancer by 1–2 years in about two-thirds of cases. Patients over 40 years, particularly those with DM, are at a higher risk for a cancer, and a careful search for neoplasia is warranted in such patients.

■ Laboratory Features

Elevated serum **muscle enzyme** levels from active muscle damage are a typical feature. Creatine kinase (CK) is the most sensitive, but aldolase, aspartate aminotransferase, glutamic pyruvic transaminase, and lactic dehydrogenase levels may also rise. The CK is high initially in 70% and eventually in 95% of patients. Rheumatoid factor occurs in 40%, and ANA in 20–60%. Antiaminoacyl tRNA synthetases and anti-signal recognition particle may define subsets. The anti-Jo 1 (histadyl tRNA synthetase) is associated with interstitial lung disease, Raynaud's phenomenon, and arthritis.

The **electromyogram** (EMG) is abnormal in 70–90% of patients. The most typical EMG feature is a short-duration, low-amplitude, polyphasic action potential with voluntary contraction. Spontaneous fibrillations, positive sawtooth potentials (denervation pattern), and insertional irritability are other patterns.

The muscle biopsy is abnormal in 75–90%. It is important to biopsy a muscle that is weakened but not atrophied. The quadriceps and deltoid muscles are biopsied most frequently. The EMG also may help select a biopsy site; however, because of electrode-induced changes, the biopsy should then be done on the opposite side. Biopsy findings include inflammation in 65% (fiber destruction and regeneration, inflammatory infiltrates); the predominantly lymphocytic infiltrate is seen between muscle fibers or around blood vessels. Muscle fibers may show necrosis and phagocytic invasion. Biopsy may be normal in 17%, given the patchy nature of the disease. Myositis associated with other connective tissue diseases or childhood more often shows vasculitis.

■ Diagnosis and Differential Diagnosis

The following criteria are useful in diagnosis:
- Symmetric proximal muscle weakness
- Characteristic EMG patterns
- Elevated muscle enzymes
- Abnormal muscle biopsy
- Typical skin rash

PM is definite if the first 4 criteria are met, and probable with 3 of the first 4. DM is definite when the skin rash occurs with 3 of the other 4 criteria, and probable with 2.

Patients with polymyalgia rheumatica have pain in proximal extremities that may be perceived as weakness, but muscle strength, CK, EMG, and biopsy are normal. Endocrinopathies (Addison's disease, Cushing's disease, thyrotoxicosis, and hypothyroidism) may mimic an inflammatory myopathy, but CK is generally normal (although it may rise in hypothyroidism). Drugs such as HMG-CoA reductase inhibitors, penicillamine, clofibrate, hydroxychloroquine, ipecac, and especially ethanol and cocaine may cause a toxic myopathy. Myositis related to sarcoidosis is distinguished by a compatible clinical picture and noncaseating granuloma on biopsy.

■ Management

Initial therapy consists of prednisone, 50–100 mg/d, continued for 1–3 months. The dosage is then gradually reduced as muscle strength improves. The CK level is the most useful biochemical index to follow; its decline often precedes improved muscle strength, and its elevation, a relapse.

Approximately 75% of patients can discontinue steroids eventually, but relapses are common. Some require maintenance steroids, either daily or every other day. Cytotoxic therapy (with methotrexate, azathioprine, and, less often, cyclophosphamide) is employed commonly for steroid-sparing or when steroids have been ineffective. Although they can control most cases of PM or DM, their onset of action is somewhat slower.

■ Prognosis

About 73% of patients will be alive after 8 years of disease. Younger age confers a better prognosis. Associated malignancy or profound weakness, especially of pharyngeal muscles, worsen the outlook. If myositis occurs as part of an overlap syndrome, the prognosis may be determined by the associated connective tissue disease. Death most commonly ensues from a malignancy or sepsis.

Systemic Sclerosis

Systemic sclerosis is characterized by hardening, thickening, or tightening of the skin (**scleroderma**) and vascular changes. It may present as **diffuse scleroderma** (proximal and distal extremity, facial and truncal skin involvement, and early onset of visceral manifestations) or as limited scleroderma (also called **CREST syndrome**—*c*alcinosis, *R*aynaud's phenomenon, *e*sophageal dysmotility, *s*clerodactyly with skin involvement usually limited to the fingers and face, and *t*elangiectasia, with delayed visceral manifestations). Other scleroderma syndromes are described subsequently. Overlaps occur with other connective tissue diseases.

Systemic sclerosis affects the skin, esophagus, and lungs and less often the joints, heart, small and large intestines, and kidneys. Its etiology is unknown. It features inflammation in tissues that evokes fibrosis. Vascular endothelial injury may be the primary abnormality, and the frequency of immunologic abnormalities supports an autoimmune etiology. The enhanced collagen synthesis seen in skin fibroblasts may be due to inflammation or locally released growth factors.

The disease affects 4–12 persons/million, often between 30 and 50 years of age. There is 3:1 predilection for women. Although the course may be variable, most persons have visceral involvement. Spontaneous remissions are rare.

■ Clinical Features

The skin is almost always involved, although in a few, visceral lesions develop without skin changes. The earliest skin changes are edema and taut hands and feet. In the next, indurated stage, the skin becomes shiny, taut, and hidebound, limiting joint motion (Figure 259.1). Skin creases and hair follicles disappear. In the atrophic phase, tight skin over joints, particularly the hands, causes contractures with ulcerations over bony prominences.

In **diffuse scleroderma,** the skin changes are most prominent in the distal extremities and gradually spread to the upper arms and legs, face, upper anterior chest, and abdomen. Hypo- or hyperpigmentation and telangiectasia may occur. Facial changes may narrow the oral aperture. In 3–15 years, the skin may enter the late phase of spontaneous softening. Skin biopsy in the classic and late stages shows increased subcutaneous collagen, epidermal thinning, and loss of rete pegs and sebaceous and sweat glands.

In **CREST syndrome,** the skin involvement is generally limited to the fingers and face. Subcutaneous calcifications of the digital pulp (Figure 259.2), extensor aspects of the forearm and olecranon, and prepatellar bursae may erode through the skin. Hand radiographs may show diffuse osteoporosis, resorption of the distal phalangeal tufts, and soft tissue calcifications.

Vascular abnormalities are a hallmark of scleroderma. Wide-field capillary microscopy of the nail-fold edge shows giant capillary loops in areas rendered avascular by loss of blood vessels. **Raynaud's phenomenon,** producing a classic triphasic color change, is virtually universal: on exposure to cold or emotional stress, the hands may first turn white or ashen (tissue anoxia), then blue (cyanosis), and finally red with

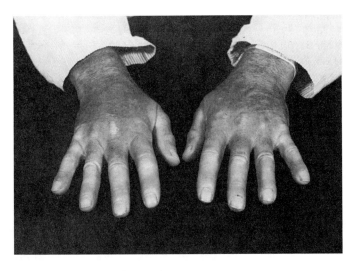

FIGURE **259.1.** Sclerodactyly in systemic sclerosis. Note the shiny skin, which is taut, hidebound and without skin creases.

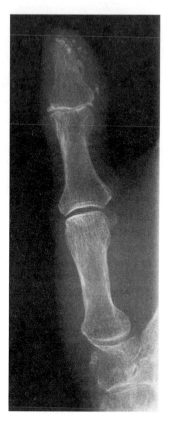

FIGURE 259.2. Roentgenogram of the thumb of a woman with CREST syndrome demonstrating soft tissue calcinosis.

the duodenum which may be widely dilated. Asymptomatic large-mouth sacculations of the large and small bowel due to atrophy of the muscularis, while rare, are distinctive. Primary biliary cirrhosis develops in some patients with CREST. Patients are at risk for severe cachexia late in the disease.

Symmetric polyarthralgias or polyarthritis and stiffness are the presenting complaints in approximately one-third and eventually develop in most patients.

Pulmonary involvement is quite common. Diffuse interstitial lung disease is most often manifested by exertional dyspnea and, less commonly, a chronic dry cough. Functional abnormalities often antedate symptoms, possibly because of decreased physical activity. Physical findings consist of tachypnea and early basilar rales. Radiographs show diffuse reticular changes predominantly involving the lower lung fields (Figure 259.3). Pulmonary function tests often show a restrictive impairment, with a low carbon monoxide diffusing capacity (DL_{CO}). Pulmonary hypertension may occur with or without interstitial disease, or as a late visceral manifestation of CREST (10%). Histologically, the major findings are interstitial and alveolar fibrosis. Patients with severe fibrotic lung disease may develop alveolar cell or other pulmonary neoplasm, the only malignancies with an excess frequency in this disease.

The **kidneys** are involved in 50% of cases of diffuse scleroderma and rarely in CREST. The lesions are slowly progressive arterial fibrinoid necrosis and intimal hyperplasia. Proteinuria, hypertension, azotemia, or low glo-

rewarming (increased blood flow). Pain, numbness, paresthesias, or a feeling of swelling as blood flow returns may be associated. Not all patients report all 3 phases. Raynaud's phenomenon has an extensive etiology, including mechanical injury (e.g., vibrating tool use), chemical exposure (e.g., vinyl chloride), certain drugs (e.g., ergot, ß-blockers, bleomycin), paraproteinemias, fibromyalgia, carpal tunnel syndrome, and thoracic outlet syndrome, but often it is idiopathic and unrelated to a connective tissue disease.

The **esophagus** is involved in 90%. Reflux symptoms are the most frequent complaints; dysphagia occurs in 50%. Stricture formation and esophageal dilatation with nearly complete loss of peristalsis are seen in later stages of the disease. The small intestine is frequently involved, with bloating, cramping, intermittent diarrhea, constipation, and adynamic ileus suggesting bowel obstruction (pseudo-obstruction). Hypomotility may cause bacterial overgrowth with subsequent malabsorption, profound weight loss, and diarrhea alternating with constipation. Radiographic studies may show delayed transit with retention in the second and third portions of

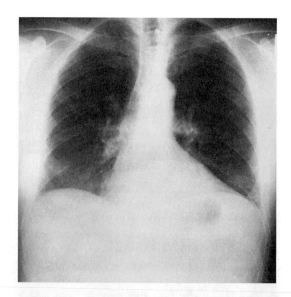

FIGURE 259.3. Chest roentgenogram of the patient in Figure 259.2 with progressive systemic sclerosis, showing the characteristic bilateral, predominantly lower-zone interstitial infiltration.

merular filtration rate are the features. Malignant hypertension may occur.

Congestive heart failure occurs in a few due to myocardial disease (contraction band necrosis) and malignant or pulmonary hypertension. Pericarditis may occur acutely or, more often, as an asymptomatic effusion. Arrhythmias and conduction defects are common.

Approximately 20% of patients with systemic sclerosis have myopathy with mild muscle weakness and mild or no elevation of muscle enzymes. A few have polymyositis with more marked weakness and abnormal biopsy and EMG. Systemic sclerosis may also be associated with Sjögren's syndrome and subclinical hypothyroidism.

■ **Laboratory Features**

About 50% of patients have a high erythrocyte sedimentation rate and polyclonal hypergammaglobulinemia. RF is seen in 25%, and ANAs (usually speckled pattern) in 75–90%. ANA with a nucleolar pattern and antibody to the Scl-70 nuclear antigen are very suggestive of systemic sclerosis. Anticentromere antibodies occur more often in CREST.

■ **Diagnosis, Management, and Prognosis**

The diagnosis of systemic sclerosis can be made when the typical skin changes occur proximal to the digits. The diagnosis can also be made if 2 of the following are present:

- Sclerodactyly
- Digital pitting scars
- Typical lung disease

The course of this disease does not appear to be altered by any treatment. General measures include avoidance of trauma (particularly to the hands) and severe cold. Tobacco smoke and vasoconstrictors such as beta-blockers should be eliminated. Vasodilators (nifedipine, phenoxybenzamine, guanethidine, methyldopa, reserpine, and prazosin) may help decrease the frequency of Raynaud's phenomenon in some patients. NSAIDs may alleviate joint symptoms. Aggressive blood pressure control and dialysis or transplantation have been used for patients with renal involvement. While penicillamine and colchicine have been used to treat skin and visceral involvement, their efficacy is uncertain. Some patients with rapidly progressive disease appear to respond to IV cyclophosphamide. Gastroesophageal reflux is treated with elevation of the head of the bed, H2 blockers and proton-pump inhibitors. Treatment for most other manifestations is symptomatic.

The 10-year survival ranges from 35–70%. Involvement of the kidneys, heart and lungs, masculine gender, and older age imply a much worse prognosis.

Other Scleroderma Syndromes

Localized scleroderma without systemic features has 2 forms. **Morphea** consists of waxy, ivory-colored, sclerotic plaques surrounded by a violaceous halo of inflammation; it occurs at any age. The lesions may be multiple and span several centimeters, and they usually heal over months to years, leaving atrophic areas of hyper- or hypopigmentation. The second form, **linear scleroderma,** usually occurs in children.

Eosinophilic fasciitis, another scleroderma syndrome, starts in the hands and feet. The extremities become swollen, painful, and tender, but induration of the skin and subcutaneous tissues follows, giving an orange peel-like, puckered appearance. The trunk and face are occasionally affected. Eosinophilia and hyperglobulinemia are usually present early. Full thickness skin biopsy down to the muscle shows inflammation and fibrosis in all layers. Response to corticosteroids is good.

The **eosinophilia-myalgia syndrome** has followed the use of L-tryptophan, with a contaminant in its manufacturing process having been implicated. The syndrome has eosinophilia and many features of scleroderma. Other diseases, most commonly diabetic cheirarthropathy (skin thickening of the hands with flexion contractures of the PIP and DIP joints), may mimic the skin changes of scleroderma.

Undifferentiated Connective Tissue and Overlap Syndromes

Some patients do not develop a defined disorder ("undifferentiated connective tissue disease") or develop an **overlap syndrome** with features that satisfy the diagnostic criteria for two or more defined disorders (e.g., "sclero-dermatomyositis" or "rhupus"). **Mixed connective tissue disease,** although its existence as a clinical entity is controversial, combines symptoms usually seen individually in systemic sclerosis, systemic lupus erythematosus, and polymyositis and is serologically defined by very high titers of antibodies to ribonucleoprotein.

The vasculitides are a group of heterogeneous conditions, which have in common inflammation and necrosis within the blood vessel walls. Although their etiology remains unknown, the similarity of vasculitis to lesions in acute experimental serum sickness suggests an immune complex pathogenesis in some. The vasculitides show features of **systemic inflammation** (e.g., weight loss, fever) and manifestations due to **vasculitic occlusion** of specific vessels (e.g., stroke, intestinal infarction, renal impairment).

Many classification schemes have been proposed, but none is entirely satisfactory. One method bases the classification on the size of the vessel involved (large-, medium-, or small-vessel vasculitis), although this schema does not seem very logical (Table 260.1). In fact, many of the vasculitides bear no clinical, histologic, or serologic resemblance to each other.

TABLE 260.1. Types and Features of Vasculitis Based on Blood Vessel Size

Medium to large arteries	
Temporal arteritis	Giant cell arteritis, affects mostly cranial arteries in the elderly
Takayasu's arteritis	Aortic arch involvement in young, usually Asian women
Small to medium arteries	
Polyarteritis group	
Polyarteritis nodosa	Necrotizing vasculitis with renal, abdominal, coronary, CNS and peripheral nerve involvement
Churg-Strauss vasculitis	Similar to above with pulmonary involvement and eosinophilia
Overlap syndrome	Features of several types of vasculitis
Small to medium arteries, veins	
Wegener's granulomatosis	Granulomatous vasculitis, involves upper and/or lower respiratory tract, eyes, ears, kidneys, skin
Arterioles, capillaries, venules	
Hypersensitivity vasculitis	Leukocytoclastic vasculitis (often with "palpable" purpura)
Rheumatoid vasculitis	
Lupus vasculitis	
Drug-induced vasculitis	
Essential mixed cryoglobulinemia	
Malignancy	
Henoch-Schönlein purpura	Purpura, joint pain, abdominal pain, glomerulitis

Polyarteritis Nodosa

Polyarteritis nodosa (PAN), a prototypic vasculitic syndrome seen predominantly in middle-aged men, usually involves the medium-sized and small muscular arteries. Histologic examination shows lesions of varying age, suggesting an evolving process. In some series, as many as 50% of such patients have evidence of persistent hepatitis B antigenemia, and antigen, immunoglobulin, and complement have been shown in involved vessels, suggesting a true immune-complex-mediated process.

■ Clinical Features

The onset of PAN is with systemic symptoms (e.g., fever, malaise, or weight loss), and the multisystem involvement often suggests the diagnosis. Coronary, renal, and mesenteric arteritis causes symptoms referable to the respective viscera and serious and potentially life-threatening complications (e.g., myocardial infarction, hypertension, abdominal pain, gastrointestinal hemorrhage, or bowel infarction). Involvement of the vasa nervorum and cranial vessels causes peripheral (e.g., mononeuritis multiplex) or central nervous system signs. Some refute pulmonary involvement, but this may simply reflect problems in distinguishing it from Churg-Strauss disease (allergic granulomatosis), a granulomatous arteritis with lung involvement and eosinophilia in asthmatics or atopic persons.

Laboratory Features

Leukocytosis, anemia of chronic disease, hypergammaglobulinemia, and an elevated erythrocyte sedimentation rate are frequent. An active urine sediment and azotemia reflect renal involvement. Cryoglobulinemia or hypocomplementemia occurs in 20–25%. Diagnosis is by demonstration of the classic lesions by histologic examination or arteriography.

Management

PAN is classically a catastrophic, often fatal illness. Despite a lack of carefully controlled studies, it is likely that **corticosteroids** and **immunosuppressive** agents (e.g., cyclophosphamide) have improved the prognosis. High-dose corticosteroids (prednisone, 80 mg/d) should be used in the severely ill, although steroids may aggravate hypertension and compromise serosal integrity in the involved bowel.

TABLE 260.2.	System Involvement and Symptoms in Wegener's Granulomatosis
General	Lower respiratory
Fever	Cough
Weight loss	Hemoptysis
Cranial	Dyspnea
Headache	Pleuritis/pleural effusion
Ophthalmic	Renal
Inflammation-conjunctiva,	Glomerulonephritis
sclera, uvea	Interstitial nephritis
Proptosis	Skin
Otologic	Purpura
Otitis	Nodules
Hearing loss	Joints
Upper respiratory	Arthralgia
Epistaxis	Arthritis
Rhinitis/obstruction	
Sinusitis	
Oral ulcers	

Wegener's Granulomatosis

Wegener's granulomatosis features sinusitis, otitis, laryngitis and lung involvement (see chapter 231), involvement of eyes, and nephritis (Table 260.2), any or all of which may be seen at presentation. The antineutrophil cytoplasmic antibody with a cytoplasmic pattern of staining (c-ANCA) is positive in most cases. Because c-ANCA is not completely specific, biopsy confirmation is essential. Another staining pattern, the perinuclear or p-ANCA, is seen in other forms of vasculitis, particularly with renal involvement.

Cyclophosphamide, usually given orally, often results in cures in this otherwise universally fatal disease. Trimethoprim-sulfamethoxazole regimen reduces relapses.

Hypersensitivity Angiitis (Leukocytoclastic Vasculitis)

This arteritis affects primarily small vessels, including arterioles and postcapillary venules. It often presents clinically as **palpable purpura.** Many of the original cases followed medication use, leading to the term "hypersensitivity." The histologic finding is hematoxyphilic debris resembling nuclear dust, predominantly in postcapillary venules. This vasculitis may be seen in association with connective tissue diseases such as systemic lupus erythematosus (see Figure 46.2), rheumatoid arthritis, and cryoglobulinemia, or with other infectious or neoplastic syndromes.

Another example is **Henoch-Schönlein purpura,** in which classically there are glomerulitis with hematuria, arthritis, fever, and gastrointestinal involvement. Circulating IgA levels may be high, and immunofluorescence of biopsy tissue usually shows IgA deposition.

Giant Cell (Temporal) Arteritis and Polymyalgia Rheumatica

These entities are related and sometimes present with overlapping features. **Giant cell arteritis** involves larger vessels, typically from the cranium to the aortic arch, although any portion of the aorta and its major branches may be involved. The typical presentation is a new-onset temporal headache in an older person, but other symptoms may include jaw or tongue claudication and, rarely, ulcers of the scalp or tongue. Although the examination can reveal entirely normal findings, thickening and tenderness of the temporal arteries, as well as decreased or absent pulses, suggest temporal arteritis. Blindness and stroke are the most common complications, the former occurring in 25% of the untreated.

No specific laboratory test exists for identifying temporal arteritis, although the erythrocyte sedimentation rate (ESR) is typically elevated above 50 and often exceeds 90 mm/hr. Diagnosis is usually by temporal artery biopsy. Because the lesions are segmental, one should biopsy a 2-3 cm section of temporal artery and sample multiple areas in order to avoid missing the lesions. Some favor obtaining bilateral temporal artery biopsies. Treatment with steroids (prednisone, m60 mg/d) can deter blindness.

Polymyalgia rheumatica is also predominantly a disease of the elderly and is unlikely in persons under age 50. A diagnosis of exclusion, it features neck, shoulder, and hip girdle pain, severe morning stiffness (with difficulty getting out of bed), and myalgias without atrophy or true weakness. These patients may also have fever, sweats, and weight loss.

The laboratory findings are nonspecific and include anemia of chronic disease and elevated serum α_2-globulin and fibrinogen. The ESR is high (at least 40 and often >90mm/hr). Rarely, the ESR may be normal, but the C-reactive protein or fibrinogen may be high. Serum muscle enzyme levels, EMG, and muscle biopsy findings are normal. Random temporal artery biopsy reveals giant cell arteritis in 20–30%.

The risk of blindness is below 1% if cranial vessel symptoms are absent. Any cranial symptoms, (e.g., headaches, jaw claudication, or visual changes) in a patient with polymyalgia rheumatica should prompt a temporal artery biopsy. The myalgias respond dramatically to prednisone in doses as low as 15 mg/day. Both temporal arteritis and polymyalgia rheumatica run a course of 2–3 years before remitting, usually permanently.

CHAPTER 261 REGIONAL (NONARTICULAR) MUSCULOSKELETAL PAIN

A glossary of key regional musculoskeletal disorders is provided in Table 261.1. Diagnosis of specific conditions is based mostly on the history and physical findings. Although trauma may play a causative role in some of these disorders, in many cases, no specific etiology may be found.

TABLE 261.1. A Glossary of Key Regional Musculoskeletal Disorders

Tendinitis	Inflammation of a tendon attachment point or another site of tendon friction.
Bursitis	Inflammation of a bursa, a sac like structure which facilitates sliding of one tissue over another.
Enthesitis	Inflammation of an enthesis, a tendon attachment point.
Reflex sympathetic dystrophy	Presumptively, a disorder of sympathetic nerve function causing chronic pain in an extremity usually following some injury.
Myofascial pain	Localized pain and tenderness in a muscle or group of muscles.
Fibromyalgia	Chronic condition of widespread pain and tenderness in characteristic trigger points.

Neck and Shoulder Pain

■ Neck Pain

Neck and shoulder pain are common symptoms, due to intrinsic lesions at either site or referred pain from one site to the other.

The neck consists of vertebrae, soft tissues (ligaments, paracervical muscles), neurovascular structures (vertebral arteries, spinal cord, nerve roots), and joints (apophyseal and lateral interbody joints and fibrocartilaginous discs). Acute neck pain, often with muscle spasm, can be triggered by ligamentous sprain (e.g.

whiplash secondary to motor vehicle accidents, falls, or athletic injuries), prolonged cold exposure, tension, activities involving repetitive neck movement, or nerve root irritation.

Disc disintegration occurs as a result of aging and probably previous cervical sprain injuries. The examination often reveals limitation of neck motion, tenderness to palpation, and spasm. Cervical nerve root irritation is usually attributable to ligamentous sprains but occasionally to a herniated cervical disc. Radiographs of the cervical spine may show disc space narrowing, osteophyte formation (bony overgrowth at the margin of a joint) and sometimes abnormalities of vertebral alignment, but these types of changes are common (seen in 50% of persons age >45 yrs) and correlate poorly with specific pain complaints.

Radicular pain and neurologic signs may accompany root irritation, which may be suggested by electrodiagnostic studies. Magnetic resonance imaging (MRI) can provide more definitive anatomic information. Occasionally, posterior osteophytes may form large bars which impinge on the spinal cord, causing cervical myelopathy with weakness and alteration in deep tendon reflexes.

Whereas chronic neck pain is often related to a myofascial pain syndrome, fibromyalgia (see below), or degenerative disc disease, **referred neck pain** may be due to thoracic outlet syndrome, brachial plexus injury or compression, intrathoracic lesions (Pancoast tumor), diaphragmatic irritation (subphrenic abscess, splenic or gallbladder disease), temporomandibular joint disorders, and coronary disease.

Initial **treatment** consists of rest (avoidance of exacerbating activities; soft cervical collar), moist heat, an NSAID for both analgesic and anti-inflammatory properties, and physical therapy (traction, deep heat, massage, exercises). Therapy for referred pain should be directed at the cause.

Shoulder Pain

The shoulder consists of three joints—the glenohumeral, acromioclavicular, and sternoclavicular—and various soft tissues (tendons, capsules, ligaments, and bursae). Shoulder pain of various types is often lumped into the category of **"bursitis,"** thus rendering this term largely meaningless (Table 261.2).

Tendinitis most commonly involves the supraspinatus; tenderness is noted on shoulder palpation along with some loss of motion. **Calcific tendinitis,** occurring beyond the fourth decade, appears radiographically as a rounded or fluffy calcific deposit of hydroxyapatite within the tendon. Most are asymptomatic, but acute calcific tendonitis with severe, disabling pain may reflect enlargement of the calcific deposit or rupture into the subacromial bursa. Persistent or recurrent cases may require needling or surgical removal of the calcific deposit.

Most shoulder problems involve the **rotator cuff,** composed of the supraspinatus, infraspinatus, teres minor, and subscapularis tendons (Table 261.2). The impingement syndrome or rotator cuff tendinitis represents a continuum of symptoms initiated by excessive overhead arm use that permits impingement of the cuff against the coracoacromial arch. Such activities may include tennis, baseball, swimming, painting, and paper hanging. In middle age, the cuff may fray (partial tear), eventually tearing completely.

Rotator cuff tears may be spontaneous or follow trauma. They also may result from various types of arthritis (e.g., rheumatoid arthritis, systemic lupus erythematosus, hydroxyapatite-associated arthropathy), metabolic conditions (e.g., renal osteodystrophy, diabetes), or repeated local injections of corticosteroid.

A tear may be suspected by the patient's inability to abduct the affected arm or by weakness of resisted abduction. Diagnosis is confirmed by arthrography or MRI. Treatment is conservative. Although surgical repair of acute tears is often necessary in younger patients, severe pain may necessitate repair even in the elderly.

Adhesive capsulitis ("frozen shoulder") often follows established tendinitis or glenohumeral arthritis, with failure to maintain shoulder range of motion. It may also be idiopathic in middle-aged women with no predisposing disorders. Patients report generalized shoulder and upper arm pain and worsening limitation of motion. Arthrography shows a small joint volume. In the absence of an underlying condition, the process tends to be self-limiting, with symptoms resolving in about a year. Physical therapy may help restore motion.

In addition to pain from primary shoulder disease, pain from neurologic conditions, such as a cervical radiculopathy (specifically C5-6) and occasionally from carpal tunnel syndrome, can be referred to the shoulder. The exact cause of shoulder pain often remains elusive. Because radiographs of the most common conditions causing shoulder pain are generally unrevealing, radiography should be reserved for those patients who fail a month of conservative management.

The initial **treatment** of most shoulder disorders is conservative, including NSAIDs and physical therapy. One or two local corticosteroid injections may be attempted. Surgical resection of the anterior third of the acromion (acromioplasty) and coracoacromial ligament may provide relief for impingement symptoms.

TABLE 261.2. Regional Musculoskeletal Disorders

Disorder	Findings
Shoulder	
Calcific tendinitis	Found on X-ray, usually asymptomatic, most often supraspinatus, occasional severe pain
Rotator cuff	
Tendinitis	Aching shoulder pain, tenderness to palpation, may have reduced ROM
Tear	Variable pain, difficulty with active shoulder abduction and resisted abduction
Adhesive capsulitis	Markedly reduced glenohumeral motion (frozen shoulder)
Primary	Usually middle-aged women, no apparent cause
Secondary	Severe loss of motion related to another shoulder problem and failure to maintain ROM (e.g. prolonged use of shoulder splint)
Bicipital tendinitis	Tenderness over biceps tendon, clicking with shoulder rotation
Elbow	
Lateral epicondylitis	Lateral elbow and forearm pain, increased with ("tennis elbow") arm use, tenderness over the lateral epicondyle
Medial epicondylitis	Medial elbow and forearm pain, increased with use, tenderness over the medial epicondyle
Wrist	
DeQuervain's tenosynovitis	Radial wrist pain; tenderness over the distal radius; pain near base of thumb (over abductor pollicis longus, extensor pollicis brevis tendons)
Hand	
Flexor tendinitis	May affect any of the flexor tendons, finger may ("trigger finger") "lock" in flexion and snap with extension, flexor tendon may be tender in distal palm, may click with finger movement
Ankle	
Achilles' tendinitis	Tenderness at the insertion of the Achilles' tendon on the calcaneous
Bursitis	
Subdeltoid	Aching shoulder pain, similar to rotator cuff tendinitis
Olecranon	Usually caused by pressure or trauma, may have fluid accumulation over olecranon
Ischial tuberosity	Pain with sitting on hard surface, tenderness over the ischial tuberosity
Greater trochanter	Patients often complain of "hip" pain, especially when lying on that side, radiation of pain down the lateral thigh, tender over the greater trochanter
Prepatellar	Tenderness and swelling anterior to the patella, may ("housemaid's knee") have fluid accumulation
Anserine	Pain in medial knee, tenderness over proximal medial tibia
Achilles'	Swelling anterior to the Achilles' tendon
Bunion	Pain and swelling over medial distal first metatarsal, usually with hallux valgus deformity

ROM = range of motion.

Reflex Sympathetic Dystrophy Syndrome

Reflex sympathetic dystrophy syndrome, seen most commonly in patients over age 50, typically features burning pain, tenderness, and swelling in a distal extremity. Predisposing conditions are trauma, fracture, cervical spine disease, hemiplegia, and myocardial infarction. Vasomotor instability (vasoconstriction or vasodilation, Raynaud's phenomenon, hyperhidrosis), tenderness and edema, altered sensation, and, in more long-standing cases, dystrophic skin changes (atrophy, scaling, increased or decreased hair, nail changes) may occur. Although bilateral involvement was noted in 18–50% of patients in older series, detailed analysis of a small cohort found it to be universal. Patchy osteopenia and heterogeneously increased radionuclide uptake may be seen on plain radiographs and bone scans, respectively.

Treatment is most effective when applied early, before atrophy and contractures develop. Basic therapy includes analgesics, local heat or cold, and therapeutic exercise to improve motion; when these therapies fail, systemic corticosteroids or sympathetic blockade is necessary.

Low Back Pain

The lumbosacral region consists of vertebrae, soft tissues (ligaments, paraspinal and abdominal muscles), nerve roots and spinal cord, and joints (apophyseal or facet joints, sacroiliac, fibrocartilaginous intervertebral disc). Low back pain may be caused by disorders involving one or more of these structures. Its neurologic aspects are discussed in chapter 185. Low back pain affects nearly 80% of the population at some time in their lives and takes a toll on worker productivity as well as health care and legal expenses.

Low back pain usually starts in the second decade and peaks in the fifth. Patients should be asked about trauma and repetitive movements related to their occupation or hobbies (especially heavy lifting). It is important to determine if the pain is local, radicular, or referred. Pain referred from pelvic and abdominal viscera (e.g., pancreas, uterus, retroperitoneum, prostate, abdominal aorta) is deep and aching, but other identifying symptoms are usually present as well.

The exact cause of back pain is often elusive. Spinal pain may be sharp or dull and localized to the affected part (e.g., ligament, muscle) but may be referred to the sacroiliac and gluteal areas and posterior thigh. It may be positional, with associated reflex paravertebral muscle spasm.

Acute sprain is self-limited and responds to rest on a firm surface, a pillow behind the knees, hot packs, NSAIDs, and antispasmodics. Early mobilization is encouraged within a few days, as outcomes are better than with prolonged bedrest. Therapeutic exercises such as Williams' flexion exercises (knees brought up to chest) may help reduce muscle tightness and spasm. After recovery, work modifications (especially of lifting or prolonged sitting), weight loss, and exercises should be initiated.

Chronic lumbosacral pain usually worsens on activity and decreases with rest. Findings include tenderness of the spine and muscles, muscle spasm, abnormal posture, and partially restricted straight leg raise and back motion.

Radicular pain arises from nerve root compression or irritation and is suggested by radiation of pain into the buttock or down the lower extremity, with or without numbness or tingling. Root compression commonly follows degenerative disc disease with herniation or lumbar spinal stenosis. The deep aching pain of disc herniation (usually L5-S1 or L4-5) is worsened by maneuvers that increase intradiscal pressure (bending, sitting, coughing) and decreased with a standing or supine position. Neurologic signs, particularly loss of a reflex or sensory loss, may help determine the level of involvement. The crossed straight leg raising test (root stretching) is nearly pathognomonic for herniation.

Root compression responds to conservative therapy, such as bedrest for 2–3 weeks and medications to relieve pain, inflammation, and muscle spasm. Thus, diagnostic tests are reserved for patients whose symptoms are atypical, persistent, or severe enough that surgery is considered. Electrodiagnostic studies may be negative in the first several weeks but may help locate the site in 80% of cases. Plain radiographs may be normal or show only nonspecific, age-related osteoarthritic changes that correlate poorly with symptoms (Figure 261.1). Computed tomography (CT), MRI, or myelography are diagnostic in 90–95% of cases.

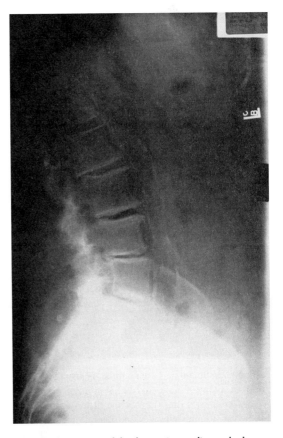

FIGURE 261.1. Lateral lumbar spine radiograph demonstrating disc space narrowing with vacuum disc phenomena, osteophyte formation, and facet joint sclerosis. Incidentally, the aorta is heavily calcified.

With midline herniation, bladder, bowel, or sexual dysfunction (cauda equina syndrome) may develop. Epidural corticosteroid injection may be tried in refractory cases before surgical intervention. Surgery is indicated for patients with unremitting pain, cauda equina syndrome, or progressive muscle weakness and neurologic deficits.

Bony entrapment of nerve roots or narrowing of the spinal canal occurs in **lumbar spinal stenosis.** Most cases of spinal stenosis occur in the elderly in the setting of degenerative disc disease, osteoarthritis and subluxation of the facet joints, ligamentous thickening, or spondylolisthesis (slippage of one vertebra in relation to another). In contrast to discogenic pain, the pain of lumbar spinal stenosis is more diffuse; it typically worsens on standing or walking (neurogenic claudication) or hyperextension of the back, radiates to the buttocks or down the legs, and decreases on sitting or with supine position. Occasionally, it presents with cauda equina syndrome. Straight leg raise is usually not markedly abnormal, and one or more dermatomal levels may be involved. CT, MRI, or myelography shows a narrowed spinal canal or nerve root entrapment. Initial therapy is conservative (back protection, NSAID, exercises). Epidural corticosteroids may be useful, but severe symptoms warrant surgery.

Other causes of low back pain are systemic inflammatory disease (spondyloarthropathy), metabolic bone disease (Paget's), infection (tuberculosis, pyogenic vertebral osteomyelitis, disc space infection), fracture, or tumor. **Diffuse idiopathic skeletal hyperostosis** (DISH, ankylosing hyperostosis, Forestier's disease) is a condition of new bone formation anterior to the vertebrae and spanning multiple vertebral levels, which causes "flowing wax" appearance on lateral spine radiographs. Disc height is normal. Most patients are older, and many have glucose intolerance. Occasionally, dysphagia may result from esophageal compression. Spinal stiffness and restricted motion are more notable than pain.

Other Regional Pain Disorders

■ Tenosynovitis

Tenosynovitis represents inflammation of a tendon sheath, often at the site where a tendon passes through a fibrous ring or narrow bony canal. Its commonest cause is injury or overuse, usually **cumulative trauma** from repetitive activity. Infection (gonococcal) or synovitis (rheumatoid arthritis, gout) are other causes.

Commonly involved sites are listed in Table 261.2. Therapy consists of cessation or modification of exacerbating repetitive activities (particularly important in work-related cases), treatment of the underlying disease, immobilization with splints, and NSAIDs. Recurrences are common. In selected cases, local corticosteroid injection and occasionally surgical excision of the fibrous constriction are indicated.

Tendinitis

Tendon inflammation, or tendinitis, is usually due to strain or injury (Table 261.2). Tendinitis commonly occurs at entheses (tendon attachment to bone) such as the medial ("tennis elbow") and lateral epicondyles of the elbow but less often at the Achilles tendon. Therapy is similar to that for tenosynovitis, although surgery is rarely indicated. Local corticosteroid injection may be used at the elbow but is more risky at the Achilles

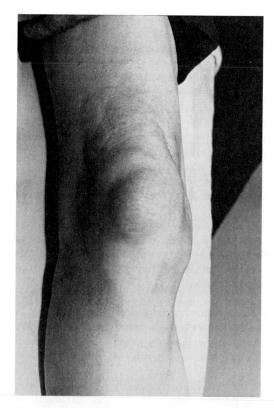

FIGURE 261.2. Prepatellar bursitis of the knee. Note the circumscribed area of swelling anterior to the patella.

tendon because of possible subsequent tears and severe disability.

Bursitis

A bursa is a sac-like structure which facilitates sliding of one tissue over another. Bursitis, or inflammation of a bursa with pain and sometimes swelling, may follow unusual use of an extremity or direct trauma. Common sites are listed in Table 261.2. Bursitis is usually recognized by tenderness to palpation over the respective bursa. Fluid accumulation may be noted in the olecranon and prepatellar bursae (Figure 261.2), but in others, there

may be little to no swelling or other inflammatory signs. Calcific bursitis tends to be of more abrupt onset. Treatment consists of modification of the inciting activity or disease, NSAIDs, local heat or cold, or ultrasound. Local corticosteroid injection is often helpful.

Septic bursitis, which usually involves the olecranon or prepatellar bursa, is recognized by swelling, erythema and tenderness; often, the swelling is fluctuant on palpation. It is nearly always due to staphylococcal or streptococcal penetration through skin abrasion. Treatment requires bursal aspiration (daily if needed) and antibiotics.

Fibromyalgia

Fibromyalgia (fibrositis) is a common musculoskeletal condition, second only to osteoarthritis in frequency. Patients report stiffness, weakness, and diffuse, poorly localized pain involving the neck, back, and extremities. Swelling or numbness are also reported, though objective evidence is often lacking. Symptoms are worse in the morning and with weather changes, stress, fatigue, or cold, and improve with heat, massage, or a vacation. Patients are chronically exhausted because of waking frequently, often due to pain, and characteristically awaken feeling unrefreshed.

Fibromyalgia is a generalized, pain-and-symptom-amplification syndrome so that its coexistence with irritable bowel syndrome and spastic bladder and its overlap with chronic fatigue syndrome are not uncommon. On examination, patients have a remarkably similar distribution of **tender points,** which are sites exquisitely sensitive on palpation; some of these tender points may not correlate with described areas of pain and thus may surprise the patient.

The American College of Rheumatology criteria for the classification of fibromyalgia identifies 18 tender points. The diagnosis of fibromyalgia rests on finding 11 of these 18 tender points, both above and below the waist and on both sides of the body, which have been present for at least 3 months (Figure 261.3). Pain in only one or a few localized areas is termed **myofascial pain,** and this is more likely to resolve over time.

Physical and laboratory studies should exclude rheumatic, endocrine, hematologic, musculoskeletal, and neurologic disorders. Although clinical data should guide laboratory tests, the complete blood count, erythrocyte sedimentation rate, and thyroid function should be examined.

Treatment is often frustrating. Patients may be defensive because they feel threatened by their symp-

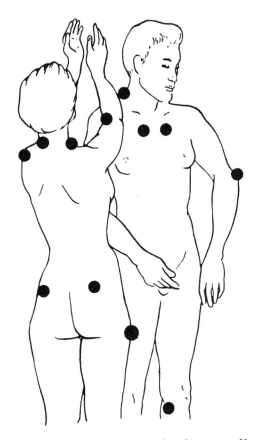

FIGURE 261.3. Location of 18 typical tender points in fibromyalgia. Tender points appear symmetrically in the body. 1) the suboccipital muscle insertions onto the base of the skull, 2) the lower lateral neck muscles, 3) the midpoint of the trapezii, 4) the medial supraspinatii, 5) the second costochondral junctions, 6) 2 cm distal to the lateral epicondyles, 7) the upper outer glutei, 8) the posterior aspect of the greater trochanters of the femur, and 9) the medial proximal tibiae.

toms and by physicians who dismiss their nonspecific symptoms as psychogenic or emotional. Explanation of a "vicious cycle" of sleep deprivation and pain magnification is the first step. Drug therapy is controversial. Many patients respond to tricyclic antidepressants (e.g., amitriptyline) taken at bedtime to improve sleep, although side effects may limit their use. Exercise, particularly aerobics (e.g., swimming or bicycling 4–6 days a week), should be started gradually and increased as tolerated. Stress management and other relaxation techniques may be important for some patients. Presented in a positive, concerned manner, these measures may alleviate the patient's fears and make symptoms more tolerable.

■ QUESTIONS

Instructions: For each question below, select only **one** lettered answer that is the **best** for that question.

1. In a 27-year-old man with back pain and limited forward spinal flexion, which of the following tests best supports the diagnosis of ankylosing spondylitis?
   A. Radiograph of the pelvis
   B. Radiograph of the lumbar spine
   C. HLA-B27 typing
   D. Erythrocyte sedimentation rate

2. A 60-year-old man has worsening back pain with no history of injury, mild paraspinal muscle tenderness, and extensive osteophyte formation with disc space narrowing on radiographs. Initial therapy should include which of the following?
   A. Bed rest for 2 weeks followed by gradually increasing activity
   B. One month trial of back exercises and an NSAID
   C. Referral to an orthopedic surgeon
   D. CT of the lumbar spine

3. A swollen right knee in a 45-year-old man is warm, red, and tender with a large effusion. The synovial fluid leukocyte count is 100,000/mm³ with 95% PMNs and extracellular monosodium urate crystals. What would you do next?
   A. Inject the joint with a corticosteroid.
   B. Start the patient on an NSAID.
   C. Start IV colchicine.
   D. Obtain Gram stain and culture the synovial fluid.

4. An 80-year-old woman reports pain in the right second DIP joint, which is very tender with synovial thickening and mild erythema. She has osteoarthritis of most PIP and DIP joints. Which of the following is most likely?
   A. Inflammatory osteoarthritis
   B. Rheumatoid arthritis

C. Septic joint
D. Pseudogout

5. The above patient improves after treatment with an NSAID. One month later, the right third DIP and left fourth PIP become inflamed. Her RF is 1:32; ANA, 1:80; ESR, 30 mm/hr; creatinine, 1.9 mg/dl; uric acid, 8 mg/dl. What is the most likely diagnosis now?
   A. Inflammatory osteoarthritis
   B. Rheumatoid arthritis
   C. Systemic lupus erythematosus
   D. Gout

6. A 25-year-old woman reports blanching and pain of her fingers on cold exposure. Arterial pulses are normal. Which of the following is possible?
   A. Idiopathic Raynaud's phenomenon
   B. Carpal tunnel syndrome
   C. Fibromyalgia
   D. All of the above

7. A 60-year-old man with scleroderma has had a 10-pound weight loss over the last 6 months. He has constipation and occasionally, diarrhea, but now has abdominal distention. What test is most likely to define his disorder?
   A. Esophagogram
   B. Upper gastrointestinal series with small bowel follow through
   C. Barium enema
   D. CT scan of the abdomen

8. Systemic lupus erythematosus (SLE) is diagnosed in a 24-year-old woman. Prednisone therapy is begun at 60 mg/day for 1 month. After 2 weeks, she has right hip pain. Limping and mildly reduced right hip motion are noted. Which of the following is most likely?
   A. Recurrence of active SLE
   B. Septic arthritis
   C. Osteonecrosis of the hip
   D. Muscle atrophy

9. A 70-year-old woman with a 20-year history of rheumatoid arthritis had an auto accident. For her upper extremity pain and a sprained neck, rest, analgesics, and a cervical collar were given. Six days later, she notes leg weakness. Mild synovitis of her hands and wrists are noted, with small knee effusions, generalized weakness, brisk reflexes, and normal sensations. What is her diagnosis?
   A. Reactivation of rheumatoid arthritis
   B. Cervical myelopathy
   C. Subdural hematoma
   D. Disuse atrophy of muscles

10. A 40-year-old woman with chest pain has a normal ECG, a high creatine kinase (all MM fraction), mildly enlarged thyroid, normal muscle strength, and no evidence of trauma, murmurs, or gallops. What is the most likely cause of the high CK?
    A. Heart attack
    B. Anxiety reaction
    C. Polymyositis
    D. Hypothyroidism

11. A 35-year-old woman reports fatigue and widespread aching pain that disrupts sleep. She has, on palpation, 14 of 18 possible tender points. Fibromyalgia is suspected. What laboratory test is most likely to be abnormal?
    A. Increased ESR
    B. Normochromic, normocytic anemia
    C. Increased C reactive protein
    D. None of the above

12. The following radiographic findings are typical of osteoarthritis EXCEPT:
    A. Periarticular osteoporosis
    B. Osteophytosis
    C. Sclerosis
    D. Geodes (subchondral cysts)

13. A 77-year-old woman has weakness with neck and shoulder stiffness. Tenderness is found in the neck and shoulder area but no definite weakness. Her ESR is 75 mm/hr, hematocrit 33%, and hemoglobin 11 g/dl. Which ONE of the following is indicated now?
    A. Surgical consult for a temporal artery biopsy
    B. Start prednisone, 15 mg/day
    C. Start prednisone, 60 mg/day
    D. Start ferrous sulfate, 325 mg tid

14. A 68-year-old woman with a new-onset headache is febrile (100° F). She has normal temporal artery pulses and an ESR of 81 mm/hr. What would you do now?
    A. Spinal tap
    B. Blood cultures
    C. CT of the head
    D. Temporal artery biopsy

■ ANSWERS

1. A	2. B	3. D	4. A	5. D
6. D	7. B	8. C	9. B	10. D
11. D	12. A	13. B	14. D	

SUGGESTED READING

Textbooks and Monographs

Kelley WN, Harris ED, Ruddy S, et al. (eds). *Textbook of Rheumatology,* 4th ed. Philadelphia: WB Saunders Co, 1993.

Klippel JH (ed). *Primer on the Rheumatic Diseases,* 11th ed. Atlanta: Arthritis Foundation, 1997.

Koopman WJ (ed). *Arthritis and Allied Conditions,* 13th ed. Baltimore: Williams & Wilkins, 1997.

Polley HF, Hunder GG. *Rheumatologic Interviewing and Physical Examination of the Joints,* 2nd ed. Philadelphia: WB Saunders Co, 1978.

Samter M (ed). *Immunological Diseases,* 3rd ed. Boston; Little, Brown & Co, 1978.

Evaluation of Joint Diseases

Dearborn JT, Jergesen HE. The evaluation and initial management of arthritis. Primary Care 1996;23:215–240.

Ostezan LB, Callen JP. Cutaneous manifestations of selected rheumatologic diseases. Am Fam Phys 1996;53:1625–1636.

Shmerling RH. Synovial fluid analysis. A critical reappraisal. Rheum Dis Clin North Am 1994;20:503–512.

Totemchokchyakarn K, Ball GV. Arthritis of systemic disease. Am J Med 1996;101:642–647.

Towheed TE, Hochberg MC. Acute monoarthritis: a practical approach to assessment and treatment. Am Fam Phys 1996;54:2239–2243.

von Muhlen CA, Tan EM. Autoantibodies in the diagnosis of systemic rheumatic diseases. Semin Arthr Rheum 1995;24:323–358.

Clinical Presentations of Rheumatic Conditions and Principles of Therapy

Baker DG, Schumacher HR, Jr. Acute monoarthritis. N Engl J Med 1993;329:1013–1020.

Crystal-Induced Synovitis

Doherty M. Calcium pyrophosphate in joint disease. Hosp Pract 1994;29:93–96.

Schumacher HR. Crystal-induced arthritis: an overview. Am J Med 1996;100:46S–56S.

Osteoarthritis

Block JA, Schnitzer TJ. Therapeutic approaches to osteoarthritis. Hosp Pract 1997;32:159–164.

Kraus VB. Pathogenesis and treatment of osteoarthritis. Med Clin North Am 1997;81:85–112.

Oddis CV. New perspectives on osteoarthritis. Am J Med 1996;100:10S–15S.

Rheumatoid Arthritis

Arend WP. The pathophysiology and treatment of rheumatoid arthritis. Arthr Rheum 1997;40:595–597.

Hummel KM, Gay RE, Gay S. Novel strategies for the therapy of rheumatoid arthritis. Br J Rheumatol 1997;36:265–267.

Jain R, Lipsky PE. Treatment of rheumatoid arthritis. Med Clin North Am 1997;81:57–84.

Pope RM. Rheumatoid arthritis: pathogenesis and early recognition. Am J Med 1996;100:3S–9S.

Youinou P, Moutsopoulos HM, Pennec YL. Clinical features of Sjögren's syndrome. Curr Opin Rheumatol 1990; 2:687–693.

Infectious Arthritis

Brower AC. Septic arthritis. Radiol Clin North Am 1996;34: 293–309.

Kramer N, Rosenstein ED. Rheumatologic manifestations of tuberculosis. Bull Rheumatic Dis 1997;46:5–8.

Mikhail IS, Alarcon GS. Nongonococcal bacterial arthritis. Rheum Dis Clin North Am 1993;19:311–331.

Norman DC, Yoshikawa TT. Infections of the bone, joint, and bursa. Clin Geriatr Med 1994;10:703–718.

Scopelitis E, Martinez-Osuna P. Gonococcal arthritis. Rheum Dis Clin North Am 1993;19:363–377.

Smith JW, Piercy EA. Infectious arthritis. Clin Infect Dis 1995;20:225–230.

Steere AC. Diagnosis and treatment of Lyme arthritis. Med Clin North Am 1997;81:179–194.

Seronegative Spondyloarthropathies

D'Cruz D, Ross E, Morrow J. Psoriatic arthritis: identifying and controlling an insidious disease. J Musculoskel Med 1998; 15:17–35.

Khan MA. An overview of clinical spectrum and heterogeneity of spondyloarthropathies. Rheum Dis Clin North Am 1992; 18:1–10.

Underwood MR, Dawes P. Inflammatory back pain in primary care. Br J Rheumatol 1995;34:1074–1077.

Systemic Lupus Erythematosus

Belmont HM, Abramson SB, Lie JT. Pathology and pathogenesis of vascular injury in systemic lupus erythematosus. Interactions of inflammatory cells and activated endothelium. Arthr Rheum 1996;39:9–22.

Lehman TJ. A practical guide to systemic lupus erythematosus. Pediatr Clin North Am 1995;42:1223–1238.

Mills JA. Systemic lupus erythematosus. N Engl J Med 1871;330:1871–1879.

Pisetsky DS, Gilkeson G, Clair EW. Systemic lupus erythematosus. Diagnosis and treatment. Med Clin North Am 1997; 81:113–128.

Von Feldt JM. Systemic lupus erythematosus. Recognizing its various presentations. Postgrad Med 1995;97:79,83,86 passim.

Other Connective Tissue Diseases

Anonymous. Case records of the Massachusetts General Hospital. Weekly clinicopathological exercises. Case 24-1995. A 46-year-old woman with dermatomyositis, increasing pulmonary insufficiency, and terminal right ventricular failure. N Engl J Med 1995;333:369–377.

Anonymous. Systemic sclerosis: current pathogenetic concepts and future prospects for targeted therapy. Lancet 1996;347: 1453–1458.

Callen JP. Relationship of cancer to inflammatory muscle diseases. Dermatomyositis, polymyositis, and inclusion body myositis. Rheum Dis Clin North Am 1994;20:943–953.

Mastaglia FL, Phillips BA, Zilko P. Treatment of inflammatory myopathies. Muscle & Nerve 1997;20:651–664.

Medsger TA, Jr., Oddis CV. Classification and diagnostic criteria for polymyositis and dermatomyositis. J Rheumatol 1995;22:581–585.

Vasculitis

Allen NB, Bressler PB. Diagnosis and treatment of the systemic and cutaneous necrotizing vasculitis syndromes. Med Clin North Am 1997;81:243–259.

Bahlas S, Ramos-Remus C, Davis P. Clinical outcome of 149 patients with polymyalgia rheumatica and giant cell arteritis. J Rheumatol 1998;25:99–104.

Gross Wl, Schmitt WH, Csernok E. Antineutrophil cytoplasmic autoantibody-associated diseases: a rheumatologist's perspective. Am J Kidney Dis 199; 18:175–179.

Hoffman GS, Kerr GS, Leavitt RY, et al. Wegener's granulomatosis: An analysis of 158 patients. Ann Intern Med 1992; 116:488–498.

Hunder G. Vasculitis: diagnosis and therapy. Am J Med 1996;100:37S–45S.

Isenberg DA, Black C. ABC of rheumatology. Raynaud's phenomenon, scleroderma, and overlap syndromes. BMJ 1995;310:795–798.

Savage CO, Harper L, Adu D. Primary systemic vasculitis. Lancet 1997;349:553–558.

Sneller MC, Fauci AS. Pathogenesis of vasculitis syndromes. Med Clin North Am 1997;81:221–242.

Watts RA, Scott DG. ABC of Rheumatology. Rashes and vasculitis. BMJ 1995;310:1128–1132.

Regional (Nonarticular) Musculoskeletal Pain

Doherty M, Jones A. ABC of rheumatology. Fibromyalgia syndrome. BMJ 1995;310:386–389.

Evans PJ, Miniaci A. Rotator cuff tendinopathy: many causes, many solutions. J Musculoskel Med 1998;15:32–36.

McClaflin RR. Myofascial pain syndrome. Primary care strategies for early intervention. Postgrad Med 1994;96:56–59.

Reiffenberger DH, Amundson LH. Fibromyalgia syndrome: a review. Am Fam Phys 1996;53:1698–1712.

Index

Page references in *italics* denote figures; those followed by "t" denote tables

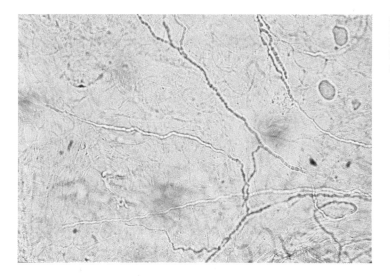

COLOR PLATE 1. Positive potassium hydroxide mount. These thin, branched, septate hyphae are characteristic of a dermatophyte infection.

(Photo courtesy of Nancy B. Esterly, MD.)

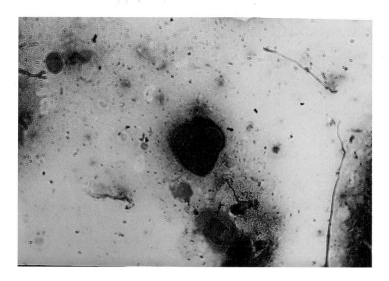

COLOR PLATE 2. Tzanck smear. The presence of multinucleated giant cells is diagnostic of a herpes virus infection.

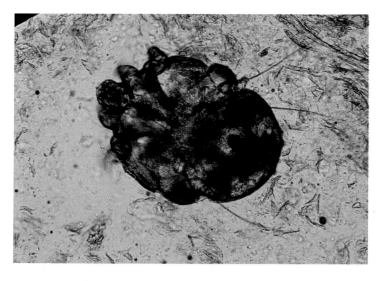

COLOR PLATE 3. Scabies prep. A female mite is readily visible in this skin scraping. Ova and feces (not shown in this mount) are also diagnostic.

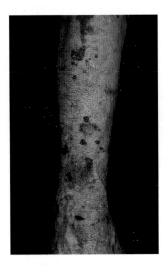

COLOR PLATE **4. Purpura secondary to topical steroid use.** This complication is most often seen in sun-exposed areas on the hands and forearms of elderly patients.

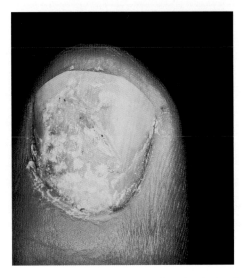

COLOR PLATE **6. Psoriasis of the nails.** Whitish discoloration of the nail with pits. Lifting of the nail from the plate (onycholysis) and subungual debris are also common findings in psoriatic nails.

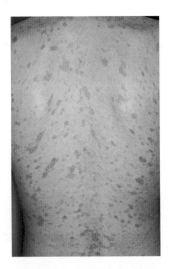

COLOR PLATE **7. Pityriasis rosea.**

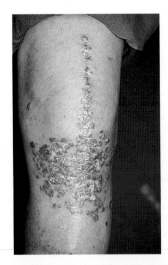

COLOR PLATE **5. Psoriasis.** A typical erythematous plaque over the knee. Koebner phenomenon, as the linear extension of the lesion above the knee, is seen in the site of a previous knee surgery.

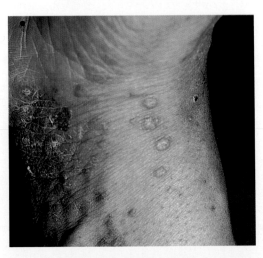

COLOR PLATE **8. Lichen planus.**

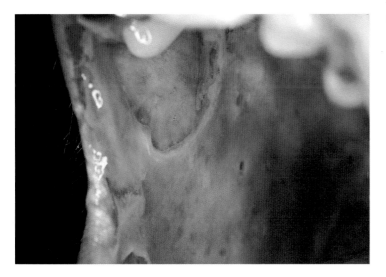

COLOR PLATE **9. Oral lichen planus.**

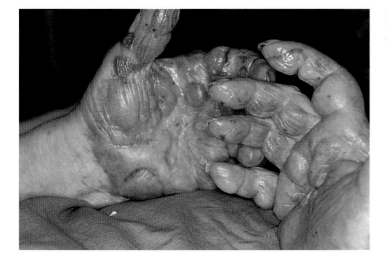

COLOR PLATE **10. Bullous pemphigoid.** Tense bullae arising on the inflamed skin of the hands of a 74-year-old woman.

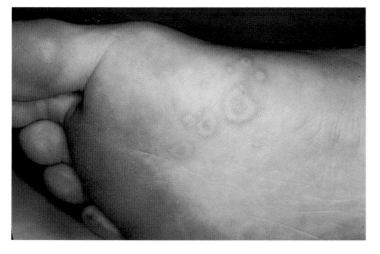

COLOR PLATE **11. Erythema multiforme.** Typical target lesions are seen on the plantar aspect of the foot.

COLOR PLATE 12. Vasculitis. Raised, purpuric lesions are seen in this patient with leukocytoclastic vasculitis secondary to lupus erythematosus.

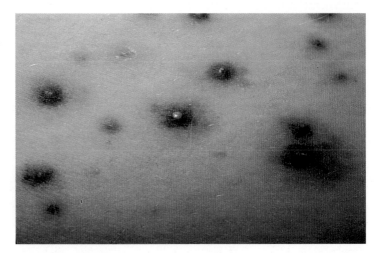

COLOR PLATE 13. Contact dermatitis secondary to poison ivy. An acutely inflamed lesion with vesicles in a linear distribution corresponding to contact area with the plant are clues to the correct diagnosis in this patient.

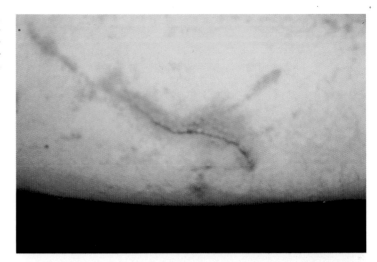

COLOR PLATE 14. Malignant melanoma, superficial spreading type.

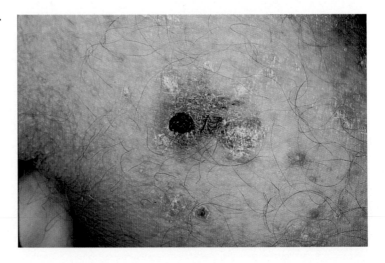

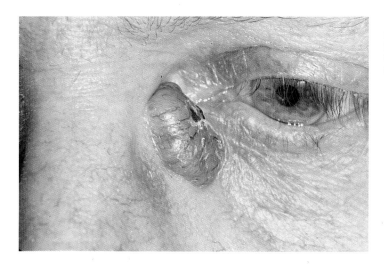

COLOR PLATE **15. Basal cell carcinoma.** The pearly quality of the lesion, telangiectases, and central ulceration are typical features of basal cell carcinoma of the skin.

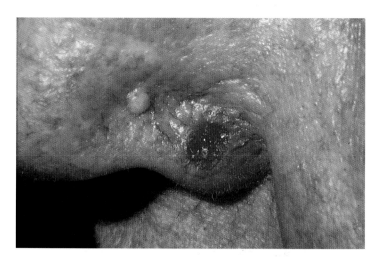

COLOR PLATE **16. Squamous cell carcinoma.**

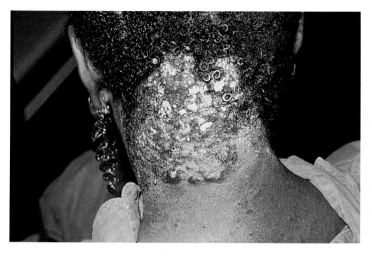

COLOR PLATE **17. Tinea capitis with kerion formation owing to *Trichophyton tonsurans.***

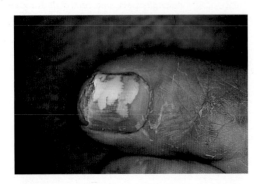

COLOR PLATE 18. Onychomycosis due to *Trichophyton rubrum*. Brownish-white discoloration of the nail plate, with accumulation of subungual debris. The findings can sometimes be difficult to differentiate from those of psoriasis, and a fungal culture may be needed.

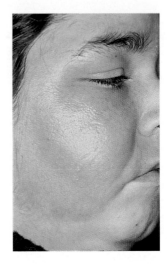

COLOR PLATE 19. Erysipelas. Facial cellulitis, with a well-demarcated border, due to group A ß-hemolytic streptococci.

COLOR PLATE 20. Secondary syphilis. Papulosquamous lesions of secondary syphilis, showing typical involvement of the palms of the hands.

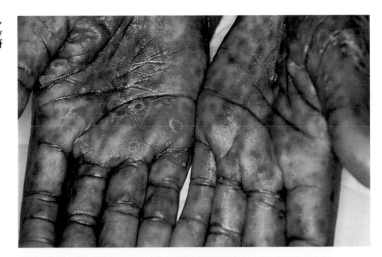

COLOR PLATE 21. Herpes simplex: Grouped vesicles with surrounding erythema.

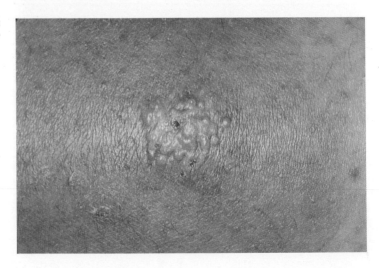